Tuberculosis

PATHOGENESIS, PROTECTION, AND CONTROL

Tuberculosis

PATHOGENESIS, PROTECTION, AND CONTROL

Editor: Barry R. Bloom, Ph.D.

(Howard Hughes Medical Research Institute / Albert Einstein College of Medicine, Bronx, New York)

ASM PRESS • WASHINGTON, DC

Copyright © 1994 American Society for Microbiology
1325 Massachusetts Avenue, N.W.
Washington, DC 20005

Library of Congress Cataloging-in-Publication Data

Tuberculosis: pathogenesis, protection, and control/edited by Barry R. Bloom.
   p.   cm.
  Includes index.
  ISBN 1-55581-072-1
  1. Tuberculosis. 2. Tuberculosis—Molecular aspects. 3. Tuberculosis—Immunological aspects. 4. Tuberculosis—Epidemiology. I. Bloom, Barry R., 1937–   .
  [DNLM: 1. Tuberculosis—pathology. 2. Tuberculosis—prevention & control. 3. Mycobacterium tuberculosis—pathogenicity. WF 215 T885 1994]
RC311.T828 1994
616.9′95—dc20
DNLM/DLC
for Library of Congress
94-2932
CIP

Cover figure: Scanning electron micrograph of the luciferase reporter phage, phAE39, absorbed to BCG cells (magnification, ×10,000). Micrograph kindly provided by R. Udani, F. Marcuso, and W. R. Jacobs, Jr. Coloration by C. Lawson.

To the generations of scientists and physicians who kept the spirit of inquiry and research on tuberculosis and leprosy alive—and especially to Karel Styblo, Philip D'Arcy Hart, Dennis Mitchison, T. Ramakrishman, Annik Rouillon, Dixie Snider, Sriram Tripathi, Jacinto Convit, S. K. Noordeen, and Tore Godal.

"Il bacillo non é ancora tutta la tuberculosi."
("The bacillus is not yet all there is to tuberculosis.")

G. Bacelli, ca. 1882

Contents

Contributors... ix

Preface xiii

Acknowledgments xv

I. INTRODUCTION TO TUBERCULOSIS

1. Global Burden of Tuberculosis. *Dixie E. Snider, Jr., Mario Raviglione, and Arata Kochi*... 3
2. History of Tuberculosis. *Thomas M. Daniel, Joseph H. Bates, and Katharine A. Downes* 13
3. Overview of Clinical Tuberculosis. *Philip C. Hopewell*..................... 25
4. Epidemiology of Tuberculosis. *P. G. Smith and A. R. Moss* 47
5. Biological Safety in the Experimental Tuberculosis Laboratory. *W. Emmett Barkley and George P. Kubica*............................... 61
6. Cultivation of *Mycobacterium tuberculosis* for Research Purposes. *Lawrence G. Wayne*.. 73
7. Current Laboratory Methods for the Diagnosis of Tuberculosis. *Leonid B. Heifets and Robert C. Good*................................... 85

II. ANIMAL MODELS OF TUBERCULOSIS

8. Mouse Model of Tuberculosis. *Ian M. Orme and Frank M. Collins*.......... 113
9. Guinea Pig Model of Tuberculosis. *David N. McMurray* 135
10. Rabbit Model of Tuberculosis. *Arthur M. Dannenberg, Jr.* 149
11. Tuberculosis in Wild and Domestic Mammals. *Charles O. Thoen*............ 157

III. GENETICS OF *MYCOBACTERIUM TUBERCULOSIS*

12. Mycobacteriophages: Cornerstones of Mycobacterial Research. *Graham F. Hatfull and William R. Jacobs, Jr.*........................... 165
13. Plasmids. *Joseph O. Falkinham III and Jack T. Crawford* 185
14. Transposition in Mycobacteria. *Ruth A. McAdam, Christophe Guilhot, and Brigitte Gicquel*... 199
15. Homologous Recombination, DNA Repair, and Mycobacterial *recA* Genes. *M. Joseph Colston and Elaine O. Davis* 217
16. Toward Mapping and Sequencing the Genome of *Mycobacterium tuberculosis*. *Stewart T. Cole and Douglas R. Smith* 227
17. Expression of Foreign Genes in Mycobacteria. *Jeanne E. Burlein, C. Kendall Stover, Shawn Offutt, and Mark S. Hanson* 239

18. Molecular Genetic Strategies for Identifying Virulence Determinants of
Mycobacterium tuberculosis. *William R. Jacobs, Jr., and Barry R. Bloom*. . . .   253

IV. PHYSIOLOGY OF *MYCOBACTERIUM TUBERCULOSIS*

19. Ultrastructure of *Mycobacterium tuberculosis*. *Patrick J. Brennan
and Philip Draper*   271
20. Lipids and Carbohydrates of *Mycobacterium tuberculosis*. *Gurdyal S. Besra
and Delphi Chatterjee*   285
21. Proteins and Antigens of *Mycobacterium tuberculosis*. *Åse Bengård Andersen
and Patrick Brennan*.   307
22. Membrane Permeability and Transport in *Mycobacterium tuberculosis*.
Nancy D. Connell and Hiroshi Nikaido.   333
23. Metabolism of *Mycobacterium tuberculosis*. *Paul R. Wheeler
and Colin Ratledge*.   353

V. IMMUNOLOGY AND PATHOGENESIS OF TUBERCULOSIS

24. Immune Mechanisms of Protection. *John Chan and Stefan H. E. Kaufmann* .   389
25. T-Cell Responses and Cytokines. *Peter F. Barnes, Robert L. Modlin,
and Jerrold J. Ellner*.   417
26. Specificity and Function of T- and B-Cell Recognition in Tuberculosis.
Juraj Ivanyi and Jelle Thole   437
27. Pathogenesis of Pulmonary Tuberculosis: an Interplay of Tissue-Damaging and
Macrophage-Activating Immune Responses—Dual Mechanisms That Control
Bacillary Multiplication. *Arthur M. Dannenberg, Jr.,
and Graham A. W. Rook*.   459
28. Mechanisms of Pathogenesis in Tuberculosis. *Graham A. W. Rook
and Barry R. Bloom*   485
29. Pathogenesis of Tuberculosis in Human Immunodeficiency Virus-Infected
People. *Sebastian Lucas and Ann Marie Nelson*.   503

VI. NEW APPROACHES TO PREVENTION AND TREATMENT OF TUBERCULOSIS

30. Molecular Approaches to the Diagnosis of Tuberculosis. *Thomas M. Shinnick
and Vivian Jonas*.   517
31. The BCG Experience: Implications for Future Vaccines against Tuberculosis.
Barry R. Bloom and Paul E. M. Fine.   531
32. Strategies for New Drug Development. *Douglas B. Young*.   559
33. Molecular Epidemiology of Tuberculosis. *Peter M. Small
and Jan D. A. van Embden*   569
34. Issues in Operational, Social, and Economic Research on Tuberculosis.
Christopher J. L. Murray   583

Index.   623

Contributors

Åse Bengård Andersen
Mycobacteria Department, Sector for Biotechnology, Statens Seruminstitut, DK-2300 Copenhagen, Denmark

W. Emmett Barkley
Howard Hughes Medical Institute, 4000 Jones Bridge Road, Chevy Chase, MD 20815

Peter F. Barnes
HMR 904, University of Southern California School of Medicine, 2025 Zonal Avenue, Los Angeles, CA 90033

Joseph H. Bates
Department of Medicine, University of Arkansas School for Medical Sciences, John L. McClellan Memorial Veterans' Hospital, 4300 West 7th Street, Little Rock, AR 72205

Gurdyal S. Besra
Department of Microbiology, Colorado State University, Fort Collins, CO 80523

Barry R. Bloom
Howard Hughes Medical Institute and Department of Microbiology and Immunology, Albert Einstein College of Medicine, Bronx, NY 10461

Patrick J. Brennan
Department of Microbiology, Colorado State University, Fort Collins, CO 80523

Jeanne E. Burlein
MedImmune Inc., 35 West Watkins Mill Road, Gaithersburg, MD 20878

John Chan
Department of Medicine, Montefiore Medical Center, Albert Einstein College of Medicine, Bronx, NY 10467

Delphi Chatterjee
Department of Microbiology, Colorado State University, Fort Collins, CO 80523

Stewart T. Cole
Unité de Génétique Moléculaire Bactérienne, Institut Pasteur, 28, rue du Docteur Roux, 75724 Paris Cedex 15, France

Frank M. Collins
The Trudeau Institute, Saranac Lake, NY 12983

M. Joseph Colston
National Institute for Medical Research, Mill Hill, London NW7 1AA, England

Nancy D. Connell
Department of Microbiology and Molecular Genetics, University of Medicine and Dentistry of New Jersey, New Jersey Medical School, 185 South Orange Avenue, Newark, NJ 07103

Jack T. Crawford
Division of Bacterial and Mycotic Diseases, National Center for Infectious Diseases, Centers for Disease Control and Prevention, Atlanta, GA 30333

Thomas M. Daniel
Center for International Health, Case Western Reserve University School of Medicine, 10900 Euclid Avenue, Cleveland, OH 44106

Arthur M. Dannenberg, Jr.
Department of Environmental Health Sciences, School of Hygiene and Public Health, The Johns Hopkins University, 615 North Wolfe Street, Baltimore, MD 21205-2179

Elaine O. Davis
National Institute for Medical Research, Mill Hill, London NW7 1AA, England

Katharine A. Downes
Center for International Health, Case Western Reserve University School of Medicine, 10900 Euclid Avenue, Cleveland, OH 44106

Philip Draper
National Institute for Medical Research, Mill Hill, London NW7 1AA, England

Jerrold J. Ellner
Division of Infectious Diseases, University Hospitals of Cleveland, Case Western Reserve University School of Medicine, 10900 Euclid Avenue, Cleveland, OH 44106-4984

Joseph A. Falkinham III
Department of Biology, Virginia Polytechnic Institute and State University, Blacksburg, VA 24061

Paul E. M. Fine
London School of Tropical Medicine and Hygiene, Keppel Street, London WC1E 7HT, United Kingdom

Brigitte Gicquel
Unité de Génétique Mycobactérienne, Département de Bactériologie et Mycologie, Institut Pasteur, 25, rue du Dr. Roux, 75724 Paris Cedex 15, France

Robert C. Good
National Center for Infectious Diseases, Centers for Disease Control and Prevention, Mailstop C-09, 1600 Clifton Road, N.E., Atlanta, GA 30333

Christophe Guilhot
Unité de Génétique Mycobactérienne, Département de Bactériologie et Mycologie, Institut Pasteur, 25, rue du Dr. Roux, 75724 Paris Cedex 15, France

Mark S. Hanson
MedImmune Inc., 35 West Watkins Mill Road, Gaithersburg, MD 20878

Graham F. Hatfull
Department of Biological Sciences, University of Pittsburgh, Pittsburgh, PA 15230

Leonid B. Heifets
National Jewish Center for Immunology and Respiratory Medicine, 1400 Jackson Street, Denver, CO 80206

Philip C. Hopewell
University of California, San Francisco, and Division of Pulmonary and Critical Care Medicine, San Francisco General Hospital, 1001 Potrero Avenue, San Francisco, CA 94110

Juraj Ivanyi
MRC Tuberculosis and Related Infections Unit, Clinical Sciences Centre, London W12 ONN, United Kingdom

William R. Jacobs, Jr.
Howard Hughes Medical Institute, Albert Einstein College of Medicine, Bronx, NY 10461
Vivian Jonas
Gen-Probe Incorporated, 9880 Campus Point Drive, San Diego, CA 92121
Stefan H. E. Kaufmann
Department of Immunology, University of Ulm, Albert-Einstein-Allee 11, D-89070 Ulm, Germany
Arata Kochi
Tuberculosis Programme, World Health Organization, CH-1211, Geneva 27, Switzerland
George P. Kubica
2323 Walton Place, Atlanta, GA 30338
Sebastian Lucas
Department of Histopathology, University College London Medical School, London WC1, United Kingdom
Ruth A. McAdam
Department of Microbiology and Immunology, Albert Einstein College of Medicine of Yeshiva University, 1300 Morris Park Avenue, Bronx, NY 10461
David N. McMurray
Department of Medical Microbiology and Immunology, Texas A&M University Health Science Center, College Station, TX 77843-1114
Robert L. Modlin
Division of Dermatology, 52-121 CHS, University of California Los Angeles School of Medicine, 10833 Le Conte Avenue, Los Angeles, CA 90024
Andrew R. Moss
Department of Epidemiology and Biostatistics, University of California, San Francisco, San Francisco, CA 94110
Christopher J. L. Murray
Harvard Center for Population and Development Studies, Harvard School of Public Health, 9 Bow Street, Cambridge, MA 02138
Ann Marie Nelson
Division of AIDS Pathology M003B, Armed Forces Institute of Pathology, Washington, DC 20306-6000
Hiroshi Nikaido
Department of Molecular and Cell Biology, c/o Stanley/Donner Administrative Services Unit, 229 Stanley Hall, Berkeley, CA 94720
Shawn Offutt
MedImmune Inc., 35 West Watkins Mill Road, Gaithersburg, MD 20878
Ian M. Orme
Mycobacteria Research Laboratories, Department of Microbiology, Colorado State University, Fort Collins, CO 80523
Colin Ratledge
Department of Applied Biology, University of Hull, Hull HU6 7RX, United Kingdom
Mario Raviglione
Tuberculosis Programme, World Health Organization, CH-1211, Geneva 27, Switzerland

Graham A. W. Rook
    Department of Medical Microbiology, School of Pathology, University College
    London Medical School, 67-73 Riding House Street, London W1P 7LD, United
    Kingdom
Thomas M. Shinnick
    Division of Bacterial and Mycotic Diseases, National Center for Infectious
    Diseases, Centers for Disease Control and Prevention, Atlanta, GA 30333
Peter M. Small
    Division of Infectious Diseases and Geographic Medicine, Beckman Center, Room
    251, Stanford University, Stanford, CA 94305-5425
Douglas R. Smith
    Collaborative Research Inc., 1365 Main Street, Waltham, MA 02154
Peter G. Smith
    Department of Epidemiology and Population Sciences, London School of Hygiene
    and Tropical Medicine, Keppel Street, London WC1E 7HT, United Kingdom
Dixie E. Snider, Jr.
    Office of the Director, Centers for Disease Control and Prevention, Atlanta, GA
    30333
C. Kendall Stover
    Department of Tuberculosis and Infectious Diseases, PathoGenesis Corp., 201
    Elliott Avenue, West, Seattle, WA 98119
Charles O. Thoen
    Department of Microbiology, Immunology, and Preventive Medicine, Iowa State
    University, Ames, IA 50011
Jelle Thole
    Department of Immunohaematology and Blood Bank, University Hospital, 2300
    RC Leiden, The Netherlands
Jan D. A. van Embden
    Unit Molecular Microbiology, National Institute of Public Health and
    Environmental Protection, P.O. Box 1, 3720 BA, Bilthoven, The Netherlands
Lawrence G. Wayne
    Tuberculosis Research Laboratory (151), Department of Veterans Affairs Medical
    Center, 5901 East Seventh Street, Long Beach, CA 90822
Paul R. Wheeler
    Department of Clinical Sciences, London School of Hygiene and Tropical
    Medicine, Keppel Street, London WC1E 7HT, United Kingdom
Douglas B. Young
    Department of Medical Microbiology, St. Mary's Hospital Medical School, Norfolk
    Place, London W2 1PG, United Kingdom

Preface

Today, as it has been for centuries, tuberculosis remains the leading cause of death in the world from infectious disease. Approximately a third of the world's population has been infected with *Mycobacterium tuberculosis* and is at risk for developing disease. Globally, tuberculosis accounts for almost 3 million deaths annually and one-fifth of all deaths of adults in developing countries. Tuberculosis is a reemergent problem in many industrialized countries. In the modern world of global interdependency, rapid transportation, expanding trade, and changing social and cultural patterns, tuberculosis in any country is a threat to people in every country. In the context of infectious diseases, there is no place in the world from which we are remote and no one from whom we are disconnected.

Current knowledge of evolutionary biology and genetics makes clear that what is at stake in the battle against infectious diseases is the survival not only of human and animal hosts but of the pathogens themselves, a confrontation that cannot be taken lightly. Human interventions serve as selections for genetic mutations, adaptations, and migrations that enable pathogens to survive. While societies traditionally deal with epidemics and outbreaks of infectious diseases in an episodic or discontinuous fashion, the evolutionary process of the pathogens is a continuous one. That elementary truth demands vigilance rather than complacency in applying the tools we have and a continuing scientific effort both to anticipate new threats from infectious pathogens and to develop new tools with which to protect the public health. In the case of tuberculosis, the demise of the disease in the industrialized world has been taken for granted and its persistence in developing countries largely ignored. Support for research dwindled, and the expertise of a generation of scientists and clinicians knowledgeable about tuberculosis was lost.

The current global reemergence of tuberculosis can be attributed to several factors. The compromise of immune mechanisms in human immunodeficiency virus (HIV)-infected individuals that leads either to reactivation of old tuberculous infections or to increased susceptibility to new infection is a major contributor to the increasing incidence of tuberculosis. Other factors are social dislocations, poverty, overcrowding, and a failure to invest in public health infrastructures. Particularly ominous is the emergence of multidrug-resistant tubercle bacilli. In the preantibiotic era, the case fatality rate of untreated tuberculosis was about 50%. With appropriate treatment, cure rates greater than 85% can now be achieved in both HIV-positive and immunocompetent individuals with conventional tuberculosis, even in developing countries. However, the case fatality rates of multidrug-resistant tuberculosis in the United States are about 40% for immunocompetent individuals and over 80% for HIV-infected individuals. Thus, tuberculosis has emerged as a major and devastating global threat to health, and many of the tools currently available for rapid diagnosis, prevention, and treatment are woefully lacking.

The aim of this book is to provide in one volume an overview of the current state of knowledge about tuberculosis and a critical appraisal of the exciting new molecular, immunological, and epidemiological approaches to understanding and controlling tuberculosis. The emphasis is on research. The authors hope to make existing knowledge and new avenues of research accessible to a new generation of researchers and clinicians. We hope to encourage scientists, clinicians, and students in many disciplines to undertake research on tuberculosis and want to facilitate the rapid generation of new knowledge, insights, and interventions.

Distinguished scientists knowledgeable in major areas of tuberculosis research and control have contributed critical reviews of current understanding and their thoughts on new approaches to each area. For most chapters in this book, I asked world experts to write collaboratively in order to provide balance, multiple perspectives on key issues, and critical delineation of the areas of consensus and contention. The authors were asked to be provocative rather than comprehensive. Our hope is that most chapters will be read with interest by anyone concerned with tuberculosis. Our intention is for the book to serve both as a challenge to scientists knowledgeable about aspects of tuberculosis and as a useful introduction to those with expertise in other disciplines who may wish to apply their knowledge and skills to the problem of tuberculosis. We hope, too, that the book will make accessible to scientists and students in developing countries, where the needs are greatest, the excitement of the new approaches to pathogenesis, resistance, and control.

This book is intended to honor rather than replace some of the classic sources of knowledge about tuberculosis. The classic studies of A. R. Rich (*The Pathogenesis of Tuberculosis*, 2nd ed., 1,028 p., Charles C Thomas, Publisher, 1951) and G. Canetti (*The Tubercle Bacillus in the Pulmonary Lesion of Man*, 226 p., Springer, 1955) on the pathogenesis of the human disease, of L. Barksdale and K.-S. Kim on the characteristics of the genus *Mycobacterium* (*Bacteriological Reviews*, **41**:217–372, 1977), of M. B. Lurie (*Resistance to Tuberculosis: Experimental Studies in Native and Acquired Defensive Mechanisms*, Harvard University Press, Cambridge, Mass., 1964) on experimental tuberculosis, and of K. Styblo (*Epidemiology of Tuberculosis*, Royal Netherlands Tuberculosis Association Selected Papers, vol. 24, The Hague, 1991) on epidemiology remain important reading for any student of the disease. The comprehensive texts edited by C. Ratledge and J. Stanford (*The Biology of the Mycobacteria*, 2 vol., Academic Press, 1981) and G. B. Kubica and L. G. Wayne (*The Mycobacteria: a Sourcebook*, 2 vol., Marcel Dekker, 1984) remain a repository of much valuable information. Yet the revolution in molecular biology, genetics, and immunology and the advances in understanding epidemiology and control of the disease in both developing and industrialized countries now offer far greater opportunities than were previously available for understanding and developing improved interventions in the disease. We hope this book will make a useful contribution to filling that gap in time and knowledge.

Acknowledgments

Because of current interest in the problem of tuberculosis, the limited number of experts on the disease are always in great demand. I wish to express my deep appreciation to each of the authors for giving so much of their valuable time and effort to this volume. I am particularly indebted to William R. Jacobs, Jr., and Patrick Brennan for providing continuing advice and wisdom in the planning of this book. Such a project would not have been possible to contemplate without the continuing support of my research from the Howard Hughes Medical Institute. Words cannot repay the dedication and heroic efforts of my secretary, Sandra Glass, for seeing to it that everything got done. I am very grateful for the commitment and care given to this project by the editorial staff of the American Society for Microbiology, particularly Patrick Fitzgerald, Susan Birch, and Marie Smith, whose contributions have been truly outstanding. Finally, I wish to express my deep appreciation for the patient understanding and support of my wife, Irene, and daughter, Inae, for the many hours I was preoccupied with this book.

I. INTRODUCTION TO TUBERCULOSIS

Tuberculosis: Pathogenesis, Protection, and Control
Edited by Barry R. Bloom
© 1994 American Society for Microbiology, Washington, DC 20005

Chapter 1

Global Burden of Tuberculosis

Dixie E. Snider, Jr., Mario Raviglione, and Arata Kochi

INTRODUCTION

The purpose of this chapter is to review the current epidemiology of tuberculosis (TB) in the world. From a global perspective, the magnitude of the TB problem is enormous. Furthermore, unless aggressive intervention is undertaken soon, the worldwide situation concerning TB will deteriorate rapidly; during this decade, nearly 90 million new cases will occur and 30 million people will die from TB. The disease is now the world's foremost cause of death from a single infectious agent.

Although in this chapter we concentrate on the number of new cases of and deaths from this disease, we recognize that these data do not fully describe the effect of the disease on the population. For example, we have not discussed the economic impact of the disease: direct and indirect costs of treatment of cases and suspected cases, costs of contact investigations, costs of TB screening and preventive therapy programs (where these are used), costs of hospital and institutional infection control programs, and costs to patients in lost income.

Dixie E. Snider, Jr. • Office of the Director, Centers for Disease Control and Prevention, Atlanta, Georgia 30333. *Mario Raviglione and Arata Kochi* • Tuberculosis Programme, World Health Organization, CH-1211, Geneva 27, Switzerland.

An increasing number of cases due to organisms multiply resistant to anti-TB drugs could escalate these costs dramatically.

Other factors we do not discuss in this chapter are the frequency of early and late complications and the impact of these complications on morbidity, mortality, and costs. There are few data on the frequency with which complications occur.

We also do not discuss the social impact of TB on the population: for example, loss of employment, decreased likelihood of marriage (especially for women), and creation of orphans and one-parent households. Again, few or no current data in the literature address these issues.

Ideally, we would like to present the exact numbers of new cases of TB and deaths from TB that occur each year. Unfortunately, disease surveillance in many countries is too incomplete to provide this information (Styblo and Rouillon, 1981). Because of this limitation, the burden of TB must be estimated indirectly by using several epidemiological parameters, including the average annual risk of TB infection, the reported incidence of smear-positive pulmonary TB, the estimated coverage of the population by health care services, the estimated proportion of all cases of TB that are smear-positive, and the estimated case-fatality rates for smear-positive and other forms of TB.

Tuberculosis Infection

The ability of the tuberculin skin test to detect the presence of *Mycobacterium tuberculosis* infection can be used to measure the prevalence of infection. A method for converting the prevalence of infection into the annual risk of infection has been developed (Styblo et al., 1969; Sutherland, 1976). The annual risk of infection is the probability that any individual will be infected with *M. tuberculosis* in 1 year. If several tuberculin surveys of the same population have been done at different times (using similar techniques and testing a representative sample of non-BCG-vaccinated subjects of the same age), the trend in the annual risk of infection can be estimated. In the absence of good surveillance systems to detect and report incident cases, calculating the annual risk of infection is a valuable technique for estimating the magnitude of the TB problem. Although there are limitations to this approach, Styblo has shown that a 1% annual risk of infection corresponds, on average, to an incidence of 50 smear-positive cases per 100,000 population (Murray et al., 1990).

Cauthen and Ten Dam (1988) have used the results of tuberculin skin test surveys done in developing countries since the 1950s to estimate the annual risks of infection in different regions of the developing world (Table 1). The annual risk of tuberculous infection is probably highest in sub-Saharan Africa, followed closely by risk in Southeast Asia.

Kochi (1991) has estimated that about one-third of the world's population, or about 1.7 billion people, is infected with *M. tuberculosis*. The great majority of the world's population, and thus the majority of infected persons, reside in developing countries. In industrialized countries, 80% of infected individuals are aged 50 years or more, while in developing countries, 75% of infected persons are less than 50 years old (Kochi, 1991).

Table 1. Estimated annual risk of TB and trends in developing countries, 1985 to 1990[a]

Area(s)	Estimated annual (%):	
	Risk of infection	Decrease in risk
Sub-Saharan Africa	1.5–2.5	1–2
North Africa and western Asia	0.5–1.5	5–6
Southeast Asia	1.0–2.0	1–3
South America	0.5–1.5	2–5
Central America and Caribbean	0.5–1.5	1–3

[a] Based on data in Cauthen and Ten Dam (1988).

Annual Incidence of Disease and Death

Table 2 shows the distribution of the present burden of cases and deaths. Over 8 million cases of TB occurred in 1992. Of these cases, 3.3 million were in the World Health Organization's (WHO's) Southeast Asian region, 1.9 million were in the western Pacific region, 1.2 million were in sub-Saharan Africa, and 1.6 million, including 199,000 cases in industrialized countries, were in the remainder of the world. TB has a devastating effect in the developing world, where 95% of cases occur. Eighty percent of these cases occur in persons who are in their productive years (ages 15 to 59). According to a 1989 WHO report, 1.3 million cases and 450,000 deaths from TB in developing countries occur in children under the age of 15 years (World Health Organization, 1989).

In the prechemotherapy era, mortality from TB was about 50 to 60% (Murray et al., 1990). Today, death rates in developing countries are not as high because a significant proportion of cases are detected and treated.

Nevertheless, an estimated 2.7 million persons died from TB in 1992: 1.1 million in the Southeast Asian region, 672,000 in the western Pacific region, 468,000 in the African region, and 426,000 in the remainder of the world (Table 2). TB causes over 25% of

Table 2. Estimated global TB incidence and mortality in 1992

Area	Incidence		Mortality	
	No. of cases	Rate[a]	No. of deaths	Rate[a]
Southeast Asia	3,263,000	240	1,142,000	84
Western Pacific[b]	1,921,000	136	672,000	48
Africa	1,182,000	214	468,000	85
Eastern Mediterranean	683,000	166	266,000	65
Americas[c]	584,000	128	117,000	26
Eastern Europe	197,000	47	29,000	7
Industrialized countries[d]	199,000	22	14,000	2
All regions	8,029,000	146	2,708,000	49

[a] Per 100,000 population.
[b] All countries of the region except Australia, Japan, and New Zealand.
[c] All countries of the region except Canada and the United States.
[d] Western Europe plus Australia, Canada, Japan, New Zealand, and the United States.

avoidable adult deaths in the developing world (Murray et al., 1990).

Impact of the HIV-AIDS Epidemic

The pandemic of human immunodeficiency virus (HIV) infection and the evidence of an association between tuberculosis and HIV infection has caused marked increases in the incidence of TB in some countries. Because of its ability to destroy the immune system, HIV has emerged as the most significant risk factor for progression of dormant TB infection to clinical disease (Selwyn et al., 1989).

The Global Programme on AIDS of the WHO estimated that in 1992 at least 13 million adults and 1 million children had been infected with HIV worldwide (World Health Organization, 1993). Nearly 85% of HIV infections have occurred in developing countries, and the vast majority have occurred in the age group 15 to 49 years.

It is estimated that about 1,700 million people are infected with *M. tuberculosis* (Kochi, 1991). The impact of HIV infection on the TB situation is greatest in those populations where the prevalence of TB infection in young adults (who are at greatest risk of HIV infection) is high. By using estimates of the prevalence of TB infection in various regions, it has been estimated that since the beginning of the HIV pandemic until mid-1993, more than 5 million persons worldwide have had dual HIV and TB infection. A great majority (3.8 million) of these patients lived in sub-Saharan Africa (Fig. 1). HIV seroprevalence rates of more than 40% are common among patients with TB in many African countries. The annual risk of progression to active TB among individuals infected with both HIV and TB is 5 to 10% (Narain et al., 1992).

The result of this increased risk is evident from the reported numbers of TB cases in several countries. After years of declining incidence of the disease, the number of reported cases of TB increased dramatically during the 1980s in many countries in sub-Saharan Africa. Within a 7-year period from 1985 to 1991, the annual number of cases in Zambia nearly tripled, that in Malawi more than doubled, and those in Tanzania and Burundi increased by about 70 and 40%, respectively. The numbers of deaths from TB have also increased in these countries (Narain et al., 1992).

The situation in some countries in Southeast Asia and the western Pacific is now similar to that in Africa several years ago. Since almost two-thirds of the world's TB-infected population is in Asia, entry of HIV into Asian communities may result in large increases in HIV-associated TB in the coming years. In Bombay, HIV seroprevalence

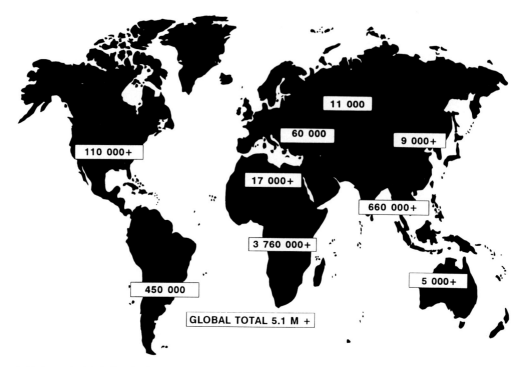

Figure 1. Estimated global distribution of adults who have been infected with HIV and TB, as of mid-1993. Source of data is WHO Tuberculosis Programme.

among TB patients increased from 2% in 1988 to 10 to 15% in 1991 and 1992. In northern Thailand, HIV seroprevalence in TB patients increased from 5% in late 1989 to 15% in 1992, and there is evidence that the incidence of TB is increasing (World Health Organization, unpublished data).

In many developing countries, TB has emerged as the most common opportunistic disease associated with HIV infection. Twenty to forty-four percent of AIDS patients in Africa, 18% of patients in Haiti, and up to 25% of patients in some Latin American countries, namely Brazil, Mexico, and Argentina, had clinical TB during the course of HIV infection (Narain et al., 1992).

It is still unclear how the increasing numbers of HIV-positive patients with TB will affect the transmission of TB in the community. It is possible that the increase in the number of TB cases will increase TB trans-

mission to both HIV-positive and HIV-negative populations. Nevertheless, preliminary data from the second round of the National Tuberculin Survey in Tanzania, where the TB control program has achieved an 80% cure rate of patients with newly diagnosed smear-positive cases during the last 5 years and a 65% case detection rate, suggest that the prevalence of infection in school children did not change appreciably from 1983–1985 to 1989–1991, despite the increase in the number of detected new smear-positive cases (Narain et al., 1992). Thus, a good control program may be able to reduce to some extent the increased chance of transmission.

HIV-infected patients with TB also have a higher incidence of noninfectious extrapulmonary forms of disease and higher mortality rates and thus may have a lesser impact on transmission than non-HIV-infected TB patients.

TUBERCULOSIS IN INDUSTRIALIZED COUNTRIES

United States

From 1953, when national surveillance began, through 1984, the United States experienced a significant decline in TB cases: from 84,304 cases in 1953 to only 22,225 cases in 1984. The average annual decline in cases was about 5.3% per year. From 1985 to 1992, however, the number of reported cases has increased by about 20%. Using the trend for 1980 to 1984 to calculate the number of expected cases, the Centers for Disease Control and Prevention (CDC) estimates that from 1985 through 1992, about 51,000 excess cases have accumulated (Fig. 2). Case rates in urban areas have increased more rapidly than those in rural areas.

Of the 26,673 TB cases reported in 1992, 71% occurred in racial and ethnic minorities. From 1985 to 1992, TB case numbers declined about 10% among non-Hispanic whites and 23% among Native Americans. However, case numbers increased 27% among blacks, 46% among Asians and Pacific Islanders, and 75% among Hispanics.

From 1985 through 1992, all age groups, except that of patients 65 years of age and older, experienced an increase in number of cases. The largest numerical and percentage increases (+3,686; +55%) were among persons 25 to 44 years of age. However, there was a 36% increase in case numbers among 0- to 4-year-old patients and a 34% increase among children 5 to 14 years old.

Of all patients with TB reported to the CDC in 1992, 27% were born in another country. The numbers and percentages of foreign-born patients increased from 4,925 and 22% in 1986 to 7,270 and 27% in 1992.

In addition to the effect of immigration on the change in the TB morbidity trend, there is evidence that the HIV epidemic is at least in part contributing to this change. The

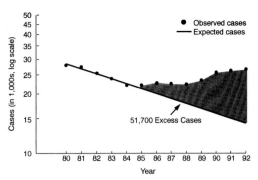

Figure 2. Numbers of expected and observed cases of TB in the United States from 1980 through 1992. Table is from the CDC (Centers for Disease Control and Prevention, 1993).

largest increases in reported TB case numbers have occurred in geographic areas and age groups heavily impacted by the HIV epidemic. TB prevalence among AIDS patients is high. Matching of TB and AIDS registries through 1990 revealed that 4.9% of reported AIDS cases were also in the TB registry (CDC, unpublished data). CDC HIV seroprevalence surveys in TB clinics have shown a high prevalence of HIV infection among TB patients. Pooled seroprevalence data from 13 cities that tested at least 50 serum samples per year for 1989, 1990, and 1991 showed seroprevalence rates of 13.1% in 1989, 17.8% in 1990, and 21.4% in 1991. Trend analysis from 1989 through 1991 also showed significant upward trends in HIV seroprevalence among black, Hispanic, and white males with TB or suspected TB. Among females, the upward trend was significant only for blacks (Onorato et al., 1993).

The United States has also experienced an increasing number of outbreaks of TB. Outbreaks have occurred in a variety of settings, including hospitals, correctional facilities, shelters for the homeless, residential care facilities for patients with AIDS, nursing homes, and even crack houses.

The most serious problem has been the outbreaks of multidrug-resistant TB (MDR-

TB), i.e., outbreaks due to organisms resistant to isoniazid and rifampin (and often other drugs as well). From 1990 through 1992, the CDC investigated outbreaks of MDR-TB in eight hospitals and a state correctional system. As of November 1992, 297 cases of MDR-TB had been identified in these outbreaks. Most but not all of the cases occurred in persons infected with HIV. Mortality was high (about 70%), and the median interval from TB diagnosis to death was short (4 to 16 weeks). The outbreak investigations demonstrated transmission of infection to health care workers. At least 17 health care and correctional workers have developed active TB with multidrug-resistant organisms (CDC, unpublished data).

Factors contributing to nosocomial outbreaks include the convergence of highly susceptible, immunocompromised patients and TB patients; the delayed recognition of TB (because of unconsidered diagnoses, nonclassical radiographic findings, and laboratory delays); the delayed recognition of drug resistance; and the delayed initiation of effective anti-TB treatment. Other factors contributing to nosocomial transmission include delayed initiation of isolation, inadequate ventilation for acid-fast bacillus (AFB) isolation, lapses in maintaining AFB isolation, inadequate duration of AFB isolation, and inadequate precautions during cough-inducing procedures.

Tuberculosis in Other Industrialized Countries

Seven of 15 Western European countries (Denmark, Ireland, Italy, Netherlands, Norway, Spain, and Switzerland) have also recently experienced increases in reported cases (Raviglione et al., 1993). The major factor responsible for most of these increases appears to be immigration from higher-prevalence countries. However, in Italy, 11.4% of AIDS patients reported during the biennium 1988 through 1989 had TB (Raviglione et al., 1993).

In Australia, death rates have remained stable at about 0.4/100,000, and notification rates of all cases have slightly increased from 5.6/100,000 in 1986 to 5.9/100,000 in 1990 (Cheah, 1992a). The HIV epidemic has had little impact on the TB situation in Australia. Two-thirds of the new patients reported in 1991 were foreign born (Cheah, 1992b).

In Canada, a similar stagnation of notifications and rates has been observed over the past 6 years. In 1991, 2,044 cases were reported (rate, 7.6/100,000). Foreign-born patients constituted 48% of all patients in 1989, and native Canadians constituted 20% of patients. TB mortality rates were stable at around 0.5/100,000 during recent years (WHO, unpublished data [from the Canadian Centre for Health Information, Ottawa]).

In Japan, the downward trend of TB notifications continues. The average decline between 1980 and 1991 has been 3.5% per year. However, this decline is smaller than that seen in previous years. Furthermore, the incidence of sputum-smear-positive cases has steadily increased since 1980. In general, mortality rates have regularly decreased at about 4.6% per year since 1980 (WHO, unpublished data [from the Japan Anti-Tuberculosis Association, Tokyo]).

In New Zealand, case notifications have recently increased from a nadir in 1988 of 295 cases reported. In 1991, 335 cases were reported (rate, 9.9/100,000). Mortality rates have decreased from 0.9 to 0.5/100,000 during the period 1980 to 1990 (WHO, unpublished data [from the New Zealand Department of Health, Wellington]).

In Israel, TB notifications, after being stable in the 1980s, recently increased to 505 in 1991 (rate, 10.2/100,000). However, if rates for Ethiopian immigrants are excluded from the data, the rate among native Jews in 1991 was 4.6/100,000 and that among native non-Jews was 3.7/100,000. Ethiopians, who generally constitute less than 25% of all cases, constituted 50% of all cases in 1985 and 55% of all cases in 1991, following two waves of migration (Operation Moses and Operation Shlomo) (WHO, unpublished data [from the Israel Ministry of Health, Jerusalem]).

In Turkey, TB notifications during the past few years have decreased, and in 1990, 24,468 cases were reported (rate, 43.8/100,000) (WHO, unpublished data [from the Turkish Ministry of Health, Ankara]).

DRUG RESISTANCE

Acquired resistance is defined as resistance to at least one anti-TB drug that arises during or after the course of treatment, usually as a result of nonadherence to the recommended regimen or of faulty prescribing. A high level of this type of resistance is a mark of a poorly functioning TB control program.

Primary resistance is defined as the presence of drug resistance to at least one anti-TB drug in a TB patient who has never received prior treatment. It is caused by infection with drug-resistant specimens from another patient excreting a drug-resistant organism; many of these patients acquired resistance as a result of inadequate treatment. Thus, primary resistance is an indicator of efficacy of TB control efforts in the past (Weyer and Kleeberg, 1992).

An accurate picture of the drug resistance problem in the world is not available, because only a limited number of countries (both industrialized and developing) have a reliable drug resistance surveillance system. However, limited available information indicates that, generally speaking, many industrialized countries that faced severe MDR-TB in the late 1950s and early 1960s successfully reduced the problem in a rather short time by improving application of the same regimen used previously and by

successfully introducing rifampin-containing short-course chemotherapy. Thus, the incidence of acquired resistance was substantially reduced, and the incidence of primary resistance remains relatively low. In many developing countries, particularly in Asia, the incidence of acquired resistance remains high and the incidence of primary resistance is higher than that in industrialized countries, because national TB control programs in the developing countries have not been able to achieve a high cure rate over a very long period, even after the introduction of short-course chemotherapy.

This already serious situation may quickly worsen as the HIV epidemic spreads. The HIV epidemic may produce increased levels of both acquired and primary resistance not only by overtaxing the national TB control programs as a result of increased caseload but also by affecting compromised immunity (Kochi et al., 1993).

FUTURE TRENDS

Without recognition of the TB crisis confronting the world and prompt, effective action, the TB epidemic can be expected to worsen for several reasons.

First, demographic forces are at work. Children born in past decades in regions with high population growth rates are now reaching the ages at which morbidity and mortality for TB are high. Even if the age-specific rates of new cases do not increase, the changing sizes of the population age groups will now begin to cause a large increase in the number of TB deaths and new cases.

Second, famine, war, and natural disasters that create large populations of displaced, malnourished people in crowded living conditions may cause increases in TB case rates.

Third, age-specific TB incidence rates can be expected to rise in those areas of the world where immunity of the population is seriously challenged by HIV infection. By mid-1993, the global cumulative number of persons coinfected with HIV and tubercle bacilli since the beginning of the HIV pandemic was estimated to be over 5 million (Fig. 1). In addition, HIV seroprevalence among TB patients is expected to increase further in areas like sub-Saharan Africa and to increase at least threefold in areas like Southeast Asia during the next decade. As a result, while about 315,000 persons are estimated to have developed HIV-associated TB in 1990, more than 700,000 people are expected to develop HIV-related TB in 1995. In the year 2000, the figure may reach 1.4 million. In 1990, 4.2% of all TB cases were associated with HIV; in the year 2000, an estimated 13.8% of all TB cases may be associated with HIV (Dolin et al., in press).

In addition, there is the threat of the increasing incidence of drug-resistant strains. This phenomenon is largely a consequence of poorly managed and inappropriately focused TB programs and is accelerated and amplified by the HIV coinfection epidemic. Drug-resistant strains are as contagious as the normal TB bacillus. The cure rates of at least 95% that can be achieved for regular TB fall to 70% or less when isoniazid and rifampin resistance occurs.

If the effectiveness and availability of TB control do not improve substantially over those existing now, more than 30 million TB deaths and 90 million new cases are expected to occur in the last decade of this century. Conservative estimates indicate that the incidence of TB can be expected to increase to 8.8 million cases annually by 1995, 10.2 million cases annually by the year 2000, and 11.9 million cases annually by 2005 (Dolin et al., in press). Demographic factors will account for three-quarters of the predicted increase in new cases. Assuming that the availability and effectiveness of treatment programs remain at the 1990 level, 3 million TB deaths can be

expected to occur annually by 1995, and 3.5 million deaths will be occurring annually by the year 2000. Action must be taken now to avert this global health disaster.

REFERENCES

Cauthen, G. M., and H. G. Ten Dam. 1988. Annual risk of tuberculosis infection. *Geneva: W.H.O./TB* **88**:154.

Centers for Disease Control and Prevention. 1993. Tuberculosis morbidity—United States, 1992. *Morbid. Mortal. Weekly Rep.* **42**:696–704.

Cheah, D. 1992a. Tuberculosis notification rates, Australia final data for 1986 to 1990. *Communicable Dis. Intell.* **16**:234–236.

Cheah, D. 1992b. Tuberculosis notification rates, Australia, 1991. *Communicable Dis. Intell.* **16**:398–400.

Dolin, P. J., M. C. Raviglione, and A. Kochi. Global tuberculosis incidence and mortality during 1990–2000. *Bull. W.H.O.*, in press.

Kochi, A. 1991. The global tuberculosis situation and the new control strategy of the World Health Organization. *Tubercle* **72**:1–6.

Kochi, A., B. Vareldzis, and K. Styblo. 1993. Multidrug-resistant tuberculosis and its control. *Res. Microbiol.* **2**:104–110.

Murray, C. J. L., K. Styblo, and A. Rouillon. 1990. Tuberculosis in developing countries: burden, intervention and cost. *Bull. Int. Union Tuberc. Lung Dis.* **65**:6–24.

Narain, J. P., M. C. Raviglione, and A. Kochi. 1992. HIV-associated tuberculosis in developing countries: epidemiology and strategies for prevention. *Tuberc. Lung Dis.* **73**:311–321.

Onorato, I., S. McCombs, M. Morgan, and E. McCray. 1993. HIV infection in patients attending tuberculosis clinics, United States, 1988–1992. *Program Abstr. 33rd Intersci. Conf. Antimicrob. Agents Chemother.*, abstr. 1363.

Raviglione, M. C., P. Sudre, H. L. Rieder, S. Spinaci, and A. Kochi. 1993. Secular trends of tuberculosis in Western Europe. *Bull. W.H.O.* **71**:297–306.

Selwyn, P. A., D. Hartel, and I. A. Lewis. 1989. A prospective study of the risk of tuberculosis among intravenous drug abusers with human immunodeficiency virus infection. *N. Engl. J. Med.* **320**:545–550.

Styblo, K., J. Meiger, and I. Sutherland. 1969. The transmission of tubercle bacilli, its trend in a human population. *Bull. Int. Union. Tuberc. Lung Dis.* **42**:5–104.

Styblo, K., and A. Rouillon. 1981. Estimated global incidence of smear-positive pulmonary tuberculosis. Unreliability of officially reported figures on tuberculosis. *Bull. Int. Union Tuberc. Lung Dis.* **56:**118–126.

Sutherland, I. 1976. Recent studies in the epidemiology of tuberculosis, based on the risk of being infected with tubercle bacilli. *Adv. Tuberc. Res.* **19:**1–63.

Weyer, K., and H. H. Kleeberg. 1992. Primary and acquired drug resistance in adult black patients with tuberculosis in South Africa: results of a continuous national drug surveillance programme involvement. *Tuberc. Lung Dis.* **73:**106–112.

World Health Organization. 1989. Childhood tuberculosis and BCG vaccine. *In EPI Update Supplement.* World Health Organization, Geneva.

World Health Organization. 1993. Global Programme on AIDS. The HIV/AIDS pandemic: 1993 overview. WHO/EPA/CNP/EVA/93.1.

Tuberculosis: Pathogenesis, Protection, and Control
Edited by Barry R. Bloom
© 1994 American Society for Microbiology, Washington, DC 20005

Chapter 2

History of Tuberculosis

Thomas M. Daniel, Joseph H. Bates, and Katharine A. Downes

EARLY HISTORY OF TUBERCULOSIS

In the paleolithic period, people lived as wanderers, did not settle in villages or permanent locations, and did not congregate in large groups. While tuberculosis may have occurred sporadically, it and other infectious diseases probably did not occur in epidemic form. Beginning in about 8000 B.C., humans developed primitive agricultural techniques that allowed settlement in permanent sites, and with this development came the domestication of cattle, swine, and sheep. In all probability, tuberculosis occurred more frequently in this setting, but it nevertheless remained rare (Clark, 1962). McGrath estimates that a social network of 180 to 440 persons is required to achieve the stable host-pathogen relationship necessary for tuberculous infection to become endemic in a community (McGrath, 1988).

Tuberculosis probably occurred as an endemic disease among animals long before it affected humans (Steele and Ranney,

Thomas M. Daniel and Katharine A. Downes • Center for International Health, Case Western Reserve University School of Medicine, 10900 Euclid Avenue, Cleveland, Ohio 44106. *Joseph H. Bates* • Department of Medicine, University of Arkansas for Medical Sciences, John L. McClellan Memorial Veterans' Hospital, 4300 West 7th Street, Little Rock, Arkansas 72205.

1958). *Mycobacterium bovis* was the most likely infecting organism, and the first human infections may have been with *M. bovis*. Since *M. tuberculosis* infects all primate species, it is also possible that this species existed in subhuman primates before it became established in humans.

As centuries and millennia passed, human beings began to live in larger and larger communities, and with this shift came environmental changes that were associated with a change in the delicate balance between humans and the tubercle bacillus. Two alternative theories have been proposed to explain the epidemic spread and subsequent decline of tuberculosis that followed. The first and widely accepted explanation involves the development of genetically determined herd immunity (Stead, 1992). As a rule, parasites are short-lived compared to their hosts, and this fact gives parasites a great advantage, since mutations can occur in them more frequently than in their hosts in response to environmental pressure. When the host generation time is much longer than that of the parasite, as is true of humans and the tubercle bacillus, the host cannot adapt as quickly as the parasite. Thus, initially the parasite has a distinct advantage and begins to eliminate the susceptible members of the species before these individuals can pass on their genes to progeny. However, since not all hosts of a species are eliminated, the progeny of the survivors form a subset of the population that is characterized by increased resistance to that particular parasite (Hamilton et al., 1990). Thus, over time, the highly advantageous position enjoyed by the parasite diminishes, and after successive generations, the once serious life-threatening infection becomes less devastating. Probably for this reason, no infectious disease has ever killed all of its host population. Many other factors, such as nutrition and overcrowding, contribute to the incidence of disease in a population, but genetic factors are of unquestioned importance in the selective mortality from infection.

Tuberculosis probably occurred as a sporadic and unimportant disease of humans in their early history. Epidemic spread began slowly with increasing population density. This spread and the selective pressure it has exerted have occurred at different times around the globe. The epidemic slowly spread worldwide as a result of infected Europeans traveling to and colonizing distant sites (Diamond, 1992). In the 1700s and early 1800s, tuberculosis prevalence peaked in Western Europe and the United States and was undoubtedly the largest cause of death (reviewed by Bloom and Murray, 1992, and Graunt, 1662), and 100 to 200 years later, it had spread in full force to Eastern Europe, Asia, Africa, and South America. Within a particular population in a defined geographic area, the tuberculosis epidemic reached its peak within 50 to 75 years after its beginning and then slowly declined, possibly as the more resistant host survivors reproduced.

Tuberculosis Epidemics in Europe and North America

It is important to recognize that tuberculosis remained an unimportant disease for humans regardless of its virulence until in feudal Europe the necessary environmental changes occurred to set off an epidemic that came to be called "The Great White Plague" (Dubos and Dubos, 1952; Castiglioni, 1933; Webb, 1936; Cummins, 1949). In the early 1600s, the incidence of tuberculosis in England began to increase sharply. The epidemic grew over the next two centuries and spread through Western Europe. During this phase of the epidemic, almost all Western Europeans became infected with *M. tuberculosis*, and about one in four deaths were due to tuberculosis. In the ever-enlarging cities, the increased population density provided the necessary environmental conditions for person-to-person spread of this airborne pathogen. Such conditions had never been met previously.

European migrants brought the tubercle bacillus with them to North America (Diamond, 1992). For example, in Boston, Massachusetts, the mortality rate from tuberculosis was as high as 650/100,000 in 1800, and it decreased to about 400/100,000 by 1860 (Grigg, 1958). In like manner, the tuberculosis death rate in New York was 750 in 1805 and decreased to 400 by 1870. In Baltimore, it was as high as 400 in 1830 and decreased to 210 by 1900. In the cities along the northeastern seaboard, each succeeding generation experienced a decreased death rate. By 1904 the tuberculosis death rate in the United States was 188; it fell to 4/100,000 by 1969. As Western Europeans moved about the globe, the epidemic of tuberculosis followed them. It moved slowly to Eastern Europe. As late as the 1880s, tuberculosis was not commonly seen in Russia, and it was relatively uncommon in India at the same time. Cummins reports that tuberculosis was almost unknown within the interior of sub-Saharan Africa as late as 1908 (Cummins, 1920). It was essentially unknown in the interior of New Guinea as late as 1920, when that area was first explored by Europeans (Brown et al., 1981).

Tuberculosis among Indigenous Peoples of the Western Hemisphere

Although tuberculosis was present in the Western Hemisphere in paleolithic times, Native Americans of North America and South America had little trouble with tuberculosis prior to the European migration. In the immediately pre-Columbian era, about 60 million persons lived in South and North Americas, with the great majority living in South America. There were few, if any, large population centers. Buikstra and Cook reported a review of 14 prehistoric human skeletons from eight population centers in Illinois dating between 100 B.C. and 1300 A.D. (Buikstra and Cook, 1981). Some of these skeletons showed deformities compatible with tuberculosis, but the lesions were not diagnostic of tuberculosis. Perzigian and Widmer (1979) described osseous changes typical of tuberculosis in the vertebral skeletal remains of 6 of 290 persons from an Ohio community dated to 1275 A.D.

Acid-fast bacilli were observed in the lungs of a mummy from southern Peru dated from about 700 A.D., and subsequent additional cases of tuberculosis have been observed in South American mummies (Allison et al., 1973). Deformities suggesting Pott's disease among skeletons dating back to 160 B.C. have been found in Peru. In his review of prehistoric skeletal deformities in Latin America, Ponce describes large numbers of prehistoric figures and drawings depicting Pott's disease (Ponce Sangines, 1969). Endemic tuberculosis in the pre-Columbian South American setting would be compatible with the fairly complex society, densely sited housing, and established agriculture that existed among the inhabitants of Peru as long as 6,000 years ago.

Despite this archaeologic evidence, tuberculosis was a rare disease among native North American Indians even early into the 19th century. Priests who explored the Great Lakes region during this time reported rare cases of glandular infection and chronic pulmonary conditions that were probably tuberculous in nature. It was only after the North American Indians were forced to settle on reservations or to live in barracks and prison camps that outbreaks of tuberculosis were observed. In these settings, contact with white settlers became frequent, and the crowding promoted airborne transmission of the bacillus. In 1887 at the Mount Vernon Barracks, several hundred Apache prisoners were kept in close confinement, and the death rate the first year was 54/1,000, rising to 143/1,000 in the fourth year. Nearly half of these deaths were due to tuberculosis (Bushnell, 1930). By 1886, the tuberculosis death rate for North American Indians reached 9,000/100,000 (Ferguson, 1955). These death rates are the highest ever recorded worldwide and exceed by 10 times the peak death rate observed in Europe in the 17th century.

Tuberculosis in Africa

Tuberculosis of the spine is depicted in several figurines dating from the predynastic era (prior to 3000 B.C.) of Nilotic North Africa (Morse et al., 1964). Some of these figurines appear to have originated from nomadic desert-living tribes. Additional similar figures and paintings clearly depicting angular spinal deformities characteristic of tuberculous spondylitis occur throughout Egyptian dynastic times. Mummies from several Egyptian sites show skeletal changes typical of tuberculosis (Morse et al., 1964), and psoas abscesses and fibrotic pulmonary disease have been observed, further supporting the impression that the skeletal changes were tuberculous in origin. Among 10 early dynastic Nubian skeletons, spinal disease typical of tuberculosis was found in 4. These four skeletons came from two graves, suggesting the familial occurrence of tuberculosis.

Despite the fact that tuberculosis was spreading rapidly in Europe, Nilotic North Africa, and the Americas, it remained essentially unknown in sub-Saharan Africa as late as the beginning of the 20th century. A number of medical observers reported the complete absence of tuberculosis in the interior of sub-Saharan Africa. Army medical officers from Great Britain noted that tuberculosis was unknown in those parts of Africa where European immigration had not occurred (Cummins, 1920). Livingstone (1857) found no tuberculosis in parts of South Africa, and Lichenstein found none as late as the first half of the 20th century (Lichenstein, 1928).

Tuberculosis in Asia and the Pacific Islands

The Hawaiian Islands had little or no tuberculosis as late as the 1850s. Wilkinson remarked upon the rarity of tuberculosis in India in the first half of the 19th century and its progressive increase in the middle years of the 19th century as industrialization increased population density (Wilkinson, 1914). Toward the end of the 19th century, India and China experienced peaks in the incidence of tuberculosis, but as late as 1951, tuberculosis was still unknown among the island populations of New Guinea (Brown et al., 1981). Finally, when the disease did reach these latter populations, it produced the typhoidal illness so characteristic of highly susceptible individuals having their first experience with tuberculosis.

TUBERCULOSIS AND THE DAWNING OF BIOMEDICAL SCIENCE

From the time of Hippocrates, tuberculosis was known as "phthisis," a term derived from the Greek for "wasting away." The swollen glands of the neck were known as "scrofula," and because newly crowned kings of England and France were believed to have special healing powers, the most desired treatment of this "King's Evil" was being touched by kings. Tuberculosis of the skin was termed lupus vulgaris, and that of the spine was termed Pott's disease. The vertebral fusion and deformity of the spine that characterize Pott's disease have enabled historians to establish the existence of tuberculosis in mummies dating from 2000 to 4000 B.C.

As Europe emerged from the Dark Ages, there was a renaissance not only of the arts but also of medical science. Observant scientists described their world and explored its nature and mechanisms. This European intellectual renaissance began in an era of extraordinarily high tuberculosis prevalence fueled by the industrial revolution and the grinding poverty it engendered in its huddled masses. Hence, it is not surprising that many fundamental concepts of biology emerged in the context of inquiry about the nature of tuberculosis. Weaving together stories of individuals whose lives were dramatically affected by tuberculosis with accounts of pioneering exploration of the pathogenesis of this disease, we will attempt to create a tapestry depicting the genesis of four areas of knowledge about tuberculosis and the human and social contexts in which the knowledge was acquired.

Infectious Etiology of Tuberculosis

Tuberculosis (consumption) was common in European cities during the first half of the 19th century, and one-fifth to one-quarter of all deaths were due to this disease (Waksman, 1964). No one knew what caused tuberculosis. Some doubted that it was a single disease, so varied were its manifestations. That it might be contagious was a notion that occurred to only a few. Thus, Frederick Chopin was not expecting hostility from the inhabitants of Majorca, where he had gone in 1839 to seek relief from his symptoms. However, his doctors alerted the residents of the island that the famous composer and musician was consumptive, public clamor ensued, and his landlord turned him out (Dubos and Dubos, 1952; Waksman, 1964).

Frederick Chopin had been a sickly youth. He first developed clinical tuberculosis at age 16. Dubos and Dubos (1952) quote Georges Sand, who accompanied Chopin to Majorca. She recounted that the landlord who expelled them sought damages for replastering the house they had occupied because it was contaminated. Their departure arrangements were complicated by the refusal of carriage drivers to transport them and their goods. They crossed the island with wheelbarrows. They sailed to Barcelona with a shipload of pigs, and the inn keeper in Barcelona charged them for Chopin's bed, which the local authorities required be burned. Chopin died of tuberculosis a decade later in 1849. He was 39 years old.

A scant 20 years prior to Chopin's ejection from Majorca, Theophile Laennec published his classic text on diseases of the chest (Laennec, 1962). While Laennec is best known to students of medicine for his description of alcoholic cirrhosis of the liver, his principal interest throughout his life was tuberculosis. Major credits Laennec with first recognizing that tuberculosis, in all of its forms and anatomic sites, is a single disease (Major, 1945). This view was not espoused by most of the pathologists of Laennec's era. Laennec died of tuberculosis in 1826. Waksman points out that this was the same year in which Chopin developed his tuberculosis (Waksman, 1964).

In 1679, Franciscus Sylvius described the characteristic lung nodules as "tubercula" or "small knots" and observed their evolution to cavities, but virtually all of the great pathologists, including Rudolf Virchow, believed the disease to be constitutional, a form of tumor or abnormal gland, rather than infectious. H. Fracastoro included phthisis in a work on contagion in 1546, but the first credible understanding that tuberculosis might be due to infectious microorganisms was made in 1722 by Benjamin Marten of London, who proposed that the cause of tuberculosis was "animaliculae or

their seed . . . inimicable to our Nature" that can be transmitted by "a Breath [a consumptive] emits from his Lungs . . . that may be caught by a sound Person" (Doetsch, 1978; Castiglioni, 1933). More than a century after Laennec's birth, Villemin performed experiments on rabbits, injecting infectious sputum and caseous material into healthy animals to produce disease. These studies, published in 1868 and cited by Major (1945), provided the first convincing evidence of the infectious nature of tuberculosis. Gradually, the infectious nature of tuberculosis became more widely recognized. As early as 1699, Italy and later Spain enacted restrictive quarantine laws, while in Northern Europe, tuberculosis was not widely viewed as a public health problem.

On March 24, 1882, a third of a century after Chopin's death, Robert Koch made a presentation to the Berlin Physiological Society that changed thinking about tuberculosis and infectious diseases forever and that can be thought of as establishing the science of microbiology. He described the tubercle bacillus, *M. tuberculosis*, an organism still known to many as Koch's bacillus, and convincingly demonstrated it to be the cause of tuberculosis (Koch, 1932; Sakula, 1982; Grange and Bishop, 1982). To carry out his pioneering studies, Koch developed staining techniques and was the first to employ culture on solid media. This landmark technical advance allowed the subculturing of individual colonies, clearly a fundamental technical advance in microbiology. His criteria for proof that the organism he discovered caused tuberculosis have been widely adopted and have become known as Koch's postulates. He specified that, "it was necessary to isolate the bacilli from the body; to grow them in pure culture . . .; and, by administering the isolated bacilli to animals, to reproduce the same morbid condition . . ." (Koch, 1932). Regrettably, in 1890 he also announced that culture filtrates cured the disease, a claim that was immediately controversial and promptly discredited. Sadly, Koch refused to divulge the nature and preparation of the curative material, an action for which he was accused of trying to give his government a monopoly and himself an institute (Bloom and Murray, 1992). Nevertheless, those filtrates, later partially purified, became the principal means of establishing the presence of infection in an individual, i.e., the tuberculin skin test.

Koch's initial presentation, made to the physiologists because Virchow refused to allow him to address the pathologists in Berlin, was received with great excitement, and his observations were rapidly confirmed by others. Among those who heard him was Paul Ehrlich, who hastened to develop improved staining techniques; Ziehl and Neelson quickly made further refinements, upon which diagnostic sputum smears are still based today. Subsequently, Ehrlich stained acid-fast bacilli in his own sputum to establish his personal diagnosis of tuberculosis. Edward Livingston Trudeau, whose own youthful, nearly fatal bout with tuberculosis led him to devote his life to the study and treatment of this disease, learned of Koch's work. He established his laboratory at Saranac Lake, New York, and repeated and extended Koch's observations. Fundamental work on tuberculosis continued at that laboratory for decades, and when Trudeau's cottage sanatorium finally closed, its endowment was used to establish the Trudeau Institute, where research on the immunology of tuberculosis continues to this day.

With the infectious nature of tuberculosis firmly established and the tubercle bacillus a pathogen that could be identified in laboratories, public health officials urged actions to interdict its spread: the beginning of the public health movement in the United States. Coughing and spitting in public were the subject of regulations and became socially unacceptable. In hospitals,

the burning of Chopin's bed linen was repeated again and again as concern over fomites grew. In the 1930s, William Wells injected both common sense and reason into controlling the transmission of infectious particles when he pointed out that the tubercle bacillus is an airborne, inhaled pathogen. He emphasized the role of infectious droplet nuclei and undertook studies of their aerial spread. This work culminated in the classic study by Riley, a pupil of Wells (Riley et al., 1962). In this study, air from a tuberculosis ward was delivered untreated to an animal exposure chamber and, after UV irradiation, to a control chamber. Each chamber housed 120 guinea pigs. No infections occurred in guinea pigs receiving irradiated air, while 63 animals receiving untreated air became infected. Thus, the aerial spread of tuberculosis was firmly established. By matching microbial drug susceptibility patterns, one patient with tuberculosis laryngitis was identified as particularly infectious. Modern parallels are presented by microepidemics in poorly ventilated areas, of which few are more dramatic than the one described by Catanzaro just 100 years after Koch's demonstration of the tubercle bacillus (Catanzaro, 1982). Among hospital personnel caring for a patient with unrecognized infectious tuberculosis in an intensive care unit, primary infections occurred in 31% of susceptible exposed individuals, with the attack rate reaching 77% in persons attending a bronchoscopy. The patient was estimated to be generating 249 infectious units per h, and the ventilation in the patient area provided only 1.2 air turnovers per h.

Resistance to Tuberculosis

The romantic age of the 19th century glamorized the sallow, wan physical appearance typical of patients with tuberculosis. Thus, when Daniel Chester French began his work on the statue of John Harvard that remains a notable feature of the

Harvard Yard, he seized upon the fact that John Harvard was known to have had tuberculosis to model a face "delicate-. . . and sensitive in expression" (Richman, 1977). But this romantic view of tuberculosis belies the facts. The variable course of tuberculosis makes it evident to all observers that some individuals are much more susceptible to the ravages of this disease than others. Some tuberculous patients are hardy and robust while still diseased; others suffer more.

John Keats was a remarkable poet who died of tuberculosis in 1821 at the age of 26. He met tuberculosis in his family at an early age; his mother died of this disease when he was 14, and his brother later developed tuberculosis. Keats studied medicine and was torn between it and poetry, for which he was acclaimed in his lifetime. In the summer of 1820 he developed hemoptysis, which he recognized as his death warrant, and from that point his course was steadily downhill. His short life ended in Italy in February 1821. During his final weeks, his treatment included phlebotomies, the same ineffective therapy used for Laennec. Although Keats succumbed rather rapidly to what must have been fulminant disease, it is incorrect to think of him as weak or asthenic. As a youth he was robust and athletic. He enjoying wrestling, mountain climbing, and long walking trips over rough terrain.

Robert Louis Stevenson's life and death contrast with those of Keats. Also a writer acclaimed in his time, Stevenson traveled across the world seeking a benevolent climate where he would find relief from his tuberculosis. He wrote *The Master of Ballantrae* and other stories published as the Scribner series while a patient at Trudeau's cottage sanatorium in Saranac Lake. His Saranac Lake home is open today as a museum. Chronically but never acutely ill, debilitated by disease of relatively stability, he continued writing and traveling, finally dying in the South Pacific in 1894 of vascular disease probably unrelated to his tuberculosis.

Perhaps the most illustrative example of familial tendency toward tuberculosis is the Brontë family. This literary British family shared a passion for learning and writing and a strong predisposition for acquiring tuberculosis. The Reverend Brontë and his wife Maria had six children in less than 7 years: Maria (1813), Elizabeth (1815), Charlotte (1816), Patrick Branwell (1817), Emily (1818), and Anne (1820) (Chadwick, 1914). All six children died of tuberculosis before they reached their 40th birthdays.

Less than a year after the birth of Anne, Mrs. Brontë died at age 39 in 1821. It is unclear whether she died from cancer, a postpartum complication, or septicemia. Three years later, in July 1824, Reverend Brontë found himself unable to care for his young daughters, and he sent the four eldest to a boarding school for the daughters of clergy at Cowan Bridge. The harsh regimen, poor diet, and walks in the freezing rain did not agree with the young girls' "delicate constitutions." In April of 1825, the eldest daughter, Maria, developed the symptoms of tuberculosis and was sent home, only to die in May at the age of 12. Elizabeth followed, returning home in May to die of the same disease in less than a month at the age of 11.

The Brontë family then enjoyed a 23-year hiatus from tuberculosis, during which each of the children wrote pieces that became cornerstones of British literature. In 1848, however, the opium-addicted poet Branwell Brontë died from tuberculosis at the age of 31 (Fraser, 1988). According to Fraser, he might have contracted tuberculosis in the village, "where it was endemic, which would explain the speed with which it killed Emily and Anne" (Fraser, 1988). Other possible sources "were either Emily or Charlotte herself, who was carrying a form of chronic fibrotic tuberculosis which periodically flared up, or Mr. Brontë, who is believed to have suffered from chronic tubercular bronchitis'' (Fraser, 1988). At her brother's funeral, Emily Brontë, author of *Wuthering Heights*, caught a cold that was said to have weakened her in her bereaved state, and in December 1848 she succumbed to "galloping consumption" at the age of 30. After losing her only brother and older sister in less than 3 months, Anne Brontë sadly soon followed, dying in May of 1849 at the age of 29, leaving behind her novel *Agnes Grey*. Only Charlotte Brontë remained. Six years later, on July 29, 1854, she married for the first time at the age of 38. Her marriage lasted less than a year. While walking on the moors with her husband, she caught a cold that developed into full tuberculosis, and she died on March 31, 1855, at the age of 39. The Reverend Brontë outlived his entire family, dying in 1861 at the age of 85.

Max Lurie emigrated from Lithuania to the United States in 1908 at the age of 15. He entered medical school at Cornell University and graduated in 1921, but he did not practice medicine, for he developed tuberculosis, making his own diagnosis. Although medical students were at increased exposure risk of tuberculosis in that time, Lurie felt that he was disposed to this disease by his family history. His mother had tuberculosis; her father and grandmother had died of it.

Beginning his studies while a patient at the National Jewish Hospital in Denver and continuing at the Phipps Institute of the University of Pennsylvania, Lurie dedicated his life to studies of the experimental pathology of tuberculosis. He recognized the central role of monocytes and their tissue forms (macrophages) in host resistance. He understood clearly the differences between host responses to initial and subsequent infections with mycobacteria. He became intrigued with the factors that made some individuals and some kindreds susceptible and others resistant to the ravages of this infection.

Lurie chose bovine tuberculosis in rabbits for his studies, feeling it to be the animal model that best approximated the pathogenesis of human tuberculosis. He undertook studies with inbred families of rabbits, developing strains that "exhibit varying characteristic inherited resistance to tuberculosis, generation after inbred generation" (Lurie, 1964). This work set the stage for the widespread use of inbred laboratory animals to elucidate genetic aspects of many diseases. Studies in twins have shown that Lurie's concepts are applicable to humans (Comstock, 1978), an observation not surprising to clinicians and other observers of people, who have long recognized the occurrence of tuberculosis in families.

Immunology of Tuberculosis

Samuel Johnson suffered from scrofula, the King's Evil. In 1712 he was touched by Queen Anne, whose ancestors, beginning with King Clovis of France in the fifth century, claimed the divine power to heal this affliction. Knowing that tuberculosis adenitis usually represents primary infection, that its course is often benign, and that primary infection confers immunity against reinfection, it is easy to understand how royal claims of a cure might have gained widespread acceptance.

In 1891, Robert Koch, already famous for his discovery of the tubercle bacillus, described experiments with guinea pigs that extended his earlier observations and clearly demonstrated acquired immunity following primary infection, and the term "Koch phenomenon" has been applied to the results he described (Bothamley and Grange, 1991). Koch noted that healthy guinea pigs inoculated cutaneously with tubercle bacilli healed the primary inoculation lesion, only to die later of disseminated infection. However, a second inoculation of virulent organisms produced a very different result. The wound became indurated in 1 or 2 days and then ulcerated; dissemination did not result. When tubercle bacilli killed by boiling were used for the initial inoculation, the same result followed. Koch noted that a sterile culture filtrate of bacilli, which he named tuberculin, evoked the cutaneous induration as well as whole organisms did, and he attributed the hypersensitivity thus demonstrated to something in this filtrate. Indeed, he proposed treating tuberculous patients with tuberculin, a measure that failed to have therapeutic benefit.

The warp thread of acquired immunity was deftly woven into the fabric of the history of tuberculosis by Albert Calmette and Camille Guérin (Sakula, 1983). Calmette, a French physician with extensive experience in infectious and tropical diseases, was appointed to the directorship of the newly founded Pasteur Institute of Lille in 1895. He was joined there by Guérin, his assistant and a veterinarian, in 1897. They knew of Koch's experiments, of early work done by von Pirquet and others on tuberculin hypersensitivity, and of the apparent success of Pasteur in vaccinating against rabies. With great hope, they began in 1908 to attenuate a strain of *M. bovis* by serial passage. By 1919 they had completed 230 passages, and their vaccine strain was found to be avirulent in guinea pigs, rabbits, cattle, and horses. It was first given to a human in 1921. Without detailing the long history of conflicting results from clinical trials, the efficacy of bacille Calmette-Guérin (BCG) remains unknown today. However, it is currently in widespread use throughout the world.

Today, the immunology of tuberculosis is well known. While many important questions are yet to be answered, it is clear that T lymphocytes responding to protein antigens of mycobacteria and lymphokines, prominently including interleukins 1 and 2, gamma interferon, and tumor necrosis factor alpha, are major mediators of protective immune responses in tuberculosis. Among the contributions of many, the seminal observations of Merrill Chase deserve special note (Chase, 1985, 1988). Chase was engaged in the study of contact dermatitis in the laboratory of Karl Landsteiner. Landsteiner was convinced that cell-fixed antibodies were responsible for this and other forms of delayed hypersensitivity. In 1941 and 1942, partly by accident, Chase found that dermal-contact hypersensitivity could be transferred by cell suspensions. Two years later, the observation was extended to tuberculin reactivity induced with mycobacteria. The science of cellular immunology was born, rising from these experiments with guinea pigs infected with tubercle bacilli.

Treatment of Tuberculosis

Alice Marble was born on September 28, 1913, in a settlement named Dutch Flat in Plumas County, California, the daughter of a lumberman and a nurse (Davidson and Jones, 1971). By her early teenage years, her athletic prowess was manifest, and she enjoyed the privilege of participating in pregame warm-ups of the San Francisco Seals, a minor league baseball team. Her oldest brother, Dan, concerned about his 15-year-old tomboy sister, returned home one evening with a gift for Alice—a tennis racquet. He hoped that she would apply herself to a more ladylike sport than baseball.

Eight months later, Alice Marble won her first tournament, and in 1931 she traveled to the East Coast to participate in the national tennis championships. In less than a year, she was ranked seventh in the national senior rankings. A new coach, Eleanor "Teach" Tennant, helped her become accustomed to the grass courts of the east, and in 1933 she traveled to Great Britain to represent the United States in the Wightman Cup. Her skills improved, and her game, marked by a masculine and powerful style exhibited in volleys and serves, seemed near perfection. Then tragedy struck. In 1934, Alice Marble collapsed during competition on the tennis court in Stade Roland Garros in Paris. She awoke in a hospital to a diagnosis of tuberculosis and the disheartening medical opinion that her tennis career was over (Marble and Leatherman, 1991).

Alice Marble left Paris by wheelchair and sailed on the S.S. *Aquitania* to New York, where she was greeted by a physician's assessment that she "would never play tennis again." She returned to her home in California and then entered Pottenger's Sanitorium in Monrovia, California. Dr. Pottenger examined her weekly with the conclusion that she was "doing nicely" (Marble and Leatherman, 1991). After 6 weeks, Pottenger declared that she need to stay for at least another 6 weeks and forbade any physical activity. Just before her 21st birthday, she received a letter from actress Carol Lombard, urging her to fight the medical odds to recover from her disease.

After 8 months of hospitalization and with the covert aid of her tennis coach, Alice Marble fled the sanatorium and refused to return. She initiated a gradual exercise program and within less than a year had returned to the tennis circuit. She won the U.S. women's singles tennis championship in each of the three ensuing years. She died in 1990 at the age of 77 without having suffered subsequent relapses of tuberculosis.

While rest resulted in the cure of some patients with tuberculosis, not all of those afflicted were so lucky. In the prechemotherapy era, the ultimate mortality of patients admitted to New York State sanatoria with tuberculosis in 1938 through 1948 was 69% for those with far-advanced disease, 23% for those with moderately advanced disease, and 13% for those with minimal disease (Alling and Bosworth, 1960). Pottenger, who treated Alice Marble, notes in his text published in 1948 that "tuberculosis shows great tendency to heal and, even though quantitatively and quali-

tatively severe, it may heal spontaneously" (Pottenger, 1948).

The grim prognosis of tuberculosis changed dramatically in November 1944, when a 21-year-old woman with progressive, far-advanced pulmonary tuberculosis who had failed to respond to both rest and thoracoplasty received the first injection of streptomycin, isolated only 11 months previously by Selman Waksman (Pfuetze et al., 1955). She improved during the ensuing 5 months and was discharged from the hospital in 1947. She was evaluated in 1954 and found to be well and the happy mother of three children.

Equally or more dramatic were the results of the first use of isoniazid reported by Robitzek and Selikoff in 1952 (Robitzek and Selikoff, 1952). Of 44 febrile patients, the temperatures of 42 "subsided promptly and sometimes precipitously." Weight gains in the treated patients were "most spectacular," with the average weight gain 19.7 lb (1 lb = 453.6 g). Appetites of treated patients were described as "ravenous," and a 50% increase in food consumption on the treatment ward was noted. Clearing of tubercle bacilli from the sputum was noted in most but not all patients, and radiographic clearing was observed in half. Side effects were minimal. With these dramatic therapeutic results, the era of successful chemotherapy for tuberculosis was launched. The conquest of tuberculosis seemed imminent.

EBB AND FLOW: THE FAILED CONQUEST

That tuberculosis was disappearing from the United States was recognized by Wade Hampton Frost in a landmark paper published posthumously in 1939 (Frost, 1939). He used Massachusetts public health data from several preceding decades to project epidemiologic trends and to explain changing age-specific tuberculin reactor rates. Clearly, tuberculosis had been on the wane

long before effective therapy was introduced. National individual tuberculosis
case reporting was introduced in the United
States in 1953, and annual data thereafter
documented a steady decline in tuberculosis incidence. Beginning in 1985, that trend
changed, and on Sunday, July 15, 1990, the
headline of the lead story on the front page
of the New York Times read, "Tuberculosis germ resurges as peril to public health;
Highest threat in cities; Re-emergence
borne on tide of AIDS, homelessness,
drugs and alcohol abuse." In fact, rising
tuberculosis case rates since 1985 mean
that more than 40,000 cases have occurred
that would not have happened had historical trends continued.

There are many reasons for the resurgence of tuberculosis in the United States.
The AIDS epidemic is an important factor,
and infection with human immunodeficiency virus is the single greatest risk factor
known for progression from primary infection to disease. The lymphocytes first identified by Chase are, of course, destroyed by
this virus. The entry into the United States
of large numbers of persons from countries
with high tuberculosis prevalence rates has
substantially changed the epidemiology of
tuberculosis in this country. Tuberculosis
remains the number one infectious disease
cause of death in the world (Kochi, 1991),
and immigrants bring with them the epidemiology of their homelands. Finally, in
some parts of this country, public health
measures have collapsed or been abandoned, and facilities to serve high-risk individuals are inadequate. Thus, 89% of patients with active tuberculosis discharged
from Harlem Hospital were found to be
noncompliant with their prescribed therapy
(Brudney and Dobkin, 1991).

Not only does the United States face the
gloomy scenario of increasing tuberculosis
incidence, but multidrug-resistant tuberculosis has emerged in several major urban
centers (Frieden et al., 1993). Patients infected with such organisms face the same

prospects for cure or progressive disease
that Alice Marble did, and our country
lacks facilities to provide for their chronic
care and for protection of others from airborne spread of their virulent bacilli.
Clearly, there is a need for major strides
forward both in tuberculosis control and in
tuberculosis research.

REFERENCES

Alling, D. W., and E. B. Bosworth. 1960. The after-
history of pulmonary tuberculosis. VI. The first
fifteen years following diagnosis. *Am. Rev. Respir.
Dis.* **81:**839–849.

Allison, M. R., O. Mendoza, and A. Pezzia. 1973.
Documentation of a case of tuberculosis in pre-
Columbian America. *Am. Rev. Respir. Dis.* **107:**
985–991.

Bloom, B. R., and C. J. L. Murray. 1992. Tuberculosis: commentary on a reemergant killer. *Science*
257:1055–1064.

Bothamley, G. H., and J. M. Grange. 1991. The Koch
phenomenon and delayed hypersensitivity: 1891–
1991. *Tubercle* **72:**7–11.

Brown, P., F. Cathala, and D. C. Gajdusek. 1981.
Mycobacterial and fungal sensitivity patterns among
remote population groups in Papua New Guinea and
in the Hebrides, Solomon and Caroline Islands. *Am.
J. Trop. Med. Hyg.* **30:**1085–1093.

Brudney, K., and J. Dobkin. 1991. Resurgent tuberculosis in New York City. Human immunodeficiency
virus, homelessness, and the decline of tuberculosis
control programs. *Am. Rev. Respir. Dis.* **144:**745–
749.

Buikstra, J. E., and D. C. Cook. 1981. Pre-Columbian
tuberculosis in West-Central Illinois: prehistoric dis-
ease in biocultural perspective, p. 115–139. *In* J. E.
Buikstra (ed.), *Prehistoric Tuberculosis in the
Americas.* Northwestern University Archeological
Program, Evanston, Ill.

Bushnell, G. E. 1930. *Epidemiology of Tuberculosis*,
p. 157. William Wood and Co., Baltimore.

Castiglioni, A. 1933. History of tuberculosis. *Med. Life*
40:1–96.

Catanzaro, A. 1982. Nosocomial tuberculosis. *Am.
Rev. Respir. Dis.* **125:**559–562.

Chadwick, E. 1914. *In the Footsteps of the Brontës.*
Sir Isaac Pitman & Sons, London.

Chase, M. W. 1985. Immunology and experimental
dermatology. *Annu. Rev. Immunol.* **3:**1–29.

Chase, M. W. 1988. Early days in cellular immunology. *Allergy Proc.* **9:**683–687.

Clark, G. 1962. *World Prehistory.* Cambridge University Press, Cambridge.

Comstock, G. W. 1978. Tuberculosis in twins: a re-analysis of the Prophit survey. *Am. Rev. Respir. Dis.* **117**:621–624.

Cummins, S. L. 1920. Tuberculosis in primitive tribes and its bearing on the tuberculosis of civilized communities. *Int. J. Public Health* **1**:137–171.

Cummins, S. L. 1949. *Tuberculosis in History*. The Williams & Wilkins Co., Baltimore.

Davidson, O., and C. M. Jones. 1971. *Great Women Tennis Players*. Pelham Books, London.

Diamond, J. M. 1992. The arrow of disease. *Discover* **13**(10):64–73.

Doetsch, R. N. 1978. Benjamin Marten and his "new theory of consumptions." *Microbiol. Rev.* **42**:521–528.

Dubos, R., and J. Dubos. 1952. *Tuberculosis, Man, and Society: the White Plague*. Little, Brown & Co., Boston.

Ferguson, R. G. 1955. *Studies in Tuberculosis*, p. 6. University of Toronto Press, Toronto.

Fraser, R. 1988. *The Brontës: Charlotte Brontë and Her Family*. Crown Publishers, Inc., New York.

Frieden, T. R., T. Sterling, A. Pablos-Mendez, J. O. Kilburn, G. M. Cauthen, and S. W. Dooley. 1993. The emergence of drug-resistant tuberculosis in New York City. *N. Engl. J. Med.* **328**:521–526.

Frost, W. H. 1939. The age selection of mortality from tuberculosis in successive decades. *Am. J. Hyg.* **30**:91–96.

Grange, J. M., and P. J. Bishop. 1982. "Uber Tuberkulose": a tribute to Robert Koch's discovery of the tubercle bacillus, 1882. *Tubercle* **63**:3–17.

Graunt, J. 1662. *Natural and Political Observations Mentioned in a Following Index and Made upon the Bills of Mortality*. [Reprint, Ayer, Salem, N.H., 1975.]

Grigg, E. R. 1958. The arcana of tuberculosis. *Am. Rev. Tuberc. Respir. Dis.* **78**:151–172, 426–453, 583–603.

Hamilton, W. D., R. Axelrod, and R. Tanese. 1990. Sexual reproduction as an adaptation to resist parasites. *Proc. Natl. Acad. Sci. USA* **87**:3566–3573.

Koch, R. 1932. Die Aetiologie der Tuberculose. *Am. Rev. Tuberc.* **25**:285–323. [Translated from the original 1882 article by Berna Pinner and Max Pinner.]

Kochi, A. 1991. The global tuberculosis situation and the new control strategy of the World Health Organization. *Tubercle* **72**:1–6.

Laennec, R. T. H. 1962. *A Treatise on the Disease of the Chest*. Hafner Publishing Co., New York. [Reprint of original 1821 edition.]

Lichenstein, H. 1928. *Travels in Africa, 1803, 1804, 1805, 1806*. [Reprint of translation by A. Plumptre from the original German, The Van Rierberck Society, Cape Town, South Africa.]

Livingstone, D. 1857. *Missionary Travels and Researches in South Africa*. Ward Lock, London.

Lurie, M. B. 1964. *Resistance to Tuberculosis*. Harvard University Press, Cambridge, Mass.

Major, R. H. 1945. *Classic Descriptions of Disease*, 3rd ed. Charles C Thomas Publishing, Springfield, Ill.

Marble, A., and D. Leatherman. 1991. *Courting Danger: My Adventures in World-Class Tennis, Golden Age Hollywood, and High Stakes Spying*. St. Martin's Press, New York.

McGrath, J. W. 1988. Social networks of disease spread in the lower Illinois valley: a simulation approach. *Am. J. Phys. Anthropol.* **77**:483–496.

Morse, D., D. R. Brothwell, and P. J. Ucko. 1964. Tuberculosis in ancient Egypt. *Am. Rev. Respir. Dis.* **90**:524–541.

Perzigian, A. J., and L. Widmer. 1979. Evidence for tuberculosis in a prehistoric population. *JAMA* **241**:2643–2646.

Pfuetze, K. H., M. M. Pyle, H. C. Hinshaw, and W. H. Feldman. 1955. The first clinical trial of streptomycin in human tuberculosis. *Am. Rev. Tuberc.* **71**:752–754.

Ponce Sangines, C. 1969. *Tunupa y Ekako: Estudio Archeologico Acerca de las Efigies Percolombinas de Dorso Adunco*. Los Amigos del Libro, La Paz, Bolivia.

Pottenger, F. M. 1948. *Tuberculosis: a Discussion of Phthisiogenesis, Immunology, Pathogenic Physiology, Diagnosis, and Treatment*. The C.V. Mosby Co., St. Louis.

Richman, M. 1977. The man who made John Harvard. *Harvard Mag.* **80**:46–51.

Riley, R. L., C. C. Mills, F. O'Grady, L. U. Sultan, F. Wittstadt, and D. N. Shivpuri. 1962. Infectiousness of air from a tuberculosis ward. Ultraviolet irradiation of infected air. Comparative infectiousness of different patients. *Am. Rev. Respir. Dis.* **85**:511–525.

Robitzek, E. H., and I. J. Selikoff. 1952. Hydrazine derivatives of isonicotinic acid (Rimifon, Marsilid) in the treatment of active progressive caseous-pneumonic tuberculosis. *Am. Rev. Tuberc.* **65**:402–428.

Sakula, A. 1982. Robert Koch: centenary of the discovery of the tubercle bacillus, 1882. *Bull. Int. Union Tuberc.* **57**:111–116.

Sakula, A. 1983. BCG: who were Calmette and Guérin? *Thorax* **38**:806–812.

Stead, W. W. 1992. Genetics and resistance to tuberculosis. *Ann. Int. Med.* **116**:937–94.

Steele, J. H., and A. F. Ranney. 1958. Animal tuberculosis. *Am. Rev. Tuberc.* **77**:908–922.

Waksman, S. A. 1964. *The Conquest of Tuberculosis*. University of California Press, Berkeley.

Webb, G. B. 1936. *Tuberculosis*. Paul B. Hoeber Inc., New York.

Wilkinson, E. 1914. Notes on the prevalence of tuberculosis in India. *Proc. R. Soc. Med.* **8**:195–225.

Tuberculosis: Pathogenesis, Protection, and Control
Edited by Barry R. Bloom
© 1994 American Society for Microbiology, Washington, DC 20005

Chapter 3

Overview of Clinical Tuberculosis

Philip C. Hopewell

The clinical expression of infection with *Mycobacterium tuberculosis* is quite varied and depends on a number of identified factors. Table 1 lists both host- and microbe-related characteristics as well as the consequences of their interactions that influence the manifestations of tuberculous infection. Among generally healthy persons, infection with *M. tuberculosis* is highly likely to be asymptomatic. Data from a variety of sources suggest that the lifetime risk of developing clinically evident tuberculosis after being infected is approximately 10%, with a 90% likelihood of the infection remaining latent (Comstock, 1982). Only a positive tuberculin skin test indicates the presence of the organism in persons with latent infections. In specific subpopulations, for example, in persons with immunodeficiency states or in infants, the proportions who develop evident tuberculosis are much higher (Allen et al., 1992; Comstock, 1982; Selwyn et al., 1992).

Immunization with bacillus of Calmette and Guérin (BCG) in persons with intact cell-mediated immunity minimizes the risk of early disseminated tuberculosis, especially in children. In addition to host fac-

tors, there probably are factors related to the organism itself, such as its virulence or predilection for specific tissues, that influence the outcome and features of the infection; however, these features of the organism have not been characterized.

The most obvious and important factor influencing the clinical features of tuberculosis is the site of involvement. Prior to the beginning of the epidemic of infection with the HIV, approximately 85% of reported tuberculosis cases were limited to the lungs, with the remaining 15% involving only nonpulmonary sites or both pulmonary and nonpulmonary sites (Farer et al., 1979) (Fig. 1). This proportional distribution is substantially different among persons with HIV infection. Although there are no national data that describe the sites of involvement in HIV-infected persons with tuberculosis, in one large retrospective study of tuberculosis in patients with advanced HIV infection, it was reported that 38% had only pulmonary involvement, 30% had extrapulmonary sites, and 32% had both pulmonary and nonpulmonary involvement (Small et al., 1991). The multiplicity of sites in HIV-infected persons is typical of what is seen in an individual having an immune system that is limited in its ability to contain infection with *M. tuberculosis*. Included in this category are infants, the elderly, and persons with pri-

Philip C. Hopewell • University of California, San Francisco, and Division of Pulmonary and Critical Care Medicine, San Francisco General Hospital, 1001 Potrero Avenue, Room 5K1, San Francisco, California 94110.

Table 1. Factors influencing the clinical features of tuberculosis

Host factors	Microbial factors	Host-microbe interaction

Age
   Immune status
      Specific immunodeficiency states
      Malnutrition
      Genetic factors (?)
   Coexisting diseases
   Immunization with bacillus of Calmette and
      Guérin (BCG)
	Virulence of organism (?)
	Predilection (tropism) for
	   specific tissues (?)
		Sites of involvement
		Severity of disease

mary or secondary immunodeficiency states resulting from coexisting diseases or malnutrition.

SYSTEMIC AND REMOTE EFFECTS OF TUBERCULOSIS

Tuberculosis occurring at any site may produce symptoms and findings that are not specifically related to the organ or tissue involved but, rather, are systemic in nature or are remote from the site of disease. Systemic manifestations of the disease, including fever, malaise, and weight loss, are likely mediated by cytokines, especially tumor necrosis factor alpha (TNF-α). Experimental data suggest that TNF-α is an important mediator of the systemic effects of the disease (Takashima et al., 1990; Valone et al., 1988). Of the systemic effects, fever is the most easily quantified. The frequency with which fever has been observed in patients with tuberculosis varies from approximately 37 to 80% (Arango et al., 1978; Kiblawi et al., 1981). In a study by Kiblawi and coworkers (Kiblawi et al., 1981) in which the fever response was specifically examined, 21% of patients had no fever at any point in the course of hospitalization for tuberculosis. Of the febrile patients, 34% were afebrile within 1 week and 64% were afebrile within 2 weeks. The median duration of fever after beginning treatment was 10 days, with a range of 1 to

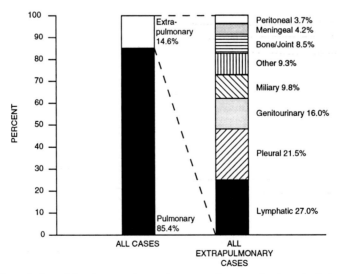

Figure 1. Distribution of sites of involvement in newly reported cases of tuberculosis in 1978 prior to the epidemic of infection with HIV.

109 days. Weight loss, weakness, and malaise appear to be less common but are more difficult to quantify.

In addition to these generalized effects of tuberculosis, there are remote manifestations that are not a result of the anatomic site of involvement. These include hematologic abnormalities, hyponatremia, and psychological disorders. The most common hematologic manifestations of tuberculosis are increases in the peripheral blood leukocyte count and anemia, each of which occurs in approximately 10% of patients with apparently localized tuberculosis (Cameron, 1974; Carr et al., 1964). The increase in leukocyte counts is usually slight, but leukemoid reactions may occur. Leukopenia has also been reported. An increase in the peripheral blood monocyte and eosinophil counts also may occur with tuberculosis. Anemia is common when the infection is disseminated. In some instances, anemia or pancytopenia may result from direct involvement of the bone marrow and thus be a local rather than a remote effect.

Other than weight loss, the most frequent metabolic effect of tuberculosis is hyponatremia, which in one series was found to occur in 11% of patients (Chung and Hubbard, 1969). Hyponatremia is caused by production of an antidiuretic hormone-like substance found within affected lung tissue (Vorken et al., 1970). The poor prognosis that in the prechemotherapy era was associated with hyponatremia was probably related simply to the amount of lung involved and perhaps to adrenal involvement. In addition, because the syndrome of inappropriate secretion of antidiuretic hormone is also associated with central nervous system disorders, hyponatremia may be a feature of central nervous system tuberculosis.

The psychological effects of tuberculosis are very poorly defined but were commonly recognized prior to the advent of effective therapy. These effects include depression and, on occasion, hypomania. The best descriptions of the psychological alterations in patients with tuberculosis are found in literary works, such as Thomas Mann's *The Magic Mountain*, rather than in medical writings.

In many patients, tuberculosis is associated with other serious disorders, including HIV infection, alcoholism, chronic renal failure, diabetes mellitus, neoplastic diseases, and drug abuse, to name but a few. The signs and symptoms of these diseases and their complications can easily obscure or modify those of tuberculosis and can result in considerable delays in diagnosis or in misdiagnoses for extended periods, especially in patients with HIV infection (Kramer et al., 1990). For this reason it is important that clinicians have an understanding of the diseases with which tuberculosis may coexist and have a high index of suspicion for a combination of the two disorders.

TUBERCULIN SKIN TESTING

As noted above, a positive tuberculin skin test is usually the only evidence of latent tuberculous infection (Sbarbaro, 1986). Among persons with symptoms or clinical findings of tuberculosis, the tuberculin skin test may provide useful diagnostic information. However, in an individual patient a positive test (usually defined as an induration of ≥10 mm in immunocompetent persons and ≥5 mm in persons with HIV infection) does not establish a diagnosis and a negative test does not exclude tuberculosis. Up to 25% of apparently immunocompetent persons will have negative tuberculin skin tests at the time of diagnosis of tuberculosis (Nash and Douglas, 1980). Among patients with tuberculosis and HIV infection, the frequency of positive tuberculin reactions varies considerably depending on the degree of immune compromise (Reider et al., 1989).

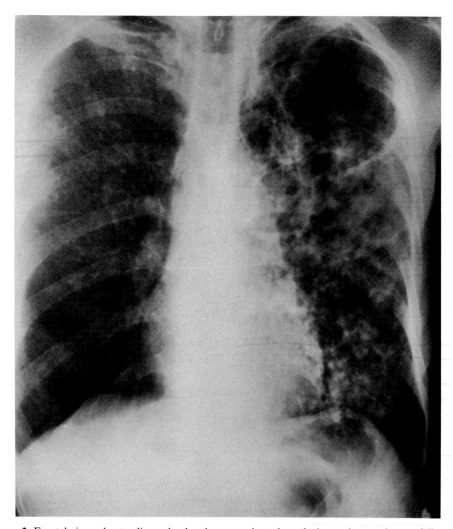

Figure 2. Frontal view, chest radiograph, showing extensive tuberculosis causing respiratory failure.

PULMONARY TUBERCULOSIS

Symptoms and Physical Findings

Cough is the most common symptom of pulmonary tuberculosis. Early in the course of the illness, the cough may be nonproductive, but subsequently, as inflammation and tissue necrosis ensue, sputum is usually produced. Inflammation of the lung parenchyma adjacent to a pleural surface may cause pleuritic pain. Spontaneous pneumothorax may also occur, often causing chest pain and perhaps dyspnea. Dyspnea (difficulty in breathing) as a result of parenchymal lung involvement is unusual unless there is extensive disease. Tuberculosis may, however, cause severe respiratory failure (Huseby and Hudson, 1976; Murray et al., 1978) (Fig. 2). Hemoptysis (coughing blood) may also be a presenting symptom but does not necessarily indicate an active tuberculous process. Hemoptysis may result from residual tuberculous bronchiectasis, rupture of a dilated vessel in the

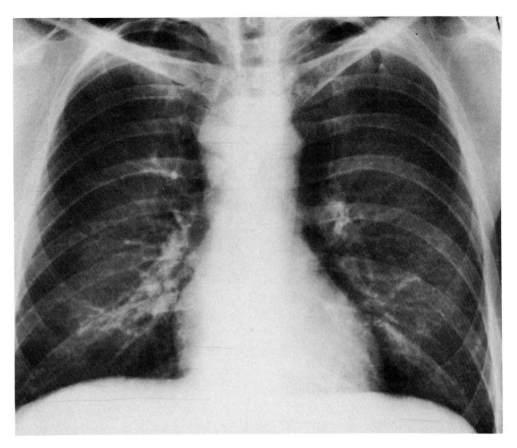

Figure 3. Frontal view, chest radiograph, showing right paratracheal adenopathy as a manifestation of recently acquired tuberculous infection.

wall of an old cavity (Rasmussen's aneurysm), bacterial or fungal infection (especially aspergillus in the form of a fungus ball or mycetoma) in a residual cavity, or erosion of calcified lesions into the lumen of an airway (broncholithiasis).

Physical findings in pulmonary tuberculosis are generally not particularly helpful in defining the disease. Rales may be heard in the area of involvement, and bronchial breath sounds may also be heard if there is lung consolidation. Amphoric breath sounds may be indicative of a cavity.

Radiographic Features of Pulmonary Tuberculosis

In developed countries, radiographic examination of the chest is usually the first diagnostic study undertaken after history and physical examination. Pulmonary tuberculosis nearly always causes abnormalities on the chest film, although an endobronchial lesion may not be associated with a radiographic finding. In primary tuberculosis occurring as a result of recent infection, the process is generally seen as a middle or lower lung zone infiltrate, often associated with ipsilateral hilar adenopathy (Fig. 3). Atelectasis (partial lung collapse) may result from compression of airways by enlarged lymph nodes. If the primary process persists beyond the time when specific cell-mediated immunity develops, cavitation may occur (so-called "progressive primary" tuberculosis).

Tuberculosis that develops as a result of

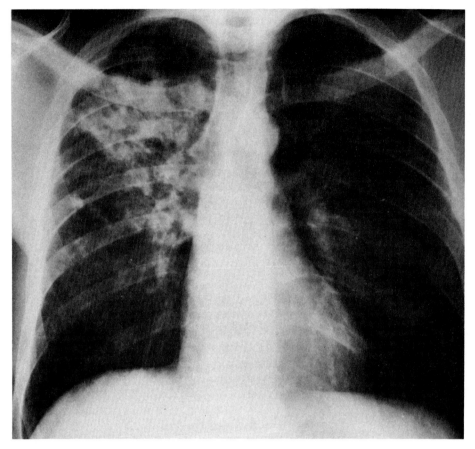

Figure 4. Frontal view, chest radiograph, showing the typical findings of endogenous reactivation tuberculosis in an immunocompetent patient. Note the upper lobe location and cavitation.

endogenous reactivation of latent infection usually causes abnormalities in the upper lobes of one or both lungs. Cavitation (destruction of lung tissue) is common in this form of tuberculosis. The most frequent sites of involvement are the apical and posterior segments of the right upper lobe and the apical-posterior segment of the left upper lobe (Fig. 4). Healing of the tuberculous lesions usually results in development of a scar with loss of lung parenchymal volume and, often, calcification. In the immunocompetent adult with tuberculosis, intrathoracic adenopathy is uncommon but may occur, especially with primary infection. As tuberculosis progresses, infected material may be spread via the airways into the lower portions of the lung or to the other lung. Erosion of a parenchymal focus of tuberculosis into a blood or lymph vessel may result in dissemination of the organism and a "miliary" (evenly distributed small nodules) pattern on the chest film (Fig. 5).

In patients with HIV infection, the nature of the radiographic findings depends to a certain extent on the degree of immunocompromise produced by the infection. Tuberculosis that occurs relatively early in the course of HIV infection tends to have the typical radiographic findings described above (Chaisson et al., 1987; Pitchenik and

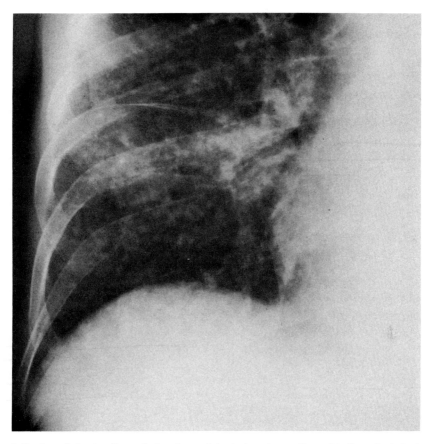

Figure 5. Portion of chest radiograph showing nodular lesions in a patient with disseminated tuberculosis.

Rubinson, 1985). With more advanced HIV disease, the radiographic findings become more "atypical": cavitation is uncommon, and lower lung zone or diffuse infiltrates and intrathoracic adenopathy are frequent (Fig. 6).

Bacteriologic Evaluation

At present, a definitive diagnosis of tuberculosis can be established only by isolation of tubercle bacilli in culture, although tests that identify specific *M. tuberculosis* DNA should soon be available for clinical use. When the lung is involved, sputum is the initial diagnostic specimen of choice. Sputum specimens should be collected at the time of the initial evaluation. Single early-morning specimens have a higher yield and a lower rate of contamination than pooled specimens. The sensitivity of sputum examination increases with the number of specimens, but there is no increase in cumulative recovery of organisms with more than five specimens, and the increased yield between three and five specimens is slight (Kubica et al., 1975).

There are several ways of obtaining specimens from patients who are not producing sputum. The first and most useful is inducing sputum production by the inhalation of a mist of hypertonic (3 to 5%) saline generated by an ultrasonic nebulizer. This is a benign and well-tolerated procedure, al-

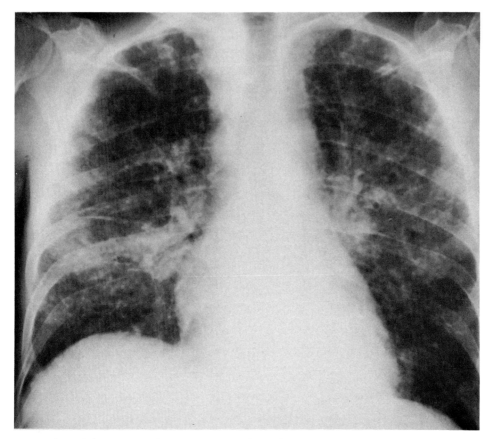

Figure 6. Frontal view, chest radiograph, showing diffuse infiltration caused by *M. tuberculosis* in a patient with HIV infection.

though bronchospasm may occasionally be precipitated in asthmatics. Samples of gastric contents obtained via a nasogastric tube have lower yields than induced sputum, and the procedure is more complicated and uncomfortable for the patient. However, in children and some adults, gastric contents may be the only specimen that can be obtained.

Usually, fiberoptic bronchoscopy is the next diagnostic step if the sputum is negative or cannot be obtained by induction. In general, the bronchoscopic procedure should include bronchoalveolar lavage and transbronchial lung biopsy. The yield of bronchoscopy has been high both for miliary tuberculosis and for localized disease

(Burk et al., 1978; Danek and Bower, 1979; So et al., 1982). For larger nodular lesions, needle aspiration biopsy may also provide specimens from which *M. tuberculosis* can be isolated. This technique is more suited to the evaluation of lesions when there is a suspicion of malignancy.

In some situations, a therapeutic trial of antituberculosis chemotherapy may be indicated before more invasive studies are undertaken (Gordin et al., 1989). Improvement in the chest film concomitant with antituberculosis treatment would be sufficient reason for making a diagnosis of tuberculosis and continuing with a full course of therapy. If a response is going to occur, it should be seen within 3

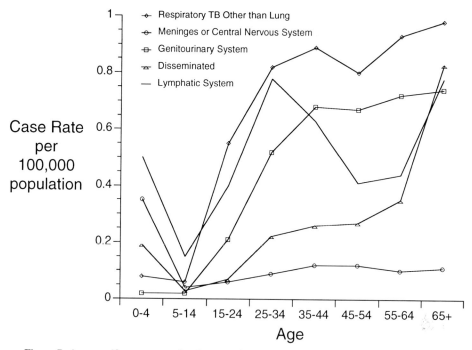

Figure 7. Age-specific case rates for the most frequent forms of extrapulmonary tuberculosis.

months of starting treatment. In the United States, the criteria for defining a case of tuberculosis allow for culture negativity if the patient in question has a positive tuberculin skin test and responds to multidrug chemotherapy.

EXTRAPULMONARY TUBERCULOSIS

As noted above, prior to the epidemic of HIV infection, approximately 15% of newly reported cases of tuberculosis involved only extrapulmonary sites (Farer et al., 1979). For reasons that are not understood, as rates of pulmonary tuberculosis decreased, rates of extrapulmonary disease remained constant, resulting in an increasing proportion of cases being extrapulmonary. With the onset of the HIV epidemic, however, both absolute and relative rates of extrapulmonary involvement have increased.

Extrapulmonary tuberculosis presents

more of a diagnostic and therapeutic problem than pulmonary tuberculosis. In part, this problem relates to its being less common and therefore less familiar to most clinicians (Alvarez and McCabe, 1984; Weir and Thornton, 1985). In addition, extrapulmonary tuberculosis involves relatively inaccessible sites, and because of the nature of the sites involved, fewer bacilli can cause much greater damage. The combination of small numbers of bacilli and inaccessible sites makes bacteriologic confirmation of a diagnosis more difficult, and invasive procedures are frequently required to establish a diagnosis.

The relative frequencies of tuberculosis at various sites in persons without immunocompromise are shown in Fig. 1, and distribution by age is shown in Fig. 7 (Farer et al., 1979). As can be seen, in general, the incidence for each extrapulmonary site increases with increasing age, except for lymphatic and meningeal tuberculosis, which

Table 2. Recovery of *M. tuberculosis* from various sites in patients with tuberculosis and HIV infection[a]

Specimen	No. positive/no. tested (%)	
	Smear	Culture
Sputum	43/69 (62)	64/69 (93)
Bronchoalveolar lavage	9/44 (20)	39/44 (89)
Transbronchial biopsy	1/10 (10)	7/10 (7)
Lymph node	21/44 (48)	39/44 (91)
Blood		15/46 (33)
Bone marrow	4/22 (18)	13/22 (62)
Cerebrospinal fluid		4/21 (19)
Urine		12/17 (71)
Other[b]	5/31 (16)	24/31 (76)

[a] Data are from Small et al. (1991).
[b] Pleural fluid or tissue, pericardial fluid or tissue, liver peritoneal fluid, abscess drainage, or bone.

are relatively more common in young children.

Extrapulmonary Tuberculosis in HIV-Infected Patients

Presumably, the basis for the frequency of extrapulmonary tuberculosis among patients with HIV infection is the failure of the immune response to contain *M. tuberculosis*, thereby enabling hematogenous dissemination and subsequent involvement of single or multiple nonpulmonary sites. As evidence of this sequence, tuberculosis bacillemia has been documented in HIV-infected patients on a number of occasions (Handwerger et al., 1987; Kramer et al., 1990; Shafer et al., 1989). Because of the frequency of extrapulmonary tuberculosis among HIV-infected patients, diagnostic specimens from any suspected site of disease should be examined for mycobacteria. Moreover, cultures of blood and bone marrow may reveal *M. tuberculosis* in patients who do not have an obvious localized site of disease but who are being evaluated because of fever. Table 2 lists the sites from which *M. tuberculosis* was recovered in a group of patients with advanced HIV infection (Small et al., 1991).

Disseminated Tuberculosis

The epidemic of HIV infection has considerably altered the frequency and de-scriptive epidemiology of disseminated tuberculosis. Disseminated or miliary tuberculosis occurs because of the inadequacy of host defenses in containing tuberculous infection. This failure of containment may occur in either latent or recently acquired tuberculous infection. Because of HIV or other causes of immunosuppression, the organism proliferates and disseminates throughout the body. Multiorgan involvement is probably much more common than is recognized, because generally, once *M. tuberculosis* is identified in any specimen, other sites are not evaluated. The term ''miliary'' is derived from the visual similarity of the lesions to millet seeds. Grossly, these lesions are 1- to 2-mm-diameter yellowish nodules that, histologically, are granulomas. Persons with HIV infection may not be able to form granulomas; thus, the individual lesions may not be present. Instead, a diffuse uniform pattern of lymphocytic infiltration and edema is seen.

Although disseminated tuberculosis nearly always involves the lungs, it is considered among the extrapulmonary forms of the disease because of the multiplicity of organs affected. In the past, miliary tuberculosis occurred mainly in young children; currently, however, except among HIV-infected persons, it is more common among older persons (Farer et al., 1979). The shift in age-specific incidence presumably has been caused by the paucity of new infections relative to the number of endogenous reactivations that take place in the United States. The sex incidence is nearly equal except in the HIV-infected population, wherein men predominate.

Because of the multisystem involvement in disseminated tuberculosis, the clinical manifestations are protean. The presenting symptoms and signs are generally nonspecific and are dominated by the systemic effects, particularly fever, weight loss, anorexia, and weakness (Grieco and Chmel, 1974; Munt, 1971; Prout and Benatar, 1980; Sahn and Neff, 1974; Slavin et al., 1980). Other symptoms depend on the relative severity of disease in the organs involved. Cough and shortness of breath are common; headache and mental status changes are less frequent and are usually associated with meningeal involvement (Munt, 1971). Physical findings are likewise variable. Fever, wasting, hepatomegaly, pulmonary findings, lymphadenopathy, and splenomegaly occur in descending order of frequency. The only physical finding that is specific for disseminated tuberculosis is the choroidal tubercle, a granuloma located in the choroid of the retina (Massaro et al., 1964).

Initial screening laboratory studies are not particularly helpful for the diagnosis of miliary tuberculosis. Both leukopenia and leukocytosis may be seen, but the majority of patients have normal leukocyte counts. Anemia is common and may be normocytic, normochronic, or microcytic and hypochromic. Coagulation disorders are unusual, but disseminated intravascular coagulation has been reported in association with miliary tuberculosis in severely ill patients (Huseby and Hudson, 1976; Murray et al., 1978). Hyponatremia also occurs, as discussed above. The most frequent abnormality of liver function is an increased alkaline phosphatase concentration. Bilirubin and alanine aminotransferase levels may also be increased.

The chest film is abnormal in most but not all patients with disseminated tuberculosis. In the series reported by Grieco and Chmel (1974), only 14 (50%) of 28 patients had a miliary pattern on chest film, whereas 90% of 69 patients reported by Munt (1971) had a miliary pattern. Overall, it appears that at the time of diagnosis, approximately 85% of patients have the characteristic radiographic findings of miliary tuberculosis. Other radiographic abnormalities may be present as well. These include upper lobe infiltrates with or without cavitation, pleural effusion, and pericardial effusion. In patients with HIV infection, the radiographic pattern is one of diffuse infiltration rather than discrete nodules.

The tuberculin skin test is positive less frequently in patients with disseminated tuberculosis than in those with other forms of the disease. The rate of positivity at the time of diagnosis in apparently immunocompetent persons ranges from approximately 50 to 75% (Grieco and Chmel, 1974; Munt, 1971; Sahn and Neff, 1974; Slavin et al., 1980). As the disease is treated, tuberculin reactivity tends to return unless there is systemic immunocompromise.

Autopsy series have shown the liver, lungs, bone marrow, kidneys, adrenals, and spleen to be the organs most frequently involved in miliary tuberculosis, but any organ can be the site of disease (Slavin et al., 1980). Because of the multiplicity of sites involved, there are many potential sources of material used to provide a diagnosis. Acid-fast smears of sputum are positive in 20 to 25% of patients, and *M. tuberculosis* is isolated from sputum in 30 to 65% of patients (Grieco and Chmel, 1974; Munt, 1971; Sahn and Neff, 1974; Slavin et al., 1980). Gastric washings or induced sputum may be positive when the patient is not expectorating spontaneously. In a patient with an abnormal chest film and negative sputum examinations, bronchoscopy should be the next step. Combinations of bronchoalveolar lavage and transbroncheal biopsy would be expected to have a high yield. Other potential sites for biopsy include liver and bone marrow, each of which has a high likelihood of showing granulomas (70 to 80%) but only a 25 to 40% chance of providing bacteriologic confirmation (Sahn and Neff, 1974). Urine is easy to obtain and may be positive in up to 25% of patients (Sahn and Neff, 1974). Selection of other potential sources of diagnostic material should be guided by specific findings.

Lymph Node Tuberculosis

Prior to the HIV epidemic, lymph node tuberculosis made up approximately 20% of the cases of extrapulmonary tuberculosis in the United States (Farer et al., 1979). Although the basic descriptive epidemiology of tuberculosis applies to lymphatic tuberculosis, there are two main differences: lymphatic tuberculosis is relatively more common among children, and it occurs more frequently in women. It also appears to be more common among Asians and Pacific Islanders than among blacks and whites. Among HIV-infected persons, the demographic features of tuberculous lymphadenitis parallel those of HIV infection.

Tuberculous lymphadenitis usually presents as painless swelling of one or more lymph nodes. The nodes most commonly involved are those of the posterior or anterior cervical chain or those in the supraclavicular fossa. Frequently, the process is bilateral, and other noncontiguous groups of nodes can be involved (Kent, 1967). At least initially, the nodes are discrete and the overlying skin is normal. With continuing disease, the nodes may become matted and the overlying skin inflamed. Rupture of the node can result in formation of a sinus tract, which may be difficult to heal. Intrathoracic adenopathy may compress bronchi, causing atelectasis and leading to lung infection and perhaps bronchiectasis.

In non-HIV-infected persons with tuberculous lymphadenitis, systemic symptoms are not common unless there is concomitant tuberculosis elsewhere. The frequency of pulmonary involvement in reported series of patients with tuberculous lymphadenitis is quite variable, ranging from approximately 5 to 70%. In HIV-infected persons, lymphadenitis is commonly associated with multiple-organ involvement, although localized lymphadenitis, as described above, may occur as well.

The diagnosis of tuberculous lymphadenopathy is established by lymph node biopsy or aspiration with histologic examination, including stains for acid-fast organisms, and culture of the material. Smears show acid-fast organisms in approximately 25 to 50% of biopsy specimens, and *M. tuberculosis* is isolated in roughly 70% of instances in which the diagnosis is tuberculosis (Huhti et al., 1975). Caseating granulomas are seen in nearly all biopsy samples from immunocompetent patients. In immunodeficiency states, granulomas may be poorly formed or absent (Marchevsky et al., 1985).

Pleural Tuberculosis

The epidemiology of pleural tuberculosis parallels that of the overall pattern for tuberculosis, with the disease being more common among males and increasing in incidence with increasing age between ages 5 and 45 (Farer et al., 1979). As noted above, this epidemiologic pattern is modified by the occurrence of HIV infection, although pleural involvement seems relatively less frequent among HIV-infected persons.

There are two mechanisms by which the pleural space becomes involved in tuberculosis, and the difference in pathogenesis results in different clinical presentations, approaches to diagnosis, treatment, and sequelae. Early in the course of a tuberculous infection, a few organisms may gain access to the pleural space, and in the presence of cell-mediated immunity, they can cause a hypersensitivity response (Berger and Mejia, 1973; Ellner, 1978). Commonly, this form of tuberculous pleuritis goes unnoticed, and the process resolves spontaneously. In some patients, however, tuberculous involvement of the pleura is manifested as an acute illness with fever and pleuritic pain. If the effusion is large enough, dyspnea may occur, although the effusions generally are small and rarely are bilateral. In approximately 30% of patients, there is no radiographic evidence of involvement of the lung parenchyma; however, parenchymal disease is nearly always present, as evidenced by findings by lung dissections (Stead et al., 1955).

The diagnosis of pleural tuberculosis is generally established by analysis of pleural fluid and/or pleural biopsy. A thoracentesis (aspiration of fluid from the chest) should be performed, and sufficient fluid for cell count, cytologic examination, biochemical analysis, and microbiologic evaluation should be obtained, leaving enough to allow a needle biopsy to be performed if the fluid is exudative and no diagnosis is evident. The fluid is nearly always straw colored, although it may be slightly bloody. Cell counts are usually in the range of 100 to 5,000/µl (Jay, 1985). Early in the course of the process, polymorphonuclear leukocytes may predominate, but mononuclear cells soon become the majority. The fluid is exudative, with a protein concentration greater than 50% of the serum protein concentration, and the glucose level may be normal to low.

Because few organisms are present in the pleural space, smears of pleural fluid are rarely positive, and M. tuberculosis is isolated by culture in only 20 to 40% of patients with proved tuberculous pleuritis (Levine et al., 1970; Scharer and McClement, 1968). A single blind needle biopsy of the pleura will confirm the diagnosis in approximately 65 to 75% of patients in whom tuberculous pleuritis is ultimately diagnosed (Levine et al., 1970; Scharer and McClement, 1968). In a patient who has a pleural effusion that remains undiagnosed after a full evaluation, including pleural biopsy, and who has a positive tuberculin skin test reaction, antituberculosis treatment should be initiated.

The second variety of tuberculous involvement of the pleura is a true empyema (pus in the pleura). This condition is much less common than tuberculous pleurisy with effusion and results from a large number of organisms spilling into the pleural space, usually from rupture of a cavity or an adjacent parenchymal focus via a bronchopleural fistula (Johnson et al., 1973). A tuberculous empyema is usually associated with evident pulmonary parenchymal disease on chest films, and air may be seen in the pleural space. In this situation, the fluid is generally thick and cloudy and may contain cholesterol, causing the fluid to look like chyle (pseudochylous effusion). The fluid is exudative and usually has a relatively high leukocyte count, with nearly all of the leukocytes being lymphocytes. Acid-fast smears and mycobacterial cultures are usually positive, making pleural biopsy unnecessary. This type of pleural involvement has a tendency to burrow through soft tissues and may drain spontaneously through the chest wall. An example of this type of tuberculosis is shown in Fig. 8.

Genitourinary Tuberculosis

As with pleural tuberculosis, the epidemiologic pattern of genitourinary tuberculosis parallels that of tuberculosis in general except that the incidence is nearly equal in men and women. The pathogenesis appears to be one of seeding of the kidney at the time of the initial infection and bacillemia.

In patients with genitourinary tuberculosis, local symptoms predominate, and systemic symptoms are less common (Christensen, 1974; Simon et al., 1977). Dysuria,

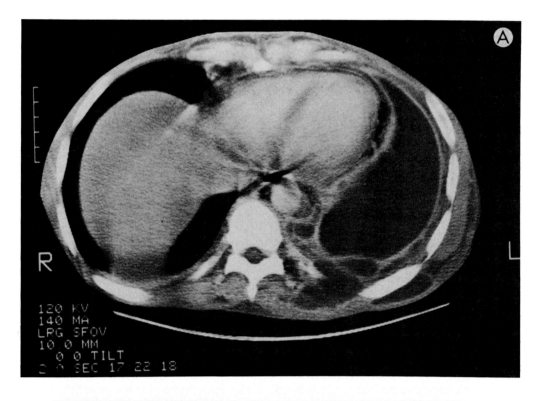

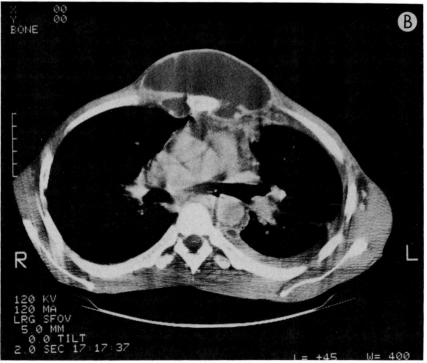

hematuria, and frequent urination are common, and flank pain may also be noted. However, the symptoms may be very subtle, and often there is advanced destruction of the kidneys by the time a diagnosis is established (Lattimer, 1965). Genital involvement without renal tuberculosis is more common in women than in men and may cause pelvic pain, menstrual irregularities, and infertility as presenting complaints (Simon et al., 1977). In men, a painless or only slightly painful scrotal mass is probably the most common presenting symptom of genital involvement, but symptoms of prostatitis, orchitis, or epididymitis may also occur (Christensen, 1974). A substantial number of patients with any form of genitourinary tuberculosis are asymptomatic and are detected because of an evaluation for an abnormal routine urinalysis. In more than 90% of patients with renal or genital tuberculosis, urinalyses are abnormal, with the main finding being pyuria and/or hematuria. The finding of pyuria (pus in urine) in an acid urine with no organisms isolated from a routine urine culture should prompt an evaluation for tuberculosis. The suspicion of genitourinary tuberculosis should be heightened by the presence of abnormalities on the chest film. In most series, approximately 40 to 75% of patients have chest radiographic abnormalities, although in many patients, these abnormalities may be the result of previous, not current, tuberculosis (Christensen, 1974; Simon et al., 1977).

When genitourinary tuberculosis is suspected, at least three first-voided early-morning urine specimens should be collected for acid-fast stains and cultures. *M. tuberculosis* is isolated from the urine in 80 to 95% of cases of genitourinary tuberculosis (Christensen, 1974; Simon et al., 1977). Diagnosis of isolated genital lesions usually requires biopsy, because the differential diagnosis often includes neoplasia as well as other infectious processes.

Significant effects of tuberculosis on renal function are unusual, but renal failure may occur, especially in patients with pre-existing renal disease. Nephrolithiasis and recurrent bacterial infections in seriously damaged kidneys also occur. Hypertension that responds to nephrectomy has also been described but is rare.

Skeletal Tuberculosis

The incidence of tuberculosis involving the joints and bones increases with increasing age and is equally frequent among men and women, overall making up approximately 9% of cases of extrapulmonary tuberculosis (Farer et al., 1979). Compared to blacks and whites, other racial groups are less likely to have skeletal involvement. Skeletal tuberculosis does not appear to be frequent among persons with HIV infection.

It is presumed that most osteoarticular tuberculosis results from endogenous reactivation of foci of infection seeded during the initial bacillemia, although spread from paravertebral lymph nodes has been postulated to account for the common localization of spinal tuberculosis to the lower thoracic and upper lumbar vertebrae (Burke, 1950). It is also postulated that the predilection for tuberculosis to localize in the metaphyses of long bones is due to the relatively rich blood supply and the scarcity of phagocytic cells in this portion of the bone (Berney et al., 1972). After beginning in the subchondral region on the bone, the infection spreads to involve the cartilage, synovium, and joint space. This produces the typical findings of metaphyseal erosion and cysts and the loss of cartilage, with

Figure 8. Computed tomographic scan of the chest showing a tuberculous empyema with adjacent chest wall involvement (A) and a large chest wall abscess overlying the sternum with mediastinal involvement (B).

narrowing of the joint space. Typically, in the spine these changes involve two adjacent vertebrae and the intervertebral disk. Paravertebral or other para-articular abscesses may develop, with occasional formation of sinus tracts. Although weight-bearing joints are the most common sites for skeletal tuberculosis, any bone or joint may be involved (Berney et al., 1972). In most series, tuberculosis of the spine (Pott's disease) makes up 50 to 70% of the cases reported. In adults, the lower thoracic and upper lumbar vertebrae are most commonly involved, whereas in children, the upper thoracic spine is the most frequent site of vertebral tuberculosis. The hip or knee is involved in 15 to 20% of cases, and shoulders, elbows, ankles, wrists, and other bones or joints are also involved in 15 to 20% of cases. Usually only one bone or joint is involved, but occasionally the process is multifocal (Cremin et al., 1970; McTammany et al., 1963). Evidence of either previous or current pulmonary tuberculosis is found in approximately one-half of the reported patients, and other extrapulmonary sites may also be involved.

The usual presenting symptom of skeletal tuberculosis is pain (Berney et al., 1972). Swelling of the involved joint may be noted, as may limitation of motion and occasionally sinus tracts. Systemic symptoms of infection are not common. Because of the subtle nature of the symptoms, diagnostic evaluations often are not undertaken until the process is advanced. Delay in diagnosis can be especially catastrophic in vertebral tuberculosis, in which compression of the spinal cord may cause severe and irreversible neurologic sequelae, including paraplegia.

The first diagnostic test undertaken is usually a radiograph of the involved area. The typical findings just described represent the more severe end of the spectrum. Early in the process, the only abnormality noted may be soft tissue swelling. Subsequently, subchondral osteoporosis, cystic changes, and sclerosis may be noted before the joint space is actually narrowed. The early changes of spinal tuberculosis may be particularly difficult to detect by standard films of the spine. Computed tomographic scans and magnetic resonance imaging of the spine are considerably more sensitive than routine films and should be obtained when there is a high index of suspicion of an infectious process.

Confirmation of the diagnosis is obtained by aspiration of joint fluid or periarticular abscesses or by biopsy of bone or synovium with histologic and microbiologic evaluation of the material obtained. Acid-fast stains of joint fluid are positive in 20 to 25% of those examined, and *M. tuberculosis* is isolated in approximately 60 to 80% (Berney et al., 1972). Biopsies of synovium or bone have a higher yield and allow histologic examination as well. Evidence of granulomatous inflammation even in the absence of bacteriologic proof of the diagnosis is sufficient evidence of tuberculosis to begin therapy unless another etiology is found.

Central Nervous System Tuberculosis

Meningitis is the most frequent form of central nervous system tuberculosis; solitary or multiple tuberculomas occur less commonly. The epidemiologic pattern of central nervous system tuberculosis is quite different from either pulmonary or other forms of extrapulmonary tuberculosis in that the peak incidence is in children in the zero- to 4-year age group, but an appreciable number of cases occur in adults (Barrett-Connor, 1967; Farer et al., 1979). Central nervous system disease accounts for only approximately 5% of all cases of extrapulmonary tuberculosis, and the cases are equally divided between males and females.

Central nervous system involvement, especially tuberculomas, seems to occur with greater frequency among HIV-infected persons. Tuberculomas have been reported even in patients who are receiving what should be adequate chemotherapy (Bishberg et al., 1986). The findings produced by tuberculomas may be indistinguishable on computed tomographic scan from those of toxoplasmosis. For this reason, a specific diagnosis should be sought when such lesions are noted.

Meningitis presumably can result from direct meningeal seeding and proliferation during a tuberculous bacillemia either at the time of initial infection or at the time of breakdown of an old pulmonary focus, or it can result from breakdown of an old parameningeal focus with rupture into the subarachnoid space. The consequences of the subarachnoid space contamination include diffuse meningitis, a localized arteritis, encephalitis, or myelitis. With meningitis, the process takes place primarily at the base of the brain (Auerbach, 1951). Symptoms therefore include those related to cranial nerve involvement in addition to headache, decreased level of consciousness, and neck stiffness. The duration of illness prior to diagnosis is quite variable and relates in part to the presence or absence of other sites of involvement. In most series, over 50% of patients with meningitis have abnormalities on chest film that are consistent with an old or current tuberculous process, often miliary tuberculosis. At autopsy, disseminated disease is found in a very high percentage of patients with meningitis (Auerbach, 1951). In patients with tuberculous meningitis, sputum cultures have been positive in 40 to 50%; thus, a substantial number of patients will have pulmonary and systemic symptoms in addition to those referable to the central nervous system. Arteritis may be the predominant manifestation of meningitis and can result in a variety of focal ischemic syndromes in addition to the symptoms already described.

Physical findings and screening laboratory studies are not particularly helpful in establishing a diagnosis. In the presence of meningeal signs on physical examination, lumbar puncture is usually the next step in the diagnostic sequence. If there are focal findings on examination or if there are suggestions of increased intracranial pressure, a computerized tomographic scan of the head, if it can be obtained expeditiously, should be performed before the lumbar puncture. With meningitis, the scan may be normal, but it can also show diffuse edema or obstructive hydrocephalus. Tuberculomas are generally seen as ring-enhancing mass lesions.

In tuberculous meningitis, the lumbar puncture usually shows increased opening pressure and the cerebrospinal fluid usually contains between 100 and 1,000 cells per μl. In approximately 65 to 75% of patients, lymphocytes predominate, whereas polymorphonuclear leukocytes predominate in the remainder of patients, generally early in the course of the illness. The protein concentration is elevated in nearly all patients. Very high (>300 mg/dl) protein concentrations have been associated with a poor prognosis (Weiss and Flippin, 1961). The glucose concentration in cerebrospinal fluid is usually low but not as low as concentrations that occur during pyogenic bacterial meningitis. Acid-fast organisms are seen on smears of cerebrospinal fluid in only 10 to 20% of patients, and the rate of culture positivity varies from 55 to 80% (Barrett-Connor, 1967). A substantial number of patients will have *M. tuberculosis* isolated from other sources, and in the presence of compatible cerebrospinal fluid findings, such isolation is sufficient to diagnose tuberculous meningitis. Given the severity of tuberculous meningitis, a presumptive diagnosis justifies empiric treatment if no other diagnosis can be established promptly.

The other major central nervous system form of tuberculosis, the tuberculoma, presents a more subtle clinical picture than tuberculous meningitis (Damergis et al., 1979). The usual presentation is that of a slowly growing focal lesion, although a few patients have increased intracranial pressure and no focal findings. The cerebrospinal fluid is usually normal, and the diagnosis is established by computed tomographic or magnetic resonance scanning and subsequent resection, biopsy, or aspiration of any ring-enhancing lesion.

Abdominal Tuberculosis

Tuberculosis can involve any intra-abdominal organ as well as the peritoneum. The age distribution of abdominal tuberculosis shows a relatively higher incidence in young adults and a second peak in older persons. Males and females have a similar incidence. Intra-abdominal tuberculosis has not been common in HIV-infected persons.

Abdominal tuberculosis presumably results from seeding at the time of initial infection and then either direct or late progression to clinical disease. Peritonitis can also be caused by rupture of tuberculous lymph nodes within the abdomen. Intestinal tuberculosis may also result from ingested tubercle bacilli with direct implantation in the gut. Before chemotherapy, tuberculous enteritis was quite common in patients with advanced pulmonary tuberculosis, presumably being caused by bacilli from the lungs that were swallowed. In a prospective study conducted between 1924 and 1949, intestinal abnormalities compatible with tuberculous enteritis were found by contrast radiography in 1, 4.5, and 24.7% of patients with minimal, moderately advanced, and far advanced pulmonary tuberculosis, respectively (Mitchell and Bristol, 1954).

The clinical manifestations of abdominal tuberculosis depend on the areas of involvement. In the gut itself, tuberculosis may occur in any location from the mouth to the anus, although lesions proximal to the terminal ileum are unusual. The most common sites of involvement are the terminal ileum and the cecum, with other portions of the colon and the rectum involved less frequently (Bhansali, 1977). In the terminal ileum or cecum, the most common manifestations are pain, which may be misdiagnosed as appendicitis, and intestinal obstruction. A palpable mass may be noted and, together with the appearance of the abnormality on barium enema or small-bowel films, may easily be mistaken as a carcinoma. Rectal lesions usually present as anal fissures or fistulae or as perirectal abscesses. Because of the concern with carcinoma, the diagnosis often is made at surgery.

For tuberculous peritonitis, pain, often accompanied by abdominal swelling, is commonly the presenting manifestation (Bhansali, 1977; Borhanmanesh et al., 1972; Burack and Hollister, 1960; Singh et al., 1968). Fever, weight loss, and anorexia are also common. Active pulmonary tuberculosis is uncommon in patients with tuberculous peritonitis. Because the process frequently coexists with other disorders, especially hepatic cirrhosis with ascites, the symptoms of tuberculosis may be obscured. The combination of fever and abdominal tenderness in a person with ascites should always prompt an evaluation for intra-abdominal infection, and a paracentesis should be performed. Ascitic fluid in tuberculous peritonitis is exudative (fluid protein content greater than 50% of serum protein concentration) and contains between 50 and 10,000 leukocytes per μl, the majority of them being lymphocytes, although polymorphonuclear leukocytes occasionally predominate (Borhanmanesh et al., 1972; Singh et al., 1968). Acid-fast organisms are rarely seen on smears of the fluid, and cultures are positive in only approximately 50% of patients. Because of the generally low yield from culture of the fluid, laparoscopic biopsy is often necessary to confirm the diagnosis.

Microscopic evidence of liver involvement is common in patients with all forms of tuberculosis, but actual hepatic tuberculosis of functional consequence is rare. A variety of histologic abnormalities may be seen, but none is specific for tuberculosis unless *M. tuberculosis* is isolated from hepatic tissue (Frank and Raffensperger, 1965). For this reason, all liver biopsy specimens should be cultured for mycobacteria.

Pericardial Tuberculosis

The descriptive epidemiology of pericardial tuberculosis is not well defined, but in general the disease tends to occur among older persons, with approximately 50% of the patients being older than 55 years (Farer et al., 1979). Nonwhites and men have a relatively higher frequency of tuberculous pericarditis. Before the use of antituberculosis chemotherapy, tuberculous pericarditis was found in 0.4 to 1.0% of all autopsied patients and in 3 to 8% of autopsied patients in whom there was other evidence of tuberculosis (Schepers, 1962). A clinical diagnosis of tuberculous pericarditis was made in 0.35% of approximately 10,000 patients with any form of tuberculosis admitted to Kings County Hospital Center, Brooklyn, N.Y., between 1 January 1960 and 31 December 1966 (Rooney et al., 1970).

The pericardium may become involved during the initial bacillemia, with early progression to clinically evident disease or recrudescence following a quiescent period. Hematogenous seeding may also occur during the course of endogenous reactivation. Alternatively, there may be direct extension of an adjacent focus of disease into the pericardium. This focus may be in lung parenchyma, pleura, or tracheobronchial lymph nodes. In fact, all of these mechanisms probably occur and may account for some of the variability in the characteristics of the pericardial fluid, severity of the process, and prognosis (Schepers, 1962). It is likely that tuberculin hypersensitivity plays a role in producing the inflammatory response in the pericardium, as presumably occurs in the pleura. On the other hand, rupture of a caseous lymph node into the pericardium may cause contamination with a much greater number of organisms; a greater inflammatory response with thicker, more purulent fluid; and a greater likelihood of either early or late hemodynamic effects.

The most common form or stage of tuberculous pericarditis is characterized by pericardial effusion with little pericardial thickening or epicardial involvement. The fluid itself is usually serosanguineous or occasionally grossly bloody, is exudative, and has a leukocyte count of 500/mm^3 to as high as 50,000/mm^3, with an average of 5,000 to 7,000/mm^3 (Harvey and Whitehill, 1937). The cells are predominantly mononuclear, although polymorphonuclear leukocytes occasionally predominate. Tubercle bacilli have been identified in pericardial fluid in approximately 25 to 30% of cases (smear and culture combined) (Rooney et al., 1970). Biopsy of the pericardium with both histologic and bacteriologic evaluation is much more likely to provide a diagnosis, although a nonspecific histologic pattern and failure to recover the organisms do not exclude a tuberculous etiology.

With persistence of the inflammation, there is thickening of the pericardium and progressive epicardial involvement. Granulomas, various amounts of free or loculated fluid, and fibrosis may be present during this stage, and evidence of cardiac constriction may begin to appear. The necrosis associated with the granulomatous inflammation may involve the myocardium, with consequent functional and electrocardiographic manifestations.

Although it is not well documented, it appears that if the patient survives the subacute phase without treatment, chronic fibrotic pericarditis nearly always follows. Prior to the advent of antituberculous therapy, 88% of one series of patients who had tuberculous pericarditis developed evidence of chronic constriction (Harvey and White-hill, 1937). Constriction has also been observed to develop during the course of antituberculous chemotherapy, although this development appears to be uncommon in patients who have had symptoms for less than 3 months. In the series reported by Hageman and coworkers (Hageman et al., 1964), 11 of 13 patients who had symptoms for more than 6 months required pericardiectomy.

The fibrotic reaction noted above progresses to complete fusion of visceral and parietal pericardium and encasement of the heart in a rigid scar. There are various amounts of calcium within the fibrotic mass. Impairment of coronary circulation is common. At this point, the histologic pattern is usually nonspecific; thus, confirmation of a tuberculous etiology is infrequent.

The symptoms, physical findings, and laboratory abnormalities associated with tuberculous pericarditis may be the result of either the infectious process per se or the pericardial inflammation causing pain, effusion, and eventually hemodynamic effects. The systemic symptoms produced by the infection are quite nonspecific. Fever, weight loss, and night sweats are common in reported series (Harvey and Whitehill, 1937; Rooney et al., 1970; Schepers, 1962). Symptoms of cardiopulmonary origin tend to occur later and include cough, dyspnea, orthopnea, ankle swelling, and chest pain. The chest pain may occasionally mimic angina but usually is described as being dull, aching, and often affected by position and by inspiration.

Apart from fever, the most common physical findings are those caused by the pericardial fluid or fibrosis-cardiac tamponade or constriction. Various proportions of patients in reported series have signs of full-blown cardiac constriction when first evaluated. It is assumed that in these patients, the acute phase of the process was unnoticed.

The definitive diagnosis of tuberculous pericarditis requires identification of tubercle bacilli in pericardial fluid or tissue. Although not conclusive, demonstration of caseating granulomata in the pericardium and consistent clinical circumstances is convincing evidence of a tuberculous etiology. Less conclusive but still persuasive evidence is the finding of another form of tuberculosis in a patient with pericarditis of undetermined etiology. Approximately 25 to 50% of patients with tuberculous pericarditis have evidence of other organ involvement, particularly pleuritis, at the time pericarditis is diagnosed (Gooi and Smith, 1978; Harvey and Whitehill, 1937). Still less direct and more circumstantial evidence of a tuberculous etiology is the combination of a positive intermediate-strength tuberculin skin test reaction and pericarditis of unproven etiology.

REFERENCES

Allen, S., J. Batungwanayo, K. Kerlikowske, A. R. Lifson, W. Wolf, R. Granich, H. Taelman, P. Van De Perre, A. Serufilira, J. Bogaerts, G. Slutkin, and P. C. Hopewell. 1992. Prevalence of tuberculosis in HIV-infected urban Rwandan women. *Am. Rev. Respir. Dis.* **146**:1439–1444.

Alvarez, S., and W. R. McCabe. 1984. Extrapulmonary tuberculosis revisited: a review of experience at Boston City and other hospitals. *Medicine* **63**:25–55.

Arango, L., A. W. Brewin, and J. F. Murray. 1978. The spectrum of tuberculosis as currently seen in a metropolitan hospital. *Am. Rev. Respir. Dis.* **108**:805–812.

Auerbach, O. 1951. Tuberculous meningitis: correlation of therapeutic results with the pathogenesis and pathologic changes. II. Pathologic changes in untreated and treated cases. *Am. Rev. Tuberc.* **64**:419–429.

Barrett-Connor, E. 1967. Tuberculous meningitis in adults. *South. Med. J.* **60**:1061–1067.

Berger, H. W., and E. Mejia. 1973. Tuberculous pleurisy. *Chest* **63**:88–92.

Berney, S., M. Goldstein, and F. Bishko. 1972. Clinical and diagnostic features of tuberculous arthritis. *Am. J. Med.* **53**:36–42.

Bhansali, S. K. 1977. Abdominal tuberculosis: experiences with 300 cases. *Am. J. Gastroenterol.* **67**:324–337.

Bishberg, E., G. Sunderam, L. B. Reichman, and R.

Kapila. 1986. Central nervous system tuberculosis with the acquired immunodeficiency syndrome and its related complex. *Ann. Intern. Med.* **105:**210–213.

Borhanmanesh, F., K. Hekmat, K. Vaezzadeh, and H. R. Rezai. 1972. Tuberculous peritonitis: prospective study of 32 cases in Iran. *Ann. Intern. Med.* **76:**567–572.

Burack, W. R., and R. M. Hollister. 1960. Tuberculous peritonitis: a study of forty-seven proved cases encountered by a general medical unit in twenty-five years. *Am. J. Med.* **28:**510–523.

Burk, J. R., J. Viroslav, and L. J. Bynum. 1978. Miliary tuberculosis diagnosed by fiberoptic bronchoscopy and transbronchial biopsy. *Tubercle* **59:**107–108.

Burke, H. E. 1950. The pathogenesis of certain forms of extrapulmonary tuberculosis. *Am. Rev. Tuberc.* **62:**48–67.

Cameron, S. J. 1974. Tuberculosis and the blood. *Tubercle* **55:**55–72.

Carr, W. P., Jr., R. A. Kyle, and E. J. W. Bowie. 1964. Hematologic changes in tuberculosis. *Am. J. Med. Sci.* **248:**709–714.

Chaisson, R. E., G. F. Schecter, C. P. Theuer, G. W. Rutherford, D. F. Echenberg, and P. C. Hopewell. 1987. Tuberculosis in patients with the acquired immunodeficiency syndrome: clinical features, response to therapy and survival. *Am. Rev. Respir. Dis.* **136:**570–574.

Christensen, W. I. 1974. Genitourinary tuberculosis: review of 102 cases. *Medicine* **53:**377–390.

Chung, D.-K., and W. W. Hubbard. 1969. Hyponatremia in untreated active pulmonary tuberculosis. *Am. Rev. Respir. Dis.* **99:**595–597.

Comstock, G. W. 1982. Epidemiology of tuberculosis. *Am. Rev. Respir. Dis.* **125**(Suppl.):8–16.

Cremin, B. J., R. M. Fisher, and M. W. Levinsohn. 1970. Multiple bone tuberculosis in the young. *Br. J. Radiol.* **43:**638–645.

Damergis, J. A., E. Lefterich, and J. A. Curtin. 1979. Tuberculoma of the brain. *JAMA* **239:**413–415.

Danek, S. J., and J. S. Bower. 1979. Diagnosis of pulmonary tuberculosis by flexible fiberoptic bronchoscopy. *Am. Rev. Respir. Dis.* **119:**677–679.

Ellner, J. J. 1978. Pleural fluid and peripheral blood lymphocyte function in tuberculosis. *Ann. Intern. Med.* **89:**932–933.

Farer, L. S., L. M. Lowell, and M. P. Meador. 1979. Extrapulmonary tuberculosis in the United States. *Am. J. Epidemiol.* **109:**205–217.

Frank, B. R., and E. C. Raffensperger. 1965. Hepatic granulomata: report of a case with jaundice improving on antituberculous chemotherapy and review of the literature. *Arch. Intern. Med.* **115:**223–233.

Gooi, H. C., and J. M. Smith. 1978. Tuberculous pericarditis in Birmingham. *Thorax* **33:**94–96.

Gordin, F. M., G. Slutkin, G. F. Schecter, P. C.

Goodman, and P. C. Hopewell. 1989. Presumptive diagnosis and treatment of pulmonary tuberculosis based on radiographic findings. *Am. Rev. Respir. Dis.* **139:**1090–1093.

Grieco, M. H., and H. Chmel. 1974. Acute disseminated tuberculosis as a diagnostic problem: a clinical study based on twenty-eight cases. *Am. Rev. Respir. Dis.* **109:**554–560.

Hageman, J. H., N. D. D'Esopo, and W. W. L. Glenn. 1964. Tuberculosis of the pericardium: a long-term analysis of forty-four proved cases. *N. Engl. J. Med.* **270:**327–332.

Handwerger, S., D. Mildvan, R. Sennie, and F. W. McKinley. 1987. Tuberculosis and the acquired immunodeficiency syndrome at a New York City hospital: 1978–1985. *Chest* **91:**176–180.

Harvey, A. M., and M. R. Whitehill. 1937. Tuberculous pericarditis. *Medicine* **16:**45–94.

Huhti, E., E. Brander, and S. Plohumo. 1975. Tuberculosis of the cervical lymph nodes: a clinical, pathological and bacteriological study. *Tubercle* **56:**27–36.

Huseby, J. S., and L. D. Hudson. 1976. Miliary tuberculosis and the adult respiratory distress syndrome. *Ann. Intern. Med.* **85:**609–611.

Jay, S. J. 1985. Diagnostic procedures for pleural disease. *Clin. Chest Med.* **6:**33–48.

Johnson, T. M., W. McCann, and W. H. Davey. 1973. Tuberculous bronchopleural fistula. *Am. Rev. Respir. Dis.* **107:**30–41.

Kent, D. C. 1967. Tuberculous lymphadenitis: not a localized disease process. *Am. J. Med. Sci.* **254:**866–874.

Kiblawi, S. S. O., S. J. Jay, R. B. Stonehill, and J. Norton. 1981. Fever response of patients on therapy for pulmonary tuberculosis. *Am. Rev. Respir. Dis.* **123:**20–24.

Kramer, F., T. Modelewsky, A. R. Walinay, J. M. Leedom, and P. F. Barnes. 1990. Delayed diagnosis of tuberculosis in patients with human immunodeficiency virus infection. *Am. J. Med.* **89:**451–456.

Kubica, G. P., W. M. Gross, J. E. Hawkins, H. M. Sommers, A. L. Vestal, and L. G. Wayne. 1975. Laboratory services for mycobacterial diseases. *Am. Rev. Respir. Dis.* **112:**773–787.

Lattimer, J. K. 1965. Renal tuberculosis. *N. Engl. J. Med.* **273:**208–211.

Levine, H., W. Metzger, and D. Lacera. 1970. Diagnosis of tuberculous pleurisy by culture of pleural biopsy specimen. *Arch. Intern. Med.* **126:**268–271.

Marchevsky, A., M. J. Rosen, G. Chrystal, and J. Kleinerman. 1985. Pulmonary complications of the acquired immunodeficiency syndrome: a clinicopathologic study of 70 cases. *Hum. Pathol.* **16:**659–670.

Massaro, D., S. Katz, and M. Sachs. 1964. Choroidal

tubercles: a clue to hematogenous tuberculosis. *Ann. Intern. Med.* **60:**231–241.

McTammany, J. R., K. M. Moser, and V. N. Houk. 1963. Disseminated bone tuberculosis: review of the literature and presentation of an unusual case. *Am. Rev. Respir. Dis.* **87:**888–895.

Mitchell, R. S., and L. J. Bristol. 1954. Intestinal tuberculosis: an analysis of 346 cases diagnosed by routine intestinal radiography on 5529 admissions for pulmonary tuberculosis, 1924–1949. *Am. J. Med. Sci.* **227:**241–249.

Munt, P. W. 1971. Miliary tuberculosis in the chemotherapy era with a clinical review in 69 American adults. *Medicine* **51:**139–155.

Murray, H. W., C. U. Tuazon, N. Kirmani, and J. H. Sheagren. 1978. The adult respiratory distress syndrome associated with miliary tuberculosis. *Chest* **73:**37–43.

Nash, D.-R., and J. E. Douglas. 1980. Anergy in active pulmonary tuberculosis: a comparison between positive and negative reactors and an evaluation of 5 TU and 250 TU skin test doses. *Chest* **77:**32.

Pitchenik, A. E., and H. A. Rubinson. 1985. The radiographic appearance of tuberculosis in patients with the acquired immune deficiency syndrome (AIDS) and pre-AIDS. *Am. Rev. Respir. Dis.* **131:**393–396.

Prout, S., and S. R. Benatar. 1980. Disseminated tuberculosis: a study of 62 cases. *S. Afr. Med. J.* **58:**835–842.

Reider, H. H., G. M. Cauthen, A. B. Bloch, et al. 1989. Tuberculosis and the acquired immunodeficiency syndrome—Florida. *Arch. Intern. Med.* **149:**1268.

Rooney, J. J., J. A. Crocco, and H. A. Lyons. 1970. Tuberculous pericarditis. *Ann. Intern. Med.* **72:**73–78.

Sahn, S. A., and T. A. Neff. 1974. Miliary tuberculosis. *Am. J. Med.* **56:**495–505.

Sbarbaro, J. A. 1986. Skin testing in the diagnosis of tuberculosis. *Semin. Respir. Infect.* **1:**234.

Scharer, L., and J. H. McClement. 1968. Isolation of tubercule bacilli from needle biopsy specimens of parietal pleura. *Am. Rev. Respir. Dis.* **97:**466–468.

Schepers, G. W. H. 1962. Tuberculous pericarditis. *Am. J. Cardiol.* **9:**248–276.

Selwyn, P. A., B. M. Sckell, P. Alcabes, G. H. Friedland, R. S. Klein, and E. E. Schoenbaum. 1992. High risk of active tuberculosis in HIV-infected drug users with cutaneous anergy. *JAMA* **268:**504–509.

Shafer, R. W., R. Goldberg, M. Sierra, and A. E. Glatt. 1989. Frequency of *Mycobacterium tuberculosis* bacteremia in patients with tuberculosis in an area endemic for AIDS. *Am. Rev. Respir. Dis.* **140:**1611–1613.

Simon, H. B., A. J. Weinstein, M. S. Pasternak, M. N. Swartz, and L. J. Lunz. 1977. Genitourinary tuberculosis: clinical features in a general hospital. *Am. J. Med.* **63:**410–420.

Singh, M. M., A. M. Bhargova, and K. P. Jain. 1968. Tuberculous peritonitis: an evaluation of pathogenetic mechanisms, diagnostic procedures and therapeutic measures. *N. Engl. J. Med.* **281:**1091–1094.

Slavin, R. E., T. J. Walsh, and A. D. Pollack. 1980. Late generalized tuberculosis: a clinical pathologic analysis of 100 cases in the preantibiotic and antibiotic eras. *Medicine* **59:**352–366.

Small, P. M., G. F. Schecter, P. C. Goodman, M. A. Sande, R. E. Chaisson, and P. C. Hopewell. 1991. Treatment of tuberculosis in patients with advanced human immunodeficiency virus infection. *N. Engl. J. Med.* **324:**289–294.

So, S. Y., W. K. Lam, and D. Y. C. Yu. 1982. Rapid diagnosis of suspected pulmonary tuberculosis by fiberoptic bronchoscopy. *Tubercle* **63:**195–200.

Stead, W. W., A. Eichenholtz, and H. K. Strauss. 1955. Operative and pathologic findings in 24 patients with the syndrome of idiopathic pleurisy with effusion presumably tuberculous. *Am. Rev. Respir. Dis.* **71:**473–502.

Takashima, T., C. Ueta, I. Tsuyuguchi, and S. Kishimoto. 1990. Production of tumor necrosis factor alpha by monocytes from patients with pulmonary tuberculosis. *Infect. Immun.* **58:**3286–3292.

Valone, S. E., E. Rich, R. S. Wallis, and J. J. Ellner. 1988. Expression of tumor necrosis factor in vitro by human mononuclear phagocytes stimulated with whole *Mycobacterium tuberculosis*, BCG, and mycobacterial antigens. *Infect. Immun.* **56:**3313–3315.

Vorken, H., S. G. Massy, R. Fallat, L. Kaplan, and C. R. Kleeman. 1970. Antidiuretic principle in tuberculous lung tissue of a patient with pulmonary tuberculosis and hyponatremia. *Ann. Intern. Med.* **72:**383–387.

Weir, M. R., and G. F. Thornton. 1985. Extrapulmonary tuberculosis: experience of a community hospital and review of the literature. *Am. J. Med.* **79:**467–478.

Weiss, W., and H. F. Flippin. 1961. The prognosis of tuberculous meningitis in the isoniazid era. *Am. J. Med.* **242:**423–430.

Tuberculosis: Pathogenesis, Protection, and Control
Edited by Barry R. Bloom
© 1994 American Society for Microbiology, Washington, DC 20005

Chapter 4

Epidemiology of Tuberculosis

P. G. Smith and A. R. Moss

Clinical medicine is concerned, generally, with how a disease progresses within patients. Clinical research seeks to better understand factors that influence the progression of disease in order to develop therapeutic interventions to prevent or lessen the severity of the pathology associated with the disease. Epidemiological research is complementary to this goal and aims to study the occurrence and determinants of disease in populations. The epidemiologist is as interested in those who do not get the disease as in those who do, since by seeking differences between these two groups, the epidemiologist hopes to identify the determinants of the disease and then with this knowledge seek ways of preventing the disease.

For an understanding of the etiology and transmission dynamics of most infectious diseases, it is important to distinguish between infection and disease. Disease may represent the tip of an iceberg with respect to the overall level of infection in a community. Also, the factors that affect the risk of infection may be quite different from the factors that determine whether an infection is followed by clinical disease or is asymptomatic. The distinction is of less importance for a disease such as measles, in which disease follows infection in the vast majority of cases and the epidemiology of infection is much the same as that of disease. For other diseases, however, and generally those in which the infectious agent has evolved a better symbiotic relationship with the human host, a relatively small proportion of those who are infected go on to develop clinical disease. Such is the case for tuberculosis.

Study of the epidemiology of tuberculosis has been greatly assisted by the availability of a test for infection, the tuberculin test, that enables us to distinguish those who are infected but without disease from those who are uninfected. The absence of such a test for leprosy, for which it is also assumed that infection with the causative agent is much more common than occurrence of the disease, has greatly impeded the development of knowledge of the natural history and transmission dynamics of that disease.

An indication that the tubercle bacillus has enjoyed a long period of evolution with the human host is the ability of the organism to survive in a latent state and then reactivate many years after the original infection. This ability has enabled the bacillus to survive in small population groups

P. G. Smith • Department of Epidemiology and Population Sciences, London School of Hygiene and Tropical Medicine, Keppel Street, London WC1E 7HT, United Kingdom. *A. R. Moss* • Department of Epidemiology and Biostatistics, University of California, San Francisco, San Francisco, California 94110.

for long periods and is a significant impediment to the eradication of the disease from a community.

TRANSMISSION OF TUBERCULOSIS

The principal risk for acquiring infection with *Mycobacterium tuberculosis* is breathing (Bloom and Murray, 1992). The concept that microbes may exist in sufficient concentration in the air to cause airborne infection and disease was controversial until the middle of this century. The classic studies of Wells (1955) and his student Riley (Riley and O'Grady, 1961) established beyond doubt that infectious particles containing *M. tuberculosis* were emitted in coughs and sneezes and even in speaking. A sneeze may contain over a million particles with diameters of less than 100 μm, the mean being 10 μm. These particles form droplet nuclei in which evaporation continues until the vapor pressure of the droplet equals the atmospheric pressure. The droplet nucleus is very stable, settles very slowly (about 12 mm/min), and remains suspended in the air for long periods. A 10-μm droplet nucleus may carry perhaps 3 to 10 tubercle bacilli. Dust-associated particles may also carry *M. tuberculosis*. These particles are larger than droplets, but they can be transiently resuspended by air convection and may serve as a reservoir for infectious bacilli.

The infectious capability of droplet nuclei was formally established by Wells (1955) and Riley (Riley et al., 1959), who showed that the number of tubercles in the lungs was equivalent to the number of live bacilli inhaled on droplet nuclei with a settling velocity of about 9 mm/min. Of the inhaled bacilli, only 6% reached the alveoli and produced tubercles; the majority of larger particles settled in the upper respiratory mucosa and were expelled by the ciliated respiratory escalator. Infection can take place by ingestion of tubercle bacilli but is about 10,000-fold less effective than inhalation of droplets in transmitting tuberculosis, probably because tubercle bacilli are very sensitive to gastric acid (Gaudier and Gernez-Rieux, 1962). The clearest demonstration that droplet nuclei were important for transmission was the finding that when air from the ventilating system of a hospital ward for tuberculosis patients was ducted through an exposure chamber that housed guinea pigs, 71 of 156 animals became infected with tuberculosis (Riley et al., 1959). Interestingly, in the same experiments, UV irradiation of the air from the same ward prevented transmission to guinea pigs.

The number and concentration of bacilli present in the source case, estimated to be between 10^2 and 10^4 in solid or nodular lesions but of the order of 10^7 to 10^8 in cavitary lesions (Canetti, 1965), are major variables in transmission, as are the duration of exposure and the aerodynamics of the exhaled particles. While many health care workers exposed for long periods to patients with tuberculosis remain uninfected, there are dramatic examples of several hundred people being infected from a single index case.

EPIDEMIOLOGICAL MODEL OF TUBERCULOSIS

Disease due to tuberculosis in populations is influenced by three distinct risks: the risk of an individual in the community being infected with tubercle bacilli in a given time period, the risk of disease following shortly after such infection, and the risk of disease occurring long after the original infection owing to the reactivation of latent bacilli. Epidemiological investigations have sought to measure these risks and to identify factors that modify them, particularly those factors that might be susceptible to change through specific intervention measures.

Most of the disease burden from tuberculosis is suffered by those living in developing countries, but in the recent past, the disease was one of the major causes of morbidity and mortality in the now-developed countries. In the 1940s in those countries, the priority of tuberculosis as a public health problem was perhaps comparable to the priority of cancer today. Consequently, the epidemiology of the disease was subjected to extensive investigation, and most of our present knowledge derives from the studies conducted in developed countries. To what extent the findings in developed countries are generalizable to those countries where the disease load is now focused remains, in some respects at least, open to question, but a reasonable first approach may be to assume that the general aspects of the epidemiology are similar until proven otherwise. It should be stressed, however, that there is an urgent need for well-conducted epidemiological investigations of the disease in those parts of the world where the disease burden is greatest.

Figure 1 is a diagrammatic representation of the natural history of tuberculosis within individuals as they age and are exposed to infection and reinfection. Disease is generally thought to develop in an individual as a consequence of one of three processes:

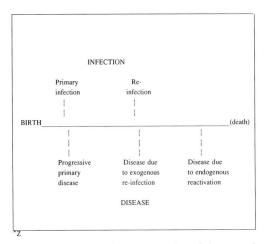

Figure 1. Diagrammatic representation of the natural history of tuberculosis within individuals as they age.

progression of primary infection, exogenous reinfection, or endogenous reactivation.

At some time after birth, an individual may be infected with *M. tuberculosis* for the first time. This infection is usually acquired through airborne infection from someone who has active pulmonary tuberculosis, i.e., from whom a smear of sputum suitably stained with an acid-fast dye can be shown to contain tubercle bacilli (so called smear-positive tuberculosis). The age at which this primary infection is acquired depends on how common active tuberculosis is in the community. In many developed countries now, there is a good chance that most individuals will escape infection for their whole lives, whereas in developing countries, many such infections occur in childhood, and a high proportion of individuals are infected by the time they are young adults.

Following primary infection, a small proportion of individuals develop progressive primary disease. This is the kind of disease usually seen in children. In 80% of those who develop this form of the disease, it is manifest within 2 years of infection, and nearly all cases occur within 5 years of infection (Medical Research Council, 1972). Children who develop progressive primary tuberculosis are usually smear negative and are therefore not an important source of infection in the community. Estimates of the magnitude of the risk of progressive primary disease following infection vary considerably, but the risk is of the order of 5 to 10%.

Most people do not develop disease following infection and are assumed to mount an effective immune response to the initial infection that limits proliferation of the bacilli and leads to long-lasting partial immunity both to further infection and to reactivation of latent bacilli remaining from the original infection. Such individuals can be identified by a positive response to a tuberculin skin test (although in some circumstances, infections with other mycobacteria in the environment may lead to false-positive skin test responses to the tuberculin test).

At later ages, the immunity of persons who have been previously infected may wane, and they are then at risk of developing active tuberculosis as a consequence of either exogenous reinfection (i.e., acquiring a new infection from another infectious individual) or endogenous reactivation of latent bacilli (i.e., reactivation of a preexisting dormant infection). The relative contributions of these two disease routes, and even the existence of one or the other, have been the subject of considerable controversy over the years. Unfortunately, until very recently, the possibility of distinguishing between the two types of disease in individual patients has not existed, and it has been necessary to employ epidemiological modeling techniques to estimate their respective contributions to the total disease load in a population (Sutherland, 1976). With the development of molecular methods of characterizing strains of tubercle bacilli, using restricted fragment length polymorphisms (RFLPs), the potential exists for determining whether disease in a patient is due to an a "new" infection (one that is currently circulating) or the reactivation of an "old" infection (one that was circulating some time previously) (see chapter 33 in this volume).

Much of the work, i.e., estimating the relative contributions of exogenous reinfection and endogenous reactivation to the total tuberculosis disease load, has been done by using historical data from The Netherlands, where for many years all new recruits to military service were skin tested with tuberculin to assess their previous exposure to *M. tuberculosis*. The proportion found to be tuberculin positive at a specific time measures their cumulative risk of infection up to their current age. By studying such data from successive cohorts of recruits, it is possible to estimate annual risks of infection and the changes in these risks over time. By also relating changes in infection rates over time to changes in the occurrence of cases of clinical disease, it is possible to estimate the contributions of the different forms of disease at different times (Sutherland, 1976). A broad general conclusion from these studies is that in populations in which infection is common, such as in The Netherlands in the earlier part of the century and in developing countries now, exogenous reinfection is likely to be responsible for a high proportion of new cases of adult disease, whereas when the risk of infection is low, as in developed countries now, the relative contribution of endogenous reactivation is greater, and most disease in adults may have this etiology (Styblo, 1984).

Tuberculosis due to reactivation of latent bacilli is presumed to result from a failure in immune surveillance. For example, immunosuppressive treatment is known to increase the risk of reactivation, and the great increase in the risk of tuberculosis in persons with human immunodeficiency virus (HIV) infection is thought to be attributable mainly, though not exclusively, to reactivation of earlier infections. However, in the great majority of cases, the specific cause of reactivation is unknown and, with the exception of HIV infection, those factors that have been identified can account for only a small proportion of all cases of disease (Rieder et al., 1989).

Disease in adults, whether due to a primary infection, reinfection, or reactivation, is sputum positive in about 50% of cases (Styblo, 1984), and it is these cases that are the main source of infection, or reinfection, in the population (Shaw and Wynn-Williams, 1954). It is for this reason that attempts to reduce the transmission of tubercle bacilli in a population through the treatment of cases focus primarily on the identification and treatment of sputum-positive patients so as to render them sputum negative as rapidly as possible and thus restrict the number of others whom they have the opportunity to infect.

The natural history of tuberculosis following the onset of clinical symptoms is difficult to study because of the availability of very effective treatments, but studies conducted in Britain (Springett, 1971) and in India (National Tuberculosis Institute, 1974) before chemotherapy was widely introduced have produced similar findings. In these studies of sputum-positive patients, about 50% died within 5 years of diagnosis, 30% "self-cured," and the remaining 20% remained alive. In many developing countries, less than half of tuberculosis patients who start treatment are cured or complete their course of chemotherapy (Snider, 1993b), and worldwide, death may still be the most common way in which patients cease to be infectious to others. Poor treatment programs may even worsen the situation by keeping infectious patients alive longer and thus prolonging the period of transmission (Grzybowski, 1991).

TRENDS IN TUBERCULOSIS RATES

Until relatively recently, rates of tuberculosis in developed countries had shown large and consistent declines for many decades. Although it is likely that effective chemotherapy speeded the decline (Styblo, 1989), the major decreases occurred before effective therapy or vaccines were available (McKeown, 1979). Part of the decrease may have been due to the segregation of infectious patients in sanatoria, and the introduction of tuberculin testing of dairy herds and the pasteurization of milk dramatically reduced the incidence of bovine tuberculosis, but the major cause of the decline was related to socioeconomic development. It is not clear exactly what components of socioeconomic development were the determining factors, but as transmission occurs almost exclusively in enclosed environments, improvements in

housing, with better ventilation and reduction of crowding, are likely to have been important changes, as were better levels of nutrition.

The rapidity of the decline in tuberculosis infection rates has been best documented by using the data on annual tuberculin testing of military recruits in The Netherlands. Between 1910 and 1939, the average annual risk of infection in The Netherlands is estimated to have decreased by 5.4% annually, and the rate of decline increased to 12.9% annually between 1940 and 1969 (Styblo et al., 1969), with the change around 1940 coinciding with the introduction of compulsory pasteurization of milk. The later development and use of adequate chemotherapy further accelerated the decrease in the annual risk of tuberculosis infection (Styblo, 1989). In many developed countries, the annual risk of infection is now well below 0.1% per year, although pockets of high transmission remain, mainly among socially deprived groups and in immigrants from developing countries. In 1978, Styblo estimated that the rate of infection in developed countries was halving about every 5 years (Styblo, 1978).

Few recent data on the risks of infection in developing countries are available, but in a large number of tuberculin surveys that were conducted by the World Health Organization in the 1950s through the 1970s in different African counties (the continent with probably the highest rates of infection [Murray et al., 1990]), annual risks of infection varied from about 2 to 5%, and in countries where repeat tuberculin surveys were done at later dates, there was little evidence of declining rates (Stott et al., 1973). Given the economic crises of the last two decades and the deterioration in many tuberculosis control programs, it seems unlikely that infection rates will have declined since then, and indeed, with the onset of the HIV epidemic, increases in the rates of infection seem very likely. What is clear is that HIV infection greatly increases the risk of tuberculosis due to reactivation of latent infection. What has yet to be determined is the magnitude of the impact on tuberculosis transmission rates in the community of the large increases in the numbers of cases of tuberculosis among HIV-infected individuals.

Socioeconomic development has been consistently associated with declining rates of tuberculosis. However, such changes generally take place over long periods, and in the short term, more rapid interventions are required. The medical intervention that has been most effective in reducing tuberculosis in a community is improved case finding and treatment. Whether the trend in the annual risk of infection is up or down will depend on how many individuals a case of tuberculosis infects on average and how many of these go on to develop clinical disease. If each case on average infects fewer people than would be necessary for one further case to be expected, the incidence of the disease will decline. If the average number of secondary cases is greater than one, the disease incidence will rise. Modern chemotherapy rapidly renders infectious cases sterile for infecting others but obviously has no impact on the number of infections transmitted before the disease was diagnosed, and this number will be critical in determining the trend in the risk of infection in a community. It has been estimated that in developed countries, two or three persons on average may be infected by a smear-positive case before its detection, whereas in developing countries, the number may be four or five because of higher numbers of close contacts (Murray et al., 1990). These numbers vary greatly according to local cultural and treatment conditions. In the absence of treatment, an untreated smear-positive person might infect on average 10 to 14 persons per year (Styblo, 1984). A first priority in control programs must be to ensure the rapid diagnosis and the effective and complete treatment of patients who report to clinics with symptoms of active tuberculosis (especially smear-positive disease), and once this is achieved, the second priority is to strengthen case detection activities to shorten the average interval between the time a case becomes infectious and the time of diagnosis and treatment (see chapter 33 in this volume).

Contact tracing is used in many control programs to identify those person a case of tuberculosis may have infected or the person from whom the infection was acquired. Generally, this tracing involves examining adults in the same household or the same workplace as a diagnosed patient and examining tuberculin-positive child contacts. While numerous epidemiological studies have demonstrated that close contacts of patients, particularly of those who are sputum positive, are at increased risk of tuberculosis, the majority of tuberculosis patients in the community have probably acquired their disease from an unknown, nonintimate contact (Grzybowski et al., 1975; Raj Narain et al., 1966; Andersen and Geser, 1960). Studies in India (Raj Narain et al., 1966) and Africa (Andersen and Geser, 1960) have illustrated the limited value of tuberculin testing child contacts of patients as a means of case detection because of the relatively high proportions of persons who have been infected with *M. tuberculosis* without evidence of having lived in the same household as an infectious person. For example, in the community study by Raj Narain et al. in India, 41% of children aged less than 15 years in the households of bacillary cases were infected and 19% of children in the households of cases diagnosed by X ray only were infected compared to 12% of children in households without a case of tuberculosis. However, the first two groups accounted for only 15% of all infected children in the community (Raj Narain et al., 1966).

INTERACTION WITH HIV

The epidemic of HIV infection has radically changed the epidemiology of tuberculosis. The overlap of HIV infection and *M. tuberculosis* infection, in developing countries in particular, threatens to produce a public health crisis of the first magnitude. HIV infection is, as Styblo and Enarson (1991) have noted, "the strongest risk factor for tuberculosis disease observed in the last hundred years in subjects infected with tubercle bacilli." To date, the major effect of HIV infection has been to affect the rate of progression to clinical disease in those already infected with *M. tuberculosis*. However, the relationship between the two pathogens is complex, and HIV infection is probably also responsible for increased rates of primary transmission of *M. tuberculosis* in some parts of the world. The overall effect on tuberculosis incidence is enormous, and there is little doubt that HIV will force a reconsideration of tuberculosis control policies in general.

The intimate connection between HIV infection and tuberculosis was demonstrated early in Africa and among intravenous drug users in the United States (De Cock et al., 1992; Stoneburner et al., 1987). It has become clear that, worldwide, tuberculosis is the most common opportunistic infection occurring in patients with AIDS. Of AIDS patients in Latin America, 20 to 30% have tuberculosis, and at least a third of all AIDS patients in African countries present with tuberculosis (De Cock et al., 1992). Among drug users with AIDS in the United States, 21% were reported to develop tuberculosis in one study (Sunderam et al., 1986). However, tuberculosis is rare as an opportunistic infection among HIV-infected homosexual men (Pulmonary AIDS Complications Study, unpublished data). These differences reflect the background prevalence of infection with *M. tuberculosis* in different populations. In African populations and in populations of developing countries in other parts of the world, about one half are infected with *M. tuberculosis*, reflecting the high annual infection rates that lead to the infection of most of the population by older ages. In the United States, about 7% of homosexual men and 15 to 25% of intravenous drug users are tuberculin positive (Markowitz et al., 1993; Selwyn et al., 1989). Thus, where *M. tuberculosis* infection is prevalent, clinical tuberculosis is common as a complication of AIDS; where it is rare, clinical tuberculosis is also rare in AIDS patients. Tuberculosis as a clinical opportunistic infection appears relatively early in the course of HIV infection, with median CD4 counts at diagnosis of 200 to 300/mm^3 in U.S. studies. De Cock suggests that pulmonary tuberculosis occurs at higher CD4 counts and is followed by localized extrapulmonary disease, tuberculosis meningitis, and miliary tuberculosis as the CD4 count falls progressively (De Cock et al., 1992).

In areas where HIV infection is common, a high proportion of cases of tuberculosis are coinfected with HIV. In some African countries, 15 to 70% of patients presenting with tuberculosis are HIV infected (De Cock et al., 1992; Bermejo et al., 1992), and a rate of 40% has been reported in Haiti (Pape et al., 1989). One quarter of all tuberculosis cases in Haiti were estimated to be attributable to HIV infection, and the rate in Abidjan was 35% (De Cock et al., 1992). Bermejo et al. (1992) estimated that if HIV prevalence reaches 13% of adults in a developing country, tuberculosis rates will double, and Pape et al. (1989) predict that at an HIV prevalence of 10%, tuberculosis rates will triple. Rates of HIV infection in U.S. tuberculosis clinics vary from 5 to 40%, the variation reflecting primarily the proportion of intravenous drug users among AIDS cases. In New York City, about 40% of tuberculosis patients are HIV infected (Shafer et al., 1991; New York City Department of Health, 1993).

Table 1. Risk of clinical tuberculosis in HIV-infected persons in six prospective studies

Study	Subjects[a]	Tuberculosis rate/yr (%)	Risk ratio[b]
Selwyn et al., 1989	HIV$^+$ PPD$^+$ IVDU	7.9	Inf
	HIV$^-$ PPD$^+$ IVDU	0	
	HIV$^+$ PPD$^-$ IVDU	0.3	Inf
	HIV$^-$ PPD$^-$ IVDU	0	
Selwyn et al., 1992	HIV$^+$ anergic IVDU	6.6	Inf
	HIV$^-$ anergic IVDU	0	
	HIV$^+$ PPD$^+$ IVDU (no prophylaxis)	9.7	10
	HIV$^-$ PPD$^+$ IVDU (no prophylaxis)	1.0	
Allen et al., 1992	HIV$^+$ women, Rwanda	2.5	50
	HIV$^-$ women, Rwanda	0.05	
Braun et al., 1991	HIV$^+$ women, Zaire	3.1	26
	HIV$^-$ women, Zaire	0.12	
Moreno et al., 1993	HIV$^+$ PPD$^+$, Spain	10.4	NA
	HIV$^+$ anergic, Spain	12.4	
	HIV$^+$ PPD$^-$ nonanergic, Spain	5.4	
Hawken et al., 1993	HIV$^+$ Kenyan tuberculosis patients	16.7	34
	HIV$^-$ Kenyan tuberculosis patients	0.5	

[a] PPD, purified protein derivative; IVDU, intravenous drug user.
[b] Inf, infinite risk ratio; NA, not applicable.

Worldwide, tuberculosis as a clinical complication of HIV infection is thought to be due usually to endogenous reactivation of *M. tuberculosis* resulting from the loss of immune control of a latent infection acquired earlier in life. However, recent evidence suggests that the risk of primary transmission of tuberculosis is also increased in both African and U.S. populations (Hawken et al., 1993; Bloom and Murray, 1992).

In HIV-infected groups, the decline in CD4 counts as the infection progresses is associated with increasing anergy (Markowitz et al., 1993), and consequently, skin testing with tuberculin may underestimate the proportion of the population infected with *M. tuberculosis*. In a large study in the United States, about 75% of HIV-infected persons with CD4 counts of less than 200/mm^3 were anergic, as were about half of those with CD4 counts between 200 and 400 and about 20% of those with CD4 counts greater than 400. Similar findings were obtained for intravenous drug users and homosexual men (Markowitz et al., 1993). Anergy in the HIV-infected patient compli-

cates decisions about prophylaxis and BCG vaccination, the two principal tuberculosis control measures other than treatment of active cases.

Rapid Progression to Clinical Disease

HIV infection "telescopes" the natural history of tuberculosis infection (Hopewell, 1992). Coinfected persons show short-term progression rates to active disease that are far higher than those among persons who are tuberculin positive but HIV negative, as shown in the studies summarized in Table 1. Among those coinfected, the probability of progression to clinical tuberculosis is 2 to 10%/year, which is 3 orders of magnitude higher than the classic estimates of the rate of developing clinical tuberculosis among the skin test positive (10 to 20/100,000/year). No studies have yet monitored coinfected individuals for a long period, so it is not clear how long the rates of Table 1 persist. If they do persist, the overall risk of tuberculosis in the coinfected (as well as the speed of progression to active tuberculosis) is clearly much increased over the classic estimate of an approximately 10% lifetime risk, and a very high proportion of coinfected persons are at risk of active tuberculosis.

Reported progression rates in the African studies noted in Table 1 appear to be lower than those in the U.S. and Spanish studies, which may reflect an increased probability of primary infection among the intravenous drug users who make up the latter studies. Primary *M. tuberculosis* infection associated with HIV may be relatively rare in African populations, because prevalent *M. tuberculosis* infection rates are very high in adults. Table 1 also suggests, surprisingly, that anergic persons who are HIV positive have the same progression rates to clinical diseases as purified protein derivative-positive patients. Although anergy is common in intravenous drug users for reasons other than HIV, anergic persons will tend to have relatively low CD4 counts and therefore relatively high rates of progression to clinical disease, which may explain this result. It has been recommended that anergic and HIV-positive persons be given chemoprophylaxis against tuberculosis (Selwyn et al., 1992).

Increased Risk of Primary *M. tuberculosis* Infection

Recent outbreaks of multiple-drug-resistant (MDR) tuberculosis in AIDS units and other congregate settings (Centers for Disease Control, 1991) suggest an increased risk of primary infection with *M. tuberculosis*. However, this phenomenon can be distinguished from rapid progression among the infected only when denominator data are available, that is, when it is known how many people were exposed to *M. tuberculosis* infection in the outbreak. It should be remembered that classic studies show infection rates as high as 80 to 100% in some outbreaks in the absence of HIV (Hopewell, 1986). So far, no denominator studies have been published in the HIV era.

Daley et al. (1992), in a study of outbreak in an AIDS patient residence in San Francisco, speculate that at least in late-stage HIV-positive patients, susceptibility to infection was high.

While it is possible that HIV-infected persons are more susceptible to infection with *M. tuberculosis*, there is no evidence that HIV-infected tuberculosis patients are more infectious than tuberculosis cases in general. In a study in Africa, the risk to close contacts of an HIV-positive index case of tuberculosis was not different from the risk to the contacts of an HIV-negative case (Elliott et al., 1993).

Exogenous Reinfection

In the absence of HIV infection, infection with *M. tuberculosis* provides some long-lasting protective immunity against a second infection. However, using RFLP fingerprinting of *M. tuberculosis* isolates (see chapter 33), Small and colleagues have recently demonstrated reinfection by a second *M. tuberculosis* strain in 4 of 19 tuberculosis patients for whom two cultures were available (Small et al., 1993). All were HIV positive. It is likely that in AIDS patients in particular, reinfection with a second strain is a relatively common occurrence. Thus, the view that in developed countries exogenous reinfection plays a very minor role in the etiology of clinical tuberculosis (Styblo, 1984) may not hold for those who are HIV infected.

Primary Transmission

The demonstration of exogenous reinfection raises the issue of the effect of HIV on primary transmission of *M. tuberculosis* in developed countries. Historically, as tuberculosis rates have declined, the burden of tuberculosis in the population has shifted away from primary transmission toward reactivation of old disease. Thus, tuberculosis in developed countries has become increasingly a disease of the old, and childhood tuberculosis has become rare. However, the recent increase in the incidence of tuberculosis in New York (New York City Department of Health, 1993) together with the outbreak studies reported by the Centers for Disease Control and Prevention (CDC) (CDC, 1991), suggests that primary tuberculosis as well as tuberculosis due to endogenous reactivation may be on the increase. Several descriptive and analytic studies support this conclusion. First, although tuberculosis as a whole has increased in the United States and elsewhere in the last decade, the age distribution of tuberculosis in both New York and the United States as a whole has shifted, with the major increase coming in blacks and Hispanics in the 25- to 44-year-old age group, that is, in the group at highest risk for HIV infection. In addition, a recent CDC analysis showed that the largest increases in tuberculosis in recent years in the United States have been in states with the highest incidence of AIDS (Snider, 1993a). In another analysis, Bloom and Murray (1992) estimate that about one quarter of the recent rise in tuberculosis incidence in the United States is due to active transmission in hospitals, homeless shelters, prisons, and other communal living situations; about one third was estimated to be due to HIV. Also, a recent study with DNA fingerprinting techniques in New York (Alland et al., submitted) (see chapter 33) suggests that 30 to 40% of tuberculosis is clonal, that is, in grouped strains, which is likely to be the result of active transmission rather than reactivation of old infection (which would be expected to produce many unique strains). Clonality, that is, active transmission, was associated with HIV infection in this study. It seems likely that a significant part of the rise in tuberculosis incidence in recent years, at least in New York and perhaps elsewhere in the United States, is attributable to active transmission, probably in association with HIV infection.

Drug Resistance

A rise in the proportion of all tuberculosis that is MDR has been observed along with the recent upturn in tuberculosis incidence in the United States. This phenomenon is particularly marked in New York. In April 1991, 19% of all prevalent strains in the city were resistant to two or more drugs (Frieden et al., 1993). There are dramatic increases in drug-resistant tuberculosis in surveys in Africa, Asia, and Latin America (Vareldis et al., 1993). Multiple resistance was strongly associated with AIDS and HIV seropositivity. The spread of drug resistance is likely to be related to HIV infection in two separate ways. First, noncompliant populations such as drug users and the homeless have a high risk for HIV infection; thus, individual MDR strains are likely to be generated in these populations as a result of noncompliance with tuberculosis treatment. Second, active transmission is likely among HIV-positive persons and AIDS patients, particularly in congregate settings, as a result of the telescoping phenomenon, i.e., the rapid generation of new infectious cases from new infections among people who may themselves be unusually susceptible. Since these noncompliant populations have a high risk of HIV infection and AIDS, the creation and active transmission of MDR strains are likely to be taking place in the same populations. MDR problems in association with HIV have not been reported from developing countries, but there is clear potential for a similar overlap in countries with intravenous drug use problems and high background rates of tuberculosis, such as Thailand and Brazil.

The "New" Tuberculosis

HIV has profoundly changed the epidemiology of tuberculosis, disrupting the balance between tuberculosis infection and control in both developing and developed countries. In developing countries, and particularly in Africa, coinfection with *M. tuberculosis* and HIV threatens to double or triple the clinical burden of tuberculosis. De Cock notes that "with current resources, existing tuberculosis programs in sub-Saharan Africa will not cope with the increased tuberculosis burden" (De Cock et al., 1992). In the United States, HIV is a major reason for the increase in tuberculosis nationwide since 1985 and is also responsible for structural changes in the epidemiology of the disease that may require a rethinking of control strategies: of prophylaxis and vaccination issues and of the relationship between reactivation and primary disease. Among the urban poor, where HIV and *M. tuberculosis* infections and poor compliance overlap, tuberculosis has become almost a "new disease," as Snider put it, in which the telescoping of the pathological process and the high prevalence of MDR strains combine to produce a dangerous form of active transmission, particularly among late-stage HIV-seropositive patients and AIDS patients (Snider and Roper, 1992). While active transmission has so far been demonstrated mainly in HIV-infected individuals, it should be remembered that *M. tuberculosis* infection in HIV-infected persons is also what shows up first as a result of rapid progression to disease. Thus, although active transmission and transmission of MDR strains are currently thought of as AIDS-associated phenomena, it is possible that both will be eventually be seen in broader populations.

REFERENCES

Alland, D., G. E. Kalkut, A. Moss, R. A. McAdam, J. A. Hahn, W. Bosworth, E. Drucker, and B. R. Bloom. Transmission of tuberculosis in New York City: an analysis by DNA fingerprinting and conventional epidemiologic methods. Submitted for publication.

Allen, S., J. Batungwayo, K. Kerlikowske, A. R. Lifson, W. Wolf, R. Granich, H. Taelman, P. Van De Perre, A. Serufilira, J. Bogaerts, G. Slutkin, and P. Hopewell. 1992. Two-year incidence of tuberculosis in cohorts of HIV-infected and uninfected urban Rwandan women. *Am. Rev. Respir. Dis.* **146:**1439–1444.

Andersen, S., and A. Geser. 1960. The distribution of tuberculosis infection among households in African communities. *Bull. W.H.O.* **22:**39–60.

Bermejo, A., H. Veeken, and A. Berra. 1992. Tuberculosis incidence in developing countries with high prevalence of HIV infection. *AIDS* **6:**1203–1206.

Bloom, B. R., and C. J. L. Murray. 1992. Tuberculosis: commentary on a reemergent killer. *Science* **257:**1055–1064.

Braun, M., N. Badi, R. Ryder, E. Baende, Y. Mukadi, M. Nsuami, B. Matela, J. C. Williams, M. Kaboto, and W. Heyward. 1991. A retrospective cohort study of the risk of tuberculosis among women of childbearing age with HIV infection in Zaire. *Am. Rev. Respir. Dis.* **143:**501–504.

Canetti, G. 1965. *Am. Rev. Respir. Dis.* **92:**687.

Centers for Disease Control. 1991. Nosocomial transmission of multidrug resistant tuberculosis among HIV-infected persons: Florida and New York, 1988–91. *Morbid. Mortal. Weekly Rep.* **40:**585–591.

Daley, C. L., P. M. Small, G. S. Schecter, G. K. Schoolnik, R. A. McAdam, W. R. Jacobs, and P. C. Hopewell. 1992. An outbreak of tuberculosis with accelerated progression among persons infected with the human immunodeficiency virus. An analysis using restriction-fragment-length polymorphisms. *N. Engl. J. Med.* **326:**231–235.

De Cock, K. M., B. Soro, I. M. Coulibaly, and S. B. Lucas. 1992. Tuberculosis and HIV infection in sub-Saharan Africa. *JAMA* **268:**1581–1587.

Di Perri, G., M. Cruciani, M. C. Danzi, et al. 1989. Nosocomial epidemic of active tuberculosis among HIV-infected patients. *Lancet* **ii:**1502–1504.

Elliott, A. M., R. J. Hayes, et al. 1993. The impact of HIV on infectiousness of pulmonary tuberculosis: a community study in Zambia. *AIDS* **7:**981–987.

Frieden, T. R., T. Sterling, A. Pabloc-Mendez, J. Kilburn, G. M. Cauthen, and S. W. Dooley. 1993. The emergence of drug-resistant tuberculosis in New York City. *N. Engl. J. Med.* **328:**521–526.

Gaudier, B., and C. Gernez-Rieux. 1962. Ètude experimentale de la vitalitè du B.C.G. au cours de la traversèe gastro-intestinale chez des enfants non allergiques vaccinès par voie digestive. *Ann. Inst. Pasteur Lille* **13:**77–87.

Grzybowski, S. 1991. Tuberculosis in the third world. *Thorax* **46:**689–691.

Grzybowski, S., G. D. Barnett, and K. Styblo. 1975. Contacts of cases of active pulmonary tuberculosis. *Bull. Int. Union Tuberc.* **50:**90–106.

Hawken, M., P. Nunn, S. Gathua, R. Brindle, P. Godfrey-Faussett, W. Githi, J. Odhiambo, B. Batchelor, C. Gilks, J. Morris, and K. McAdam. 1993. Increased recurrence of tuberculosis in HIV-1-infected patients in Kenya. *Lancet* **342**:332–337.

Hopewell, P. C. 1986. Factors influencing the transmission and infectivity of Mycobacterium tuberculosis: implications for public health and clinical management, p. 191–216. *In* M. A. Sande, L. D. Hudson, and R. K. Root (ed.), *Respiratory Infections.* Churchill Livingstone, New York.

Hopewell, P. C. 1992. Impact of human immunodeficiency virus infection on the epidemiology, clinical features, management and control of tuberculosis. *Clin. Infect. Dis.* **18**:540–546.

Markowitz, N., N. I. Hansen, T. C. Wilcosky, P. Hopewell, J. Glassroth, P. A. Kvale, B. T. Mangura, D. Osmond, J. M. Wallace, M. J. Rosen, and L. B. Reichman. 1993. Tuberculin and anergy testing in HIV-seropositive and HIV-seronegative persons. *Ann. Intern. Med.* **119**:185–193.

McKeown, T. 1979. *The Role of Medicine: Dream, Mirage or Nemesis?* Basil Blackwell, Oxford.

Medical Research Council. 1972. BCG and vole bacillus vaccines in the prevention of tuberculosis in adolescence and early adult life. *Bull. W.H.O.* **46**:371–385.

Moreno, S., J. Baraia-Extaburu, E. Bopuza, F. Parras, M. Perez-Tascon, P. Miralles, T. Vicente, J. C. Alberdi, J. Cosin, and D. Lopez-Gay. 1993. Risk for developing tuberculosis among anergic patients infected with HIV. *Ann. Intern. Med.* **119**:194–198.

Murray, C. J. L., K. Styblo, and A. Rouillon. 1990. Tuberculosis in developing countries: burden, intervention and cost. *Bull. Int. Union Tuberc.* **65**:2–19.

National Tuberculosis Institute. 1974. Tuberculosis in a rural population in South India: a five years epidemiological study. *Bull. W.H.O.* **51**:473–488.

New York City Department of Health. 1993. *Tuberculosis 1992.* New York City Department of Health, New York.

Pape, J. W., M. E. Stanback, M. Pamphile, M. Boncy, M. M. H. Deschamps, R. I. Verdier, M. E. Beaulieu, W. Blattner, B. Liautaud, and W. D. Johnson, Jr. 1989. Prevalence of HIV infection and high-risk activities in Haiti. *J. Acquired Immune Defic. Syndr.* **3**:995–1001.

Pulmonary AIDS Complications Study. Unpublished data.

Raj Narain, S., S. Nair, G. Ramanatha Rao, and P. Chandrasekhar. 1966. Distribution of tuberculosis infection and disease among households in a rural community. *Bull. W.H.O.* **34**:639–654.

Rieder, H. L., G. M. Cauthen, G. W. Comstock, and D. E. Snider. 1989. Epidemiology of tuberculosis in the United States. *Epidemiol. Rev.* **11**:79–97.

Riley, R. L., C. L. Mills, W. Nyka, N. Weinstock, P. B. Storey, L. K. Sultan, M. C. Riley, and W. F. Wells. 1959. Aerial dissemination of pulmonary tuberculosis: a two year study of contagion in a tuberculosis

ward. *Am. J. Hyg.* **70**:185.

Riley, R. L., and F. O'Grady. 1961. *Airborne Infection: Transmission and Control.* The Macmillan Co., New York.

Selwyn, P. A., D. Hartel, V. A. Lewis, E. E. Schoenbaum, S. H. Vermund, R. S. Klein, A. T. Walker, and G. H. Friedland. 1989. A prospective study of the risk of tuberculosis among intravenous drug users with human immunodeficiency virus infection. *N. Engl. J. Med.* **320**:545–550.

Selwyn, P. A., B. M. Sckell, P. Alcabes, G. H. Friedland, R. S. Klein, and E. E. Schoenbaum. 1992. High risk of active tuberculosis in HIV-infected drug users with cutaneous anergy. *JAMA* **268**:504–509.

Shafer, R. W., K. D. Chirgwin, A. E. Glatt, M. Dahdouh, S. Landesman, and B. Suster. 1991. HIV prevalence, immunosuppression and drug resistance in patients with tuberculosis in an area endemic for AIDS. *AIDS* **5**:399–405.

Shaw, J. B., and N. Wynn-Williams. 1954. Infectivity of pulmonary tuberculosis in relation to sputum status. *Am. Rev. Tuberc.* **69**:724.

Small, P. M., R. W. Shafer, P. C. Hopewell, S. P. Singh, M. J. Murphy, E. Desmond, M. F. Sierra, and G. K. Schoolnik. 1993. Exogenous reinfection with multidrug-resistant Mycobacterium tuberculosis in patients with advanced HIV infection. *N. Engl. J. Med.* **328**:1137–1144.

Snider, D. E. 1993a. The impact of tuberculosis on women, children and minorities in the United States. Paper presented at the World Congress on Tuberculosis, Bethesda, Md., 1993.

Snider, D. E. 1993b. Tuberculosis: the world situation. History of the disease and efforts to combat it. *In* J. Porter and K. McAdam (ed.), *Tuberculosis: Back to the Future.* John Wiley and Sons, Chichester, United Kingdom.

Snider, D. E., and W. L. Roper. 1992. The new tuberculosis. *N. Engl. J. Med.* **326**:703–705.

Springett, V. H. 1971. Tuberculosis control in Britain 1945–1970–1985. *Tubercle* **52**:136–147.

Stoneburner, R. L., M. M. Ruiz, J. A. Milberg, S. Schultz, A. Vennema, and D. L. Morse. 1987. Tuberculosis and acquired immunodeficiency syndrome—New York City. *Morbid. Mortal. Weekly Rep.* **36**:786–790.

Stott, H., A. Patel, I. Sutherland, I. Thorup, P. G. Smith, P. W. Kent, and Y. P. Rykushin. 1973. The risk of tuberculosis infection in Uganda, derived from the findings of national tuberculin surveys in 1958 and 1970. *Tubercle* **54**:1–22.

Styblo, K. 1978. Recent advances in tuberculosis epidemiology with regard to the formulation or readjustment of control programmes. *Bull. Int. Union Tuberc.* **53**:283–299.

Styblo, K. 1984. *Epidemiology of Tuberculosis.* VEB

Gustav Fischer Verlag Jena, The Hague, The Netherlands.

Styblo, K. 1989. Overview and epidemiologic assessment of the current global tuberculosis situation with an emphasis on control in developing countries. *Rev. Infect. Dis.* **2**(Suppl. 2):S339–S346.

Styblo, K., and D. A. Enarson. 1991. Epidemiology of tuberculosis in HIV prevalent countries, p. 116–136. *In Selected Papers*, vol. 24. Royal Netherlands Tuberculosis Association, The Hague.

Styblo, K., J. Meijer, and I. Sutherland. 1969. The transmission of tubercle bacilli: its trend in a human population. Tuberculosis Surveillance Research Unit report no. 1. *Bull. Int. Union Tuberc.* **42**:5–104.

Sunderam, G., R. J. McDonald, T. Maniatis, J. Oleske, R. Kapila, and L. B. Reichman. 1986. Tuberculosis as a manifestation of the acquired immunodeficiency syndrome (AIDS). *JAMA* **256**:362–366.

Sutherland, I. 1976. Recent studies in the epidemiology of tuberculosis, based on the risk of being infected with tubercle bacilli. *Adv. Tuberc. Res.* **19**:1–63.

Vareldis, B. P., J. Grosset, I. de Kantor, J. Crafton, A. Laszlo, M. Felton, M. C. Ranglione, and A. Kochi. 1993. *Laboratory Evaluations of Drug Resistant Tuberculosis.* WHO/TB/93.171. World Health Organization, Geneva.

Wells, W. F. 1955. *Airborne Contagion and Air Hygiene.* Harvard University Press, Cambridge, Mass.

Tuberculosis: Pathogenesis, Protection, and Control
Edited by Barry R. Bloom
© 1994 American Society for Microbiology, Washington, DC 20005

Chapter 5

Biological Safety in the Experimental Tuberculosis Laboratory

W. Emmett Barkley and George P. Kubica

The reemergence of tuberculosis as a potential public health threat, the high susceptibility of human immunodeficiency virus-infected persons to the disease, and the proliferation of multiple-drug-resistant strains have created both a national expectation for and much scientific interest in expanding current research programs in experimental tuberculosis and starting new ones. As a result of these circumstances, a large new group of laboratory workers will be exposed to the risk of occupationally acquired tuberculosis. Fortunately, there are effective methods for controlling laboratory hazards that could cause accidental or inadvertent exposures to *Mycobacterium tuberculosis*. However, laboratory safety habits that enable laboratory workers to protect themselves from this risk are not easily acquired, and the efficacy of engineering controls may be unknowingly compromised (Kubica, 1990).

The decline in the incidence of tuberculosis observed from 1963 to 1985 (Centers for Disease Control, 1988) has had the adverse consequence of reducing the number of workers experienced with experimental tuberculosis. As a result, the hazard for inhalation of *M. tuberculosis* will be a new challenge for almost every scientist and technician who will now conduct research with this agent. The purpose of this chapter is to provide for these scientists and technicians a basic orientation to health and safety practices appropriate for the control of hazards associated with the handling of *M. tuberculosis* in the research laboratory.

No written guidance, however, can adequately prepare even the most conscientious technical person to work safely with a microorganism that is transmitted by droplet nuclei (airborne particles of ≤ 5-μm diameter) and is very capable of causing infection by the inhalation route. Protecting oneself is dependent on the use of scrupulous technique and the exercise of enough self-discipline to maintain proficiency at all times when handling the agent. These skills are acquired through practice under the careful observation of experienced workers. The most important message in this chapter is that *M. tuberculosis* should be handled only by those who have mastered basic safe practices. All workers in the experimental tuberculosis laboratory must have confidence in everyone's ability to maintain this level of practice. Specifically,

W. Emmett Barkley • Howard Hughes Medical Institute, 4000 Jones Bridge Road, Chevy Chase, Maryland 20815. *George P. Kubica* • 2323 Walton Place, Atlanta, Georgia 30338.

because of the aerosol threat of disease transmission, the health and safety of one's colleagues are dependent on maintaining this level of performance.

SAFETY GUIDELINES

The Centers for Disease Control and Prevention and the National Institutes of Health recommend that research activities involving *M. tuberculosis* be performed at biosafety level 3 (U.S. Department of Health and Human Services, 1993). This level of containment requires the use of special practices and containment equipment that when used properly can protect the laboratory worker from direct contact and inhalation exposures to the agent. The laboratory in which this work is carried out has certain design and operational features that provide protection from exposure to *M. tuberculosis* for those other facility occupants who do not require access to the laboratory. The facility safeguards include both administrative directives and architectural and engineering systems that collectively prevent microorganisms that were accidentally or inadvertently released into the laboratory space from moving either with air currents or on contaminated surfaces to other occupied areas of the facility.

PRIMARY LABORATORY RISK

Tuberculosis is transmitted in the laboratory primarily through exposure to infectious droplet nuclei. A susceptible person can acquire an infection with *M. tuberculosis* by inhaling fewer than 10 bacilli (Riley, 1957). This low infectious dose suggests a high risk for laboratory-acquired infection with *M. tuberculosis*.

A comprehensive review of laboratory-acquired infections through 1974 found that tuberculosis was the fifth most frequently reported infection among laboratory workers in the United States (Pike, 1976). Non-

pulmonary tuberculosis accounted for only 23% of the cases, and the probable cause of these infections was overt contact exposures. The majority of infections with *M. tuberculosis* were associated with aerosols. This conclusion is supported by observations that most common laboratory techniques, when used to handle microorganisms, are capable of producing infectious aerosols (Dimmick et al., 1973; Kenny and Sabel, 1968; Stern et al., 1974). The actual number of cases of laboratory-acquired pulmonary tuberculosis is thought to be much higher than that reported (Pike, 1979). When experiments involving *M. tuberculosis* are being planned, it is prudent to consider that every procedure can produce an infectious aerosol and that additional precautions may be necessary to avoid inhalation exposures.

CONTROLLING THE RISKS OF LABORATORY-ACQUIRED TUBERCULOSIS

Training, technique, and containment are essential elements for controlling the risks of laboratory-acquired tuberculosis. Equally important is the need to establish a community standard whereby all laboratory workers engaged in experimental tuberculosis share a commitment to protect colleagues and neighbors from exposure to *M. tuberculosis*. Only in this way can the risk of laboratory-acquired infections be adequately controlled.

Scientists, technicians, and support staff in experimental tuberculosis laboratories, unlike their clinical health care colleagues, have the opportunity to precisely control the events that could lead to occupational exposure. They decide when, where, and how to handle the agent. Reasonable practices and containment equipment that can isolate the microorganism from those who handle it have been devised. Laboratory workers can significantly reduce the inadvertent release of *M. tuberculosis* into their breathing zones by their own techniques and actions. The ability to control all experimental processes involving *M. tuberculosis* enables research with this agent to be performed safely.

Training

Safety training must precede the first encounter with *M. tuberculosis* in the laboratory. The ability to recognize hazards, assess risks, and select appropriate practices and the skill to handle *M. tuberculosis* safely must be learned through careful instruction and experience supervised by expert and responsible mentors. The training must be relevant to the experimental tuberculosis research program of the laboratory. No experimental procedure involving *M. tuberculosis* should be performed until the laboratory worker can demonstrate proficiency with the procedure when handling a less serious pathogen or a recognized saprophytic species of the genus. The laboratory director should establish the standard for proficiency, but the spirit of community commitment could be enhanced if consensus criteria for determining proficiency were set by the laboratory staff. In addition to learning safe techniques, the laboratory worker must be trained in emergency procedures before being allowed to work unsupervised in the laboratory.

Initial safety training might involve the study of *Biosafety in Microbiological and Biomedical Laboratories* (U.S. Department of Health and Human Services, 1993) and other useful references on biological safety (National Research Council, 1989; Miller et al., 1986). The Department of Health and Human Services publication is a consensus code of practice and presents valuable discussions on the principles of laboratory safety, risk assessment, and laboratory hazards associated with human pathogens, including *M. tuberculosis*. It also describes practices, equipment, and facility design features that are necessary to control the risks of laboratory-acquired infections. The other two references provide more detail regarding specific laboratory practices.

It is imperative, however, that supervised training in laboratory methods and aseptic technique be provided to the laboratory worker who has no experience in working with *M. tuberculosis*. Modeling experimental procedures that will be carried out in the laboratory while using BCG or other low-risk organism can be a relevant strategy for acquiring the necessary laboratory skills.

Training in laboratory safety within the experimental tuberculosis laboratory must be a dynamic process. It can be done most effectively in the normal setting of the laboratory with the careful guidance of the laboratory director or the shared responsibility of laboratory colleagues. Laboratory meetings are a valuable way for sharing information, introducing new practices, addressing concerns, correcting problems, and evaluating safety performance. Opportunities to encourage and enhance informal training through collegial interactions should be vigorously pursued. This can create an atmosphere in which colleagues reinforce good patterns. Continuing training will help foster the attitude that safety is an inseparable part of the laboratory routine. Good laboratory practice will eventually become laboratory habit.

Basic Laboratory Practices

The consistent use of good laboratory practices is of fundamental importance in controlling the risk of laboratory-acquired infection. Techniques must be learned so that they can be executed with ease. Abrupt or jerky movements should be consciously avoided, as they will compromise safety. All actions must be planned and carried out in a deliberate and disciplined manner. Focused attention must be given to every movement when handling *M. tu-*

berculosis. Nothing should be left to happenstance. This discipline should become routine and should be constantly reinforced by the laboratory director and all laboratory colleagues.

The practices listed below, when followed by everyone in the laboratory, will enable research in experimental tuberculosis to be conducted safety.

- When in the laboratory, wear a solid-front or wraparound gown or a scrub suit.
- Always wear protective gloves. If gloves become soiled or contaminated, remove them carefully, wash the hands immediately, and put on a new pair of gloves.
- Perform all procedures that involve the handling of *M. tuberculosis* in open vessels in a certified and properly functioning biological safety cabinet. Always carry out procedures carefully to reduce aerosol formation and avoid splashes and spills. Important precautions regarding the use of this equipment are discussed below in the section on containment.
- Wash the hands as soon as the procedure is completed and always before leaving the laboratory.
- When pipetting, always use a mechanical pipetting device; *never* mouth pipette.
- Do not eat, drink, smoke, or handle contact lenses in the laboratory.
- Keep the laboratory scrupulously clean, and decontaminate work surfaces daily with a tuberculocidal detergent solution.
- Avoid use of syringes, needles, Pasteur pipettes, capillary tubes, scalpels, and other sharp instruments whenever possible. When these items must be used, handle them with caution to avoid accidental punctures or cuts.
- Discard used needles and disposable cutting instruments into a puncture-re-

sistant container with a lid. Used needles should not be resheathed, bent, broken, removed from the disposable syringe, or otherwise manipulated by hand.
- Keep all laboratory doors closed when experiments are in progress, because safety can be compromised by disruptions to the ventilation system.
- Use tongs or forceps to handle broken glassware; never handle broken glassware directly by hand.
- Use secondary leak-proof containers to move or transfer cultures and other research materials containing *M. tuberculosis* between areas where they are kept when not being handled, such as incubators or freezers, and biological safety cabinets.
- Decontaminate waste cultures and all other waste materials that are potentially contaminated with *M. tuberculosis* before disposal. Steam sterilization is the method of choice.

Containment

Biological safety cabinets and engineering controls associated with the laboratory facility provide primary and secondary levels of containment, respectively, against the accidental or inadvertent release of *M. tuberculosis*. Primary containment protects the laboratory worker from exposure. Engineering controls associated with the facility provide additional protection to prevent the escape of *M. tuberculosis* to other occupied areas of the facility in which the biosafety level 3 laboratory is located.

Biological safety cabinets

Any procedure that involves the manipulation of liquid suspensions or culture of *M. tuberculosis* must be carried out within a biological safety cabinet or a physically contained enclosure designed to prevent leakage of experimental materials. The control of aerosols is the principal objective in

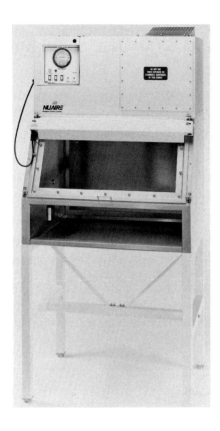

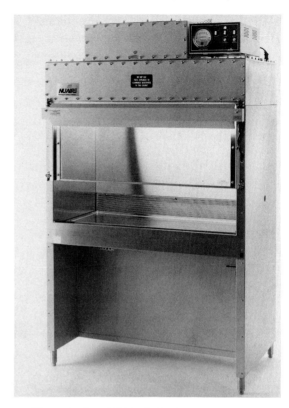

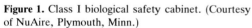

Figure 2. Class II biological safety cabinet. (Courtesy of NuAire, Plymouth, Minn.)

Figure 1. Class I biological safety cabinet. (Courtesy of NuAire, Plymouth, Minn.)

the use of this equipment in the experimental tuberculosis laboratory. Class I (Fig. 1) and class II (Fig. 2) biological safety cabinets are most commonly used in the biosafety level 3 facility and are appropriate for use with *M. tuberculosis*. Both types of cabinets offer similar protection for the laboratory worker when they are operating properly and prudent practices are being used by the worker. Containment of aerosols is provided by room air that is drawn into the cabinet through its front opening. This room air is generally referred to as intake airflow. The intake airflow entrains or captures aerosols that may have been released by the experimental techniques conducted within the cabinet and transports them to a high-efficiency particulate

air (HEPA) filter, where the aerosolized particles are removed from the airstream before it is discharged from the cabinet. Detailed descriptions of biological safety cabinets are available in several review articles (Kruse et al., 1991; Chatigny, 1986) and in specifications provided by manufacturers. The following discussion will emphasize important safety considerations and precautions that will help the user understand both the limitations and the benefits of this equipment.

In the class I cabinet, the intake airflow passes through the work space of the cabinet. The airflow path may be undesirable when the experimental procedure may be compromised by fungi, bacteria, and other airborne contaminants that are commonly found in room air.

Class II cabinets can protect experimental materials from airborne contamination. In these cabinets, intake airflow is drawn into an exhaust grill located between the cabinet opening and the front edge of the work surface. Airborne contamination within the room air is prevented from reaching the work space by the downward airflow of HEPA-filtered air, which is supplied at the top of the cabinet's interior work space. Approximately one-third of the downward airflow is captured by the front grill; the remainder is removed by the longitudinal grill located at the back edge of the work surface. The downward airflow, however, can have a profound adverse effect on worker protection. The balance between downward airflow and intake airflow is critically important. A dramatic loss of containment can occur when the intake airflow falls below the airflow parameters set by the cabinet manufacturer (Jones et al., 1990). This effect was first demonstrated in a cabinet that was configured to have a 100-ft/min (1 ft = 30.48 cm) downward airflow with a range of intake airflows (Barkley, 1972). At a calculated intake air velocity of 75 linear ft/min (lfpm), a test aerosol was fully contained, whereas less than 20% was contained when the intake velocity was 55 lfpm. In contrast to this significant loss in containment, less than 0.003% loss in containment was observed when the intake velocity for a similarly configured class I cabinet was reduced from 75 to 55 lfpm.

The critical importance of air balance in class II cabinets requires that this type of biological safety cabinet be purchased from a responsible manufacturer and be certified in accordance with nationally recognized consensus standards (United States National Sanitation Foundation standard no. 49, Ann Arbor, Michigan, 1983) and that the operational parameters be confirmed after installation by a knowledgeable testing group or experienced staff. Operational parameters should also be verified periodically (every 6 to 12 months) and whenever the cabinet is moved to a new location. It is also prudent to select a class I biological safety cabinet for containing procedures involving *M. tuberculosis* when product protection is not a major concern.

Containment performance of class I and II cabinets is also influenced by the technique of the laboratory worker. It has been estimated that poor technique can increase leakage across the cabinet opening by a factor of as much as 1,000 (Chatigny, 1986). Always carry out procedures carefully to reduce the generation of aerosols. Avoid erratic movements, because they will disrupt the intake airflow and cause reverse air currents that can draw aerosols out of the cabinet. Reduce both lateral and in-and-out motions across the front opening of the cabinet to an absolute minimum. When such motions are required, perform them with extreme care. Disruption of the intake airflow can also be caused by the movement of colleagues near the cabinet, the opening and closing of the laboratory door, and poor distribution of supply air to the laboratory. Always be conscious of the fact that class I and II cabinets are not absolute containment devices. Airflow alone cannot prevent the escape of aerosols from the front opening of the cabinet.

A simple method has been devised to help assess good technique and containment when using a class I safety cabinet (Smithwick, personal communication). A cotton ball soaked with an odor-distinctive compound, like perfume, is placed inside the cabinet. The odor serves as a sentinel for indicating loss of containment. If the odor becomes a permanent presence, as opposed to an occasional fast-disappearing odor, it suggests either poor technique or inadequate intake airflow.

The following additional practices are considered excellent techniques when using class I and II biological safety cabinets.

- Plan the experiment in advance.
- Designate areas on the work surface where clean supplies, the experimental agent, disinfectants, and contaminated waste will be placed. Do not handle contaminated materials over areas designated for clean materials.
- A disinfectant-soaked towel placed on the work surface can reduce the hazards of splatter and surface contamination caused by droplets or minor spills.
- Place all materials needed for the experiment into the cabinet before beginning the experiment. When this is not possible, use a cart or bench adjacent to the cabinet only for excess clean material.
- Use slow and deliberate motions when bringing items into or out of the cabinet after the experiment has been started.
- Place a sign on the laboratory door that informs colleagues that an experiment is in progress. Avoid opening and closing the door during this period.
- When using a class I cabinet, always conduct the experiment at least 4 in. (1 in. = 2.54 cm) inside the cabinet's front opening. When using a class II cabinet, always work beyond the front exhaust grill.
- Always disinfect the surfaces of containers before removing them from the cabinet.
- Remove protective gloves carefully before leaving the cabinet. Double-gloving can offer a practical benefit when working in the cabinet. If the outer glove becomes contaminated before a task is completed, the glove can be removed in the cabinet and replaced with a new outer glove. The work activity can continue without having to wash hands.
- Never place anything on the cabinet or occlude its intake or exhaust grills.
- Use a disinfectant trap and air filter to protect the cabinet vacuum source from contamination.

- Disinfect the work surface after the experiment has been completed and all items have been removed from the cabinet.
- Know the operational parameters of the cabinet, and do not use the cabinet if any deficiency is suspected.
- Immediately stop any manipulation of the agent if the blower or exhaust ventilation system fails.
- Always handle a bunsen burner with care. The flame can disrupt downward airflow; its use may not be necessary for contamination control in class II cabinets.
- Make sure that periodic certification tests are performed and performance parameters are confirmed.

Physically contained enclosures such as centrifuge cups with O-rings (Fig. 3) provide primary containment for experimental procedures that cannot be confined to biological safety cabinets unless the cabinets have been customized for this purpose. However, the biological safety cabinet should be used when centrifuge tubes are put into the safety cups and when they are removed after centrifugation. It is also prudent to place small contained equipment designed for hand-performed operations, such as the Stomacher (Colworth Stomacher Lab-Blender; Cook Laboratory Products Division, Dynatech Lab Products, Inc., Alexandria, Va.) in the biological safety cabinet. This is particularly important when further processing of the sample can generate aerosols.

Confining aerosol-producing procedures to biological safety cabinets or physically contained enclosures will generally make reliance on respirators for primary protection against inhalation exposure unnecessary in the experimental tuberculosis laboratory. However, it may be prudent to consider the use of a disposable dust and mist respirator (3M Dust/Mist Respirator; 3M Co., St. Paul, Minn.) when handling

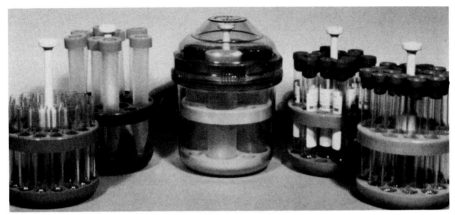

Figure 3. Centrifuge containment cannister. (Courtesy of Beckman, Fullerton, Calif.)

cultures of *M. tuberculosis* within the biological safety cabinet. This type of respirator is capable of filtering droplet-nuclei-size particles (Chen et al., 1992) and would provide a further barrier to airborne infection should an infectious aerosol escape containment of the cabinet. It is important that the wearer properly fit the respirator to reduce face seal leakage (Lowry et al., 1977).

Facility safeguards

The design of a biosafety level 3 containment laboratory is complex and beyond the scope of this chapter. Two facility design features, however, will be highlighted here because of their importance to the prevention of occupationally acquired tuberculosis. These features are directional airflow and access control. The safety function of these features is to prevent exposure of persons who occupy areas of the laboratory facility that are outside the perimeter of the biosafety level 3 laboratory. Directional airflow greatly minimizes the possibility that aerosols generated in the laboratory will migrate to other occupied areas of the building. Access control provisions prevent unauthorized people from entering the laboratory. These factors do not provide additional protection for the laboratory worker. Poor design and operation of the directional

airflow system, however, can compromise the safety of the laboratory worker.

A biosafety level 3 laboratory should have a dedicated exhaust ventilation system that creates and maintains directional airflow. Air supplied to the laboratory should move from areas where *M. tuberculosis* will not be handled to areas where experimental procedures will be performed. For this to happen, the laboratory will be at a relative air pressure lower than those of adjacent spaces. The air pressure differential should be very small (<0.05 in. on a water gauge) so as not to create turbulent air currents when doors are opened and closed (Keene and Sansone, 1984). Directional airflow can easily be maintained by infiltration between the closed door and door jambs. Where large volumes of air may be required, special devices like louvers or barometric dampers should be provided. It is imperative, however, that turbulent conditions be avoided.

Only persons who are directly involved with the scientific and technical activities of the experimental tuberculosis program and who have been advised of administrative policies controlling access should be allowed to enter the laboratory. In most research facilities, it is difficult to control access unless the laboratory is set apart from other areas of the facility. This is usually accomplished by constructing an access foyer or special entrance area through which people must pass before entering the laboratory. Passage always requires traversing two sets of closed doors. A list of access control procedures that incorporates the universal biohazard symbol should be affixed to the first entrance door. The access control area will serve as a visual warning to staff who do not need to gain access that they should not enter the laboratory.

Further discussion on the design of a biosafety level 3 laboratory can be found in other references (Lunsford and Barkley, 1990; West and Chatigny, 1986).

Community Standards

Rules governing laboratory safety performance are followed best by those who participate in their creation. This is particularly important in the collegial setting of a research laboratory, where independent experiments may be performed in the same laboratory. Safety in the experimental tuberculosis laboratory will be enhanced if all laboratory workers become involved in establishing and enforcing operational practices and procedures. The risk of laboratory-acquired infection with *M. tuberculosis* will be shared by everyone who works in the laboratory. The magnitude of the risk, however, can be significantly reduced when the laboratory workers join together in fostering an attitude for promoting safe practices.

The laboratory group should also encourage the support staff who provide institutional safety services and operate the building systems to participate in establishing community standards. Communication among these groups must be constant and sincere. Good relations can only enhance the operational integrity and safety of the biosafety level 3 laboratory.

EMERGENCY RESPONSE GUIDELINES

Every laboratory should have a plan for responding to emergency situations. The plan should address fire, medical emergencies, personal injury, and spills of hazardous research materials. It is imperative that such plans be in place in experimental tuberculosis laboratories. The first priority in any response is to safeguard the laboratory worker from a life-threatening situation or from the most immediate danger to his or her health. This may require overriding some of the access control procedures of the laboratory. Guidance is provided below for responding to spills of research materials involving *M. tuberculosis*.

Spills within Biological Safety Cabinets

A prerequisite for handling cultures of *M. tuberculosis* is to know how to decontaminate minor spills in the biological safety cabinet. Materials necessary for this task should always be readily available.

The immediate response to a spill in the cabinet is to keep the cabinet turned on. The functioning cabinet will contain the aerosol and prevent significant contamination of the laboratory environment that could otherwise occur if the cabinet blower were turned off. Persons in the area of the cabinet should be alerted to the spill and advised to either leave the laboratory or stay away from the cabinet. The decontamination procedure should then proceed. The cabinet should never be turned off during the decontamination procedure. Spray or wipe the interior cabinet walls, work surfaces, and equipment with a tuberculocidal detergent such as a phenolic derivative or iodophor. Flood the catch basin in class II cabinets with the disinfectant. Allow a 30-min contact period. Place the disposable disinfected items into double autoclavable bags. Tie the bags shut, and carry them to the autoclave. All reusable items should either be autoclaved or thoroughly wiped again with disinfectant. Gloves and protective clothing should also be decontaminated at the end of the decontamination procedure. Finally, allow the cabinet to run for 10 min before using it again or turning it off.

If a large spill has occurred within the cabinet, consider decontaminating the cabinet with paraformaldehyde. This procedure should be carried out by experienced staff or professional consultants who perform this work.

Spills in the Biosafety Level 3 Laboratory

Biological spills outside biological safety cabinets generate aerosols that can be dispersed in the air throughout the laboratory. These spills are very serious when they involve *M. tuberculosis*. To reduce the risk of inhalation exposure in such an incident, occupants should hold their breath and leave the laboratory *immediately*. The door should be closed as they leave the laboratory. The laboratory *should not* be reentered to decontaminate and clean up the spill until the aerosol has been removed from the laboratory by the exhaust air ventilation system. This will take approximately 30 min for a well-designed ventilation system that provides 10 changes of fresh air per h. It would be prudent to stay out for 2 h if the status of the ventilation system is unknown. Appropriate protective equipment is particularly important in decontaminating spills involving *M. tuberculosis*. This equipment includes a back-fastening gown or jumpsuit, disposable gloves, disposable shoe covers, and respirator with full face shield. Use of this equipment will prevent contact with contaminated surfaces, protect eyes and mucous membranes from exposure to splattered materials, and prevent secondary inhalation exposure.

Before reentering the laboratory, put on protective equipment. Assess the extent of the spill, and determine whether more-extensive procedures are required to decontaminate the affected area. Cover the spill with paper towels or other absorbent materials. Carefully pour a freshly prepared 1 in 10 dilution of household bleach around the edges of the spill and then into the spill. Avoid splashing. Allow a 20-min contact period. Use paper towels to wipe up the spill, working from the edges into the center. Clean the spill area with fresh towels soaked in disinfectant. Place the towels in a plastic bag, and decontaminate them in an autoclave.

MEDICAL SURVEILLANCE

A program to screen for and evaluate potential laboratory-acquired infections should be instituted. This program should include an initial tuberculin skin test for all personnel who plan to work in the experimental tuberculosis laboratory. Tuberculin-positive individuals should be evaluated by a physician. It may be prudent to perform a periodic chest X ray for tuberculin-positive individuals.

The tuberculin test should be repeated every 6 months for individuals whose initial test results are tuberculin negative. Periodic chest X rays should be considered by the physician for monitoring previously tuberculin-positive individuals. If a conversion or symptoms of disease are noted, the individual should be evaluated for preventive therapy.

A person who experiences an overt exposure in the laboratory to *M. tuberculosis* should report the occurrence to the laboratory director. A repeat tuberculin test should be obtained within 1 week following the exposure if the individual was previously tuberculin negative. Nonconverters should be retested in 12 weeks (Centers for Disease Control, 1990). If a conversion has been documented, a medical evaluation for active disease and treatment should be carried out. A symptom check should be provided by a physician for all exposed individuals who were previously tuberculin positive. It is imperative that the tuberculin skin test always be placed and interpreted by an expert.

REFERENCES

Barkley, W. E. 1972. Ph.D. thesis. University of Minnesota, Minneapolis.

Centers for Disease Control. 1988. Tuberculosis, final data—United States, 1986. *Morbid. Mortal. Weekly Rep.* **36**:817.

Centers for Disease Control. 1990. Guidelines for preventing the transmission of tuberculosis in healthcare settings, with special focus on HIV-related issues. *Morbid. Mortal. Weekly Rep.* **39**:19.

Chatigny, M. A. 1986. Primary barriers, p. 144–163. *In* B. M. Miller, D. H. M. Gröschel, J. H. Richardson, D. Vesley, J. R. Songer, R. D. Housewright, and W. E. Barkley (ed.), *Laboratory Safety: Principles and Practices*. American Society for Microbiology, Washington, D.C.

Chen, C. C., M. Lehtimäski, and K. Willeke. 1992. Aerosol penetration through filtering face pieces and respirator cartridges. *Am. Ind. Hyg. Assoc. J.* **53**:566–574.

Dimmick, R. L., W. F. Vogl, and M. A. Chatigny. 1973. Potential for accidental microbial aerosol transmission in the biological laboratory, p. 246–266. *In* A. Hellman, M. N. Oxman, and R. Pollack (ed.), *Biohazards in Biological Research*. Cold Spring Harbor Laboratory, Cold Spring Harbor, N.Y.

Jones, R. L., D. G. Stuart, D. Eagelson, T. J. Greenier, and J. M. Eagelson, Jr. 1990. The effects of changing intake and supply air flow on biological safety cabinet performance. *Appl. Occup. Environ. Hyg.* **5**:370–377.

Keene, J. H., and E. B. Sansone. 1984. Airborne transfer of contaminants in ventilated spaces. *Lab. Anim. Sci.* **34**:453–457.

Kenny, M. T., and F. L. Sabel. 1968. Particle size distribution of *Serratia marcescens* aerosols created during common laboratory procedures and simulated laboratory accidents. *Appl. Microbiol.* **16**:1146–1150.

Kruse, R. H., W. H. Puckett, and J. H. Richardson. 1991. Biological safety cabinetry. *Clin. Microbiol. Rev.* **2**:207–241.

Kubica, G. P. 1990. Your tuberculosis laboratory: are you really safe from infection? *Clin. Microbiol. Newsl.* **11**:85–87.

Lowry, P. L., P. R. Hesch, and W. H. Revoir. 1977. Performance of single use respirators. *Am. Ind. Hyg. Assoc. J.* **38**:462–467.

Lunsford, E. G., and W. E. Barkley. 1990. Specialized facilities: biohazard containment, p. 620–627. *In* T. Ruys (ed.), *Handbook of Facilities Planning*, vol. 1. Van Nostrand Reinhold, New York.

Miller, B. M., D. H. M. Gröschel, J. H. Richardson, D. Vesley, J. R. Songer, R. D. Housewright, and W. E. Barkley (ed.). 1986. *Laboratory Safety: Principles and Practices*. American Society for Microbiology, Washington, D.C.

National Research Council. 1989. *Biosafety in the Laboratory*. National Academy Press, Washington, D.C.

Pike, R. M. 1976. Laboratory-associated infections: summary and analysis of 3921 cases. *Health Lab. Sci.* **13**:105–114.

Pike, R. M. 1979. Laboratory-associated infections: incidence, fatalities, causes, and prevention. *Annu. Rev. Microbiol.* **33**:41–66.

Riley, R. L. 1957. Aerial dissemination of pulmonary tuberculosis. *Am. Rev. Tuberc.* **76**:931–941.

Smithwick, R. W. (Centers for Disease Control and Prevention). Personal communication.

Stern, E. L., J. W. Johnson, D. Vesley, M. M. Halbert, L. E. Williams, and P. Blume. 1974. Aerosol production associated with clinical laboratory procedures. *Am. J. Clin. Pathol.* **62**:591–600.

U.S. Department of Health and Human Services. 1993. *Biosafety in Microbiological and Biomedical Laboratories*. U.S. Department of Health and Human Services publication no. (CDC) 93-8395. U.S. Government Printing Office, Washington, D.C.

West, D. L., and M. A. Chatigny. 1986. Design of microbiological and biomedical research facilities, p. 124–137. *In* B. M. Miller, D. H. M. Gröschel, J. H. Richardson, D. Vesley, J. R. Songer, R. D. Housewright, and W. E. Barkley (ed.), *Laboratory Safety: Principles and Practices*. American Society for Microbiology, Washington, D.C.

Tuberculosis: Pathogenesis, Protection, and Control
Edited by Barry R. Bloom
© 1994 American Society for Microbiology, Washington, DC 20005

Chapter 6

Cultivation of *Mycobacterium tuberculosis* for Research Purposes

Lawrence G. Wayne

Individual investigators have different reasons for cultivating *Mycobacterium tuberculosis* in their laboratories; the medium to be used and the conditions of incubation should be tailored to the specific goals, taking into account the physiologic characteristics of this organism. The most common reason for cultivating tubercle bacilli is to confirm a clinical diagnosis of tuberculosis. Procedures for isolating *M. tuberculosis* from clinical specimens are well documented in many good clinical laboratory manuals, and that aspect of their cultivation will not be discussed further in this review. I shall concentrate instead on those aspects of the growth characteristics of *M. tuberculosis* that may influence the methods used to cultivate the organism in a research setting. Other species of mycobacteria will not be considered except in passing or by contrast, although the comments will usually be applicable to other members of the *M. tuberculosis* complex, which encompasses *M. tuberculosis*, *M. bovis* (including bacillus Calmette-Guérin [BCG]), *M. africanum*, and *M. microti* (Wayne and Kubica, 1986).

Among the nondiagnostic activities that require cultivation of tubercle bacilli are the following: (i) the study of dynamics of growth and survival and the in vitro study of drug susceptibility and mechanisms of action, which may employ growth calculations based on colorimetric or turbidimetric methods and/or actual plating and counting of colonies; (ii) preparation of whole bacilli for immunology or the study of pathogenesis; and (iii) preparation of bacillary products for immunologic, chemical, physiologic, or genetic study.

This chapter is not a cookbook of all possible media or methods but instead is intended to point the reader in the right direction within a very large body of information, much of which was developed during a "golden age" of tuberculosis research, i.e., the early days of chemotherapy, when the study of tuberculosis had not yet fallen from favor and when lung associations and their journals still had the word tuberculosis in their titles.

GENERAL CHARACTERISTICS OF *M. TUBERCULOSIS*

Because things change slowly in mycobacteriology, the reader will find information that is still relevant and useful in *The*

Lawrence G. Wayne • Tuberculosis Research Laboratory (151), Department of Veterans Affairs Medical Center, 5901 East Seventh Street, Long Beach, California 90822.

Mycobacteria—a Sourcebook, a comprehensive sourcebook on mycobacteriology that goes into great detail on the physiology, chemistry, immunology, and pathogenicity of this genus and encompasses the state of the art up to 1984 (Kubica and Wayne, 1984). The present review is of narrower scope, expanding on those characteristics that influence the selection of methods and conditions to be used for growing *M. tuberculosis* in the research or applied biotechnology laboratory. The most important point to be made here is that the physiology, antigenicity, pathogenicity, and chemical composition of tubercle bacilli are all influenced by the composition of the culture medium and the conditions under which the organisms are grown. If results from different experiments within a given laboratory or from experiments conducted in different laboratories are to be compared, it is essential that these parameters be comparable or at least defined.

A classic description of *M. tuberculosis*, which would be only partially accurate, might characterize this organism as a fastidious, slowly growing, strictly aerobic, lipid-rich, hydrophobic, acid-fast bacterial rod.

It is true that tubercle bacilli are best isolated from clinical specimens on rich and fairly complex media, but the apparent fastidiousness of some such isolates may be a consequence of their injury by conditions in host tissue or by the treatment employed for processing the clinical specimen. Once isolated, *M. tuberculosis* is capable of adapting to growth on extremely simple medium, i.e., one containing a simple source of carbon and nitrogen plus some buffer salts and trace elements. The functions of various ingredients of simple and complex media will be further discussed below in the section on culture media.

It is true that tubercle bacilli have a long generation time compared to that of most commonly studied bacteria. Under optimal conditions, *M. tuberculosis* requires 16 to 18 h to undergo one cycle of replication (Wayne, 1977). With a generation time in that range, a single bacillus can yield a visible colony on solid medium within 2 weeks or less after inoculation. The excessively long time of 6 to 10 weeks required for detection of colonies on media planted with some clinical specimens (Krasnow and Wayne, 1969) is, again, probably the result of a need to repair injury of the bacilli in the specimen, as suggested above.

It is true that tubercle bacilli grow most rapidly when well aerated and do not appear to multiply under completely anaerobic conditions. The overwhelming bulk of research done on the chemistry and physiology of *M. tuberculosis* has been conducted with bacilli grown as pellicles or as agitated dispersed cultures. However, the choice of highly aerobic growth conditions was usually dictated by a desire for rapid production of good crops of cells without an adequate appreciation of the physiologic characteristics associated with a particular degree of aeration. As Segal has noted in his review of the physiology of tubercle bacilli grown under different conditions (Segal, 1984), *M. tuberculosis* has many of the enzymes required for anaerobic metabolism, and indeed, the virulence of this organism appears to be in part a function of its ability to survive and/or grow under the wide range of variation in partial O_2 pressures that may occur in healthy, inflamed, or necrotic tissue. Furthermore, there are marked differences in biochemical, antigenic, and pathogenic behaviors between tubercle bacilli grown in vitro and those grown in host tissues (Segal, 1984).

It is true that tubercle bacilli, like all other mycobacteria, are very rich in lipid. Furthermore, unlike some other mycobacterial species (Barrow et al., 1980), *M. tuberculosis* does not produce a hydrophilic outer sheath; it is indeed hydrophobic and grows as a waxy pellicle in unagitated medium and with extensive clumping in stirred culture unless a detergent is included in the medium. The tendency for pellicle formation reinforced the perception of this organism as a strict aerobe. However, except in the early veil-like stage of surface growth, the thick clumps that form in a pellicle or agitated culture appear to enclose bacilli in various degrees of O_2 deprivation, and the bacilli within a single culture undoubtedly represent a physiologically heterogeneous population (Wayne and Sramek, 1979).

MEDIA

Liquid Media

Much of the early research on the tubercle bacillus was directed toward production of tuberculin or other crude chemical products of the bacilli, such as unique lipids or polysaccharides. Media containing very simple and defined ingredients were developed to allow recovery of bacillary products free of macromolecular medium components and to yield very high yields of the slowly growing bacilli and their products. These media, including those attributed to Sauton, Long, Kirchner, Wong, and Proskauer and Beck, were quite similar to one another in composition. All contained phosphate salts, citrate, $MgSO_4$, glycerol, and either asparagine or an ammonium salt as nitrogen source (Soltys, 1952). Most were supplemented with iron, and all contained unrecognized trace minerals as impurities in the defined ingredients; these trace elements were essential to satisfactory growth (Affronti et al., 1990; Baisden, 1951). The glycerol was a carbon source considered essential for copious growth as a pellicle or as clumps in agitated medium. As will be discussed below, the presence of glycerol may have directed the metabolism into a pathway that is not representative of the physiologic state of the bacilli as they occur in tissues of the infected host and thus may have been counterproductive in

the in vitro study of *M. tuberculosis* as it may occur in tissues.

One specialized use of this type of medium is for maintenance of the virulence of a strain of *M. tuberculosis*. It has been reported that cultivation of this organism in detergent-containing medium results in diminution of virulence for the experimental mouse. Bacilli obtained from a thin veil of early pellicle growth from a detergent-free synthetic medium, on the other hand, are reported to be more virulent; when the pellicle thickens and becomes bumpy with age, virulence is again diminished (Youmans, 1979, p. 332). Collins and colleagues have presented evidence that the ages and physiologic states of dispersed cultures influence the distribution between lung and spleen of tubercle bacilli inoculated intravenously into mice (Collins et al., 1974). For methods of preparing well-dispersed bacilli for inoculation of mice, see the section on inocula below.

The formulation for a representative example of a simple synthetic medium for cultivation of *M. tuberculosis*, the modified Proskauer and Beck medium recommended by Youmans (Youmans, 1979, p. 25), follows. Into 1 liter of glass distilled water are dissolved, in the sequence listed, 5 g of asparagine, 5 g of KH_2PO_4, 5 g of K_2SO_4, and 20 g of glycerol. Each ingredient must be dissolved before the next ingredient is added. The pH is then adjusted to 6.8 to 7.0 with 40% NaOH, after which 1.5 g of magnesium citrate is added, and the medium is dispensed as needed and autoclaved at 15 lb for 20 min. The asparagine or glycerol used should not be of the highest purity, as trace metal contaminants have been reported to be necessary to support growth of *M. tuberculosis* (Affronti et al., 1990; Baisden, 1951; Youmans, 1979). On the other hand, traces of fatty acids or heavy metals may be inhibitory if they are introduced from inadequately cleaned or some dry sterilized glassware. If the presence of albumin does not interfere with the use for which the medium is intended, introduction of a sterile stock solution to yield a final concentration of 0.5% will result in binding of traces of toxic materials, permitting the bacilli to grow.

The growth of tubercle bacilli in the synthetic media cited is difficult to follow in quantitative terms, since it cannot be measured optically and since simple plating is not accurate because of the severe clumping of the bacilli. This problem was solved by the introduction of detergents into culture medium by Dubos and colleagues during the 1940s (Dubos, 1945; Dubos and Davis, 1946; Dubos and Middlebrook, 1948). Dubos liquid medium contains (per liter) asparagine, 2 g; Casitone (Difco), 0.5 g; Na_2HPO_4, 2.5 g; KH_2PO_4, 1 g; ferric ammonium citrate, 50 mg; $MgSO_4$, 10 mg; $CaCl_2$, 0.5 mg; $ZnSO_4$, 0.1 mg; $CuSO_4$, 0.1 mg; Tween 80, 0.2 g; bovine albumin fraction V, 5 g; and glucose, 7.5 g, at a final pH of 6.6 ± 0.2. To prepare a liter of the medium, all ingredients except the albumin and glucose are dissolved in 900 ml of distilled water, and this basal medium is autoclaved. The albumin fraction V and the glucose are dissolved in 100 ml of saline and filter sterilized; this supplement is added to the basal medium aseptically, and the complete medium is distributed to appropriate sterile culture containers. In practice, dehydrated basal medium (Dubos broth base) and sterile glucose-albumin supplement are available commercially to facilitate preparation of this medium.

The most commonly used detergent, Tween 80, is a polyoxyethylene derivative of sorbitan monooleate, and it permits growth of M. tuberculosis in liquid medium in a diffuse form, as single cells or small clusters of cells that are easily dispersed by agitation. One problem associated with the use of Tween 80 is that traces of free oleic acid are released into the medium as a result of either spontaneous hydrolysis or specific enzymatic action of some species of mycobacteria (Davis and Dubos, 1948).

Free oleate is toxic to M. tuberculosis, but the problem is gotten around by adding bovine serum albumin to the medium (Dubos, 1950). The oleate is complexed to the albumin and thus is no longer inhibitory to the bacilli; the oleate complexed to the albumin can, however, be metabolized by the bacilli (Dubos, 1950; Dubos and Middlebrook, 1948). Media based on a Tween 80-albumin formulation are satisfactory for cultivation of tubercle bacilli for studies of growth rates and kinetics and, in most cases, for preparation of bacilli for chemical extraction. Furthermore, the basal media and supplements needed to prepare such media as Dubos Tween-albumin broth are readily available from commercial sources.

The disadvantage of using a Tween 80-albumin medium is that the albumin supplement represents an unwanted extrinsic protein that complicates the detection of the small amounts of mycobacterial antigens that are produced. Thorough washing of the bacilli before their disruption and extraction can minimize this problem when intracellular proteins are the substances of interest. The problem associated with introduction of the foreign albumin becomes more serious when one is searching for traces of extracellular proteins secreted by the bacilli themselves into the medium.

Although most studies of diffuse growth of M. tuberculosis in liquid medium have relied on the presence of Tween 80 and albumin, it is possible to obtain diffuse growth with a detergent in the absence of albumin. Wayne and Sramek used a dialysate of the peptide-rich TB Broth Base (Difco, Detroit, Mich.) as a base for a Tween 80 medium that supported growth of fairly large inocula of M. tuberculosis without the addition of albumin (Wayne and Sramek, 1979). Various Triton detergents, which do not contain fatty acids, have been employed to permit dispersed growth of tubercle bacilli in the absence of albumin (Dubos and Middlebrook, 1948); optimal growth in the presence of Triton detergent required the incorporation of the phospholipid sphingomyelin in the medium.

Glycerol has commonly been used in media when large crops of bacilli are desired, since this carbohydrate markedly stimulates growth of *M. tuberculosis* (note that glycerol inhibits growth of fresh isolates of the closely related *M. bovis* [Wayne and Kubica, 1986]). However, there are disadvantages to the use of glycerol. For one, glycerol causes production of excessive amounts of lipids and polysaccharides in mycobacteria (Tepper, 1968), which may interfere with isolation and purification of other products of interest such as proteins or nucleic acids (Hill et al., 1972). Additionally, since it greatly stimulates oxygen consumption by *M. tuberculosis*, the presence of glycerol may cause such severe depletion of dissolved oxygen as to lead to death and autolysis of the bacilli in diffuse culture when oxygen becomes limiting (Wayne and Diaz, 1967).

Solid Media

A number of inspissated egg-based solid media, including Lowenstein-Jensen, Wallenstein, Petragnani, and variants thereof, have been used widely for primary isolation of tubercle bacilli from clinical specimens. They tend to yield a higher proportion of positives from direct clinical specimens than do semisynthetic agar media (Krasnow and Wayne, 1969). The egg media are very rich and contain phospholipids and proteins that tend to bind and/or neutralize toxic products in clinical specimens. They are not especially useful for research purposes, being very complex and not reproducible because of variation in the quality of ingredients and the effects of heat in their preparation.

Agar-based media

Agar media for growth of *M. tuberculosis* are usually prepared from semisynthetic

basal media enriched with supplements. They offer better defined components than egg-based media. Furthermore, they are transparent, permitting early microscopic detection of colonies and the observation of morphologic detail. Agar media are used mainly for the quantification of viable bacilli in growth and survival studies and for determination of drug susceptibility. Generally, growth of tubercle bacilli on agar plates is stimulated by inclusion of a 5 to 10% CO_2 supplement to the air in the incubator.

Dubos oleic albumin agar is almost equivalent to Dubos Tween 80-albumin medium that has been solidified with agar (Dubos and Middlebrook, 1947). The major differences are that the Tween 80 is omitted from the agar base and oleic acid is substituted for the glucose in the albumin complex supplement. Middlebrook introduced a number of small modifications (i.e., the 7H series) to Dubos oleic albumin agar to enhance repair and accelerate detection of damaged bacilli in clinical specimens (Roberts et al., 1991). Both the original Dubos and the modified Middlebrook types of media are available commercially, either already prepared or as dehydrated products and sterile supplements.

Other media

Among the other "culture media" that have been used for preparation of crops of *M. tuberculosis* is the mouse lung. Bacilli isolated in large amounts from the lungs of infected mice have been compared biochemically, physiologically, and immunologically to bacilli isolated from conventional culture, and striking differences have been observed. It is beyond the scope of this chapter to explore this subject further, but the reader is referred to a comprehensive review by one of the pioneers in the field, William Segal (Segal, 1984).

INOCULA

Once a strain or strains of *M. tuberculosis* have been selected for study, a large seed pool should be prepared, subdivided into small aliquots, and maintained at −70°C. That is, the culture should not be maintained by serial passage from experiment to experiment, as such passage would cause it to undergo physiologic changes. A fresh seed vial should be thawed and used to inoculate a single-passage subculture to provide a large inoculum for each experiment, or it may be used directly without subculture to inoculate the experimental culture or to inoculate animals.

The seed pool can be prepared from a dispersed, detergent-containing liquid medium; from a young, thin veil of pellicle; from an unagitated synthetic medium; or from typical corded colonies from solid medium. If the last two types of preparations are to be used, they should be well suspended in medium containing a detergent (e.g., 0.02% Tween 80) by use of a tissue grinder or agitation in a sealed tube with a few glass beads in a vortex-type mixer (Wayne, 1962). For safety reasons, an open tissue grinder is not recommended; if it is necessary to use one, stringent precautions, including working in a biosafety hood, must be taken to prevent escape of infectious aerosols into the laboratory.

When the suspension is to be used to inoculate experimental animals, especially by the intravenous route, it is especially important that the bacilli be very uniformly dispersed, preferably as single cells with a minimum of clumping. The deposition of the bacilli in different organs of intravenously inoculated mice is known to be strongly affected by the degree of dispersion of the bacteria in the inoculum. Optimal dispersion for this purpose may be achieved by brief exposure of the suspension to a burst of moderate energy in a sonicator. Care must be taken to avoid too

great an exposure, which may disrupt some of the bacilli (Lefford, 1984).

TEMPERATURE

M. tuberculosis has a narrower range of growth temperatures than most other mycobacteria (Wayne and Kubica, 1986). I have studied the growth of different species of mycobacteria in tubes of Dubos Tween-albumin broth incubated in an aluminum gradient temperature block (Wayne, 1970). Incubation, with a single brief, daily shake, of cultures of *M. tuberculosis* in this block yielded little if any growth at temperatures below 29°C (unpublished data) (Fig. 1). The growth rate increased in a temperature-dependent fashion over the 10° range up to about a 39°C maximum and underwent a precipitous decline at higher temperatures, with no significant growth seen at 42°C. For most practical purposes, *M. tuberculosis* should be cultivated at 37°C to allow for slight drifts in temperature without serious impact on the growth.

AERATION AND AGITATION

For many years, when large crops of tubercle bacilli were needed, they were

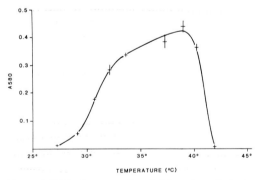

Figure 1. Eight-day growth of *M. tuberculosis* in Tween-albumin broth incubated in a gradient temperature block. Growth is expressed as optical absorbance (A_{580}). Triplicate tubes were incubated at each temperature, and the results were plotted as the mean A_{580}, with vertical bars spanning ±1 standard deviation.

grown as pellicles on the surfaces of un-agitated shallow layers of one of the synthetic media cited above. Alternatively, they were stirred or aerated with a sparger, resulting in distribution of large clumps of growth throughout the medium. This latter method is suitable for production of masses of cells for extraction of a variety of the chemical components of tubercle bacilli for different purposes. It must be recognized, however, that old, thickened pellicles and large dispersed clumps do not represent physiologically homogeneous populations of cells. Oxygen and components of the culture medium do not penetrate into the center of the hydrophobic clumps, so these cultures represent mixtures of cells in a wide range of physiologic conditions from rapidly replicating cells to dormant ones or even dead, autolyzing cells. Nevertheless, these preparations are good sources of DNA, lipids, and polysaccharides. The proteins, on the other hand, may be present in various degrees of degradation, as they are released from some bacilli that may be autolyzing due to inadequate nutrition or aeration (Turcotte, 1969a, b). This is probably true of RNA as well.

Far better control of aeration and the physiologic state of tubercle bacilli in culture may be achieved through the use of detergent-containing medium as described above. Most published work in this area has employed 0.02% Tween 80 as the detergent and 0.5% bovine serum albumin fraction V as a scavenger to protect the bacilli from toxic effects of traces of oleate released from the Tween 80.

Although *M. tuberculosis* obviously grows most rapidly with maximum exposure to air, as on the surface of an agar plate, an anomalous inhibition of growth has been observed consistently when cultures in flasks of Tween 80-containing media are aerated on a rotary shaker-incubator (Lyon et al., 1961). It has been proposed that excess oleate production was the cause of this phenomenon and that addition of glycerol reversed the effect by esterification (Lyon et al., 1961). This seems an unlikely explanation, since albumin is present in the medium in an adequate amount to protect against oleate. Although I also observed the growth inhibition in flasks on a rotary shaker, I have always been able to grow *M. tuberculosis* in Tween-albumin medium in culture tubes on a rotary shaker or in flasks that were aerated by magnetic stirring. On careful observation of the contents of flasks agitated on a rotary shaker and on a magnetic mixer, I have come to the following conclusions about the cause of the anomalous failure of tubercle bacilli to grow on the rotary shaker (unpublished observations). Since the flasks are mounted in positions around the center of rotation of these shakers, centrifugal force creates a wave motion of the medium, with a crest of medium, followed by a contralateral trough, sweeping around the perimeter of the flask. The bacilli in the culture tend to accumulate at the triphasic interface of air, glass, and culture medium. As a crest of medium sweeps past a given point on the glass wall, some of the cells are deposited on the glass and marooned there as the crest passes. The next pass of the crest deposits more cells, which physically push the previous deposit up the flask wall until, on successive revolutions, most of the bacilli in the medium become trapped in a veil of cells on the flask wall out of reach of fresh medium. The apparent protective role of glycerol may thus be an effect on surface tension of the medium. Behling and colleagues (Behling et al., 1993) have recently demonstrated that when trehalose 6,6'-dimycolate (cord factor) extracted from *M. tuberculosis* is coated onto inert particles and suspended in saline in a test tube, the particles aggregate in veils that climb the wall of the container. This cord factor effect suggests a mechanism for the peculiar tendency of tubercle bacilli to accumulate at the triphasic interface and climb the walls of shaken flasks.

In contrast to the failure of flasks of medium on a rotary shaker to support growth of *M. tuberculosis*, luxuriant growth occurs when a magnetic stirrer is used to agitate the contents of a flask. The crest-and-trough wave effect is absent in the magnetically stirred medium; instead, a vortex forms and continuously transports the tubercle bacilli back into the aerated medium, where they are bathed in nutrients and grow rapidly. In test tubes on a rotary shaker, the surface-to-volume ratio seems to be so low that the wave effect is inconsequential, and the bacilli remain suspended in the medium and grow rapidly. Similarly good growth is obtained in roller bottle cultures in Tween-containing 7H9 medium.

VIABILITY

The viability of mycobacterial cultures varies greatly with conditions. In the case of BCG vaccines, the total number of organisms present in a culture is generally determined by microscopic counting in special bacterial counting chambers, e.g., Petroff-Hauser chambers, and the number of viable organisms is determined by counting the CFU on solid agar medium. As described in chapter 31, BCG vaccines prepared as pellicle cultures have viabilities generally between 5 and 20% (Mackaness et al., 1973; Gheorghiu et al., 1988). Bacteria grown under optimal conditions (for example, in roller bottles) can yield cultures in which virtually every physical bacillary particle is viable and is a CFU (Mackaness et al., 1973). Mycobacteria survive freezing at $-70°C$ with little loss in viability, but they lose 50% or more viable CFU by freeze-drying.

MEASUREMENT OF GROWTH AND GROWTH DYNAMICS

Measurement of Growth

When tubercle bacilli are grown in detergent-free medium, it is very difficult to measure rates of growth, since different-sized clumps contain bacilli in different physiologic states. Optical or colony-counting methods are essentially useless with hydrophobic clumps. The major approach has been filtration or centrifugation and measurement of wet or dry weight of the crop (Bowles and Segal, 1965).

When accurate measures of growth dynamics are needed, it is far better to use diffuse cultures in a detergent-containing medium. The simplest method of measuring growth rates is determination of the optical absorbance of cultures in tubes or sidearm flasks, since these flasks do not require the opening of the culture at each reading and therefore diminish the risk of contamination. It has been my practice to distribute Dubos Tween-albumin broth in 10-ml amounts to screw-cap culture tubes (20 by 125 mm) for agitated or stationary culture (see below). The growth is measured by determining the A_{580} in a Coleman Jr. spectrophotometer (Coleman Instruments, Maywood, Ill.). In this system, an A_{580} of 0.100 corresponds to a count of 6.3×10^7 CFU of *M. tuberculosis* H37R$_v$ per ml (Wayne, 1976). The A_{580} of a culture is a linear function of cell concentration over a range of readings up to $A_{580} = 0.200$. At higher cell concentrations, particle coincidence effects cause a departure from linearity. However, it is not difficult to prepare a correction curve by using dilutions of a barium sulfate suspension of known concentrations, which allows adjustment of observed to true A_{580} readings. This permits plotting of growth curves of *M. tuberculosis* of remarkable reproducibility and excellent correlation with plate counts over a wide range of growth (Wayne, 1976).

While optical measurements are usually sufficient for following growth dynamics once a correlation has been established with actual counts of CFU per milliliter, studies of survival or of very early growth of tubercle bacilli can be done accurately only by plating dilutions of liquid cultures or suspensions to solid medium and determining CFU per milliliter by direct colony counts. If the original culture material has been prepared in detergent-containing medium, serial 10-fold dilutions may be made directly from the culture into detergent-containing diluent. One can use the complete Dubos Tween-albumin broth as a diluent, or if the dilutions are made and plated rapidly, it is more economical to use the Dubos broth base with Tween 80 but without albumin as diluent. If the original culture material is not in a well-dispersed form, it is necessary to grind it gently in the detergent-containing media by vortex-type mixing in a sealed tube with glass beads (Wayne, 1962) or in a tube-and-pestle type of tissue grinder; in the latter case, stringent precautions must be taken to prevent escape of infectious aerosols into the air of the laboratory. Optimal dispersion of tubercle bacilli may be achieved by brief, moderate-energy sonication of the suspension (Lefford, 1984). The upper end of the range of dilutions needed for a given experiment may be estimated from the turbidity of the original suspension on the basis of a previously established constant correlating A_{580} in the 0.10 to 0.20 range with dilution plate counts.

After the dilutions have been made, they should be inoculated to one of the conventional solid media, such as Dubos oleic-albumin agar or one of its derivative media. The medium is dispensed in 5-ml amounts to each of the segments of a quadrant petri dish or in 3-ml amounts to the wells of a 24-well tissue culture plate and allowed to gel. If petri plates are used, each quadrant should receive 50 μl of one of the dilutions of inoculum dotted about the surface by a calibrated micropipettor fitted with sterile disposable tips; if tissue culture plates are used, the inoculum should not exceed 20 μl per well. The agar should be incubated at 37°C in a well-humidified chamber, and colonies should be counted at 10× to 100× power twice a week until counts have sta-

bilized. Colonies of *M. tuberculosis* first appear as dense dots but soon produce corded fringes that are characteristic of the species. The original concentration of viable bacilli is calculated from the size of the inoculum plated and the number of colonies seen in those dilutions that yield a final count of 10 to 100 colonies per quadrant or 10 to 50 colonies per well.

Growth Dynamics

The decision as to whether to use stirred or unagitated cultures should be made according to the purposes to which the culture is to be put and an understanding of the different physiologic phases that *M. tuberculosis* manifests under various conditions of aeration.

When *M. tuberculosis* is grown dispersed in continuously agitated liquid medium, it exhibits the expected logarithmic growth, with doubling times of 16 to 18 h (Wayne, 1976). Unexpectedly, when comparable cultures are not agitated continuously but are simply shaken briefly to permit turbidimetric determination of growth, the growth appears to conform to a simple arithmetic mode (Fisher and Kirchheimer, 1952) rather than merely shifting to a slower rate of geometric growth; this phenomenon is difficult to understand when dealing with organisms that replicate by binary fission. Volk and Myrvik (1953) suggested that this could be explained by a slowing down of the replication of tubercle bacilli in oxygen-limiting unstirred culture until the rate of settling of bacilli equaled the rate of replication, with the bacilli that had settled to the bottom of the tube having ceased replicating entirely. My colleagues and I subsequently confirmed this explanation and established a number of physiologic events that characterize this phenomenon (Wayne, 1976, 1977; Wayne and Lin, 1982; Wayne and Sramek, 1979). When small inocula of tubercle bacilli were dispersed in tubed media and incubated without any agitation, the initial growth occurred at a logarithmic rate, with doubling every 16 to 18 h until the cell density approached 4×10^7 CFU/ml. Thereafter, dissolved oxygen became limiting. By the use of inocula stably labeled with ^{14}C, it was established that replication in the unstirred culture slowed down until it reached a doubling time of 33 h, at which time the logarithmic doubling in the upper layers was exactly balanced by the rate at which bacilli settled to the bottom of the tube (Wayne, 1976). Thus, there was a constant population of slowly dividing cells in suspension and an arithmetically increasing mass of bacilli in the sediment. Furthermore, the bacilli that accumulated in the sediment had undergone a discrete metabolic shiftdown during their transition through the self-generated oxygen gradient in the tube and were in a uniform state of dormancy. When the bacilli in the sediment were resuspended and diluted into fresh aerated medium, they immediately initiated RNA synthesis. Between hours 8 and 12 after reconstitution, the bacilli underwent a cycle of synchronized division, and only then did they initiate DNA synthesis (Wayne, 1977). Synchronized replication was sustained through at least three 20-h cycles. The dormant bacilli that accumulated in unstirred cultures were far more resistant to the bactericidal effects of anaerobiosis than were actively aerated cultures after being abruptly deprived of oxygen (Wayne and Lin, 1982). As tubercle bacilli in unstirred cultures shifted down while settling through their self-generated oxygen gradient, they accumulated an antigen that was not found in aerated cultures (Wayne and Sramek, 1979) and exhibited a 4-fold increase in isocitrate lyase and later a 10-fold increase in a glycine dehydrogenase that may have been instrumental in scavenging sufficient NAD for completion of the final round of DNA synthesis before dormancy was established (Wayne and Lin, 1982).

Inasmuch as tubercle bacilli in the mammalian host occur in intracellular environments and in conditions of inflammation and necrosis, the highly aerobic in vitro conditions of shaken cultures or the surfaces of solid medium do not reflect the state of the bacilli as they occur in the infected host. *M. tuberculosis* is known to produce enzymes of anaerobic metabolism, and these are especially prominent when bacilli are tested after direct harvest from host tissues; there is a general shift away from O_2-dependent pathways to anaerobic or facultative anaerobic pathways in host-derived bacilli compared to cultured organisms (Segal, 1984). The availability of the in vitro model of shiftdown to dormancy and of synchronized shiftup from dormancy to rapid replication of *M. tuberculosis* through manipulation of the degree of aeration of cultures, as described above, should make it possible to study the physiology, immunology, and chemistry of these bacilli in phases that reflect their condition in various stages of activity and dormancy (latency) in human disease.

REFERENCES

Affronti, L. F., V. Porrello, and S. Gupta. 1990. Trace elements incorporated into the culture medium of *Mycobacterium tuberculosis* promote the presence of tuberculoprotein C in the preparation of purified protein derivatives. *Microbios* **63:**101–107.

Baisden, L. A. 1951. Trace element supplements for asparagine brands found to be deficient for the growth of tubercle bacilli. *Am. J. Vet. Res.* **12:**254–256.

Barrow, W. W., B. P. Ullom, and P. J. Brennan. 1980. Peptidoglycolipid nature of the superficial cell wall sheath of smooth-colony-forming mycobacteria. *J. Bacteriol.* **144:**814–822.

Behling, C. A., B. Bennett, K. Takayama, and R. L. Hunter. 1993. Development of a trehalose 6,6′-dimycolate model which explains cord formation by *Mycobacterium tuberculosis*. *Infect. Immun.* **61:** 2296–2303.

Bowles, J. A., and W. Segal. 1965. Kinetics of utilization of organic compounds in the growth of *Mycobacterium tuberculosis*. *J. Bacteriol.* **90:**157–163.

Collins, F. M., L. G. Wayne, and V. Montalbine. 1974. The effect of cultural conditions on the distribution of *Mycobacterium tuberculosis* in the spleens and lungs of specific pathogen-free mice. *Am. Rev. Respir. Dis.* **110:**147–156.

Davis, B. D., and R. J. Dubos. 1948. The inhibitory effect of lipase on bacterial growth in media containing fatty acid esters. *J. Bacteriol.* **55:**11–23.

Dubos, R. J. 1945. Rapid and submerged growth of mycobacteria in liquid media. *Proc. Soc. Exp. Biol. Med.* **58:**361–362.

Dubos, R. J. 1950. The effect of organic acids on mammalian tubercle bacilli. *J. Exp. Med.* **92:**319–332.

Dubos, R. J., and B. D. Davis. 1946. Factors affecting the growth of tubercle bacilli in liquid media. *J. Exp. Med.* **83:**409–423.

Dubos, R. J., and G. Middlebrook. 1947. Media for tubercle bacilli. *Am. Rev. Tuberc.* **56:**334–345.

Dubos, R. J., and G. Middlebrook. 1948. The effect of wetting agents on the growth of tubercle bacilli. *J. Exp. Med.* **88:**81–88.

Fisher, M. W., and W. Kirchheimer. 1952. Studies on the growth of mycobacteria. I. The occurrence of arithmetic linear growth. *Am. Rev. Tuberc.* **66:**758–761.

Gheorghiu, M., P. H. Lagrange, and C. Fillastre. 1988. The stability and immunogenicity of a dispersed-grown freeze-dried Pasteur BCG vaccine. *J. Biol. Stand.* **16:**15–26.

Hill, E. G., L. G. Wayne, and W. M. Gross. 1972. Purification of mycobacterial deoxyribonucleic acid. *J. Bacteriol.* **112:**1033–1039.

Krasnow, I., and L. G. Wayne. 1969. Comparison of methods for tuberculosis bacteriology. *Appl. Microbiol.* **18:**915–917.

Kubica, G. P., and L. G. Wayne. 1984. *The Mycobacteria—a Sourcebook.* Marcel Dekker, Inc., New York.

Lefford, M. J. 1984. Diseases in mice and rats, p. 947–977. *In* G. P. Kubica and L. G. Wayne (ed.), *The Mycobacteria: a Source Book.* Marcel Dekker, Inc., New York.

Lyon, R. H., H. C. Lichstein, and W. H. Hall. 1961. Factors affecting the growth of *Mycobacterium tuberculosis* in aerobic and shake culture. *Am. Rev. Respir. Dis.* **83:**255–260.

Mackaness, G. B., D. J. Auclair, and P. H. Lagrange. 1973. Immuno-potentiation with BCG: immune response to different strains and preparations. *J. Natl. Cancer Inst.* **51:**1655–1667.

Roberts, G. D., E. W. Koneman, and Y. K. Kim. 1991. *Mycobacterium*, p. 304–339. *In* A. Balows, W. J. Hausler, Jr., K. L. Herrmann, H. D. Isenberg, and H. J. Shadomy (ed.), *Manual of Clinical Microbiology*, 5th ed. American Society for Microbiology, Washington, D.C.

Segal, W. 1984. Growth dynamics of in vivo and in vitro grown mycobacterial pathogens, p. 547–573. *In* G. P. Kubica and L. G. Wayne (ed.), *The Mycobacteria—a Sourcebook.* Marcel Dekker, Inc., New York.

Soltys, M. A. 1952. *Tubercle Bacillus and Laboratory Methods in Tuberculosis.* E. & S. Livingstone Ltd., Edinburgh.

Tepper, B. S. 1968. Differences in the utilization of glycerol and glucose by *Mycobacterium phlei*. *J. Bacteriol.* **95:**1713–1717.

Turcotte, R. 1969a. Yield of non-dialyzable mycobacterial constituents during the growth cycle. *Can. J. Microbiol.* **15:**35–41.

Turcotte, R. 1969b. The variations in the antigenic composition of *Mycobacterium tuberculosis* during the growth cycle as measured by the passive hemagglutination and precipitation reactions. *Can. J. Microbiol.* **15:**681–687.

Volk, W. A., and Q. N. Myrvik. 1953. An explanation for the arithmetic linear growth of mycobacteria. *J. Bacteriol.* **66:**386–388.

Wayne, L. G. 1962. Preparation of suspensions of tubercle bacilli on a Vortex mixer. *Am. J. Clin. Pathol.* **37:**328–329.

Wayne, L. G. 1970. Temperature adaptations and biochemical activities of group III mycobacteria. *Pneumonology* **142:**278–283.

Wayne, L. G. 1976. Dynamics of submerged growth of *Mycobacterium tuberculosis* under aerobic and microaerophilic conditions. *Am. Rev. Respir. Dis.* **114:**807–811.

Wayne, L. G. 1977. Synchronized replication of *Mycobacterium tuberculosis*. *Infect. Immun.* **17:**528–530.

Wayne, L. G., and G. A. Diaz. 1967. Autolysis and secondary growth of *Mycobacterium tuberculosis* in submerged culture. *J. Bacteriol.* **93:**1374–1381.

Wayne, L. G., and G. P. Kubica. 1986. Section 16. *Mycobacteria*, p. 1436–1457. *In* P. H. A. Sneath, N. S. Mair, M. E. Sharpe, and J. G. Holt (ed.), *Bergey's Manual of Systematic Bacteriology*, vol. 2. The Williams & Wilkins Co., Baltimore.

Wayne, L. G., and K.-Y. Lin. 1982. Glyoxylate metabolism and adaptation of *Mycobacterium tuberculosis* to survival under anaerobic conditions. *Infect. Immun.* **37:**1042–1049.

Wayne, L. G., and H. A. Sramek. 1979. Antigenic differences between extracts of actively replicating and synchronized resting cells of *Mycobacterium tuberculosis*. *Infect. Immun.* **24:**363–370.

Youmans, G. P. 1979. *Tuberculosis*. The W.B. Saunders Co., Philadelphia.

Tuberculosis: Pathogenesis, Protection, and Control
Edited by Barry R. Bloom
© 1994 American Society for Microbiology, Washington, DC 20005

Chapter 7

Current Laboratory Methods for the Diagnosis of Tuberculosis

Leonid B. Heifets and Robert C. Good

One of the goals of research in the field of mycobacteriology is development of new methods that will improve and expedite the diagnosis and treatment of tuberculosis and other mycobacterial infections. The value of any new method can be estimated on the basis of comparison with technologies currently available in clinical laboratories. Therefore, the goal of this chapter is to present a broad picture of activities in a diagnostic mycobacteriology laboratory. We address the methodology currently available in most laboratories as well as the techniques that require further standardization and therefore have been implemented in only a few laboratories, mostly in conjunction with research and development. Detailed descriptions of these new methods can be found in other chapters of this volume, and we therefore provide only short descriptions in order to review their possible application in clinical laboratories. Biosafety in the mycobacteriology laboratory is an important part of any method or procedure, and a section of this chapter

contains a condensed description of biosafety practices. Detailed descriptions can be found in chapter 5 of this volume.

In an attempt to present a comprehensive review of all activities that take place in a clinical mycobacteriology laboratory, we have divided this chapter in four sections: (i) biosafety in the mycobacteriology laboratory; (ii) specimen collection, smear examination, and inoculation of primary culture media; (iii) methods for identification of *Mycobacterium tuberculosis*; and (iv) drug susceptibility testing for detection of initial and acquired drug resistance.

While anticipating practical implementation of new methods in the future, most clinical laboratories will have to rely in the meantime on currently available technology. Therefore, we have made all possible efforts to address various ways of implementing these conventional methods, with emphasis on the options that can provide physicians with test results in the shortest turnaround time, especially when the reported information is essential for proper management of the patient.

Leonid B. Heifets • National Jewish Center for Immunology and Respiratory Medicine, 1400 Jackson Street, Denver, Colorado 80206. *Robert C. Good* • Centers for Disease Control and Prevention, 1600 Clifton Road, N.E., Mailstop C-09, Atlanta, Georgia 30333.

BIOSAFETY IN THE MYCOBACTERIOLOGY LABORATORY

The threat of contracting an infection in the laboratory is as old as the history of microbiology. Numerous reports of laboratory-associated infection have been published throughout this century, but in less than one-fifth of the cases was a known accident recalled. In the overview of these publications, a report from the Centers for Disease Control and Prevention (CDC) (Richmond and McKinney, 1993) suggested that infection in the laboratory was most commonly acquired through aerosols, mouth pipetting, and the use of syringes (Pike et al., 1965; Pike, 1976; Skinholj, 1974). Although tuberculosis was rarely found among the most frequent laboratory-related infections, some reports (Harrington and Shannon, 1976; Reid, 1957; Smithwick, 1976) suggest that tuberculosis occurs more frequently in laboratory personnel than in the general population. Recent increases in the number of tuberculosis cases in the United States and expanded funding for research have resulted in laboratory work being done by persons who may not have had previous training or experience in working with tubercle bacilli. This can result in *M. tuberculosis* infection being overreported or underreported by laboratories because of insufficient or inappropriate application of the available diagnostic technology. On the other hand, unjustified publicity about the higher virulence or contagiousness of multidrug-resistant strains ("killer strains") from recent outbreaks has led to the creation of some laboratory facilities that far exceed any reasonable necessity of containment. In fact, this "overkill" may have a negative effect on real biosafety, since the environment created by some of the implemented measures can be highly uncomfortable and tiring, increasing the probability of an accident or a breach of technique. Sometimes such a facility becomes just a "showroom," while the actual work is done outside of this containment area. It is clear that along with the necessary specific protection measures, an appropriate work environment that is comfortable for personnel

should be considered among the most important principles of biosafety guidelines.

The most recent summary of biosafety guidelines for microbiology laboratories was published in 1993 (Richmond and McKinney, 1993), and the requirements for biosafety levels 2 and 3 are very clear. *M. tuberculosis* and *M. bovis* require special considerations because of the proven hazard encountered in handling these species. Biosafety level 2 practices, containment equipment, and facilities are required for preparation of smears and culturing of clinical specimens such as sputum, and these activities must be performed in class I or II biological safety cabinets (Richmond and McKinney, 1993). It is recommended that biosafety level 3 practices be applied to some other procedures, but "it is the responsibility of the laboratory director to establish standard procedures in the laboratory which realistically address the issue of the infective hazard . . ." (Richmond and McKinney, 1993).

Biosafety Level 2

Basic requirements for biosafety level 2 include standard microbiological practices, training in biosafety, protective laboratory clothing, protective gloves, annual tuberculin skin test, limited access, decontamination of all infectious waste, and class I or II biosafety cabinets for some manipulative procedures.

Biosafety Level 3

Level 3 practices require containment facilities (American Thoracic Society, 1974; Kubica et al., 1975). Other requirements, in addition to those for level 2, are special laboratory clothing, controlled access, and biosafety cabinets for all manipulations of infectious materials.

The protection of personnel and the laboratory environment (primary containment) can be achieved by observing standard laboratory practices and techniques, selecting appropriate safety equipment and using it properly, and designing a reasonably safe laboratory layout, including proper air handling. If the laboratory is located in a hospital, protection of the environment outside the laboratory (secondary containment) is an additional design issue.

Design

High-quality service by well-trained and experienced personnel who have modern equipment at their disposal can be achieved at its best in a clinical laboratory specializing in mycobacteriology. Such a laboratory minimizes turnaround time by receiving raw specimens and performing all necessary tests in one place. This laboratory implements biosafety measures properly because it must handle materials and cultures of various hazard potentials: sputum specimens that may or may not contain *M. tuberculosis*; blood and other specimens from human immunodeficiency virus (HIV)-infected individuals; and pure cultures of *M. tuberculosis* and nontuberculous mycobacteria referred from other laboratories. The modern specialized mycobacteriology laboratory should have areas of different biosafety levels for handling different materials and performing procedures with various potential hazard levels. Some parts of the laboratory can be designated biosafety level 2, and some can be biosafety level 3. Cultures of *M. tuberculosis* should be handled in a biosafety level 3 facility. The laboratory director may designate actual safeguards such as an access zone, sealed penetrations, or directional airflow, but the safety and well-being of personnel must be placed ahead of other factors.

The director's office, a receiving room (for arriving specimens and mail), a storage room for arriving supplies, and a lounge for personnel should be separated from spaces where the laboratory functions are actually performed and should preferably be outside the access doors. The mycobacteriology laboratory should be separated from the rest of the building. Some areas within the laboratory proper (locker room, computer and communications systems, medium preparation room, supervisor's office) must be physically separated from those where procedures with infectious materials are performed. The following laboratory activities require specific biosafety level practices and appropriate designs: unpacking and inspection of arriving specimens and cultures; processing of specimens, including preparing smears and inoculating media; subcultivating isolates for species identification and drug susceptibility testing; using BACTEC instruments and walk-in incubator; examining grown cultures; and reading results of the susceptibility and biochemical tests.

A full-scale biosafety level 3 facility or its simplified modification is necessary only for procedures associated with preparing *M. tuberculosis* bacterial suspensions for various tests. Such a facility is more important in research laboratories than in clinical laboratories, particularly in those handling large volumes of bacterial suspensions or broth cultures. Currently, many laboratories must handle *M. tuberculosis* isolates resistant (or suspected of being resistant) to two or more antituberculosis drugs. These multidrug-resistant strains are no different from susceptible strains in their virulence or contagiousness, but these strains must be handled with extra care because of fewer treatment choices for potential laboratory-associated infection. For the same reason, laboratories that receive a substantial number of specimens containing multidrug-resistant strains should use a biosafety level 3 facility for initial processing of the raw specimens as well.

Taking into account these considerations, a specialized mycobacteriology laboratory should have at least two or three appropriately designed facilities of this level. Each of them should comfortably accommodate one or two people and should contain one or two laminar-flow hoods. With these size limitations, an accident will not compromise the safety of many people or interrupt the work of the rest of the laboratory. If the mycobacteriology laboratory is not separated from the rest of the building by an airlock, an anteroom should be added to each biosafety level 3 facility within the laboratory. This type of access is not necessary if the entrance is from the general open-bench area of the laboratory, instead of the hallway. However, even when the biosafety level 3 facility is accessed from the main laboratory, a small intermediate room separating the main laboratory from this special facility is desirable. Additional important features of such a facility include negative air pressure, so that exhaust air is discharged to the outside; floor, ceiling, walls, and other surfaces accessible for cleaning; and access doors that are self-closing and have windows.

Other parts of the mycobacteriology laboratory should be designed for laboratory practices at biosafety level 2. This includes special furniture design, sealed windows, a sink for hand washing, and an eye wash area. The mycobacteriology laboratory should also incorporate autoclaves that decontaminate infectious waste.

Safety Equipment

Proper design by itself is not enough to provide a safe environment in the mycobacteriology laboratory. Safety equipment must be appropriate for the mycobacteriology laboratory and must be used properly. It serves mainly to prevent the dissemination of bacterial aerosols. Class I or II biological safety cabinets equipped with a high-efficiency particulate air (HEPA) filter are the most important equipment in the mycobacteriology laboratory, since any manipulation of cultures or specimens must be conducted only in these cabinets. Exhaust air from the cabinet should be dis-

charged outside the building, or it can be recirculated if the cabinet is tested and certified at least once a year.

All centrifuges must have safety caps for each bucket or sealed aerosol containment or both. Centrifuges should be placed in the sterile rooms where other manipulations with the cultures or specimens are performed. Another piece of safety equipment for the mycobacteriology laboratory is a heating plate, which replaces flaming for inactivation of smears. Use of disposable (instead of metallic) loops prevents aerosol formation and cross-contamination. Proper use of syringes, pipettes, and dispensers also prevents aerosols.

Safety Practices

The most important principle of biosafety in the mycobacteriology laboratory is the observance of standard and special practices. These practices start with the instructions given by the laboratory for collection, delivery, and shipment of the specimens. Interstate shipment of diagnostic specimens and etiologic agents is subject to the Interstate Shipment of Etiologic Agents Regulations (42 CFR, Part 72). The specific requirements for collection and delivery or shipment of the specimens are described in another section of this chapter.

Standard microbiological practices include restricted access to the laboratory, especially to the areas where work is in progress; decontamination of the work surfaces every day; prohibition of mouth pipetting; prohibition of eating, drinking, smoking, and applying cosmetics; and washing hands after handling infectious material and before leaving the laboratory.

In addition, special practices in the mycobacteriology laboratory include the following: doors of the rooms where the work is in progress must be closed; all manipulations with cultures or specimens should be done with gloved hands; gloves should not be worn outside the areas where the procedures are performed; personnel should wear special clothing while handling infectious materials; protective clothing should not be worn outside of the laboratory; tubes with specimens or cultures should be removed from the shipping containers in a biosafety level 2 room equipped with a biosafety class I cabinet; the surfaces of these tubes should be disinfected before they are placed in a rack; all other manipulations with specimens or cultures should be performed in a properly maintained class 2 biosafety cabinet. Appropriate masks to be used immediately after any spill or accident should be readily available at every station and in laboratory wear pockets; a spill area should be covered with paper towels and then generously soaked with a tuberculocidal disinfectant (for example, Clorox); after an accident or spill, all persons present must leave the room, which should be sealed for 24 h and cleaned later according to the instructions incorporated in the laboratory manual. Spills and accidents should be reported to the laboratory director or supervisor, and appropriate medical surveillance should be implemented for exposed individuals. All waste from the laboratory should be collected in cannisters, baskets, or bags that are autoclaved within the confines of the laboratory. Only disposable syringe and needle units should be used, and they must be disposed of in the sharps containers placed in the hoods. No animals or plants not related to the work are allowed in the laboratory; a hazard warning should be posted on all laboratory doors that access the areas where infectious materials are being handled.

Reading closed plates or tubes for appearance of growth and examining the results of biochemical or drug susceptibility tests can be done safely at the bench. Plates should be kept closed, stored in baskets or boxes. BACTEC vials can be stored in their compartmented boxes. Tubes must be stored in racks. Workbenches should be cleaned at the end of the day, and all surfaces should be cleaned with a tuberculocidal disinfectant.

The personnel working in the mycobacteriology laboratory should be skin tested and given chest X rays on a regular schedule. Tuberculin-positive persons should be trained to identify the disease symptoms. Systematic training of personnel in biosafety issues and policy updates, all of which should be documented in the laboratory safety manual, is a necessary task in a safe laboratory. The laboratory director is responsible for specific application of the general principles of biosafety and for selecting any additional measures needed in each individual situation.

SPECIMEN COLLECTION, SMEAR EXAMINATION, AND INOCULATION OF PRIMARY CULTURE MEDIA

There is an adage as true today as it was many years ago: the laboratory report is only as good as the specimen submitted. Therefore, collection and delivery of specimens for processing are basic to the definitive diagnosis of tuberculosis, to the determination of drug susceptibility patterns, and hence to the ability to make an informed decision regarding diagnosis and therapy.

Specimen Collection and Delivery

Specimens must be collected in clean, sterile containers and held under conditions that inhibit the growth of contaminants, since most specimens will contain bacteria other than mycobacteria. Certain specimen collection procedures are optimal for *M. tuberculosis*. Sputum is the specimen most often collected and processed, but other specimens such as induced sputum, fluids collected by gastric or bronchial lavage, urine, tissue from any organ, spinal fluid, blood, and aspirates from lesions may be collected. All specimens from nonsterile sites are similar in that they must be decontaminated before culture on a rich, supportive medium that encourages overgrowth of the rapidly growing microorganisms present in most specimens.

A series of three to six early-morning sputum specimens should be collected on successive days before the start of chemotherapy and sent to the laboratory without delay. The patient should be placed in a well-ventilated area for the collection of the specimen and be instructed in the difference between saliva and sputum. Five to 10 ml of sputum brought up by a deep, productive cough is collected most conveniently in a sterile, disposable, 50-ml conical screw-cap centrifuge tube. If the patient is unable to produce an acceptable sputum specimen, inhalation of a warm, sterile, aerosolized solution of saline (5 to 10%) will induce coughing for the collection of a thin, watery specimen. This must be identified as induced for the laboratory, or it may be discarded as inadequate. All specimens should be sent to the laboratory immediately. Interstate shipments of diagnostic specimens must be packaged in accordance with interstate quarantine regulations (Federal Register, Title 42, Chapter 1, part 72, revised July 30, 1972). Adequate specimens obtained by other procedures or from different sites are handled in a similar manner. Specimens collected from normally sterile sites may be placed directly into a liquid medium without the decontamination step described below. For example, blood may be cultured directly into BACTEC 13A medium (Becton Dickinson Diagnostic Instrument Systems, Sparks, Md.) following the manufacturer's recommendations.

Processing

Upon arrival in the laboratory, most specimens are homogenized with a mucolytic agent, but tissues and similar specimens may be ground in Teflon-to-glass or glass-to-glass homogenizers. Along with homogenization, specimens must be treated to kill contaminating organisms that may be present. Mycobacteria resist the bactericidal action of selected chemicals that will kill contaminating bacteria; however, because even the mildest agents will reduce the numbers of viable tubercle bacilli, all procedures must be carried out as quickly and as gently as possible in order to preserve the numbers of viable bacilli (Kent and Kubica, 1985). Many agents or combinations such as zephiran-trisodium phosphate, Petroff's sodium hydroxide, oxalic acid, sulfuric acid, and cetylpyridinium chloride-sodium chloride have been used for digestion and decontamination of specimens; however, the N-acetyl-L-cysteine–sodium hydroxide (NALC-NaOH) method is preferred in most laboratories (Kubica et al., 1963, 1964). Current descriptions of the method (Kent and Kubica, 1985; Roberts et al., 1991), basically unchanged from the original, depend on preparation of the digestant by mixing 50 ml of 2.94% aqueous trisodium citrate · $3H_2O$ solution with 50 ml of 4% NaOH. Immediately before use, 0.5 g of the mucolytic agent NALC is added. An equal amount of this digestant solution is added to 10 ml or less of sputum in a 50-ml plastic centrifuge tube. Caps are tightened, and the contents are mixed with a vortex or similar tube mixer for 5 to 20 s until the specimen is liquefied; tubes are held for 15 min at room temperature. The digested mixture is then diluted to 50 ml with sterile distilled water or 0.067 M phosphate buffer (pH 6.8), mixed, and centrifuged at 3,000 × g for 15 min, preferably at 4°C, using aerosol-free, sealed centrifuge cups. The supernatant fluid is discarded into a splash-proof discard pan containing a tuberculocidal disinfectant, and a portion of the sediment is collected with either an applicator stick, a 3-mm-diameter bacteriological loop, or a capillary pipette and is spread over an area 1 by 2 cm on a microscope slide. The remaining sediment is resuspended in 1 to 2 ml of a sterile 0.2% solution of bovine albumin fraction V for inoculation of the culture medium.

Staining and Smear Examination

Procedures for smear preparation and staining as well as the theoretical background of the stain reactions have been described elsewhere (Kent and Kubica, 1985; Smithwick, 1976). Smears may be made directly from untreated specimen or from concentrated specimen. If a smear is made directly from sputum, select those areas that will be most likely to contain mycobacteria, i.e., cheesy, necrotic particles, or areas that are tinged with blood. Smears of concentrates prepared as directed above are most often used when the specimen will be cultured. If it will not be cultured, add an equal volume of a 5% hypochlorite solution such as a common household bleach for a few minutes to kill bacilli before making the smear. Spread the treated specimen evenly over an area 1 by 2 cm on a clean glass slide. After the smear air dries, heat fix it by passing the slide through the blue cone of the Bunsen flame three or four times, or heat it on an electric slide warmer at 65 to 75°C for at least 2 h.

The acid-fast staining procedure depends on the ability of mycobacteria and some other microorganisms to retain dye even when treated with mineral acid or an acid-alcohol solution. The procedure may involve application of heat or inclusion of a surfactant to allow penetration of the dye into the cell. Each method has its advantages and its ardent adherents. Two procedures, those using the Ziehl-Neelsen and the auramine O fluorescence acid-fast stains, are the most widely used (Fig. 1 and 2). For the Ziehl-Neelsen procedure, flood the fixed smear with a solution prepared by dissolving 0.3 g of basic fuchsin in 10 ml of ethanol and then diluting it to 100 ml with aqueous 5% phenol. Gently heat the smear to steaming on an electric rack or with the

flame from a Bunsen burner for 5 min. Wash the slides in tap water, and then flood the smears with 3% hydrochloric acid in 95% ethanol. Wash the smear with tap water to halt the action of the acid alcohol, and finally, counterstain the smear by flooding it with 3% aqueous methylene blue for 1 or 2 min. Rinse with water, drain, air dry, and examine under the oil immersion objective. Mycobacteria will appear as red-stained rods or coccobacilli on a blue background.

The auramine O fluorescence acid-fast stain procedure is similar to the Ziehl-Neelsen procedure. Flood the fixed smear for 15 min with a solution of 0.1 g of auramine O dissolved in 10 ml of 95% ethanol which has been diluted with 90 ml of 3% aqueous phenol. Rinse the smear with chlorine-free water and drain. Flood with 70% ethanol containing 0.5% hydrochloric acid. Rinse, drain, and then cover for 2 min with aqueous 0.5% potassium permanganate. Rinse, drain, air dry, and examine under a fluorescence microscope. Mycobacteria appear as yellow fluorescing rods on a dark background. Often debris will fluoresce, but experienced microscopists can differentiate tubercle bacilli from the "clutter."

Smears must be examined carefully, and a preparation cannot be considered negative until the microscopist has examined the equivalent of 300 oil immersion fields. The smear must be examined in a standardized manner, which is best accomplished by making three sweeps along its longest dimension. Alternatively, make nine sweeps along the narrowest dimension. Reports of the results of smear examination should include a measure of quantitation, such as actual number of bacilli seen per field or a 1 to 4+ rating, which roughly estimates the same numbers (Tenover et al., 1993). This quantitation is important to the clinician for following the results of therapy and for estimating the condition of the patient. Between 5×10^3 and 1×10^4 acid-fast bacilli

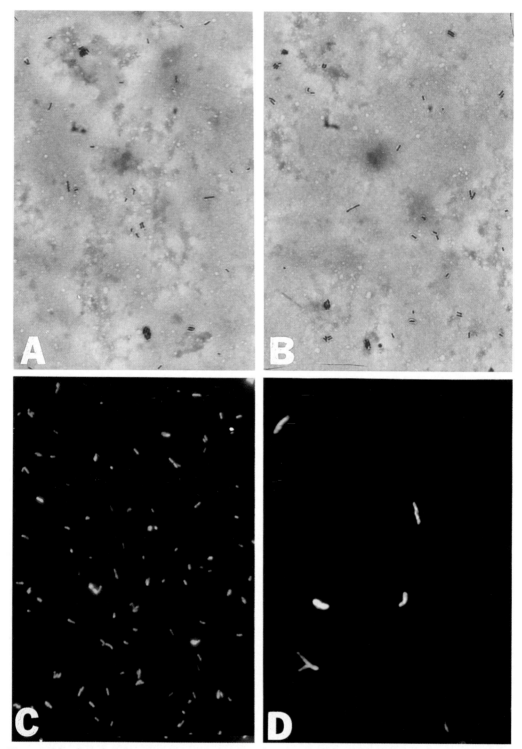

Figure 1. *M. tuberculosis* in a smear from a concentrated sputum specimen. Photography by N. Mor. (A and B) Ziehl-Nielsen stain; Olympus microscope model BH2 with 100× objective. Total magnification, ×1,125. (C) Auramine O stain; fluorescence microscope, Olympus model BH2 with 40× objective. Total magnification, ×1,440. (D) Auramine O stain; fluorescence microscope, model Leitz-Wetzlar with 40× objective. Total magnification, ×2,000.

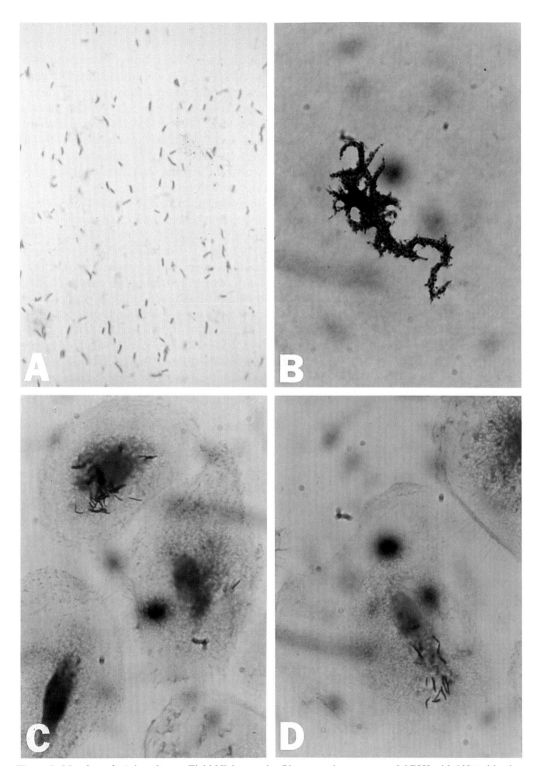

Figure 2. *M. tuberculosis* in cultures. Ziehl-Nielsen stain; Olympus microscope model BH2 with 100× objective. Total magnification, ×1,125. Photography by N. Mor. (A) Smear from a culture grown on 7H11 agar; (B) "cord" formation in 7H12 broth; (C and D) intracellular growth in human-monocyte-derived macrophages.

(AFB) per ml of sputum must be present to be detected by microscopy. Those specimens that contain only three or fewer AFB in 300 oil immersion fields are considered doubtful and should be retested.

A sputum smear positive for AFB may represent either *M. tuberculosis* or some nontuberculous mycobacterium. In conjunction with clinical and radiological data indicating that the patient has tuberculosis, the report of a positive smear result indicates that the patient is definitely infectious. In this case, a number of prevention and control steps must be taken. Therefore, it is suggested that the results of the acid-fast stain be reported to the physician or clinic within 24 h of specimen collection (Tenover et al., 1993). This is the first report issued following receipt of a specimen, and it can be instructive regarding the adequacy of therapy; i.e., if AFB are not detected on the smear, the physician may want to consider another diagnosis.

Primary Isolation of *M. tuberculosis*

Historically, the egg-based media (Lowenstein-Jensen, Ogawa, and American Trudeau Society) are the best known among the solid media used for isolation of *M. tuberculosis*. The agar-based media (Middlebrook-Cohn 7H10 agar [Middlebrook et al., 1960; Middlebrook and Cohn, 1958] and 7H11 agar [Cohn et al., 1968]) allow a more rapid recovery of growth (within 2 to 4 weeks) and offer a better opportunity to study colonial morphology than the egg-based media. Selective 7H11 agar, containing four incorporated antibiotics, inhibits growth of the nonmycobacterial contaminants, some of which may survive digestion-decontamination of nonsterile specimens such as sputum (McClatchy et al., 1976). Liquid medium can be used for primary isolation of *M. tuberculosis* from sputum only if it is a selective medium. The most popular medium of this type is Middlebrook 7H12 broth (Middle-

brook et al., 1977), currently manufactured as BACTEC 12B vials by Becton Dickinson Diagnostic Instrument Systems for the radiometric detection of growth in the BACTEC TB-460 system. Five antimicrobial agents, under the acronym PANTA, may be added to this medium to prevent growth of nonmycobacterial contaminants. The growth of *M. tuberculosis* on this medium can be detected within 1 or 2 weeks depending on the number of bacteria in the specimen. Another option of a selective 7H9 broth, also with PANTA, is a biphasic medium system (the Septi-Chek AFB system), which represents a combination in one unit of a selective liquid medium with two types (egg based and agar based) of solid media (Isenberg et al., 1991).

A slant with any type of solid medium is inoculated with 0.1 ml of the original suspension and with a 1:10 dilution of the resuspended sediment from the digested and decontaminated sputum specimen. Plain and selective 7H11 agars may be prepared as half-plates rather than slants. Prepare the media as directed in more detailed manuals (Kent and Kubica, 1985; Nash and Krenz, 1991), or purchase them from suppliers such as Difco (Detroit, Mich.), Becton Dickinson Microbiology Systems (Cockeysville, Md.), Carr-Scarborough Microbiologicals, Inc. (Atlanta, Ga.), or Remel (Lenexa, Kans.). Incubate inoculated tubed media in a slanted position with the tube's screw cap loosened for at least the first week at 35 to 37°C in an atmosphere of 10% CO_2 and 90% air. Place the plates containing media in CO_2-permeable plastic bags for incubation. Examine all inoculated media at weekly intervals for at least 8 weeks to select positive cultures as soon as growth is visible and to recognize contaminated cultures, which are removed immediately. Additional specimens should be requested to replace those that were contaminated. Inoculated media may be held for up to 12 weeks or more before being discarded as negative. Inoculate

BACTEC liquid medium (12B or 13A) as specified in instructions supplied by the manufacturer, and test it daily for the evolution of radiolabeled CO_2, an indicator of cell metabolism and growth.

According to the experience of the Mycobacteriology Laboratory at National Jewish Center for Immunology and Respiratory Medicine in Denver, a combination of four units of medium is most efficient for the primary isolation of mycobacteria from a processed sputum specimen. The BACTEC 12B vial (with PANTA) is inoculated along with a biplate containing plain and selective 7H11 agars and a Lowenstein-Jensen slant. While BACTEC broth allows rapid growth, the agar plate provides an opportunity to examine the colonial morphology and detect mixed cultures. Selective 7H11 agar is useful as a backup when digestion-decontamination of the specimen does not prevent the nonmycobacterial contaminants from growing in 12B vials and on plain 7H11 agar. Lowenstein-Jensen medium in this combination is an important backup for rare *M. tuberculosis* strains that may not grow on the other three media. Even if no growth is detected in the BACTEC 12B vials and on agar plates, the final report that the specimen is culture negative can be issued only after 8 weeks of incubation of the Lowenstein-Jensen slants.

METHODS FOR IDENTIFICATION OF *M. TUBERCULOSIS*

Detection of AFB in a sputum smear in conjunction with certain clinical symptoms and X-ray findings leads to the suspicion of tuberculosis, the initiation of public health measures, and the start of therapy as early as 24 to 48 h after the sputum specimen was obtained from the patient. The AFB smear was an important tool in the past, but the current epidemiological situation has greatly diminished its diagnostic value. It is now recognized that an AFB-positive smear is not sufficient evidence for the bacteriological diagnosis of tuberculosis. The probability that the AFB seen in a sputum smear are *M. tuberculosis* depends on the frequency with which the laboratory isolates various nontuberculous mycobacteria. With the increasing rates of tuberculosis among HIV-infected persons, who frequently develop extrapulmonary tuberculosis, sputum may not be available, and specimens from other sources are frequently submitted for mycobacterial isolation. Additionally, HIV-infected persons may be coinfected with *M. avium* complex or other nontuberculous mycobacteria.

Differentiation of *M. tuberculosis* from other mycobacteria represents an important health issue, since only tuberculosis is transmissible from person to person. In the near future, clinical laboratories may be able to reliably identify *M. tuberculosis* in patients' raw specimens. In the meantime, to expedite the answer to a question ("TB or not TB"), the laboratory must rely on today's methods: DNA-RNA hybridization with a culture grown in BACTEC 7H 12 broth (12B medium) or a *p*-nitro-α-acetyl-amino-β-hydroxypropiophenone (NAP) test with the same culture. Either of these tests tells, with a high level of sensitivity and specificity, whether or not the culture belongs to the *M. tuberculosis* complex, which includes four species: *M. tuberculosis*, *M. bovis* (and BCG), *M. africanum*, and *M. microti*. Therefore, differentiation of *M. tuberculosis* from other species of the complex requires further confirmation by some biochemical tests.

Rarely, some of the nontuberculous mycobacteria may cause a false-positive signal for *M. tuberculosis* even in the highly specific DNA-RNA hybridization and BACTEC NAP tests, requiring confirmation of *M. tuberculosis* by the conventional methods. Other methods used to identify *M. tuberculosis* are based on the chromatographic analysis of cell wall lipids:

high-performance liquid chromatography (HPLC), gas-liquid chromatography (GLC), or thin-layer chromatography. These methods not only help differentiate between *M. tuberculosis* and other mycobacteria but also expedite determination of the species of the nontuberculous mycobacteria. However, these methods usually require a substantial bacterial harvest from solid media that can hardly be achieved in the BACTEC medium. Preliminary identification of *M. tuberculosis* complex can be reported for most isolates within 2 weeks of receipt of the specimen when DNA-RNA hybridization is used with a culture grown in BACTEC 12B medium, whereas HPLC, thin-layer chromatography, or GLC assay may take 3 weeks or longer to report. Final identification of *M. tuberculosis* by a few biochemical tests requires 2 weeks or more. In the United States, the other members of the complex are rarely found in human specimens. BCG is usually isolated as the result of BCG vaccine treatment of malignant tumors. A patient's history, therefore, can be helpful in alerting the laboratory that the isolate may not be *M. tuberculosis*. *M. bovis* usually grows poorly on agar medium and produces dysgonic colonies on egg-based media, sometimes showing a wet surface rather than a dry one. The growth of *M. bovis* on 7H11 agar can be improved if the medium is prepared without glycerol and contains 0.4% pyruvate (Dixon and Guthbert, 1967). Despite the rare occurrence of other members of the complex in the United States, it is necessary to confirm, in most cases just for legal reasons, that an isolate indeed is *M. tuberculosis*. Practically, a laboratory report that the isolate belongs to the *M. tuberculosis* complex is sufficient to justify immediate public health measures and to start therapy, which can be adjusted later on those rare occasions when the isolate is *M. bovis*. Two weeks is a reasonable period for laboratory identification of *M. tuberculosis* complex if specimens have been submitted to a labo-

ratory that uses the BACTEC medium (among others) for primary isolation and is properly equipped to perform DNA-RNA hybridization with a BACTEC broth culture. Introduction of polymerase chain reaction (PCR) technology will shorten this period to a few days, but even now some additional procedures can help obtain, in very short periods, data indicating whether the growing culture is *M. tuberculosis* rather than one of the nontuberculous mycobacteria. One such tool is examination of a smear made from BACTEC broth of growth index (GI) greater than 200 to detect the cording typical of *M. tuberculosis* but not typical of other mycobacteria (except *M. kansasii*) (Fig. 2). However, the lack of cording does not necessarily exclude *M. tuberculosis*, since some strains may produce cords only after prolonged incubation. These data cannot be used for precise bacteriological diagnosis, but they can help in making decisions about necessary preventive and treatment measures.

Nontuberculous Mycobacteria

More than 25 mycobacterial species other than *M. tuberculosis* can be found in specimens from humans. It is not the aim of this chapter to address the features of these organisms or the methods of determining their species, descriptions of which can be found in special reviews (Roberts et al., 1991; Wolinsky, 1979; Woods and Washington, 1987). Though our goal is identification of *M. tuberculosis*, it is important to mention briefly some of the characteristics of the nontuberculous mycobacteria, because some of these species may have quite a high likelihood of being human pathogens. They include rapidly growing *M. fortuitum* and *M. chelonae* and slowly growing *M. kansasii*, *M. avium*, *M. intracellulare*, *M. scrofulaceum*, *M. xenopi*, *M. malmoense*, *M. simiae*, *M. szulgai*, *M. marinum*, *M. haemophilum*, and *M. ulcerans*. Pathogenicity for humans for some of the following bacteria is questionable: *M. gordonae*, *M. asiaticum*, *M. terrae*, *M. triviale*, *M. nonchromogenicum*, *M. gastri*, *M. flavescens*, and *M. phlei*. These species may be found in sputum specimens, except for *M. marinum*, *M. haemophilum*, and *M. ulcerans*, which are typical of specimens from skin lesions. Any of these species can be found in blood specimens obtained from HIV-infected individuals, although *M. avium* is most often isolated. Since *M. tuberculosis* can also be isolated from blood specimens, one must give special attention to the possibility of a mixed culture. The frequency of finding more than one mycobacterial species in sputum specimens from non-HIV patients is increasing as well. *M. tuberculosis* can be detected in mixed culture if special measures are taken. One of these measures is the use of 7H10 or 7H11 agar plates, along with other media (BACTEC, Lowenstein-Jensen), for primary isolation. These plates should be incubated at 37°C for at least 3 weeks even if the colonies of other mycobacteria, especially of rapidly growing mycobacteria, grow faster. Lowenstein-Jensen slants should be incubated up to 8 weeks, since some *M. tuberculosis* strains may grow very slowly and only on this medium, while the growth of some other mycobacterial species may be inhibited. In some cases, the mycobacteria may not have grown on any of the solid media yet the BACTEC broth may contain a mixed culture, including some nontuberculous mycobacteria that will overgrow *M. tuberculosis*. Therefore, if the growth is obtained only in BACTEC broth, a subculture on agar plates can be used to examine colonial morphology, growth rate, temperature preference, and chromogenicity, and it will provide a harvest for other characteristics.

Nucleic Acid Probes

The DNA probe most widely used in the United States for identification of *M. tuber-*

culosis complex is the commercially available AccuProbe (Gen-Probe, San Diego, Calif.). Tests with this probe are based on the ability of complementary nucleic acid strands to align and associate with bacterial RNA to form a stable, specific, double-stranded complex. The chemiluminescent acridinium ester-labeled single-stranded DNA probe is complementary to the rRNA of the target species, so that the association of the two strands forms a stable hybrid. Chemiluminescence is developed by the addition of hydrogen peroxide, and the response is measured in a luminometer (Arnold et al., 1989; Tenover, 1991). Other probes are available for identification of *M. avium*, *M. intracellulare*, *M. kansasii*, and *M. gordonae*. The manufacturer describes tests with cultures grown on solid media or in Middlebrook 7H9 broth. Obtaining cultures on solid media requires at least 3 weeks, and 7H9 broth is usually used for subculture but not for primary isolation. Therefore, strict adherence to the manufacturer's instruction does not allow truly rapid identification of *M. tuberculosis* despite the fact that the test itself can be completed in a few hours. A test of adequate sensitivity has not been developed with bacilli harvested in 12B BACTEC broth. However, based on our experience at National Jewish Center for Immunology and Respiratory Medicine in Denver, the following protocol is recommended for using the AccuProbe with BACTEC 12B broth cultures. The sensitivity of the test is very high with the *M. tuberculosis* complex probe but less so with the *M. avium* complex probe. Since the unknown isolates are usually tested with both probes, the procedure should be adjusted to decrease as much as possible the probability of false-negative results in *M. avium* complex isolates. Two measures should be implemented. First, the 12B broth cultures should be used when the GI is as high as possible. The best results have been achieved when the GI is greater than 500, and practically, we use the cultures when there are no more daily increases in GI. The best results with the *M. avium* probe were achieved when the growth reached a GI of 900 or greater. Second, centrifugation of the culture at 11,000 × *g* for 15 min increases the sensitivity of the test. For this purpose, we use a Beckman centrifuge (Microfuge 12) that has an aerosol containment rotor. After centrifugation of the culture (800 μl in a sterile 2.0-ml microcentrifuge tube [Sarstedt, Inc., Newton, N.C.]), the pellet is resuspended in 100 μl of the lysis reagent (reagent 1), after which 100 μl of the hybridization buffer (reagent 2) is added. Only 200 μl of the suspension is transferred to the lysing reagent tube containing glass beads. After the water is adjusted to 50°C, the recapped and vortexed tubes are placed in the sonicator bath for 15 min. The tubes are then placed in a heating block at 95°C for 10 min. These manipulations should result in the release of the RNA from the bacterial cells.

Hybridization takes place in the probe reagent tubes, to which 100 μl of the lysed specimen is added; tubes are then placed in a heating block or water bath at 60°C for 15 min. After incubation, 300 μl of the selection reagent (reagent 3) is added, and the recapped and vortexed tubes are placed at 60°C for 5 min. The tubes are cooled and cleaned before each is placed in the luminometer. Luminescence readings with the BACTEC cultures are lower than with cultures from other media. The manufacturer suggests that positive hybridization with cultures other than BACTEC produces 30,000 relative luminescence units (RLU) and a repeat range of 20,000 to 29,000 RLU when the Leader luminometer (Gen-Probe) is used. We found that 10,000 RLU can be safely used as a cutoff point for a positive result with the *M. tuberculosis* probe and BACTEC cultures. The repeat zone is 8,000 to 10,000 RLU, and negative and positive quality controls must give satisfactory results. Reliable results with the *M.*

avium complex probe can be obtained with a cutoff at 5,000 RLU.

Special attention should be given to the BACTEC cultures inoculated with blood specimens, even if such specimens were lysed and the bacterial contents were concentrated before inoculation. The BACTEC broth cultures inoculated with blood specimens processed for 12B medium or not processed but cultured in 13A medium always cause false-positive results in controls in the AccuProbe test. To prevent this, inoculate 0.1 ml of the original culture into a new 12B vial for subcultivation. Small amounts of blood still may cause false-positive results, so process these subcultures twice with sodium dodecyl sulfate (SDS). The first process consists of mixing 0.8 to 1.0 ml of the culture with 100 μl of 10% SDS solution containing 50 mM EDTA (pH 7.2). The second process is done with 1% SDS solution. After centrifugation in a microcentrifuge tube at 11,000 × *g* for 5 min, discard the supernatant, and resuspend the pellet in 0.8 ml of sterile distilled water. The next centrifugation at 11,000 × *g* for 15 min is the first step of the procedure described above for blood-free BACTEC broth cultures. An alternative to this procedure is to wait until the colonies on 7H11 agar plates, inoculated along with the 12B vials, are mature enough to be used for the AccuProbe test. Bacterial suspensions made from these colonies do not cause false-positive results if the blood specimens used to inoculate these plates were processed by blood cell lysis and centrifugation.

PCR

The details about PCR are given in chapter 30 of this volume, and therefore we have limited this paragraph to a few comments regarding the clinical application of this test. The PCR is based on hybridization between a particular region of the mycobacterial DNA or RNA and a single-stranded DNA probe (Eisenstein, 1990; Remic et al., 1990; chapter 30 of this volume). Though the principle of this reaction is the same as that of the RNA-DNA hybridization procedure described above, an important difference is that hybridization is performed after amplification of a particular segment of the bacterial DNA by PCR, a process of exponentially doubling the amount of targeted DNA. PCR as a diagnostic test for mycobacteria is currently being developed in various technological modifications, but to date none is fully standardized as a clinical laboratory test. The attraction of this approach is that PCR can detect just a few bacterial cells in a raw specimen, which means that a bacteriological (or rather, molecular) diagnosis of tuberculosis can be completed in a few days or perhaps hours after arrival of the specimen in the laboratory instead of in the 7 to 14 days required currently. Another advantage of this test is the possibility of diagnosis with specimens having a number of bacteria below the levels of sensitivity of culture methods. Will such a test, even standardized and fully automated, eliminate the necessity of cultivation? That is very unlikely, at least in the foreseeable future, because cultivation is necessary for monitoring the response to therapy, the conversion to bacillus-negative status at a level that should be much less sensitive than detection of a few DNA molecules in the specimen, and the changes in the drug susceptibility patterns of the patient's bacterial population.

BACTEC NAP Differentiation Test

The NAP test employs p-nitro-α-acetylamino-β-hydroxypropiophenone, which inhibits the growth of *M. tuberculosis* complex but does not inhibit growth of nontuberculous mycobacteria (Roberts et al., 1991). The test can be performed with the initial 12B broth culture when the growth reaches a daily GI reading of 50.

Three milliliters of 12B broth is removed from a new BACTEC vial, and 1.0 ml of the original culture is added. If the GI in the original vial is greater than 100, less medium is removed from the new vial to provide greater dilution of the culture: for a GI of 100 to 400, 2.8 ml is removed and replaced with 0.8 ml of the original culture; for a GI of 400 to 800, 2.6 ml is removed, and 0.6 ml of the culture is added; for a GI of >800, 2.2 ml is removed, and 0.2 ml of the culture is added. By this means, the final volume of bacterial suspension in the new vial is 2.0 ml, of which 1.0 ml should be transferred, after vortexing, into the NAP vial that contains a paper disk impregnated with 5 mg of the reagent. Both vials, with and without NAP, are incubated at 37°C for 4 to 5 days, and the daily GI is recorded. Substantial inhibition of growth in the NAP vial in comparison with clear GI increases in the NAP-free vial indicates the presence of *M. tuberculosis* complex. Substantial growth without any significant difference between vials indicates nontuberculous mycobacteria. These results are valid if positive and negative quality controls with *M. tuberculosis* and *M. avium* are performed simultaneously with the test and show expected results.

HPLC

HPLC uses a liquid mobile phase at high pressure to carry a sample through a column packed with particulate material or stationary phase, where the separation into components takes place (Butler and Kilburn, 1988; Butler et al., 1991; Susser and Wichman, 1991). Mycolic acids extracted from saponified mycobacterial cells are converted to the p-bromophenacyl esters, and the unique mycolic acid pattern associated with each species is detected by chromatographic separation of the esters. The method has been used for accurate (98.6%) identification of eight slowly growing mycobacterial species: *M. tuberculosis*,

M. bovis, M. kansasii, M. szulgai, M. gordonae, M. asiaticum, M. marinum, and *M. gastri* (Butler et al., 1991). The analysis is based on a comparison of retention time of the peaks and of their height ratios. Simplification of the method has made it feasible to examine a large number of cultures in one working day, but approximately 10^6 CFU are required to perform the test. However, HPLC is a "rapid, accurate and cost-effective alternative to the genetic probes and conventional biochemical tests" (Butler et al., 1991). There is no doubt that this method can be very helpful for identification of *M. kansasii, M. asiaticum, M. marinum, M. szulgai, M. gordonae, M. gastri,* and probably *M. avium* complex, as reported previously (Butler and Kilburn, 1988), as well as of some other species, pending further development of the appropriate standards. The question is whether this method can be considered a rapid alternative to the AccuProbe technique for identification of *M. tuberculosis*. To date, BACTEC cultures have not been used in HPLC, but the usual harvest of *M. tuberculosis* from 12B broth cultures may not be sufficient for this procedure even at their maximum level of growth. Preliminary data (Butler and Warren, 1993) suggest that the addition of oleic acid-albumin-dextrose-catalase (OADC) enrichment (Difco, Detroit, Mich.) to the BACTEC cultures when it attains a GI of 999 results in stimulation of growth and a harvest sufficient for HPLC analysis after 3 to 4 days of additional cultivation. The mycolic acid patterns are similar among the members of the *M. tuberculosis* complex (*M. tuberculosis, M. bovis, M. africanum, M. microti*) with one important exception: the pattern for BCG is quite different. This distinction cannot be made by the AccuProbe technique. Regarding species other than *M. tuberculosis*, HPLC techniques cannot distinguish between *M. avium* and *M. intracellulare*, but the AccuProbe method can do so if separate *M. avium* and *M. intracellulare* probes

are used. HPLC technology is an important addition to the mycobacteriology reference laboratory for better determination of the species of nontuberculous mycobacteria and BCG. It is also a possible alternative to the AccuProbe for rapid diagnosis of tuberculosis. Determination of the mycolic acid patterns is the primary step in identification of referred cultures at the CDC.

GLC

GLC uses gas (hydrogen) in the mobile phase and liquid in the stationary phase. The analysis of the microbial short-chain fatty acids (methyl esters) by GLC is based on the comparison of the retention time of the tested sample to the retention times of known standards. GLC analysis of the cell wall lipids for mycobacterial identification has been successfully used in several laboratories (Larsson et al., 1989; Maliwan et al., 1988; Tisdall et al., 1982) by employing a commercially available chromatograph and a computer (Hewlett-Packard Co., Palo Alto, Calif.). The software for this technology, the Microbial Identification System, is also commercially available (Microbial ID, Inc., Newark, Del.). The library of aerobic bacteria includes the cell wall lipid patterns of 26 or more mycobacterial species. Profiles of the tested cultures are compared with those in the library, and the results are presented by a computer-generated report giving the actual parameters of the chromatogram as well as percentages of probability that the isolate belongs to a certain species. This method can be a very important tool in better determination of the species of the nontuberculous mycobacteria, especially if it is used in conjunction with some conventional biochemical tests. The procedure requires about 60 mg of bacterial harvest obtained only from solid media after 3 to 6 weeks of cultivation. Bacterial harvest accumulated in the BACTEC 12B broth cultures is not sufficient for chromatographic analysis; therefore, the test cannot be performed in as short a turnaround time as the AccuProbe technique.

Conventional Tests

When the determination of *Mycobacterium* species is required after a preliminary report of *M. tuberculosis* complex, only a limited number of tests are necessary for differentiation from other species in the complex. *M. tuberculosis* colonies grow on 7H10 or 7H11 agar plates in 2 to 3 weeks during incubation at 35 to 37°C, while no growth appears at 25, 32, or 42°C. The buff-colored colonies are always nonpigmented and have a rough, dry surface and irregular edges; the colonies often have a wrinkled surface. It is typical to find serpentine cording in smears made from a broth culture (Fig. 2). A combination of the following four tests results may be used for final identification of *M. tuberculosis* and its differentiation from *M. bovis*: positive niacin production, positive nitrate reduction, resistance to 5 μg of thiophene-2-carboxylic acid hydrazide (TCH) per ml incorporated into 7H11 agar, and positive pyrazinamidase test. The results of these four tests are reversed for *M. bovis*. A negative heat-stable catalase test and production of a <45-mm column of foam in the room temperature catalase tests are also important for final identification, but they do not differentiate between *M. tuberculosis* and *M. bovis*. The niacin test can be negative for some *M. tuberculosis* strains, especially those resistant to isoniazid. The same applies to the nitrate reduction test. The pyrazinamidase test with *M. tuberculosis* can be negative if the patient has been treated with pyrazinamide (PZA) and resistance to this agent has developed. In addition, false-negative results with any of these tests may appear owing to the quite common deviation from the prescribed technique.

Niacin test

Formerly the niacin test was relied upon for identification of *M. tuberculosis* (Konno, 1956; Runyon et al., 1959), but rapid methods have greatly diminished its value. It should be recognized that the niacin test can be positive with some mycobacterial species other than *M. tuberculosis*, such as *M. simiae*, some BCG strains, and some rapidly growing mycobacteria. Many laboratories use 3- to 4-week-old cultures grown on Middlebrook 7H10 or 7H11 agar, and the test works well in most cases. However, some *M. tuberculosis* strains do not produce sufficient niacin on this medium for detection. The frequency of these false-negative results can be decreased if the agar medium is enriched with L-asparagine (0.25%) or its potassium salt (0.1%) (Kilburn et al., 1968). False-negative results can be almost completely eliminated by using 6-week-old or older cultures on Lowenstein-Jensen medium containing L-asparagine, but more than 50 well-grown colonies must be present. Therefore, a slant of Lowenstein-Jensen medium inoculated with the raw specimen, along with other media, can serve as a backup if results with the agar-grown culture after 3 weeks of cultivation are negative. The presence of some contaminants in the culture may cause false-positive results; therefore, it is necessary to confirm the purity of the culture by examining a smear stained by the Ziehl-Nielson method.

The test is based on detection of niacin in the medium, not in the bacteria. Therefore, in cases of confluent growth that may prevent the extraction of niacin, it is necessary to pierce through the bacterial growth with a pipette to expose the medium. To extract niacin, place sterile distilled water or saline on the surface of the medium for 30 min or longer (up to 2 h) at room temperature. Incubation at 37°C can improve the extraction, but the amount of fluid placed on the medium should be sufficient to compensate for evaporation. Transfer the extract (0.6 ml) to a screw-cap tube. Most laboratories in the United States use commercially available paper strips (Kilburn and Kubica, 1968; Young et al., 1970). Insert the niacin strip into the tube containing the extract, with the end of the strip, indicated by an arrow, immersed in the fluid. Tighten the cap, and leave the tube at room temperature for 20 min. The test is positive if the liquid turns yellow. Use an *M. tuberculosis* laboratory strain for a positive quality control and an *M. avium* strain for a negative control.

Nitrate reduction test

The second most important test for identifying *M. tuberculosis*, and particularly for differentiating it from *M. bovis* if the isolate already has been identified as *M. tuberculosis* complex, is the nitrate reduction test (Virtanen, 1960). Besides *M. tuberculosis*, other species (*M. kansasii*, *M. szulgai*, *M. flavescens*, *M. fortuitum*, *M. terrae*, *M. triviale*, *M. phlei*, *M. smegmatis*, and *M. vaccae*) produce nitrate reductase. The test is negative with *M. bovis*, but it can be weakly positive with some BCG strains. Like the niacin test, the best results can be obtained with a culture grown on egg-based medium at least 4 weeks old, but it can be done with a culture on agar medium if the growth is sufficient. Two techniques are commonly used: one with liquid reagents and another with commercially available paper strips (Quigley and Elston, 1970). For either of these techniques, make a heavy bacterial suspension in 0.2 ml of distilled water or 7H9 broth in a 13- by 100-mm screw-cap tube or in 0.5 ml of the same in a 16- by 125-mm tube. Perform the test after adding 2.0 ml of a 0.01 M sodium nitrate solution made in phosphate buffer (pH 7.0) to the tube and incubating it in a 37°C water bath for 2 h. Add the following three reagents in order: 1 drop of hydrochloric acid solution (made by adding concentrated HCl

to an equal volume of distilled water), 2 drops of a 0.2% aqueous solution of sulfanilamide, and 2 drops of a 0.1% aqueous solution of *N*-naphthylethylenediamine dihydrochloride. Color development with *N*-naphthylethylenediamine ranges from pale pink (±) to deep red (++++) and should be compared with color plate standards and with the reactions of three quality controls (positive *M. tuberculosis*, negative *M. avium*, inoculated reagent control). Color graded as +++ or greater indicates a positive nitrate reduction test. Additional quality controls can be used if there are any doubts about the correctness of the negative results. A pinch of zinc dust should result in the appearance of a red color, indicating the presence of unreacted nitrate and confirming that the negative reading was valid. If color does not develop, repeat the test. False-negative results may occur if the culture was too old, the inoculum was insufficient, or the reagents were not active or were added in the wrong sequence.

The Difco nitrate paper strip, when used instead of liquid reagents, is inserted arrow down into the tube containing the bacterial suspension, avoiding contact with fluid on the side of the tube. After a 2-h incubation at 37°C in a vertical position, tilt the tube several times to wet the entire strip. After 10 min, the appearance of a blue area at the top of the strip indicates a positive reaction. Other nitrate reduction tests have been described elsewhere (Kubica, 1964; Warren et al., 1983), some of them as a combined niacin-nitrate test. Use a drug-susceptible *M. tuberculosis* strain as a positive quality control and *M. bovis* or *M. avium* as a negative control.

Pyrazinamidase test

The pyrazinamidase test detects the presence of the enzyme that converts PZA to pyrazinoic acid (Wayne, 1974). Pyrazinamidase can be found in cultures of *M. tuber-*

culosis strains susceptible to PZA, but PZA-resistant *M. tuberculosis* strains do not possess detectable amounts of the enzyme. All *M. bovis* strains including BCG are resistant to PZA; therefore, this drug is not used in therapy for *M. bovis* infection, and the organism shows negative results in the pyrazinamidase test. This test, as well as the PZA susceptibility test (described in another section of this chapter), is useful for differentiation between *M. tuberculosis* and *M. bovis*. Positive results confirm *M. tuberculosis*, while a negative test indicates *M. bovis*. One must be alert to negative reactions with *M. tuberculosis* strains resistant to PZA that were isolated from patients previously treated with this drug. *M. africanum* is susceptible to PZA and is positive in the pyrazinamidase test. All nontuberculous mycobacteria are resistant to PZA, but some of them are pyrazinamidase positive (*M. marinum*, *M. avium*, *M. intracellulare*, *M. xenopi*, *M. malmoense*, *M. flavescens*), and some are negative (*M. kansasii*, *M. simiae*, *M. szulgai*, *M. gastri*). Therefore, this test can be used for differentiation between some of these species, for example, between *M. kansasii* and *M. marinum*.

For differentiation between *M. tuberculosis* and *M. bovis*, the test is performed after 4 days of incubation at 37°C of a special semisolid agar medium heavily inoculated with a bacterial harvest scraped from the surface of a culture on solid media. The inoculum should be visible to the naked eye. The PZA medium contains (per liter of distilled water) 6.5 g of Dubo broth base, 2.0 g of sodium salt of pyruvic acid, 0.1 g of PZA, and 15.0 g of agar. After the ingredients have been dissolved and autoclaved, dispense the medium in screw-cap tubes (16 by 125 mm), and allow it to harden in an upright position to form a butt. Inoculate the butt, and add 1.0 ml of a 1% ferrous ammonium sulfate solution to each tube after 4 days of incubation. Examine the reaction after 30 min, and if negative, examine the tubes again after 4 h of refrig-

eration. A positive reaction is indicated by a pink band in the subsurface of the agar medium. Usually, two tubes of PZA medium are inoculated with an unknown culture. If the first is negative at 4 days, incubate the other tube for 3 more days and use it to identify the species of nontuberculous mycobacteria. Use a drug-susceptible *M. tuberculosis* strain as a positive control and an *M. bovis* strain as a negative control.

TCH

The test for susceptibility to TCH (Bönicke, 1958; Vestal and Kubica, 1967) is especially useful for differentiation between *M. bovis* and multidrug-resistant strains of *M. tuberculosis*, since these strains can produce negative results in the three other differentiation tests described above. Only *M. bovis* strains (including BCG) are susceptible to 1.0 and 5.0 µg of TCH per ml incorporated into Middlebrook 7H10 or 7H11 agar medium. This test is performed in the same way as an indirect susceptibility test, and all mycobacterial species other than *M. bovis* produce growth in the presence of TCH that greatly exceeds the required 1% in comparison with that in the drug-free medium. Some strains of *M. bovis* may produce minimal growth in the presence of 1.0 µg of TCH per ml, but no growth appears in the presence of 5.0 µg/ml. Use an *M. tuberculosis* strain as a positive control and *M. bovis* as a negative control.

Heat-stable catalase test

The heat-stable (68°C) catalase test (at pH 7.0) aids in identification of *M. tuberculosis* complex (Kent and Kubica, 1985), but it has no role in differentiating *M. tuberculosis* from *M. bovis*, since both species produce negative results. The test is also negative for *M. gastri* and *M. malmoense* and is useful for differentiating between these species and other slowly growing nonchromogenic mycobacteria. When the isolate is identified as *M. tuberculosis* complex by one of the rapid methods, the differentiation between members of the complex can be limited to the four other biochemical tests described above.

DRUG SUSCEPTIBILITY TESTING FOR DETECTION OF INITIAL AND ACQUIRED DRUG RESISTANCE

The following is a description of procedures and interpretations for tests as conducted in the Mycobacteriology Laboratory at National Jewish Center for Immunology and Respiratory Medicine in Denver. For other approaches, see detailed descriptions in publications specifically devoted to the drug susceptibility testing of mycobacteria (Hawkins, 1984; Heifets, 1991; Kent and Kubica, 1985; Sommers and Good, 1985).

Definitions

Drug-susceptible strains of *M. tuberculosis* (wild strains) are those that have been isolated from patients before treatment and that contain less than 1% of the bacterial population resistant to any of the antituberculosis drugs. For *M. tuberculosis*, all wild strains that have never come into contact with the antituberculosis agent have a uniform degree of susceptibility, showing narrow ranges of MICs. At the same time, the wild strains always contain some spontaneous resistant mutants, and their frequencies range from 10^{-7} to 10^{-11} for different drugs. Mutations for resistance to each drug are independent, and the frequency of a mutant resistant to two drugs is the multiple of the frequencies determined for each, usually ranging from 10^{-14} to 10^{-20}. The probability of having triple and quadruple mutatants is even smaller. Monotherapy for tuberculosis leads to the selective multiplication of the corresponding resistant mutants. This realization led to the establishment of the multiple-drug regimens as a basic principle

of tuberculosis therapy in preventing the emergence of drug resistance.

A resistant *M. tuberculosis* strain is usually defined as one that differs significantly from wild strains in its degree of susceptibility because of the increased proportion of resistant mutants. The proportion of the bacterial population resistant to a so-called critical concentration of drug can be determined by the proportion method of drug susceptibility testing, which is described below. The critical concentrations are usually those that are significantly higher than the highest MICs found for wild strains, and they are different for different culture media. By United States standards for most of the drugs (Bailey et al., 1984; David, 1971; Hawkins, 1984; Heifets, 1991; Kent and Kubica, 1985; Sommers and Mc-Clatchy, 1983; Sommers and Good, 1985; Vestal, 1977), a strain is considered resistant if the proportion of mutants is 1% or greater, which indicates that their presence in the patient's bacterial population has increased 10^7-fold or more. For PZA the accepted cutoff is 10%. It is assumed that a diminished clinical response may occur if the patient is treated with the drug to which resistance has been demonstrated in the laboratory.

A multidrug-resistant *M. tuberculosis* strain is currently defined as one resistant to two or more antituberculosis drugs. The emergence of such strains is a result of insufficient or inappropriate chemotherapy associated with either noncompliance by the patient or administration of inadequate drug regimens. Sometimes it is caused by the malabsorption of medications by patients who are malnourished or immunocompromised. In a typical scenario of an inadequate regimen, no attempts have been made to determine the drug susceptibility or resistance of the initial pretreatment isolate, changes in the failing regimen were made without monitoring changes in drug susceptibility, and only one drug was added to a failing regimen, often with no drug susceptibility tests being done.

Acquired resistance to one or several drugs emerges during therapy because of selective multiplication of resistant mutants. Initial (or primary) drug resistance is not associated with the emergence of resistance during therapy but is the result of infection with a resistant strain from another patient. Detection of initial drug resistance in a pretreatment isolate from a patient with newly diagnosed tuberculosis is essential for proper and timely adjustment of initial therapy. Previously, such testing was not mandatory (American Thoracic Society, 1974; Bass et al., 1990), but recently, CDC has changed the official policy, and now it is recommended that the pretreatment isolates from all patients be tested (Tenover et al., 1993). Systematic monitoring of the susceptibility of strains isolated during the course of therapy detects emerging acquired drug resistance and allows appropriate and timely changes in the drug regimen.

Principles of Detection of Drug Resistance

There are two basic approaches to drug susceptibility testing of *M. tuberculosis*, the direct and the indirect methods. In the direct test, the drug-containing media are directly inoculated with the patient's smear-positive specimen. The indirect test is performed with a bacterial suspension made from a pure culture. Most patients with pulmonary tuberculosis have a substantial number of AFB in their sputum when they first appear in the physician's office. Therefore, it is quite feasible to rely on the direct susceptibility test at the time of the initial diagnosis of tuberculosis. The greatest advantage of the direct test over the indirect is the turnaround time. With the direct test, the results can be anticipated within the time necessary for isolation: 3 weeks for almost all new strains isolated on 7H10 or 7H11 agar plates. The

indirect test requires initial isolation followed by preparation of a bacterial suspension (or a broth subculture) to inoculate the drug-containing media. The indirect test requires 6 to 7 weeks when both isolation and the test itself are done on 7H10 or 7H11 agar medium, and the time can be shortened to 4 to 5 weeks if the test itself is performed on agar plates but the inoculum is prepared from a BACTEC 12B broth culture. Finally, if the indirect test is performed in the BACTEC 12B broth from a culture also grown in 12B broth, the turnaround time can be shortened to 3 to 4 weeks. The only advantage of the indirect test is that it allows more accurate calibration of the inoculum size than the direct test. Some results of the direct test may not be valid because of overinoculation or, more often, insufficient growth on the drug-free medium. Excess contamination may also invalidate the results of a direct test.

The strategy in selection of the direct or indirect test and the medium used depends on the type of patients, the specimen sources, and the bacterial contents of the specimens. The direct test on agar plates should be set up for all AFB smear-positive specimens. The 7H11 agar is preferred over 7H10 at the Mycobacteriology Laboratory at National Jewish Center for Immunology and Respiratory Medicine because it promotes better growth, especially of the drug-resistant strains. Experience in this laboratory has shown that the direct test on 7H11 agar plates can provide valid results in 95% of the smear-positive sputum specimens. We perform the direct test with 10 drugs, as described below. This gives a more complete picture of the drug susceptibility pattern of the isolate than a test with first-line drugs only. The difference in cost of testing 10 drugs versus 3 or 4 drugs is minimal, and such an approach can, in fact, be cost-effective if resistance to one or more first-line drugs means that the test would have to be repeated with the second-line drugs. The indirect test is performed on cultures isolated from smear-negative specimens or in cases of failure of the direct test (about 5% of the smear-positive specimens). The necessity of an indirect test can be decided in most cases after 2 weeks of cultivation of the direct-test plates. Although about half of the results of the direct test are not reportable at 2 weeks, examination of the plates with a dissecting microscope can indicate whether the direct test may not be valid. The inoculum for the indirect test may be taken from any of the media (12B broth, 7H11 plain or selective agar, Lowenstein-Jensen) that had been inoculated simultaneously with the direct test plates. However, when failure of the direct test is determined after 2 weeks of incubation, 12B culture may be the only source available at this point. The indirect test can be set up on 7H11 agar plates or in the BACTEC 12B broth vials.

At the 4-week turnaround time, additional susceptibility information can be obtained on two more drugs that are not included in the direct test: PZA and ofloxacin. The only currently reliable method for assessing susceptibility to these drugs is determination of their MICs in 12B broth, as described below. These are indirect tests for which the original isolate in 12B broth can be used as an inoculum.

Overall, the strategy described above provides information on susceptibility to 12 drugs within 4 weeks from the time of arrival of the raw specimen. The methods briefly described below are only those pertinent to the optimal protocol suggested in this chapter. Detailed descriptions of other methods can be found in a recently published monograph on drug susceptibility (Heifets, 1991).

Direct or Indirect Test on 7H11 Agar Plates by the Proportion Method

The agar medium for the proportion drug susceptibility test incorporates critical concentrations (in micrograms per milliliter) of isoniazid, 0.2 and 1.0; rifampin, 1.0; ethambutol, 7.5; streptomycin, 2.0; kanamycin, 6.0; amikacin, 4.0; capreomycin, 10.0; ethionamide, 10.0; p-amino salicylate, 8.0; and D-cycloserine, 30.0. On the basis of experience in our laboratory, we include some additional higher concentrations to ensure the reliability of the test or to determine the degree of resistance in more detail. More information regarding preparation of the medium and the drug solutions is given in the CDC manual (Kent and Kubica, 1985). The medium is made from commercially available 7H10 agar base. The powder is suspended in distilled water with 5 ml of glycerol added per 1,000 ml of medium, autoclaved at 121°C for 10 min, and cooled to 50 to 52°C in a water bath. The appropriate drug solutions and OADC (10% of the total volume) are added, and the medium (about 5.0 ml per quadrant) is dispensed into three of the four compartments of the quadrant plastic plates. The fourth compartment contains drug-free control. After overnight incubation at 37°C to dry the surface and for sterility control, the plates are stored in the refrigerator in brown paper bags to protect them from light; they must be used within 4 weeks of preparation. For the direct test, the concentrated decontaminated specimen is inoculated undiluted and diluted 10^{-2} if the smear contains less than 1 AFB per field under 1,000× magnification. When a very low number of AFB are seen on the smear, 0.2 ml per quadrant can be used to ensure a sufficient inoculum. Specimens containing 1 to 10 AFB per field should be inoculated with 10^{-1} and 10^{-3} dilutions, and those having more than 10 AFB per field should be diluted 10^{-2} and 10^{-4} before inoculation. This approach can be modified according to the experience of each laboratory.

The indirect test can be performed with a bacterial suspension made from growth on solid media and adjusted to the optical density of McFarland standard no. 1. Two dilutions of this suspension, 10^{-2} and 10^{-4}

or 10^{-3} and 10^{-5}, are used to inoculate respective sets of plates. When BACTEC 12B broth cultures are the source of inoculum, dilutions of 10^{-2} and 10^{-4} can be used when the daily GI reaches 800 or higher.

The inoculated plates are incubated for 3 weeks at 37°C in an atmosphere of 5 to 10% CO_2. The results can be reported in 2 weeks if they show that the strain is resistant. The percentage of resistant bacteria in the population is reported on the basis of comparison of the number of CFU on drug-containing and drug-free quadrants. For quality control, one drug-susceptible strain and one multidrug-resistant *M. tuberculosis* strain are included. More details on these techniques can be found in the CDC manual (Kent and Kubica, 1985).

BACTEC Indirect Qualitative Test in 12B Broth

The BACTEC indirect qualitative test in 12B broth is performed with the following critical concentrations (in micrograms per milliliter): isoniazid, 0.1; rifampin, 0.5; ethambutol, 4.0; streptomycin, 4.0; kanamycin, 5.0; amikacin, 4.0; capreomycin, 5.0; ethionamide, 2.5 (Heifets, 1991). Susceptibility of *M. tuberculosis* to cycloserine cannot be tested in 12B broth (Heifets, 1991). The original 12B culture can be used undiluted as an inoculum (0.1 ml per vial) if the GI is between 300 and 800. Two drug-free controls are necessary: one vial inoculated with the same suspension as for the drug-containing vials and one with a 1:100 dilution. The vials are incubated at 36 ± 1°C for a minimum of 4 days and a maximum of 12 days and are read daily in the BACTEC instrument. In the first 2 days, no growth should appear in the diluted control, while the daily GI reading in drug-containing vials can be as high as that in the undiluted control (usually less than 200, and it should not exceed 300). In the subsequent period, the daily GIs in drug-free controls grow substantially. In the presence of a drug to

which the strain is resistant, the increase in daily GI readings can be faster than in the diluted 1:100 control. The daily GI readings in the presence of drugs to which the strain is susceptible remain the same or decrease. The strain is considered resistant if the daily increase in GI in a drug-containing vial is greater than that in the 1:100 control. This relationship should be evaluated after the GI in the 1:100 control reaches 30, which should occur no sooner than after 4 days of incubation if the inoculum did not exceed the established limits. More details about this method were given in a review published recently (Heifets, 1991).

Quantitative BACTEC Test for Determining MICs

The quantitative BACTEC test for determining MICs can be especially useful in evaluating new drugs for which no critical concentrations have been established. The susceptibility to conventional drugs can also be expressed quantitatively as MICs. This alternative to the qualitative BACTEC test can be considered for clinical trials and in resolving conflicting reports of the susceptibility of multidrug-resistant strains.

Unlike in the qualitative test described above, a minimum of three concentrations of each drug is necessary for MIC determination; the lowest among them is the highest MIC found in our studies for wild strains (Heifets, 1991). The tested strain is considered susceptible if the MIC is equal to or less than this concentration. The cutoff point for resistance is a concentration that is equal to or higher than the maximum concentration attainable in humans, which is the highest concentration included in the procedure. A concentration in the intermediate position detects moderately susceptible strains. The following concentrations (in micrograms per milliliter) have been developed for MIC determination with *M. tuberculosis* strains (Heifets, 1991): isoniazid, 0.1, 0.5, 2.5; rifampin, 0.5, 2.0, 8.0;

ethambutol, 2.0, 4.0, 8.0; streptomycin, 2.0, 4.0, 8.0; kanamycin, 2.0, 4.0, 8.0; amikacin, 2.0, 4.0, 8.0; capreomycin, 2.5, 5.0, 10.0; ethionamide, 1.0, 2.0, 4.0; ofloxacin, 2.0, 4.0, 8.0; and rifabutin, 0.12, 0.25, 0.5.

Inclusion of more than one concentration helps avoid misinterpretation in cases of the permissible twofold drug dilution errors. The test is performed by a technique similar to the qualitative method. The MIC is defined as the lowest drug concentration in the presence of which no increase in the daily GI takes place, while in the 1:100 control the daily increases above a GI of 30 are observed for a minimum of three consecutive days of cultivation. The radiometric technique for determining the MIC as the lowest drug concentration inhibiting more than 99% of the bacterial population was validated by a parallel determination of the number of viable bacteria in the same 12B broth (Heifets, 1991).

PZA MIC Determination

The MIC of PZA can be determined in 12B broth in which the pH has been adjusted to 6.0. This drug has high sterilizing activity against the portion of the patient's bacterial population that persists in the acidic environment (pH 5.0) of the early acute inflammation sites and within the phagolysosomes of macrophages. The bacteria can be affected if they are susceptible to the concentration of PZA achievable in these sites (usually less than 25.0 μg/ml). *M. tuberculosis* strains do not grow in vitro at pH 5.0. Therefore, it is very hard to determine susceptibility to 25.0 μg of PZA per ml under these conditions. At pH 6.0, *M. tuberculosis* strains grow well, but the drug concentration required to inhibit growth of the susceptible strains is three to five times greater than that at pH 5.0 (Salfinger and Heifets, 1988). Therefore, at pH 6.0, the suggested breakpoint for susceptible is 100.0 μg/ml. The PZA-resistant strains are those for which the MIC is equal to or greater than 900.0 μg/ml. Strains for which the MIC is 300.0 μg/ml are in the transient phase of becoming resistant, and we call them moderately susceptible (Heifets, 1991). Using three concentrations instead of one for determining susceptibility to PZA avoids misinterpretation when the strain is in this intermediate position. In this test, dilution of the two drug-free controls is different from that in the MIC determination with other drugs: they are diluted 1:10 instead of 1:100, which is the basis for determining the MIC as the lowest concentration that inhibits more than 90% of the bacterial population. The radiometrically determined MIC is the lowest PZA concentration in the presence of which there is practically no daily increase in GI, while a substantial increase in the 1:10 control takes place within three consecutive days (starting after a GI of 30 is reached). At the end of the observation, the GI in this control is usually greater than that in the presence of the concentration considered the MIC. The test requires 6 to 12 days.

REFERENCES

American Thoracic Society. 1974. Policy statement: quality of the laboratory for mycobacterial disease. *Am. Rev. Respir. Dis.* **110:**376–377.

Arnold, L. J., P. W. Hammond, W. A. Wiese, and N. C. Nelson. 1989. Assay formats involving acridinium-ester-labeled DNA probes. *Clin. Chem.* **35:** 1588–1594.

Bailey, W. C., J. B. Bass, J. E. Hawkins, G. P. Kubica, and R. J. Wallace. 1984. Drug susceptibility testing for mycobacteria. *Am. Thorac. Soc. News* **Winter:** 9–10.

Bass, J. B., L. S. Farer, P. C. Hopewell, R. F. Jacobs, and D. E. Snider. 1990. Diagnostic standards and classification of tuberculosis (joint statement of ATS and CDC). *Am. Rev. Respir. Dis.* **142:**725–735.

Bönicke, R. 1958. Die Differenzierung humaner und boviner Tuberkelterien mit Hilfe von Thiophen-2-carbonsaure-hydrazid. *Naturwissenschaften* **46:**329–393.

Butler, W. R., K. C. Jost, and J. O. Kilburn. 1991. Identification of mycobacteria by high-performance liquid chromatography. *J. Clin. Microbiol.* **29:**2468–2472.

Butler, W. R., and J. O. Kilburn. 1988. Identification of major slowly growing pathogenic mycobacteria and *Mycobacterium gordonae* by high-performance liquid chromatography of their mycolic acids. *J. Clin. Microbiol.* 26:50–53.

Butler, W. R., and N. Warren. 1993. Personal communication.

Cohn, M. L., R. F. Waggoner, and J. K. McClatchy. 1968. The 7H11 medium for the culture of mycobacteria. *Am. Rev. Respir. Dis.* 98:295–296.

David, H. L. 1971. Fundamentals of drug susceptibility testing in tuberculosis. U.S. Department of Health, Education, and Welfare publication no. 00-2165. Center for Disease Control, Atlanta.

Dixon, J. M. S., and E. H. Guthbert. 1967. Isolation of tubercle bacilli from uncentrifuged sputum on pyruvic acid medium. *Am. Rev. Respir. Dis.* 96:119–127.

Eisenstein, B. I. 1990. The polymerase chain reaction: a new method of using molecular genetics for medical diagnosis. *N. Engl. J. Med.* 322:178–183.

Harrington, J. M., and H. S. Shannon. 1976. Incidence of tuberculosis, hepatitis, brucellosis, and shigellosis in British medical laboratory workers. *Br. Med. J.* 1:759–762.

Hawkins, J. E. 1984. Drug susceptibility testing, p. 177–193. *In* G. P. Kubica and L. G. Wayne (ed.), *The Mycobacteria: a Sourcebook.* Marcel Dekker, Inc., New York.

Heifets, L. B. (ed.). 1991. *Drug Susceptibility in the Chemotherapy of Mycobacterial Infections.* CRC Press, Boca Raton, Fla.

Isenberg, H. D., R. F. D'Amato, L. Heifets, et al. 1991. Collaborative feasibility study of biphasic media systems (Roche Septi-Chek AFB) for the rapid detection and isolation of mycobacteria. *J. Clin. Microbiol.* 29:1719–1722.

Kent, P. T., and G. P. Kubica. 1985. *Public Health Mycobacteriology: a Guide for the Level III Laboratory.* Centers for Disease Control, Atlanta.

Kilburn, J. O., and G. P. Kubica. 1968. Reagent impregnated paper strips for detection of niacin. *Am. J. Clin. Pathol.* 50:530–532.

Kilburn, J. O., K. D. Stottmeier, and G. P. Kubica. 1968. Aspartic acid as a precursor for niacin synthesis by tubercle bacilli grown on 7H11 agar medium. *Am. J. Clin. Pathol.* 50:582–586.

Konno, K. 1956. New chemical method to differentiate human-type tubercle bacilli from other mycobacteria. *Science* 124:985.

Kubica, G. P. 1964. A combined niacin-nitrate reduction test for use in the identification of mycobacteria. *Acta Tuberc. Pneumol. Scand.* 45:161–167.

Kubica, G. P., W. E. Dye, M. L. Cohn, and G. Middlebrook. 1963. Sputum digestion and decontamination with *N*-acetyl-L-cysteine-sodium hydroxide for culture of mycobacteria. *Am. Rev. Respir. Dis.* 87:775–779.

Kubica, G. P., W. Gross, J. E. Hawkins, H. M. Sommers, A. L. Vestal, and L. G. Wayne. 1975. Laboratory services for mycobacterial diseases. *Am. Rev. Respir. Dis.* 112:773–787.

Kubica, G. P., A. J. Kaufmann, and W. E. Dye. 1964. Comments on the use of the new mycolytic agent, *N*-acetyl-L-cysteine, as a sputum digestant for the isolation of mycobacteria. *Am. Rev. Respir. Dis.* 89:284–286.

Larsson, L., J. Jiminez, A. Sonesson, and F. Portaels. 1989. Two-dimensional gas chromatography with electron capture detection for the sensitive determination of specific mycobacterial lipid constituents. *J. Clin. Microbiol.* 27:2230–2231.

Maliwan, N. R., W. Reid, S. R. Pliska, T. J. Bird, and J. R. Zvetina. 1988. Identifying *Mycobacterium tuberculosis* cultures by gas-liquid chromatography and a computer-aided pattern recognition model. *J. Clin. Microbiol.* 26:182–187.

McClatchy, J. K., R. F. Waggoner, W. Kanes, M. S. Arnick, and T. L. Bolton. 1976. Isolation of mycobacteria from clinical specimens by use of a selective 7H11 medium. *Am. J. Clin. Pathol.* 65:412–415.

Middlebrook, G., and M. L. Cohn. 1958. Bacteriology of tuberculosis: laboratory methods. *Am. J. Public Health* 48:844–853.

Middlebrook, G., M. L. Cohn, W. E. Dye, W. F. Russell, Jr., and D. Levy. 1960. Microbiologic procedures of value in tuberculosis. *Acta Tuberc. Scand.* 38:66–81.

Middlebrook, G., Z. Riggiardo, and W. D. Tigertt. 1977. Automatable radiometric detection of growth of *M. tuberculosis* in selective media. *Am. Rev. Respir. Dis.* 115:1066–1069.

Nash, P., and M. M. Krenz. 1991. Culture media, p. 1226–1228. *In* A. Balows, W. J. Hausler, Jr., K. L. Herrmann, H. D. Isenberg, and H. J. Shadomy (ed.), *Manual of Clinical Microbiology,* 5th ed. American Society for Microbiology, Washington, D.C.

Pike, R. M. 1976. Laboratory-associated infections: summary and analysis of 3,921 cases. *Health Lab. Sci.* 13:105–114.

Pike, R. M., S. E. Sulkin, and M. L. Schulze. 1965. Continuing importance of laboratory-acquired infections. *Am. J. Public Health* 55:190–199.

Quigley, H. S., and H. R. Elston. 1970. Nitrite strips for detection of nitrate reduction by mycobacteria. *Am. J. Clin. Pathol.* 53:663–665.

Reid, D. D. 1957. Incidence of tuberculosis among workers in medical laboratories. *Br. Med. J.* 2:10–14.

Remic, D. G., S. L. Kunkel, E. A. Holbrook, and C. A. Hanson. 1990. Theory and applications of the polymerase chain reaction. *Am. J. Clin. Pathol.* 93:S49–S54.

Richmond, J. Y., and R. W. McKinney (ed.). 1993.

Biosafety in microbiological and biomedical laboratories, 3rd ed. Health and Human Services publication no. (CDC) 93-8395. U.S. Government Printing Office, Washington, D.C.

Roberts, G. D., E. W. Koneman, and Y. K. Kim. 1991. *Mycobacterium*, p. 304–339. *In* A. Balows, W. J. Hausler, Jr., K. L. Herrmann, H. D. Isenberg, and H. J. Shadomy (ed.), *Manual of Clinical Microbiology*, 5th ed. American Society for Microbiology, Washington, D.C.

Runyon, E. H., M. J. Selin, and H. W. Harris. 1959. Distinguishing mycobacteria by the niacin test. *Am. Rev. Tuberc.* **79**:663–665.

Salfinger, M., and L. B. Heifets. 1988. Determination of pyrazinamide MICs for *Mycobacterium tuberculosis* at different pHs by the radiometric method. *Antimicrob. Agents Chemother.* **32**:1002–1004.

Skinholj, P. 1974. Occupational risks in Danish clinical chemical laboratories. II. Infections. *Scand. J. Clin. Lab. Invest.* **33**:27–29.

Smithwick, R. W. 1976. *Laboratory Manual for Acid-Fast Microscopy.* Center for Disease Control, Atlanta.

Sommers, H. M., and R. C. Good. 1985. *Mycobacterium*, p. 216–248. *In* E. H. Lennette, A. Balows, W. J. Hausler, Jr., and H. J. Shadomy (ed.), *Manual of Clinical Microbiology*, 4th ed. American Society for Microbiology, Washington, D.C.

Sommers, H. M., and J. K. McClatchy. 1983. *Cumitech 16, Laboratory Diagnosis of the Mycobacterioses.* Coordinating ed., J. A. Morello. American Society for Microbiology, Washington, D.C.

Susser, M., and M. D. Wichman. 1991. Identification of microorganisms through use of gas chromatography and high-performance liquid chromatography, p. 111–118. *In* A. Balows, W. J. Hausler, Jr., K. L. Herrmann, H. D. Isenberg, and H. J. Shadomy (ed.), *Manual of Clinical Microbiology*, 5th ed. American Society for Microbiology, Washington, D.C.

Tenover, F. C. 1991. Molecular methods for the clinical microbiology laboratory, p. 119–127. *In* A. Balows, W. J. Hausler, Jr., K. L. Herrmann, H. D.

Isenberg, and H. J. Shadomy (ed.), *Manual of Clinical Microbiology*, 5th ed. American Society for Microbiology, Washington, D.C.

Tenover, F. C., J. T. Crawford, R. E. Heubner, L. J. Geiter, C. R. Horsburgh, and R. C. Good. 1993. The resurgence of tuberculosis: is your laboratory ready? *J. Clin. Microbiol.* **31**:767–770.

Tisdall, P. A., D. R. DeYoung, G. D. Roberts, and J. P. Anhalt. 1982. Identification of clinical isolates of mycobacteria with gas-liquid chromatography: a 10-month follow-up study. *J. Clin. Microbiol.* **16**:400–402.

Vestal, A. L. 1977. Procedures for the isolation and identification of mycobacteria. U.S. Department of Health, Education, and Welfare publication no. (CDC) 77:8320-115. Center for Disease Control, Atlanta.

Vestal, A. L., and G. P. Kubica. 1967. Differential identification of mycobacteria. III. Use of thiacetazone, thiophen-2-carboxylic acid hydrazide and triphenyltetrazolium chloride. *Scand. J. Respir. Dis.* **48**:142–148.

Virtanen, S. 1960. A study of nitrate reduction by mycobacteria. *Acta Tuberc. Scand. Suppl.* **48**:1–119.

Warren, N. G., B. A. Body, and H. P. Dalton. 1983. An improved reagent for mycobacterial nitrate reductase tests. *J. Clin. Microbiol.* **18**:546–549.

Wayne, L. G. 1974. Simple pyrazinamidase and urease tests for routine identification of mycobacteria. *Am. Rev. Respir. Dis.* **109**:147–151.

Wolinsky, E. 1979. Nontuberculous mycobacteria and associated diseases. *Am. Rev. Respir. Dis.* **119**:107–159.

Woods, G. L., and J. A. Washington. 1987. Mycobacteria other than *Mycobacterium tuberculosis*: review of microbiologic and clinical aspects. *Rev. Infect. Dis.* **9**:275–294.

Young, W. D., Jr., A. Maslansky, M. S. Lefar, and D. P. Kronish. 1970. Development of a paper strip test for detection of niacin produced by mycobacteria. *Appl. Microbiol.* **20**:939–945.

II. ANIMAL MODELS OF TUBERCULOSIS

Tuberculosis: Pathogenesis, Protection, and Control
Edited by Barry R. Bloom
© 1994 American Society for Microbiology, Washington, DC 20005

Chapter 8

Mouse Model of Tuberculosis

Ian M. Orme and Frank M. Collins

The mouse is one of several animal models that can be used in the study of experimental tuberculosis infection. The mouse is cost-effective to use and (biosafety considerations aside) relatively easy to handle. Like the majority of healthy humans, the mouse is able to generate a strong immune response to *Mycobacterium tuberculosis*; hence, the animal is generally resistant to low-dose inocula and can contain the infection without developing active, disseminating disease. Again, as in humans, this infection is likely to recrudesce as the animal grows old.

The usefulness of the mouse model has grown in parallel with the explosion of knowledge over the past 25 years in the field of immunology. Thus, those studying immunity or immunopathology associated with tuberculosis in the mouse model have profited greatly from the large number of immunological reagents now available. Of these reagents, the great majority are monoclonal antibodies, which have allowed us to study the key protein and lipoglycan molecules of the bacillus, to measure cytokines secreted by activated macrophages and T cells, and to characterize the pheno-

types of responding cell populations, including the very structure of the T-cell receptor itself.

In this chapter, we briefly describe how the mouse model has evolved over the past century from the simple but beautiful experiments of Koch to present-day models based on sophisticated gene targeting. In the process, we describe the course of the infection in the mouse after inoculation by various routes and our growing picture of how the host immune response is mobilized against the infecting organism. Finally, we describe various mouse models that involve immunodeficiency; these may prove useful not only in the further dissection of the cellular immune response but also in applied strategies of chemotherapy and immunotherapy. Given the present disastrous combination of tuberculosis (much of it drug resistant) and human immunodeficiency virus infection, such new models are badly needed.

EVOLUTION OF THE MOUSE MODEL FOR TUBERCULOSIS

The discoverer of the tubercle bacillus, Robert Koch, was also the first to use the mouse as an experimental tool, and indeed, Koch was able to apply his own famous set of postulates to this animal by showing that inoculation with *M. tuberculosis* induced

Ian M. Orme • Mycobacteria Research Laboratories, Department of Microbiology, Colorado State University, Fort Collins, Colorado 80523. *Frank M. Collins* • The Trudeau Institute, Saranac Lake, New York 12983.

lesions ("tubercles") similar to those seen in the natural disease in humans (Collins, 1982). Most of these mice were "field mice," but some studies were conducted with white mice. These latter animals had been given to his daughter Gertrud as pets; they were housed in a cage constructed like a doll's house, where they of course rapidly multiplied and from whence Koch removed some of the "excess" mice for his experiments.

In fact, a number of early investigators in the field quickly established that infections could be actively induced in a variety of rodents, including rabbits, guinea pigs, rats, and mice, when the animals were inoculated with pure cultures of *M. tuberculosis*. Because of interest in the progressive pulmonary infection, these studies tended to involve guinea pigs and rabbits because of their high degree of susceptibility to the disease (Collins, 1984). However, poineering studies by Romer in 1903, Weber and Bofinger in 1904, and Browning and Gulbransen in 1926 began to define the pattern of disease in the more resistant mouse model (Browning and Gulbransen, 1926), while an appreciation of this model for investigating the strong immune response to tuberculosis that mice obviously possessed also began to slowly emerge (Gunn et al., 1933).

In the 1940s another use for the mouse model began to emerge. At this time the first effective chemotherapy for tuberculosis was under active development, and it was quickly realized, most notably by Youmans and his colleagues (Youmans and McCarter, 1945; Raleigh and Youmans, 1949; Youmans, 1949) that the mouse provided an excellent cost-effective model for the evaluation of drugs such as streptomycin. In addition, evidence also emerged at this time to indicate that the mouse model was more accurate as a readout of drug protection than other models such as the guinea pig (McKee et al., 1949).

This era soon became a Golden Age for tuberculosis research. In 1945, Chase found evidence for a cellular rather than a humoral limb of immunity, using as an example the passive transfer of tuberculin hypersensitivity with lymphoid cells (Chase, 1945), and this method was later applied by Suter (1961) to demonstrate the transfer of resistance to tuberculosis infection. In addition, a classic series of protection studies carried out by Dubos and his colleagues showed that mice that had been vaccinated with a number of substrains of BCG were subsequently resistant to tuberculosis, with this protection clearly demonstrated in terms of changes in bacterial numbers in vivo (Pierce et al., 1956; Dubos and Pierce, 1956). This approach, in which serial enumeration of bacteria present in organs harvested from sublethally challenged animals can be used to provide evidence for the emergence of protective immunity, remains a mainstay of vaccine evaluation (Weigeshaus and Smith, 1968).

The 1970s saw the development of concepts that continue to guide our thinking to the present day. Collins and Mackaness (1970) began to dissect the basis of the relationship between protective immunity and tuberculin hypersensitivity, while work by Lefford (1975) further developed the mouse model of adoptive immunity (passive cell transfer). In a beautiful series of experiments, North and colleagues (North et al., 1972) described in careful detail the immunologic and histologic development of the immune response to an intravenous inoculum of *M. tuberculosis*, while a pivotal paper by North a year later confirmed the role of T cells in these events (North, 1973).

The last two decades have seen the continued development of the concept that acquired immunity to tuberculosis is mediated by T cells that secrete cytokines that lead to the activation of parasitized macrophages and accumulating mononuclear phagocytes. The fact that we have continued to amass large amounts of information from the mouse regarding these events is a testament to the usefulness of this animal model in the dissection of the acquired immune response to this disease (Mackaness, 1968; Collins, 1979; Kaufmann and Hahn, 1981; Orme et al., 1993a).

EXPERIMENTAL INFECTION OF MICE WITH TUBERCULOSIS

Monitoring the course of tuberculosis infections in mice is a very straightforward procedure that uses a highly reproducible series of techniques. The evolution of these procedures, however, given the fastidious and hazardous nature of this organism, serves as a tribute to the tenacity of early workers in the field who were involved in the thorough, painstaking development of these methods.

An excellent review of the technical aspects of growing and infecting mice with inocula of *M. tuberculosis* can be found elsewhere (Brown, 1983). Briefly, the major technical advances in the field in the past few decades include (i) techniques for growing bacilli in liquid media (Dubos, 1945), (ii) the development of reproducible methods for counting bacterial colonies on solid agar (Fenner et al., 1949; Fenner, 1951), (iii) the influence of the choice of nutrient media on the virulence of cultures of *M. tuberculosis* (Collins and Smith, 1969; Collins et al., 1974), and (iv) improved methods of bacterial storage (Kim and Kubica, 1972, 1973).

In fact, the virulence of a given strain of *M. tuberculosis* can vary extensively depending on the experimental conditions. In particular, the route of infection (Collins et al., 1974; Collins and Montalbine, 1975), the manner of preparation of the suspension, and the dispersion and size of the suspension (Shier and Long, 1971; Collins and Montalbine, 1976) can affect the apparent virulence of the test organism. Host-associated factors such as severe malnutri-

tion, stress, terminal cancer, diabetes, kidney failure, silicosis, degenerative lung disease, and even chronic vitamin D deficiency can also influence virulence (Davies, 1985; McMurray et al., 1986; Khansari et al., 1990).

Course of Experimental Infections

The growth of *M. tuberculosis* in mice has been extremely well characterized (Collins, 1979), with the organism giving rise to highly characteristic distribution patterns in target organs after inoculation (Collins and Montalbine, 1976; Orme, 1987a). There are multiple routes of inoculation, but the most commonly used are the intravenous and aerogenic routes (the latter, of course, most closely mimicking reality) (Fig. 1 through 4).

The course and rate of mycobacterial infections are modulated by a number of factors recently reviewed by Lefford (Lefford, 1984). These factors are as follows.

(i) The virulence of the organism. Virulence itself obviously involves a number of factors, although in the context of the tubercle bacillus, these factors remain poorly defined. The lipoglycans of *M. tuberculosis* are certainly one group of interest, given their induction of cytokines by infected macrophages (see below) and their ability to scavenge oxygen radicals (Chan et al., 1991). What is not a factor is the rate of growth of the organism; fast growers such as the H37Ra strain are actually readily killed in vivo (Collins and Montalbine, 1976).

(ii) The organ in which bacilli are lodged. Bacilli in the liver, for example, do not grow as fast as bacilli in the spleen. Another, recently recognized issue (Flynn et al., 1992; Cooper et al., submitted) is the fate of bacteria that may erode into nonphagocytic cells in the lungs and in tissues such as the kidney. These bacteria may grow barely at all in immunocompetent mice but may eventually cause abscessing,

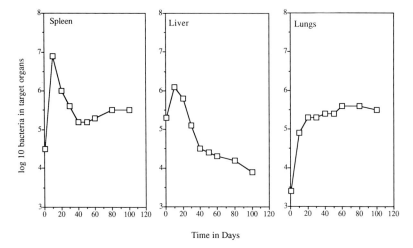

Time in Days

Figure 1. Course of *M. tuberculosis* infection in mice given 10^5 viable bacilli intravenously. The infection grows quickly in the spleen over the first 10 to 14 days, triggering the emergence of protective immunity. The liver is more resistant to the infection; it does not permit rapid growth initially and continues to slowly clear the infection (in contrast, the disease remains chronic in both the spleen and lungs). Note the characteristic distribution of the inoculum: about 90% is taken up in the liver, about 10% is taken up in the spleen, and about 1% is taken up in the lungs (uptake that exceeds 5% in the lungs is a sure sign that the inoculum is clumped).

as seen in gene-disrupted mouse models (see below).

(iii) The size of inoculum (threshold effect). This phenomenon, first noted by Lefford (1971), refers to the inverse relationship between the inoculum size and the delay before the inoculum grows in the mouse to a size that triggers acquired immunity.

(iv) The intensity of the immune response. Some have suggested that mouse strains may differ in their susceptibilities to tuberculosis infections; in fact, differences between mouse strains have occasionally been reported (Lefford, 1984), but in our experience, these differences are minimal in mice given sublethal immunizing doses. An *H-2*-controlled difference in mice in the later stages of chronic pulmonary infection has been reported, however (Brett et al., 1992), as have changes in the serologic response (Huygen et al., 1993). There is a clear difference between mouse strains infected with very low doses of the Montreal strain of BCG (Gros et al., 1981). We stress the strain designation here, because these

differences, which led to the identification of the *Bcg* gene locus, have tended to creep into the current literature as a major factor influencing BCG growth in general. In fact, as is documented in the literature (Orme and Collins, 1984a; Orme et al., 1985), the gene effect is clearly seen in action only against BCG Montreal and is not seen at all if most of the currently available BCG vaccines are tested.

HOST RESPONSE TO TUBERCULOSIS IN THE MOUSE

It has become increasingly apparent over the past few years that all three subsets of T cells, namely, CD4, CD8, and γδ cells, play some sort of role in the acquired cellular immune response to experimental *M. tuberculosis* infection in the mouse (Orme et al., 1993a). These observations, for example, that T cells could transfer immunity to tuberculosis to sublethally irradiated recipients (Lefford, 1975; Orme, 1987a) or that a particular T-cell clone might be cytolytic

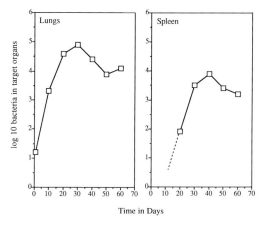

Figure 2. Course of *M. tuberculosis* infection in mice given approximately 20 viable bacilli by aerosol. The infection progresses in the lungs over the first 20 to 30 days before being contained by the emerging immune response. At around this time, significant numbers of bacteria can be detected in the spleen (and liver); these bacilli probably arose from a few organisms that eroded early from the lungs into the bloodstream (hematogenous spread).

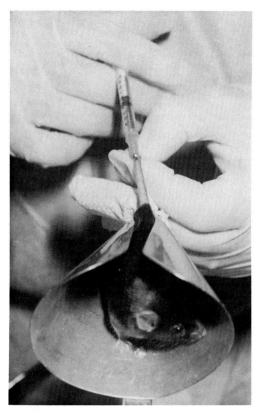

Figure 3. Intravenous injection of mice. Following warming under a heat lamp for a few minutes to induce vasodilation, the mouse is gently positioned in this simple restraining device. The bacterial inoculum is injected into a lateral tail vein with a 26-gauge needle.

(DeLibero et al., 1988; Orme et al., 1992b), were at first purely functional, but we are now moving into a more analytical era in which the T-cell subset can be more readily identified by its expression of an increasingly larger array of various cell surface markers, by its use of certain gene elements needed to construct the T-cell receptor, and by its secretion profile of certain important cytokines. As a result, we are inching closer and closer to a more precise definition of the T-cell subsets that respond to tuberculosis infection.

Having said that, however, it must be conceded that much of the activity of T cells in tuberculosis-infected mice is still defined in purely functional or operational terms. Several years ago, for example, we applied the term "protective T cell" to those cells (mentioned above) that transfer protection against an acute challenge infection.

Likewise, depending on the type of experiment or type of assay, we can invoke the presence of "delayed-type hypersensi-

tivity (DTH) effector T cells" and "memory T cells." In addition, the activities of such cells can be further defined in terms of cytokine secretion and the presence or absence of cytolytic activity. As a result, we are drawing a very complex picture of events, but much of this picture is still poorly defined (Orme, 1993b). Another complicating factor is the fact that tuberculosis is a chronic disease, and hence any understanding of the T-cell response has to be couched in terms of the kinetics of the response. In fact, there is now good evidence that different stages of the experimental infection involve the activity of different T-cell subset responses (Orme et al., 1993a).

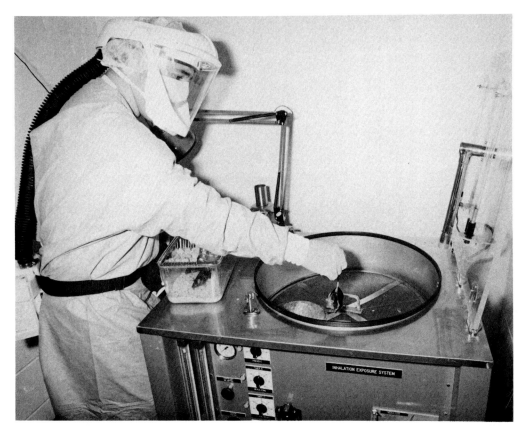

Figure 4. Aerosol infection of mice. The venturi unit at the front of the generator creates an aerosol that is pumped into a central sealed chamber containing the animals. The operator is wearing a Racal AC3 helmet for added protection (this device includes a small HEPA filter, worn on a waist belt, that blows sterilized air up and through the helmet). The aerosol generator suite is negative with respect to atmospheric pressure, and all air leaving the room is HEPA filtered.

Nor is this concept limited to the host response. The tubercle bacillus cannot be regarded by the immunologist in the same way as a soluble protein antigen (unfortunately, in some cases, it has been) when in fact it is an extremely complex living organism. Again, evidence now accumulating suggests that one particular class of mycobacterial proteins is presented to the immune response when the infection is initially thriving, and other, completely different classes of antigen become targets as the infecting bacteria are gradually killed off (Orme et al., 1993a, b). To the novice reading this text, this latter point may seem somewhat trivial, but in reality, a failure by some workers in the field to appreciate the intrinsic difference between live, metabolically active bacilli and dead or killed bacilli, leading as it has to experimental designs in which immunity to dead bacilli suspended in adjuvant has been confidently believed by these workers to be fully equivalent to cellular immunity to the live infection, has in our opinion added an extra layer of confusion to what is already a difficult and complex field. In mice infected with live bacilli by the intravenous route, a highly reproducible sequence of events ensues, starting with the appearance of activated

CD4 T cells. Hence, we will begin this section by looking at our current knowledge of the CD4 T-cell response.

CD4 Response in Experimental Tuberculosis

A week or so after inoculation of mice with a sublethal intravenous dose of *M. tuberculosis*, a population of CD4 cells that are capable of adoptively transferring protective immunity emerges in the spleen (Orme, 1987a). The majority of these protective T cells appear to be within a minor subset (approximately 5 to 10%) of CD4 cells that concomitantly increase expression of the CD44 marker and decrease expression of the CD45RB marker over the next 15 to 20 days or so (a common phenotype of activated T cells). By collecting these cells with a cell sorter and culture in vitro, it can be demonstrated that these CD44^{hi}/CD45RB^{lo} cells are a potent source of the key protective cytokine gamma interferon (IFN-γ) (Griffin et al., submitted). In contrast, such cells do not produce interleukin 4 (IL-4), classifying them (in the present vernacular) as Th1-type CD4 cells (Mosmann and Coffman, 1989).

By analogy to plasma cells that secrete large amounts of antibody and then die, the early emerging CD4 protective T cell is also probably short-lived. Two lines of evidence suggest this: (i) if these cells are transferred into recipients but the challenge infection is delayed by a few days, then transferred resistance decreases substantially (Orme, 1988a); (ii) the kinetics of IFN-γ-secreting CD4 cells reveals a dramatic falloff after about 20 days of the infection (Orme et al., 1992b, 1993c).

The disappearance of this population at this time may reflect the reduction in presentation of key "protective antigens" (which we believe are among the secreted/export proteins of the bacillus; see below) as most of the mycobacteria are killed off.

Moreover, a preprogrammed (apoptotic) mechanism may also be involved in removing these cells at this point (Lui and Janeway, 1990), so that they no longer continue to secrete cytokines such as IFN-γ, IL-2, and tumor necrosis factor (TNF), all of which may be detrimental to the host if allowed to accumulate to high concentrations (Fig. 5).

At this time, however, at least three (functionally defined) CD4 populations still remain. The first are cells that mediate DTH (which we refer to as DTH effector T cells). This population is rather elusive, because in the mouse, at least, the ability to elicit a DTH reaction in infected animals seems to wane about 30 to 40 days postinoculation (Orme and Collins, 1984b). Whether these cells also gradually die or whether they sequestrate in lymphoid tissues and await secondary infections or recrudescence of the original remains far from clear at this time.

Another cell that expresses CD4 can be detected in mice 20 to 40 days postinoculation. This cell possesses cytolytic activity and seems to recognize the same class of mycobacterial antigens that protective T cells react to (Orme et al., 1992b). Although this population is still poorly characterized, our current idea is that it represents some form of surveillance mechanism, wandering through granulomas searching for residual live bacteria. These bacteria will reveal their presence by continuing to produce key protective antigens, and hence the host cell containing them becomes recognized by this CD4 population and is lysed.

When the existence of cytolytic cells in mycobacterial infections was first described, many of us could not accept the idea that these cells would have a protective function, because we felt it was more likely that such activity would directly disseminate the disease. Our finding in a kinetic study (Orme et al., 1992b) that such cells peak in activity about a month into the

Infected macrophage presents
secreted/export mycobacterial
protein antigens to CD4 T cell

Some immune cells
remain in lesion and
hence continue to be
exposed to antigen. These
"protective T cells" are
short-lived [as a result of
apoptosis ?]

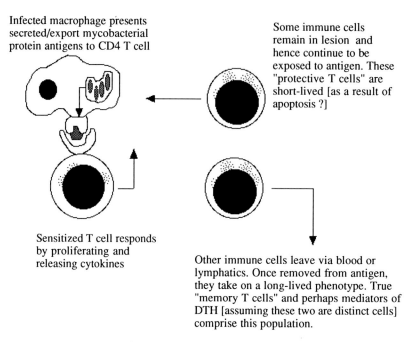

Sensitized T cell responds
by proliferating and
releasing cytokines

Other immune cells leave via blood or
lymphatics. Once removed from antigen,
they take on a long-lived phenotype. True
"memory T cells" and perhaps mediators of
DTH [assuming these two are distinct cells]
comprise this population.

Figure 5. The potential fate of immune CD4 T cells. Sensitized protective T cells release cytokines (IFN-γ, migration inhibition factor, TNF, etc.) that activate the parasitized macrophage to contain the intracellular *M. tuberculosis* infection. In addition, these materials recruit monocytes into the lesion to initiate granuloma formation. We currently speculate that memory T cells arise from the same lineage but express a longer-lived phenotype as a result of emigration from the infectious site. Of course, it is equally possible that memory cells arise from a completely separate lineage. This issue remains to be resolved.

experimental infection now dispels these concerns, because it shows that cell lysis and bacterial release will occur after an intact, extensive granuloma has formed at the site of the infection, making it much less likely that bacteria can escape.

It has been suggested (Kumararatne et al., 1990) that this cytolytic CD4 population may be very important for the long-term outcome of the infection. Thus, if you have a strong cytolytic CD4 response, this population is more likely to track down bacteria that may have escaped the attentions of the initial protective T-cell response. If the CD4 response is weak, however, then residual bacteria may remain and give rise to recrudescent disease at some later date.

A third cell expressing CD4, the memory T cell, is the most enigmatic of the three. In this era of intensive development of poten-

tial new vaccines for tuberculosis control, it is obviously the cell population that we most want to target with such vaccines, but it is also the CD4 population that we know the least about.

In fact, work on this population has a substantive history, going back to observations by Gray and Cheers on the "steady state" of immunity in tuberculosis (Gray and Cheers, 1967) and the pioneering work of Lambert, who was the first to use chemotherapy in mice to establish a true state of memory (Lambert, 1960). It was not until the late 1980s, however, that memory immunity to *M. tuberculosis* (Orme, 1988a) and *M. bovis* (Orme, 1988b) was formally shown to be mediated by CD4 cells.

Unlike protective CD4 T cells, which are sensitive to irradiation or to the DNA-alkylating drug cyclophosphamide, memory CD4 cells are not affected by these agents, indicating that they are a resting-nondividing population of recirculating lymphocytes. Because of these properties, they could be distinguished from residual protective T cells in passive cell transfer experiments in which the donor animals were treated just prior to T-cell harvest (Orme, 1988a). In such assays, a gradual emergence of these cells can be observed about 20 to 40 days postinoculation.

It is not clear how the intensity of the initial response to *M. tuberculosis* influences the subsequent longevity or size of the memory T-cell pool (although one study using a very high dose of BCG vaccine suggested that the pool might be diminished under such conditions [Orme, 1988b]). It is also unclear whether memory is sustained by periodic recrudescence of the disease from individual granulomas; it is quite possible that the integrity of these structures benefits from occasional reactivation by cytokine-secreting memory cells. It should be noted that one school of thought holds that memory immunity relies on constant restimulation by antigen; however, the reader should also note that this idea has mainly arisen from workers studying the T-cell response in humoral immunity (Sprent, 1993).

What is obvious about memory immune T cells is that their response to secondary challenge infections is quite rapid. This implies two things: (i) they probably act straightaway and do not have to clonally expand or interact with other intermediary cells, and (ii) the antigens they see must be presented very quickly by infected cells. It has been shown that heat-killed *M. tuberculosis* cannot generate memory (Orme and Collins, 1986), and hence the secreted export proteins of the bacillus again seem likely targets. In fact, recent evidence from Andersen and his colleagues directly confirms this hypothesis (Andersen and Heron, 1993).

CD8 Cells in Experimental Tuberculosis

With the availability of the highly lytic antibody Lyt-2.43 in the mid-1980s, a possible role for CD8 T cells in infections with nonviral intracellular pathogens became increasingly observed. In the mouse model of tuberculosis, enriched populations of immune CD8 T cells transferred some degree of resistance (Orme, 1987a), albeit rather weakly, and in vivo depletion of CD8 T cells by intravenous administration of monoclonal antibody was shown to diminish resistance to some extent (Muller et al., 1987; Cox et al., 1989). Together, therefore, these studies seemed to suggest that CD8 has a minor protective role, but just how important this role might be was unclear.

Perhaps because of the observation that CD4 T cells expressed most of the initial immunity to tuberculosis infection in the mouse, studies of the role of CD8 T cells underwent a hiatus for a few years in the recent literature. Then, in 1992, a study was published that resurrected the entire question. This study, by Flynn and her colleagues (Flynn et al., 1992) at the Albert Einstein College of Medicine in the Bronx, showed that mice that had had their β2-microglobulin (β2m) genes disrupted by homologous recombination died from a normally sublethal injection of *M. tuberculosis*. Because β2m is an integral component of the class I major histocompatibility complex (MHC) molecule, these mice are unable to sensitize CD8 T cells, because the class I MHC molecule cannot form properly and hence cannot properly present antigenic peptides. These data for the infected mice thus provided the startling information that not only are CD8 T cells important, but their sensitization appears to be essential to surviving a tuberculosis infection.

A common denominator of these observations was the fact that the lungs seemed to be particularly important in terms of CD8 function, and this fact seems to present an obvious clue as to what these cells may be doing. During hematogenous spread of the infection (or intravenous inoculation), bacteria in the blood are highly likely to be picked up within a very short time by macrophages lining the venous sinusoids in the spleen and liver. A few of these bacteria, however, can be detected in homogenates of the lungs, and histologically some of these seem to have eroded into blood vessel endothelial cells. Likewise, if an aerosol inoculum is given, many bacteria are cleared by lung alveolar macrophages and carried to draining lymph nodes, but some clearly erode directly into alveolar endothelial cells.

Within 10 to 15 days or so, small granulomas begin to develop around the alveolar cells, but whether the monocytes directly release the mycobacteria prior to digestion themselves is unclear. CD8 class I-restricted cells seem to be obvious candidates in this action, and hence it is possible that their principal role is to detect "nonprofessional" cells (as opposed to "professional" class II-expressing phagocytes) that can express only mycobacterial antigens using class I molecules. If we presume that these cells are lytic (this has been shown with cloned CD8 cells from mice injected with dead mycobacteria [DeLibero et al., 1988] but not as yet with the living infection), then destruction of the infected cell by CD8 cytolytic cells would release the intracellular bacilli for ingestion and destruction by the surrounding monocytes.

Obviously, if the infected mouse lacked these CD8 T cells, then *M. tuberculosis* bacilli might survive and grow in these tissues, causing abscess formation and increasingly necrotic destruction. Such histopathology was indeed seen in the β2m-deficient mouse model, and it appears that these specific events in the lung tissues were ultimately fatal to these animals.

The question remains as to how the CD8 cells become sensitized in the first place. One possible scenario is as follows (Orme,

1993a). As the infection progresses, the bacterial load in infected macrophages increases, but eventually T-cell-mediated immunity is generated and infected cells are triggered by cytokines to become bactericidal. Some macrophages may be damaged by the high bacterial load, however, while others may be completely refractory to cytokine activation. Under these conditions, it is reasonable to speculate that the phagosomal membrane surrounding the mycobacteria may become damaged, enabling mycobacterial proteins to leak into the cytoplasm and hence into the class I MHC processing pathway. In fact, recent evidence (McDonough et al., 1993) indicates that whole bacteria themselves may protrude into the cytoplasm to some extent.

If this is true, then CD8 T cells may be an essential backup to protective CD4 T cells (Fig. 6). These latter cells can interact with and activate infected macrophages, but they cannot detect the probably small number of residual bacteria hiding in tissues that cannot express class II molecules. Under these conditions, the CD8 cells would become essential to the detection and resolution of these surviving pockets of bacterial infection.

γδ Cells in Experimental Tuberculosis

The discovery a few years ago of a third major subset of T cells, the γδ T-cell-receptor-bearing cell population (γδ cells), has generated considerable interest in the possible role of these cells in combating infectious diseases, including those caused by mycobacteria (Born et al., 1991).

Two observations are particularly noteworthy. First, γδ cells appear to have a higher percentage of sessile cells than their recirculating αβ T-cell cousins. Moreover, the distribution of γδ cells in areas such as the skin, gut, and upper respiratory tract seems to suggest that these cells represent some form of initial immunologic barrier to

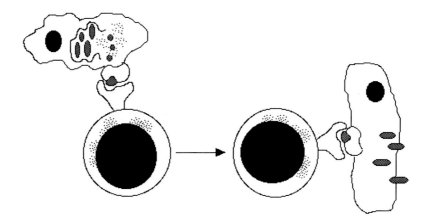

An infected macrophage is damaged by its intracellular burden, leading to bursting of the phagosome and introduction of mycobacterial antigens into the cytoplasm. These are processed and presented by Class I molecules to CD8 cells.

The CD8 cell detects the presence of mycobacteria in association with "nonprofessional" cells [bacteria eroding into alveolar or blood vessel endothelial cells, for example]. The cell is lysed, releasing the bacteria for passing monocytes to engulf.

Figure 6. Possible role of CD8 T cells. These cells become sensitized by presentation of mycobacterial antigens in association with class I MHC molecules. As the infection progresses in the lungs, these cells may play a vital role in releasing bacteria that have eroded into local tissues (such as the lung endothelial cells). This speculative model is based on the work of Flynn and her colleagues (Flynn et al., 1992).

invading microorganisms that attempt to penetrate such tissues (Haas et al., 1993).

The second important observation is that $\gamma\delta$ cells appear to accumulate in relatively large numbers in tissues that are infected with mycobacteria. In one early report (Inoue et al., 1991), a rapid and preferential accumulation of $\gamma\delta$ cells was observed in the peritoneal cavities of mice injected with BCG. These observations led this group to propose that an early and rapid response by $\gamma\delta$ cells to mycobacterial infection, prior to any involvement by $\alpha\beta$ cells, acts as an important first line of defense in such infections.

In contrast, Griffin and colleagues (Griffin et al., 1991) documented the accumulation of $\gamma\delta$ cells in mice infected intravenously with *M. tuberculosis* and found that the accumulation of such cells in infected tissues tended to parallel the accumulation of $\alpha\beta$ cells, peaking at about day 20, with

the $\gamma\delta$ cell numbers always representing about 10 to 15% of the total CD3 population. In a further rechallenge experiment, a very rapid $\alpha\beta$ response with no $\gamma\delta$ involvement was seen, indicating that if the primary $\gamma\delta$ response did have an antigen-specific basis, then no anamnestic response was subsequently generated. This latter observation is consistent with work showing that stimulation of $\gamma\delta$ cells can lead to apoptosis (Janssen et al., 1991).

In addition to the observations above, several groups have shown that isolated $\gamma\delta$ cells proliferate in vitro in response to mycobacterial antigen; expand in large numbers when cocultured with dead preparations of the avirulent H37Ra strain of *M. tuberculosis*; and release cytokines, including IL-2, IFN-γ, and granulocyte macrophage–colony-stimulating factor (GM-CSF) (Munk et al., 1990; Follows et al., 1992). Thus, on the basis of all this information, it seems very reasonable to assume that γδ cells are an important component of the overall cellular response to mycobacterial infections.

Having stated that, let us inject some notes of caution. First, early studies that precipitated the interest in γδ cells in antimycobacterial immunity were in fact performed with nonliving materials. Thus, an early paper (Augustin et al., 1989) documented an accumulation of γδ cells in the lungs of mice exposed to aerosols of purified protein derivative, a rather inflammatory material, while a further study (Janis et al., 1989) showed a very potent accumulation of γδ cells in the lymph nodes of mice immunized with heat-killed *M. tuberculosis* H37Ra emulsified in incomplete Freund's adjuvant. In this latter study, the accumulation of γδ cells was believed to model a primary immune response in tuberculosis, but a more recent study (Griffin et al., 1991) showed that this accumulation was purely in response to the adjuvant vehicle alone.

In view of this, the question remains as to whether γδ cells respond in an antigen-specific manner to mycobacterial infections or whether they accumulate in response to local tissue signals induced by the highly inflammatory mycobacteria. Similarly, in vitro, the adjuvantive qualities of the bacilli could induce cytokine secretion by macrophages present, driving proliferation and cytokine release by γδ cells. In this regard, it has been recently shown that the lipoglycan lipoarabinomannan (LAM) derived from the H37Ra strain of *M. tuberculosis*, which is usually used to expand γδ cells in vitro, is a particularly potent inducer of macrophage cytokine secretion (Moreno et al., 1989; Chatterjee et al., 1992; Barnes et al., 1992).

On the other hand, some evidence for antigen-specific responses also exists, mainly based on the observation that γδ cells responding to stimulation with mycobacteria tend to use a very restricted pattern of V-region genes, namely, Vδ2, Vγ2,

and Vγ9. That the specificity of epitope recognition is not extremely limited, however, is suggested by the extensive use of N-region junctional diversification that is also observed in these cell populations (Panchamoorthy et al., 1991; Ohmen et al., 1991).

Target Antigens in the Immune Response to Tuberculosis in the Mouse

Most early experiments with bacterial antigens consisted of immunizing mice with dead (usually heat-killed) *M. tuberculosis* or BCG, usually emulsified in some form of adjuvant (usually incomplete Freund's). Two methods were then used to identify recognized antigens: (i) T cells from the draining nodes were cloned in vitro by using sonicates of dead mycobacteria as antigen and then tested in proliferation assays against isolated mycobacterial proteins; or (ii) B cells were fused to form hybridomas, and the specificities of the monoclonal antibodies thus derived were determined by immunoblotting. In both cases, it was hypothesized that the major antigens that would be identified by these methods would be those of key importance to protective immunity. Unfortunately, because of the lack of appreciation at the time that live mycobacteria are intrinsically different from dead mycobacteria, this hypothesis now appears to be fundamentally incorrect.

The reason for this is that the constitutive proteins of *M. tuberculosis*, which are of course still present in dead mycobacterial preparations, are not the major targets of protective immunity in the mouse. Instead, several laboratories now believe that proteins that are exported or secreted by the actively dividing mycobacterium within the phagosome are removed by the macrophage and used to signal T cells that an intracellular invader is present (Orme et al., 1993a) (Fig. 7).

These ideas arose in the mid-1980s in

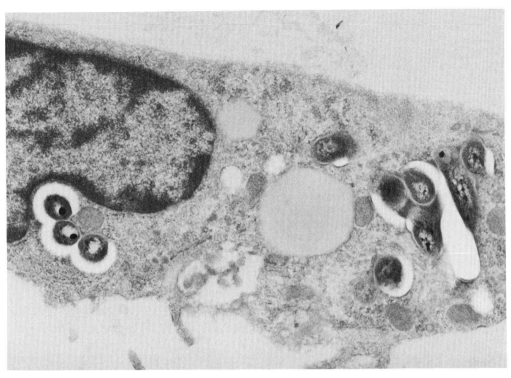

Figure 7. Mouse macrophage containing several intact bacterial particles. The apparent paradox whereby the bacteria are healthy and intact yet strong immunity can be generated can be explained by the hypothesis that the macrophage is presenting secreted/export proteins of the bacillus rather than constitutive proteins. The ability of the bacilli to survive under such conditions is also a matter of debate; recent data (Sturgill-Koszycki et al., submitted) now suggests that the mycobacteria have an unknown property that prevents the fusion of proton-ATPase complex-containing vesicles to the bacterial phagosome, thus preventing acidification of this compartment. (Photo courtesy of David Russell.)

experiments (Rook et al., 1986; Orme, 1988c) that suggested that immunity to the live organism was not preferentially directed against the constitutive proteins of the bacillus. As a result, since that time much emphasis has been directed toward the characterization of bacterial proteins appearing in the culture filtrate.

In fact, the protein profile of the *M. tuberculosis* culture filtrate can vary considerably and depends on the precise culture conditions in which the bacteria are grown (Abou-Zeid et al., 1988; De Bruyn et al., 1989; Verbon et al., 1990; Andersen et al., 1991). In addition, continued growth past mid-log phase results in an increasing contamination of the filtrate with cytoplas-

mic antigens, such as hsp60 and isocitrate dehydrogenase (Abou-Zeid et al., 1988; Andersen et al., 1991). An example of a culture filtrate preparation is shown in Fig. 8; for a comprehensive description of known mycobacterial proteins, the reader should consult a recent review by Young and his colleagues (Young et al., 1992).

Very little is known about the antigenic targets of CD8 T cells. As described above, there is growing evidence that these cells may be very important in identifying pockets of infection where mycobacterial antigens are expressed only in association with class I MHC molecules (Flynn et al., 1992). Moreover, the kinetics of emergence of such cells may occur a little later than the

M S

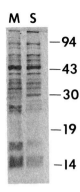

—94

—43

—30

—19

—14

Figure 8. Culture filtrate proteins of *M. tuberculosis* Erdman. This protein pool contains multiple targets of IFN-γ-secreting protective CD4 T cells harvested from infected mice. Note the differing protein content depending on whether the filtrate is harvested at mid-log phase (M) or several days earlier (short-term filtrate; S). Numbers at right are molecular sizes in kilodaltons. (Courtesy of John Belisle.)

first wave of CD4 protective T cells (Orme, 1987a) when large amounts of mycobacterial antigens have been processed; hence, the spectrum of antigens that may possibly be recognized could well be large.

Work by DeLibero and his colleagues has attempted to address this question (DeLibero et al., 1988). Cloned CD8 T cells were shown to be cytolytic, and they lysed cells pulsed with mycobacterial antigens but not listerial antigens, indicating some degree of antigen specificity. MHC restriction of such clones was not absolute, but most produced IFN-γ upon stimulation with mycobacterial sonicates. These studies showed clearly, therefore, that cytolytic CD8 T cells could be sensitized against mycobacterial antigens, although exactly what these antigens were remains unclear.

As for γδ T cells, there is evidence to suggest that they are indeed antigen specific, but the question remains as to which mycobacterial antigen(s) they recognize. In fact, at the time of writing, this is a very controversial area because of considerable inconsistency between studies in the mouse and in humans. Since this chapter deals with the former, we should note that most

current evidence tends to indicate that the hsp60 stress protein of *M. tuberculosis* is a primary target of such cells in the mouse (O'Brien et al. 1989, 1992; Born et al., 1990a, b), while a recent study (Fu et al., 1993) provides evidence for strong recognition in vivo of a 16-amino-acid peptide within the hsp60 heat shock protein sequence.

Cytokine Response in Mice to Tuberculosis Infection

The cytokine response to *M. tuberculosis* probably begins almost immediately after infection of host macrophages, as these cells begin to transcribe message from a number of early response genes (Roach et al., 1993). Within 24 h, infected-macrophage culture supernatants begin to contain sizable quantities of proinflammatory cytokines (IL-1, IL-6), colony stimulation factors (macrophage-CSF, GM-CSF), and other cytokines that may be regarded as effector cytokines (Orme et al., 1993c). These latter include TNF, which has antimicrobial properties, and IL-10, which probably acts to downregulate the physiological effects of the former.

The probable purposes of this early response are to prepare an inflammatory site and to initiate the events that lead eventually to the recruitment of mononuclear phagocytes and the formation of a granuloma. Some of these cytokines (IL-1 and IL-12, for example) also probably have positive effects on incoming T cells.

All intact live mycobacteria have these effects on murine macrophages (especially if one uses bone marrow-derived macrophages, which are very permissive to mycobacterial ingestion), but the intensity and content of the overall response may differ from isolate to isolate. One event that is subject to considerable variation is the quantity of TNF that is secreted. Recent work (Moreno et al., 1989; Chatterjee et al., 1992) suggests that the primary culprit involved in the induction of TNF secretion is the cell wall-associated lipoglycan LAM. Not only is this material present on the bacterium in copious amounts, but it is also shed from the surface of the bacillus in substantial quantities, even within the macrophage phagosome (Russell et al., 1993).

As described elsewhere in this volume, Chatterjee and her colleagues have recently made the interesting observation (Chatterjee et al., 1992) that LAM isolated from the avirulent H37Ra strain of *M. tuberculosis*, which is characterized by extensive side chains composed of arabinose, is an extremely potent elicitor of TNF secretion by mouse bone marrow macrophages. In contrast, LAM isolated from the virulent Erdman strain, which differs only in the fact that the arabinose chains are "capped" at the ends by one or more units of mannose, is a very poor inducer of TNF secretion. These observations thus raise the intriguing possibility that a primary reason that the virulent Erdman strain can infect and begin to grow inside macrophages is the fact that its LAM structure does not induce the production of any significant amount of the antimicrobial cytokine TNF. On the other hand, the LAM from the avirulent strain induces large amounts of this cytokine, which activates the infected host macrophage to inhibit its growth and also acts to promote a granulomatous response at the site of infection (Kindler et al., 1989).

Turning to the T-cell response, recent evidence indicates that live infection with BCG (Huygen et al., 1992) or with *M. tuberculosis* (Orme et al., 1992b, 1993c) induces an early Th1-like T-cell response associated with the production of IL-2 and IFN-γ. In the study using BCG, this response was very strong in C57BL/6 mice but much weaker in BALB/c mice. In these latter animals, a stronger secretion of IL-4 was seen, suggesting more of a Th2-like T-cell response.

Similar findings were made with *M. tuberculosis* (Orme et al., 1993c). In this study, CD4 T cells were harvested from mice at various times after infection and overlaid on macrophages pulsed either with mycobacterial antigens or with live or dead bacilli. Seventy-two hours later, supernatants were harvested and assayed for cytokine content. An early, Th1-like response was seen by IFN-γ-secreting CD4 cells stimulated in vitro with culture filtrate proteins or with macrophages infected with live bacilli. Later, 40 or so days into the course of the infection, a second wave of Th2-like IL-4-secreting CD4 T cells could be identified. The antigen spectrum recognized by these cells was broader, including the major heat shock protein of *M. tuberculosis*, hsp60 (65-kDa protein) (Fig. 9). This latter observation is of interest because it may explain why T-cell reactivity is

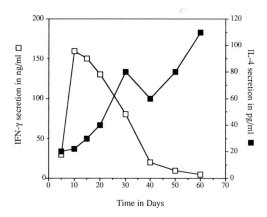

Figure 9. IFN-γ and IL-4 responses by CD4 T cells to *M. tuberculosis* antigens. In this experiment, CD4 T cells were harvested from infected mice at the times indicated and overlaid in vitro on macrophages presenting filtrate protein antigens. Three days later, the supernatants were harvested and tested for IFN-γ or IL-4 by enzyme-linked immunosorbent assay. These data indicate that the CD4 response consists of an early Th1-like response associated with containment and initial clearance of the infection followed after about a month by the emergence of a Th2-like response that presumably drives the humoral response to dead bacteria. In addition, while the Th1 response seems to be preferentially directed against the secreted/export proteins, the Th2 response is broader, including strong recognition of the hsp60 antigen (see text).

so strongly expressed against the hsp60 protein if dead mycobacteria in adjuvant is used to immunize mice, leading as it did to the designation of hsp60 as the "immunodominant" antigen of tuberculosis (Kaufmann, 1990; Kaufmann et al., 1990).

These observations indicate, therefore, that both Th1- and Th2-like responses occur in tuberculosis in the mouse. The early arising Th1 response mediates protective immunity by the release of IFN-γ and other cytokines, while the later emerging Th2 response drives a helper T-cell response that mediates antibody production to accumulating antigens processed from (now) dead mycobacteria.

TUBERCULOSIS IN IMMUNODEFICIENT MOUSE MODELS

Because immunity to tuberculosis is T cell mediated, considerable interest has focused on spontaneously occurring mouse mutants that cannot generate this population of cells. Two such models are currently in use: the nude mouse and the severe combined immunodeficiency (scid) mouse.

The nude mouse was discovered in Scotland in the mid-1960s; it is furless (hence the name) and suffers from thymic aplasia. As a result of this defect, it contains no functional T cells and hence has substantially less resistance to tuberculosis and other mycobacterial infections. A similar lack of resistance is seen in the scid mouse, which lacks both T cells and B cells as a result of a defect in variable-region gene recombination (Bosma et al., 1983). This model is being used increasingly to test the capacities of isolated cell populations to protect against mycobacterial infections.

While these models have arisen from spontaneous events, other models of immunodeficiency have been contrived. One of the earliest examples is the TXB mouse model, which took advantage of the knowledge that the thymus gland was essential to

T-cell production. In this model, a young mouse (about 4 weeks old, while the thymus gland is still large and productive) is thymectomized. Then, a week or so later, when the animal has recovered from the surgery, it is exposed to a dose of ionizing gamma irradiation that kills all dividing cells, including bone marrow stem cells. The mouse is then reconstituted with an infusion of syngeneic bone marrow cells. This inoculum contains functional B cells, but in the absence of the thymus gland, the mouse cannot now generate new mature T cells. As a result of this deficiency, TXB mice are substantially less resistant to an intravenous M. tuberculosis infection (North, 1973).

A recent further development of the TXB model is the TxCD4⁻ mouse model, or thymectomized, CD4 T-cell-deficient mouse. This model, which was originally developed in this laboratory to mimic events in mycobacterium-infected AIDS patients (Furney et al., 1990; Orme et al., 1992a), involves thymectomy as mentioned above followed by infusion of monoclonal anti-CD4 antibody. This model seems to be particularly efficient in that as little as 200 to 250 μg of purified antibody can cause severe CD4 depletion (Fig. 10) and that as a result of the thymectomy, repeated antibody administration is not required. Upon infection with M. tuberculosis, this animal eventually dies from disseminated disease (Ordway and Orme, 1993).

Retroviral Infections

Decreased resistance to M. tuberculosis infection can be induced in mice by using the murine retrovirus LP-BM5. This virus induces severe lymphadenopathy and profound T-cell depression (Mosier et al., 1985; Hartley et al., 1989) and hence may prove useful in the general development of models for opportunistic infections in AIDS. When LP-BM5-infected mice are

C57BL/6 Control

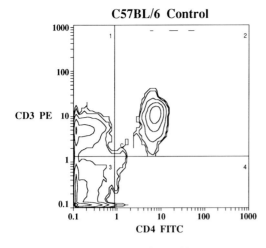

C57BL/6 Tx/CD4-

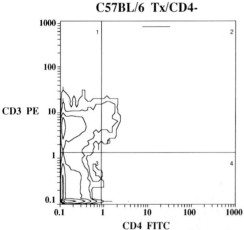

Figure 10. CD4 T-cell depletion of thymectomized mice by in vivo administration of monoclonal antibody. One injection of 250 μg of highly purified anti-CD4 (clone GK1.5) almost completely eliminates the host CD4 T-cell population. The data are expressed as contour maps following analysis of $CD3^+$ $CD4^+$ cells in the spleen by flow cytometry. FITC, fluorescein isothiocyanate.

exposed to *M. tuberculosis*, the mycobacterial infection grows progressively, resulting in death of the animal. In addition, the viral infection can induce the recrudescence of low-dose pulmonary tuberculosis infections in the mouse that were established by prior exposure of the mice in an aerosol generation device (Ordway and Orme, 1993).

Gene-Disrupted Mice

The first new model of tuberculosis using targeted gene disruption, involving deactivation of the β2m gene, was discussed above. As we saw, this model provided important information indicating a potentially vital role for CD8 T cells in the successful resolution of tuberculosis infections.

A second new model, which has provided equally important and interesting information, was developed by Dyana Dalton and her colleagues (Dalton et al., 1993). In this model, the IFN-γ gene was specifically disrupted by the insertion of a neomycin resistance gene after the second exon.

Work in this laboratory (Cooper et al., 1993) and similar studies by Flynn and her colleagues (Flynn et al., 1993) have recently shown that these "IFN-γ knockout" mice (GKO mice) are extremely susceptible to *M. tuberculosis* and eventually die from a disseminated form of tuberculosis in which multiple organs are heavily infected with bacilli. These studies therefore demonstrate the pivotal role of IFN-γ in the control of *M. tuberculosis* infections in the mouse.

At the time of this writing, much effort is being put into the targeted gene disruption type of approach, and it will be interesting to see what this "new wave" of animal modeling will tell us about the immunopathology of tuberculosis. Newly appearing models include the IL-4 KO mouse (raising the question of whether this mouse might be even more resistant to tuberculosis as a result of losing possible downregulatory Th2-type activity) and the γδ-KO mouse, which should help answer some the questions regarding whether the γδ T cell is a "curious onlooker" or an "essential element" in tuberculosis infection, as discussed above.

Immunosenescent Mice

A form of immunodeficiency that we are all prone to is the gradual weakening of the immune response that occurs as a result of aging. Indeed, in the developed nations, aside from the growing incidence of tuberculosis in younger people (many of whom, of course, are immunocompromised), recrudescence of latent tuberculosis in the elderly is still a major source of new cases.

Given the great difficulties involved in animal modeling of this scenario, including the biosafety aspects and the enormous cost of maintaining mice throughout their life span (2 to 2.5 years on average), it is hardly surprising that only a relatively small amount of information is available.

As described above, young mice infected intravenously with a sublethal dose of 10^5 *M. tuberculosis* bacilli contain and control the infection. In mice that are 24 to 28 months old, however, this inoculum size is fatal (Orme, 1987b).

It was initially believed that this mortality was simply due to a lack of protective T cells in old animals, but more recent work now shows that this hypothesis is incorrect (Orme et al., 1993b). Instead, it appears that T cells that are capable of recognizing mycobacterial antigens in old animals have very low or negligible expression of adhesion-homing markers such as L-selectin and CD11a and hence focus poorly at sites of infection.

CONCLUDING REMARKS

In the past 2 decades in particular, the mouse model of tuberculosis has provided us with a wealth of information regarding the host immune response to this infection. Moreover, technical developments in mainstream immunology continue to provide new tools and approaches to this problem; as a specific example, the cytokine response to mycobacterial infections, which was mostly only a "black box" a decade ago, is now being defined in considerable detail.

However, there is no doubt that we still have an incomplete picture of the disease process and the host response to it. As another example, just a year or so ago it would have been true to say that CD8 T cells were not considered particularly important in the response in the mouse, but the use of CD8-deficient mice, in which the infection is fatal, not only disproves this point but also warns us not to take anything for granted in this clearly complex immune response.

Having said that, we feel that these are exciting times. New technologies, such as the use of gene-disrupted mice and the use of tissue-specific promoter genes to define the role of cytokines in defined tissues, promise much in terms of the new information they may provide.

Finally, however, it must be remembered that tuberculosis is a chronic disease in the mouse model, and for this reason we need more longer-term studies to look at the precise nature of memory immunity, given its essential relationship to the efficacy of vaccination strategies, and the effects of other variables, including aging itself.

Acknowledgments. We thank our colleagues at the Trudeau Institute and at Colorado State University for their contributions to many of the ideas contained in this review.

This work was supported by NIH grants AI27156 and AI27288.

REFERENCES

Abou-Zeid, C., I. Smith, J. M. Grange, T. L. Ratliff, J. Steele, and G. A. W. Rook. 1988. The secreted antigens of *Mycobacterium tuberculosis* and their relationship to those recognized by the available antibodies. *J. Gen. Microbiol.* **134:**531–538.

Andersen, P., D. Askgaard, L. Ljungqvist, J. Bennedsen, and I. Heron. 1991. Proteins released from *Mycobacterium tuberculosis* during growth. *Infect. Immun.* **59:**1905–1910.

Andersen, P., and I. Heron. 1993. Specificity of a protective memory immune response against *Mycobacterium tuberculosis*. *Infect. Immun.* **61:**844–851.

Augustin, A., R. T. Kubo, and G. Sim. 1989. Resident pulmonary lymphocytes expressing the γδ T cell receptor. *Nature* (London) **340:**239–241.

Barnes, P. F., D. Chatterjee, J. S. Abrams, S. H. Lu, E.

Wang, M. Yamamura, P. J. Brennan, and R. L. Modlin. 1992. Cytokine production induced by *Mycobacterium tuberculosis* lipoarabinomannan—relationship to chemical structure. *J. Immunol.* **149:**541–547.

Born, W., L. Hall, A. Dallas, J. Boymel, T. Shinnick, D. Young, P. Brennan, and R. O'Brien. 1990a. Recognition of a peptide antigen by heat shock reactive γδ T lymphocytes. *Science* **249:**67–69.

Born, W., M. P. Happ, A. Dallas, C. Reardon, R. Kubo, T. Shinnick, P. Brennan, and R. O'Brien. 1990b. Recognition of heat shock proteins and γδ cell function. *Immunol. Today* **11:**40–43.

Born, W. K., R. L. O'Brien, and R. L. Modlin. 1991. Antigen-specificity of γδ T lymphocytes. *FASEB J.* **5:**2699–2705.

Bosma, G. C., R. P. Custer, and M. J. Bosma. 1983. A severe combined immunodeficiency mutation in the mouse. *Nature* (London) **301:**527–530.

Brett, S., J. M. Orrell, J. Swanson Beck, and J. Ivanyi. 1992. Influence of H-2 genes on growth of *Mycobacterium tuberculosis* in the lungs of chronically infected mice. *Immunology* **76:**129–132.

Brown, I. N. 1983. Animal models and immune mechanisms in mycobacterial infection, p. 173–234. *In* C. Ratledge and J. Stanford (ed.), *Biology of Mycobacteria*, vol. 2. Academic Press Ltd., London.

Browning, C. H., and R. Gulbransen. 1926. Studies on experimental tuberculosis in mice. The susceptibility of mice to inoculation with tubercle bacilli. *J. Hyg.* **25:**323–332.

Chan, J., X. Fan, S. W. Hunter, P. J. Brennan, and B. R. Bloom. 1991. Lipoarabinomannan: a possible virulence factor involved in persistence of *Mycobacterium tuberculosis* within macrophages. *Infect. Immun.* **59:**1755–1761.

Chase, M. W. 1945. The cellular transfer of cutaneous hypersensitivity to tuberculin. *Proc. Soc. Exp. Biol. Med.* **59:**134–146.

Chatterjee, D., A. D. Roberts, K. Lowell, P. J. Brennan, and I. M. Orme. 1992. Structural basis of capacity of lipoarabinomannan to induce secretion of tumor necrosis factor. *Infect. Immun.* **60:**1249–1253.

Collins, F. M. 1979. Cellular antimicrobial immunity. *Crit. Rev. Microbiol.* **7:**27–91.

Collins, F. M. 1982. Immunology of tuberculosis. *Am. Rev. Respir. Dis.* **125:**S42–S49.

Collins, F. M. 1984. Protection against mycobacterial disease by means of live vaccines tested in experimental animals, p. 787–839. *In* G. P. Kubica and L. G. Wayne (ed.), *The Mycobacteria: a Sourcebook*. Marcel Dekker, Inc., New York.

Collins, F. M., and G. B. Mackaness. 1970. The relationship of delayed hypersensitivity to acquired antituberculous immunity. I. Tuberculin sensitivity and resistance to reinfection in BCG-vaccinated

mice. *Cell. Immunol.* **1:**253–265.

Collins, F. M., and V. Montalbine. 1975. Relative immunogenicity of streptomycin-resistant and -sensitive strains of BCG. II. Effect of route of inoculation on growth and immunogenicity. *Am. Rev. Respir. Dis.* **111:**43–51.

Collins, F. M., and V. Montalbine. 1976. Distribution of in vivo grown mycobacteria in the organs of intravenously infected mice. *Am. Rev. Respir. Dis.* **113:**281–286.

Collins, F. M., and M. M. Smith. 1969. A comparative study of the virulence of *Mycobacterium tuberculosis* measured in mice and guinea pigs. *Am. Rev. Respir. Dis.* **100:**631–639.

Collins, F. M., L. G. Wayne, and V. Montalbine. 1974. The effect of cultural conditions on the distribution of *Mycobacterium tuberculosis* in the spleens and lungs of specific pathogen-free mice. *Am. Rev. Respir. Dis.* **110:**147–156.

Cooper, A. M., D. K. Dalton, T. A. Stewart, J. P. Griffin, D. G. Russell, and I. M. Orme. 1993. Disseminated tuberculosis in interferon-γ gene-disrupted mice. *J. Exp. Med.* **178:**2243–2247.

Cox, J. H., B. C. Knight, and J. Ivanyi. 1989. Mechanisms of recrudescence of *Mycobacterium bovis* BCG infection in mice. *Infect. Immun.* **57:**1719–1724.

Dalton, D. K., S. Pitts-Meek, S. Keshaw, I. S. Figari, A. Bradley, and T. A. Stewart. 1993. Multiple defects of immune cell function in mice with disrupted interferon γ genes. *Science* **259:**1739–1742.

Davies, P. D. O. 1985. A possible link between vitamin D deficiency and impaired host defense to *Mycobacterium tuberculosis*. *Tubercle* **66:**301–306.

De Bruyn, J., R. Bosmans, J. Nyabenda, and J. P. Van Vooren. 1989. Effect of zinc deficiency on the appearance of two immunodominant protein antigens (32 kDa and 65 kDa) in culture filtrates of mycobacteria. *J. Gen. Microbiol.* **135:**79–84.

DeLibero, G., I. Flesch, and S. H. E. Kaufmann. 1988. Mycobacteria-reactive Lyt-2+ T cell lines. *Eur. J. Immunol.* **18:**59–66.

Dubos, R. J. 1945. Rapid and submerged growth of mycobacteria in liquid media. *Proc. Soc. Exp. Biol. Med.* **58:**361–362.

Dubos, R. J., and C. H. Pierce. 1956. Differential characteristics in vitro and in vivo of several substrains of BCG. IV. Immunizing effectiveness. *Am. Rev. Tuberc.* **74:**699–717.

Fenner, F. 1951. The enumeration of viable tubercle bacilli by surface plate counts. *Am. Rev. Tuberc.* **64:**353–380.

Fenner, F., S. P. Martin, and C. H. Pierce. 1949. The enumeration of viable tubercle bacilli in cultures and infected tissues. *Ann. N.Y. Acad. Sci.* **52:**751–764.

Flynn, J. L., J. Chan, K. J. Triebold, D. K. Dalton, T. A. Stewart, and B. R. Bloom. 1993. An essential role for IFN-γ in resistance to *M. tuberculosis* infection. *J. Exp. Med.* **178**:2248–2253.

Flynn, J. L., M. M. Goldstein, K. J. Triebold, B. Koller, and B. R. Bloom. 1992. Major histocompatibility complex class I-restricted T cells are required for resistance to *Mycobacterium tuberculosis* infection. *Proc. Natl. Acad. Sci. USA* **89**:12013–12017.

Follows, G. A., M. E. Munk, A. J. Gatrill, P. Conradt, and S. H. E. Kaufmann. 1992. Gamma-interferon and interleukin-2, but not interleukin-4, are detectable in gamma-delta T-cell cultures after activation with bacteria. *Infect. Immun.* **60**:1229–1231.

Fu, X.-Y., R. Cranfill, M. Vollmer, R. Van Der Zee, R. L. O'Brien, and W. Born. 1993. In vivo response of murine γδ T cells to a heat shock protein-derived peptide. *Proc. Natl. Acad. Sci. USA* **90**:322–326.

Furney, S. K., A. D. Roberts, and I. M. Orme. 1990. Effect of rifabutin on disseminated *Mycobacterium avium* infections in thymectomized, CD4 T-cell-deficient mice. *Antimicrob. Agents Chemother.* **34**:1629–1632.

Gray, D. F., and C. Cheers. 1967. The steady state in cellular immunity. *Aust. J. Exp. Biol. Med. Sci.* **45**:407–416.

Griffin, J. P., M. H. Fox, L. W. Armstrong, and I. M. Orme. Phenotypic identification of a IFN-γ-secreting CD4+ T cell subset in the spleens of mice infected with mycobacteria that appears concomitantly with the expression of protective immunity. Submitted for publication.

Griffin, J. P., K. V. Harshan, W. K. Born, and I. M. Orme. 1991. Kinetics of accumulation of γδ receptor-bearing T lymphocytes in mice infected with live mycobacteria. *Infect. Immun.* **59**:4263–4265.

Gros, P., E. Skamene, and A. Forget. 1981. Genetic control of natural resistance to *Mycobacterium bovis* (BCG) in mice. *J. Immunol.* **127**:2417–2421.

Gunn, F. D., W. J. Nungester, and E. T. Hougen. 1933. Susceptibility of the white mouse to tuberculosis. *Proc. Soc. Exp. Biol. Med.* **31**:527–529.

Haas, W., P. Pereira, and S. Tonegawa. 1993. Gamma/delta cells. *Annu. Rev. Immunol.* **11**:637–685.

Hartley, J. W., T. N. Fredrickson, R. A. Yetter, M. Makino, and H. C. Morse. 1989. Retrovirus-induced murine acquired immunodeficiency syndrome: natural history of infection and differing susceptibility of inbred mouse strains. *J. Virol.* **63**:1223–1231.

Huygen, K., D. Abramowicz, P. Vandenbussche, F. Jacobs, J. De Bruyn, A. Kentos, A. Drowart, J. P. Van Vooren, and M. Goldman. 1992. Spleen cell cytokine secretion in *Mycobacterium bovis* BCG-infected mice. *Infect. Immun.* **60**:2880–2886.

Huygen, K., A. Drowart, M. Harboe, R. ten Berg, J. Cogniaux, and J.-P. Van Vooren. 1993. Influence of genes from the major histocompatibility complex on the antibody repertoire against culture filtrate anti-

gens in mice infected with live *Mycobacterium bovis* BCG. *Infect. Immun.* **61**:2687–2693.

Inoue, T., Y. Yoshikai, G. Matsuzaki, and K. Nomoto. 1991. Early appearing γδ-bearing T cells during infection with Calmette Guerin bacillus. *J. Immunol.* **146**:2754–2762.

Janis, E. M., S. H. E. Kaufmann, R. H. Schwartz, and D. M. Pardoll. 1989. Activation of γδ T cells in the primary immune response to *Mycobacterium tuberculosis*. *Science* **244**:2754–2762.

Janssen, O., S. Wesselborg, B. Heckl-Ostreicher, K. Pechhold, A. Bender, A. Schondelmaier, G. Moldenhauer, and D. Kabelitz. 1991. T cell receptor/CD3 signalling induces death by apoptosis in human T cell receptor γδ+ T cells. *J. Immunol.* **146**:35–39.

Kaufmann, S. H. E. 1990. Heat shock proteins and the immune response. *Immunol. Today* **11**:129–136.

Kaufmann, S. H. E., and H. Hahn. 1981. The role of cell-mediated immunity in bacterial infections. *Rev. Infect. Dis.* **3**:1221–1250.

Kaufmann, S. H. E., B. Schoel, A. Wand-Wurttenberger, U. Steinhoff, M. E. Munk, and T. Koga. 1990. T-cells, stress proteins, and pathogenesis of mycobacterial infections. *Curr. Top. Microbiol. Immunol.* **155**:125–141.

Khansari, D. N., A. J. Murgo, and R. E. Faith. 1990. Effects of stress on the immune system. *Immunol. Today* **11**:170–175.

Kim, T. H., and G. P. Kubica. 1972. Long-term preservation and storage of mycobacteria. *Appl. Microbiol.* **24**:311–317.

Kim, T. H., and G. P. Kubica. 1973. Preservation of mycobacteria: 100% viability of suspensions stored at −70°C. *Appl. Microbiol.* **25**:956–960.

Kindler, V., A. P. Sappino, G. E. Grau, P. F. Piguet, and P. Vassilli. 1989. The inducing role of tumor necrosis factor in the development of bactericidal granulomas during BCG infection. *Cell* **56**:731–740.

Kumararatne, D. S., A. S. Pithie, P. Drysdale, J. S. H. Gaston, R. Kiessling, P. B. Iles, C. J. Ellis, J. Innes, and R. Wise. 1990. Specific lysis of mycobacterial antigen-bearing macrophages by class II MHC-restricted polyclonal T cell lines in healthy donors or patients with tuberculosis. *Clin. Exp. Immunol.* **80**:314–323.

Lambert, H. P. 1960. The influence of chemoprophylaxis on immunity in experimental tuberculosis. *Am. Rev. Respir. Dis.* **82**:619–626.

Lefford, M. J. 1971. The effect of inoculum size on the immune response to BCG infection in mice. *Immunology* **21**:369–381.

Lefford, M. J. 1975. Transfer of adoptive immunity to tuberculosis in mice. *Infect. Immun.* **11**:1174–1181.

Lefford, M. J. 1984. Diseases in mice and rats, p. 947–977. *In* G. P. Kubica and L. G. Wayne (ed.), *The Mycobacteria: a Sourcebook.* Marcel Dekker, Inc., New York.

Lui, Y., and C. A. Janeway. 1990. Interferon γ plays a critical role in induced cell death of effector T cells: a possible third mechanism of self-tolerance. *J. Exp. Med.* **172:**1735–1739.

Mackaness, G. B. 1968. The immunology of anti-tuberculous immunity. *Am. Rev. Respir. Dis.* **97:**337–344.

McDonough, K. A., Y. Kress, and B. R. Bloom. 1993. Pathogenesis of tuberculosis: interaction of *Mycobacterium tuberculosis* with macrophages. *Infect. Immun.* **61:**2763–2773.

McKee, C. M., G. Rake, R. Donovick, and W. P. Jambor. 1949. The use of the mouse in a standardized test for antituberculous activity of compounds of natural or synthetic origin. *Am. Rev. Tuberc.* **60:**90–108.

McMurray, D. N., C. L. Mintzer, C. L. Tetzlaff, and M. A. Carlomagno. 1986. The influence of dietary protein on the protective effect of BCG in guinea pigs. *Tubercle* **67:**31–39.

Moreno, C., J. Taverne, A. Mehlert, C. A. W. Bate, R. J. Brealey, A. Meager, G. A. W. Rook, and J. H. L. Playfair. 1989. Lipoarabinomannan from *Mycobacterium tuberculosis* induces the production of tumor necrosis factor from human and murine macrophages. *Clin. Exp. Immunol.* **76:**240–245.

Mosier, D. E., R. A. Yetter, and H. C. Morse. 1985. Retroviral induction of acute lymphoproliferative disease and profound immunosuppression in adult C57BL mice. *J. Exp. Med.* **161:**766–784.

Mosmann, T. R., and R. E. Coffman. 1989. Heterogeneity of cytokine secretion patterns and functions of helper T cells. *Adv. Immunol.* **46:**111–147.

Muller, I., S. Cobbold, H. Waldmann, and S. H. E. Kaufmann. 1987. Impaired resistance to *Mycobacterium tuberculosis* infection after selective in vivo depletion of L3T4$^+$ and Lyt-2$^+$ T cells. *Infect. Immun.* **55:**2037–2041.

Munk, M. E., A. J. Gatrill, and S. H. E. Kaufmann. 1990. Target cell lysis and IL-2 secretion by γδ T lymphocytes after activation with bacteria. *J. Immunol.* **145:**2434–2439.

North, R. J. 1973. Importance of thymus-derived lymphocytes in cell-mediated immunity to infection. *Cell. Immunol.* **7:**166–176.

North, R. J., G. B. Mackaness, and R. W. Elliott. 1972. The histogenesis of immunologically committed lymphocytes. *Cell. Immunol.* **3:**680–694.

O'Brien, R., M. P. Happ, A. Dallas, E. Palmer, R. Kubo, and W. K. Born. 1989. Stimulation of a major subset of lymphocytes expressing T cell receptor γδ by an antigen derived from *Mycobacterium tuberculosis*. *Cell* **57:**667–674.

O'Brien, R. L., Y. Fu, R. Cranfill, A. Dallas, C. Ellis, C. Reardon, J. Lang, S. R. Carding, R. Kubo, and W. Born. 1992. Heat shock protein Hsp60-reactive γδ cells: a large, diversified T-lymphocyte subset with highly focused specificity. *Proc. Natl. Acad. Sci. USA* **89:**4348–4352.

Ohmen, J. D., P. F. Barnes, K. Uyemura, S. Z. Lu, C. L. Grisso, and R. L. Modlin. 1991. The T-cell receptors of human γδ T-cells reactive to *Mycobacterium tuberculosis* are encoded by specific-V genes but diverse V-J junctions. *J. Immunol.* **147:**3353–3359.

Ordway, D. J., and I. M. Orme. 1993. Unpublished observations.

Orme, I. M. 1987a. The kinetics of emergence and loss of mediator T lymphocytes acquired in response to infection with *Mycobacterium tuberculosis*. *J. Immunol.* **138:**293–298.

Orme, I. M. 1987b. Aging and immunity to tuberculosis: increased susceptibility of old mice reflects a decreased capacity to generate mediator T lymphocytes. *J. Immunol.* **138:**4414–4418.

Orme, I. M. 1988a. Characteristics and specificity of acquired immunologic memory to *Mycobacterium tuberculosis* infection. *J. Immunol.* **140:**3589–3593.

Orme, I. M. 1988b. Evidence for a biphasic memory T cell response to high dose BCG vaccination in mice. *Tubercle* **69:**125–131.

Orme, I. M. 1988c. Induction of nonspecific acquired resistance and delayed-type hypersensitivity, but not specific acquired resistance, in mice inoculated with killed mycobacterial vaccines. *Infect. Immun.* **56:**3310–3312.

Orme, I. M. 1993a. The role of CD8+ T cells in immunity to tuberculosis infection. *Trends Microbiol.* **1:**77–78.

Orme, I. M. 1993b. Immunity to mycobacteria. *Curr. Opin. Immunol.* **5:**497–502.

Orme, I. M., P. Andersen, and W. H. Boom. 1993a. T cell response to *Mycobacterium tuberculosis*. *J. Infect. Dis.* **167:**1481–1497.

Orme, I. M., and F. M. Collins. 1984a. Demonstration of acquired resistance in *Bcg*^{r} inbred mouse strains infected with a low dose of BCG Montreal. *Clin. Exp. Immunol.* **56:**81–88.

Orme, I. M., and F. M. Collins. 1984b. Passive transfer of tuberculin sensitivity from anergic mice. *Infect. Immun.* **46:**850–853.

Orme, I. M., and F. M. Collins. 1986. Crossprotection against nontuberculous mycobacterial infections by *Mycobacterium tuberculosis* memory immune T lymphocytes. *J. Exp. Med.* **163:**203–208.

Orme, I. M., S. K. Furney, and A. D. Roberts. 1992a. Dissemination of enteric *Mycobacterium avium* infections in mice rendered immunodeficient by thymectomy and CD4 depletion or by prior infection with murine AIDS retroviruses. *Infect. Immun.* **60:**4747–4753.

Orme, I. M., J. P. Griffin, A. D. Roberts, and D. N. Ernst. 1993b. Evidence for a defective accumulation of protective T cells in old mice infected with

Mycobacterium tuberculosis. Cell. Immunol. **147:** 222–229.

Orme, I. M., E. S. Miller, A. D. Roberts, S. K. Furney, J. P. Griffin, K. M. Dobos, D. Chi, B. Rivoire, and P. J. Brennan. 1992b. T lymphocytes mediating protection and cellular cytolysis during the course of *Mycobacterium tuberculosis* infection. *J. Immunol.* **148:**189–196.

Orme, I. M., A. D. Roberts, J. P. Griffin, and J. S. Abrams. 1993c. Cytokine secretion by CD4 T lymphocytes acquired in response to *Mycobacterium tuberculosis* infection. *J. Immunol.* **151:**518–525.

Orme, I. M., R. W. Stokes, and F. M. Collins. 1985. Only two out of fifteen BCG strains follow the *Bcg* pattern, p. 285–290. *In* E. Skamene (ed.), *Genetic Control of Host Resistance to Infection and Malignancy.* Alan R. Liss, Inc., New York.

Panchamoorthy, G., J. McLean, R. L. Modlin, C. T. Morita, S. Isikawa, M. B. Brenner, and H. Band. 1991. A predominance of the T-cell receptor Vγ2/Vδ2 subset in human mycobacteria-responsive T-cells suggests germline gene encoded recognition. *J. Immunol.* **147:**3360–3369.

Pierce, C. H., R. J. Dubos, and W. B. Schaefer. 1956. Differential characteristics in vitro and in vivo of substrains of BCG. III. Multiplication and survival in vivo. *Am. Rev. Tuberc.* **74:**683–688.

Raleigh, G. W., and G. P. Youmans. 1949. The use of mice in experimental chemotherapy of tuberculosis. *J. Infect. Dis.* **82:**197–204.

Roach, T. I. A., C. H. Barton, D. Chatterjee, and J. M. Blackwell. 1993. Macrophage activation: lipoarabinomannan from avirulent and virulent strains of *Mycobacterium tuberculosis* differentially induces the early genes c-fos, KC, JE, and tumor necrosis factor-α. *J. Immunol.* **150:**1886–1896.

Rook, G. A. W., J. Steele, S. Barnass, J. Mace, and J. L. Stanford. 1986. Responsiveness to live *M. tuberculosis*, and common antigens, of sonicate-stimulated T cell lines from normal donors. *Clin. Exp. Immunol.* **63:**105–110.

Russell, D. G., A. M. Cooper, D. Chatterjee, and I. M. Orme. 1993. Unpublished observation.

Shier, D. R., and M. W. Long. 1971. The relation between infecting dosage and mean survival in tuberculous guinea pigs. *Am. Rev. Respir. Dis.* **104:** 206–214.

Sprent, J. 1993. Lifespans of naive, memory and effector lymphocytes. *Curr. Opin. Immunol.* **5:**433–438.

Sturgill-Koszycki, S., P. H. Schlesinger, P. Chakraborty, P. L. Haddix, H. L. Collins, S. Gluck, A. K. Fok, R. D. Allen, J. Heuser, and D. G. Russell. Mycobacteria resist acidification of their phagosomes by selectively blocking incorporation of the vesicular proton-ATPase. *Science*, in press.

Suter, E. 1961. Passive transfer of acquired resistance to infection with *Mycobacterium tuberculosis* by means of cells. *Am. Rev. Respir. Dis.* **83:**535–543.

Verbon, A., S. Kuijper, H. M. Jansen, P. Speelman, and A. H. Kolk. 1990. Antigens in culture supernatant of *Mycobacterium tuberculosis*: epitopes defined by monoclonal and human antibodies. *J. Gen. Microbiol.* **136:**955–964.

Wiegeshaus, E. H., and D. W. Smith. 1968. Experimental models for study of immunity to tuberculosis. *Ann. N.Y. Acad. Sci.* **154:**194–199.

Youmans, G. P. 1949. The use of the mouse for the testing of chemotherapeutic agents against *Mycobacterium tuberculosis. Ann. N.Y. Acad. Sci.* **52:** 662–670.

Youmans, G. P., and J. C. McCarter. 1945. Streptomycin in experimental tuberculosis. *Am. Rev. Tuberc.* **52:**432–439.

Young, D. B., S. H. E. Kaufmann, P. W. M. Hermans, and J. E. R. Thole. 1992. Mycobacterial protein antigens: a compilation. *Mol. Microbiol.* **6:**133–145.

Tuberculosis: Pathogenesis, Protection, and Control
Edited by Barry R. Bloom
© 1994 American Society for Microbiology, Washington, DC 20005

Chapter 9

Guinea Pig Model of Tuberculosis

David N. McMurray

HISTORICAL PERSPECTIVE

It is not by chance that the term "guinea pig" in the modern lexicon has come to denote an experimental subject. In the 1800s and early 1900s, the guinea pig was perhaps the most widely used experimental animal for the study of infectious diseases. Indeed, the classic experiments that led to the establishment of the criteria that must be satisfied to identify a microorganism as the etiologic agent of a disease, known as Koch's postulates, were carried out with guinea pigs infected with *Mycobacterium tuberculosis* (Koch, 1882). Koch's discovery of the tubercle bacillus as the causative agent of human tuberculosis was facilitated by the animal model that this pioneer scientist chose to employ in his studies. Koch's principal reason for choosing the guinea pig for experimental infection with *M. tuberculosis* in the 1890s is every bit as valid today, namely, the exquisite susceptibility of this species to infection with human tubercle bacilli (Dannenberg, 1984).

More recent studies of the comparative biology of the guinea pig have revealed a number of remarkable similarities between this species and humans (Sisk, 1976). Many of those fundamental similarities bear directly or indirectly on the relevance of the guinea pig as a species in which to model human infectious disease. Thus, like human infants, newborn guinea pigs possess a very mature lymphomyeloid complex (Ernstrom, 1970). Hormonally and immunologically, guinea pigs are much more similar to humans than are rodents (Shewell and Long, 1956). Guinea pigs share with human beings the rather unusual need for exogenously supplied ascorbic acid in the diet (Collins and Elvehjem, 1958). Like humans and nonhuman primates, the guinea pig is considered a corticosteroid-resistant species (Calman, 1972). The physiology of the pulmonary tract, especially the response of the lung to inflammatory stimuli, is quite similar to that of humans (Lechner and Banchero, 1982), as is the dermal response to both acute and chronic inflammatory mediators (Ediger, 1976). Recent phylogenetic analyses indicate that the guinea pig may not be part of the order Rodentia (Graur et al., 1991).

APPLICATIONS TO CLINICAL AND EXPERIMENTAL TUBERCULOSIS

For more than 100 years, the guinea pig has contributed to the battle against tuberculosis in both the clinical and research arenas. Prior to the formulation of conve-

David N. McMurray • Department of Medical Microbiology and Immunology, Texas A&M University Health Science Center, College Station, Texas 77843-1114.

nient artificial media that presently allow the identification of *M. tuberculosis* by culture of clinical specimens, the material from the suspected patient was injected directly into guinea pigs. The innate susceptibility of the guinea pig to infection with human tubercle bacilli allowed even a few viable bacteria to produce progressive disease that would be detected at necropsy several weeks later. Although this method remains at least as sensitive as culture in vitro, the cost and biohazard risk of maintaining infected animals resulted in the demise of this diagnostic test.

Guinea pigs have also been employed in the testing of both biological reagents and drugs for use in human beings with tuberculosis. Since Koch's original observation of a delayed hypersensitivity reaction following the intradermal injection of tubercle bacilli into an infected guinea pig, this animal has been the "gold standard" for the potency testing and biological standardization of tuberculins for use in human skin testing (Tolderland et al., 1967; Ladefoged et al., 1976). Likewise, the development and preclinical testing of BCG vaccine by Calmette and Guérin in the first quarter of this century relied heavily on the guinea pig (Calmette et al., 1924). Indeed, much of the data relating to differing potencies among BCG vaccines and the quality control procedures used to ensure the continued attenuation of BCG were determined or carried out in guinea pigs (Smith et al., 1979). Finally, guinea pigs respond quite well to many of the antibiotics currently used to treat tuberculosis patients. Evidence for the efficacy of new drugs or drug combinations has been obtained with this model (Cohn et al., 1962; Smith et al., 1991). This application of the model will undoubtedly become more important as the specter of multidrug-resistant strains of *M. tuberculosis* drives the search for new and better antimycobacterial drugs (Collins, 1993).

Perhaps the most important application of the guinea pig model in the past 50 years has been in understanding the fundamental relationship between the tubercle bacillus and its mammalian host. The determinants of microbial virulence on the one hand and the mechanisms of host resistance on the other have been studied quite successfully in the guinea pig by a number of investigators. Early workers focused on the kinetics of spread of virulent tubercle bacilli following injection or inhalation of widely varying doses of *M. tuberculosis* into naive or previously sensitized guinea pigs (Jensen et al., 1935; Long et al., 1931; Ratcliffe and Palladino, 1953). These studies of the pathogenesis of experimental tuberculosis in vaccinated and nonvaccinated guinea pigs revealed that previous exposure to mycobacterial antigens often resulted in the acquisition of delayed hypersensitivity and an ability to retard the accumulation of tubercle bacilli in the tissues (Schwabacher and Wilson, 1938; Palmer and Hopwood, 1962; Liebow et al., 1940). The interaction between deficiencies of essential nutrients such as protein, vitamin C, and vitamin D and resistance to experimental tuberculosis was examined many years ago in the guinea pig (Leichentritt, 1924; McConkey and Smith, 1933; Rao and Gopalan, 1958). Early observations on the interaction between tubercle bacilli and host phagocytic cells were made with guinea pigs (Berthrong and Hamilton, 1959). The potential role of mycobacterial constituents, such as "cord factor," as virulence factors because of their toxicity for host cells was suggested by early investigations using guinea pigs (Middlebrook et al., 1947; Bloch and Noll, 1953). In spite of these seminal observations, it was difficult to obtain a comprehensive understanding of the pathogenesis of tuberculosis in the guinea pig prior to 1965 because of major variations in crucial test variables between laboratories. Perhaps the most important of these was the lack of an adequately controlled, reproducible procedure for infecting guinea pigs with very small inocula of virulent *M. tuberculosis* by the respiratory route.

GUINEA PIG MODEL OF PULMONARY TUBERCULOSIS

Experiments in the 1950s demonstrated that guinea pigs were exquisitely susceptible to infection by both natural and artificial aerosols containing low levels of virulent *M. tuberculosis* (Riley et al., 1959; Middlebrook, 1952). The rationale for exposing animals under these conditions has been discussed by Smith and his colleagues (Smith and Harding, 1977; Smith and Wiegeshaus, 1989). The concept of a "rational" animal model of tuberculosis was based upon the selection of test system variables that mimic the important aspects of human disease (Smith and Harding, 1977; Smith, 1985). Thus, Smith and co-workers demonstrated that guinea pigs could be infected reproducibly with very small inocula (1 to 2 CFU) of a single-cell suspension of *M. tuberculosis* and that the frozen inoculum could be stored for several years at −70°C without altered viability (Smith et al., 1966; Grover et al., 1967). The characteristics of an aerosol chamber that made it possible to achieve such realistic pulmonary exposure were described in detail in 1970 (Wiegeshaus et al., 1970). The chamber was shown to produce a cloud of droplet nuclei that resulted in the inhalation and retention in the alveolar spaces of very small inocula. Experiments involving culture of the whole lung immediately following infection with highly virulent mycobacteria demonstrated that the number of viable organisms recovered was nearly identical to the number of primary tubercles that developed 4 weeks later (unpublished observations).

Initial studies with this model attempted to define the early events in the pathogenesis of pulmonary tuberculosis (Smith et al., 1970). Following exposure to a few

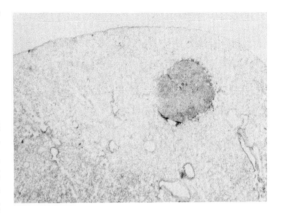

Figure 1. Primary tubercle in the lung of a guinea pig 4 weeks following inhalation of a few virulent *M. tuberculosis* H37Rv bacilli (Mainali and McMurray, submitted).

viable virulent *M. tuberculosis* bacilli, guinea pigs developed primary pulmonary lesions that histologically resembled typical human tubercles (Fig. 1). The number of viable mycobacteria recovered from the lungs increased exponentially between days 3 and 21 postinfection, when levels in lung plateaued at 10^5 to 10^6 viable organisms. Sometime between 14 and 18 days following pulmonary exposure, the first organisms appeared in the bronchotracheal lymph nodes draining the lung fields. Somewhat later (at 18 to 21 days), the first mycobacteria were detected in the spleen. Concomitant with evidence of detectable bacillemia, the guinea pigs converted their tuberculin skin tests to positive. Infected guinea pigs mount a delayed hypersensitivity reaction to low doses of tuberculin (1 to 5 tuberculin units of purified protein derivative [PPD]) that is macroscopically and histologically indistinguishable from the reactions of infected humans.

Vaccination has a dramatic effect on the course and ultimate outcome of pulmonary tuberculosis in the guinea pig. A variety of vaccines have been tested in this model, including nonviable bacilli (Fregnan and Smith, 1963), attenuated mycobacteria (Smith et al., 1972), many strains of BCG

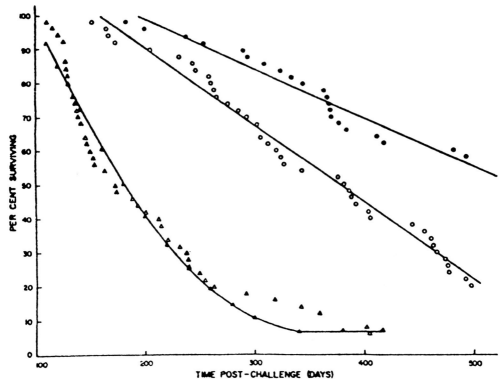

Figure 2. Survival curves for groups of guinea pigs vaccinated with either BCG (●), nonviable defatted bacilli (○), or placebo (△) and infected with a few virulent *M. tuberculosis* H37Rv bacilli (from Wiegeshaus et al., 1970, with permission).

(Smith et al., 1979; Wiegeshaus and Smith, 1989), and, more recently, recombinant vaccines (Wiegeshaus and Smith, 1989). Early studies demonstrated that BCG was quite effective even at very low doses when given by the subcutaneous or intradermal route (Jespersen, 1956). Aerosol vaccination with BCG is also at least as effective if not more so than parenteral immunization (Legranderie et al., 1993).

The effect of successful vaccination is to significantly increase the survival of guinea pigs infected with a low dose of virulent *M. tuberculosis* by the respiratory route. In terms of both percent survival 500 days postchallenge and mean survival time of animals dying before the termination of the experiment, BCG-vaccinated guinea pigs benefitted significantly (Fig. 2) (Wiegeshaus et al., 1970). Necropsy evidence from ani-

mals dying during the experiment confirmed that extensive pulmonary pathology and compromised respiratory function were probably the causes of death. Many of the surviving BCG-vaccinated guinea pigs had evidence of healed or regressing pulmonary lesions (unpublished observations).

The protracted course of disease following low-dose pulmonary exposure made the routine use of survival as an experimental readout impractical. Therefore, groups of guinea pigs in the survival experiment just described were euthanized at early intervals (3 and 5 weeks) postinfection, and the number of viable mycobacteria recoverable from the lung, spleen, and bronchotracheal lymph nodes was determined. The numbers of viable *M. tuberculosis* in the lung at the two intervals were highly correlated statistically with survival. Therefore, bacterial

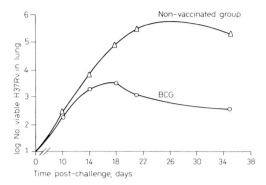

Figure 3. Influence of BCG vaccination on the early course of pulmonary infection with virulent *M. tuberculosis* H37Rv in the lungs of vaccinated and nonvaccinated guinea pigs (from Smith et al., 1970, with permission).

enumeration 3 to 5 weeks postinfection was established as a relevant measure of acquired resistance in this model (Wiegeshaus et al., 1970).

Comparison of the course of pulmonary disease in BCG-vaccinated and nonvaccinated guinea pigs at frequent intervals during the first 5 weeks following low-dose aerosol exposure revealed that although vaccinated animals exhibited a strong PPD reaction at the time of virulent infection, the effect of this preexisting immunity on events in the lung did not appear immediately (Fig. 3). In fact, bacillary loads in the lung reached 10^3 CFU (2 weeks postchallenge) before differences between the two groups became statistically significant (Smith et al., 1970). The principal effects of BCG were a dramatic restriction of the accumulation of virulent mycobacteria in the lung and spleen and the occurrence of primary tubercles that were histologically smaller and less necrotic than those observed in nonvaccinated guinea pigs (Smith and Wiegeshaus, 1989).

One important advantage of the low-dose aerosol model is that when guinea pigs are exposed under these conditions, some lung lobes do not receive an inoculum via the airway and therefore do not contain myco-

bacteria initially. Utilizing an X-ray machine, Smith and colleagues were able to select lung lobes containing primary lesions and others that were free of primary lesions and compare the events in these two regions of the lung at intervals following pulmonary infection (Harding and Smith, 1977; Ho et al., 1978). They demonstrated that lung lobes that were not initially infected remained free of mycobacteria for more than 2 weeks. Coincident with the extrapulmonary spread of tubercle bacilli via the bloodstream to the spleen, mycobacteria began to appear in primary-lesion-free lung lobes. Over the next several weeks, the levels of viable *M. tuberculosis* in those lobes rose to approximate the levels detected in lobes containing primary lesions (Ho et al., 1978). Thus, reseeding of the lung by the hematogenous route is an important component of pulmonary disease in this model, as it clearly is in human beings (Stead, 1989). In fact, experiments conducted with clinical isolates of *M. tuberculosis* that varied in virulence revealed a high correlation between the extent of gross disease in the tissues and the ability of that strain to disseminate to the spleen (Prabhakar et al., 1987). Thus, the bacillemic capacity of an isolate may be an intrinsic characteristic, and the guinea pig is clearly capable of discriminating between isolates on that basis. Additional studies proved that among the beneficial effects of BCG vaccination are reduction of the extent of extrapulmonary dissemination to the spleen and prevention or retarding of hematogenous infection of areas of the lung originally not involved in the disease process (Fok et al., 1976; Harding and Smith, 1977; Smith and Harding, 1978).

Much of the work with this model has involved the use of outbred guinea pigs. However, for some experimental applications, the inclusion of inbred animals could have significant advantages. Experiments involving adoptive transfer of lymphocytes between donors and recipients or the coculture in vitro of populations of cells derived from donors treated in different ways require syngeneic animals. Anecdotal evidence suggested that the two commercially available inbred strains of guinea pigs, strains 2 and 13, differed in their susceptibilities to infection with *M. tuberculosis*. However, direct comparison of the response of outbred Hartley, inbred strain 2, and inbred strain 13 guinea pigs to low-dose pulmonary infection revealed no significant differences in the bacillary loads in the lung and spleen 4 to 6 weeks postinfection. Prior vaccination with BCG protected all three strains equally well. Parameters of T-lymphocyte reactivity to mycobacterial antigens in vivo and in vitro were essentially the same in all three strains (Cohen et al., 1987). On the basis of these results, it appears that inbred guinea pigs may be quite useful for experiments in which syngeneic hosts are required. The results of examples of such experiments are described later in this chapter.

A useful generic approach to the elucidation of mechanisms of resistance to an infectious agent is to treat the host in such a way that the immune status is altered (either enhanced or suppressed) in some predictable and reproducible fashion and then to determine the effect of that alteration on disease resistance. The human immunodeficiency virus epidemic has made it very clear that reduced T-cell-mediated immunity is a potent risk factor for tuberculosis (Chaisson and Slutkin, 1989). Even in the pre-AIDS era, a proportion of patients infected with *M. tuberculosis* were immunologically unresponsive and experienced difficulty controlling their disease (Zeitz et al., 1974; McMurray and Echeverry, 1978). Tuberculosis presents in a large population of patients as a spectrum of clinical conditions, ranging from the reactive patient at one extreme to the unreactive or anergic patient at the other (Lenzini et al., 1977). Studies of anergic tuberculosis patients have revealed a num-

Table 1. Impact of chronic, moderate protein deficiency on immunity to experimental pulmonary tuberculosis in the guinea pig model

1. Partial to complete loss of BCG vaccine-induced protection
2. Failure of low-virulence primary infection to protect against exogenous reinfection
3. Loss of PPD-induced lymphocyte responses in vivo and in vitro
4. Temporal reduction in circulating erythrocyte rosette-forming (CD2) T cells
5. Alteration in the production and activity of IL-2
6. Significant shifts in the proportions of Tμ- and Tγ-cell subsets
7. Increased levels of circulating anti-PPD antibody
8. Complete and rapid reversal of immune dysfunction upon renutrition

ber of immunological abnormalities that might explain their failure to respond appropriately to mycobacterial infection (McMurray, 1980).

Since malnutrition has long been known to exert a deleterious effect on T-cell-mediated immune functions (McMurray, 1984), the impact of chronic, moderate dietary protein deprivation on resistance to tuberculosis has been examined in the guinea pig model (McMurray and Yetley, 1983; McMurray et al., 1986a, b). These studies demonstrate that the protein-malnourished animal infected with mycobacteria exhibits several immunological deficits, the most important of which is the loss of protection following vaccination with BCG (Table 1) (McMurray et al., 1985, 1990). These results have obvious implications for control of tuberculosis in malnourished populations. They also reveal that protein deficiency mimics the nonresponder pole of the clinical spectrum of tuberculosis. Like anergic human patients, malnourished guinea pigs infected with *M. tuberculosis* mount poor T-cell responses to mycobacterial antigens in vivo (tuberculin skin test) and in vitro (PPD-driven lymphoproliferation), have high levels of circulating antimycobacterial antibodies or immune complexes,

Table 2. Diet-induced immunological spectrum of experimental pulmonary tuberculosis in the guinea pig[a]

Criterion	Diet	
	Control	Low protein
Delayed hypersensitivity	+++	+
Lymphocyte proliferation	+++	+
BCG-induced resistance	+++	+
Antimycobacterial antibodies	+	+++

[a] The degree of reactivity is expressed in level of intensity: +++, very intense; +, low intensity.

and do not control replication of the organisms in the tissues (Table 2) (McMurray and Bartow, 1992). Histologic examination of the lungs of normally nourished and protein-deficient guinea pigs demonstrates that malnutrition interferes with normal granuloma formation, leaving deprived animals with smaller, more numerous, less well circumscribed tubercles in the lung (Fig. 4) (Mainali and McMurray, submitted). Thus, the malnourished guinea pig may be a useful model for the anergic tuberculosis patient in attempts to dissect the crucial determinants of resistance to pulmonary tuberculosis.

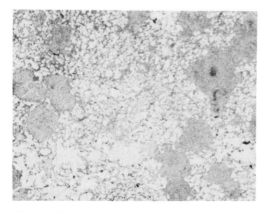

Figure 4. Primary and secondary tubercles in the lung of a protein-malnourished guinea pig 4 weeks following inhalation of a few virulent *M. tuberculosis* H37Rv bacilli (Mainali and McMurray, submitted).

APPLICATION OF MODERN IMMUNOLOGICAL TECHNIQUES IN THE GUINEA PIG

For all its clinical relevance, the guinea pig as a model for human tuberculosis has one major disadvantage: the lack of reagents necessary to perform sophisticated studies of the immune system. Compared to the mouse or human, guinea pigs lag far behind in terms of the development of monoclonal antibodies specific for phenotypic markers on lymphocytes, immunochemical assays for cytokines, or genetic probes for genes of interest. In recent years, however, some advances have been made in the application of modern immunological tools to the study of mechanisms of resistance to tuberculosis in the guinea pig.

Prior to the availability of monoclonal antibodies for CD markers, the CD2 molecule on guinea pig T cells was detected by the binding of heterologous (rabbit) erythrocytes in a classic rosette-forming assay (Stadecker et al., 1973; Bartow and McMurray, 1990). By modifying that procedure to include erythrocytes coated with either immunoglobulin M (IgM) or IgG antibodies, T-cell subsets expressing Fc receptors for IgM (Tμ) or IgG (Tγ) were studied (Shigeki et al., 1982; Bartow and McMurray, 1989; McMurray et al., 1990). A few laboratories have pioneered the development and characterization of monoclonal antibodies directed against guinea pig major histocompatibility complex molecules, the T-cell receptor, and analogs of CD3, CD4, and CD8 (Elias et al., 1985; Tan et al., 1985; McPhee et al., 1988; Schafer et al., 1989; Payne and Thomson, 1989; Schafer and Burger, 1992; Hart et al., 1992). Some of these antibodies are now available commercially and have been used in flow cytometric analyses of the anatomical distribution of T-cell subsets in guinea pigs infected with *M. tuberculosis* (Mainali and McMurray, unpublished data). These studies reveal that one of the mechanisms by which protein deprivation reduces disease resistance is by causing the pooling or sequestration of T cells in the bronchotracheal lymph nodes draining the site of implantation (Mainali and McMurray, 1992).

A second recent improvement in the application of the model has been the development of an adoptive transfer paradigm. Inbred guinea pigs have been used to study the role of adoptively transferred cells in resistance to other infectious diseases but not to tuberculosis (Pavia and Niederbuhl, 1985; Wicher et al., 1987). This system involves the generation of lymphocyte or column-purified T-cell populations from immune strain 2 guinea pigs and their injection into syngeneic recipient animals by the intraperitoneal or intravenous route. The level of passive resistance to virulent infection achieved in these experiments is equivalent to that obtained with active immunization with BCG in terms of reductions in mycobacterial loads in the lung 4 weeks following respiratory exposure (Mainali and McMurray, submitted). More important, experiments involving reciprocal transfer of lymphocytes from protein-deprived or well-nourished immune donors and recipients suggest that protein-malnourished guinea pigs can be protected quite effectively by normal immune lymphocytes but cannot themselves generate a protective population of cells (McMurray et al., 1993; Mainali and McMurray, submitted).

Although the lack of purified guinea pig cytokines or antibodies against such cytokines has restricted the study of cytokine involvement in this model, recent progress has been made. Biological assays for some cytokines have been employed successfully in the guinea pig. These include the CTLL-2 cell line proliferation assay for interleukin-2 (IL-2) (McMurray et al., 1989b) and the L929 cytotoxicity assay for tumor necrosis factor (Phalen and McMurray, 1993a). Guinea pig IL-1 was reported to be active in the standard comitogenic stimulation assay using C3H/HeJ mouse thymocytes (Zhao et al., 1992). In addition, the macrophage migration inhibition factor assay has been used in guinea pigs infected with mycobacteria (Kramer and Good, 1978; Carlomagno et al., 1985). Some recombinant cytokines from other species have activity for guinea pig cells. Murine recombinant IL-2 can stimulate guinea pig T cells to proliferate and under some circumstances can rescue the PPD-induced proliferative response of lymphocytes derived from protein-deficient guinea pigs infected with *M. tuberculosis* (McMurray et al., 1989b). Other investigators have demonstrated that guinea pig eosinophils are responsive to recombinant human IL-8 in vivo and in vitro (Collins et al., 1993) and that recombinant murine IL-5 induced airway hyperreactivity and eosinophil accumulation in guinea pigs (Oosterhaut et al., 1993). Thus, some currently available recombinant murine and human cytokines may be useful in dissecting the participation of those mediators in the pathogenesis of tuberculosis in the guinea pig model.

The cloning of genes encoding important cell receptors or soluble mediators is a powerful approach to elucidating the functions of these receptors and mediators. Little such work has been done to date in the guinea pig for molecules that might be involved in resistance to tuberculosis. The constant-region genes for the guinea pig $\alpha\beta$ T-cell receptor have been cloned (Schenkel et al., 1992), as have the genes for three isoforms of the guinea pig Fc receptor for IgG1 and IgG2 (Yamashita et al., 1993). Other investigators have reported cloning the genes for guinea pig neutrophil activation protein-1 and monocyte chemoattractant protein-1 (Yoshimura, 1993). The latter protein has been produced in recombinant form, and its activity has been tested in vivo and in vitro (Yoshimura, 1993). It is conceivable that the selection of highly conserved regions in the sequences of other cloned murine or human genes would allow the synthesis of probes for the homologous guinea pig genes. The availability of such reagents would greatly enhance the value of the guinea pig in the study of pulmonary tuberculosis and would bring a degree of experimental sophistication to an already highly relevant disease model.

Another very useful approach to defining the immunological mechanisms involved in resistance to tuberculosis in the guinea pig model would be T-cell lines or clones reactive with mycobacterial antigens. Early literature described some success at cloning guinea pig T cells (Malek et al., 1981; Polak and Scheper, 1983). Recently, the generation of guinea pig T-cell lines reactive to culture filtrate antigens from *M. tuberculosis* H37Rv was reported (Haslov and Heron, 1989).

MODELING OTHER CLINICAL FORMS OF TUBERCULOSIS IN THE GUINEA PIG

In addition to primary, pulmonary tuberculosis, there are other forms of disease caused by *M. tuberculosis* that are important clinically and for which experimental models would be extremely valuable. These include tuberculous meningitis, tuberculous pleuritis, exogenous reinfection, and endogenous reactivation. The guinea pig has been used in preliminary studies to develop models of these clinical manifestations of mycobacterial disease.

Pleuritis can be induced in previously immunized guinea pigs by the intrapleural injection of either living BCG (Windstrom and Nilsson, 1982) or heat-killed *M. tuberculosis* (Phalen and McMurray, 1993a). The cellular nature of the effusion, with particular reference to the enrichment of T lymphocytes that proliferate in response to mycobacterial antigens, has been shown to be quite similar to human tuberculous pleural effusion (Phalen and McMurray, 1993a). Recently, the relevance of the guinea pig

model was enhanced by the report of elevated tumor necrosis factor alpha levels in effusion fluid as well as in supernatant fluids from pleural effusion lymphocytes stimulated with PPD (Phalen and McMurray, 1993b). Similar increases in tumor necrosis factor alpha activity have been reported in cases of human tuberculous pleuritis (Barnes et al., 1990).

Exogenous reinfection has been studied in the guinea pig. Reinfection by the pulmonary route with virulent *M. tuberculosis* of guinea pigs previously infected with either nontuberculous mycobacteria or low-virulence clinical isolates did not result in more severe disease as has been reported in humans (Nardell et al., 1986) but actually resulted in protection (Ziegler et al., 1985; Edwards et al., 1982). Reinfected guinea pigs controlled the second (virulent) challenge more successfully than guinea pigs infected for the first time under identical conditions, and the protective effect of a prior pulmonary exposure to a low-virulence isolate was significantly impaired by protein malnutrition (McMurray et al., 1989a). Further development of this model will be important, since the design of vaccination strategies for tuberculosis may be quite different in areas where exogenous reinfection is prevalent (Smith and Wiegeshaus, 1989).

Endogenous reactivation tuberculosis is seen frequently in elderly populations whose primary exposure may have occurred decades previously. A model of endogenous reactivation disease would contribute to our understanding of the factors associated with persistence of *M. tuberculosis* in the tissues as well as of the events that allow the dormant mycobacteria to reappear in large numbers. Although no experimental data on endogenous reactivation in the guinea pig exist, Smith and Wiegeshaus (1989) have presented a clear rationale for how such a model might be developed.

SUMMARY

In summary, the advantages of the guinea pig model of tuberculosis are as follows: (i) animals can be infected reproducibly by the pulmonary route with very small numbers of virulent human tubercle bacilli; (ii) the course of disease following pulmonary infection, which includes bacillemia and hematogenous reseeding of the lung, is similar to that in humans; (iii) the similarities between the granulomatous and hypersensitivity responses of guinea pigs and humans to *M. tuberculosis* are remarkable; (iv) the degree of protection induced by vaccination with BCG is excellent, and we can discriminate between various degrees of protection; and (v) there is the potential for modeling other clinical forms of tuberculosis in the guinea pig.

The disadvantages of this model are primarily related to the current paucity of readily available reagents with which to perform sophisticated studies of cell phenotypes and cytokine involvement, the high cost of guinea pigs compared to rodents, and the requirement for excellent husbandry of this species. On balance, the unquestioned biological relevance of the guinea pig model of tuberculosis more than justifies the effort required to improve the model and enhances its usefulness.

REFERENCES

Barnes, P. F., S.-J. Fong, P. J. Brennan, P. E. Twomey, A. Mazumder, and P. L. Modlin. 1990. Local production of tumor necrosis factor and IFNγ in tuberculous pleuritis. *J. Immunol.* **145:**149–154.

Bartow, R. A., and D. N. McMurray. 1989. Vaccination with *Mycobacterium bovis* BCG affects the distribution of Fc receptor-bearing T lymphocytes in experimental pulmonary tuberculosis. *Infect. Immun.* **57:**1374–1379.

Bartow, R. A., and D. N. McMurray. 1990. Erythrocyte receptor (CD2)-bearing T lymphocytes are affected by diet in experimental pulmonary tuberculosis. *Infect. Immun.* **58:**1843–1847.

Berthrong, M., and M. A. Hamilton. 1959. Tissue culture studies on resistance in tuberculosis. II. Monocytes from normal and immunized guinea pigs

infected with virulent human tubercle bacilli. *Am. Rev. Tuberc.* **79:**221–231.

Bloch, H., and H. Noll. 1953. Studies on the virulence of tubercle bacilli. Variations in the virulence effect elicited by Tween 80 and thiosemicarbazone. *Br. J. Exp. Pathol.* **97:**1–16.

Calman, H. N. 1972. Corticosteroids and lymphoid cells. *N. Engl. J. Med.* **287:**388–397.

Calmette, A., A. Boquet, and L. Negre. 1924. Essais de vaccination contre l'infection tuberculeuse par voie buccale chez les petits animaux de laboratorie. *Ann. Inst. Pasteur* **38:**399–404.

Carlomagno, M. A., C. L. Mintzer, C. L. McFarland, and D. N. McMurray. 1985. Differential effect of protein and zinc deficiencies on delayed hypersensitivity and lymphokine activity in BCG-vaccinated guinea pigs. *Nutr. Res.* **5:**959–968.

Chaisson, R., and G. Slutkin. 1989. Tuberculosis and human immunodeficiency virus infection. *J. Infect. Dis.* **159:**96–100.

Cohen, M. K., R. A. Bartow, C. L. Mintzer, and D. N. McMurray. 1987. Effects of diet and genetics on *Mycobacterium bovis* BCG vaccine efficacy in inbred guinea pigs. *Infect. Immun.* **55:**314–319.

Cohn, M. L., C. L. Davis, and G. Middlebrook. 1962. Chemoprophylaxis with isoniazid against aerogenic tuberculosis infection with the guinea pig. *Am. Rev. Respir. Dis.* **86:**95–97.

Collins, F. M. 1993. Tuberculosis: the return of an old enemy. *Crit. Rev. Microbiol.* **19:**1–16.

Collins, M., and C. A. Elvehjem. 1958. Ascorbic acid requirement of the guinea pig using growth and tissue ascorbic acid concentrations as criteria. *J. Nutr.* **64:**503–511.

Collins, P. D., V. B. Weg, L. H. Faccioli, M. L. Watson, R. Moqbel, and T. J. Williams. 1993. Eosinophil accumulation induced by human interleukin-8 in the guinea pig *in vivo*. *Immunology* **79:**312–318.

Dannenberg, A. M., Jr. 1984. Pathogenesis of tuberculosis: native and acquired resistance in animals and humans, p. 344–354. *In* L. Leive and D. Schlessinger (ed.), *Microbiology—1984*. American Society for Microbiology, Washington, D.C.

Ediger, R. D. 1976. Care and management, p. 5–12. *In* J. E. Wagner and P. J. Manning (ed.), *The Biology of the Guinea Pig*. Academic Press, Inc., New York.

Edwards, M. L., J. M. Goodrich, D. Muller, A. Pollack, J. E. Ziegler, and D. W. Smith. 1982. Infection with *Mycobacterium avium-intracellulare* and the protective effects of bacille-Calmette-Guerin. *J. Infect. Dis.* **145:**733–741.

Elias, J. M., J. Chiba, E. M. Shevach, and H. P. Godfrey. 1985. Guinea pig T lymphocyte development analyzed by enzyme histocytochemistry, monoclonal antibodies and flow cytometry. *Lab. Invest.* **52:**270–277.

Ernstrom, U. 1970. Hormonal influences on thymic release of lymphocytes into the blood. *CIBA Found. Study Group* **36:**53–65.

Fok, J. S., R. S. Ho, P. K. Arora, G. E. Harding, and D. W. Smith. 1976. Host-parasite relationships in experimental airborne tuberculosis. V. Lack of hematogenous dissemination of *Mycobacterium tuberculosis* to the lungs of animals vaccinated with bacille-Calmette-Guerin. *J. Infect. Dis.* **133:**137–144.

Fregnan, G. B., and D. W. Smith. 1963. Immunogenicity and allergenicity in guinea pigs of a defatted mycobacterial vaccine and its fractions. *Am. Rev. Respir. Dis.* **87:**877–888.

Graur, D., W. A. Hide, and L. Wen-Hsiung. 1991. Is the guinea pig a rodent? *Nature* **351:**649–652.

Grover, A. A., H. K. Kim, E. H. Wiegeshaus, and D. W. Smith. 1967. Host-parasite relationships in experimental airborne tuberculosis. II. Reproducible infection by means of an inoculum preserved at −70°C. *J. Bacteriol.* **94:**832–835.

Harding, G. E., and D. W. Smith. 1977. Host-parasite relationships in experimental airborne tuberculosis. VI. Influence of vaccination with bacille-Calmette-Guerin on the onset and/or extent of hematogenous dissemination of virulent *Mycobacterium tuberculosis* to the lungs. *J. Infect. Dis.* **136:**439–443.

Hart, I. J., H. Schafer, R. J. Scheper, and G. T. Stevenson. 1992. Subpopulations of guinea pig T lymphocytes defined by isoforms of the leukocyte common antigen. *Immunology* **77:**377–384.

Haslov, K., and I. Heron. 1989. The generation of guinea pig T-cell lines reactive to antigens from *Mycobacterium tuberculosis*. Selected lines induce erythematous skin reactions. *Scand. J. Immunol.* **29:**281–288.

Ho, R. S., J. S. Fok, G. E. Harding, and D. W. Smith. 1978. Host-parasite relationships in experimental airborne tuberculosis. VII. Fate of *Mycobacterium tuberculosis* in primary lung lesions and in primary lesion-free lung tissue infected as a result of bacillemia. *J. Infect. Dis.* **138:**237–241.

Jensen, K. A., G. Bindslev, and J. Holm. 1935. Experimental studies on the development of tuberculosis infection in allergic and nonallergic animals. I. Development of tuberculous infection in the lungs after inhalation of virulent tubercle bacilli. *Acta Tuberc. Scand.* **9:**27–46.

Jespersen, A. 1956. Studies on tuberculin sensitivity and immunity in guinea pigs induced by vaccination with varying doses of BCG vaccine. *Acta Pathol. Microbiol. Scand.* **38:**203–209.

Koch, R. 1882. Aetiologie der Tuberculose. *Berlin Klin. Wochenschr.* **19:**221–230.

Kramer, T. R., and R. A. Good. 1978. Increased *in vitro* cell-mediated immunity in protein-malnour-ished guinea pigs. *Clin. Immunol. Immunopathol.* **11:**212–228.

Ladefoged, A., K. Bunch-Christensen, and J. Guld. 1976. Tuberculin sensitivity in guinea pigs after vaccination with varying doses of BCG of 12 different strains. *Bull. W.H.O.* **53:**435–443.

Lechner, A. J., and N. Banchero. 1982. Advanced pulmonary development in newborn guinea pigs (*Cavia porcellus*). *Am. J. Anat.* **163:**235–246.

Legranderie, M., P. Ravisse, G. Marchal, M. Gheorghiu, V. Balasubramanian, E. H. Wiegeshaus, and D. W. Smith. 1993. BCG-induced protection in guinea pigs vaccinated and challenged via the respiratory route. *Tuberc. Lung Dis.* **74:**38–46.

Leichentritt, B. 1924. Tuberkulose und Ernahrung. I. Mitteilung. *Z. Hyg. Infektionskr.* **102:**388–407.

Lenzini, L., P. Rottoli, and L. Rottoli. 1977. The spectrum of human tuberculosis. *Clin. Exp. Immunol.* **27:**230–237.

Liebow, A. A., C. G. Burn, and W. B. Soper. 1940. BCG immunization. A comparison of the effects of BCG and of heat-killed organisms on the course of a subsequent infection with virulent tubercle bacilli in the guinea pig. *Am. Rev. Tuberc.* **41:**592–604.

Long, E. R., A. J. Vorwald, and L. Donaldson. 1931. Early cellular reaction to tubercle bacilli: a comparison of this reaction in normal and tuberculous guinea pigs and in guinea pigs immunized with dead bacilli. *Arch. Pathol.* **12:**956–969.

Mainali, E. S., and D. N. McMurray. Unpublished data.

Mainali, E. S., and D. N. McMurray. 1992. Influence of infection route in the generation of immune lymphocytes by guinea pigs infected with virulent *Mycobacterium tuberculosis. FASEB J.* **6:**A1335.

Mainali, E. S., and D. N. McMurray. Adoptive transfer of resistance to pulmonary tuberculosis in guinea pigs is altered by protein deficiency. Submitted for publication.

Malek, T. R., R. B. Clark, and E. M. Shevach. 1981. Alloreactive T cells from individual soft agar colonies specific for guinea pig Ia antigens. *J. Immunol.* **127:**616–621.

McConkey, M., and D. T. Smith. 1933. The relation of vitamin C deficiency to intestinal tuberculosis in the guinea pig. *J. Exp. Med.* **58:**503–512.

McMurray, D. N. 1980. Mechanisms of anergy in tuberculosis. *Chest* **77:**4–5.

McMurray, D. N. 1984. Cell-mediated immunity in nutritional deficiency. *Prog. Food Nutr. Sci.* **8:**193–228.

McMurray, D. N., and R. A. Bartow. 1992. Immunosuppression and alteration of resistance to pulmonary tuberculosis in guinea pigs by protein undernutrition. *J. Nutr.* **122:**738–743.

McMurray, D. N., R. A. Bartow, and C. L. Mintzer. 1989a. Impact of protein malnutrition on exogenous reinfection with *Mycobacterium tuberculosis. Infect. Immun.* **57**:1746–1749.

McMurray, D. N., R. A. Bartow, and C. L. Mintzer. 1990. Protein malnutrition alters the distribution of $Fc_\gamma R^+$ (Tγ) and $Fc_\mu R^+$ (Tμ) T lymphocytes in experimental pulmonary tuberculosis. *Infect. Immun.* **58**:563–565.

McMurray, D. N., M. A. Carlomagno, C. L. Mintzer, and C. L. Tetzlaff. 1985. *Mycobacterium bovis* BCG vaccine fails to protect protein-deficient guinea pigs against respiratory challenge with virulent *Mycobacterium tuberculosis. Infect. Immun.* **50**:555–559.

McMurray, D. N., and A. Echeverry. 1978. Cell-mediated immunity in anergic patients with pulmonary tuberculosis. *Am. Rev. Respir. Dis.* **118**:827–834.

McMurray, D. N., M. S. Kimball, C. L. Tetzlaff, and C. L. Mintzer. 1986a. Effects of protein deprivation and BCG vaccination on alveolar macrophage function in pulmonary tuberculosis. *Am. Rev. Respir. Dis.* **133**:1081–1085.

McMurray, D. N., E. S. Mainali, and S. Phalen. 1993. Malnutrition, immunoregulatory defects and the white plague. *Adv. Biosci.* **86**:19–28.

McMurray, D. N., C. L. Mintzer, R. A. Bartow, and R. L. Parr. 1989b. Dietary protein deficiency and *Mycobacterium bovis* BCG affect interleukin 2 activity in experimental pulmonary tuberculosis. *Infect. Immun.* **57**:2606–2611.

McMurray, D. N., C. L. Mintzer, C. L. Tetzlaff, and M. A. Carlomagno. 1986b. Influence of dietary protein on the protective effect of BCG in guinea pigs. *Tubercle* **67**:31–39.

McMurray, D. N., and E. A. Yetley. 1983. Response to *Mycobacterium bovis* BCG vaccination in protein- and zinc-deficient guinea pigs. *Infect. Immun.* **39**:755–761.

McPhee, C. A., J. I. Milton, and A. W. Thomson. 1988. Flow cytometric analysis of lymphocyte populations in guinea pig blood and spleen. *Int. Arch. Allergy Appl. Immunol.* **87**:275–280.

Middlebrook, G., R. J. Dubos, and C. H. Pierce. 1947. Virulence and morphological characteristics of mammalian tubercle bacilli. *J. Exp. Med.* **86**:175–184.

Middlebrook, G. M. 1952. An apparatus for airborne infection of mice. *Proc. Soc. Exp. Biol. Med.* **80**:105–110.

Nardell, E., B. McInnis, B. Thomas, and S. Weidhaas. 1986. Exogenous reinfection with tuberculosis in a shelter for the homeless. *N. Engl. J. Med.* **315**:1570–1575.

Oosterhaut, A. J. M. V., A. R. C. Ladenius, H. F. J. Savelkoul, I. V. Ark, K. C. Delsman, and F. P. Nijkamp. 1993. Effect of anti-IL-5 and IL-5 on airway hyperreactivity and eosinophils in guinea pigs. *Am. Rev. Respir. Dis.* **147**:548–552.

Palmer, C. E., and L. Hopwood. 1962. Effect of previous infection with unclassified mycobacteria on survival of guinea pigs challenged with virulent tubercle bacilli. *Bull. Int. Union Tuberc.* **32**:389–398.

Pavia, C. S., and C. J. Niederbuhl. 1985. Experimental infections of inbred guinea pigs with *Treponema pallidum*: development of lesions and formation of antibodies. *Genitourin. Med.* **61**:75–81.

Payne, S. N. L., and A. W. Thomson. 1989. Immunohistochemical analysis of contact sensitivity reactions in the guinea pig using novel monoclonal antibodies: the influence of topical cyclosporin A. *Clin. Exp. Immunol.* **75**:444–450.

Phalen, S. W., and D. N. McMurray. 1993a. T lymphocyte response in a guinea pig model of tuberculous pleuritis. *Infect. Immun.* **61**:142–145.

Phalen, S. W., and D. N. McMurray. 1993b. Production of tumor necrosis factor (TNFα) in experimental tuberculous pleuritis. *J. Immunol.* **150**:66A.

Polak, L., and R. J. Scheper. 1983. Antigen-specific T cell lines in DNCB-contact sensitivity in guinea pigs. *J. Invest. Dermatol.* **80**:398–402.

Prabhakar, R., R. Ventkataraman, R. S. Vallishayee, P. Reeser, S. Musa, R. Hashim, Y. Kim, C. Dimmer, E. Wiegeshaus, M. Edwards, and D. W. Smith. 1987. Virulence for guinea pigs of tubercle bacilli isolated from the sputum of participants in the BCG trial, Chingleput district, south India. *Tubercle* **68**:3–17.

Rao, B. S. N., and C. Gopalan. 1958. Nutrition and tuberculosis. II. Studies on nitrogen, calcium and phosphorus metabolism in tuberculosis. *Indian J. Med. Res.* **46**:93–112.

Ratcliffe, H. L., and V. S. Palladino. 1953. Tuberculosis induced by droplet nuclei infection: initial homogeneous response of small mammals (rats, mice, guinea pigs and hamsters) to human and to bovine bacilli and the rate and pattern of tubercle development. *J. Exp. Med.* **97**:61–68.

Riley, R. L., C. C. Mills, W. Nyka, N. Weinstock, P. B. Storey, L. U. Sultan, M. C. Riley, and W. F. Wells. 1959. Aerial dissemination of pulmonary tuberculosis. A two year study of contagion in a tuberculosis ward. *Am. J. Hyg.* **70**:185–196.

Schafer, H., and R. Burger. 1992. Analysis of mature guinea pig T cells with a monoclonal antibody directed against a framework determinant of the T-cell receptor for antigen. *Scand. J. Immunol.* **36**:587–595.

Schafer, H., B. Muller, A. Bader, J. Schenke, and R. Burger. 1989. Analysis of guinea pig leukocyte antigens using interspecies T cell hybrids. *J. Immunol. Methods* **118**:169–177.

Schenkel, J., H. Schafer, U. Baron, B. Muller, and R. Burger. 1992. cDNA cloning of the constant region genes of the guinea pig α/β T-cell receptor. *Dev. Comp. Immunol.* **16**:221–227.

Schwabacher, H., and G. S. Wilson. 1938. The vaccination of guinea pigs with living BCG, together with observations on tuberculous superinfection in rabbits. *J. Pathol. Bacteriol.* **46**:535–547.

Shewell, J., and D. A. Long. 1956. A species difference with regard to the effect of cortisone acetate on body weight, γ-globulin and circulating antitoxin levels. *J. Hyg.* **54**:452–460.

Shigeki, K., K. Itoh, I. Kurane, and K. Kumagai. 1982. Detection of guinea pig Tγ and Tμ cells by a double rosette assay. *J. Immunol. Methods* **51**:89–100.

Sisk, D. B. 1976. Physiology, p. 63–98. *In* J. E. Wagner and P. J. Manning (ed.), *The Biology of the Guinea Pig.* Academic Press, Inc., New York.

Smith, D. W. 1985. Protective effect of BCG in experimental tuberculosis. *Adv. Tuberc. Res.* **22**:1–93.

Smith, D. W., V. Balasubramanian, and E. H. Wieges-haus. 1991. A guinea pig model of experimental airborne tuberculosis for the evaluation of the response to chemotherapy: the effect on bacilli in the initial phase of treatment. *Tubercle* **72**:223–321.

Smith, D. W., and G. E. Harding. 1977. Animal model: experimental airborne tuberculosis in the guinea pig. *Am. J. Pathol.* **89**:273–276.

Smith, D. W., and G. E. Harding. 1978. Influence of BCG vaccination on the bacillemic phase of experimental airborne tuberculosis in guinea pigs, p. 85–90. *In* R. J. Montali (ed.), *Mycobacterial Infections of Zoo Animals.* Smithsonian Institution Press, Washington, D.C.

Smith, D. W., G. E. Harding, and J. K. Chan. 1979. Potency of 10 BCG vaccines as evaluated by their influence on the bacillemic phase of experimental airborne tuberculosis in guinea pigs. *J. Biol. Stand.* **7**:179–197.

Smith, D. W., D. N. McMurray, E. H. Wieges-haus, A. A. Grover, and G. E. Harding. 1970. Host-parasite relationships in experimental airborne tuberculosis. IV. Early events in the course of infection in vaccinated and nonvaccinated guinea pigs. *Am. Rev. Respir. Dis.* **102**:937–949.

Smith, D. W., and E. H. Wiegeshaus. 1989. What animal models can teach us about the pathogenesis of tuberculosis in humans. *Rev. Infect. Dis.* **11**:S385–S393.

Smith, D. W., E. H. Wiegeshaus, R. Navalkar, and A. A. Grover. 1966. Host-parasite relationships in experimental airborne tuberculosis. I. Preliminary studies in BCG-vaccinated and nonvaccinated animals. *J. Bacteriol.* **91**:718–724.

Smith, D. W., E. H. Wiegeshaus, R. H. Stark, and G. E. Harding. 1972. Models for potency assays of tuberculosis vaccines. *Fogarty Int. Cent. Proc.* **14**:205–218.

Stadecker, M., G. Bishop, and H. Wartis. 1973. Rosette formation by guinea pig thymocytes and thymus-derived lymphocytes with rabbit red blood cells. *J. Immunol.* **111**:1834–1837.

Stead, W. W. 1989. Pathogenesis of tuberculosis: clinical and epidemiological perspective. *Rev. Infect. Dis.* **11**:366–368.

Tan, B. T. G., F. Ekelaar, J. Luirink, G. Rimmelzwaan, A. J. R. DeJonge, and R. J. Scheper. 1985. Production of monoclonal antibodies defining guinea pig T cell surface markers and a strain 13 Ia-like antigen: the value of immunohistological screening. *Hybridoma* **4**:115–124.

Tolderland, K., K. Bunch-Christensen, and J. Guld. 1967. Duration of allergy and immunity in BCG-vaccinated guinea pigs. A five-year study. *Bull. W.H.O.* **36**:759–769.

Wicher, V., K. Wicher, A. Jakubowski, and S. M. Nakeeb. 1987. Adoptive transfer of immunity to *Treponema pallidum* Nichols infection in inbred strain 2 and C4D guinea pigs. *Infect. Immun.* **55**:2502–2508.

Wiegeshaus, E. H., D. N. McMurray, A. A. Grover, G. E. Harding, and D. W. Smith. 1970. Host-parasite relationships in experimental airborne tuberculosis. III. Relevance of microbial enumeration to acquired resistance in guinea pigs. *Am. Rev. Respir. Dis.* **102**:422–429.

Wiegeshaus, E. H., and D. W. Smith. 1989. Evaluation of the protective potency of new tuberculosis vaccines. *Rev. Infect. Dis.* **11**:S484–S490.

Windstrom, O., and B. S. Nilsson. 1982. Pleurisy induced by intrapleural BCG in immunized guinea pigs. *Eur. J. Respir. Dis.* **63**:425–434.

Yamashita, T., K. Shinohara, and Y. Yamashita. 1993. Expression cloning of complementary DNA encoding three distinct isoforms of guinea pig Fc receptor for IgG1 and IgG2. *J. Immunol.* **151**:2014–2023.

Yoshimura, T. 1993. cDNA cloning of guinea pig monocyte chemoattractant protein-1 and expression of the recombinant protein. *J. Immunol.* **150**:5025–5032.

Zeitz, S. J., J. H. Ostrow, and P. P. Van Arsdel. 1974. Humoral and cellular immunity in the anergic tuberculosis patient. *J. Allergy Clin. Immunol.* **53**:20–26.

Zhao, J., V. Wicher, R. Burger, H. Schafer, and K. Wicher. 1992. Strain- and age-associated differences in lymphocyte phenotypes and immune responsiveness in C4-deficient and Albany strains of guinea pigs. *Immunology* **77**:165–170.

Ziegler, J. E., M. L. Edwards, and D. W. Smith. 1985. Exogenous reinfection in experimental airborne tuberculosis. *Tubercle* **66**:121–128.

Tuberculosis: Pathogenesis, Protection, and Control
Edited by Barry R. Bloom
© 1994 American Society for Microbiology, Washington, DC 20005

Chapter 10

Rabbit Model of Tuberculosis

Arthur M. Dannenberg, Jr.

The most extensive studies on tuberculosis in rabbits were made by Max B. Lurie (1932, 1938, 1941, 1964; Lurie and Dannenberg, 1965). He inbred different rabbit families for resistance and susceptibility to tuberculosis. When infected with the virulent Ravenel strain of *Mycobacterium bovis*, the resistant rabbit families developed cavitary tuberculosis resembling that found in adult immunocompetent human beings. The susceptible rabbit families developed hematogenously spread tuberculosis resembling that found in infants and immunocompromised individuals.

Lurie's rabbit families were of various breeds. His most resistant family, strain III, and his most susceptible family, strain C, were both albinos. His FC family was Dutch; his A family (which was highly resistant and then with time became intermediately resistant) was mainly English. The names referred mostly to the characteristics and color distribution of the rabbits' fur and had no correlation with their resistance to tuberculosis. In general, III and A rabbits were large, C rabbits were of intermediate size, and FC rabbits were relatively small (about 30 to 40% the weight of

the largest). All of Lurie's rabbit families have been extinct for about 25 years because the inbreeding resulted in infertility (Altman and Katz, 1979).

Please realize, however, that the response among the rabbits within each of Lurie's rabbit families was not completely uniform (Lurie, 1964). After aerosol exposure to human-type tubercle bacilli (which are of reduced virulence for rabbits), the number of tubercles produced in the lungs varied over about a sevenfold range with a standard error of the mean of approximately 15%. Similar data on market New Zealand White rabbits are not available, but I would expect their resistance to tuberculosis to show about three times the variability of Lurie's inbred rabbits.

Most commercially available rabbits are of intermediate resistance to tuberculosis. Therefore, many will develop cavities when infected with virulent bovine tubercle bacilli, but some will die early from hematogenous spread of the disease. Since the rabbits are not inbred, considerable variation in resistance to tubercle bacilli is to be expected. There are many types of rabbits on the market: New Zealand (White), English Spot, Dutch, Flemish Giant, Polish, Silver Marten, and English Lop(-eared), for example. The American Rabbit Breeders Association (1991) keeps track of the pedigrees of each type of rabbit. It would be

Arthur M. Dannenberg, Jr. • Department of Environmental Health Sciences, School of Hygiene and Public Health, The Johns Hopkins University, 615 North Wolfe Street, Baltimore, Maryland 21205-2179.

prudent to check these breeds for resistance to tuberculosis, but this has never been done. The resistance to tuberculosis of some of these breeds may be more uniform than that of the New Zealand White rabbits on the market today, and among such breeds, new resistant or susceptible strains may be discovered.

A completely inbred, distant relative of Lurie's resistant strain III rabbits, however, is still alive in The Netherlands. Also in The Netherlands is a nearly completely inbred strain of rabbits, AX, the resistance of which remains to be tested. These two inbred strains are in the laboratory of L. F. M. van Zutphen, Faculty of Veterinary Medicine, University of Utrecht, Yalelaan 2, De Uithof-Utrecht (phone, 31-30-532033; FAX, 31-30-531407).

The Jackson Laboratory at Bar Harbor, Maine, had several inbred rabbit races with unknown resistance to tuberculosis (Fox, 1974, 1975; Altman and Katz, 1979) but has stopped inbreeding rabbits. A few of these inbred strains, however, have been preserved as early embryos in a frozen state (at the 4- to 8-cell stage). These embryos could be brought back to life by implanting them into the uteri or Fallopian tubes of living female rabbits primed with chorionic gonadotropin. Richard R. Fox (Fox, 1974) (phone, 207-288-3366; FAX, 207-288-5385) can provide more information on the Jackson Laboratory embryos to interested investigators.

The remainder of this report contrasts the responses of Lurie's natively resistant and susceptible rabbit families to tuberculosis (summarized in Table 1). From the description of these extremes, the reader can gather what to expect from market rabbits.

RESISTANCE TO THE ESTABLISHMENT OF TUBERCULOSIS

Resistance to the establishment of an infectious disease is distinct from resistance to its progress (Lurie, 1944; Henderson et al., 1963; Lurie et al., 1955; Allison et al., 1962; Dannenberg, 1991, 1993). "Establishment" refers to the initial multiplication of an infectious agent in the host. "Progress" refers to the agent's continued multiplication in the host. Inapparent infection represents host resistance to progress (rather than resistance to establishment), because the infectious agent has multiplied long enough to stimulate a serologic or cellular immune response. It is only by such an immune response that a previous inapparent infection can be detected.

Two factors influence resistance to the establishment of tuberculosis: (i) the trapping of tubercle bacilli in the lung and (ii) the initial inactivation of these bacilli. The trapping is partly dependent on the ability of the alveolar macrophages to phagocytize the bacilli. When tested in vitro, alveolar macrophages from certain resistant rabbits were able to ingest twice as many bacilli as alveolar macrophages from certain susceptible rabbits were able to ingest (Henderson et al., 1963).

These findings could explain why resistant rabbits developed tuberculosis sooner than did susceptible rabbits when both groups breathed infected air in a closed room over a period of many months (Lurie, 1944). Highly virulent *bovine-type* bacilli were used in this experiment. When trapped in the pulmonary alveoli, each of these bacilli is capable of producing a tuberculous lesion in resistant as well as susceptible rabbits (Lurie et al., 1950).

In contrast, for every inhaled *human-type* tubercle bacillus that produced a lesion, many of the inhaled bacilli were inactivated (Lurie et al., 1952a, 1955; Allison et al., 1962; Dannenberg, 1991, 1993). Resistant rabbits inactivated more bacilli than did susceptible rabbits. Thus, in spite of trapping more bacilli, resistant rabbits resisted the establishment of the primary lesion better than did susceptible rabbits (Lurie et al., 1952a).

Table 1. Characteristics of resistance and susceptibility to tuberculosis in Phipps rabbits[a]

Characteristic	Resistance		Susceptibility	
	Degree[b]	Family (reference)	Degree[b]	Family (reference)
Bacilli				
Trapping of tubercle bacilli in lung	++++	A (1), T (2–4)	++	F (1), C (1–4), FCCa (2)
Initial inactivation of inhaled bacilli	+++	T (3, 4)	+	C (3, 4)
Subsequent inhibition of bacillary accumulation	++++	T (3, 4)	++	C (3, 4)
Drainage of bacilli to tracheobronchial lymph nodes	++++	T (3, 4)	+	C (3, 4)
Histopathology				
Rate of mobilization of mononuclear cells (in early pulmonary lesions)	+++	T (3)	+	C (3)
Rate of epithelioid cell maturation	++++	A (5), T (3, 6, 7)	+	C (3, 5–7), F (5)
Pneumonic inflammation	+	T (3)	++++	C (3)
Interstitial inflammation	++++	T (3)	+	C (3)
Maturation of caseous process	++++	T (3)	++	C (3)
Gross pathology				
No. of gross tubercles 5 wk after inhalation of human bacilli	+	T (3, 6–8)	++++	C (3, 8), Ca (6), FC (3, 6, 7)
Sizes of tubercles and sizes of their caseous centers	++	T (3)	++++	C (3), FC (3)
Cavity formation	++	A (5), T (3)	±	F (5), C (3, 5)
Spread of disease to kidneys and other organs	+	A (5), T (4, 9)	+++	F (5), C (5)
Rate of healing of lesions	++++	A (5), T (6)	+	F (5), C (5), FC (6)
Other factors				
Amount of acquired immunity	++++	A (5), T (7)	+	F (5), C (5), FC (7)
Longevity after infection with virulent bovine bacilli	++++	A (1, 5), T (6)	+	F (1, 5), C (1, 5), FC (4, 9)

[a] Data are from Lurie and Dannenberg (1965). References are given in parentheses as follows: 1, Lurie (1944); 2, Henderson et al. (1963); 3, Lurie et al. (1955); 4, Allison et al. (1962); 5, Lurie (1941); 6, Lurie et al. (1952a); 7, Lurie et al. (1952b); 8, Lurie et al. (1952c); 9, Lurie (1964).
[b] Symbols: +, low; ++ and +++, intermediate; ++++, high; ±, usually absent.

In human beings, both human and bovine types of tubercle bacilli seem to be of intermediate virulence. One would therefore expect many inhaled tubercle bacilli to be initially inactivated by the alveolar macrophages, although the exact percentage has never been determined.

RESISTANCE TO THE PROGRESS OF TUBERCULOSIS

After infection with virulent *bovine-type* tubercle bacilli, the resistant rabbits lived about twice as long as susceptible rabbits (Lurie, 1941, 1944, 1964). Progression of the disease was slow because the resistant rabbits rapidly developed acquired cellular resistance: the caseous center of each tubercle became surrounded by activated macrophages that ingested and inhibited or destroyed many of the bacilli escaping from the caseous center. Lurie (1932, 1964; Lurie et al., 1955) called such effective macrophages "mature epithelioid cells." We showed histochemically that mature epithelioid cells were rich in β-galactosidase (Dannenberg, 1968; Dannenberg et al., 1968; Ando et al., 1977) and other oxidative enzymes (Dannenberg et al., 1968). The β-galactosidase histochemical test is therefore an excellent way to identify microbicidal macrophages in tissue sections of rabbit tuberculous lesions.

The susceptible rabbits formed few mature epithelioid cells (activated macrophages). Therefore, bacilli (escaping from the caseous center of each tubercle) multiplied in the macrophages that ingested them. The host then proceeded to destroy the bacilli-laden macrophages along with nearby lung tissue, and the disease progressed more rapidly (Dannenberg, 1991, 1993; see also chapter 27 in this volume).

The spread of bacilli from the pulmonary lesions to the hilar lymph nodes (via lymphatics) was greater in the resistant animals (Lurie et al., 1955), but the growth of the bacilli once they had reached these nodes was more inhibited (Lurie, 1964; Lurie et al., 1955). Conversely, there was less spread of bacilli to the hilar nodes in susceptible animals (Lurie et al., 1955), but once there, the bacilli multiplied sufficiently to produce caseous lesions that are typical of the primary childhood type of tuberculosis (Lurie, 1941, 1944).

Bacilli invaded the bloodstreams of both resistant and susceptible rabbits. In early lesions of resistant rabbits, interstitial inflammation was more pronounced than in those of susceptible rabbits (Lurie et al., 1955), and more bacilli entered the bloodstream and lymphatics. In older lesions of susceptible rabbits, more blood vessels and lymphatics were injured by the caseous process than in those of resistant rabbits (Lurie, 1941), and more bacilli entered these channels (Lurie, 1941; Lurie et al., 1955). Thus, attributes of both resistance and susceptibility contributed to the dissemination of bacilli from the primary lesion. The decisive factor, however, was not the number of bacilli disseminated but the fate of these bacilli in their new environment. The macrophages of resistant rabbits inhibited the intracellular growth of many of the bacilli that reached the lymph nodes, spleen, and kidneys, whereas the macrophages of susceptible rabbits were less inhibitory (Lurie, 1941; Lurie et al., 1955; Allison et al., 1962).

PATHOGENESIS OF TUBERCULOSIS CAUSED BY BOVINE-TYPE BACILLI

The severity of tuberculosis was determined by both the susceptibility of the host and the virulence of the infecting bacilli. Fully virulent bovine-type bacilli produced one pulmonary lesion for every bacillus that reached the alveolar spaces (Lurie et al., 1950), regardless of the native resistance of the host.

In Lurie's *susceptible* rabbits, these bacilli initially multiplied to a much greater degree than in his resistant animals (Lurie, 1964; Allison et al., 1962), and this multiplication continued until acquired immunity developed (Allison et al., 1962). Caseation necrosis resulted from sensitivity to the tuberculin-like products of the bacilli. It began at the centers of the tubercles and spread centrifugally, destroying the surrounding lung tissue along with the macrophages (immature epithelioid cells) that attempted to localize the disease (Lurie, 1941). Blood vessels and lymphatics became necrotic, and bacilli entered their lumens and spread throughout the body. In the lungs, many secondary tubercles developed, became confluent, and killed the host. Cavity formation was rare. At autopsy, progressive caseous tuberculosis was also present in the tracheobronchial lymph nodes, kidneys, spleen, and bone marrow (Lurie, 1941).

In Lurie's *resistant* rabbits, there was less initial multiplication of bovine-type bacilli than in susceptible rabbits (Allison et al., 1962). After acquired immunity developed (Lurie, 1941, 1964; Allison et al., 1962), the lesions were usually epithelioid-cell granulomas, and caseation was less extensive. Secondary lesions of hematogenous and lymphogenous origin were infrequent in the lungs and other organs. The caseous lesions were surrounded by tuberculous granulation tissue consisting of macrophages, lymphocytes, fibroblasts, capillaries, and lymphatics. In time, some of the lesions developed fibrous capsules, and their caseous centers sometimes calcified. More frequently, however, the lesions underwent liquefaction, a process in which the caseous material softens as fluid is absorbed. In the liquefied caseum, the bacilli multiplied in tremendous numbers, causing further destruction of tissue. They entered the peripheral branches of the bronchial tree and spread to other parts of the lung. There, the bacilli and their tuberculin-like products produced areas of caseous pneumonia or new lesions, which often liquefied. The large number of bacilli overwhelmed the existing immunity, high as it was, and the ulcerative pulmonary phthisis progressed until death. Without the process of liquefaction, the genetically resistant rabbits would have conquered their disease. At autopsy, the other organs of the body, including the tracheobronchial lymph nodes, showed few if any progressive lesions (Lurie, 1941).

PATHOGENESIS OF TUBERCULOSIS CAUSED BY HUMAN-TYPE BACILLI

Human strains of tubercle bacilli are less virulent for rabbits than the bovine strains. Recovery from infection with them is the rule, even in genetically susceptible rabbits. The use of these strains of bacilli has made possible the development of one of the most precise tests available for native and acquired resistance to tuberculosis. Briefly, natively resistant and susceptible rabbits are exposed to an aerosol of the bacilli (usually strain H37Rv). After 5 weeks, the rabbits are sacrificed, and the primary tubercles in the lungs are counted. Since human strains of tubercle bacilli are of reduced virulence for the rabbit, many microorganisms reaching the alveolar spaces are inactivated for every one that multiplies. In other words, because of phenotypic variations among the bacilli aerosolized and among the alveolar macrophages that ingest them, only the most virulent bacilli in the aerosol are able to grow in the most susceptible alveolar macrophages of the host. The natively resistant rabbits apparently have more resistant alveolar macrophages and fewer susceptible alveolar macrophages than do susceptible rabbits (Dannenberg, 1991, 1993; Lurie et al., 1952a).

If the alveolar macrophage did not eventually destroy the tubercle bacillus (or a cluster of two or three bacilli) that it ingested, the bacillus would multiply and the macrophage would in time die and release its bacillary load. Then, nonactivated monocytes (macrophages) would enter the lesion from the bloodstream. In these nonactivated macrophages, the bacilli multiply logarithmically (Lurie et al., 1955; Allison et al., 1962) until the immune processes, especially the tissue-damaging delayed-type hypersensitivity response, kill the bacilli-laden macrophages, forming the caseous center of the tubercle (Dannenberg, 1991, 1993; see also chapter 27 in this volume).

In natively *resistant* rabbits, such early tubercles became surrounded by many highly activated macrophages, owing to the acquired cellular resistance (produced by the T lymphocytes responsible for cell-mediated immunity) (Dannenberg, 1991, 1993; see also chapter 27 in this volume). *Susceptible* rabbits did not activate macrophages to the same degree. To control the intracellular growth of tubercle bacilli in these weakly activated macrophages, the susceptible host had to destroy the macrophages and surrounding lung tissue. There-fore, the caseous centers in tubercles in susceptible rabbits were larger than those in resistant rabbits (Lurie et al., 1955; Dan-nenberg, 1991, 1993; see also chapter 27 in this volume).

Lurie also studied the eventual fate of pulmonary lesions produced in rabbits by human-type tubercle bacilli. Five to 6 months (Lurie, 1964; Lurie et al., 1952a) and 11 to 12 months (Lurie, 1964) after infection, primary lesions in the *resistant* rabbits had either healed completely or formed cavities that were healing without producing appreciable bronchial spread of the disease. There were few if any grossly visible secondary lesions (Lurie, 1964; Lu-rie et al., 1952a, 1955). At these times, primary lesions in the *susceptible* rabbits were healing slowly, without cavitation, and secondary lesions of hematogenous or-igin were often present (Lurie, 1964; Lurie et al., 1952a, 1955). In both groups of rabbits, however, the disease seemed to be well controlled because of the relative avir-ulence of human-type bacilli for the rabbit species.

In general, the primary tubercles in the *resistant* rabbits were smaller and more interstitial in character and contained fewer bacilli (Lurie et al., 1955). Their caseous centers were more mature, in that they contained more completely disintegrated nuclear debris (Lurie et al., 1955) (Table 1). In contrast, the primary tubercles in the *susceptible* rabbits were more intra-alveo-lar in character and contained far more bacilli. Their caseous centers showed in-complete digestion of nuclear debris (Lurie et al., 1955).

The number of primary pulmonary tuber-cles produced by an aerosol of human-type tubercle bacilli was used by Lurie as an index of both native and acquired resis-tance of the rabbit host. He sacrificed the rabbits 5 weeks after exposure and counted the number of tubercles. The number of tubercles was a quantitative measure of

host resistance. In fact, Lurie used this number to measure (i) the native resistance of each of his rabbit families (Lurie et al., 1952a) and (ii) the acquired resistance re-sulting from BCG vaccination. Immuniza-tion with BCG increased the resistance of natively resistant rabbits fivefold (Lurie et al., 1952b). We strongly recommend this method (i.e., the use in rabbits of human-type tubercle bacilli by aerosol) to assess all newly developed vaccines for tuberculosis, using appropriate equipment to protect per-sonnel from infection. The number of grossly visible primary tubercles at 5 weeks is an excellent measure of the combination of both native and acquired resistance, be-cause in both of these cases, many devel-oping primary lesions apparently healed while they were still microscopic in size.

Note that BCG vaccination would not be expected to increase resistance to the es-tablishment of the disease. Vaccination would control the disease only after a small tubercle had been established. In both vac-cinated and nonvaccinated hosts, the alve-olar macrophages are nonspecifically acti-vated by the dust and microbial particles they have ingested (Dannenberg et al., 1963). Only after the tubercle bacillus has multiplied in an early (microscopic) tuber-cle is sufficient antigen produced to cause the expanded population of specific lym-phocytes to activate (via their cytokines) the local macrophages (Dannenberg, 1990; see also chapter 27 in this volume).

BCG INFECTION

BCG is even less virulent for rabbits than human bacilli. The inhalation of an aerosol of thousands of viable BCG bacilli was required to produce in rabbits a single pri-mary pulmonary tubercle, which was quite small and healed rapidly (Abramson, un-published data). However, following the intravenous injection of 1 mg (wet weight) of BCG, rabbits developed small lesions in many organs of the body, e.g., lung, liver, spleen, and lymph nodes (Lurie, 1934). After 2 weeks, these lesions rapidly healed. This healing was associated with the development of cell-mediated immunity and delayed-type hypersensitivity (to tuberculin). Caseous necrosis developed in the tracheobronchial lymph nodes, and viable BCG sometimes persisted in these (and other) nodes for many months.

BCG is usually given intradermally, so the response of Lurie's resistant and susceptible rabbits to this route of infection will be described herein. Compared to those in susceptible rabbits, the dermal BCG lesions of resistant rabbits grew more rapidly, reached a peak more quickly, ulcerated more frequently, and healed sooner (Lurie et al., 1952b). The bacilli multiplied for a shorter time and were subsequently more rapidly inactivated (Lurie et al., 1952b). The associated histological responses were also accelerated: epithelioid cells matured faster, and plasma cells and fibroblasts appeared sooner (Lurie et al., 1952b). The rapid development of BCG lesions in resistant animals was associated with a rapid development of tuberculin sensitivity (Lurie et al., 1952b).

The BCG lesions of susceptible rabbits showed the opposite characteristics: the lesions developed more slowly, reached their peak tardily, did not usually ulcerate, and took longer to heal (Lurie et al., 1952b).

The acquired immunity from BCG vaccination was higher in resistant than susceptible animals (Lurie et al., 1952b). After such vaccination, at 5 weeks after the inhalation of virulent human-type tubercle bacilli, the number of primary tubercles in resistant rabbits was decreased by 80%, whereas the number in susceptible rabbits was decreased only 15%. In other words, BCG vaccination increased the resistance of resistant animals 5-fold and increased the resistance of susceptible animals only 1.2-fold. Thus, vaccination helped most those rabbits that needed it least and, conversely, helped least those rabbits that needed it most.

These results were not surprising. The ability of the host to inhibit the growth of tubercle bacilli in its tissues was largely due to the cellular resistance acquired by macrophages as a result of the infection. (Such highly activated microbicidal macrophages are produced by T lymphocytes and their lymphokines [Dannenberg, 1991, 1993; see also chapter 27].) Natively resistant animals acquired more resistance than did susceptible animals during either a virulent infection or an attenuated one, e.g., one produced by BCG. The level of acquired resistance is therefore determined by the level of native resistance.

GENETIC STUDIES

Lurie obtained a hybrid strain of rabbits (F_1) by crossing one of his highly resistant strains with one of his highly susceptible strains (Lurie et al., 1952c). The degree of resistance to tuberculosis of this F_1 generation was intermediate between that of the two parent strains. A backcross of the F_1 hybrid to its resistant ancestors produced F_2 strains of the same high resistance as the original resistant strain. A backcross of the F_1 hybrid to susceptible ancestors produced F_2 strains that were more resistant than the original susceptible strain. Therefore, either factors determining resistance were more dominant in the phenotype than factors determining susceptibility, or susceptible individuals lacked certain factors that resistant individuals possessed. Lurie concluded, therefore, that determinants of resistance to tuberculosis were multiple, complex, and additive (Lurie et al., 1952c).

Acknowledgments. We are grateful to the late Max B. Lurie, of the University of Pennsylvania, for the fundamental understanding of tuberculosis that he personally gave to me. Part of this chapter was already published in Lurie and Dannenberg, 1965. Ilse M. Harrop provided excellent editorial assistance.

Financial support for the studies in my laboratory came from the following grants: AI-27165, from the National Institute of Allergy and Infectious Diseases;

ES-03819, for the Johns Hopkins Environmental Health Sciences Center, from the National Institute of Environmental Health Sciences, Research Triangle Park, N.C.; and HL-10342, from the National Heart, Lung and Blood Institute, Bethesda, Md.

REFERENCES

Abramson, S. Unpublished data.

Allison, M. J., P. Zappasodi, and M. B. Lurie. 1962. Host-parasite relationships in natively resistant and susceptible rabbits on quantitative inhalation of tubercle bacilli. *Am. Rev. Respir. Dis.* **85**:553–569.

Altman, P. L., and D. D. Katz. 1979. Rabbit, p. 565–606. *In Inbred and Genetically Defined Strains of Laboratory Animals*, vol. 3, part 2. *Hamster, Guinea Pig, Rabbit, and Chicken.* Federation of American Societies for Experimental Biology, Bethesda, Md.

American Rabbit Breeders Association, Inc. 1991. *Official Guide Book.* American Rabbit Breeders Association, Inc., Bloomington, Ill.

Ando, M., A. M. Dannenberg, Jr., M. Sugimoto, and B. S. Tepper. 1977. Histochemical studies relating the activation of macrophages to the intracellular destruction of tubercle bacilli. *Am. J. Pathol.* **86**:623–634.

Dannenberg, A. M., Jr. 1968. Cellular hypersensitivity and cellular immunity in the pathogenesis of tuberculosis: specificity, systemic and local nature, and associated macrophage enzymes. *Bacteriol. Rev.* **32**:95–102.

Dannenberg, A. M., Jr. 1990. Controlling tuberculosis: the pathologist's point of view. *Res. Microbiol.* **141**:192–196, 262–263.

Dannenberg, A. M., Jr. 1991. Delayed-type hypersensitivity and cell-mediated immunity in the pathogenesis of tuberculosis. *Immunol. Today* **12**:228–233.

Dannenberg, A. M., Jr. 1993. Immunopathogenesis of pulmonary tuberculosis. *Hosp. Pract.* **28**:33–40 (or 51–58).

Dannenberg, A. M., Jr., M. S. Burstone, P. C. Walter, and J. W. Kinsley. 1963. A histochemical study of phagocytic and enzymatic functions of rabbit mononuclear and polymorphonuclear exudate cells and alveolar macrophages. I. Survey and quantitation of enzymes, and states of cellular activation. *J. Cell Biol.* **17**:465–486.

Dannenberg, A. M., Jr., O. T. Meyer, J. R. Esterly, and T. Kambara. 1968. The local nature of immunity in tuberculosis, illustrated histochemically in dermal BCG lesions. *J. Immunol.* **100**:931–941.

Fox, R. R. 1974. Taxonomy and genetics, p. 1–22. *In* S. H. Weisbroth, R. E. Flatt, and A. L. Kraus (ed.), *The Biology of the Laboratory Rabbit.* Academic Press, Inc., New York.

Fox, R. R. (ed.). 1975. *Handbook on Genetically Standardized JAX Rabbits.* The Jackson Laboratory, Bar Harbor, Maine.

Henderson, H. M., A. M. Dannenberg, Jr., and M. B. Lurie. 1963. Phagocytosis of tubercle bacilli by rabbit pulmonary alveolar macrophages and its relation to native resistance to tuberculosis. *J. Immunol.* **91**:553–556.

Lurie, M. B. 1932. The correlation between the histological changes and the fate of living tubercle bacilli in the organs of tuberculous rabbits. *J. Exp. Med.* **55**:31–54.

Lurie, M. B. 1934. The fate of BCG and associated changes in the organs of rabbits. *J. Exp. Med.* **60**:163–178.

Lurie, M. B. 1938. Nature of inherited resistance to tuberculosis. *Proc. Soc. Exp. Biol. Med.* **39**:181–187.

Lurie, M. B. 1941. Heredity, constitution and tuberculosis. An experimental study. *Am. Rev. Tuberc.* **44**(Suppl.):1–125.

Lurie, M. B. 1944. Experimental epidemiology of tuberculosis. Hereditary resistance to attack by tuberculosis and to the ensuing disease and the effect of the concentration of tubercle bacilli upon these two phases of resistance. *J. Exp. Med.* **79**:573–589.

Lurie, M. B. 1964. *Resistance to Tuberculosis: Experimental Studies in Native and Acquired Defensive Mechanisms.* Harvard University Press, Cambridge, Mass.

Lurie, M. B., S. Abramson, and A. G. Heppleston. 1952a. On the response of genetically resistant and susceptible rabbits to the quantitative inhalation of human-type tubercle bacilli and the nature of resistance to tuberculosis. *J. Exp. Med.* **95**:119–134.

Lurie, M. B., and A. M. Dannenberg, Jr. 1965. Macrophage function in infectious disease with inbred rabbits. *Bacteriol. Rev.* **29**:466–476.

Lurie, M. B., A. G. Heppleston, S. Abramson, and I. B. Swartz. 1950. An evaluation of the method of quantitative airborne infection and its use in the study of the pathogenesis of tuberculosis. *Am. Rev. Tuberc.* **61**:765–797.

Lurie, M. B., P. Zappasodi, E. Cardona-Lynch, and A. M. Dannenberg, Jr. 1952b. The response to the intracutaneous inoculation of BCG as an index of native resistance to tuberculosis. *J. Immunol.* **68**:369–387.

Lurie, M. B., P. Zappasodi, A. M. Dannenberg, Jr., and G. H. Weiss. 1952c. On the mechanism of genetic resistance to tuberculosis and its mode of inheritance. *Am. J. Hum. Genet.* **4**:302–314.

Lurie, M. B., P. Zappasodi, and C. Tickner. 1955. On the nature of genetic resistance to tuberculosis in the light of the host-parasite relationships in natively resistant and susceptible rabbits. *Am. Rev. Tuberc. Pulm. Dis.* **72**:297–323.

Tuberculosis: Pathogenesis, Protection, and Control
Edited by Barry R. Bloom
© 1994 American Society for Microbiology, Washington, DC 20005

Chapter 11

Tuberculosis in Wild and Domestic Mammals

Charles O. Thoen

Different animal species vary in their susceptibilities to infection by the different types of virulent tubercle bacilli: *Mycobacterium tuberculosis*, *Mycobacterium africanum*, *Mycobacterium bovis*, and *Mycobacterium avium*. The most comprehensive studies of tuberculosis in different animals were reported by Francis (1958) and are summarized in Table 1, which is excerpted from Francis's book. This table was slightly modified by the late Alfred G. Karlson of the Mayo Clinic, who had extensive experience with tuberculosis (Karlson, 1960). There is considerable variation among mammals in the number of bacilli within lesions, degree of tuberculin sensitivity (allergy), and amounts of caseation, fibrosis, and calcification. Not included in the table are the extents of liquefaction of solid caseous foci and cavity formation, which are the main mechanisms by which tuberculosis is spread in human beings (Dannenberg, 1984). Liquefaction promotes extracellular multiplication of tubercle bacilli to tremendous numbers, and cavity formation allows these bacilli to spread through the air passages to other parts of the lung and to other people.

The importance of transmission of tuber-cle bacilli (*M. bovis*) from animals to humans was recognized in the early 1900s; therefore, compulsory pasteurization ordinances were adopted by Chicago and New York City in 1910 and 1913, respectively. When pasteurization was adopted, there was usually a concomitant decrease in tuberculosis in children. Outbreaks of *M. bovis* infection remain an important public health problem in children and adults originating from developing countries in which pasteurization of milk is not uniformly practiced (Dankner et al., 1993). Reports on the isolation of *M. bovis* from human beings in developed countries are also available (Grange, in press).

Tubercle bacilli that are inhaled usually lodge in alveolar spaces, where they are ingested by alveolar macrophages. The reaction of wild mammals to infection by mammalian or avian tubercle bacilli is basically similar to that observed in cattle (Thoen et al., 1988, 1992). Development or elimination of disease depends on the microbicidal activities of the ingesting macrophages in destroying the tubercle bacilli (Thoen and Chiodini, 1993). When the organism multiplies within the phagocyte, the host cell may die, resulting in the development of a microscopic tubercle. Initially, the lesion is composed of sensitized leukocytes and specialized macrophages, referred to as epithelioid cells. The cellular

Charles O. Thoen • Department of Microbiology, Immunology and Preventive Medicine, Iowa State University, Ames, Iowa 50011.

Table 1. Main features of tuberculosis in a variety of species[a]

Group	Species	Allergy	No. of bacilli in lesions	Caseation	Calcification	Fibrosis	Giant cells	Susceptibility to infection with three types of tubercle bacilli			Spread	Route
								Bovine	Human	Avian		
1	Primitive humans	5	1	5	3	2	3	5	5	1	5	R90
	Monkeys	2	2	5	3	1	5	5	5	1	5	R90
	Guinea pigs	3	1	5	2	1	4	5	5	2	1	Expr
	Rabbits	2	2	5	2	1	4	5	1	4	1	Expr
	Voles	1	3	4	2	1	2	5	1	1	1	Expr
	Avg	2.6	1.8	4.8	2.4	1.2	3.6	5	3.4	1.8	2.6	
2	Modern humans	5	1	5	5	5	5	2	2	1	5	R90
	Elephants	1	3	4	1	5	1	3	3	1	?	R100
	Cattle	2	1	4	5	4	5	4	1	1	5	R90
	Buffalo	2	1	4	4	4	4	4	1	1	4	R90
	Goats	2	1	4	4	3	4	4	1	2	1	R90
	Sheep	2	1	4	4	4	2	3	1	2	1	R80
	Camels	2	1	3	4	4	1	3	1	1	1	R90
	Pigs	3	1	4	4	4	2	4	2	2	1	A90
	Avg	2.4	1.3	4	3.9	4.1	3	3.4	1.5	1.4	2.6	
3	Fowl	2	4	4	1	3	2	1	1	3	4	A100
4	Horses	1	3	3	1	2	4	2	1	1	1	A90
	Asses and mules	1	3	3	1	2	4	2	1	1	1	A90
	Avg	1	3	3	1	2	4	2	1	1	1	
5A	Dogs	2	2	3	1	2	1	2	2	0	0	R60
5B	Cats	1	3	3	1	2	1	4	1	2	1	A70
	Mink	0	5	3	1	1	1	5	1	1	0	A90
	Ferrets	0	5	3	0	2	1	5	1	2	0	A90
5C	Hamsters	0	4	0.5	0	0	0	5	5	1	0	Expr
5D	Mice	1	4	0.5	0	0	0	2	2	1	0	Expr
	Rats	1	3	0.5	0	0	0	1	1	0.5	0	Expr
	Avg	0.71	3.9	1.9	0.43	1	0.57	3.4	1.9	1.1	0.14	
6	Chicken embryo	0	5	1	0	1	1	5	4	2		
	Tissue culture	0	5	1	0	1	0	5	4	2		
	Avg	0	5	1	0	1	0.5	5	4	2		

[a] The maximum value for each feature in this table is 5. Obviously, the figures represent a somewhat arbitrary approximation, and the table should be studied in conjunction with the text. The use of boldface numbers indicates that little evidence is available. A zero in a column does not completely preclude the existence of these features in any given species. No species is completely resistant to tuberculosis, and consequently, in the columns on susceptibility to various types of tubercle bacilli, a 1 has been used for those species that are virtually resistant to infection with a given type. The figures for susceptibility are roughly comparable vertically as well as horizontally; thus, those for rabbits are 5, 1, and 4, and those for mice are 2, 2, and 1. The values for spread represent the ease with which tuberculosis spreads naturally between members of any one species, and the figures under "Route" show the percentages of all natural infections acquired by the most important route; obviously, if 90% of infections are respiratory (R), nearly 10% will be alimentary (A). Expr is used when nearly all our information on tuberculosis in these species is based on experimentally induced disease. (Compiled by Francis [1958] and slightly modified. Reproduced by permission of Cassell & Co. Ltd., London.)

debris of degenerated macrophages sensi-tizes local lymphocytes, which may in turn produce lymphokines that attract and im-mobilize other macrophages. Subse-quently, there is a dynamic turnover of engulfment of bacteria and degeneration of phagocytes at the lesion site. As the lesion develops, necrosis occurs and multinucle-ated giant cells usually appear in the lesion. As the tubercle progresses, a zone of lym-phocytes and mononuclear cells surrounds the site; often there is a proliferation of connective tissue at the periphery that ap-pears as a capsule. As lesions increase in size, caseous necrosis becomes apparent and mineralization may occur.

Clinical signs of tuberculosis in exotic mammals are variable. The extensiveness of disease is often related to the virulence of the organism, the route of infection, the stage of infection, and several host-related factors. Tubercles are often found in bron-chial, mediastinal, and portal lymph nodes. Other tissues commonly affected include lung, liver, spleen, and the surfaces of body cavities. When tuberculous lesions are located in the parenchyma of a lung, a productive bronchopneumonia may be present; dyspnea and emaciation are often apparent. In some cases of generalized tu-berculosis, lesions in the genital tract have been reported.

Wild mammals found to have tubercu-lous lesions at necropsy after natural death are usually without prior suspicion of tuber-culosis. Gross lesions may be extensive, involving entire organs of one or both body cavities; however, the anatomical sites of lesions, the extensiveness of pathologic in-volvement, and the consistency of nodular formations with some caseous necrosis are not usually different from those seen in domestic animals (Thoen, 1993). Tubercu-lous lesions observed at necropsy usually have yellowish, caseous, necrotic areas in nodules of firm white to light gray fibrous tissue. Tubercles may not appear discrete where lesions diffuse into existing tissues.

Some lesions have a purulent consistency, whereas others are partially dry with case-ation or have extensive fibrosis. Mineral-ization or caseocalcification may occur in lesions but is often slight when present in wild mammals.

A tubercle is characteristically composed of a caseous, necrotic center bordered by a zone of epithelioid cells (some of which may have formed multinucleated giant cells), an accumulation of lymphocytes, a few granulocytes, and a capsule of fibrous connective tissue of variable thickness. There is considerable variation in the ap-parent abilities of some wild mammals to form tubercles associated with connective tissue and of epithelioid cells to form multi-nucleated giant cells, which are common-place in tubercles of domestic bovines. Multinucleated cells are not often present in tubercles in the lungs of some Indian elephants (Thoen et al., 1988; Thoen and Himes, 1981). This may be histologic evi-dence for species- or individual-animal-as-sociated factors that influence host-parasite relationships. However, other reports indi-cate that the lung from an elephant with tuberculous lesions exhibited multinucle-ated giant cells (Langhans type), epithelioid cells, and an area of caseation with no recognizable connective tissue cells. Other tuberculous lesions from this elephant were conspicuously lacking in connective tissue proliferation. Several lung tubercles from yet another elephant with *M. tuberculosis* revealed lesions with thick zones of fibrous connective tissue, but multinucleated giant cells were absent.

Tuberculous lesions from camelines, cervines, and wild bovines closely resem-ble those of domestic bovines. A central area of caseation and slight calcification is surrounded by a zone of epithelioid cells and lymphocytes encapsulated by a thick zone of fibrous connective tissue. Also, lesions from antelopines such as oryxes, kudus, nilgais, and a sable horned antelope closely resemble those in Bovidae. Nodular areas of caseation and epithelioid cells exhibit an apparent lack of connective tissue involvement.

In nonhuman primates, *M. bovis*, *M. africanum*, and *M. tuberculosis* can produce extensive disease involving the parenchyma of the lung as well as extrapulmonary tissues. When animals cough, the disease may be transmitted by aerosol or droplets of exudate containing the bacilli. Animals may also be infected by ingestion of feed and water contaminated with urine, fecal material, or pulmonary exudates from diseased animals that contain tubercle bacilli.

Tuberculous lesions from baboons and several species of monkeys usually demonstrate microscopic similarities to those in other wild mammals; however, the spleens of large apes infected with *M. bovis* may exhibit numerous tubercles of uniform size and, microscopically, an absence of multinucleated cells. Tubercles from nonhuman primates infected with *M. bovis* do not have significant histologic differences to differentiate them from lesions caused by *M. tuberculosis*.

Naturally acquired infections with *M. avium* are reported to be rare in nonhuman primates. However, epizootics of *M. avium* serovars 1, 2, and 8 have been reported in several species of macaques. The clinical features of this disease include diarrhea and debilitation. Gross lesions were often absent, but in some animals, the mucosas of the small intestine and colon were irregularly thickened and the mesenteric lymph nodes were enlarged. Microscopically, the intestinal mucosa was diffusely infiltrated with epithelioid cells that extended into the submucosa. Foci of epithelioid cells were also encountered in the liver, lung, kidney, spleen, bone marrow, and myocardium. Necrosis, calcification, or fibrosis was not usually observed. Multinucleated giant cells were only occasionally observed.

Swine have been reported to be the most susceptible of all domestic animals to *M. bovis* (Thoen, 1992). Progressive lesions are usually observed in the lungs; well-defined tubercles may be present in the liver, spleen, and lymph nodes in the thoracic and abdominal cavities. Microscopically, granulomas may contain caseated centers with some mineralization. Giant cells and epithelioid cells are usually present in lesions in the lung. Although acid-fast bacilli can be demonstrated in appropriately stained sections, it should be emphasized that only a few tubercle bacilli may be observed.

The horse can be infected with *M. bovis*, *M. avium*, or *M. tuberculosis*; however, information from experimental inoculations suggests that the horse is relatively resistant (Francis, 1958). Lesions often are present in the liver and mesenteric lymph nodes. Tubercles are seldom seen in the spleen and kidneys; however, the spleen may be enlarged and several times the normal size. Lung lesions are usually present in *M. bovis* infections. Skeletal lesions have been reported. Microscopically, the granulomas in lymph nodes and lung are characterized by accumulations of epithelioid cells and Langhans-type giant cells. Mineralization is rarely observed; however, necrosis may be present.

Goats are susceptible to *M. bovis* but quite resistant to *M. tuberculosis*. In natural and experimental infections with *M. bovis*, lesions are usually present in the lungs and associated lymph nodes. Tubercles may be present in the liver and spleen. Histologically, these lesions are similar to those observed in cattle. Well-defined granulomas are observed and are characterized by the presence of epithelioid cells and numerous giant cells. Acid-fast bacilli are usually present; however, the number of organisms varies greatly for different animals.

M. bovis may cause lesions in sheep similar to those observed in cattle (Karlson, 1960). Evidence for generalization of disease includes the presence of lesions in lung and in bronchial and mediastinal lymph nodes as well as in spleen and kidney. The lesions are often large and calcified.

Generally, it is believed that the susceptibility of dogs to *M. bovis* and *M. tuberculosis* is similar to that of humans (Francis, 1958). The occurrence of disease is usually related to exposure to a human patient or to infected cattle. In the dog, lesions are most often found in the lungs, liver, and kidney; however, tubercles may also be observed in the pleura and peritoneum (Francis, 1958). The lesions are invariably exudative in type and appear gray. The absence of calcification has been considered characteristic of tuberculosis in dogs; however, exceptions do occur, as other reports reveal liver lesions with extensive fibrosis and calcification. Microscopic examination of the lung tissue may reveal coalescing lesions with central areas of caseation. Numerous leukocytes and macrophages are present; however, giant cells are not usually observed. Acid-fast bacilli are often seen.

Cats appear to be very resistant to *M. tuberculosis* but are susceptible to *M. bovis* and *M. avium*. Milk from tuberculous cows has been incriminated as the most common source of infection for cats (Francis, 1958); therefore, the primary site of infection is considered to be the alimentary tract. The mesenteric lymph nodes become enlarged and necrotic, and in some cases, they adhere to the adjacent intestinal wall or the mesentery. Hematogenous spread of bacilli results in progressive disease in other organs, including the lungs. Microscopic examination shows accumulations of nonspecific granulation tissue. Numerous epithelioid cells are present, but few giant cells develop. Central necrosis is often present, but calcification rarely occurs. The bronchial and mediastinal lymph nodes often are involved.

M. avium serovars 1, 2, 4, and 8 are the acid-fast organisms most frequently isolated from granulomatous lesions in swine and other mammals. Tuberculosis lesions in mammals usually involve lymph nodes of the cervical regions and the mesentery; however, other tissues, including lungs, kidney, brain, intestinal mucosa, tonsils, muscle, ovaries, and the skin, may be involved. The lesions range from small, yellowish white, caseous foci a few millimeters in diameter to involvement of an entire node. The disease may be localized or may involve a number of lymph nodes along the intestinal tract. Lesions have also been reported to occur in the wall of the intestine. On necropsy, the lesions due to *M. avium* complex are not easily enucleated. Diffuse granulomas with large areas of caseation may be present; however, usually there is little or no evidence of mineralization.

It should be noted that some differences in cellular composition of tuberculous lesions, including the presence or absence of acid-fast bacilli, occur for different mammals. However, it must be emphasized that considerable variation in lesions may be observed in animals within a particular species. Therefore, it is important to consider tuberculosis in a differential diagnosis whenever granulomatous lesions are observed.

Experimental infections may be induced in susceptible animals by aerosol or by intratracheal, intravenous, subcutaneous, or intramuscular inoculation of virulent *M. bovis*, *M. africanum*, or *M. tuberculosis*. *M. avium* is usually given by the oral route. In conducting pathogenicity studies, the dose of organisms varies depending on the age of the animal, the age of the mycobacterial culture, and the route of inoculation. Cultures more than 6 weeks old may produce variable results. It is recommended that 10- to 14-day-old subcultures grown in liquid media be used for animal inoculations. The organisms should be harvested by centrifugation. All culture manipulations and slide preparations should be done in a biological safety cabinet with negative air supply and suitable filters. A phenolic or substituted phenolic disinfectant should be used for decontaminating the work area of the safety cabinet and the outer surfaces of tubes containing inoculum. Screw-cap tubes are to be used, and the caps should be wrapped with Parafilm to minimize the possibility of leakage during transport to the animal area.

Most strains of mammalian tubercle bacilli are highly virulent and remain so for considerable periods of time on subculture (Thoen and Chiodini, 1993). However, attenuated strains of *M. bovis* have been reported. One such example is bacillus Calmette-Guérin (BCG). Variations in the relative degree of virulence have been described for each of the 16 or more strains of BCG used in experimental investigations.

M. avium strains often become attenuated following subculture on egg-enriched or synthetic culture media (Thoen, 1993). Reports indicate that the reduction in virulence is associated with changes in colony morphology from rough and transparent to smooth and opaque dome-shaped forms. Upon passage in animals, certain attenuated strains become more virulent. Three main colony forms are present on initial isolation. Virulence appears to be associated with the rough and smooth transparent colonies, since few smooth, dome-shaped, opaque colonies are observed on primary culture from animal tissues.

Recently, there has been increased interest in the isolation of *M. avium* complex serovars 1, 4, and 8 from patients with AIDS and from nonimmunocompromised patients (Cook, 1992). Some of the same serovars have been isolated from domestic and wild animals (Thoen, in press). Although *M. avium* has been isolated from environmental specimens (i.e., soil and water), no definitive information on a common source(s) of these bacteria for animals and humans is available.

REFERENCES

Cook, J. L. 1992. *M. avium*, the modern epidemic. *Med. Sci. Update* 19(6):1–7.

Dankner, W. M., N. J. Waecker, M. A. Essey, K. Moser, M. Thompson, and C. E. Davis. 1993. *Mycobacterium bovis* infections in San Diego: a clinicoepidemiologic study of 73 patients and a historical review of a forgotten pathogen. *Medicine* 72:11–37.

Dannenberg, A. M., Jr. 1984. Pathogenesis of tuberculosis: native and acquired resistance in animals and humans, p. 344–354. *In* L. Leive and D. Schlessinger (ed.), *Microbiology—1984*. American Society for Microbiology, Washington, D.C.

Francis, J. 1958. *Tuberculosis in Animals and Man: a Study in Comparative Pathology*. Cassell and Co., Ltd., London.

Grange, J. M. Human aspects of bovine tuberculosis. *In* J. M. Steele and C. O. Thoen (ed.), *Bovine Tuberculosis in Animals and Man*. Iowa State University Press, Ames, in press.

Karlson, A. G. 1960. Tuberculosis caused by human, bovine and avian tubercle bacilli in various animals. *Proc. U.S. Livestock Sanitary Assoc.* 64:194–201.

Thoen, C. O. 1992. Tuberculosis, p. 617–626. *In* A. D. Leman, B. E. Straw, W. L. Mengeling, S. D'Allaire, and D. J. Taylor (ed.), *Diseases of Swine*, 7th ed. Iowa State University Press, Ames.

Thoen, C. O. 1993. Tuberculosis and other mycobacterial diseases in captive wild animals, p. 45–49. *In* M. E. Fowler (ed.), *Zoo and Wild Animal Medicine*. The W. B. Saunders Co., Philadelphia.

Thoen, C. O. *Mycobacterium avium* infections in animals. *Res. Microbiol.*, in press.

Thoen, C. O., and R. Chiodini. 1993. *Mycobacterium*, p. 44–56. *In* C. L. Gyles and C. O. Thoen (ed.), *Pathogenesis of Bacterial Infections in Animals*. Iowa State University Press, Ames.

Thoen, C. O., and E. M. Himes. 1981. Tuberculosis, p. 263–274. *In* J. W. Davis, L. H. Karstad, and D. O. Trainer (ed.), *Infectious Diseases of Captive Wild Mammals*, 2nd ed. Iowa State University Press, Ames.

Thoen, C. O., W. J. Quinn, L. K. Miller, L. L. Stackhouse, B. F. Newcomb, and J. M. Ferrell. 1992. *Mycobacterium bovis* infection in North American elk (*Cervus elephus*). *J. Vet. Diagn. Invest.* 4:423–427.

Thoen, C. O., K. J. Throlson, L. D. Miller, E. M. Himes, and R. L. Morgan. 1988. Pathogenesis of *Mycobacterium bovis* infection in American bison. *Am. J. Vet. Res.* 49:1861–1865.

III. GENETICS OF *MYCOBACTERIUM TUBERCULOSIS*

Tuberculosis: Pathogenesis, Protection, and Control
Edited by Barry R. Bloom
© 1994 American Society for Microbiology, Washington, DC 20005

Chapter 12

Mycobacteriophages: Cornerstones of Mycobacterial Research

Graham F. Hatfull and William R. Jacobs, Jr.

Some may think it presumptuous to refer to mycobacteriophages as cornerstones of mycobacterial research. After all, these creatures are metabolically inert entities consisting mainly of DNA and protein. For some, phages are nothing more than anachronistic curiosities that share a name with a human cell whose profession it is to engulf foreign objects. Despite their seemingly lifeless existence outside a host cell, when phages interact with host cells, a marvelous transformation occurs: the phages come alive. They redirect the focus of a cell selectively to expressing their proteins, replicating their genomes, and directing the synthesis of a complex macromolecular virion. In an analogous fashion, phages have brought new life to the biological sciences as experimental tools. Phages played pivotal roles in elucidating the nature of bacterial mutation, establishing that DNA was the genetic material, unveiling the genetic code, and defining systems of recombination, gene expression, and regulation. Mycobacteriophages have played key roles in establishing molecular genetic systems for mycobacteria.

The first mycobacteriophage was described in 1947 (Gardner and Weiser, 1947). There are over 250 known mycobacteriophages, and much of the early work on mycobacteriophages has been reviewed extremely well by others (Redmond, 1963; Barksdale and Kim, 1977; Mizuguchi, 1984). A number of genetic phenomena have been described for the mycobacteriophages, including transfection (Tokunaga and Sellers, 1964) and transduction (Sundaraj and Ramakrishnan, 1971). Mycobacteriophages have for many years been used to classify mycobacteria by phage typing (Tokunaga et al., 1968; Baess, 1969; Snider et al., 1984). Although most mycobacteriophages have a relatively broad host range, there are useful phages with highly restricted specificities; e.g., DS6A will form plaques on *Mycobacterium tuberculosis* and no other species (Redmond and Cater, 1960). In this chapter, we describe the ways that a systematic use of phages led to the development of novel cloning vectors and ultimately transformation of mycobacteria. In addition, we will describe how the detailed characterization of one phage, L5, has provided an abundance of novel insights into and genetic tools for mycobac-

Graham F. Hatfull • Department of Biological Sciences, University of Pittsburgh, Pittsburgh, Pennsylvania 15230. *William R. Jacobs, Jr.* • Howard Hughes Medical Institute, Albert Einstein College of Medicine, 1300 Morris Park Avenue, Bronx, New York 10461.

terial molecular genetics. Last, we will describe how the combination of a reporter gene with a mycobacteriophage has breathed new life into rapid assessment of drug susceptibilities in clinical samples of *M. tuberculosis* and is also providing a useful tool for screening novel antituberculosis compounds.

MYCOBACTERIOPHAGES: KEYS TO DEVELOPING MOLECULAR GENETIC SYSTEMS FOR MYCOBACTERIA

The full promise of recombinant DNA technology for the genetic analysis of mycobacteria could be achieved only with the development of systems to stably introduce recombinant molecules into mycobacterial cells (see also chapter 18). Despite many attempts by many investigators over many years, transformation of mycobacteria had not been achieved. The contributing potential barriers to successful transformation were numerous and included (i) inability to introduce DNA through the lipid cell wall into the mycobacterial cell, (ii) restriction of the foreign DNA by the mycobacterial host cell, (iii) unstable replication or maintenance of the plasmid, (iv) failure to express the selectable marker gene, and/or (v) inability to regenerate intact cells from protoplasts. In fact, unsuccessful transformation may have resulted from any or all of the above possibilities. Mycobacteriophages provided the basic tools with which we could test these possibilities and also were a means by which we could overcome specific barriers. More specifically, phages provided a means whereby the process of transformation of foreign DNA could be dissected into a number of discrete steps, including (i) DNA entry, (ii) avoidance of restriction systems, (iii) stable integration of foreign DNA, and (iv) expression of selectable marker genes. Only by systematically evaluating these possibilities was successful transformation of mycobacteria ultimately achieved.

OPTIMIZING DNA UPTAKE

Successful DNA transfer events are recognized by assays that measure the successful introduction of a DNA molecule into a bacterial cell. For organisms such as *Escherichia coli* or *Bacillus subtilis*, the DNA transfer event is usually a transformation in which a selectable marker gene is introduced into the bacterial cell and relatively infrequent transformants are then selected for. This assay is rapid, since a plasmid or a chromosomal gene carrying a selectable marker gene can be introduced into a single cell and the cell can give rise to a colony in less than 8 h. In contrast, after transformation, even a fast-growing mycobacterium, such as *M. smegmatis*, would require 3 to 4 days to yield colonies on a plate. Even worse, after transformation, the slow-growing mycobacterium *M. tuberculosis* would require 2 to 3 weeks to form colonies on a plate. The first important benefit of a phage transformation assay, i.e., transfection, was that it provided a relatively rapid assay for quantitating DNA entry. The successful introduction of a phage genome into a bacterial cell or a cell wall-deficient form of a mycobacterium results in a productive phage infection. The cells that are transfected with a phage DNA molecule are termed infectious centers, as they will give rise to the generation of viable phage particles capable of infecting nearby phage-sensitive cells. When infectious centers are mixed with phage-sensitive mycobacterial cells, they generate plaques. In contrast to the generation of mycobacterial colonies that can require from 3 days to 3 weeks to form, mycobacterial phage plaques resulting from a transfection event could be formed in as little as 12 to 48 h. Thus, transfection provided a rapid assay for evaluating sets of parameters designed to optimize DNA entry into cells. Although transfection was first reported by Tokunaga and Sellers in 1964, the efficiency was very low. To improve the efficiency, a method employing protoplasts and polyethylene glycol that had been successful in optimizing the introduction of DNA into *Streptomyces* spp. was attempted (Jacobs et al., 1987). Successful generation of protoplasts is a fairly empirical procedure that is affected by the strain, growth media, culture conditions, growth state of the cells, and various treatments with lysozyme and lipases. The DNA uptake event is similarly an empirical procedure affected by the buffer into which the protoplasts are resuspended and even the batch of polyethylene glycol used. By using a transfection assay, we were able to rapidly explore a large number of variables to obtain conditions that enabled us to obtain transfection frequencies of 10^4 to 10^5 PFU/μg of D29 phage DNA in a cloned isolate of *M. smegmatis*, mc^{2}6 (Jacobs et al., 1987). These studies established that the transfection event was true transfection of protoplasts, as the assay was sensitive to both DNase and osmotic shock. Having achieved such frequencies, we attempted to achieve transformation of *M. smegmatis* with a hybrid plasmid library that had been constructed using the *M. fortuitum* plasmid pAL5000 (Labidi et al., 1984). All of our initial attempts at achieving transformation of *M. smegmatis* were disappointingly unsuccessful. However, the phage transfection experiments demonstrated that DNA entry was not the limiting factor to achieving transformation.

INTRODUCTION OF FOREIGN DNA INTO MYCOBACTERIA USING A MYCOBACTERIOPHAGE CLONING VECTOR

Phages such as lambda and M13 have provided some of the most useful and versatile cloning vectors employed in recombinant DNA methodologies for *E. coli*. Thus, it was reasonable to create mycobacteriophage cloning vectors. As mentioned above, numerous phages that were capable of replicating on a broad range of mycobacterial hosts had been identified. In evaluating which mycobacteriophage to develop into a mycobacteriophage cloning vector, properties similar to those of bacteriophage λ were sought: (i) possession of a double-stranded DNA genome with cohesive ends, (ii) ability to stably lysogenize mycobacteria, (iii) presence of nonessential regions, and (iv) a broad host range.

Genomes for phages are fairly diverse entities consisting of either RNA or DNA in single strands or double strands. The most useful phage cloning vectors would be those that possess a double-stranded DNA genome so that phage genomes isolated directly from phage particles could be digested with the large collection of restriction endonucleases. Although a number of *E. coli* phages that possess genomes consisting of single-stranded RNA or DNA have been described, all mycobacteriophage genomes examined to date contain double-stranded DNAs. Double-stranded DNA genomes isolated from phage particles exist only rarely as supercoiled circles, as in PM2 from *Pseudomonas* spp., and most often as linear DNA molecules. All mycobacteriophage genomes examined to date exist as linear double-stranded DNA molecules of greater than 35 kb. A linear DNA molecule, depending on the phage's strategy for replication and packaging into phage heads, might possess cohesive ends such as those of λ, exhibit terminal redundancy such as that of T4, or have irregular ends such as those of phage Mu. We examined a large variety of mycobacterial genomes and found a rapid way for determining the nature of the ends by running pulsed-field gels on the phage genomes isolated from phage particles (Fig. 1) (Tuckman and Jacobs, unpublished result). If the phage possesses cohesive ends, it characteristically will form a ladder of genome lengths ranging from a monomer to many genome lengths. This analysis allowed us to

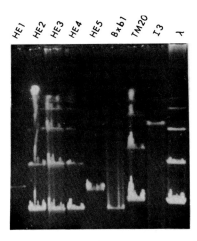

Figure 1. Contour-clamped homogeneous electric field (CHEF) analysis of mycobacteriophage genomes. A set of mycobacteriophage genomes were analyzed using the CHEF electrophoresis system. Genomes that have cohesive ends tend to form ladders, whereas phages that are terminally redundant or have irregular ends yield single bands. Thus, I3 and BxbI appear to have irregular ends, while the rest of the phages have cohesive ends.

demonstrate that the majority of mycobacteriophages possess cohesive ends. Some phages, such as I3 or BxbI (Barletta et al., 1991), produce single bands on the pulsed-field gel, suggesting that they either have terminally redundant ends characteristic of phages that can act as generalized transducing phages or have irregular ends. Indeed, I3 has been shown to be a generalized transducing phage (Sundaraj and Rama-krishnan, 1971). In choosing a phage for development of a phage vector, it was simplest to choose a phage that possessed cohesive ends, as the DNA molecules isolated from phage particles were a homogeneous population. This quality facilitated further genetic manipulation.

Initially, we chose the phage TM4 (Timme and Brennan, 1984) to work with, as it resembles bacteriophage lambda in that it is approximately 50 kb in length and possesses cohesive ends. In addition, it had been isolated from *M. avium*, where it was thought to be a temperate phage. The trick

to constructing a phage cloning vector was to introduce a foreign DNA fragment into a nonessential region of the phage. In order to do this, we took advantage of the observation that genes from mycobacteria, which characteristically possess a high guanine-plus-cytosine content, are generally not expressed in *E. coli* (Jacobs et al., 1986a, b). Thus, it seemed plausible that one could clone an entire mycobacteriophage in *E. coli* and not lyse or kill the *E. coli* cell. Furthermore, if the *E. coli* plasmid could be inserted into a nonessential region of the phage, the resulting construct would be a shuttle phasmid, a hybrid *E. coli* plasmid-mycobacteriophage recombinant that could replicate in *E. coli* as a plasmid and replicate in mycobacteria as a phage (Fig. 2). Since nothing was known about the existence or location of a nonessential region of TM4, a novel strategy was used to generate a library of constructs in which an *E. coli*-bacteriophage λ cosmid was inserted at random sites around the TM4 genome (Jacobs et al., 1987). The generation of plaques following transfection of the library into *M. smegmatis* allowed for the selection of TM4 recombinant phages into which the cosmid was inserted in a nonessential region. These resulting shuttle phasmids represented the generation of the first mycobacteriophage cloning vectors and the first demonstration that recombinant DNA could be introduced into mycobacterial cells. Furthermore, shuttle phasmids provided a means of testing whether foreign DNA was being degraded by a host restriction system of *M. smegmatis*, since we could compare the transfection frequencies of shuttle phasmid DNA isolated from *E. coli* to those of shuttle phasmid DNA isolated from mycobacteriophage particles. The observation that the *E. coli* plasmid form of a shuttle phasmid yielded as many PFU per microgram of DNA or more than the linear mycobacteriophage form of the shuttle phasmid suggested that *M. smegmatis* had no restriction system that recog-

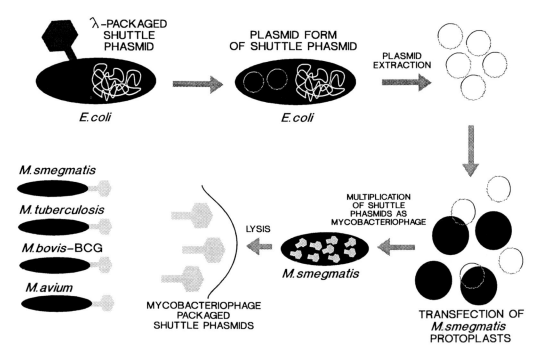

Figure 2. Schematic of shuttle phasmid transfer. Shuttle phasmids have pleiotropic properties. First, they are cosmids, and they can be packaged into λ heads and can replicate in *E. coli* as cosmids. Alternatively, the shuttle phasmid DNAs can be transfected into *M. smegmatis*, where they express mycobacteriophage genes and undergo lytic growth. These mycobacteriophage-packaged DNAs can be efficiently introduced into a broad range of mycobacteria, including the slow-growing mycobacteria (reprinted from Jacobs et al., 1989).

nized *E. coli* DNA as foreign. These experiments suggested that restriction of foreign DNA was not the limiting factor to achieving transformation of mycobacteria.

STABLE EXPRESSION OF A SELECTABLE MARKER GENE USING A TEMPERATE SHUTTLE PHASMID

TM4 shuttle phasmids are versatile cloning vectors. They contain unique restriction endonuclease sites in the *E. coli* plasmid portion of the nonessential region of the TM4 phage that facilitate the introduction of additional DNA. These shuttle phasmids also contain bacteriophage λ cohesive ends (different from the TM4 cohesive ends) that permit these large molecules to be packaged into bacteriophage λ particles in vitro. This property greatly facilitated the cloning

of additional DNA fragments (Jacobs et al., 1989). Initially, we sought to determine whether the aminoglycoside phosphotransferase gene (*aph*) could be expressed and would confer resistance via lysogeny upon *M. smegmatis*. Although the *aph* gene could be readily cloned into a shuttle phasmid vector, we failed to observe the ability of the TM4 shuttle phasmids to confer kanamycin resistance upon *M. smegmatis*. At this point, we did not know whether the failure to express the kanamycin resistance gene was due to the fact that the *aph* gene was not being expressed or the fact that the phage was not being stably maintained. Analysis of putative TM4 lysogens of *M. smegmatis* demonstrated that the TM4 phage genome was in fact not being stably maintained. Although it appeared that TM4 might be able to stably lysogenize *M.*

avium, we failed to find it capable of stably lysogenizing *M. smegmatis*. TM4 is similar to many mycobacteriophages that form pseudolysogens, and we believe it is not a true temperate phage (Baess, 1971). At this point, we screened a set of phages that generated turbid and partially turbid plaques on *M. smegmatis* for their ability to site specifically integrate into the *M. smegmatis* chromosome. Phage L1 was shown to possess this ability (Snapper et al., 1988), and shuttle phasmids generated from phage L1 retained their ability to site specifically integrate into the chromosome of *M. smegmatis* (Snapper et al., 1988). This was the first demonstration that foreign DNA could be stably integrated and replicated in mycobacteria. Armed with this knowledge, we proceeded to clone selectable marker genes into the L1 shuttle phasmids and were delighted to see that the *aph* gene conferred kanamycin resistance upon lysogenizing *M. smegmatis* cells. Having established that kanamycin resistance could be expressed in *M. smegmatis* and used as a selectable marker in mycobacteria, we once again undertook to attempt to transform *M. smegmatis* with a library of hybrid plasmid constructs in which the kanamycin resistance gene had been introduced at random sites around the pAL5000 plasmid. Numerous attempts using this library were made, but all were unsuccessful. However, based on our expression of kanamycin resistance with the L1 shuttle phasmids, we predicted that the failure to transform was due either to the fact that the plasmid was unable to stably replicate in *M. smegmatis* or to the fact that we were unable to regenerate protoplasts. In order to bypass the protoplast regeneration step, electroporation, which had just been developed, was employed. Fortunately, this procedure was efficient enough that we could select for a rare mutant of *M. smegmatis* that permitted efficient plasmid transformation (Snapper et al., 1990). The nature of these mutations that permit efficient plasmid replication re-

mains a mystery, but they appear to be specific for plasmid replication. Ultimately, the discovery that *M. smegmatis* could not be transformed with a plasmid at any reasonable efficiency unless it acquired a specific mutation that permitted plasmid replication explained why so many attempts had failed. Fortunately, the systematic employment of phages enabled transformation to be achieved, not only for *M. smegmatis* but also for *M. tuberculosis* and BCG.

MYCOBACTERIOPHAGE I3

I3 was first described by Sundaraj and Ramakrishnan (1971) and is the first transducing mycobacteriophage described. It has a large hexagonal head and a long tail that can contract up to 60% when injecting DNA into host cells. The phage has a latent period of 1,803 h, an eclipse period of 2 h, and a rise period of 1 h. The burst size is 30 to 60, and the low burst size appears to be due to the limitation of available nutrients. The genome is circularly permuted, and DNA is packaged by a "headful" mechanism. Most curiously, the genomic DNA of I3, when denatured, dissociates into heterogenous-sized single-stranded fragments smaller than the expected genomic length (Reddy and Gopinathan, 1986). The biologically active I3 DNA harbors 13 or 14 single chain interruptions, each of about 6 to 10 nucleotides, that are host cell independent. It has been suggested that the interruptions facilitate the compaction and packaging of the genomic DNA into the phage heads. I3, in contrast to other phages, requires continuous function of host cell RNA polymerase. Its replication is blocked by rifampin in conventional host cells but not in rifampin-resistant mutants. Transduction activity was first reported by Sundaraj and Ramakrishnan (1971), who showed that I3 mediated transduction of several auxotrophic markers in *M. smegmatis* that was completely inhibited by treatment of the bacteria with antiserum to I3 but not with DNase. Antibiotic resistance has also been transduced (Saroja and Gopinathan, 1973).

MYCOBACTERIOPHAGE L5

Mycobacteriophage L5 is the best characterized of the mycobacteriophages. It was originally isolated in 1960 by Doke (1960) in Japan from a lysogenic strain of *M. smegmatis*. It is a temperate phage and forms turbid plaques on *M. smegmatis* from which stable lysogens can be recovered. Phage L1, isolated at the same time, is essentially identical to L5, the only apparent difference being the inability of L1 to form plaques at 42°C (Lee et al., 1991). A third phage, D29, also falls into this general class of phages, since it strongly cross-hybridizes to L5 DNA. D29 is subject to L5 superinfection immunity, although D29 is a lytic phage and is not able to form lysogens (Donnelly-Wu et al., 1993). Another phage resembling L1 and L5 at the level of restriction enzyme mapping has been isolated from a completely independent source in France (McAdam and Jacobs, unpublished results), which is consistent with the idea that L5 represents one member of a family of related phages. In this section, we will review the principal features of L5 and this family of phages and discuss several unresolved questions that demand further attention.

The complete host range of mycobacteriophage L5 is uncertain, though it appears to form plaques on a number of fast-growing mycobacterial species. L5 appears to infect the slow-growing mycobacteria such as BCG or *M. tuberculosis*, though it is difficult to obtain plaques on lawns of these strains. In addition, L5 does not form plaques on *Streptomyces* spp. (Jacobs, unpublished results). In contrast, phage D29 efficiently infects both fast- and slow-growing mycobacterial species and has also been shown to adsorb to *M. leprae* (David et al., 1984).

L5 is a true temperate phage and forms stable lysogens in *M. smegmatis* (Snapper et al., 1988; Lee et al., 1991). L5 plaques have a turbid morphology due to the growth and survival of lysogenic cells within the plaque. These lysogens can be recovered and cultured and have the properties expected of true lysogens; i.e., they are immune to superinfection by L5 particles, release virion particles into the medium when grown in rich broth, and contain a single copy of the L5 genome integrated into a specific location in the bacterial chromosome (Lee et al., 1991).

The most appropriate paradigm for L5 studies is the well-characterized phage λ, a temperate phage of *E. coli* (Hendrix et al., 1983). As discussed below, the two phages have considerable commonality in their life cycles, morphology, and some aspects of genome organization, even though they are unrelated at the DNA sequence level (Hatfull and Sarkis, 1993). It thus seems reasonable that they have a common ancestry but have undergone a considerable period of independent evolution in their distantly related host organisms (Casjens et al., 1992). In view of the abundant knowledge accrued from studies of λ and its central role in molecular biology, a detailed study of L5 should provide a similar genetic toolbox for the molecular analysis of its mycobacterial hosts.

L5 Genome Structure

Early studies indicated that L5 particles contained a linear double-stranded DNA genome of approximately 50 kb (Oyaski and Hatfull, 1992). Each end of the L5 genome contains a 9-base single-stranded 3′ extension, and the two extensions are complementary; presumably, these cohesive termini are sealed by a DNA ligase following DNA injection into the cell.

The complete DNA sequence of the 52,297-bp L5 genome has been determined, and a map of the genome organization has been proposed (Hatfull and Sarkis, 1993). Protein-coding genes were located using codon usage biases, and a total of 85 putative protein-coding genes were identified, accounting for over 90% of the size of the genome; these putative genes are numbered sequentially, with gene 1 being closest to the left end of the DNA (Fig. 3). Database comparisons with each of these putative proteins indicated that genes 33 and 44 encode an integrase and a DNA polymerase, respectively, but few other gene functions were identifiable. Poor similarities were observed between gp58 and DNA primases and between gp59 and T4 *Exo*VII, but it is not clear whether they represent true homologs. Other weak similarities that have yet to be discovered may exist.

DNA sequence analysis also showed that L5 encodes three tRNA genes located in a cluster about 4 kb from the left end. The genes encode $tRNA^{Asn}$, $tRNA^{Trp}$, and $tRNA^{Gln}$ and are in the 430-bp region between protein-coding genes 6 and 10. The genes are reasonably evenly spaced, with 50 bp between gene 6 and $tRNA^{Asn}$, 80 bp between $tRNA^{Asn}$ and $tRNA^{Trp}$, 60 bp between $tRNA^{Trp}$ and $tRNA^{Gln}$, and 30 bp between $tRNA^{Gln}$ and gene 10. The role of the tRNAs in L5 growth is not clear; however, since structural genes are located both upstream and downstream, it seems reasonable that they would be expressed at similar times. Examination of the tRNA anticodons suggests that they recognize common codons ($tRNA^{Trp}$ presumably recognizes only a single codon), arguing against a role in increasing rates of biosynthesis of genes possessing rare codons. They could, however, play a role in compensating for bacterial tRNA species that are of insufficient abundance for the high levels of phage gene expression demanded in late lytic growth; this may be important for growth in particular mycobacterial hosts. Alternatively, the tRNAs may be active in any number of regulatory roles in which tRNAs have been postulated.

During the formation of L5 lysogens, the L5 genome becomes integrated site specifically into the *M. smegmatis* genome (Hatfull and Sarkis, 1993). The attachment site in the phage genome (*attP*) is located near the center of the genome and effectively separates it into a left and right arm (Fig. 3). In the left arm, all of the genes, with the exception of gene 33, are transcribed in the rightward direction, i.e., toward *attP*. At least seven of these left-arm genes encode proteins involved in virion structure or assembly, suggesting a functional relationship to the left arm of phage lambda, which also encodes structure and assembly proteins. A closer examination suggests some underlying similarities in the organization of this segment of the two genomes in spite of the complete lack of similarity even at the protein sequence level (Fig. 4). These genes in L5 are close together with little or no space between the open reading frames; presumably, they are transcribed from only a few transcriptional promoters (or even a single one) (Fig. 3). The only left-arm gene transcribed in the opposite direction is gene 33, which encodes the phage integrase protein and is located next to its site of action, *attP* (Fig. 3).

The right-arm genes of L5 are all transcribed in the leftward direction, toward *attP*. This represents a significant departure from the lambda paradigm, where divergently transcribed RNA originates from the operator site, O_R. However, L5 does encode a repressor-like protein, the product of gene 71, which occupies an approximately collinear position to the *c*I gene of λ. The genes to the right of gene 71 do not appear to be essential for L5 lytic growth (Hatfull, unpublished results). While the functional role of other right-arm genes is not known (although gene 44 encodes a DNA polymerase), it seems likely that they act as regulatory functions for DNA replication and gene expression.

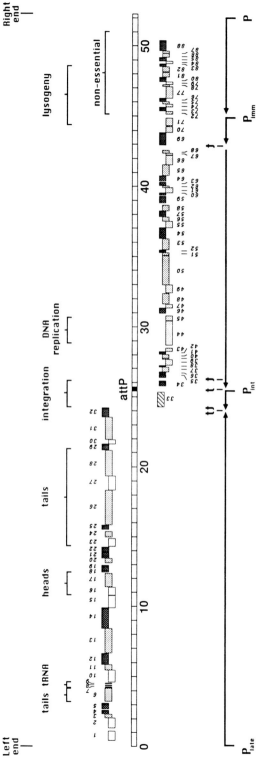

Figure 3. Map of the phage L5 genome. The 52,297-bp genome of L5 is shown as the horizontal bar, with vertical bars spaced 1 kb apart; the attachment site (*attP*) is located near the center of the genome. The shaded boxes represent the putative L5 genes, with those above the genome being transcribed rightward and those below the genome being transcribed leftward; the different shadings and vertical heights depict the reading frame for each gene. The functions of some of the genes are indicated. At the bottom, the locations of putative promoters are shown, although the positions are not precise and in some cases are inferred from the genome organization. It is not known whether genes 68 to 34 are transcribed from a separate promoter located between genes 68 and 69 or by antitermination of transcripts originating upstream. Putative transcription terminators are also shown, affecting either rightward (t) or leftward (ꓕ) transcription. A terminator is presumed to exist between genes 68 and 69 in order to prevent transcription of downstream genes (68 to 34) during lysogeny.

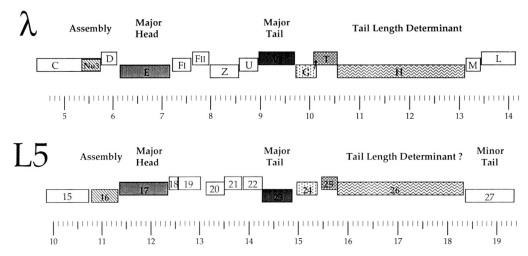

Figure 4. Comparison of regions of lambda and L5 left arms. Segments of the L5 and lambda left arms aligned by the 5' ends of the major head subunit genes (E and 17 in lambda and L5, respectively) are shown; the coordinates of each segment in the whole genome are given below the genes. Note the similarity of the organization of genes with similar functions despite the lack of sequence similarity. In lambda, gpT is not made, but gpG-T is synthesized as a result of a translational frameshift at the 3' end of the G gene (↑); genes 24 and 25 of L5 are organized such that gp24-25 could also be made by a related mechanism.

L5 Virion Structure and Assembly

Electron microscopy reveals the general morphology of L5 to be a common form among bacteriophages of which λ is an example. The L5 head is icosahedral and similar in size to that of lambda, whereas the tail is somewhat shorter. No side tail fibers are observed, and a unique structure, presumably responsible for specific recognition of the phage's mycobacterial hosts, is seen at the tip of the tail. Visualization of the virion protein components by sodium dodecyl sulfate (SDS)-gel electrophoresis reveals a curious aspect of the L5 head structure. Like those of related phages, the head is composed of multiple copies (approximately 415 protomers) of the major head subunit, the product of gene 17. However, gp17, which is predicted to be 35 kDa in size, is not found in the monomeric form in the head. Instead, it appears to be extensively covalently cross-linked such that most of the material is too large to enter the gel. However, pentameric and hexameric cross-linked forms are observed as high-molecular-weight species. This pattern is remarkably similar to that found in the lambdoid phage HK97, where the chemistry of the cross-link and its role in head assembly have been well characterized (Popa et al., 1991). Interestingly, although L5 and HK97 both employ similar wholesale covalent cross-linking strategies, there is no amino acid sequence similarity between their major head subunit proteins. There are some other notable differences in that unlike HK97, the L5 major head subunit is not proteolytically processed and the L5 head assembly utilizes an additional protein, gp16, that is present in purified head-like particles but is absent from intact virions.

N-terminal sequence analysis of individual virion proteins demonstrates that these genes are encoded in the L5 left arm. Four of the tail genes (genes 23, 26, 27, and 28) are located in a cluster to the right of the head genes (genes 16 and 17), and one tail gene (gene 6) is in a separate location to the left of the tRNA genes. It is likely that

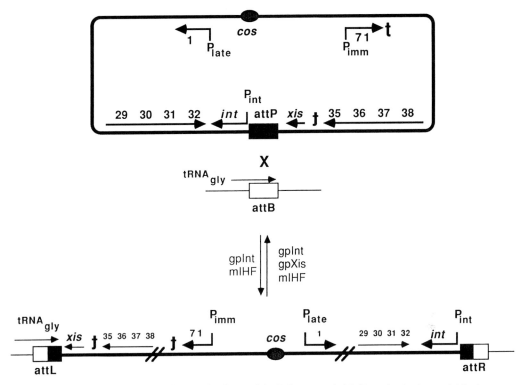

Figure 5. Integration of phage L5. The circular form of the L5 genome (with ligated cohesive ends) is shown at the top. Some notable features, such as the positions of sites *cos* and *attP*, the putative promoters ^{P}late, ^{P}imm, and ^{P}int (located upstream of genes 1, 71, and 33, respectively), and the genes 29 to 32, 35 to 38, *int*, and *xis*, are indicated. The directions of transcription of the genes are indicated by arrows. At the bottom is shown a segment of the mycobacterial chromosome representing the *attB* site that overlaps the 3′ end of the tRNA^{Gly} gene. Integration of the L5 genome involves a site-specific recombination event between the *attP* and *attB* sites, which share a 43-bp sequence, that is catalyzed by integrase (gpInt) and a mycobacterial integration host factor (mIHF); excision requires excisionase (gpXis) in addition to these two proteins. We propose that in the integrated prophage state, a small amount of gpInt is constantly synthesized by the autoregulated promoter ^{P}int and that excision is prevented by tight regulation of gpXis expression. Although a terminator between genes 68 and 69 (Fig. 1) may stop most transcripts from ^{P}imm getting through to *xis*, a second terminator downstream of gene 35 may further prevent *xis* expression, thus ensuring the integrated state.

many of the other L5 left-arm genes encode proteins that are involved in virion structure and assembly but either are absent from intact virions or are present in such low abundance that they are not seen by SDS-gel electrophoresis.

Site-Specific Integration of L5

L5 lysogens of *M. smegmatis* contain a copy of the L5 prophage integrated site specifically into the bacterial chromosome

(Snapper et al., 1988; Lee et al., 1991). The general mechanism of this integration is closely related to that described for other temperate phages, in which the phage-encoded integrase enzyme catalyzes a conservative site-specific recombination event between attachment sites on the phage (*attP*) and bacterial (*attB*) genomes (Fig. 5). Assuming that recombination involves a circular phage genome (as a result of ligation of the cohesive genome termini), the result is the insertion of the L5 prophage flanked by attachment junction sites *attL* and *attR* (Fig. 5).

Analysis of the DNA sequences of the attachment sites shows a region of 43 bp that is identical between *attP* and the *M. smegmatis attB* sites; recombination must occur within this common "core" region (Hatfull and Sarkis, 1993). The 43-bp core that defines *attB* actually overlaps the 3' end of a bacterial tRNA^{Gly} gene, one of two divergently transcribed genes in this region (Lee et al., 1991); one consequence of this relationship is that the tRNA^{Gly} gene is "reconstructed" following L5 integration. It is not known whether the tRNA gene is the only one in *M. smegmatis* that encodes tRNA^{Gly}, although it does appear to be well conserved among mycobacterial species (Lee et al., 1991). This conservation raises the possibility that L5 may be able to integrate into the chromosomes of a broad range of mycobacterial species. However, the only other *attB* region that has been characterized is that of BCG, which does contain both tRNA genes and the *attB* core, although there is a 1-base difference between it and the *M. smegmatis attB* site (Hatfull and Sarkis, 1993). This single base change corresponds to a position in the variable loop of the tRNA structure and does not appear to influence integration.

The L5 integrase (gp33) is a member of the large family of integrase-related proteins and contains the three absolutely conserved amino acid residues that contribute to the active site (Lee and Hatfull, 1993). However, it is only a distant relative of the other members of the family, with the closest relative being the integrase from the *Staphylococcus* phage L54a (Lee et al., 1991). The L5 integrase has been overexpressed and purified from *E. coli* and shown to catalyze integrative recombination in vitro, although there is strong dependence on a stimulatory activity encoded by *M. smegmatis*.

Integration-proficient plasmid vectors that contain a segment of L5 DNA containing the *attP* site and the integrase gene have been constructed (Lee et al., 1991; Stover et al., 1991). Such vectors also carry an antibiotic resistance gene (*aph*) for selection of transformants but do not have mycobacterium-specific replication sequences. These vectors transform both *M. smegmatis* and BCG at a remarkably high efficiency, producing recombinant strains in which the plasmid DNA is inserted at the bacterial *attB* site. Moreover, provided that the phage genes to the right of *attP* are not included in the vector, the integrated sequences are stably inherited even in the absence of antibiotic selection. The simple interpretation of this observation is that the phage excisionase gene, a required component of prophage excision, lies adjacent to and to the right of *attP* (perhaps the product of gene 34). Curiously, although inclusion of this segment does not influence the transformation frequency of *M. smegmatis*, it greatly reduces the frequency of transformation of BCG (Lee et al., 1991), an observation that mirrors that observed with L1-derived phasmids (Snapper and Jacobs, unpublished result). The transformants that do appear at low frequency contain plasmids integrated at *attB* but have extensive deletions of the vector DNAs. A plausible explanation is that the excisionase gene is poorly regulated in BCG such that the integrated plasmids are substrates for efficient and immediate excision. Nevertheless, integration-proficient vectors containing just *attP* and the *int* gene (a region of about 1.3 kb) have the desirable features of high transformation frequency in both *M. smegmatis* and BCG and generation of recombinants that are genetically stable. Such traits are desirable for a variety of purposes, including the construction of recombinant BCG vaccine strains (Stover et al., 1991).

Little is known about how the overall processes of L5 integration and excision are regulated. However, the simple order of the genes, *int-attP-xis*, raises some important questions (Fig. 5). For example, since gpInt is needed for prophage excision, how is it synthesized at the appropriate time? Since *attP* separates *int* from the "upstream" (i.e., right-arm) DNA, late phage promoters in the right arm cannot serve this function (Fig. 5). Furthermore, the tRNA^{Gly} gene at *attB* is expressed in the wrong direction to account for synthesis of gpInt (Fig. 3). We therefore favor an alternative explanation that a promoter for *int* expression is located between the *attP* core and the coding region, a hypothesis that is supported by preliminary observations (Hatfull, unpublished results) using an in vitro transcription system (Fig. 5). Moreover, the arrangement is such that gpInt could regulate its own synthesis by acting as a transcriptional repressor when bound at the attachment sites. If this scenario is correct, then maintenance of the integrated state must be tightly controlled by availability of excisionase, since gpInt will always be bound at the recombination sites. This possibility is supported by the observation that a putative strong transcription terminator (a 17-bp stem-loop followed by UUUUUUU) is located between genes 34 and 35; this terminator could serve to protect excisionase expression from transcripts originating upstream in the right arm, such as from the gene 71 repressor (see below and Fig. 3). Synthesis of the excisionase gene during prophage induction could be achieved by use of an antitermination apparatus similar to that of the N-mediated system in phage lambda (Hendrix et al., 1983). These hypotheses can be readily tested, and the model can be evaluated.

Regulation of Lysogeny

Several lines of evidence suggest that gene 71 encodes a repressor-like protein that is a key regulator of the lytic and lysogenic life cycles (Donnelly-Wu et al., 1993). For example, recombinant plasmids containing gene 71 are competent to confer superinfection immunity to L5 and also to its relative D29. The majority of clear-plaque mutants of L5 (i.e., that are not able to form lysogens) result from mutations with gene 71, including those that confer a temperature-sensitive clear-plaque phenotype. These latter mutants are also thermoinducible, such that lysogens formed at the permissive temperature (30°C) immediately enter lytic growth when shifted to the nonpermissive temperature (42°C); gp71 is thus required for maintenance of the lysogenic state. Since gp71 contains a helix-turn-helix DNA-binding structural motif, it seems probable that it acts similarly to other phage repressors by binding to operator sites and repressing promoters needed for lytic growth. However, the DNA-binding properties of gp71 and the location of putative operator sites have yet to be described.

Two clear-plaque mutants that behave as though they are defective in the establishment of lysogeny have been isolated (Donnelly-Wu et al., 1993); the plaques appear much less turbid than those of wild-type L5, but stable lysogens can be recovered from infected cells. Although the genes affected by the mutations are not known, we have recently observed that deletion of a region containing the genes 73 to 83 results in a similar phenotype, indicating that one or more of these genes influences the frequency with which lysogeny occurs (Hatfull, unpublished result) (Fig. 1). If gene 71 is a functional analog of *c*I in λ, then one of these L5 genes may act similarly to either *c*II or *c*III of lambda.

Characterization of the phage immunity genes not only offers insights into the regulation of L5 gene expression but also provides tools for mycobacterial genetic manipulation. For example, since plasmids expressing L5 gene 71 are immune to superinfection, they can be directly selected for by using a clear-plaque mutant of L5 or D29; these phages efficiently kill mycobacteria if gene 71 is absent. Such a scheme provides not only an additional selectable marker but also one that does not require the use of antibiotic selection (Donnelly-Wu et al., 1993). This should be useful for the construction of recombinant BCG strains in which the incorporation of antibiotic resistance genes in live vaccines is undesirable or for the manipulation of mycobacterial strains that are naturally antibiotic resistant.

L5 Gene Expression

Unfortunately, the locations of transcriptional promoters that are active in lytic growth of L5 have yet to be identified. However, the patterns of protein synthesis in lytic growth were observed by [^{35}S]methionine labeling following a temperature shift of a thermoinducible lysogen (Hatfull and Sarkis, 1993). Two important phenomena were seen. First, within 5 to 10 min after the induction, a change in the pattern of protein synthesis was observed. This change involved the appearance of some novel, presumably phage-encoded early lytic proteins and an apparent reduction in the background of host synthesis. A simple interpretation is that L5 encodes early lytic functions that inhibition the expression of bacterial genes while permitting expression of phage genes. Second, approximately 20 to 25 min after the induction, a second transition was seen in which synthesis of the early proteins was reduced and a novel set of late lytic proteins were made. The pattern remained unaltered until cell lysis about 2 to 3 h after induction.

Little is known about the correlation between the proteins observed by radiolabeling and the L5 genetic map. Since nonsense suppressor strains of mycobacteria have yet to be isolated or constructed, a collection of amber mutants that would simplify this correlation does not yet exist. However, some limited information is available. The most highly labeled late protein is about 35 kDa and is probably the primary gene product of gene 17, which encodes the major head subunit. This is supported by the observation in a pulse-chase experiment that the 35-kDa product is converted into higher-molecular-weight (presumably cross-linked) forms (Hatfull, unpublished results). It seems likely that other structural and assembly left-arm genes are also made in late lytic growth. By extrapolation, we suggest that the right-arm genes are expressed in the early phase of lytic growth (Fig. 3).

L5 uses the host RNA polymerase for transcription of both early and late genes. Evidence for this comes from the observation that rifampin inhibits synthesis of both early and late phage proteins coupled with the fact that there are no open reading frames that are large enough to encode an RNA polymerase like that of bacteria. If the shutdown of host gene expression includes the inhibition of host transcription, the phage may modify the host RNA polymerase or substitute alternative phage-encoded sigma factors in order to redirect it toward phage promoters. However, L5 genes that encode transcription factors (such as sigma-like proteins) have yet to be identified.

Essential and Nonessential Regions of the L5 Genome

The description of L1 shuttle phasmids was the first indication that there may be small regions of L5 (and L1) that could be manipulated or removed (Snapper et al., 1988). We now know that the insertion of the plasmid moiety in these phasmids was in a region close to the right end of the genome (Hatfull, unpublished results). More recently, we have isolated two deletion mutants that have lost part of the region to the right of gene 71 (Hatfull, unpublished results) (Fig. 3). Although we do not know the precise end points of the deleted regions, one removes genes 72 to 88 (a deletion of about 4.5 kb), while the other removes genes 83 to 88 (about 2.5 kb is lost). Both of the mutants form normal-sized plaques, but the one with the larger deletion produces lysogens only at low frequency (see above). A region of up to about 2.5 kb can also be removed from the gene 71 region, although these have a clear-plaque phenotype and cannot form lysogens. Last, a segment including the *attP* and integrase genes can apparently be removed, although integration is presumably abolished.

The isolation and characterization of temperature-sensitive mutants of L1 (Chaudhuri et al., 1993) and L5 (Hatfull, unpublished result) show that L5 encodes functions necessary for DNA replication and bacterial lysis, although these latter functions could arise from any mutations that block entry into late lytic gene expression. However, the mutations appear to map to numerous parts of the genome, suggesting that most of the L5 genes are essential for viral growth.

LUCIFERASE REPORTER PHAGES

Clinical Need for Rapid Tests of Drug Susceptibility to *M. tuberculosis* Infections

The use of bacteriophages as genetic toolboxes for bacterial systems should be generally applicable to all or most bacterial species. However, the special role of bacteriophages in analysis of slow-growing bacteria such as *M. tuberculosis* is nicely illustrated by the development of luciferase reporter mycobacteriophages, a system that has the potential to greatly decrease the time currently required for clinical determination of diagnosis and drug susceptibilities of tuberculosis.

To appreciate the potential role of luciferase reporter phages, we will briefly revisit some of the clinical problems associated with the extremely slow growth of *M. tuberculosis*. After collection of a clinical sample suspected of containing *M. tu-*

berculosis (e.g., sputum), a portion of the sample is incubated in growth medium to amplify the bacteria for identification and characterization; if solid media are used, it usually takes about 3 to 4 weeks to obtain bacterial colonies that are large enough for further analysis, and at this point, it is possible to determine whether the organism is present. To determine drug susceptibilities, the bacteria must then be incubated in the presence of various antibiotics, and the effects of these antibiotics on growth must be determined; this requires at least another 2 to 4 weeks. In practical terms, it frequently takes more than 12 weeks to determine *M. tuberculosis* drug susceptibilities and report the results (Centers for Disease Control, 1992). Unfortunately, by this time, the initial tuberculosis infection may well have acquired new or different drug susceptibilities, especially in the face of inadequate treatment or poor compliance. However, the need for determining drug susceptibilities has become critical with the emergence of drug-resistant and multidrug-resistant strains of *M. tuberculosis*.

The introduction of the BACTEC system for clinical analysis of *M. tuberculosis* has considerably shortened the time needed for drug susceptibility determination. The system operates by measurement of metabolic products (usually $^{14}CO_2$) released from growing bacteria under conditions that favor growth of *M. tuberculosis*. It is possible to determine *M. tuberculosis* drug susceptibilities in less than 2 weeks with BACTEC (Heifets, 1991), but its widespread use is restricted by its cost and the generation of radioactive wastes.

Luciferase Reporter Phage Idea

Luciferase reporter mycobacteriophages (Fig. 6) have the potential of greatly reducing the time needed for *M. tuberculosis* analysis in a simple and relatively inexpensive assay. The basis of this assay is

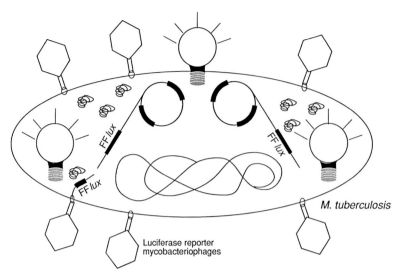

Figure 6. Luciferase reporter phage idea. The idea is to introduce into a mycobacteriophage the luciferase gene from fireflies (FF *lux*) that has been fused to a mycobacterial promoter as a reporter gene. The phage will find mycobacterial cells and inject their DNAs, and the injected luciferase gene will be expressed. Upon addition of the luciferin substrate, the bacteria will glow. Thus, the test has tremendous sensitivity based on the luciferase reaction that yields light and exquisite specificity based on the host specificity of the mycobacteriophage.

the construction of recombinant bacteriophages that carry a so-called "reporter gene," whose activity can be easily monitored (Ulitzer and Kuhn, 1987). Genes encoding a luciferase enzyme, such as that from the firefly, *Pnotinus pyralis*, are ideal reporters, since the activity of the gene product can be easily monitored by addition of a substrate (luciferin) and measurement of emitted light in the presence of ATP. The availability of sensitive light detection systems makes possible the detection of small amounts of luciferase enzyme and consequently small numbers of bacterial cells. It is this potential for assaying small numbers of cells that is at the basis of the phage assay, since it eliminates the need for extensive bacterial growth; moreover, light-producing organisms are rarely found in clinical specimens, and the phage particle contains only the luciferase gene and not the enzyme and thus gives no light in the absence of the host. Therefore, the specificity of the phage-host interaction and the sensitivity of luciferase detection

should provide a powerful combination for detection of *M. tuberculosis* in clinical samples.

The production of light following reporter phage infection of *M. tuberculosis* requires a live bacterial cell, since the enzyme requires ATP to emit photons. More specifically, the cell must be competent to synthesize and translate the mRNA to produce enzyme and be able to produce the ATP that is required for luciferase action. It is thus a good assay for discriminating between drug-resistant and drug-susceptible cells, since a resistant organism is expected to produce light in the presence of antibiotic, whereas a susceptible organism is not. We call such an assay the "turn on the light assay" (Fig. 7), as it provides a relatively simple test for the effects of drugs on *M. tuberculosis* strains.

Choice of Mycobacteriophages

There are several important considerations in choosing phages for constructing

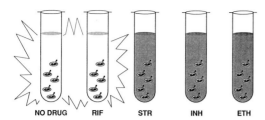

NO DRUG   RIF   STR   INH   ETH

Figure 7. "Turn on the light assay." This assay is based on the observation that luciferase reporter phages will make *M. tuberculosis* cells glow. Light production requires that the phage DNA be injected and replicated and that the luciferase gene be expressed and have sufficient ATP present within the cell. Anything that interferes with any of these steps, such as contact with drugs, will prohibit light production. Drug screening can be performed by dividing the *M. tuberculosis* cells into aliquots and incubating each aliquot with a different drug. If the strain is drug susceptible, the cell will become sick and no light will be produced. However, if the strain is drug resistant, the *M. tuberculosis* cells will be unaffected and light will be produced. Thus, in this figure, the strain is resistant to rifampin (RIF) but susceptible to isoniazid (INH), streptomycin (STR), and ethambutol (ETH).

luciferase recombinants. First, a suitable host range must be employed, since it is desirable to obtain signals from a restricted subset of bacteria that may be present in a clinical specimen. Second, the life cycles available to the phage may be important, since lytic and temperate phages may behave differently. Third, the possibility of constructing recombinant phages must be considered, and this is influenced by the size of the phage genome and the identification of suitable locations at which additional DNA can be inserted and nonessential regions can be removed. Construction should be simplified if DNA sequence information is available.

Demonstration of Feasibility

The first luciferase reporter phage to be constructed was based on phage TM4, which infects both fast- and slow-growing mycobacterial species. The firefly luciferase gene was inserted into the TM4 genome by using the shuttle phasmid strat-

egy described above to produce the recombinant phage phAE40 (Jacobs et al., 1993). Characterization of this phage demonstrated that the reporter phage system behaves entirely as anticipated. Infection of *M. tuberculosis* or BCG results in the production of light that can be easily monitored and used to discriminate between drug-resistant and drug-susceptible strains of *M. tuberculosis*, at least for the antibiotics isoniazid, rifampin, and streptomycin (Jacobs et al., 1993). It also became apparent from the characterization of this phage that mycobacteria can take up the luciferin substrate from solution, thus greatly simplifying the assay, since no lysis procedure is required. This observation is significant, since lysis of mycobacteria can be not only problematic and irreproducible but also undesirable with pathogenic organisms.

The principal limitations to the use of phAE40 are its relatively broad host specificity and poor sensitivity compared to those of plasmids expressing luciferase. Its low sensitivity may derive from poor expression of the luciferase gene, although the lack of any detailed characterization of TM4 makes this difficult to assess. Thus, while phAE40 can be used to analyze *M. tuberculosis* grown in the laboratory, it is not yet optimal for direct analysis of clinical samples. Presumably, the sensitivity could be improved by increasing the efficiency of transcription and translation of the gene during phage infection.

TM4 is a lytic bacteriophage that does not form stable lysogens. Consequently, infection of the bacteria results in light production that peaks after about 2 to 3 h and then diminishes to background levels as the cells lyse. Preliminary observations with luciferase recombinants derived from phage L5 show that temperate phages may improve the sensitivity of the system by extending the time for light output. Temperate luciferase phages that efficiently infect the slow-growing mycobacteria such as

M. tuberculosis have not yet been described.

A Rapid Method for Identifying New Antituberculosis Drugs

Luciferase reporter mycobacteriophages have an important utility beyond the analysis of clinical isolates. Since they can provide a rapid readout of the viability of the cell, they can be used to rapidly screen for new antimycobacterial drugs (Jacobs et al., 1993). The attractions in using luciferase reporter phages for drug screening are many. First, they can provide a readout of results in as little as 2 h. Second, they can be easily adapted to an automated system that uses microtiter plates. In this manner, it becomes possible to screen large numbers of compounds at several concentrations in a non-labor-intensive manner that can be readily automated. The finding of even a single new antituberculosis drug could have an important impact on the control of tuberculosis, and we believe that the search for such a drug warrants efforts to develop luciferase reporter antibiotic screening systems for *M. tuberculosis.*

REFERENCES

Baess, I. 1969. Subdivision of *M. tuberculosis* by means of bacteriophages. *Acta Pathol. Microbiol. Scand.* **76:**464–474.

Baess, I. 1971. Report on pseudolysogenic *Mycobacterium* and a review of the literature concerning pseudolysogeny. *Acta Pathol. Microbiol. Scand.* **79:**428–434.

Barksdale, L., and K.-S. Kim. 1977. *Mycobacterium. Bacteriol. Rev.* **41:**217–372.

Barletta, R. G., D. D. Kim, S. B. Snapper, B. R. Bloom, and W. R. Jacobs, Jr. 1991. Identification of expression signals of the mycobacteriophages Bxb1, L1, and TM4 using the *Escherichia-Mycobacterium* shuttle plasmids pYUB75 and pYUB76 designed to create translational fusions to the *lacZ* gene. *J. Gen. Microbiol.* **138:**23–30.

Casjens, S., G. F. Hatfull, and R. W. Hendrix. 1992. Evolution of dsDNA tailed-bacteriophage genomes. *Semin. Virol.* **3:**383–397.

Centers for Disease Control. 1992. *Morbid. Mortal. Weekly Rep.* **41:**507.

Chaudhuri, B. S., S. Sau, H. J. Datta, and N. C. Mandel. 1993. Isolation, characterization, and mapping of temperature sensitive mutations in the genes essential for lysogenic or lytic growth of mycobacteriophage L1. *Virology* **194:**166–172.

David, H., F. Clement, S. Clavel-Seres, and N. Rastogi. 1984. Abortive infection of *Mycobacterium leprae* by the mycobacteriophage D29. *Int. J. Lepr.* **52:**515–523.

Doke, S. 1960. Studies on mycobacteriophages and lysogenic mycobacteria. *J. Kunamoto Med. Soc.* **34:**1360–1373.

Donnelly-Wu, M. K., W. R. Jacobs, Jr., and G. F. Hatfull. 1993. Superinfection immunity of mycobacteriophage L5: applications for genetic transformation of mycobacteria. *Mol. Microbiol.* **7:**407–417.

Gardner, G. M., and R. S. Weiser. 1947. A bacteriophage for *Mycobacterium smegmatis. Proc. Soc. Exp. Biol. Med.* **66:**205–206.

Hatfull, G. F. Unpublished results.

Hatfull, G. F., and G. J. Sarkis. 1993. DNA sequence, structure, and gene expression of mycobacteriophage L5: a phage system for mycobacterial genetics. *Mol. Microbiol.* **7:**407–417.

Heifets, L. 1991. Drug susceptibility test in the management of chemotherapy of tuberculosis, p. 89–122. *In* L. Heifets (ed.), *Drug Susceptibility in the Chemotherapy of Mycobacterial Infections.* CRC Press, Inc., Boca Raton, Fla.

Hendrix, R. W., J. W. Roberts, F. W. Stahl, and R. A. Weisberg. 1983. *Lambda II.* Cold Spring Harbor Press, Cold Spring Harbor, N.Y.

Jacobs, W. R., Jr. Unpublished results.

Jacobs, W. R., Jr., R. Barletta, R. Udani, J. Chan, G. Kalkut, G. Sarkis, G. F. Hatfull, and B. R. Bloom. 1993. Rapid assessment of drug susceptibilities of *Mycobacterium tuberculosis* by means of luciferase reporter phages. *Science* **260:**819–822.

Jacobs, W. R., J. F. Barrett, J. E. Clark-Curtiss, and R. Curtiss III. 1986a. In vivo repackaging of recombinant cosmid molecules for analysis of *Salmonella typhimurium, Streptococcus mutans,* and mycobacterial genomic libraries. *Infect. Immun.* **52:**101–109.

Jacobs, W. R., M. A. Docherty, R. Curtiss III, and J. E. Clark-Curtiss. 1986b. Expression of *Mycobacterium leprae* genes from a *Streptococcus mutans* promoter in *Escherichia coli* K-12. *Proc. Natl. Acad. Sci. USA* **83:**1926–1930.

Jacobs, W. R., Jr., S. B. Snapper, M. Tuckman, and B. R. Bloom. 1989. Mycobacteriophage vector systems. *Rev. Infect. Dis.* **11**(Suppl. 2):404–410.

Jacobs, W. R., Jr., M. Tuckman, and B. R. Bloom. 1987. Introduction of foreign DNA into mycobacteria using a shuttle phasmid. *Nature* (London) **327:**532–536.

Laibidi, A., C. Dauguet, K. S. Goh, and H. L. David. 1984. Plasmid profiles of *Mycobacterium fortuitum* complex isolates. *Curr. Microbiol.* **11:**235–240.

Lee, M. H., and G. F. Hatfull. 1993. Mycobacteriophage L5 integrase-mediated site-specific integration in vitro. *J. Bacteriol.* **175:**6835–6841.

Lee, M. H., L. Pascopella, W. R. Jacobs, Jr., and G. F. Hatfull. 1991. Site-specific integration of mycobacteriophage L5: integration-proficient vectors for *Mycobacterium smegmatis*, BCG, and *M. tuberculosis*. *Proc. Natl. Acad. Sci. USA* **88:**3111–3115.

McAdam, R., and W. R. Jacobs, Jr. Unpublished result.

Mizuguchi, Y. 1984. Mycobacteriophages, p. 641–662. *In* G. P. Kubica and L. G. Wayne (ed.), *The Mycobacteria: a Sourcebook*, part A. Marcel Dekker, Inc., New York.

Oyaski, M., and G. F. Hatfull. 1992. Characterization of the cohesive ends of mycobacteriophage L5 DNA. *Nucleic Acids Res.* **20:**3251.

Popa, M. P., T. A. McKelvey, J. Hempel, and R. W. Hendrix. 1991. Bacteriophage HK97 structure: wholesale covalent cross-linking between the major head shell subunits. *J. Virol.* **65:**3227–3237.

Reddy, A. B., and K. P. Gopinathan. 1986. Presence of random single-stranded gaps in mycobacteriophage I3 DNA. *Gene* **44:**227–234.

Redmond, W. B. 1963. Bacteriophages of mycobacteria: a review. *Adv. Tuberc. Rev.* **12:**191–229.

Redmond, W. B., and J. C. Cater. 1960. A bacteriophage specific to *Mycobacterium tuberculosis* varieties *hominis* and *bovis*. *Am. Rev. Respir. Dis.* **82:**781–786.

Saroja, D., and K. P. Gopinathan. 1973. Transduction of isoniazid susceptibility-resistance and streptomycin resistance in mycobacteria. *Antimicrob. Agents Chemother.* **4:**643–645.

Snapper, S. B., and W. R. Jacobs, Jr. Unpublished result.

Snapper, S. B., L. Lugosi, A. Jekkel, R. Melton, T. Kieser, B. R. Bloom, and W. R. Jacobs, Jr. 1988. Lysogeny and transformation of mycobacteria: stable expression of foreign genes. *Proc. Natl. Acad. Sci. USA* **85:**6987–6991.

Snapper, S. B., R. E. Melton, S. Mustafa, T. Kieser, and W. R. Jacobs, Jr. 1990. Isolation and characterization of efficient plasmid transformation mutants of *Mycobacterium smegmatis*. *Mol. Microbiol.* **4:**1911–1919.

Snider, D. E., W. D. Jones, Jr., and R. C. Good. 1984. The usefulness of phage typing *Mycobacterium tuberculosis* isolates. *Am. Rev. Respir. Dis.* **130:**1095–1099.

Stover, C. K., V. F. de la Cruz, T. R. Fuerst, J. E. Burlein, L. A. Benson, L. T. Bennett, G. P. Bansal, J. F. Young, M. H. Lee, G. F. Hatfull, S. B. Snapper, R. G. Barletta, W. R. Jacobs, Jr., and B. R. Bloom. 1991. New use of BCG for recombinant vaccines. *Nature* (London) **351:**456–460.

Sundaraj, C. V., and T. Ramakrishnan. 1971. Transduction in *Mycobacterium smegmatis*. *Nature* (London) **228:**280–281.

Timme, T. L., and P. J. Brennan. 1984. Induction of bacteriophage from members of the *Mycobacterium avium*, *Mycobacterium intracellulare*, *Mycobacterium scrofulaceum* serocomplex. *J. Gen. Microbiol.* **130:**2059–2066.

Tokunaga, T., Y. Maruyama, and T. Murohashi. 1968. Classification of subtypes of human tubercle bacilli by phage susceptibility. *Am. Rev. Respir. Dis.* **97:**469–471.

Tokunaga, T., and M. I. Sellers. 1964. Infection of *Mycobacterium smegmatis* and D29 phage DNA. *J. Exp. Med.* **119:**139–149.

Tuckman, M., and W. R. Jacobs, Jr. Unpublished result.

Ulitzer, S., and J. Kuhn. 1987. Introduction of *lux* genes into bacteria: a new approach for specific determinants of bacteria and their antibiotic susceptibilities, p. 463–472. *In* J. Sclomerick, R. R. Andersen, A. Kapp, M. Ernst, and W. G. Woods (ed.), *Bioluminescence and Chemiluminescence: New Perspectives*. John Wiley & Sons, Inc., New York.

Tuberculosis: Pathogenesis, Protection, and Control
Edited by Barry R. Bloom
© 1994 American Society for Microbiology, Washington, DC 20005

Chapter 13

Plasmids

Joseph O. Falkinham III and Jack T. Crawford

In spite of the fact that representatives of the species *Mycobacterium* are among the oldest known microorganisms, until recently there had been very few studies of their genetics. Information concerning the distribution and characteristics of plasmids of mycobacteria has been accumulating since the first description of the plasmids in 1979 (Crawford and Bates, 1979). Much of the research on mycobacterial plasmids has been directed at the *Mycobacterium avium* complex (*M. avium* and *M. intracellulare*), *M. scrofulaceum*, and the *M. fortuitum* complex. Plasmids are common in strains of these species, with many strains carrying multiple plasmids. The functions of many plasmids are unknown; i.e., the plasmids are cryptic.

Plasmids frequently carry genes that confer a selective advantage on the organism. For example, in environmental microorganisms, plasmid-encoded functions include resistance to heavy-metal ions or other toxic compounds and the ability to utilize uncommon carbon sources. In pathogenic microorganisms, plasmids carry genes (frequently located in transposons) conferring

resistance to a number of antibiotics and genes encoding a number of virulence factors such as toxins, hemolysins, and proteases. In addition, plasmids are frequently self-transmissible and promote genetic exchange among strains of the same or related species. The species of mycobacteria in which plasmids have been demonstrated are not only common environmental organisms but also important opportunistic pathogens. Thus, studies of naturally occurring mycobacterial plasmids are important because of the possibility that they encode virulence factors, drug resistance, or other significant features.

Plasmids are also important because of the central role they play in recombinant DNA technology. Because plasmids replicate independently from the bacterial chromosome, plasmid origins can be combined with genes encoding selectable phenotypes (usually drug resistance) to create vectors for molecular cloning. The potential for using mycobacterial plasmids as vectors in mycobacteria was recognized early on (Crawford and Bates, 1984), but research efforts were thwarted by the lack of a simple method for introducing plasmids into mycobacteria. The development of electroporation, its application to mycobacteria, the identification of selectable markers expressed in mycobacteria (Snapper et al., 1988), and the isolation of high-fre-

Joseph O. Falkinham III • Department of Biology, Virginia Polytechnic Institute and State University, Blacksburg, Virginia 24061.   *Jack T. Crawford* • Division of Bacterial and Mycotic Diseases, National Center for Infectious Diseases, Centers for Disease Control and Prevention, Atlanta, Georgia 30333.

quency transformation mutants (Snapper et al., 1990) have led to an explosion of research utilizing plasmid vectors. Much of this work has used the *M. fortuitum* plasmid pAL5000 (Labidi et al., 1984).

In this chapter we will review what is known concerning plasmids of the genus *Mycobacterium*. This review includes methods for plasmid isolation, analysis of plasmid distribution, and identification of plasmid-encoded genes. We will also discuss the background for use of mycobacterial plasmids as vectors.

METHODS FOR ISOLATION OF PLASMIDS FROM MYCOBACTERIA

General Principles

There are several obstacles to isolation and characterization of mycobacterial plasmids. The first is the slow growth rate of most mycobacteria. Second, all mycobacterial cells are difficult to lyse, making efficient isolation of intact circular plasmid DNA difficult. Third, mycobacterial cell walls contain complex lipids and polysaccharides that can contaminate DNA preparations, rendering them unsuitable for molecular biologic techniques.

Growth of Strains for Plasmid Isolation

Because plasmid DNA is lost during steps required for removal of chromosomal DNA and other contaminants, a large cell mass is required for high yields of plasmid DNA. Mycobacterial cells are most susceptible to lysis during logarithmic growth phase, and stationary-phase cells contain higher levels of polymers that can interfere with DNA isolation. Thus, for plasmid DNA isolation, it is best to grow large volumes of cells to mid- to late logarithmic phase. Because of the relative oxygen sensitivity of many slowly growing mycobacterial species, it is best to stage cultures, using as inoculum 1/10 the culture volume. Inoculation with less than 1/10 the volume

of the culture usually results in an abnormally long lag period.

Successful isolation of intact plasmid DNA requires gentle lysis of cells, which precludes the use of mechanical methods employed to release fragmented chromosomal DNA. Enzymatic digestion and detergent lysis are generally used, but mycobacteria are fairly resistant to such treatments. One of the best methods to facilitate lysis is to grow cells in the presence of inhibitors of cell wall synthesis such as D-cycloserine or glycine (Mizuguchi and Tokunaga, 1970). Cycloserine at a concentration of 1 mg/ml is most effective. Ampicillin is also effective for *M. avium* complex strains that do not produce significant amounts of β-lactamase. Active growth of the cells is required for effectiveness. The length of cycloserine treatment is determined by the growth rate. For *M. smegmatis*, 2 to 3 h is sufficient, whereas slow-growing mycobacteria require 18 h or longer. Addition of fresh medium to late-log-phase cultures enhances the effect (Meissner and Falkinham, 1986). Once the cells are weakened, they are susceptible to lysis with sodium dodecyl sulfate (SDS) or other detergents.

Though there are distinct advantages to studies of rapidly growing mycobacteria, e.g., *M. fortuitum* and *M. chelonae*, these organisms are still difficult to lyse. Consequently, methods have been employed to reduce the barrier to lysis before plasmid DNA isolation. Wall-deficient cells were prepared as described by Rastogi and David (1981) as a preliminary step before lysis and plasmid DNA isolation (Labidi et al., 1984). Wall-deficient cells were lysed by using 4% SDS and incubation at 65°C for 20 min.

Large-Scale Isolation of Plasmid DNA

Plasmids were first demonstrated in *M. avium* complex strains by using the salt-cleared-lysate method, which takes advantage of the observation that the bacterial chromosome is found in a large, dense, easily pelleted aggregate in the presence of high salt, while plasmid DNA is not aggregated and is found in solution (Crawford and Bates, 1979). Cycloserine-treated cells are lysed with SDS, and then salt precipitation of the chromosomal DNA is done. Crude plasmid DNA can be obtained from these lysates by precipitation with polyethylene glycol (Humphreys et al., 1975). Highly purified plasmid DNA is prepared from these crude lysates by cesium chloride-ethidium bromide density gradient centrifugation. The covalently closed circular plasmid DNA molecules bind less ethidium bromide than the linear chromosomal DNA fragments and separate into a band of greater density that is detected by illumination with UV light. If care is taken to minimize shearing, this method allows isolation of even very large plasmids. Unfortunately, considerable plasmid DNA is lost in the salt-cleared-lysate step, and large volumes of culture are required for this approach.

As an alternative to the cleared-lysis technique, Meissner and Falkinham (1986) modified the Kado and Liu (1981) alkaline lysis procedure for isolation of plasmid DNA from *M. avium*, *M. intracellulare*, and *M. scrofulaceum*. Further modifications (Jucker and Falkinham, 1990) were required to provide plasmid DNA suitable as a substrate for restriction endonucleases. In this method, cells are treated with alkaline-SDS and elevated temperature, which provides efficient lysis of mycobacteria. Chromosomal DNA is fragmented, denatured, and removed by phenol extraction. Cells are grown to late exponential phase (10 to 14 days at 37°C); oleic acid-albumin-dextrose complex enrichment, D-cycloserine, and ampicillin are added to final concentrations of 5%, 1 mg/ml, and 100 μg/ml, respectively; and incubation is continued for 3 days at 37°C. Cells from two 250-ml cultures are harvested by

centrifugation and suspended in 12 ml of E buffer (40 mM Tris-acetate [pH 7.9], 2 mM Na$_2$EDTA) in a 250-ml phenol-resistant centrifuge bottle. Cell clumps are dispersed completely, 24 ml of lysing solution (50 mM Tris [pH 12.3], 3% SDS) is added, and the suspension is gently mixed by rolling the bottle across the tabletop. Heating the viscous lysate to 60°C for 20 min and then cooling it to room temperature for 10 min reduce the amount of contaminating chromosomal DNA and increase the extent of lysis. Next, 40 ml of phenol equilibrated with 50 mM NaCl is added, and extraction is performed by gently rotating the bottle on a roller drum at 5 rpm for 10 min. Best results are obtained when extraction is carried out in bottles with volumes at least three times the total liquid volume. The mixture is centrifuged, and the upper phase is removed with a wide-bore pipette. At this point, an agarose gel can be run to determine whether any plasmid DNA is present. The sample is extracted again with an equal volume of phenol-chloroform-isoamyl alcohol. If the aqueous phase contains an appreciable amount of phenol, the sample is extracted with an equal volume of water-saturated ether (Maniatis et al., 1982). Contaminants can be removed by ammonium acetate precipitation (Maniatis et al., 1982). One-half volume of cold 7.5 M ammonium acetate is added, and the sample is mixed without strong agitation and incubated on ice for 30 min. The precipitate is eliminated by centrifugation at $10,000 \times g$ for 30 min at 4°C. Plasmid DNA is precipitated with 2 volumes of 95% ethanol (-20°C). The DNA is dissolved in Tris-EDTA (TE) buffer in a volume no smaller than one-half the volume of the initial lysate. The DNA is precipitated again with ethanol and dissolved in a small volume of TE.

Rapid Screening Methods

Rapid determination of the plasmid content of a large number of strains requires a simple small-scale screening method. Because of the difficulty in lysing mycobacteria, many of the rapid procedures applied to *Escherichia coli* do not work well with mycobacteria. The alkaline extraction procedure of Birnboim and Doly (1979) has been used with both *M. avium* and *M. fortuitum* strains, although treatment of the cultures with cycloserine is required for efficient lysis (Crawford and Bates, 1986; Villar and Benitez, 1992). This method is particularly useful for small-scale preparation of plasmid DNA for restriction digestion, which would include analysis of recombinant plasmids in *M. smegmatis*. However, this method is not suitable for detection of large plasmids and thus is not useful for screening purposes. The alkaline lysis method of Kado and Liu (1981) is the most efficient screening method for mycobacteria (Crawford and Bates, 1986; Hellyer et al., 1991). This method can be applied to 5-ml cultures treated with cycloserine. The cells are harvested by centrifugation and then processed in microcentrifuge tubes essentially as described by Kado and Liu (1981), using 60°C for 20 min in the heat denaturation step. This procedure provides reliable detection of plasmids of all sizes. Unfortunately, these crude preparations are not suitable for restriction digestion, and we have not found any satisfactory, simple procedure for purifying the plasmid DNA from such samples.

Detection of Plasmid DNA by Dot-Blot Hybridization

The presence of plasmids can also be demonstrated by hybridization assays, the simplest being the dot-blot format (Jucker and Falkinham, 1990). Total DNA samples are prepared as follows. Cells are grown to exponential phase and collected by centrifugation. Cells are suspended in 1 ml of TE buffer–0.3 ml of 2 N NaOH, 1 g of 0.1-mm-diameter glass beads is added, and the cells are broken by 90 s of shaking in a mini-bead

beater (BioSpec Products, Bartlesville, Okla.). The tubes are centrifuged, and 0.4 ml of the supernatant is added to a well of a dot-blot apparatus containing Zeta-Probe membrane (Bio-Rad Laboratories, Richmond, Calif.) previously wet with 2× SSC (1× SSC is 0.15 M NaCl plus 0.015 M sodium citrate). The membrane is removed from the apparatus, placed on a piece of filter paper soaked with 0.4 N NaOH, thoroughly rinsed with 2× SSC, and then dried. Whole plasmids are radiolabeled with ^{35}S-dCTP by using the Random-Primer DNA Labeling kit (Boehringer-Mannheim, Indianapolis, Ind.). As a control, the plasmid cloning vectors are labeled and used as probes.

FREQUENCY AND DISTRIBUTION OF MYCOBACTERIAL PLASMIDS

M. tuberculosis

There is no strong evidence for naturally occurring circular plasmids in *M. tuberculosis*. An early report of a satellite DNA band in cesium chloride-ethidium bromide gradients of *M. tuberculosis* H37Rv DNA appears to have been an artifact (Crawford and Bates, 1979). Zainuddin and Dale (1990) reported apparent extrachromosomal DNA bands on agarose gels but were unable to isolate plasmid DNA on CsCl-ethidium bromide gradients. They suggested that these might be single-stranded DNA plasmids. This finding has not been confirmed.

M. avium Complex

Plasmids are common in *M. avium* complex isolates recovered from infected humans, including both isolates from patients with pulmonary infections and isolates from AIDS patients with disseminated infections. The plasmids in *M. avium* complex isolates are primarily small (<30 kb) or very large (>150 kb), although some intermediate-sized plasmids have been demonstrated. Two groups of small plasmids have been identified. Group 1 is represented by pVT2, a plasmid carried by an *M. avium* isolate (Jucker and Falkinham, 1990). Group 2 is represented by pLR7, which is carried by a serotype 4 *M. avium* strain (Crawford et al., 1981a; Crawford and Bates, 1984). Both of these plasmids have been cloned and used as hybridization probes to detect related plasmids from other strains.

Meissner and Falkinham (1986) described a large study of the plasmid content of *M. avium* complex and *M. scrofulaceum* strains. In this study, 64 (55%) of 116 *M. avium* complex strains recovered from non-AIDS patients in the United States carried plasmids. In strains with plasmids, multiple plasmids of different sizes were common. In fact, strains with single plasmids were rare. Franzblau et al. (1986) reported that 16 (52%) of 31 *M. avium* complex isolates recovered from patients in Japan carried one to three plasmids.

In a study of 26 *M. avium* complex isolates of serotypes 4 and 8 recovered from U.S. AIDS patients, all were found to carry plasmids (Crawford and Bates, 1986). Each of the 26 isolates carried a small plasmid related to pLR7, as demonstrated by hybridization with pJC20, a pLR7::pBR322 chimera. There was considerable heterogeneity in these pLR7-related plasmids. Digestion with endonuclease *Sal*I and probing with pJC20 demonstrated heterogeneity in the restriction fragment patterns. Most of the serotype 4 isolates but none of the serotype 8 isolates carried a second small plasmid. One of these plasmids was cloned (Hellyer et al., 1991) and was subsequently shown to be related to pVT2. Ten of the isolates also carried large (>150 kb) plasmids. In another study of *M. avium* strains, six of six isolates from AIDS patients had a plasmid that hybridized with pLR7, and five had a plasmid that hybridized with pVT2 (Jucker and Falkinham, 1990). Ten (59%) of 17 isolates from non-AIDS pa-

tients had a plasmid that hybridized to pVT2, and 6 (35%) had a plasmid that hybridized to pLR7. Again, a great range of sizes was observed among plasmids hybridizing to either pLR7 or pVT2.

The data given above suggest that the small plasmids, especially those related to pLR7, might play some role in the ability of *M. avium* strains of serotype 4 and 8 to infect AIDS patients. Additional results, primarily with strains isolated outside of the United States, indicate that the plasmids are not a consistent feature of AIDS-associated isolates. Hellyer and coworkers (1991), studying isolates from the United Kingdom, found that only 34 of 71 isolates from AIDS patients carried plasmids. Plasmids related to pLR7 were most common, but eight isolates carried only a single large plasmid. Overall, they observed no difference between the strains isolated from AIDS patients and those from other patients. In a study performed in Denmark, 31% (5 of 16) of *M. avium* complex strains isolated from AIDS patients were found to carry plasmids, and 27% (4 of 15) of isolates from children with cervical lymphadenitis carried plasmids (Jensen et al., 1989).

Though there have been no widespread, comprehensive studies of plasmids in *M. avium* strains of animal origin, plasmids were found in 4 (20%) of 20 *M. avium* complex strains isolated from swine (Masaki et al., 1989). Further, those plasmids displayed the wide size range characteristic of *M. avium* plasmids isolated from strains recovered from other sources (Meissner and Falkinham, 1986). Plasmids were not detected in five *M. avium* strains recovered from pig organs or in one strain recovered from cattle organs (Jensen et al., 1989). In another study, 2 of 14 veterinary isolates were shown to carry a small plasmid (Hellyer et al., 1991).

Because the source of infection by members of the *M. avium* complex is thought to be environmental, surveys of the incidence and numbers of these organisms in different environmental compartments (e.g., water, soil, aerosols, dust) have been performed and the plasmid content of each isolate has been determined. In the United States, 25 of 135 environmental isolates of the *M. avium* complex yielded plasmids (Meissner and Falkinham, 1986). The highest percentage of plasmid-carrying strains was among aerosol isolates (12 of 16 [75%]), with a lower percentage among water isolates (10 of 48 [21%]). In another study focusing on *M. avium* environmental isolates that carry plasmids, 4 of 16 carried a pLR7-hybridizing plasmid, and 8 (50%) of 16 harbored a plasmid that hybridized with pVT2 (Jucker and Falkinham, 1990). In Denmark, only one (11%) of nine environmental *M. avium* isolates yielded plasmids (Jensen et al., 1989). The only strain yielding plasmids was isolated from sawdust.

M. scrofulaceum

Plasmids were detected in 9 (60%) of 15 U.S., non-AIDS clinical isolates (Meissner and Falkinham, 1986). As is the case with the related *M. avium* complex, the source of infection by *M. scrofulaceum* is thought to be environmental. Twelve (20%) of 61 U.S. environmental *M. scrofulaceum* isolates yielded plasmids. Of these isolates, 31% (11 of 36) of isolates from water yielded plasmids.

Evolution of *M. avium* Complex Plasmids

The demonstration of related plasmids in different *M. avium*, *M. intracellulare*, and *M. scrofulaceum* strains suggests that mycobacterial plasmids are capable of horizontal transfer. Further, the facts that related plasmids are of widely different sizes and contain discrete, unique regions in addition to the common, conserved regions suggest that mycobacterial plasmids have accumulated novel fragments. Specifically, those plasmids that hybridize with pVT2 have discrete sizes of 12.9, 13.5, and 15.3 kb (Jucker and Falkinham, 1990; Jucker,

1991). Restriction endonuclease mapping coupled with hybridization demonstrated that the group 1 plasmids shared discrete regions that hybridized under stringent conditions. In the larger plasmids, those regions of similarity were separated by inserted sequences. The conserved regions of two plasmids were shown to have identical sequences. Thus, it appears that *M. avium* plasmids have evolved by insertion of large DNA sequences. The origins of those inserted DNA sequences are not known.

M. fortuitum Complex

The prevalence of plasmids has been determined in clinical isolates of the *M. fortuitum* complex (Labidi et al., 1984). Plasmids were detected in seven of seven *M. fortuitum* subsp. *fortuitum* isolates, five of five *M. fortuitum* subsp. *peregrinum* isolates, five of five *M. chelonae* subsp. *chelonae* isolates, and a single *M. chelonae* subsp. *abscessus* isolate. Interestingly, a 32-kb plasmid was found in 17 of 18 isolates.

PLASMID-ENCODED FUNCTIONS

Background

Historically, determination of plasmid-encoded genes has followed from analysis of characteristics of plasmid-free variants of plasmid-carrying strains (i.e., cured derivatives) or of strains that have inherited plasmids from other strains. This analysis has permitted comparison of characteristics of strains isogeneic except for the plasmids and the correlation of characteristics to the presence of plasmids. To perform these studies, it is necessary to guess a probable plasmid-encoded phenotype in order to allow selection of cured derivatives or plasmid recipients. Unfortunately for mycobacteriologists, naturally occurring mycobacterial plasmids are extremely stable, and there exist few instances of cured strains. Lengthy unsuccessful attempts to cure *M.*

avium complex isolates have included growth in the presence of intercalating agents such as acriflavin and ethidium bromide and the DNA gyrase inhibitor novobiocin, growth at elevated temperature, and spheroplasting and reversion. Thus, the number of identified plasmid-associated characteristics is limited.

Plasmid-Encoded Restriction and Modification

Crawford and coworkers (1981b) characterized strain LR25, an isolate from a patient with pulmonary disease. This strain, which carries plasmids of 16.8, 27.5, and 150 kb, would now be classified as *M. avium*. The strain possesses a restriction-modification system, as was demonstrated in the classic manner by infection with phage JF2 and demonstration of a restriction enzyme activity. The enzyme produced by this and some other plasmid-containing *M. avium* isolates is an isoschizomer of *Xho*I and was designated *Mav*I (Crawford and Falkinham, 1990). It was also reported that a cured derivative of LR25 produced by exposure to neutral acriflavin and designated LR163 lacked the restriction-modification system. Kunze and McFadden (personal communication) demonstrated by restriction fragment length polymorphism typing that LR25 is an *M. avium* strain, whereas LR163 is an *M. intracellulare* strain, proving that LR613 could not have been derived from LR25. This observation has been confirmed by testing the oldest available isolates with the Gen-Probe Accuprobe assay (Crawford, unpublished data). Thus, data obtained with LR25 may be useful, but any conclusions based on comparisons of LR25 and LR163 are invalid (Crawford et al., 1981b; Gangadharam et al., 1988; Pethal and Falkinham, 1989).

Plasmid-Encoded Mercury and Copper Resistance

A spontaneous mercury-sensitive (Hg^s) segregant of a waterborne isolate of a mercury-resistant (Hg^r) *M. scrofulaceum* strain, W262, lost mercuric reductase activity and a 170-kb plasmid, one of four (13.3, 150, 170, and 300 kb) found in the parent strain (Meissner and Falkinham, 1984). Strain W262 was isolated from the Chester River in the Delaware-Maryland peninsula where a fish-canning plant had been located. Like other mercury-resistant bacteria, the mercuric reductase activity was soluble and resulted in the loss of ^{54}HgCl$_2$ added to medium containing the resistant strain (i.e., volatilization). No volatilization activity was detected in the mercury-sensitive segregant lacking the 170-kb plasmid.

The same spontaneous, mercury-sensitive segregant of W262 also lost copper resistance (Erardi et al., 1987). Thus, the 170-kb plasmid encodes mercury and copper resistance. The mechanism of copper resistance appeared novel, because the resistant parent was found to accumulate copper in the insoluble cell fractions, e.g., the membranes, while the majority of copper was found in the soluble fraction of the copper-sensitive strain. Because the cell pellets of the resistant strain were black and the resistance phenotype required sulfate, it was hypothesized that the copper was precipitated in the membrane of the resistant cells as copper sulfide. That was confirmed on the basis of the solubility of the black precipitate.

Further, it is likely that mercuric sulfide is formed in *M. scrofulaceum* W262 (Hg^r Cu^r) in the presence of mercuric ion, because cell pellets of cultures grown in the presence of mercuric ion are also black (Meissner and Falkinham, 1984). The ability to partition mercury into the insoluble fraction is likely to contribute to the mercury resistance of *M. scrofulaceum* W262.

Growth at 43°C and without Oleic Acid

In a study of human (non-AIDS) and environmental *M. avium* complex and *M. scrofulaceum* isolates, high correlations between the presence of plasmids and growth at 43°C or without oleic acid were discovered (R = 0.833 and 0.737, respectively [Fry et al., 1986]). Those data suggest that these phenotypes are due to plasmid-encoded genes.

Virulence and Catalase Activity

The higher frequency of plasmids among both AIDS and non-AIDS clinical isolates compared to environmental *M. avium* isolates led to the hypothesis that plasmids are involved in virulence (Crawford and Bates, 1986; Meissner and Falkinham, 1986; Jucker and Falkinham, 1990). Because of the difficulty in curing or transferring *M. avium* plasmids, the hypothesis has not been directly tested. As indicated above, results obtained from comparisons of strains LR25 and LR163 in the mouse model and in catalase assays were flawed (Gangadharam et al., 1988; Pethal and Falkinham, 1989).

Antibiotic Resistance

In addition to the reasons cited above that have prevented ready identification of plasmid-encoded genes, the relatively high background of antibiotic resistance of all mycobacteria, especially members of the *M. avium* complex, has confounded identification of plasmid-encoded antibiotic resistance (Franzblau et al., 1986). Drug resistance in mycobacteria is generally attributed to mutations that alter the targets of drug action, and one would not expect such genes to be found on plasmids. Plasmid-encoded drug resistance usually entails production of an enzyme that modifies the drug or the drug target. One study found no correlation between intrinsic aminoglycoside resistance and the presence of aminoglycoside acetyltransferase and plasmids in *M. fortuitum* (Hull et al., 1984).

PLASMID pAL5000

Characterization of pAL5000

The most thoroughly studied mycobacterial plasmid is pAL5000. This plasmid, which is carried by an *M. fortuitum* subsp. *fortuitum* strain, was originally described by Labidi and coworkers (1984). Because of its small size (about 5,000 bp), the plasmid was a good candidate for analysis and exploitation as a vector for molecular cloning. Although this plasmid has been extensively investigated, its function in the original *M. fortuitum* strain is unclear.

Initially, pAL5000 was cloned into *E. coli*, and a restriction map was generated (Labidi et al., 1985a). The complete sequence of pAL5000 and an analysis of the organization of plasmid genes have been reported elsewhere (Rauzier et al., 1988; Labidi et al., 1992). The data of Rauzier et al. indicated a sequence of 4,837 bp with five open reading frames (ORFs) and a putative origin of replication. Labidi et al. reported a sequence of 4,821 bp. Analysis of the plasmid sequence revealed only two ORFs that would encode proteins of 20 and 67 kDa. This result is consistent with the results of analysis of plasmid-encoded proteins in *E. coli* minicells carrying pBR322::pAL5000 chimeras (Labidi et al., 1985b).

The primary interest in pAL5000 has centered on use of the plasmid in construction of cloning vectors for mycobacteria. The feasibility of using pAL5000 for this purpose was demonstrated by Snapper et al. (1988). Plasmid DNA was linearized at random sites by partial digestion with endonuclease *Mbo*I. The positive *E. coli* selection vector pIJ666 was inserted into pAL5000, and the recombinants were introduced into *E. coli*. This vector carries the neomycin-kanamycin phosphotransferase gene derived from Tn5. Recombinant plasmids isolated from *E. coli* were electroporated into *M. smegmatis* and BCG, and the transformants were selected by plating on kanamycin. Analysis of 56 recombinants obtained from *E. coli* indicated that pIJ666 was inserted at an essentially random distribution of sites in pAL5000. However, clones obtained from *M. smegmatis* were limited to insertions in one half of pAL5000. It was subsequently demonstrated that the 2.6-kb *Eco*RV-*Hpa*I fragment of pAL5000 was sufficient for replication of recombinants. The same result was reported by Ranes et al. (1990). The 2.6-kb *Eco*RV-*Hpa*I fragment contains ORF1, ORF2, ORF5, and the putative origin of replication. Similar results were obtained by Villar and Benitez (1992). In addition, Villar and Benitez showed that stable plasmid inheritance required only ORF2 in *M. fortuitum* but ORF1, ORF2, and ORF5 in *M. smegmatis*.

Temperature-Sensitive Inheritance of pAL5000

Plasmid mutants unable to replicate at high temperature have been isolated (Gilhot et al., 1992). The shuttle plasmid pB4, derived from pAL5000, was mutagenized with hydroxylamine and transformed into *M. smegmatis* mc^{2}155. Transformants were selected at 30°C. Six hundred transformants were screened for plasmid-encoded antibiotic resistance following replica plating at 37 and 39°C, and six that exhibited temperature sensitivity were found. Among the six, four had temperature-sensitive antibiotic resistance, one had temperature-sensitive plasmid inheritance, and one had both. The pAL5000 inserts of both temperature-sensitive plasmids were subcloned, and the recombinant plasmids were shown to retain the temperature sensitivity. It was not known whether the mutations affected plasmid replication or plasmid partition. This approach can be used to identify plasmid genes involved in stable inheritance of mycobacterial plasmids. The temperature sensitivity plasmid will also be useful as a vehicle for transposon mutagenesis.

TRANSFER OF MYCOBACTERIAL PLASMIDS

Problems of Plasmid Transfer in Mycobacteria

The permeability barrier of mycobacteria that results in resistance to antibiotics, intracellular killing by macrophages, and environmental stresses is likely to limit the ability of DNA to traverse the cell wall and membrane. Because of this formidable barrier, the slow growth of mycobacteria of widespread public health interest, and the possibility of laboratory-acquired infection by pathogenic mycobacteria, development of plasmid transfer systems has focused on the rapidly growing mycobacteria of low pathogenicity (Jacobs et al., 1987; Snapper et al., 1988). In addition, because of interest in developing superior mycobacterial vaccines (Gheorghiu, 1990) and polyvalent vaccines with BCG (Jacobs et al., 1987, 1989), BCG plasmid transfer systems have been developed. Reviews of genetic systems of mycobacteria are presented by Jacobs et al. (1989) and Konicek et al. (1991), and an excellent comprehensive presentation of methodology is given by Jacobs et al. (1991).

Plasmid Transformation of *M. smegmatis*

Transformation, the acquisition of DNA by intact cells, was initially not readily achieved in even the fast-growing mycobacteria. The introduction of mycobacteriophage DNA could be efficiently accomplished in cell wall-deficient forms of *M. smegmatis* (spheroplasts or protoplasts) by using polyethylene glycol (Jacobs et al., 1987). Further, by using this protoplast-polyethylene glycol system, it was first possible to introduce and express foreign DNA in mycobacteria, suggesting that *M. smegmatis* and BCG had no insuperable restriction-modification systems. Stable transformation of protoplasts requires reversion of the cells to normal bacilli and replication.

While reversion of protoplasts is possible with *M. smegmatis*, stable maintenance of plasmids during this process appears to be difficult. Despite these difficulties, transient transformation of spheroplasts using the plasmids pIJ666 and pSGMU37 was reported by Zainuddin et al. (1989).

Numerous attempts to introduce pAL5000-based plasmids into *M. smegmatis* protoplasts have been unsuccessful (Gicquel-Sanzey et al., 1989); using electroporation resulted only in transient transformation (Zainuddin et al., 1989). Stable transformation of *M. smegmatis* was obtained by Snapper et al. (1990), who, after careful analysis of transformants, realized that successful transformation of the cloned *M. smegmatis* strain mc^{2}6 had occurred in only rare mutant cells within the population. One of these efficient plasmid transformation mutants, mc^{2}155, has been extensively characterized and widely used as a plasmid cloning host. Although the precise nature of the mutation conferring the efficient plasmid transformation phenotype is not known, the mutation appears not to affect DNA uptake or restriction-modification systems but rather to specifically affect plasmid replication (Snapper et al., 1990).

Plasmid Electroporation

The problem of introduction of DNA into mycobacteria has been overcome by the use of electroporation in the highly efficient plasmid transformation mutant of *M. smegmatis*. In this technique, cells are suspended in a nonelectrolyte solution (usually distilled water or 10% glycerol for mycobacteria) and subjected to a short, high-voltage pulse. This results in the formation of transient pores and the entry of DNA into cells. Though pAL5000-based shuttle plasmid pAL8 was not inherited by transformation using a polyethylene glycol-mediated uptake system, electroporation led to the formation of pAL8-carrying derivatives of *M. smegmatis* (Gicquel-Sanzey et

al., 1989). Optimization of transformation in mc^{2}155 has resulted in yields of greater than 10^6 transformants per μg of plasmid DNA (Cirillo et al., 1993).

Efficient electroporation appears to be limited by cell permeability barriers and genetic factors. Inheritance of the shuttle plasmid pAL8 by electroporation in *M. aurum* was enhanced by pretreatment of cells with 0.2 M glycine, 1 mg of lysozyme per ml, or 4 μg of isoniazid per ml (Hermans et al., 1990). Exposure of *M. aurum* cells to both glycine and isoniazid did not further enhance electroporation efficiency, i.e., the number of transformants per microgram of DNA per 10^9 cells electroporated.

A detailed method for preparation of *M. smegmatis* and BCG cells for electroporation is presented by Jacobs et al. (1991). Herein we present a simplified method that provides washed, electroporation-ready cells with high efficiency for electroporation of plasmid DNA (Falkinham, unpublished data). Cultures of strain VT307, an electroporation-proficient mutant of *M. smegmatis*, are cultured to exponential phase (6 days) in 100 ml of 7H9 broth with shaking at 37°C in 1-liter screw-cap flasks. Cells are harvested by centrifugation (7,000 × *g* for 10 min at 4°C), washed twice by suspension in an equal volume of sterile distilled water, and suspended in 1/10 the volume of sterile distilled water. The viable count is determined, and the suspensions are divided into 1-ml aliquots and frozen at −70°C.

Methods for electroporation are described by Snapper et al. (1988) and Jacobs et al. (1991). Low transformation yields have been increased by (i) exposing the washed electroporation-ready cell–plasmid DNA mixture to two electrical pulses of the same voltage and time constant, with a 10-s interval between pulses; (ii) decreasing the volume of cells and hence the reaction mixture; and (iii) increasing the length of incubation of cells under nonselective conditions to 12 to 18 h at 37°C before plating them on selective medium.

Plasmid Electroduction

Plasmid electroduction is the transfer of plasmid DNA between intact strains catalyzed by electroporation. The shuttle plasmid pRR3 was shown to be capable of electroduction from *M. smegmatis* to BCG and from either *M. smegmatis* or BCG to *E. coli* (Baulard et al., 1992). The advantage of electroduction is that there is no requirement for isolation of plasmid DNA from the donor strain.

Conjugation

The gram-negative, broad-host-range plasmid RSF1010 was transferred from *E. coli* to the electroporation-proficient *M. smegmatis* strain mc²155 by conjugation, i.e., by direct contact between the donor and recipient cells (Gormley and Davies, 1991). The mechanism is unknown.

PLASMID CLONING VECTORS FOR MYCOBACTERIA

pAL5000 Vectors

A variety of pAL5000 vectors have been developed since the description of pYUB12 (Snapper et al., 1988; see also chapter 17 of this volume). A polymerase chain reaction-generated 1.8-kb minimal origin was used in the construction of pMV261 (Stover et al., 1991). This vector is intended for expression of inserted genes and contains the *hsp60* promoter upstream from a multiple cloning site. For example, this plasmid has been used to express the firefly luciferase gene in *M. tuberculosis* and *M. smegmatis* (Cooksey et al., 1993). Other shuttle plasmids include pRR3 (Ranes et al., 1990), pMY10 (Lazraq et al., 1990), and pMSC1 (Hinshelwood and Stoker, 1992).

M. scrofulaceum Plasmid pMSC262-Based Vectors

A shuttle plasmid was constructed by using the 13.3-kb plasmid pMSC262 found in *M. scrofulaceum* W262. The shuttle plasmid pYT72 was constructed by inserting an 11.3-kb *Bam*HI fragment of pMSC262 into the *Bam*HI site of *E. coli* cloning vector pACYC177 (Goto et al., 1991). This plasmid was capable of replication in both *E. coli* and BCG. Deletion mutants of pYT72 generated by cleavage with *Pst*I resulted in identification of a region required for inheritance in BCG, and that knowledge was used to guide construction of a smaller, 5.9-kb shuttle plasmid, pYT937.

Corynebacterium-Based Shuttle Vectors

A novel set of *Mycobacterium-E. coli* shuttle vectors was constructed by using either a kanamycin or a hygromycin resistance gene and the replication region from a *Corynebacterium* plasmid (Radford and Hodgson, 1991). The plasmids replicated to a high copy number in both *M. smegmatis* and BCG.

L5-Based Integrating Plasmids

A novel type of plasmid vector was constructed by utilizing the L5 phage integration system (see chapter 12 in this volume). These vectors contain the *att*P site of phage L5 and the L5 integrase gene. Upon electroporation, these vectors, lacking a mycobacterial origin of replication, site specifically integrate into a single *att*B site in the chromosomes of *M. smegmatis*, BCG, and *M. tuberculosis* (Lee et al., 1991). These integrating vectors, e.g., pMV361, have proven useful for stably introducing recombinant plasmids and antigens into recombinant BCG vaccine strains (Stover et al., 1991; see chapter 17 in this volume).

Vectors Based on the Mycobacteriophage D29 Origin

Shuttle vectors that use an apparent origin of replication from mycobacteriophage D29 have been reported (Lazraq et al., 1991; David et al., 1992). One of these vectors was used to express vibrio bioluminescence genes in *M. smegmatis*.

Gram-Negative Plasmids Inherited Stably by Mycobacteria

Investigators have discovered that a number of gram-negative plasmid cloning vectors are able to transform strains of mycobacteria. Plasmid vectors pIJ666 and pSGMU37 are capable of transforming *M. smegmatis* (Zainuddin et al., 1989), and Hermans et al. (1991) demonstrated that the gram-negative cosmid pJRD215 was capable of transforming *M. aurum* and *M. smegmatis*. The broad-host-range gram-negative plasmid RSF1010 was also shown to replicate in *M. smegmatis* (Gormley and Davies, 1991).

SUMMARY

Despite recent success in using plasmids in recombinant methodology, there is still relatively little knowledge of the functions of naturally occurring mycobacterial plasmids. It has not been possible to either cure or transfer mycobacterial plasmids by using an inherent selectable phenotypic marker. Introduction of kanamycin resistance or other antibiotic resistance genes into various mycobacterial plasmids and the use of electroporation to introduce the plasmids into other strains may allow analysis of plasmid functions. Although plasmid surveys have been adequately initiated in the *M. avium* complex, analysis of the plasmid content of various other mycobacterial species, including *M. tuberculosis*, is justified. Additional studies may provide a fuller understanding of the role of plasmids in mycobacterial pathogenesis, physiology, ecology, and epidemiology.

REFERENCES

Baulard, A., C. Jourdan, A. Mercenier, and C. Locht. 1992. Rapid mycobacterial plasmid analysis by electroduction between *Mycobacterium* spp. and *Escherichia coli*. *Nucleic Acids Res*. **20**:4105.

Birnboim, H. C., and J. Doly. 1979. A rapid alkaline extraction procedure for screening recombinant plasmid DNA. *Nucleic Acids Res*. **7**:1513–1523.

Cirillo, J. D., T. R. Weisbrod, and W. R. Jacobs, Jr. 1993. Efficient electro-transformation of *M. smegmatis*. *BioRad Tech. Bull*. 1360.

Cooksey, R. C., J. T. Crawford, W. R. Jacobs, Jr., and T. M. Shinnick. 1993. A rapid method for screening antimicrobial agents for activity against a strain of *Mycobacterium tuberculosis* expressing firefly luciferase. *Antimicrob. Agents Chemother*. **37**:1348–1352.

Crawford, J. T. Unpublished data.

Crawford, J. T., and J. H. Bates. 1979. Isolation of plasmids from mycobacteria. *Infect. Immun*. **24**:979–981.

Crawford, J. T., and J. H. Bates. 1984. Restriction endonuclease mapping and cloning of *Mycobacterium intracellulare* plasmid pLR7. *Gene* **27**:331–333.

Crawford, J. T., and J. H. Bates. 1986. Analysis of plasmids in *Mycobacterium avium-intracellulare* isolates from persons with acquired immunodeficiency syndrome. *Am. Rev. Respir. Dis*. **134**:659–661.

Crawford, J. T., M. D. Cave, and J. H. Bates. 1981a. Characterization of plasmids from strains of *Mycobacterium avium-intracellulare*. *Rev. Infect. Dis*. **3**:949–951.

Crawford, J. T., M. D. Cave, and J. H. Bates. 1981b. Evidence for plasmid-mediated restriction-modification in *Mycobacterium avium-intracellulare*. *J. Gen. Microbiol*. **127**:333–338.

Crawford, J. T., and J. O. Falkinham III. 1990. Plasmids of the *Mycobacterium avium* complex, p. 97–119. *In* J. McFadden (ed.), *Molecular Biology of the Mycobacteria*. Harcourt Brace Jovanovich Publishers, London.

David, M., S. Lubinsky-Mink, A. Ben-Zvi, S. Ulitzur, J. Kuhn, and M. Suissa. 1992. A stable *E. coli*-*Mycobacterium smegmatis* plasmid shuttle vector containing the mycobacteriophage D29 origin. *Plasmid* **28**:267–271.

Erardi, F. X., M. L. Failla, and J. O. Falkinham III. 1987. Plasmid-encoded copper resistance and precipitation by *Mycobacterium scrofulaceum*. *Appl. Environ. Microbiol*. **53**:1951–1954.

Falkinham, J. O., III. Unpublished data.

Franzblau, S. G., T. Takeda, and M. Nakamura. 1986. Mycobacterial plasmids: screening and possible relationship to antibiotic resistance in *Mycobacterium avium/Mycobacterium intracellulare*. *Microbiol. Immunol.* **30:**903–907.

Fry, K. L., P. S. Meissner, and J. O. Falkinham III. 1986. Epidemiology of infection by nontuberculous mycobacteria. VI. Identification and use of epidemiologic markers for studies of *Mycobacterium avium*, *Mycobacterium intracellulare*, and *Mycobacterium scrofulaceum*. *Am. Rev. Respir. Dis.* **134:**39–43.

Gangadharam, P. R. J., V. K. Perumal, J. T. Crawford, and J. H. Bates. 1988. Association of plasmids and virulence of *Mycobacterium avium* complex. *Am. Rev. Respir. Dis.* **137:**212–214.

Gheorghiu, M. 1990. The present and future role of BCG vaccine in tuberculosis control. *Biologicals* **18:**135–141.

Gicquel-Sanzey, B., J. Moniz-Pereira, M. Gheorghiu, and J. Rauzier. 1989. Structure of pAL5000, a plasmid from *M. fortuitum* and its utilization in transformation of mycobacteria. *Acta Leprol.* **7**(Suppl. 1):208–211.

Gilhot, C., B. Gicquel, and C. Martin. 1992. Temperature-sensitive mutants of the *Mycobacterium* plasmid pAL5000. *FEMS Microbiol. Lett.* **98:**181–186.

Gormley, E. P., and J. Davies. 1991. Transfer of plasmid RSF1010 by conjugation from *Escherichia coli* to *Streptomyces lividans* and *Mycobacterium smegmatis*. *J. Bacteriol.* **173:**6705–6708.

Goto, Y., H. Taniguchi, T. Udou, Y. Mizuguchi, and T. Tokunaga. 1991. Development of a new host vector system in mycobacteria. *FEMS Microbiol. Lett.* **83:**277–282.

Hellyer, T. J., I. N. Brown, J. W. Dale, and C. S. F. Easmon. 1991. Plasmid analysis of *Mycobacterium avium-intracellulare* (MAI) isolated in the United Kingdom from patients with and without AIDS. *J. Med. Microbiol.* **34:**225–231.

Hermans, J., J. G. Boschloo, and J. A. M. de Bont. 1990. Transformation of *Mycobacterium aurum* by electroporation: the use of glycine, lysozyme and isonicotinic acid hydrazide in enhancing transformation efficiency. *FEMS Microbiol. Lett.* **72:**221–224.

Hermans, J., C. Martin, G. N. M. Huijberts, T. Goosen, and J. A. M. de Bont. 1991. Transformation of *Mycobacterium aurum* and *Mycobacterium smegmatis* with the broad host-range Gram-negative cosmid vector pJRD215. *Mol. Microbiol.* **5:**1561–1566.

Hinshelwood, S., and N. G. Stoker. 1992. An *Escherichia coli-Mycobacterium* shuttle cosmid vector, pMSC1. *Gene* **110:**115–118.

Hull, S. I., R. J. Wallace, D. G. Bolbey, K. E. Price, R. A. Goodhines, J. M. Swenson, and V. A. Silcox. 1984. Presence of aminoglycoside acetyltransferase and plasmid in *Mycobacterium fortuitum*, lack of correlation with intrinsic aminoglycoside resistance. *Am. Rev. Respir. Dis.* **129:**614–618.

Humphreys, G. O., G. A. Willshaw, and E. S. Anderson. 1975. A simple method for the preparation of large quantities of pure plasmid DNA. *Biochim. Biophys. Acta* **383:**457–463.

Jacobs, W. R., Jr., G. V. Kalpana, J. D. Cirillo, L. Pascopella, S. B. Snapper, R. A. Udani, W. Jones, R. G. Barletta, and B. R. Bloom. 1991. Genetic systems for mycobacteria. *Methods Enzymol.* **204:** 537–555.

Jacobs, W. R., Jr., S. B. Snapper, L. Lugosi, A. Jekkel, R. E. Melton, T. Kieser, and B. R. Bloom. 1989. Development of genetic systems for the mycobacteria. *Acta Leprol.* **7**(Suppl. 1):203–207.

Jacobs, W. R., Jr., M. Tuckman, and B. R. Bloom. 1987. Introduction of foreign DNA into mycobacteria using a shuttle plasmid. *Nature* (London) **327:** 532–535.

Jensen, A. G., J. Brennedsen, and W. T. Rosdahl. 1989. Plasmid profiles of *Mycobacterium avium/intracellulare* isolated from patients with AIDS or cervical lymphadenitis and from environmental samples. *Scand. J. Infect. Dis.* **21:**645–649.

Jucker, M. T. 1991. Ph.D. dissertation. Virginia Polytechnic Institute and State University, Blacksburg.

Jucker, M. T., and J. O. Falkinham III. 1990. Epidemiology of infection by nontuberculous mycobacteria. IX. Evidence for two DNA homology groups among small plasmids in *M. avium*, *M. intracellulare*, and *M. scrofulaceum*. *Am. Rev. Respir. Dis.* **142:**858–862.

Kado, C. I., and S. T. Liu. 1981. Rapid procedure for detection and isolation of large and small plasmids. *J. Bacteriol.* **145:**1365–1373.

Konicek, J., M. Konickova-Radochova, and M. Slosarek. 1991. Gene manipulation in mycobacteria. *Folia Microbiol.* **36:**411–422.

Kunze, Z. M., and J. J. McFadden. Personal communication.

Labidi, A., C. Dauget, K. S. Goh, and H. L. David. 1984. Plasmid profiles of *Mycobacterium fortuitum* complex isolates. *Curr. Microbiol.* **11:**235–240.

Labidi, A., H. L. David, and D. Roulland-Dussoix. 1985a. Restriction endonuclease mapping and cloning of *Mycobacterium fortuitum* var *fortuitum* plasmid pAL5000. *Ann. Inst. Pasteur/Microbiol.* **136B:** 209–215.

Labidi, A., H. L. David, and D. Roulland-Dussoix. 1985b. Cloning and expression of mycobacterial plasmid DNA in *Escherichia coli*. *FEMS Microbiol. Lett.* **30:**221–225.

Labidi, A., E. Mardis, B. A. Roe, and R. J. Wallace, Jr. 1992. Cloning and DNA sequence of the *Mycobacterium fortuitum* var. *fortuitum* plasmid pAL5000. *Plasmid* **27:**130–140.

Lazraq, R., S. Clavel-Seres, H. L. David, and D. Roulland-Dussoix. 1990. Conjugative transfer of a shuttle plasmid from *Escherichia coli* to *Mycobacterium smegmatis*. *FEMS Microbiol. Lett.* **69**:135–138.

Lazraq, R., M. Houssaini-Iraqui, S. Clavel-Seres, and H. L. David. 1991. Cloning and expression of the origin or replication of mycobacteriophage D29 in *Mycobacterium smegmatis*. *FEMS Microbiol. Lett.* **80**:117–120.

Lee, M. H., L. Pascopella, W. R. Jacobs, Jr., and G. F. Hatfull. 1991. Site-specific integration of mycobacteriophage L5: integration-proficient vectors for *Mycobacterium smegmatis*, *Mycobacterium tuberculosis*, and bacille Calmette-Guérin. *Proc. Natl. Acad. Sci. USA* **88**:3111–3115.

Maniatis, T., E. F. Fritsch, and J. Sambrook. 1982. *Molecular Cloning: a Laboratory Manual.* Cold Spring Harbor Laboratory, Cold Spring Harbor, N.Y.

Masaki, S., T. Konishi, G. Sugimori, A. Okamoto, Y. Hayashi, and F. Kuze. 1989. Plasmid profiles of *Mycobacterium avium* complex isolated from swine. *Microbiol. Immunol.* **33**:429–433.

Meissner, P. S., and J. O. Falkinham III. 1984. Plasmid-encoded mercuric reductase in *Mycobacterium scrofulaceum*. *J. Bacteriol.* **157**:669–672.

Meissner, P. S., and J. O. Falkinham III. 1986. Plasmid DNA profiles as epidemiological markers for clinical and environmental isolates of *Mycobacterium avium*, *Mycobacterium intracellulare*, and *Mycobacterium scrofulaceum*. *J. Infect. Dis.* **153**:325–331.

Mizuguchi, Y., and T. Tokunaga. 1970. Method for isolation of deoxyribonucleic acid from mycobacteria. *J. Bacteriol.* **104**:1020–1021.

Pethal, M. L., and J. O. Falkinham III. 1989. Plasmid-influenced changes in *Mycobacterium avium* catalase activity. *Infect. Immun.* **57**:1714–1718.

Radford, A. J., and A. L. M. Hodgson. 1991. Construction and characterization of a *Mycobacterium-Escherichia coli* shuttle vector. *Plasmid* **25**:149–153.

Ranes, M. G., J. Rauzier, M. LaGranderie, M. Gheorghiu, and B. Gicquel. 1990. Functional analysis of pAL5000, a plasmid from *Mycobacterium fortuitum*: construction of a "mini" mycobacterium-*Escherichia coli* shuttle vector. *J. Bacteriol.* **172**:2793–2797.

Rastogi, N., and H. L. David. 1981. Ultrastructural and chemical studies on wall-deficient forms, spheroplasts and membrane vesicles from *Mycobacterium aurum*. *J. Gen. Microbiol.* **124**:71–79.

Rauzier, J., J. Moniz-Pereira, and B. Gicquel-Sanzey. 1988. Complete nucleotide sequence of pAL5000, a plasmid from *Mycobacterium fortuitum*. *Gene* **71**:315–321.

Snapper, S. B., L. Lugosi, A. Jekkel, R. E. Melton, T. Kieser, B. R. Bloom, and W. R. Jacobs, Jr. 1988. Lysogeny and transformation in mycobacteria: stable expression of foreign genes. *Proc. Natl. Acad. Sci. USA* **85**:6987–6991.

Snapper, S. B., R. E. Melton, S. Mustafa, T. Kieser, and W. R. Jacobs, Jr. 1990. Isolation and characterization of efficient plasmid transformation mutants of *Mycobacterium smegmatis*. *Mol. Microbiol.* **4**:1911–1919.

Stover, C. K., V. F. de la Cruz, T. R. Fuerst, J. E. Burlein, L. A. Benson, L. T. Bennett, G. P. Bansal, J. F. Young, M. H. Lee, G. F. Hatfull, S. B. Snapper, R. G. Barletta, W. R. Jacobs, Jr., and B. R. Bloom. 1991. New use of BCG for recombinant vaccines. *Nature* (London) **351**:456–460.

Villar, C. A., and J. Benitez. 1992. Functional analysis of pAL5000 plasmid in *Mycobacterium fortuitum*. *Plasmid* **28**:166–169.

Zainuddin, Z. F., and J. W. Dale. 1990. Does *Mycobacterium tuberculosis* have plasmids? *Tubercle* **71**(1):43–49.

Zainuddin, Z. F., Z. M. Kunze, and J. W. Dale. 1989. Transformation of *Mycobacterium smegmatis* with *E. coli* plasmids carrying a selectable resistance marker. *Mol. Microbiol.* **3**:29–34.

Tuberculosis: Pathogenesis, Protection, and Control
Edited by Barry R. Bloom
© 1994 American Society for Microbiology, Washington, DC 20005

Chapter 14

Transposition in Mycobacteria

Ruth A. McAdam, Christophe Guilhot, and Brigitte Gicquel

TRANSPOSABLE ELEMENTS IN EUBACTERIA

Insertion elements and transposons are mobile genetic elements that are present in most living organisms. They were first discovered by B. McClintock in the 1940s as "controlling elements," i.e., chromosomal elements able to move, affect gene expression, and cause chromosomal rearrangements during the development of maize (*Zea mays*) (McClintock, 1956a, b). Mobile genetic elements were rediscovered in *Escherichia coli* 20 years later, when molecular genetics allowed their isolation. In this case, they were also identified by their characteristic of inducing mutations. When antibiotic-resistant transposons were discovered and designated "translocatable drug-resistance elements" (Kleckner et al., 1977), a whole new era in molecular genetics began, leading to the extensive use of transposons in the genetic analysis of bacteria.

All mobile elements have common char-

acteristics. They are discrete DNA fragments encoding their own transposition functions and are able to move from one site in the DNA strand to another independently of host recombination functions. Recombination by transposition also occurs without homology between the sequences of the transposon and the target sequence. Many mobile elements insert randomly; however, several have preferred or even specific target sites.

Structure and Occurrence

A large number of different mobile genetic elements have been discovered in prokaryotes. The most basic are known as insertion sequences (ISs). These are usually 0.8 to 2.5 kb in length, possess inverted repeats at their termini, and contain at least one open reading frame (ORF) encoding the transposase (see Galas and Chandler [1989] for a full review). Transposons are larger elements containing additional genes such as those for antibiotic resistance or virulence determinants. The best characterized include those from gram-negative members of the family *Enterobacteriaceae*, and most of these transposons belong to one of two groups according to their structure: class I, which is compound transposons, and class II, or Tn3-like elements. Compound, or class I, transposons also contain several genes not involved in the transposition pro-

Ruth A. McAdam • Department of Microbiology and Immunology, Albert Einstein College of Medicine of Yeshiva University, 1300 Morris Park Avenue, Bronx, New York 10461. ***Christophe Guilhot and Brigitte Gicquel*** • Unité de Génétique Mycobactérienne, Département de Bactériologie et Mycologie, Institut Pasteur, 25, rue du Dr. Roux, 75724 Paris Cedex 15, France.

cess (usually encoding antibiotic resistance) that are flanked by ISs in direct or inverse orientation. In the cases of Tn5 and Tn10, only one of the ISs can mediate transposition. Tn3, from class II, encodes a transposase and a resolvase for transposition, a β-lactamase gene providing ampicillin resistance, and inverted repeats at its termini.

Some elements do not fall into either class. The transposon Mu is a phage infecting a range of *Enterobacteriaceae* that replicates lytically but is also able to lysogenize the host, inserting at random into host DNA. Some of the more unusual transposons originate in gram-positive organisms. These include Tn916 and Tn1545, conjugative transposons from *Enterococcus faecalis* and *Streptococcus pneumoniae*, respectively. For a full review, see selected chapters in Berg and Howe (1989).

Transposition Mechanisms and Consequences

Many different chromosomal rearrangements can occur because of transposition. Transposons normally cause inactivation of genes when they insert into host DNA. However, some IS elements, such as IS3 (Charlier et al., 1982), are also capable of activating genes through an outward reading promoter. On insertion into a new site, usually a duplication of between 2 and 13 bp of the target sequence occurs, giving rise to direct repeats appearing on either side of the element. The length of the target duplication is a characteristic of the particular

mobile element, as is the transposition mechanism.

Transposable elements can move by either conservative or replicative mechanisms. These mechanisms are represented in Fig. 1. Conservative transposition leads to the insertion of the element into its new site without replication of the element. In this case, the donor molecule is generally lost and DNA repair occurs, leading to a repetition of the target site. Replicative transposition leads to a duplication of the element and the formation of a cointegrate consisting of the transposon donor molecule with an extra copy of the element. The two copies of the transposon are then in direct orientation. These mechanisms have been well studied in in vitro systems (for a review, see Mizuuchi [1992]). Some transposons contain a resolvase able to perform site-specific recombination of the cointegrate, resulting in restoration of the transposon donor molecule and insertion of one transposable element into the recipient molecule.

After transposition, chromosomal rearrangements other than a simple insertion can occur. Deletions or inversions can be seen when transposition occurs on the same DNA molecule. When replicative transposition involves two DNA molecules and the cointegrate is not resolved, a fusion of replicons results. When a DNA fragment is located between two transposable elements, this segment can be mobilized by the flanking mobile elements, which act as a compound transposable element. When

---

Figure 1. Model (according to Shapiro [1979]) of two different mechanisms of transposition. The three possible outcomes are illustrated. (I) The transposon, represented by a black arrow, is cleaved at its 3′ extremities. A staggered cleavage of the target site leads to 5′ protruding ends. (The specific cuts are indicated by small arrows.) (II) Joining the 3′ ends of the transposon to the 5′ ends of the target forms a transposition intermediate called the Shapiro intermediate. This structure can be resolved in the following two ways: (III) specific cleavage of the 5′ ends of the transposon and filling in of the target site (white box) leads to a simple insertion of the transposon in the recipient by "conservative transposition," or (IV) replication of the target site and the transposon by using the recipient as primer (white boxes and dashed arrows) leads to the formation of a cointegrate. This is called "replicative transposition." (V) This structure can be resolved either by a site-specific resolvase or by the general homologous recombination pathway of the host.

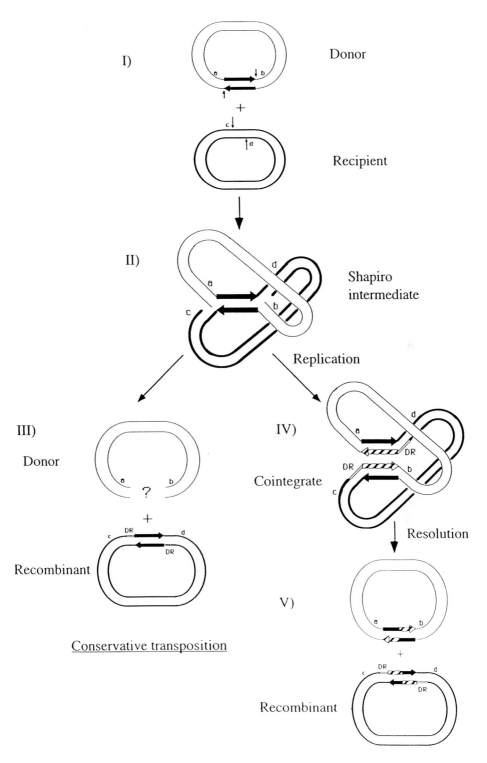

this segment is adjacent to conjugative sequences or is on a plasmid or a phage, the transfer of transposons containing new DNA to other bacteria can occur. This event is largely responsible for the dissemination of drug resistance genes among streptococcal and staphylococcal strains responsible for widespread hospital infections.

TRANSPOSABLE ELEMENTS AS GENETIC TOOLS

General Uses

Many transposons, or slightly modified derivatives of them, have been widely exploited as genetic tools in bacteria such as *E. coli*, since they can be used to insert a marker gene into target DNA (see Berg et al. [1989] and Kleckner et al. [1991] for details on uses). Thus, selectable markers can be placed next to or within a gene of interest to provide regions of homology and restriction sites for DNA rearrangements, sequencing, and mapping.

The insertion of a transposable element into a gene can logically lead to inactivation of the gene. Owing to the ability of some transposons to insert randomly into DNA, they are important in creating mutants to identify genes by selecting for the loss of a certain phenotype. The region containing the insertion can easily be recovered for further analysis. Modified transposons have been constructed to investigate specific biological problems. For example, transposons bearing truncated reporter genes are used to locate promoters and to examine the condition of that gene's expression. They can also be constructed with portable, regulatable promoters for manipulation of gene expression. Exported proteins can be identified and studied by using a reporter gene encoding an enzyme that is functional only in an extracytoplasmic compartment. One example of this is Tn*phoA*, a derivative of Tn5 that carries a truncated alkaline phosphatase gene that will encode a functional enzyme after fusion with exported proteins (Manoil et al., 1990).

When an element is able to transpose in one species, for example, *E. coli*, but not in the species of study, and when the selectable marker is used by both species, shuttle mutagenesis is used. First, genes of interest, or a genomic library, are constructed in the transposon-containing *E. coli*, mutagenized, and then transferred back into the original strain, where the mutagenized fragments integrate by homologous recombination and a double crossover effects replacement of the wild-type gene with the insertion.

Use of Transposons in Pathogenic Bacteria

Transposons as genetic tools have been instrumental in uncovering virulence characteristics of bacterial pathogens. Only a few examples of such studies will be described below. Hoiseth and Stocker (1981) used Tn*10* mutagenesis to make an *aroA* strain of *Salmonella typhimurium* and showed that it was nonvirulent and protective as a vaccine. This approach was extended in an in vitro screen; mutants unable to survive in a macrophage were also avirulent. Some of these mutants mapped to *phoP*, which is responsible for resistance to macrophage defensins (Fields et al., 1986, 1989). In vitro studies allowed the cloning of the *Yersinia pseudotuberculosis* invasin (Isberg and Falkow, 1985), selected by cloning the phenotype in *E. coli*, and its identity was subsequently proven by shuttle mutagenesis using Tn5. The notion that factors involved in interaction with the host, such as toxins, enzymes, and adhesins, must be secreted led to the development of Tn*phoA* as a transposon tool and the isolation of *Vibrio cholerae* virulence factors, including *tcp*, the gene for toxin-coregulated pilus (Taylor et al., 1989). Intracellular life has also been investigated by using Tn*phoA* to identify the *Shigella flex-neri icsA* gene (Bernardini et al., 1989), whose product interacts with actin intracellularly and brings about spread of the bacterium into adjacent cells. Nonhemolytic mutants of *Listeria monocytogenes*, isolated after insertional mutagenesis with Tn*1545* (Gaillard et al., 1986), result from insertion into the listeriolysin gene (*hlyA*). These mutants can no longer escape from the phagolysosome into the cytoplasm and are avirulent (Cossart et al., 1989). When cloned into *Bacillus subtilis*, this gene allowed growth of this nonpathogen inside J774 cells (Bielecki et al., 1990). The regulators of virulence factors can also be discovered by transposon mutagenesis, as was the case with *Bordetella pertussis*. Insertion of Tn*5* into the *bvg* (or *vir*) locus eliminated expression of at least five virulence factors (Weiss and Falkow, 1983) and led to the characterization of this locus as a sensory transduction pathway. More recently, *vir*-repressed genes have also been identified and cloned by using Tn*phoA* (Beattie et al., 1993).

Relevance to Mycobacteria

Attempts to utilize the available transposons directly for insertional mutagenesis in mycobacteria have met with limited success (Gicquel and Jacobs, personal communications). One possible cause of the problem with gram-negative elements could be lack of recognition of *E. coli* promoters (Clark-Curtiss et al., 1985; Thole et al., 1985) or the absence of suitable host factors. This is evidenced in *B. subtilis*, where transposition of Tn*10* was achieved by using signals from this bacterium (Petit et al., 1990). Elements from gram-positive bacteria have been used in other gram-positive bacteria when an efficient delivery system such as conjugation was available (Murphy, 1989). Although conjugation between *E. coli* and mycobacteria has been achieved (Gormley and Davies, 1991), there are no

reports on its use to deliver transposons to mycobacteria. Reverse mutagenesis, using Tn*5*, has been successful in *Mycobacterium smegmatis*, allowing the isolation of a methionine auxotroph (Kalpana et al., 1991). However, this approach supposed that every part of the mycobacterial genome can be cloned in *E. coli*. This may be a limitation if some mycobacterial genes or fragments are toxic in this host. This approach is currently of limited use in the *Mycobacterium tuberculosis* complex, because the second step requires homologous recombination between a plasmid and the chromosome. Kalpana et al. (1991) and Aldovini et al. (1993) have shown that homologous recombination is very inefficient in the mycobacteria from the *M. tuberculosis* complex.

Transposons derived from *Streptomyces* spp., however, could be useful in mycobacteria. Both species belong to the gram-positive group *Actinomyces*, which also has a high G+C content, and some commonalities between the groups have been investigated (Keiser et al., 1986; Martín et al., 1991). It may be that transposons from G+C-rich organisms transpose more frequently in hosts that also have a high percentage of G+C. At least two different transposons have been successfully used for mutagenesis in *Streptomyces* spp. (Baltz et al., 1992; Sohaskey et al., 1992), but no study of their use in mycobacteria has been reported.

MYCOBACTERIAL TRANSPOSABLE ELEMENTS

Overview

Mycobacterial IS elements were first discovered while workers were looking for strain-specific probes in the pathogenic mycobacteria by using differential hybridization. The first such elements included IS*900*, which allowed comparison of *Mycobacterium paratuberculosis* and Crohn's disease isolates with strains of the *Myco-*

Table 1. Main features of mycobacterial ISs[a]

Mobile DNA	Length (bp)	IR (bp)	Target DR (bp)	Insertion site	Family	Copy no.	Strain specificity
IS6100	880	14	ND	Random	IS6	4	*M. fortuitum* FC1
IS6110-IS986	1,361	28	3 or 4	Random	IS3	0–23	*M. tuberculosis* complex
IS1141	1,588	23	ND	ND	IS3	ND	*M. intracellulare*
IS1137	1,364	32	3	ND	IS3	1–8	*M. smegmatis, M. chitae*
IS900	1,451	None	None	CATGN$_{(4-6)}$*CNCCTT	IS110	15–20	*M. paratuberculosis*
IS901	1,472	None	None	CATN$_{(7)}$*TTCCNTTC	IS110	2–8	*M. avium* RFLP type A/I
IS1081	1,324	15	ND	ND	IS256	5–6	*M. tuberculosis* complex
IS6120	1,486	24	9	Random	IS256	2–8	*M. smegmatis, M. aurum*
IS1096	2,260	26	8	ND	Tn3926	8–16	*M. smegmatis*
ISmyco	968	17	4	ND	IS402	1	*M. tuberculosis* complex

[a] IR, inverted repeat; DR, direct repeat; ND, not done; RFLP, restriction fragment length polymorphism.

bacterium avium complex (McFadden et al., 1987a, b), and IS6110 from *M. tuberculosis*, which was found during a search for specific or repetitive DNA for use as gene probes for diagnosis (Eisenach et al., 1988; Thierry et al., 1990a; McAdam, personal communication). Subsequently, mycobacterial IS elements have been cloned by a combination of active pursuit, the use of hybridization to drug resistance markers (Martín et al., 1990), the use of transposon traps in *Mycobacterium smegmatis* (Guilhot et al., 1992a; Cirillo et al., 1991), and simply serendipity.

Most of the elements were initially characterized as mobile elements because of their sequence similarity to known insertion elements from microorganisms other than mycobacteria, and most can be grouped with a particular family of eubacterial elements. Summaries of the main features of each element are given in Table 1 and Fig. 2.

The majority are species specific or are present in a narrow host range. Tn610 from *Mycobacterium fortuitum* was found only in that particular isolate. This makes some of the elements useful as gene probes in

determining species, as has been demonstrated for other bacteria (van der Zee et al., 1993), and IS6110 has found a special use in epidemiology (see chapter 33 in this volume). Work on constructing transposons from ISs for use as genetic tools in the mycobacteria has also been initiated.

ISs in *M. paratuberculosis*, *M. avium*, and *Mycobacterium intracellulare*: IS900, IS901, and IS1141

IS900 was isolated from a *M. paratuberculosis* DNA library (Green et al., 1989). This IS sequence is 1,451 bp long and does not exhibit inverted repeats at its extremities or direct repeats flanking the element as repetitions of the target sequence. One major open reading frame was found. It shows similarities with the potential transposases of IS110 and IS116 insertion elements from *Streptomyces* spp. (Bruton and Chater, 1987; Leskiw et al., 1990). This ORF has been expressed in *E. coli* under the control of the TAC promoter, confirming that this ORF does encode a polypeptide (Tizard et al., 1992). Significant production of this protein could open the door to in vitro

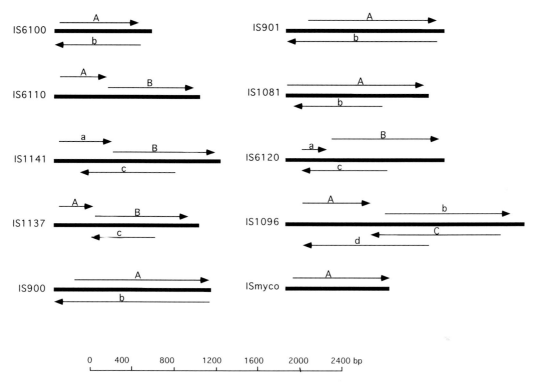

Figure 2. Main ORFs of mycobacterial insertion sequences. Capital letters indicate the putative transposases of the IS. In the elements of the IS*3* family (i.e., IS*6110*, IS*1137*, and IS*1141*), the transposase is possibly the result of a fusion of ORFA and ORFB. In the case of IS*1096*, ORFA encodes the putative resolvase, and ORFC encodes a putative transposase.

studies of the transposition mechanisms. An analysis of the sequences surrounding different copies of IS*900* has demonstrated similarities in the insertion sites of this element. These insertion sites share a consensus sequence: $CATGN_{(4-6)}$*CNCCTT (the asterisk corresponds to the insertion site). As a consequence, transposition mediated by this element is probably not random. Accordingly, no major polymorphism has been found in the location of this element in all *M. paratuberculosis* strains so far analyzed.

Analysis of the sequence upstream of an IS*900* element has revealed the presence of a promoter that drives expression of an ORF, ORF2, located on the strand complementary to that encoding the potential transposase (Murray et al., 1992). A sequence similar to a Shine-Dalgarno consensus, AAGGAG, precedes the IS*900* sequence. This sequence is homologous to the complementary sequence of the published consensus for the IS*900* insertion sites. Therefore, upon integration of IS*900* at some sites, ORF2 can be expressed under the control of an external promoter; a Shine-Dalgarno sequence possibly associated with such a promoter belongs to the consensus insertion site of IS*900*. However, the role of ORF2 is still unknown.

Transposition mediated by IS*900* was demonstrated by constructing an artificial transposon consisting of a kanamycin-resistant gene flanked by two IS*900* elements. This artificial transposon was cloned onto a vector that does not replicate in mycobacteria and was transformed into *M. smegmatis* by electroporation. A number of transformant clones resistant to kanamycin correspond to replicative transposition events (England et al., 1991).

IS901, which was found in *M. avium* strains (Kunze et al., 1991), is a sequence similar to IS900. IS901 was not found in *M. avium* isolates from AIDS patients or in strains from the environment. In contrast, this sequence was found in 48 of 55 strains isolated from infected birds. Kunze et al. (1991) hypothesize that this sequence is associated with the virulent phenotype of the strains.

IS901 possesses characteristics similar to those of IS900, i.e., a large ORF and the absence of inverted repeats at the ends of the elements and of direct repeats flanking the element. A consensus for an insertion similar to that found for IS900 was proposed: $CATN_{(7)}$*TTCCNTTC. These elements show sequences and characteristics similar to those of IS110, IS116, and IS117, which were isolated from *Streptomyces* species; IS1000, isolated from *Thermus thermophilus*; and IS492, isolated from *Pseudomonas atlantica* (Bruton and Chater, 1987; Leskiw et al., 1990; Henderson et al., 1990; Ashby and Bergquist, 1990; Barlett and Silverman, 1989). Alignment of the putative transposase of the element of this family is shown in Kunze et al. (1991). IS110, IS117, and IS1000 carry inverted repeats at their extremities and exhibit direct repeats flanking the elements. These characteristics are absent in IS116, IS900, IS901, and IS402. The mechanism of transposition of these last four elements may be different in the steps of DNA recognition and cleavage of the target sites.

IS1141 has been included recently in the GenBank database by Via and Falkinham (1993). This sequence, isolated from *Mycobacterium intracellulare*, is 1,588 bp long and contains 23-bp inverted repeats at its extremities. Sequence similarities to IS3 family elements are observed at the level of its putative transposase. This sequence is implicated in colonial variation.

ISs in *M. tuberculosis* Complex: IS6110, IS1081, and a New IS-Like Sequence

IS6110 and IS986 are two virtually identical IS elements initially sequenced by different groups (Thierry et al., 1990a, b; McAdam et al., 1990) and are now both referred to as IS6110. This sequence is found in the large majority of *M. tuberculosis* strains in a variable number of copies and at different locations. Although some strains, mainly from Asia, possess only one copy of this element, most strains investigated to date have between 5 and 20 copies (only four isolates from Vietnam were shown to lack this element [Yuen et al., 1993]). IS6110 is found in a variable number of copies and at different loci in the genomes of *M. tuberculosis* strains. Locations of these copies in the genomes are different in epidemiologically unrelated isolates, and this characteristic is effectively utilized for the typing of *M. tuberculosis* strains and in studies of tuberculosis transmission (see chapter 33). BCG (the Dutch vaccine strain) has one copy of this element, named IS987 (Hermans et al., 1991), which has also been sequenced. In addition to the 3-bp target site repeat, this element is surrounded by 20 additional direct repeat sequences, of 36 bp each. Hybridization with the direct repeat sequences showed that most *M. tuberculosis* strains also have an IS6110 copy at this same site. IS6110 is similar to elements of the IS3 family, which is the most frequently represented group, encompassing 25% of all ISs isolated. IS6110 is 1,361 bp long and contains 28-bp imperfect repeats at its extremities and 3-bp direct repeats that probably result from a duplication of the target sequence during transposition. These features are characteristic of IS3 elements. Like these elements, IS6110 contains two ORFs. The largest is similar to the IS3 family transposases. An alignment of IS3 family element transposases including mycobacterial sequences and two other IS sequences, IS3 and

IS*3411*, is shown in Fig. 3. As demonstrated for IS*911* and IS*150*, the synthesis of the IS*6110* transposase could involve a frameshifting, resulting in a fusion of the ORFA and ORFB polypeptides (Chandler and Fayet, 1993). A potential signal for ribosome slippage, TTTAAAG, is located before the end of ORFA in IS*6110*. IS*6110* and the other elements of the IS*3* family have features in common with retroviruses, including a potential −1 frameshift resulting in the production of a fusion-active protein and amino acid sequence homologies (Fayet et al., 1990).

Analysis of the regions surrounding all the IS*6110* sequences of one *M. tuberculosis* strain containing four copies has shown that all these sequences are surrounded by a different 3-bp repeat, suggesting that insertion of all IS*6110* copies in this strain were the result of random transposition events. One copy was found in the region with direct repeat sequences at the same location as the single copy found in the Dutch BCG strain (Mendiola et al., 1992). Other mycobacteria harbor IS*3* family elements. Such ISs were found in *Mycobacterium gordonae* (Hermans, personal communication), *M. smegmatis* (namely, IS*1137* [Garcia et al., submitted, discussed below]), and *M. intracellulare* (IS*1141*).

Another IS specific to *M. tuberculosis* complex, IS*1081*, was found in all strains of these species in five or six copies. In contrast to IS*6110*, no major polymorphism in the locations of this element was found in the various strains. IS*1081* is 1,324 bp long with 15-bp inverted repeats at the ends, and it contains a large ORF (Collins and Stephens, 1991). It is similar to IS*256*, IS*406*, IS*T2*, ISR*m3*, and IS*6120*. This last sequence (IS*6120*) was isolated from *M. smegmatis* (Guilhot et al., 1992a). Alignments of the putative transposases are shown in Fig. 4. Flanking sequences have been determined for one IS*1081* copy. They are similar to the target sequences of IS*900* and IS*116*. This suggests that as observed

for these elements, IS*1081* might insert at specific sites. This is in accordance with the absence of polymorphism in the locations of this sequence.

A new IS-like sequence was recently isolated from *M. tuberculosis*. It is 968 bp long with 17-bp inverted repeats (with one mismatch) at its extremities. This sequence is flanked by 4-bp direct repeats. Only one copy was detected in all *M. tuberculosis* complex strains (Mariani et al., 1993). Although transposition of this element has not yet been demonstrated, similarities to other ISs have been observed. Together with IS*427* and IS*869* from *Agrobacterium tumefaciens*, IS*402* from *Pseudomonas cepacia*, Tn*4811* from *Streptomyces lividans*, and ISR*m4* from *Rhizobium meliloti*, these sequences form a previously unrecognized family of transposable elements (Mariani et al., 1993).

ISs in *M. smegmatis*: IS*6120*, IS*1096*, and IS*1137*

IS*6120* was isolated from *M. smegmatis* by using a transposon trap system similar to that described for the isolation of *Streptomyces* transposon IS*493* (Solenberg and Burgett, 1989). A shuttle plasmid carrying an apramycin resistance gene controlled by cI, the lambda phage repressor, was replicated in *M. smegmatis* and then transferred into *E. coli*. Strains resistant to the antibiotic might correspond to cI inactivations. Such an event could be the consequence of insertion of mobile elements into this gene during replication in *M. smegmatis*. The sequence of the cI gene from plasmids extracted from *E. coli* apramycin-resistant strains revealed the presence of the same insertion sequence at different sites with no sequence similarity (Guilhot et al., 1992a). This suggests that transposition of this element occurs randomly. This element was named IS*6120*. It is 1,486 bp long and possesses 24-bp imperfect terminal repeats. A duplication of 9 bp flanks the element. On

```
            1                                                        50
       is3b ........MK YVFIEKHQAE FSIKAMCRVL R.....VARS GWY..TWCQR
    is3411b .........M MPLLDKLREQ YGVGPLCSEL H.....IAPS TYY..HCQQQ
is6110/986b .......... .......M P.....IAPS TYY..D....
    is1137b MEFITTHQHM RVGVDGLK.. WGVESMCAVL SEYGVTIAPS TYY..AHRAR
    is1141b ........VS DAAISELAPK IGVRNACDAV G.....VAQA SYYRRHRKAR
  Consensus ---------- ---------- --V---C--L ------IA-S -YY------

            51                                                       100
       is3b RT...RISTR QQFRQHC... ....DSVVLA AFTRSKQRYG APRLTDELRA
    is3411b RHHPDKRSAR AQRDDWL... ....KKQIQR VYDENHKVYG VRKVWRQLLR
is6110/986b .HINREPSRR ELRDGEL... ....KEHISR VHAANYGVYG ARKVWLTLNR
    is1137b QRLESRLGRC AGDRCDL... ....GSFANR ..RVLYRVLG ARKTWIVLRT
    is1141b HRSGRRRSRT PTGCSRVHCP AAERAAILNE LHSERFIDTS PTEVWATLLD
  Consensus -------S-R ------L--- -------I-- --------YG -R-VW--L--

            101                                                      150
       is3b QG.YPFNVKT VAASLRRQGL RAKASR.KFS PVSYRAHGLP .VSENLLEQD
    is3411b EG.IRVARCT VARLMAVMGL AG.VLRGKKV RTTISRKAVA ..AGHRVNRQ
is6110/986b EG.IEVARCT VERLMTKLGL SG.TTRGKAR RTTIADPATA R.PADLVQRR
    is1137b NG.IDVSRCV VERVMREMGW RGACKLPCGC TTTVADPGMT DCSPGSVRRN
    is1141b EGRYLGSIST FYRLLRQAGE SRERRRQATH PAT....... ......VKPE
  Consensus -G-I-V-R-T V-RLM--MGL -----R-K-- --T------- ------V---

            151                                                      200
       is3b FYASGPNQKW AGDITYLRTP E..GWLYLAV VIDLWSRAVI GWSMSPRMTA
    is3411b FVAERPDQLW VADFTYVSTW R..GFVYVAF IIDVFAGYIV GWRVSSSMET
is6110/986b FGPPAPNRLW VADLTYVSTW A..GFAYVAF VTDAYARRIL GWRVASTMAT
    is1137b FVAGAPDQLW VADFTYCRTR A..AGRYTAF VTDVYARKIV GWKVATEMTQ
    is1141b LVAFEPNQVW SWDITKLRGP AKWSWYYLYV ILDIFSRYVV GWMVASRESA
  Consensus F-A--P-Q-W --DFTYV-T- ---GF-Y-A- I-DVF---IV GW-----M--

            201                                                      250
       is3b QLACDALQMA LWRRKRPR.. ...NVIVHTD RGGQYCSADY QAQLKRHNLR
    is3411b TFVLDALEQA LWTRRPSG.. ....TVHHSD KGSQYVSLAY TQRLKEAGLL
is6110/986b SMVLDAIEQA IWTRQQEGVL DLKDVIHHTD RGSQYTSIRF SERLAEAGIQ
    is1137b KLVTDATDHA IDTRKRSGAA SLDSLIHHSD AGSQYT.... ..RSRSPNVW
    is1141b ALA....EVL IRQTCAKQDI GRDRLTIHAD RGSSMTSKPV AFLLADLGVT
  Consensus -L--DALE-A -W-R------ -----IHH-D -GSQY-S--Y ---L---G--

            251                                                      300
       is3b GSMSAKGCCY DNACVESFFH SLKVECIHGE H.FISREIMR ATVFNYIECD
    is3411b ASTGSTGDSY DNAMAESING LYKAEVIHR. KSWKNRAEVE LATLTWVD.W
is6110/986b PSVGAVGSSY DNALAETING LYKTELIKPG KPWRSIEDVE LATARWVD.W
    is1137b PLRGSVGDSF DNALAESVNS SYKTELIDRQ PLYPGATELA LGTAEWVA.F
    is1141b QSHSRPHVSD DNPFSEAQFK TLKYRPDFPD R.FDSIEAAR RHCQIFFG.W
  Consensus -S----G-SY DNA--ES--- --K-E-I--- -----R-E-- -----WVD-W

            301                                                      350
       is3b YNRWRRHSWC GGLSPEQFEN K..NLA.... .......... ..........
    is3411b YNNRRLLERL GHTPPAEAEZ .......... .......... ..........
is6110/986b FNHRRLYQYC GDVPPVELEA AYYAQRQRPA AG........ ..........
    is1137b YNRQRPNGYC RTZ....... .......... .......... ..........
    is1141b YNDEHRHTGL GLHVPADVHY GTAAIIRDKR AGVLDAAYAA HPERFVQKPP
  Consensus YN--R---R- G---P-E--- ---------- ---------- ----------

            351            373
       is3b .......... .......... ...
    is3411b .......... .......... ...
is6110/986b .......... .......... ...
    is1137b .......... .......... ...
    is1141b EPPKLPSGSW INKPDDTEEA IQ*
  Consensus ---------- ---------- ---
```

the basis of DNA sequence similarities, IS6120 belongs to a previously unrecognized family containing IS1081, IS256, IS406, IST2, and ISRm3 (Fig. 4). The sequence of IS6120 shows three ORFs. Similarities are observed between the largest ORFs (Guilhot et al., 1992a).

Another element was isolated as an insert in a lacZ gene that was integrated into the chromosome of M. smegmatis for use as a reporter gene. At a low frequency, white colonies resulting from insertion of an element at various locations in the lacZ gene were isolated (Cirillo et al., 1991). This element was named IS1096; it is 2,260 bp long and carries imperfect 26-bp repeats at its extremities. An 8-bp direct repeat likely corresponding to the target flanks the element. Eight different insertions into the lacZ gene were identified, suggesting that transposition occurs randomly. This element is specific to M. smegmatis. It is present in 8 to 16 copies, with a high polymorphism of location. Two major ORFs were found. The large one exhibits slight similarities to transposon Tn3926 and to IS1001 (Cirillo et al., 1991; van der Zee et al., 1993).

The third IS that was isolated from M. smegmatis is IS1137 (Garcia et al., submitted). It possesses homologies with IS3 family elements. This sequence is 1,364 bp long and exhibits characteristics of other IS3 family elements, a 28-bp imperfect inverted repeat at the extremities, 3-bp direct repeats flanking the element, and two ORFs that could encode a transposase after frameshifting. IS1137 is found only in M. smegmatis strains and in Mycobacterium chitae.

Transposon Tn610

Transposon Tn610 was isolated during the search for antibiotic resistance genes in a M. fortuitum strain exhibiting various antibiotic modifying enzyme activities (Martín et al., 1990). This transposon contains a sulfonamide resistance gene (sul) and a truncated site-specific integrase, int, flanked by two insertion sequences, which were both named IS6100. This central DNA fragment is nearly identical to a homologous region found in the elements related to the Tn21 transposon. Other elements of the Tn21 family harbor additional resistance genes between the integrase and the sul gene (Wohlleben et al., 1989). Thus, the fragment carried by Tn610 might have derived from an ancient transposon carrying a single antibiotic resistance gene (sul). Following successive selections in the presence of various antibiotics, the different elements of the Tn21 family may then have acquired different cassettes containing antibiotic resistance genes by means of a site-specific recombination mediated by the integrase carried by the Tn21 family elements. These elements are responsible for many nosocomial infections with antibiotic-resistant strains.

The IS6100 sequences that flank the sul and int genes are identical. The sequence IS6100 shows similarities to elements of the IS6 family (Martín et al., 1990). Like these elements, it transposes by a replicative process that leads to the formation of cointegrates. Analysis of several target sites did not reveal specificity for insertion. Transposition was demonstrated by replacing the sulfonamide resistance gene with a kanamycin resistance gene. The recombinant transposon was cloned on a nonreplicative

Figure 3. Alignment of the ORFBs of IS6110, IS1137, IS1141, IS3, and IS3411. This alignment was realized by using the Higgins and Sharp (1989) method (PILEUP; GCG, University of Wisconsin). Highly conserved amino acids related to retroviral integrase are underlined. The consensus is indicated when the amino acid is conserved in at least three sequences.

```
           1                                                  50
tnpis6120  .......... .......... .......... .......... ..........
 tnpist2   .......... .......... .......... .......... ..........
tnpis1081  MILRNDQQKS IEGNDAMTSS HL.IDTEQLL ADQLAQASPD L..LRGLLST
tnpis256   .......... ......MTQV HFTLKSEEIQ SIIEYSVKDD V..SKNILTT
tnpis406   .......... .........M AMRVETNPLE AAYAALLENG LDGAGEALRI
tnpisRm3   .......... .......... .MAIEKELLD QLLAGRDPSE VFGKDGLLDD
Consensus  ---------- ---------- ---------- ---------- -------L--

           51                                                 100
tnpis6120  .......... .......... .......... .......... ..........
 tnpist2   .......... .......... .......... .......... ..........
tnpis1081  FIAAL....M GAEADALCGA GYRERSDERS NQRNGYRHRD FDTRAATIDV
tnpis256   VFNQL....M ENQRTEYIQA KEYERTENRQ SQRNGYYERS FTTRVGTLEL
tnpis406   LVNEA....A KIERSAFLGA RPYERTETRR DYANGFKPKT VLTRHGELTF
tnpisRm3   LKKALSERIL NAELDDHLDV ERLE..GGPA NRRNGSSKKT VLTGTSKMTL
Consensus  ---------- ---------- ---E------ ---NG----- --T-------

           101                                                150
tnpis6120  .......... .......... .....MSEVL PLLYLHGLSS NDFTPALEQF
 tnpist2   .......... .......... .......... .......... ..MQEALSIL
tnpis1081  AIPKLRQGSY FPDWLLQRRK RAERALTSVV ATCYLLGVST RRMERLVETL
tnpis256   KVPRTRDGHF SPT.VFERYQ RNEKALMASM LEMYVSGVST RKVSKIVEEL
tnpis406   QVPQVRSSDF YPS.ALEKGT RTDQAVNLAL AEMYVQGVST RRVIDVLQRL
tnpisRm3   TIPRDRAGTF DPK.LIARYQ RRFPDFDDKI ISMYARGMTV REIQGHLEEL
Consensus  --P--R---F -P-------- R----L---- --MY--G-S- R-----LE-L

           151                                                200
tnpis6120  LGSGA.GLSA STITRLTAQW QDEARAFGAR DLSATDYVYL WVDGIHLKVR
 tnpist2   LGDEAKGLSP AVLGRLKAEW AQEYAHWQRR SYRKALCLLV GRRYLYEPPC
tnpis1081  GVT...KLSK SQVSIMAKEL DEAVEAFRTR PLDAGPYTFL AADALVLKVR
tnpis256   CGK...SVSK SFVSSLTEQL EPMVNEWQNR LLSEKNYPYL MTDVLYIKVR
tnpis406   LGPEI.SLSS AQVSRAAAKL DEGLRAWRER PLGETPYLFL ..DARYEKVR
tnpisRm3   YG..I.DVSP DLISAVTDTV LEAVGEWQNR PL.ELCYPLV FFDAIRVKIR
Consensus  -G-----LS- --VS-L---- -E----W--R -L----Y--L --D----KVR

           201                                                250
tnpis6120  LDQEKL..CL LVMLGVRADG RKELVAITDG YRESAESWAD LLRDCKRRGM
 tnpist2   GEDPRI..CL LVIIGVTAEG KKELVMVSDG LRESKASWLE ILRDLQARGL
tnpis1081  EAGRVVGVHT LIATGVNAEG YREILGIQVT SAEDGAGWLA FFRDLVARGL
tnpis256   EENRVLSKSC HIAIGITKDG DREIIGFMIQ SGESEETWTT FFEYLKERGL
tnpis406   LEGRIVDCAV LIAVGIEASG KRRVLGCEVA TSEAEINWRR FLESLLARGL
tnpisRm3   DEGFVRNKAV YVALAVLADG SKEILGLWIE QTEGAKFWLR VMNELKNRGC
Consensus  -E--V----- L-A-GV-ADG --EI-G---- --E----W-- FL-DL--RGL

           251                                                300
tnpis6120  .TAPVLAIGD GALGFWKAVR EVFPATKEQR CWFHKQANVL A.ALPKSAHP
 tnpist2   ETAPLLAIGD GAMGFWAALD EAYPETGQQR CWVHKTANIL N.ELPKAQQS
tnpis1081  S.GVALVTSD AHAGLVAAIG ATLPAAAWQR CRTHYAANLM A.ATPKPSWP
tnpis256   Q.GTELVISD AHKGLVSAIR KSFTNVSWQR CQVHFLRNIF T.TIPKKNSK
tnpis406   K.GVTLIIAD DHAGLKAARR AVLPSVPWQR CQFHLQQNAG ALTTRQEARK
tnpisRm3   Q.DILIAVVD GLKGFPEAIT AVFPQTIVQT CIVHLIRHSL EF.VSYKDRR
Consensus  -----L-I-D ---G---AI- --FP----QR C--HL--N-L ----PK----

           301                                                350
tnpis6120  SALAAIKEIY NAEDIDKAQI AVKAFEADFG A....KYPKA VAKITDDLDV
 tnpist2   KAKAALQEIW MAANRQAAEK ALDVFVRNYQ A....KYPKA VAKLEKDRAE
tnpis1081  WVRTLLHSIY DQPDAESVVA QYDRVLDALT D....KLPAV AEHLDTARTD
tnpis256   SFREAVKGIF KFTDINLARE AKNRLIHDYI DQ..PKYSKA CASLDDGFED
tnpis406   TVAAQMRAIF NAPD....RT EAERLLKAAL TLWCKEHPKL AEWAETAIPE
tnpisRm3   TVVPALRAIY RARDAEAGLK ALEAFEEGYW GQ...KYPAI AQSWRRNWEH
Consensus  ----AL--IY -A-D------ A---F---Y- -----KYPK- -------R--
```

```
           351                                                          400
tnpis6120  LLEFYKYPAE HWIHLRTTNP IESTFATVRL RTKVTKGPGS RAAGLAMAYK
tnpist2    LLAFYDFPAE HWRHIRTTNA IESTFATVRH RTTRTKNCVS RSSFLGLGFK
tnpis1081  LLAFTAFPKQ IWRQIWSNNP QERLNREVRR RTDVVGIFPD RASIIRLVGA
tnpis256   AFQYT.VQGN SHNRLKSTNL IERLNQEVRR REKIIRIFPN QTSANRLIGA
tnpis406   SLTVFDFPAA HRIRLRTTNG LERINRELRR RTRVASIFPN PDSCLRLVSA
tnpisRm3   VVPFFAFPEG VRRIIYTTNA IEALNSKLRR AVRSRGHFPG DEAAMKLLYL
Consensus  -L-F--FP-- -W---RTTN- IE--N--VRR RT-V---FP- --S-L-L---

           401                                                          450
tnpis6120  LIDAAAARWR AVNAPHLVAL VRAGAVFHKG RLLERPTDIT PPTSPSDGGQ
tnpist2    MLQQAEKRWI GIYAPEKVLQ LFAGVKFIDG ....IPANLT LPDDQQTAAZ
tnpis1081  VLAEQHDEWI .EGRRYLGLE VLTRARAALT STEEPAKQQT TNTPALTTZ.
tnpis256   VLMDLHDEWI YSSRKYINFD K*........ .......... ..........
tnpis406   LLAELDDEWM .TGKVYLNFN P*........ .......... ..........
tnpisRm3   VLNNAAEQWK RAPREWVEAK TQFAVIFGER FFN*...... ..........
Consensus  -L----D-W- -----Y---- ---------- ---------- ----------

           451
tnpis6120  HAGTEVAZ
tnpist2    ........
tnpis1081  ........
tnpis256   ........
tnpis406   ........
tnpisRm3   ........
Consensus  --------
```

Figure 4. Alignment of the putative transposases of IS*6120*, IS*1081*, IS*T2*, IS*256*, IS*Rm3*, and IS*406*. This alignment was realized by using the Higgins and Sharp (1989) method (PILEUP; GCG, University of Wisconsin). The consensus is indicated when the amino acid is conserved in at least three sequences.

plasmid and transferred into *M. smegmatis* by electroporation. Colonies having a kanamycin resistance phenotype corresponded to transposition events (Martín et al., 1990). Each copy of the IS*6100* part of Tn*610* can promote transposition, but this does not rule out the possibility that two copies of IS*6100* are involved in the transposition process (our unpublished results). As observed for other elements of the IS6 family, the transposition product is a cointegrate. The analysis of cointegrates isolated from different *M. smegmatis* strains each having one copy of Tn*610* inserted has demonstrated that transposition occurs randomly with no specific target sites.

IS*6100* was found only in the *M. fortuitum* strain containing the transposon but not in any other *M. fortuitum* strains or in other mycobacterial species. A recent study (Negoro et al., 1993) has shown that IS*6100* is found as multiple copies in plasmids encoding enzymes responsible for ny-

lon degradation by *Flavobacterium* species. Therefore, the IS*6100* sequence that is present in a single *M. fortuitum* species might have been transferred from other species in the environment such as *Flavobacterium* spp.

UTILIZATION OF TRANSPOSABLE ELEMENTS FOR GENETIC STUDIES IN MYCOBACTERIA

Transposable elements from mycobacteria are potentially useful sources of genetic tools for the manipulation of mycobacteria in general and for the investigation of virulence mechanisms in pathogenic strains. Ten IS-like sequences have been isolated in the last few years (Table 1). Of these elements, three (IS*900*, IS*6110*, and IS*6120*) have been shown to transpose in *M. smegmatis* (England et al., 1991; Fomukong and Dale, 1993; Guilhot et al., 1992a), and two

(IS6100 and IS1096) are able to transpose in M. smegmatis and BCG (Martín et al., 1990; Guilhot, unpublished results; Cirillo et al., 1991; McAdam, unpublished data). Useful insertion elements for the development of mutagenesis systems for mycobacteria should (i) have a high frequency of transposition, (ii) not be present in the bacterial strains in which they will be used for mutagenesis, and (iii) exhibit no site or regional specificity. IS900 has a strong specificity of insertion (Green et al., 1989) and consequently cannot be used for insertional mutagenesis. Nevertheless, this mobile element could be useful for integrating single copies of a gene into a mycobacterial chromosome. This possible use will be discussed below. IS6110 seems to transpose randomly but is present in the chromosomes of mycobacteria from the M. tuberculosis complex. This limits the use of this element in M. tuberculosis and M. bovis, but it could be useful in mutagenizing other species such as M. avium or M. paratuberculosis. Finally, three of the five elements transposing in M. smegmatis (IS6110, IS6120, and IS1096) exhibit the features required for a transposon mutagenesis system. Derivatives of these IS-carrying reporter genes will be useful for genetic studies of mycobacteria. The use of a reporter gene would allow investigation of the expression of mycobacterial genes in vivo. Some of the genes currently used in E. coli (de Lorenzo et al., 1990; Berg et al., 1989), such as lacZ, xylE, or phoA, are functional in mycobacteria (Murray et al., 1992; Stover et al., 1991; Timm et al., submitted; Guilhot, unpublished data). Transposons with reporter genes such as phoA will allow the screening of genes coding for exported proteins. Some of these proteins may play a role in protection, since proteins from culture supernatants have recently been shown to be protective in animal models (see chapter 8 in this volume). It will therefore be very important to isolate these genes and study their regulation. Mutants that do not express these exported proteins

will provide information on their in vivo role.

Several methods may be considered for delivery of these transposons. The first consists of the utilization of a plasmid unable to replicate in the species of interest. The suicide vector carrying a transposon with a selectable marker is transferred into bacterial cells. The transformants are selected for the phenotype encoded for by the transposon. Since the vector is not maintained, the transposition events can be selected. This strategy has been used extensively in bacteria other than E. coli in which the suicide vector can be transferred very efficiently either by transformation or by conjugation (for a review, see Berg et al., 1989). In mycobacteria, nonreplicative vectors have been used to demonstrate the transposition of IS6100, IS900, and IS6110 in M. smegmatis. Unfortunately, delivery of transposons by electroporation with these vectors is very inefficient.

An alternative way to deliver a transposon is to utilize conditionally replicative plasmids. The vector carrying the transposon is propagated in the species of interest under permissive conditions. Then, the vector is eliminated by shifting the culture to nonpermissive conditions. This strategy is independent of transformation frequency. A large number of conditional plasmids have been described for E. coli and other bacteria. This strategy has been used in streptomyces to develop different transposon mutagenesis systems (Solenberg and Baltz, 1991; Hahn et al., 1991; McHenney and Baltz, 1991; Sohaskey et al., 1992). In 1992, a thermosensitive shuttle plasmid that replicates at 30°C but not at 39°C in mycobacteria was isolated after random in vitro mutagenesis of an E. coli-mycobacterium shuttle plasmid (Guilhot et al., 1992b). This plasmid contains the pUC18 and pAL5000 replicons with thermosensitive mutations for replication. Transposition of Tn611, a derivative of Tn610 carrying a kanamycin resistance gene, with such a plasmid as a delivery system allowed the construction of

Table 2. Auxotrophic types

Transposon library	No. of clones tested	% of auxotrophs	Auxotroph phenotypes identified[a]
1	4,500	0.4	5 Leu⁻, 3 His⁻, 3 Val⁻ Ile⁻, 3 Ade⁻, 1 Ala⁻, 1 Trp⁻
2	4,200	0.1	2 His⁻, 1 Asp⁻
3	7,300	0.2	5 Vit⁻, 3 Leu⁻, 3 Pur⁻, 2 Trp⁻, 2 His⁻, 1 Ade⁻, 2 ND
4	10,700	0.4	8 Pur⁻, 7 Leu⁻, 6 Vit⁻, 2 Tyr⁻, 2 His⁻, 1 Asp⁻, 1 Pyr⁻, 1 Met⁻, 1 Phe⁻, 1 Thr⁻, 1 Trp⁻, 1 Ade⁻, 9 ND

[a] Abbreviations: Ade, adenine; Ala, alanine; Asp, aspartic acid; His, histidine; Ile, isoleucine; Leu, leucine; Met, methionine; Phe, phenylalanine; Pur, purines (adenine and guanine); Pyr, pyrimidines (thymidine, uracil, and cytidine); Thr, threonine; Trp, tryptophan; Tyr, tyrosine; Val, valine; Vit, vitamins (biotin, thiamine, inositol, calcium panthothene, pyridoxine); ND, undetermined requirement.

representative *M. smegmatis* insertion libraries. Of 30,000 insertion mutants tested, 80 auxotrophic mutants with 15 different phenotypes were obtained (Table 2) (Guilhot et al., 1994). Thus, this system is fully functional in *M. smegmatis*, yielding large numbers of insertional mutations, and could be adapted for slow-growing mycobacteria.

Another strategy for transposon delivery is the use of bacteriophage as a vector. In *E. coli*, lambda derivatives are powerful tools for the isolation of Tn*10* and Tn*5* insertions. The lambda derivatives are crippled by nonsense mutations in phage replication genes (nonsense suppressors to propagate the bacteriophages are required), by mutation in the repressor, and often by deletion of the phage integration system. These vehicles are then unable to replicate, kill, or integrate into the host cell to allow the selection of transposition events (Kleckner et al., 1991). Similar constructs can be envisaged with the temperate L5 mycobacteriophage, whose entire sequence is known (Hatfull and Sarkis, 1993). This bacteriophage has a broad host range and can infect *M. smegmatis*, BCG, or *M. tuberculosis*. A derivative of L5 could then be used to deliver transposons in various species of mycobacteria.

Most of the tools described here are under investigation, with the ultimate goal being efficient mutagenesis of *M. tuberculosis*. However, transposon mutagenesis remains to be perfected in this species. Auxotrophs would be useful as new vaccine candidates and for the development of strategies for the investigation of in vivo growth (Mahan et al., 1993). The mutants affected in virulence genes could be selected as clones that are unable to survive in macrophages by using a method similar to that initially used for salmonellae (Fields et al., 1986). These experiments will provide us with a set of mutants that will be further analyzed in animal models. Study of virulence genes will help in defining new drugs able to inhibit the synthesis or the functioning of the products of these genes. Studies of the mutants in animal models will provide us with information concerning their residual virulence and protective effect. This could be the basis for the construction of new vaccines against tuberculosis.

Transposons can be used for purposes other than mutagenesis. Genes of interest can be cloned in them and introduced as a stable single copy into the chromosome. This procedure will be extremely useful for genetic complementation studies and for the cloning of protective antigens in BCG vaccine strains, with the aim of developing polyvalent vaccines. In streptomycetes, IS*117* has been used to develop an integration system (Keiser and Hopwood, 1991). For mycobacteria, IS*900* or IS*901*, both of which are homologous to IS*117*, could be used in the same way.

Another application of mobile elements utilizes their specificity. Most ISs isolated from mycobacteria are species specific. Primers have been derived from these sequences and used for identification in polymerase chain reaction tests. ISs that are present in multiple copies permit results with enhanced sensitivity.

Acknowledgment. This work was supported in part by an E.C. grant (contract BIO2-CT92-0520).

REFERENCES

Ashby, M. K., and P. L. Bergquist. 1990. Cloning and sequence of IS1000, a putative insertion sequence from *Thermus thermophilus* HB8. *Plasmid* **24**:1–11.

Baltz, R. H., D. R. Hahn, M. A. McHenney, and P. J. Solenberg. 1992. Transposition of Tn5096 and related transposons in *Streptomyces species. Gene* **115**:61–65.

Barlett, D. H., and M. Silverman. 1989. Nucleotide sequence of IS492, a novel insertion sequence causing variation in extracellular polysaccharide production in the marine bacterium *Pseudomonas atlantica. J. Bacteriol.* **171**:1763–1766.

Beattie, D. T., M. J. Mahan, and J. J. Mekalanos. 1993. Repressor binding to a regulatory site in the DNA coding sequence is sufficient to confer transcriptional regulation of the *vir*-repressed genes (*vrg* genes) in *Bordetella pertussis. J. Bacteriol.* **175**:519–527.

Berg, C. M., D. E. Berg, and E. A. Groisman. 1989. Transposable elements and the genetic engineering of bacteria, p. 879–925. *In* D. E. Berg and M. M. Howe (ed.), *Mobile DNA.* American Society for Microbiology, Washington, D.C.

Berg, D. E., and M. M. Howe (ed.). 1989. *Mobile DNA.* American Society for Microbiology, Washington, D.C.

Bernardini, M. L., J. Mounier, H. d'Hauteville, M. Coquis-Rondon, and P. J. Sansonetti. 1989. Identification of *icsA*, a plasmid locus of *Shigella flexneri* that governs bacterial intra- and intercellular spread through interaction with F-actin. *Proc. Natl. Acad. Sci. USA* **86**:3867–3871.

Bielecki, J., P. Youngman, P. Connelly, and D. A. Portnoï. 1990. *Bacillus subtilis* expressing a haemolysin gene from *Listeria monocytogenes* can grow in mammalian cells. *Nature* (London) **345**:175–176.

Bruton, C. J., and K. F. Chater. 1987. Nucleotide sequence of IS110, an insertion sequence of *Streptomyces coelicolor* A3(2). *Nucleic Acids Res.* **15**:7053–7065.

Chandler, M., and O. Fayet. 1993. Translational frameshifting in the control of transposition in bacteria. *Mol. Microbiol.* **7**:497–503.

Charlier, D., J. Piette, and N. Glansdorff. 1982. IS3 can function as a mobile promoter in *E. coli. Nucleic Acids Res.* **10**:5935–5948.

Cirillo, J. D., R. G. Barletta, B. R. Bloom, and W. R. Jacobs, Jr. 1991. A novel transposon trap for mycobacteria: isolation and characterization of IS1096. *J. Bacteriol.* **173**:7772–7780.

Clark-Curtiss, J. E., W. R. Jacobs, M. A. Docherty, L. R. Ritchie, and R. Curtiss III. 1985. Molecular analysis of DNA and construction of genomic libraries of *Mycobacterium leprae. J. Bacteriol.* **161**:1093–1102.

Collins, D. M., and D. M. Stephens. 1991. Identification of an insertion sequence, IS1081, in *Mycobacterium bovis. FEMS Microbiol. Lett.* **83**:11–16.

Cossart, P., M. F. Vicente, J. Mengaud, F. Baquero, J. C. Perez-Diaz, and P. Berche. 1989. Listeriolysin O is essential for virulence of *Listeria monocytogenes*: direct evidence obtained by gene complementation. *Infect. Immun.* **57**:3629–3636.

de Lorenzo, V., M. Herrero, U. Jakubzik, and K. N. Timmis. 1990. Mini-Tn5 transposon derivatives for insertion mutagenesis, promoter probing, and chromosomal insertion of cloned DNA in gram-negative eubacteria. *J. Bacteriol.* **172**:6568–6572.

Eisenach, K. D., J. T. Crawford, and J. H. Bates. 1988. Repetitive DNA sequences as probes for *Mycobacterium tuberculosis. J. Clin. Microbiol.* **26**:2240–2245.

England, P. M., Q. Wall, and J. McFadden. 1991. IS900-promoted stable integration of a foreign gene into mycobacteria. *Mol. Microbiol.* **5**:2047–2052.

Fayet, O., P. Ramond, P. Polard, M. F. Frère, and M. Chandler. 1990. Functional similarities between retroviruses and the IS3 family of bacterial insertion sequences? *Mol. Microbiol.* **4**:1771–1777.

Fields, P. I., E. A. Groisman, and F. Heffron. 1989. A *Salmonella* locus that controls resistance to microbicidal proteins from phagocytic cells. *Science* **243**:1059–1062.

Fields, P. I., R. V. Swanson, C. G. Haidaris, and F. Heffron. 1986. Mutants of *Salmonella typhimurium* that cannot survive within the macrophage are avirulent. *Proc. Natl. Acad. Sci. USA* **83**:5189–5193.

Fomukong, N. G., and J. W. Dale. 1993. Transpositional activity of IS986 in *Mycobacterium smegmatis. Gene* **130**:99–105.

Gaillard, J. L., P. Berche, and P. Sansonetti. 1986. Transposon mutagenesis as a tool to study the role of hemolysin in the virulence of *Listeria monocytogenes. Infect. Immun.* **52**:50–55.

Galas, D. J., and M. Chandler. 1989. Bacterial insertion sequences, p. 109–162. *In* D. E. Berg and M. M. Howe (ed.), *Mobile DNA.* American Society for Microbiology, Washington, D.C.

Garcia, M. J., C. Guilhot, R. Lathigra, C. Menendez, P. Domenech, C. Moreno, B. Gicquel, and C. Martin. Insertion sequence IS1137, a new IS3 family element from *Mycobacterium smegmatis*. Submitted for publication.

Gicquel, B., and W. R. Jacobs, Jr. Personal communication.

Gormley, E. P., and J. Davies. 1991. Transfer of plasmid RSF1010 by conjugation from *Escherichia coli* to *Streptomyces lividans* and *Mycobacterium smegmatis*. *J. Bacteriol.* 173:6705–6708.

Green, E. P., M. L. V. Tizard, M. T. Moss, J. Thompson, D. J. Winterbourne, J. McFadden, and J. Hermon-Taylor. 1989. Sequence and characteristics of IS*900*, an insertion element identified in a human Crohn's disease isolate of *Mycobacterium paratuberculosis*. *Nucleic Acids Res.* 17:9063–9073.

Guilhot, C. Unpublished data.

Guilhot, C., B. Gicquel, J. Davies, and C. Martín. 1992a. Isolation and analysis of IS*6120*, a new insertion sequence from *Mycobacterium smegmatis*. *Mol. Microbiol.* 6:107–113.

Guilhot, C., B. Gicquel, and C. Martin. 1992b. Temperature-sensitive mutants of the *Mycobacterium* plasmid pAL5000. *FEMS Microbiol. Lett.* 98:181–186.

Guilhot, C., I. Otal, I. van Rompaey, C. Martin, and B. Gicquel. 1994. Efficient transposition in mycobacteria: construction of *M. smegmatis* insertional mutant libraries. *J. Bacteriol.* 176:535–539.

Hahn, D. R., P. J. Solenberg, and R. H. Baltz. 1991. Tn*5099*, a *xylE* promoter probe transposon for *Streptomyces* spp. *J. Bacteriol.* 173:5573–5577.

Hatfull, G. F., and G. J. Sarkis. 1993. DNA sequence, structure and gene expression of mycobacteriophage L5: a phage system for mycobacterial genetics. *Mol. Microbiol.* 7:395–405.

Henderson, D. J., D. F. Brolle, T. Kieser, R. E. Melton, and D. A. Hopwood. 1990. Transposition of IS*117* (the *Streptomyces coelicolor* A3(2) mini-circle) to and from a cloned target site and into secondary chromosomal sites. *Mol. Gen. Genet.* 224:65–71.

Hermans, P. W. Personal communication.

Hermans, P. W., D. van Soolingen, E. M. Bik, P. E. W. de Haas, J. W. Dale, and J. D. A. van Embden. 1991. Insertion element IS*987* from *Mycobacterium bovis* BCG is located in a hot-spot integration region for insertion elements in *Mycobacterium tuberculosis* complex strains. *Infect. Immun.* 59:2695–2705.

Higgins, D. G., and P. M. Sharp. 1989. Fast and sensitive multiple sequence alignments on a microcomputer. *Comput. Appl. Biosci.* 5:151–153.

Hoiseth, S. K., and B. A. D. Stocker. 1981. Aromatic-dependent *Salmonella typhimurium* are non-virulent and effective as live vaccines. *Nature* (London) 291:238–239.

Isberg, R. R., and S. Falkow. 1985. A single genetic locus encoded by *Yersinia pseudotuberculosis* permits invasion of cultured animal cells by *Escherichia coli* K-12. *Nature* (London) 317:262–264.

Kalpana, G., B. Bloom, and W. R. Jacobs. 1991. Insertional mutagenesis and illegitimate recombination in mycobacteria. *Proc. Natl. Acad. Sci. USA* 88:5433–5437.

Keiser, T., and D. A. Hopwood. 1991. Genetic manipulation of *Streptomyces*: integrating vectors and gene replacement. *Methods Enzymol.* 204:430–458.

Keiser, T., M. T. Moss, J. W. Dale, and D. A. Hopwood. 1986. Cloning and expression of *Mycobacterium bovis* BCG DNA in "*Streptomyces lividans.*" *J. Bacteriol.* 168:72–80.

Kleckner, N., J. Bender, and S. Gottesman. 1991. Uses of transposons with emphasis on Tn*10*. *Methods Enzymol.* 204:139–180.

Kleckner, N., J. Roth, and D. Botstein. 1977. Genetic engineering *in vivo* using translocatable drug-resistance elements. New methods in bacterial genetics. *J. Mol. Biol.* 116:125–159.

Kunze, Z. M., S. Wall, R. Appelberg, M. T. Silva, F. Portaels, and J. J. McFadden. 1991. IS*901*, a new member of a widespread class of atypical insertion sequences, is associated with pathogenicity in *Mycobacterium avium*. *Mol. Microbiol.* 5:2265–2272.

Leskiw, B. K., M. Mevarech, L. S. Barritt, S. E. Jensen, D. J. Henderson, D. A. Hopwood, C. J. Bruton, and K. F. Chater. 1990. Discovery of an insertion sequence, IS*116*, from *Streptomyces clavuligerus* and its relatedness to other transposable elements from actinomycetes. *J. Gen. Microbiol.* 136:1251–1258.

Mahan, M. J., J. M. Slauch, and J. J. Mekalanos. 1993. Selection of bacterial virulence genes that are specifically induced in host tissues. *Science* 259:686–688.

Manoil, C., J. J. Mekalanos, and J. Beckwith. 1990. Alkaline phosphatase fusions: sensors of subcellular location. *J. Bacteriol.* 172:515–518.

Mariani, F., E. Piccolella, R. Colizzi, R. Rappuoli, and R. Gross. 1993. Characterization of an IS-like element from *Mycobacterium tuberculosis*. *J. Gen. Microbiol.* 139:1767–1772.

Martín, C., P. Mazodier, M. V. Mediola, B. Gicquel, T. Smokvina, C. J. Thompson, and J. Davies. 1991. Site-specific integration of the *Streptomyces* plasmid pSAM2 in *Mycobacterium smegmatis*. *Mol. Microbiol.* 5:2499–2502.

Martín, C., J. Timm, J. Rauzier, R. Gomez-Lus, J. Davies, and B. Gicquel. 1990. Transposition of an antibiotic resistance element in mycobacteria. *Nature* (London) 345:739–743.

McAdam, R. A. Personal communication.

McAdam, R. A. Unpublished data.

McAdam, R. A., P. W. M. Hermans, D. van Soolingen, Z. F. Zainuddin, D. Catty, J. D. A. van Embden, and J. W. Dale. 1990. Characterization of a *Mycobacterium tuberculosis* insertion sequence belonging to the IS*3* family. *Mol. Microbiol.* 4:1607–1613.

McClintock, B. 1956a. Intranuclear systems controlling gene action and mutation. *Brookhaven Symp. Biol.* 8:58–74.

McClintock, B. 1956b. Controlling elements and the gene. *Cold Spring Harbor Symp. Quant. Biol.* **21**: 197–216.

McFadden, J. J., P. D. Butcher, R. J. Chiodini, and J. Hermon-Taylor. 1987a. Use of DNA probes to distinguish between mycobacterial species: Crohn's disease-isolated mycobacteria are identical to *Mycobacterium paratuberculosis*. *J. Clin. Microbiol.* **25**:796–801.

McFadden, J. J., P. D. Butcher, J. Thompson, R. Chiodini, and J. Hermon-Taylor. 1987b. The use of DNA probes identifying restriction-fragment-length polymorphisms to examine the *Mycobacterium avium* complex. *Mol. Microbiol.* **1**:283–291.

McHenney, M. A., and R. H. Baltz. 1991. Transposition of Tn*5096* from a temperature-sensitive transducible plasmid in *Streptomyces* spp. *J. Bacteriol.* **173**:5578–5581.

Mendiola, M. V., C. Martin, I. Otal, and B. Gicquel. 1992. Analysis of the regions responsible for IS*6110* RFLPs in a single *Mycobacterium tuberculosis* strain. *Res. Microbiol.* **143**:767–772.

Mizuuchi, K. 1992. Transpositional recombination: mechanistic insights from studies of Mu and other elements. *Annu. Rev. Biochem.* **61**:1011–1051.

Murphy, E. 1989. Transposable elements in gram-positive bacteria, p. 269–288. *In* D. E. Berg and M. M. Howe (ed.), *Mobile DNA*. American Society for Microbiology, Washington, D.C.

Murray, A., N. Winter, M. Lagranderie, D. F. Hill, J. Rauzier, J. Timm, C. Leclerc, K. M. Moriarty, M. Georghiu, and B. Gicquel. 1992. Expression of *Escherichia coli* b-galactosidase in *Mycobacterium bovis* BCG using an expression system isolated from *Mycobacterium paratuberculosis* which induced humoral and cellular immune responses. *Mol. Microbiol.* **6**:3331–3342.

Negoro, S., K. Kato, T. Yomo, and I. Urabe. 1993. Structural analysis of nylon oligomer degradative plasmid pOAD2. *International Conference on Pseudomonas '93*.

Petit, M.-A., C. Bruand, L. Jannière, and S. D. Ehrlich. 1990. Tn*10*-derived transposons active in *Bacillus subtilis*. *J. Bacteriol.* **172**:6736–6740.

Shapiro, J. A. 1979. Molecular model for the transposition and replication of bacteriophage Mu and other transposable elements. *Proc. Natl. Acad. Sci. USA* **76**:1933–1937.

Sohaskey, C. D., H. Im, and A. T. Schauer. 1992. Construction and application of plasmid- and transposon-based promoter-probe vectors for *Streptomyces* spp. that employ a *Vibrio harveyi* luciferase reporter casette. *J. Bacteriol.* **174**:367–376.

Solenberg, P., and R. H. Baltz. 1991. Transposition of Tn*5096* and other IS*493* derivatives in *Streptomyces griseofuscus*. *J. Bacteriol.* **173**:1096–1104.

Solenberg, P., and S. G. Burgett. 1989. Method for selection of transposable DNA and characterization of a new insertion sequence, IS*493*, from *Streptomyces lividans*. *J. Bacteriol.* **171**:4807–4813.

Stover, C. K., et al. 1991. New use of BCG for recombinant vaccines. *Nature* (London) **351**:456–460.

Taylor, R. K., C. Manoil, and J. J. Mekalanos. 1989. Broad-host-range vectors for delivery of Tn*phoA*: use in genetic analysis of secreted virulence determinants of *Vibrio cholerae*. *J. Bacteriol.* **171**:1870–1878.

Thierry, D., A. Brisson-Noël, V. Vincent-Lévy-Frébault, S. Nguyen, J. L. Guesdon, and B. Gicquel. 1990a. Characterization of a *Mycobacterium tuberculosis* insertion sequence, IS*6110*, and its application in diagnosis. *J. Clin. Microbiol.* **28**:2668–2673.

Thierry, D., M. D. Cave, K. D. Eisenach, J. T. Crawford, J. H. Bates, B. Gicquel, and J. L. Guesdon. 1990b. IS6110, an IS-like element of Mycobacterium tuberculosis. *Nucleic Acids Res.* **18**:188.

Thole, J. R., H. G. Dauwerse, P. K. Das, D. G. Groothuis, L. M. Schouls, and J. D. A. van Embden. 1985. Cloning of *Mycobacterium bovis* BCG DNA and expression of antigens in *Escherichia coli*. *Infect. Immun.* **50**:800–806.

Timm, J., et al. Transcription and expression analysis, using *lacZ* and *phoA* gene fusions, of Mycobacterium fortuitum β-lactamase genes cloned from a natural isolate and a high-level β-lactamase producer. Submitted for publication.

Tizard, M. V. L., M. T. Moss, J. D. Sanderson, B. M. Austen, and J. Hermon-Taylor. 1992. p43, the protein product of the atypical insertion sequence IS*900*, is expressed in *Mycobacterium paratuberculosis*. *J. Gen. Microbiol.* **138**:1729–1736.

van der Zee, A., C. Agterberg, M. van Agterveld, M. Peeters, and F. R. Mooi. 1993. Characterization of IS*1001*, an insertion sequence element of *Bordetella parapertussis*. *J. Bacteriol.* **175**:141–147.

Via, L. E., and J. O. Falkinham III. 1993. GenBank, L10239.

Weiss, A. A., and S. Falkow. 1983. The use of molecular techniques to study microbial determinants of pathogenicity. *Phil. Trans. R. Soc. London Ser. B* **303**:219–225.

Wohlleben, W., W. Arnold, L. Bissonnette, A. Pelletier, A. Tanguay, P. H. Roy, G. C. Gamboa, G. F. Barry, E. Aubert, J. Davies, and S. K. Kagan. 1989. On the evolution of Tn*21*-like multiresistance transposons: sequence analysis of the gene (*aacC1*) for gentamicin acetyltransferase-3-I(AAC(3)-I), another member of the Tn*21*-based expression cassette. *Mol. Gen. Genet.* **217**:202–208.

Yuen, L. K., B. C. Ross, K. M. Jackson, and B. Dwyer. 1993. Characterization of *Mycobacterium tuberculosis* strains from Vietnamese patients by Southern blot hybridization. *J. Clin. Microbiol.* **131**:1615–1618.

Tuberculosis: Pathogenesis, Protection, and Control
Edited by Barry R. Bloom
© 1994 American Society for Microbiology, Washington, DC 20005

Chapter 15

Homologous Recombination, DNA Repair, and Mycobacterial *recA* Genes

M. Joseph Colston and Elaine O. Davis

Bacterial responses to DNA damage are highly conserved. One system, the SOS response, involves the coordinately induced expression of over 20 genes through a common regulatory mechanism. The RecA protein, found in most bacteria, plays a central role in the regulation of the SOS response (Fig. 1). In addition to its regulatory function, this protein also mediates genetic recombination and DNA repair. Virtually nothing is known about these systems in mycobacteria. However, since some mycobacteria are intracellular pathogens and many of the mechanisms involved in macrophage killing of such pathogens require the production of DNA-damaging agents such as peroxide and nitric oxide, DNA repair mechanisms are likely to be particularly important for mycobacterial survival. In addition, homologous genetic recombination, a process mediated by RecA, is an important technique for the genetic manipulation of bacteria and could play an important role in our understanding of gene function. In this chapter we discuss the mechanisms involved in homologous recombination and DNA repair, what is known about these systems in mycobacteria, and recent information on the unusual structure of the *recA* gene in the pathogenic mycobacteria.

ROLE OF RecA IN DNA REPAIR AND RECOMBINATION

SOS Response

The RecA protein of *Escherichia coli* induces the expression of several genes in response to DNA damage, resulting in an increase in cell survival (for a review, see Walker [1984]). The induction is brought about by cleavage of a repressor protein, LexA. Activation of RecA by exposure to DNA damage triggers autocatalytic cleavage of the LexA repressor, resulting in increased expression of over 20 genes, including the *recA* gene itself (Fig. 2). This is known as the SOS response, and it results in increased synthesis of proteins involved in DNA repair, DNA synthesis, homologous and site-specific recombination, and cell division. The outcome of these inducible activities is an increase in the cell's ability to survive the potentially harmful effects of a wide variety of agents that interrupt the structure or normal replication of DNA. Nothing is known about the SOS response in mycobacteria, although the

M. Joseph Colston and Elaine O. Davis • National Institute for Medical Research, Mill Hill, London NW7 1AA, England.

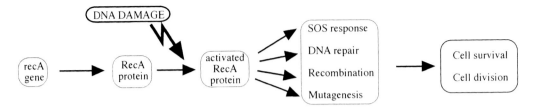

Figure 1. Multiple roles of the RecA protein following exposure to DNA damage.

gene encoding *Mycobacterium tuberculosis* RecA (Davis et al., 1991, 1992; also see below) has been identified.

Functional Role of RecA in DNA Repair

In addition to its role in the regulation of the SOS response, RecA is also involved in repair activities themselves by means of its activity as a recombinational exchange protein. The active form of RecA in this reaction is a nucleoprotein filament formed by the polymerization of RecA around single-stranded ends of DNA. The preferential binding of RecA filaments to single-stranded DNA therefore serves to target the protein to sites of damage (for a review, see Miller and Kokjohn [1990]).

RecA in Recombination

Homologous genetic recombination involves the exchange of homologous regions of DNA between two DNA molecules. The RecA protein is essential for homologous recombination in *E. coli*. It promotes homologous pairing and strand exchange in an ATP-dependent reaction (Fig. 3). This process is a complex, multistep series of events involving binding of RecA to single-stranded DNA, pairing of the RecA–single-stranded-DNA complex with double-stranded DNA, alignment of homologous sequences on the single-stranded and double-stranded DNAs, DNA strand exchange requiring local denaturation of the double-stranded DNA and exchange of the corresponding single strands of DNA, and branch migration resulting in the complete exchange of DNA single strands (reviewed in Kowalczykowski, 1987). Subsequent separation of the recombinant strands requires the nucleolytic action of RuvA, RuvB, and RuvC proteins. In addition to involving strand exchange, recombination can also involve nonreciprocal exchange between nearby sites on the chromosome;

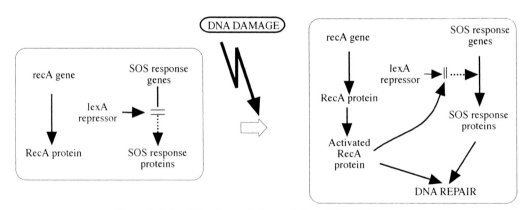

Figure 2. Role of RecA protein in regulation of the SOS response.

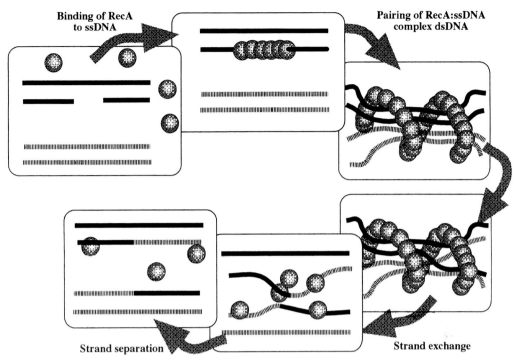

Figure 3. Role of RecA protein in homologous recombination. ds, double stranded; ss, single stranded.

such an event is termed "gene conversion." In nature, recombination is a source of genetic variation. In the laboratory, homologous recombination is a powerful technique for investigating gene function.

Homologous Recombination as a Laboratory Tool

Homologous recombination provides a tool for creating and characterizing specific mutations. "Gene knockout" techniques, for example, involve the replacement of a wild-type gene with a disrupted, nonfunctional mutated gene (Fig. 4). Such targeted mutations are widely used to study gene function in mammalian, eukaryotic, and bacterial cells (Capecchi, 1989). A typical example of such an approach in *E. coli* is provided by the *murI* gene (Baliko and Venetianer, 1993). An open reading frame of unknown function was inactivated by disruption with a kanamycin resistance gene. The corresponding chromosomal open reading frame was replaced by the inactivated gene by homologous recombination; by complementing the cells carrying the mutation with plasmids bearing the wild-type gene, it was possible to study the

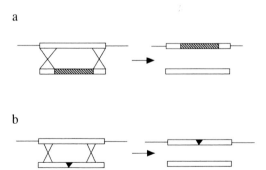

Figure 4. Homologous recombination as a laboratory tool. Homologous recombination can be used to delete genes by incorporating a disrupted gene, in which case the sequence used to disrupt the gene is usually an antibiotic resistance gene or other selectable marker (a), or to introduce a mutation by double crossover events (b).

function of the unknown open reading frame and identify its involvement in the synthesis of cell wall components. Another example is the production of recombination-deficient *Streptococcus gordonii* by disruption of the *recA* gene itself, using homologous recombination (Vickerman et al., 1993). The ability to precisely and permanently modify genes in this way would make a major contribution to the genetic analysis of mycobacteria.

Homologous Recombination in Mycobacteria

Homologous recombination has been reported in the fast-growing mycobacterium *Mycobacterium smegmatis* (Husson et al., 1990). The *pyrF* gene was disrupted by the aminoglycoside phosphotransferase gene (*aph*), and this construct was incorporated into a vector that also contained the *E. coli* origin of replication and the β-lactamase gene. The vector was capable of autonomous replication in *E. coli* and integrated into the *M. smegmatis* genome at the *pyrF* locus by homologous recombination. However, there have been no reports of successful homologous recombination in the slow-growing mycobacteria, such as *M. tuberculosis*. In one series of experiments (Kalpana et al., 1991), the DNA sequence that complemented a methionine auxotrophic mutation was disrupted and introduced into BCG and *M. tuberculosis*. Homologous recombination involving a double crossover between the chromosomal locus and the inactivated, extrachromosomal DNA should have resulted in disruption of the *met* gene. In fact, random, illegitimate recombination of the DNA fragments occurred at such a high frequency that it was impossible to ascertain whether homologous recombination had occurred. Such illegitimate recombination is uncommon in bacteria and yeast cells but is seen at high frequency in many eukaryotic and mammalian cells.

MYCOBACTERIAL *recA* GENES AND PROTEIN SPLICING

The Unusual Structure of the *M. tuberculosis recA* Gene

The *recA* gene of *M. tuberculosis* has been cloned and characterized (Davis et al., 1991), The characterization of mycobacterial RecA was important for a number of reasons. First, the development of recombination-deficient mutants of mycobacteria by inactivation of RecA function could provide strains in which cloned DNA would be more stably maintained. Second, pathogenic mycobacteria reside within macrophages, where they are exposed to a variety of DNA damage-inducing agents as part of the macrophage defense mechanism. In *E. coli*, resistance to hydrogen peroxide correlates with the *recA* genotype (Carlsson and Carpenter, 1980), while SOS induction, requiring RecA activity, increases the virulence of *Erwinia carotovora* (McEvoy et al., 1990). Thus, it is possible that the *recA* gene of pathogenic mycobacteria plays a similar role in virulence. Finally, the apparent difficulty in achieving homologous recombination in *M. tuberculosis* and BCG (Kalpana et al., 1991; also see above) suggests that RecA activity might be abnormal in these organisms.

The *recA* genes from more than 20 species of bacteria have been isolated and characterized (Miller and Kokjohn, 1990). All show a striking degree of similarity, which is consistent with the strong selective pressure imposed on a multifunctional molecule that is central to survival. Surprisingly, however, the *M. tuberculosis recA* gene was found to be unlike any other (Davis et al., 1991). Although the gene produces a protein of approximately 40 kDa, similar in size to the other RecA proteins, the gene has the coding capacity for a protein of 85 kDa. Furthermore, the predicted *M. tuberculosis* RecA protein sequence is homologous with RecA se-

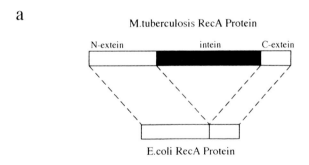

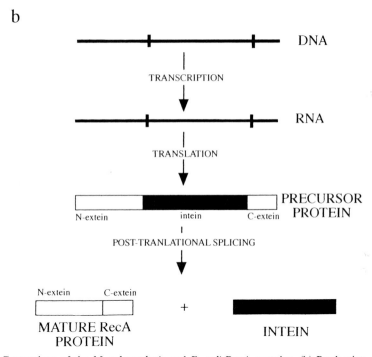

Figure 5. (a) Comparison of the *M. tuberculosis* and *E. coli* RecA proteins. (b) Production of the mature *M. tuberculosis* protein by posttranslational splicing.

quences from other bacteria, but this homology is not dispersed; rather, it is localized to the first 254 and last 96 amino acids, with the intervening 440 amino acids being unrelated (Fig. 5a).

It was subsequently shown (Davis et al., 1992) that the *M. tuberculosis* RecA protein is produced from an 85-kDa precursor protein that undergoes an unusual splicing reaction by which the 47-kDa spacer protein is excised and the N- and C-terminal domains are religated to form the mature RecA protein (Fig. 5b). This process, known as protein splicing, is an extremely unusual postranslational mechanism for the formation of a mature protein.

Protein Splicing in Other Genes

At the time that splicing of the *M. tuberculosis* RecA protein was discovered, only one other example of this mechanism of protein maturation was known. This was in VMA1, a vacuolar proton pump ATPase, of the yeast *Saccharomyces cerevisiae* (Kane et al., 1990). Subsequently, a number of other examples have emerged (for a summary, see Fig. 6), and a nomenclature has been proposed in which the protein intron is known as the "intein" and the N- and C-terminal domains are known as the "exteins" by analogy with the introns and exons of spliced mRNA (Perler et al., in press). Although on the whole the sequences of the inteins are quite different,

they have a number of features in common. In each case there is an identifiable pair of dodecamer sequences with some similarity to the LAGLIDADG motif found in some endonucleases; indeed, the yeast VMA1 and the archaebacterial inteins each have endonuclease activity, recognizing and cutting the DNA sequence into which its coding DNA is inserted (Gimble and Thorner, 1992; Perler et al., 1992). The *M. tuberculosis* intein also has endonuclease activity (Davis, unpublished data). In addition, there are conserved features around the splice sites that appear to be characteristic of this type of element (Fig. 6).

recA of *Mycobacterium leprae* Also Contains an Intein, or Protein Intron

When DNA encoding the intein of *M. tuberculosis* was used to probe genomic DNA of a range of mycobacteria, no hybridization was obtained (Davis, unpublished data). However, when the *M. leprae* recA gene was cloned and sequenced, it, too, was found to contain an intein-like sequence with homology to other *recA* genes that was split by a stretch of unrelated sequence and a well-conserved hexapeptide motif previously identified at the C termini of inteins (Davis et al., 1991; Hodges et al., 1992) (Fig. 6). However the predicted size of the *M. leprae* intein was 41 kDa, compared to 47 kDa for the *M. tuberculosis* intein. Moreover, apart from the C-terminal motif, the sequences of the two inteins were quite dissimilar (only 27% identity), whereas the RecA-like sequences were very homologous, with 92% of amino acids being identical. Most surprising, however, were the facts that the two inteins were located at different positions within the RecA coding sequences in the two species and that the nucleotide sequences into which they inserted were quite different (Fig. 7). Thus, the *recA* genes of the two species have independently acquired inteins.

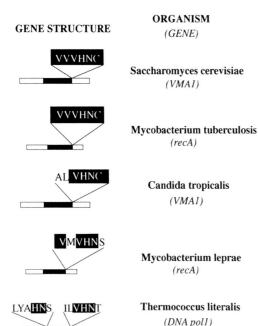

GENE STRUCTURE	ORGANISM (GENE)
VVVHNC	Saccharomyces cerevisiae (*VMA1*)
VVVHNC	Mycobacterium tuberculosis (*recA*)
AL VHNC	Candida tropicalis (*VMA1*)
VMVHNS	Mycobacterium leprae (*recA*)
LYAHNS IIVHNT	Thermococcus literalis (*DNA pol1*)

Figure 6. Known examples of inteins (protein introns). The conserved hexapeptide motif at the intein-C-extein junction is shown in expanded form, with identity to the *Saccharomyces cerevisiae VMA1* sequence highlighted. The *Candida tropicalis VMA1* gene is described in Gu et al., 1993.

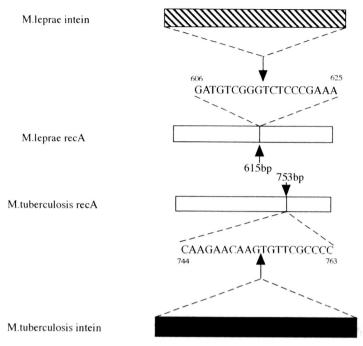

Figure 7. Schematic comparison of the *M. leprae* and *M. tuberculosis recA* gene structures. The insertion sites of the inteins within the genes are shown along with the nucleotide sequences flanking the insertion sites. The sizes, sequences, and insertion sites of the two inteins differ, indicating the independent origins of the two genetic elements.

recA Gene Structures of Other Mycobacteria

The presence of independently acquired inteins in the *recA* genes of the two major mycobacterial pathogens raised the possibility that they are a common feature of mycobacterial *recA* genes. In order to investigate this possibility, a further 14 species of mycobacteria, representing various groups, were analyzed by polymerase chain reaction (PCR), using primers based on sequences conserved between *M. leprae* and *M. tuberculosis* from near the two ends of the *recA* genes; the presence of an intein would be inferred from the size of the PCR product (Fig. 8a). In fact, only *M. leprae* and members of the *M. tuberculosis* complex contain inteins in the *recA* gene, with all other species giving products that indicate a normal *recA* locus (Fig. 8b). All clinical isolates of *M. tuberculosis* tested

did appear to contain an intein (Fig. 8c). It therefore appears that protein splicing in the production of RecA is confined to *M. leprae* and members of the *M. tuberculosis* complex.

Has There Been Selection for Protein Splicing in *recA* Genes of Pathogenic Mycobacteria?

The fact that the two major pathogenic mycobacteria have independently acquired protein splicing elements in *recA* suggests that there has been selection for splicing RecA proteins in the two species. Previously, it had been thought that inteins were an example of selfish genetic elements with no functional consequences for the host organism. If selection has occurred, then the intein itself, or the RecA splicing mechanism, must play a role in host survival. Until assays for RecA activity in mycobac-

a

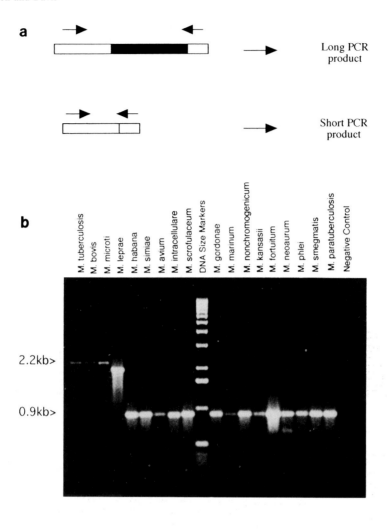

b

c

M.tb clinical isolates

teria have been developed, it will be difficult to determine what such a role might be. One clue, however, may be provided by the fact that splicing of *M. leprae* RecA may be conditionally regulated (Davis et al., in press). Since we know that the presence of unspliced RecA blocks RecA activity (Davis et al., 1992), this splicing could represent a novel, posttranslational mechanism for regulating RecA function.

SUMMARY

Virtually nothing is known about DNA repair mechanisms and genetic recombination in mycobacteria, although it seems likely that such mechanisms have played an important role in the evolution of the intracellular pathogenic species. Experiments to demonstrate homologous recombination in mycobacteria have been successful in the fast-growing species *M. smegmatis* but not in *M. tuberculosis* or BCG. This is of some practical importance, since homologous recombination is a powerful laboratory technique for the analysis of gene function and could be important in furthering our understanding of mycobacterial genetics.

The key enzyme involved in recombination and repair in bacteria is the RecA protein. Recent studies of the *recA* genes of mycobacteria have indicated that the major human pathogens *M. tuberculosis* and *M. leprae* have an unusual *recA* structure, suggesting that these organisms may have evolved novel mechanisms for dealing with DNA damage and effecting genetic recombination. As yet, we do not know the role that the unusual mechanism for RecA production plays; the development of assays for RecA activity in mycobacteria, particularly *M. tuberculosis*, should enable us to investigate the biological role of RecA splicing. Such studies, particularly the development of assays for homologous recombination, should also enable us to develop new and powerful approaches for the genetic manipulation of mycobacteria.

Acknowledgments. We thank Steve Sedgwick for his helpful comments and critical reading of the manuscript. We also thank Peter Jenner, Pat Brooks, Harry Thangaraj, and Steve Sedgwick for their important contributions on the structure of mycobacterial *recA* genes.

REFERENCES

Baliko, G., and P. Venetianer. 1993. An *Escherichia coli* gene in search of a function: phenotypic effects of the gene recently identified as *murI*. *J. Bacteriol.* **175:**6571–6577.

Capecchi, M. R. 1989. Altering the genome by homologous recombination. *Science* **244:**1288–1292.

Carlsson, J., and V. S. Carpenter. 1980. The *recA*[+] gene product is more important than catalase and superoxide dismutase in protecting *Escherichia coli* against hydrogen peroxide toxicity. *J. Bacteriol.* **142:**319–321.

Davis, E. O. Unpublished data.

Davis, E. O., P. J. Jenner, P. C. Brooks, M. J. Colston, and S. G. Sedgwick. 1992. Protein splicing in the maturation of *M. tuberculosis* RecA protein: a mechanism for tolerating a novel class of intervening sequences. *Cell* **71:**201–210.

Davis, E. O., S. G. Sedgwick, and M. J. Colston. 1991. Novel structure of the *recA* locus of *Mycobacterium tuberculosis* implies processing of gene product. *J. Bacteriol.* **173:**5653–5662.

Davis, E. O., H. S. Thangaraj, P. C. Brooks, and M. J. Colston. Evidence of selection for protein introns in the RecAs of pathogenic mycobacteria. *EMBO J.*, in press.

Gimble, F. S., and J. Thorner. 1992. Homing of a DNA endonuclease gene by meiotic gene conversion in *Saccharomyces cerevisiae*. *Nature* (London) **357:**301–306.

Gu, H. H., J. Xu, M. Gallagher, and G. E. Dean. 1993. Peptide splicing in the vacuolar ATPase subunit A

Figure 8. Inteins are confined to the *recA* genes of *M. leprae* and the *M. tuberculosis* complex. Primers to conserved sequences were used in PCR reactions on genomic DNA from the various mycobacteria. (a) The size of the PCR product reveals the presence or absence of an intein. (b) Only *M. leprae*, *M. tuberculosis*, BCG, and *M. microti* show long products. (c) All clinical isolates of *M. tuberculosis* had an intein. The primers used in panels b and c differed and hence gave products of different sizes in the two experiments.

from *Candida tropicalis. J. Biol. Chem.* **268:**7372–7381.

Hodges, R. A., F. B. Perler, C. J. Noren, and W. Jack. 1992. Protein splicing removes intevening sequences in an archaea DNA polymerase. *Nucleic Acids Res.* **20:**6153–6157.

Husson, R. N., B. E. James, and R. A. Young. 1990. Gene replacement and expression of foreign DNA in mycobacteria. *J. Bacteriol.* **172:**519–524.

Kalpana, G. V., B. R. Bloom, and W. R. Jacobs, Jr. 1991. Insertional mutagenesis and illegitimate recombination in mycobacteria. *Proc. Natl. Acad. Sci. USA* **88:**5433–5437.

Kane, P. M., C. T. Yamashiro, D. F. Wolczyk, N. Neff, M. Goebl, and T. H. Stevens. 1990. Protein splicing converts the yeast *TFP1* gene products to the 69 kd subunit of the vacuolar H$^+$-adenosine triphosphatase. *Science* **250:**651–657.

Kowalczykowski, S. C. 1987. Mechanistic aspects of the DNA strand exchange activity of *E. coli* recA protein. *Trends Biochem. Sci.* **12:**141–145.

McEvoy, J. L., H. Murata, and A. K. Chatterjee. 1990. Molecular cloning and characterization of an *Erwinia carotovora* subsp. *carotovora* pectin lyase gene that responds to DNA-damaging reagents. *J. Bacteriol.* **172:**3284–3289.

Miller, R. V., and T. A. Kokjohn. 1990. General microbiology of *recA*: environmental and evolutionary significance. *Annu. Rev. Microbiol.* **44:**365–394.

Perler, F. B., D. G. Comb, W. E. Jack, L. S. Moran, B. Qiong, R. B. Kucera, J. Brenner, B. E. Slatko, D. O. Nwankwo, S. K. Hempstead, C. K. S. Carlow, and H. Jannasch. 1992. Intervening sequences in an archaea DNA polymerase gene. *Proc. Natl. Acad. Sci. USA* **89:**5577–5581.

Perler, F. B., E. O. Davis, G. E. Dean, F. S. Gimble, W. E. Jack, N. Neff, C. J. Noren, J. Thorner, and M. Belfort. Protein splicing elements: inteins and exteins—a definition of terms and recommended nomenclature. *Nucleic Acids Res.*, in press.

Vickerman, M. M., D. G. Heath, and D. B. Clewell. 1993. Construction of recombination-deficient strains of *Streptococcus gordonii* by disruption of the *recA* gene. *J. Bacteriol.* **175:**6354–6357.

Walker, G. C. 1984. Mutagenesis and inducible responses to deoxyribonucleic acid damage in *Escherichia coli. Microbiol. Rev.* **48:**60–93.

Tuberculosis: Pathogenesis, Protection, and Control
Edited by Barry R. Bloom
© 1994 American Society for Microbiology, Washington, DC 20005

Chapter 16

Toward Mapping and Sequencing the Genome of *Mycobacterium tuberculosis*

Stewart T. Cole and Douglas R. Smith

Although there is a wealth of knowledge about the structure and organization of many bacterial chromosomes and episomes (Cole and Saint-Girons, in press; Krawiec and Riley, 1990), the study of the genome of *Mycobacterium tuberculosis* is still in its infancy. There are several reasons why this aspect of the biology of this important human pathogen has been neglected; to a great extent, the reasons result from the difficulties of working with *M. tuberculosis*. Owing to the lack of appropriate tools, classic genetic studies based on gene linkage analysis have not been undertaken. Furthermore, the slow growth rate of this mycobacterium and the significant health hazard associated with its manipulation have deterred many workers.

The advent of recombinant DNA technology in the late 1970s and the subsequent development of suitable hosts and vector systems for working with mycobacteria (Jacobs et al., 1991; Ranes et al., 1990; Rauzier et al., 1988; Snapper et al., 1988, 1990; Young et al., 1985a, b) meant that many of the difficulties encountered while working

directly with *M. tuberculosis* could be conveniently circumvented. Owing to the importance of developing an efficient protective vaccine against tuberculosis, much of the early work in molecular genetics involved screening lambda gt11 expression libraries with murine monoclonal antibodies or patient sera in the hope of finding protective antigens (Andersen et al., 1988; Young et al., 1988; Young and Cole, 1993; Young et al., 1985a, b). Subsequently, more ambitious approaches were employed to identify *M. tuberculosis* genes. These approaches took advantage of the ability of the surrogate hosts *M. smegmatis* and BCG to faithfully express cloned genes (Jacobs et al., 1991; Snapper et al., 1988; Winter et al., 1991; Young and Cole, 1993).

In the mid-1980s, as the power of new techniques such as pulsed-field gel electrophoresis (PFGE) and the polymerase chain reaction became apparent (Saiki et al., 1988; Schwartz and Cantor, 1984), the prospect of undertaking genome research directly with mycobacteria became a reality. The initial emphasis was on *M. leprae*, the etiologic agent of leprosy, and several cosmid libraries were constructed (Clark-Curtiss et al., 1985; Eiglmeier et al., 1993a, submitted). These studies culminated in the establishment of a contig map of the *M.*

Stewart T. Cole • Unité de Génétique Moléculaire Bactérienne, Institut Pasteur, 28 rue du Docteur Roux, 75724 Paris Cedex 15, France. *Douglas R. Smith* • Collaborative Research Inc., 1365 Main Street, Waltham, Massachusetts 02154.

leprae chromosome derived from sets of ordered cosmids based on both conventional and shuttle vectors (Clark-Curtiss et al., 1985; Eiglmeier et al., 1993a, submitted) and led to the identification of over 80 genetic loci.

The availability of an ordered set of clones provided ideal starting material for the systematic sequencing of the *M. leprae* genome. This work, initiated in 1991, has so far yielded over 700 kb of unique genomic sequence data (Honoré et al., 1993; Smith et al., 1993). Encouraged by the success of this project and the wealth of data that it is yielding, it was decided to extend the approach to include *M. tuberculosis*. Additional motivation for doing so was provided by the resurgence of tuberculosis in the industrialized countries as a consequence of the AIDS pandemic and the emergence of large numbers of multidrug-resistant strains (Bloom and Murray, 1992; Dooley et al., 1992; Snider and Roper, 1992). The experimental approach used to produce an integrated genetic and physical map of the *M. tuberculosis* chromosome was heavily influenced by previous work with *M. leprae*, and the strategy being employed is summarized in Fig. 1. Basically, it is hoped that a contig map will be produced by combining fingerprinting and hybridization analysis of cosmid libraries carrying large DNA fragments from the chromosome of the long-studied *M. tuberculosis* strain H37Rv. Cloned genes are being positioned by hybridization, and this information, together with knowledge of the locations of sites for rarely cutting restriction enzymes within individual clones, will allow correlation of the physical map with the contig map. Eventually, a set of selected cosmids with minimal overlaps will be subjected to multiplex sequence analysis, and the fine details of chromosome structure and organization will be deduced from the nucleotide sequence. The aims of this chapter are to present the current status of the *M. tuberculosis* genome project, to summarize

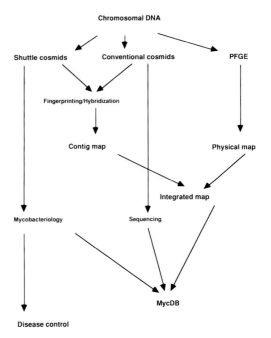

Figure 1. Integrated approach to mycobacterial genome mapping. The steps and approaches being used in analysis of the *M. tuberculosis* chromosome are shown in the form of a flow diagram. Genomic DNA is used for either PFGE analysis or cosmid cloning. The integrated map combines data from physical, contig, and gene mapping, and this map together with DNA sequences is stored in MycDB, a database dedicated to mycobacterial research.

the main findings of that project, and to discuss its potential impact on future tuberculosis research.

CHROMOSOME MAPPING BY PFGE

At the time of writing, the genome sizes of over 100 bacterial species have been established by PFGE analysis of macrorestriction fragments, and detailed physical maps of the chromosomes of 70 bacterial strains have been obtained (Cole and Saint-Girons, in press; Krawiec and Riley, 1990). As might have been expected, *M. tuberculosis* does not figure among the latter group, although several attempts have been made to estimate the size of the genome. Again, there are two reasons for this apparent lack of progress, both intimately linked to the biology of *M. tuberculosis*.

The slow growth rate of the organism can complicate the preparation of genome-sized DNA molecules, and the fact that these molecules may differ in age by several weeks means that there is significant variation in quality. In our experience, this difficulty is best overcome by using a heavy inoculum and harvesting the culture in early log phase after treatment with cycloserine (1 mg/ml for 24 h). DNA can then be prepared in agarose plugs by the standard protocol (Smith et al., 1986a), and no special modifications or additional enzymatic treatments are required. The second limitation to PFGE analysis of *M. tuberculosis* is the lack of suitable rarely cutting restriction enzymes, a constraint imposed by the dG+dC content of the chromosome, which is 66%. Generally, the genomes of microorganisms with dG+dC-rich chromosomes are readily cleaved into a limited number of fragments by restriction endonucleases with dA+dT-rich recognition sequences, as these sites are underrepresented. This is not the case with *M. tuberculosis*, since neither of the enzymes with 8-bp recognition sites, that is, *Pac*I (TTAATTAA) and *Swa*I (ATTTAAAT), cuts the chromosome, whereas all of the enzymes with 6-bp recognition sites (*Cla*I, *Hpa*I, *Nde*I, *Ssp*I, *Xba*I, etc.) yield more than 50 fragments and are thus not useful for map construction.

The most valuable enzymes are *Dra*I (TTTAAA) and *Asn*I (ATTAAT), which yield 35 and 45 fragments, respectively, although their usefulness in map construction is limited, as they generate many small fragments (<30 kb) in addition to those in the conventional PFGE resolution range (50 to 1,000 kb). It is indeed ironic to note that the chromosome of *Streptomyces lividans*, which has a similar dG+dC content but is about 8 Mb in size, has considerably fewer recognition sites for both *Asn*I and *Dra*I, i.e., only 16 and 7, respectively (Kieser et al., 1992; Leblond et al., 1993).

An estimate of the chromosome size can be obtained by summing the fragment sizes, and in both cases, this is about 4 Mb. However, until a complete map is obtained, this estimate should be treated with caution, since many fragments comigrate. PFGE maps of bacterial chromosomes are generally produced by a combination of approaches such as comparative single and double digestions, two-dimensional gel electrophoresis, indirect end labeling, or linking clone analysis. For the reasons outlined above, only the last is applicable to the *M. tuberculosis* chromosome, and thus far, 35 and 31 clones carrying independent *Asn*I and *Dra*I restriction sites, respectively, have been isolated from a cosmid library. Most of the *Dra*I linking clones have been used to identify adjacent fragments, and the chromosome can be represented as six stretches of contiguous *Dra*I fragments (Philipp et al., 1993).

PFGE Fingerprints of Mycobacterial Genomes

Different laboratory strains and clinical isolates of *M. tuberculosis* and BCG have been subjected to comparative PFGE, and in many cases, distinctive *Dra*I restriction profiles were obtained (Varnerot et al., 1992). Transposition of the insertion sequence IS*6110* (McAdam et al., 1990; Thierry et al., 1990a, b; Varnerot et al., 1992), also known as IS*986*, is believed to be responsible for these polymorphisms, as this insertion sequence element contains a unique *Dra*I site. Many copies of IS*6110* are present in *M. tuberculosis* (16 in H37Rv), but only a single copy is found in *M. bovis* (Hermans et al., 1991). Genomic fingerprints of other mycobacteria such as *M. paratuberculosis* and *M. fortuitum* have also been obtained by PFGE of *Dra*I fragments (Hector et al., 1992; Lévy-Frébault et al., 1989).

A   **B**

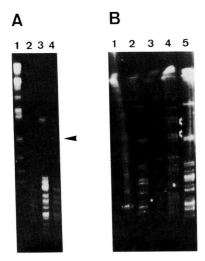

Figure 2. PFGE analysis of *M. tuberculosis* H37Rv and Ra. (A) DNA in agarose plugs from H37Ra was digested with *Asn*I (lane 2) or *Dra*I (lane 3), while H37Rv DNA was digested with *Dra*I (lane 4) and separated by field inversion gel electrophoresis as described previously (Canard and Cole, 1989). The agarose gel (1% in 0.66× Tris-borate-EDTA [TBE]) was calibrated with yeast chromosomes (lane 1) or λ concatamers (not shown) and run for 48 h at constant voltage (240 V). (B) Similar DNA samples from H37Rv were digested with *Asn*I (lane 2) and *Dra*I (lane 3), and H37Ra DNA was digested with *Asn*I (lane 4) or *Dra*I (lane 5) and separated by contour-clamped homogeneous electric field gel electrophoresis as described previously (Canard et al., 1992). The agarose gel (1.2% in 0.5× TBE) was calibrated with 1 concatamer (lane 1) and run for 50 h at constant voltage (170 V). Fragments discussed in the text are indicated by arrowheads. The black arrow indicates the 480-kb *Dra*I fragment, and the white arrows indicate 260- and 280-kb *Dra*I fragments.

A Link between Virulence and a Polymorphic *Dra*I Site?

The most striking *Dra*I polymorphism was found on comparison of the restriction profiles of the well-characterized strains of *M. tuberculosis* H37Rv and H37Ra, because the latter, an avirulent derivative of H37Rv, has apparently lost a 480-kb *Dra*I restriction fragment (Fig. 2A). As this fragment has been replaced by two novel fragments of 260 and 220 kb, it seems likely to reflect the insertion of IS*6110* into the

480-kb *Dra*I restriction fragment (Fig. 2B). Evidence against this polymorphism stemming from a chromosomal rearrangement, such as a large deletion, is provided by the identical *Asn*I restriction fragment profiles of H37Rv and H37Ra. It is tempting to attribute the attenuation of strain H37Ra to this putative insertional mutagenesis event, despite the lack of further arguments in its favor. As this explanation could provide fresh insight into the mechanisms of pathogenesis, it clearly warrants further investigation. Likewise, the availability of a genome map, coupled with PFGE analysis, will facilitate other studies aimed at dissecting mycobacterial virulence by enabling the sites of integration of transposons and phages to be rapidly localized. To further this approach, a unique *Pac*I site has been engineered into a novel transposon (Jacobs, 1993).

ORDERING CLONES COVERING THE *M. TUBERCULOSIS* GENOME

Contig Mapping Using Cosmids

As was so stunningly demonstrated by Kohara et al. (1987) for *Escherichia coli*, an ordered library of chromosomal DNA in the form of overlapping clones is an extremely valuable tool for genetic and other forms of biological research. Not only does the library represent an easily renewable resource of DNA, but it also allows instant access to given areas of the chromosome, enables genes to be mapped and identified with ease, and provides useful starting material for a genome-sequencing project.

The approach being used to construct an ordered library representing the chromosome of *M. tuberculosis* strain H37Rv involves fingerprinting and DNA hybridization analysis of two cosmid banks and assembly of the overlapping clones into contigs (Coulson et al., 1986; Sulston et al., 1988). The first library was constructed in the shuttle cosmid pYUB18 (Jacobs et al.,

1991) and, because of its versatility, will undoubtedly find many biological applications, whereas the second library is based on a novel *E. coli* cosmid, pYUB328. The chromosomal inserts carried by the latter clones can be excised by digestion with *Pac*I and are destined for systematic DNA sequence analysis. At the time of writing, over 1,500 clones have been analyzed and assembled into 15 contigs. These account for almost all of the chromosome and can be directly correlated with the physical map via the *Dra*I linking clones.

Gene Mapping

The rapid mapping of genes is achieved by hybridization of specific probes to cosmid grids, and since the distribution of cosmid clones within a contig is relatively uniform, genes can usually be positioned with a precision of 10 to 20 kb. A list of the genetic markers localized in this way and their functions is given in Table 1. A further 25 loci encoding anonymous protein antigens have also been positioned.

LARGE-SCALE GENOMIC SEQUENCING AND ITS APPLICATION TO MYCOBACTERIA

Description of the Technology

Since fall 1991, a group at Collaborative Research, Inc., has been engaged in a large-scale sequencing project to apply and improve technology for computer-assisted multiplex sequencing, a rapid DNA-sequencing approach based on sample mixing and molecular decoding by oligonucleotide hybridization (Church and Kieffer-Higgins, 1988). The current sequencing targets for this project are the genomes of two biomedically important and biologically interesting pathogens: *M. tuberculosis* and *M. leprae*. It is expected that their DNA sequences will aid in the definition of targets for rational drug design and also in the development of improved recombinant vaccines.

Multiplex sequencing (Church and Kieffer-Higgins, 1988) has received considerably less attention than the other major large-scale sequencing technologies that use automated fluorescence detection instruments (Ansorge et al., 1986; Prober et al., 1987; Smith et al., 1986b). However, with similar personnel and capital investment, the potential throughput of multiplex sequencing far exceeds that obtained with fluorescence instruments. The approach has proven robust, and the image analysis, editing, and automated sequence-reading software (Mintz et al., 1993) have improved dramatically over the past several years of development.

Significant economies of scale can be realized in multiplex sequencing projects because most of the laboratory work consists of oligonucleotide hybridization, membrane washing, and film exposure, all of which can be conveniently done in large batches by small numbers of technicians. Thus, large numbers of autoradiograms or phosphorimager screen exposures can be produced very efficiently. An overview of the sequencing approach is given in Fig. 3 and is described below.

High-purity DNA preparations are made for each cosmid to be sequenced, and a shotgun subclone library is then constructed in one of a set of 20 uniquely tagged "plex" vectors (Church and Kieffer-Higgins, 1988). Individual clones from 15 to 20 different subclone libraries (one clone from each library) are pooled, and DNA is purified from enough of these pools to guarantee final eightfold random coverage for each cosmid (typically, 10 sets of 96 pools). These samples are chemically sequenced, separated on polyacrylamide gels, and transferred onto nylon membranes by using the technique of direct transfer electrophoresis (Richterich and Church, 1993). The membranes are probed with labeled oligonucleotides to visualize sequence ladders from each subclone library individually. The membranes are

Table 1. Identities and sources of genetic markers mapped in *M. tuberculosis*[a]

Locus	Canonical cosmid	Description	Origin of probe	Source or accession no.
adh	T854	Alcohol dehydrogenase	Mb	J. Content
ahp	T183	Alkylhydroperoxide reductase	Mt	GMB
ald	T292	L-Alanine dehydrogenase	Mt	A. Andersen
aroA	T146	5-Enolpyruvylshikimate-3-P-synthase	Mt	D. B. Young
aroD	T130	Dehydroquinate synthase	Mt	D. B. Young
att-L5	T606	Putative tRNA^{Pro}; tRNA^{Gly}; attachment site for L5	Ms	M65195
attB-pSAM2	T449	Putative tRNA^{Pro}; attachment site for pSAM2	Ml	GMB
bib	T830	Biotin-binding protein	Mt	J. Dale
clpC	T485	Proteolysis regulator; chaperone	Ml	GMB
dnaA	T776	Initiation of DNA biosynthesis	Ml	H. E. Takiff
dnaJ	T369	Chaperone	Mt	D. B. Young
dnaK	T369	HSP-70; chaperone	Mt	D. B. Young
efg	T663	Elongation factor G	Ml	GMB
fbpA	T366	Fibronectin-binding protein = 85A	Mt	J. Thole
fbpB	T336	Fibronectin-binding protein = 85B	Mt	J. Thole
fbpC	T464	Fibronectin-binding protein = 85C	Mt	J. Thole
groES	T721	HSP-12; chaperone	Mt	T. Shinnick
groEL-1	T521	HSP-60; chaperone	Mt	D. B. Young
groEL-2	T721	HSP-60 homolog	Mt	GMB
gyrA	T728	DNA gyrase, A subunit	Mt	H. E. Takiff
gyrB	T416	DNA gyrase, B subunit	Mt	H. E. Takiff
hrd	T144	RNA polymerase sigma factor	Mt	S. Poulet
inhA	T20	Isoniazid resistance gene	Mt	W. R. Jacobs
katG	T116	Catalase-peroxidase	Mt	B. Heym
mtrA	T146	Response regulator	Mt	V. Deretic
oriC	T776	Origin of replication	Sc	H. Schrempf
phoS	T172	Phosphate-binding protein	Mt	D. B. Young
polA	T167	DNA polymerase I	Mt	V. Misrahi
recA	T49	Homologous recombination	Mt	M. J. Colston
recS	T252	Putative recombinase	Mt	S. Nair
regX	T449	Response regulator	Mt	M. Pallen
rpoB	T311	Beta subunit of RNA polymerase	Ml	GMB
rpoC	T663	Beta′ subunit of RNA polymerase	Ml	GMB
rpsL	T663	Ribosomal protein S12	Ml	GMB
rrn	T198	16S, 23S, and 5S rRNAs	Ml	X56657
sodA	T264	Superoxide dismutase	Ml	X16453
thyA	T31	Putative thymidylate synthetase	Mt	J. Dale
trxB	T14	Thioredoxin reductase	Ms	J. Davies
tuf	T663	Elongation factor Tu	Ml	GMB
DR-r	T684	Direct repeats flanking IS*987*	Mt	P. Hermans
IS*987*	T684	Insertion sequence	Mt	P. Hermans
IS*1081*	Several	*M. bovis* insertion sequence	Mb	GMB
IS*6110*	Many	Insertion sequence	Mt	P. Hermans

[a] Abbreviations: Ml, *M. leprae*; Mt, *M. tuberculosis*; Sc, *S. coelicolor*; Mb, *M. bovis*; Ms, *M. smegmatis*; GMB, Unité de Génétique Moléculaire Bactérienne, Institut Pasteur, Paris.

stripped and reprobed up to 40 times, providing a large number of films from each gel. The films are scanned using a CCD-based film scanner or a laser-scanning densitometer during the day, and the data are entered into computer workstations overnight, resulting in efficient use of computer time.

The digitized images thus produced are processed, and the sequences are read,

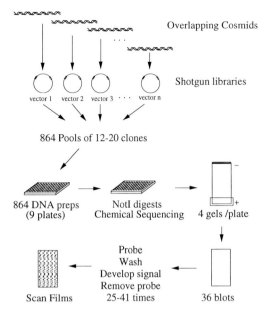

Overlapping Cosmids

Shotgun libraries

vector 1   vector 2   vector 3 · · · vector n

864 Pools of 12-20 clones

864 DNA preps
(9 plates)

NotI digests
Chemical Sequencing

4 gels /plate

Probe
Wash
Develop signal
Remove probe
25-41 times

Scan Films

36 blots

Figure 3. Schematic diagram of the multiplex cosmid sequencing process. See text for explanation.

proofread, and assembled on computer workstations using the programs REPLICA and GTAC (Mintz et al., 1993). The assembled sequences are proofread, and any ambiguous regions or regions with low coverage are resequenced by primer-directed cycled sequencing with cosmid templates.

A large amount of data is accumulated initially by shotgun sequencing of random fragments at high coverage (7- to 10-fold). This is followed by a relatively small amount of finishing that is accomplished by primer-directed cycled sequencing with cosmid templates or subclone pools. As before, data acquisition is by digital film scanning, and the sequences are reassembled and proofread in the context of the assembled shotgun sequencing data. The actual insertion/deletion error rate for the first four cosmids analyzed (GenBank accession numbers L01263, L01095, L04666, and L01536) was approximately 1.3×10^{-4} (or 1/7,500), based on frameshift analysis of 30 genes with GenBank homologies covering a total of 30.7 kb (Smith et al., 1993).

Technology Development

Technology development is focused in two areas: computational methods and sequencing biochemistry. In terms of information science, effort is concentrated on automating key steps of the data entry and sequence reading that are expected to provide a substantial increase in sequencing speed. In addition, new algorithms for sequence assembly are being developed that incorporate positional information in the starting clones to eliminate problems associated with repetitive sequences. Current biochemical method development is directed toward constructing a new and more versatile set of multiplex sequencing vectors, improving sequencing chemistry, and testing new labeling and detection methods that are amenable to automation.

Data Management and Sequence Production

Efficient data management capabilities have been developed to maintain the large amounts of data being produced in an organized and accessible format. Sequences are considered finished when both strands have been completely sequenced at an indel error rate of about 1/5,000 and when the sequence has been analyzed for genes and open reading frames. Finished sequences are submitted electronically to GenBank and a mycobacterial mapping and sequence database, MycDB (Bergh and Cole, submitted), based on the ACEDB software (Durbin and Thierry-Mieg, 1991; Dunham et al., in press).

At this writing, we have generated over 6 Mb of raw sequencing data (7- to 10-fold coverage) for 18 *M. leprae* cosmids and one *M. tuberculosis* cosmid. All of these cosmid sequences are assembled into single contigs and have been analyzed for genes and open reading frames. In addition, we have produced multiplex membranes and have begun data entry on another set of 17 cosmids. Together, the 27 *M. leprae*

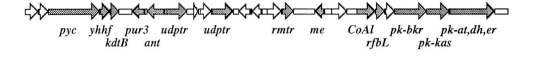

Figure 4. Map of *M. tuberculosis* cosmid TBC2. A reference scale in kilobases is given below the map. The positions and orientations of genes are indicated on the map. Shaded arrows represent genes that have homology to other genes in public databases, and open arrows represent ORFs that do not have significant homologies to any known genes. Key to gene names: *pyc*, pyruvate carboxylase; *yhhf*, 22-kDa putative cell cycle regulator; *kdtB*, homolog of a lipopolysaccharide operon gene; *pur3*, phosphoribosylglycinamide formyltransferase; *ant*, putative anion transporter; *udptr*, putative UDP-sugar transferase; *rmtr*, rRNA methyl transferase; *me*, putative methylase; *CoAl*, putative acetyl coenzyme A ligase; *rfbL*, homolog of the *V. cholerae rfbL* gene; *pk-bkr*, polyketide synthase (beta-keto reductase); *pk-kas*, polyketide synthase (ketoacyl acyl carrier protein synthase); *pk-at,dh,er*, polyketide synthase (acyl transferase, dehydratase, enoyl reductase). See text for references.

cosmids in the sequencing process are expected to cover approximately 1 Mb, or about one-third of the *M. leprae* genome.

Sequence Analysis

Primary sequence analysis is done using the large sequence analysis suite (Robison and Church, 1993). This set of programs provides a graphic representation of each cosmid, with the locations of putative reading frames, corresponding homologies to sequences in GenBank, and an indicator of organism-specific dicodon usage for each frame (a useful predictor of coding sequences). After this initial scan, more detailed information on the start sites of genes and predicted coding sequences is generated by using the GCG package (Devereux et al., 1984).

Gene Products Encoded in the First Completed *M. tuberculosis* Cosmid

Cosmid TBC2 was sequenced with 8.6-fold random shotgun coverage (approximately 400 kb of raw data) and contained a genomic insert approximately 32 kb in size (the cloning vector, pYUB18, is about 12 kb in size [Jacobs et al., 1991]). Analysis of the TBC2 sequence revealed 23 putative genes, including 14 encoding polypeptides with homologies to other known proteins and 9 open reading frames (ORFs) (the sequence will be described in detail and

published elsewhere). A map showing the positions of the identified genes and unidentified ORFs is shown in Fig. 4. Brief descriptions of the genes identified in TBC2, with their preliminary gene designations shown in Fig. 4, and their closest homologs are given in the following paragraphs.

The genes (Fig. 4) are *pk-at,dh,er*, which encodes a putative polyketide synthase and has acyl transferase, enoylreductase, and dehydratase domains homologous to those of one of the *Saccharopolyspora erythraea* genes that govern biosynthesis of the polyketide portion of erythromycin (ORF2, module 4; Donadio et al., 1991.); *pk-kas*, which encodes a putative ketoacyl acyl carrier protein synthase and is homologous to one of the *S. erythraea* erythromycin biosynthesis genes (ORF2, module 3; Donadio et al., 1991); *pk-bkr*, which codes for a putative beta-keto reductase and is homologous to the *S. erythraea* ORF1, module 2 (Donadio et al., 1991); *CoAl*, which is a homolog of BCG mycocerosic acid synthase operon ORF1 (Mathur and Kolattukudy, 1992) and shares identity with a number of coenzyme A fatty acid ligases and antibiotic synthetases; *rfbL*, whose product shows homology to *Vibrio cholerae* RfbL protein (Cheah and Manning, 1993) and a number of coenzyme A ligases and antibiotic synthetases; two putative UDP-sugar transferase genes, *udptr*, which are homologous to *E. coli* outer membrane protein MurG (Ikeda et al., 1990) and several other UDP-glucosuronyl transferases; *me*, which encodes a putative methyltransferase gene homologous to EryG (Haydock et al., 1991). The *ktdB* gene product shows homology to *E. coli* KdtB protein, an essential 18-kDa protein that is encoded in operon 3 of the lipopolysaccharide gene cluster (Roncero and Casadaban, 1992), and *pyc* encodes pyruvate carboxylase, a key gluconeogeneic enzyme that catalyzes the ATP-dependent carboxylation of pyruvate to oxaloacetate in the presence of cofactors biotin and zinc. The *M. tuberculosis* enzyme is highly homologous to yeast pyruvate carboxylase (Lim et al., 1988). The *pur3* gene encodes a phosphoribosylglycinamide formyltransferase, which catalyzes the third step in de novo purine biosynthesis: 10-formyltetrahydrofolate + 5'-phosphoribosylglycinamide → tetrahydrofolate + 5' phosphoribosyl-*N*-formylglycinamide. The *M. tuberculosis* enzyme is highly homologous to *Bacillus subtilis* PUR3 (Ebole and Zalkin, 1987). A putative transport protein, encoded by *ant*, shows weak homology to the *E. coli* ArsB proton pump (Chen et al., 1986), P-glycoprotein (Endicott et al., 1992), and other transport proteins. A putative cell division protein, coded for by *yhhf*, is homologous to *E. coli* protein YhhF encoded within a cell division operon (Gill et al., 1986). The *rmtr* gene is predicted to encode an rRNA methylase homologous to *ermK* from *Bacillus licheniformis* (Kwak et al., 1991). Nine ORFs longer than 50 codons with acceptable translation initiation sites (Shine and Dalgarno, 1975) exist, but their products show no homologies to other proteins in the database.

FUTURE PROSPECTS IN MYCOBACTERIAL GENOME RESEARCH

There is a strong chance that the integrated map of the *M. tuberculosis* chromosome will be completed in 1994 and that intensive DNA sequence analysis will then begin. Clearly, as illustrated here, completion of this project will provide a wealth of new information about this feared pathogen and will open up many new leads for research in chemotherapy and rational drug design, identify new avenues for biochemical and immunological investigation, and above all make a significant contribution to the fight against tuberculosis.

As the vast amounts of new data are obtained, they will be annotated and stored in MycDB, a database dedicated to the mycobacterial genome projects (Bergh and Cole, submitted). Ultimately, detailed comparisons of the chromosomes of *M. leprae* and *M. tuberculosis* will be possible and will allow conserved and variable regions to be identified. In turn, this offers the exciting prospect that species-specific chromosomal domains that can be correlated with characteristic traits such as tropisms, slow growth, or mycobacterial persistence in infected tissues will be identified.

Acknowledgments. We thank K. Eiglmeier, J. Grosset, B. Heym, B. Jacobs, W. Philipp, S. Poulet, and L. Pascopella for helpful discussions, strains, data, and encouragement. A large group at Collaborative Research, Inc., has contributed to the sequencing work and technology development. This group includes A. Avruch, C. Butler, N. Capparell, M. Chung, S. Drill, K. Falls, K. Gunderson, J. Imrich, H.-M. Lee, R. Lundstrom, J. Mao, J. Maher, P. Richterich, M. Rubenfield, H. Safer, A. Smyth, D. Torrey, and Q. Xu. George Church and his associates L. Mintz, G. Gryan, K. Robison, N. Lakey, and S. Kieffer-Higgins at Harvard Medical School have also contributed to the success of the sequencing effort.

These studies were supported by grants from the World Health Organisation, the National Center for Human Genome Research (NIH), the Fondation pour la Recherche Medicale, the Association Française Raoul Follereau, the Institut Pasteur, and Collaborative Research, Inc.

REFERENCES

Andersen, Å. B., A. Worsaae, and S. D. Chaparas. 1988. Isolation and characterization of recombinant lambda gt11 bacteriophages expressing eight different mycobacterial antigens of potential immunological relevance. *Infect. Immun.* **56:**1344–1351.

Ansorge, W., B. S. Sproat, J. Stegemann, and C. J. Schwage. 1986. Automated DNA sequencing; ultrasensitive detection of fluorescent bands during electrophoresis. *Nucleic Acids Res.* **15:**4593–4602.

Bergh, S., and S. T. Cole. MycDB, an integrated mycobacterial database. Submitted for publication.

Bloom, B. R., and C. J. L. Murray. 1992. Tuberculosis: commentary on a reemergent killer. *Science* **257:**1055–1064.

Canard, B., and S. T. Cole. 1989. Genome organization of the anaerobic pathogen *Clostridium perfringens*. *Proc. Natl. Acad. Sci. USA* **86:**6676–6680.

Canard, B., B. Saint-Joanis, and S. T. Cole. 1992. Genomic diversity and organisation of virulence genes in the pathogenic anaerobe *Clostridium perfringens*. *Mol. Microbiol.* **6:**1421–1429.

Cheah, K. C., and P. A. Manning. 1993. Inactivation of the *Escherichia coli* B41 (O101:K99/F41) *rfb* gene encoding an 80-kDa polypeptide results in the synthesis of an antigenically altered lipopolysaccharide in *E. coli* K-12. *Gene* **123:**9–15.

Chen, C.-M., T. K. Misra, S. Silver, and B. P. Rosen. 1986. Nucleotide sequence of the structural genes for an anion pump: the plasmid-encoded arsenical resistance operon. *J. Biol. Chem.* **261:**15030–15038.

Church, G., and S. Kieffer-Higgins. 1988. Multiplex DNA sequencing. *Science* **240:**185–188.

Clark-Curtiss, J. E., W. R. Jacobs, M. A. Docherty, L. R. Ritchie, and R. Curtiss III. 1985. Molecular analysis of DNA and construction of genomic libraries of *Mycobacterium leprae*. *J. Bacteriol.* **161:**1093–1102.

Cole, S. T., and I. Saint-Girons. Bacterial genomics. *FEMS Microbiol. Rev.*, in press.

Coulson, A., J. Sulston, S. Brenner, and J. Karn. 1986. Toward a physical map of the genome of the nematode *Caenorhabditis elegans*. *Proc. Natl. Acad. Sci. USA* **83:**7821–7825.

Devereux, J., P. Haeberli, and O. Smithies. 1984. A comprehensive set of sequence analysis programs for the VAX. *Nucleic Acids Res.* **12:**387–395.

Donadio, S., M. J. Staver, J. B. McAlpine, S. J. Swanson, and L. Katz. 1991. Modular organization of genes required for complex polyketide biosynthesis. *Science* **252:**675–679.

Dooley, S. W., W. R. Jarvis, W. J. Martone, and D. E. Snider, Jr. 1992. Multi-drug resistant tuberculosis. *Ann. Intern. Med.* **117:**257–259.

Dunham, I., R. Durbin, J. Thierry-Mieg, and D. R. Bentley. 1993. Physical mapping projects and ACEDB. *In* M. J. Bishop (ed.), *Guide to Human Genome Computing*, in press. Academic Press, London.

Durbin, R., and J. Thierry-Mieg. 1991. A *C. elegans* database. Documentation, code, and data available

from anonymous FTP servers at lirmm.lirmm.fr, cele.mrc-lmb.cam.ac.uk, and hcbi.nlm.nih.gov.

Ebole, D. J., and H. Zalkin. 1987. Cloning and characterization of a 12-gene cluster from *Bacillus subtilis* encoding nine enzymes for de novo purine nucleotide synthesis. *J. Biol. Chem.* **262:**8274–8287.

Eiglmeier, K., N. Honoré, S. A. Woods, B. Caudron, and S. T. Cole. 1993. Use of an ordered cosmid library to deduce the genomic organisation of *Mycobacterium leprae*. *Mol. Microbiol.* **7:**197–206.

Eiglmeier, K., L. Pascopella, N. Honoré, W. R. Jacobs, Jr., and S. T. Cole. An ordered collection of shuttle cosmids representing the chromosome of *Mycobacterium leprae*: some practical applications. Unpublished data.

Endicott, J. A., F. Sarangi, and V. Ling. 1992. Complete DNA sequences encoding the Chinese hamster P-glycoprotein gene family. *DNA Sequence* **2:**89–101.

Gill, D. R., G. F. Hatfull, and G. P. C. Salmond. 1986. A new cell division operon in *Escherichia coli*. *Mol. Gen. Genet.* **205:**134–145.

Haydock, S. F., J. A. Dowson, N. Dhillon, G. A. Roberts, J. Cortes, and P. F. Leadlay. 1991. Cloning and sequence analysis of genes involved in erythromycin biosynthesis in Saccharopolyspora erythraea: sequence similarities between EryG and a family of S-adenosylmethionine-dependent methyltransferases. *Mol. Gen. Genet.* **230:**120–128.

Hector, J. S. R., Y. Pang, G. H. Mazurek, Y. Zhang, A. A. Brown, and R. J. Wallace, Jr. 1992. Large restriction fragment patterns of genomic *Mycobacterium fortuitum* DNA as strain-specific markers and their use in epidemiologic investigation of four nosocomial outbreaks. *J. Clin. Microbiol.* **30:**1250–1255.

Hermans, P. W. M., D. van Soolingen, E. M. Bik, P. E. W. de Haas, J. W. Dale, and J. D. A. van Embden. 1991. Insertion element IS*987* from *Mycobacterium bovis* BCG is located in a hot-spot region for insertion elements in *Mycobacterium tuberculosis* complex strains. *Infect. Immun.* **59:**2695–2705.

Honoré, N., S. Chanteau, F. Doucet-Populaire, K. Eiglmeier, T. Garnier, C. Georges, P. Launois, P. Limpaiboon, S. Newton, K. Nyang, P. del Portillo, G. K. Ramesh, T. Reddy, J. P. Riedel, N. Sittisombut, S. Wu-Hunter, and S. T. Cole. 1993. Nucleotide sequence of the first cosmid from the *Mycobacterium leprae* genome project: structure and function of the Rif-Str regions. *Mol. Microbiol.* **7:**207–214.

Ikeda, M., M. Wachi, H. K. Jung, F. Ishino, and M. Matsuhashi. 1990. Nucleotide sequence involving *murG* and *murC* in the *mra* gene cluster region of *Escherichia coli*. *Nucleic Acids Res.* **18:**4014.

Jacobs, W. R., Jr. 1993. Personal communication.

Jacobs, W. R., Jr., G. V. Kalpana, J. D. Cirillo, L.

Pascopella, S. B. Snapper, R. A. Udani, W. Jones, R. G. Barletta, and B. R. Bloom. 1991. Genetic systems for mycobacteria. *Methods Enzymol.* **204:**537–555.

Kieser, H., T. Kieser, and D. Hopwood. 1992. A combined genetic and physical map of the *Streptomyces coelicolor* A3(2) chromosome. *J. Bacteriol.* **174:**5496–5507.

Kohara, Y., K. Akiyama, and K. Isono. 1987. The physical map of the whole *E. coli* chromosome: application of a new strategy for rapid analysis and sorting of a large genomic library. *Cell* **50:**495–508.

Krawiec, S., and M. Riley. 1990. Organization of the bacterial chromosome. *Microbiol. Rev.* **54:**502–539.

Kwak, J. H., E. C. Choi, and B. Weisblum. 1991. Transcriptional attenuation control of *ermK*, a macrolide-lincosamide-streptogramin B resistance determinant from *Bacillus licheniformis*. *J. Bacteriol.* **173:**4725–4735.

Leblond, P., M. Redenbach, and J. Cullum. 1993. Physical map of the *Streptomyces lividans* 66 chromosome and comparison with that of the related strain *Streptomyces coelicolor* A3(2). *J. Bacteriol.* **175:**3422–3429.

Lévy-Frébault, V. V., M. F. Thorel, A. Varnerot, and B. Gicquel. 1989. DNA polymorphism in *Mycobacterium paratuberculosis*, "wood pigeon mycobacteria," and related mycobacteria analyzed by field inversion gel electrophoresis. *J. Clin. Microbiol.* **27:**2823–2826.

Lim, F., C. P. Morris, F. Occhiodoro, and J. C. Wallace. 1988. Sequence and domain structure of yeast pyruvate carboxylase. *J. Biol. Chem.* **263:**11493–11497.

Mathur, M., and P. E. Kolattukudy. 1992. Molecular cloning and sequencing of the gene for mycocerosic acid synthase, a novel fatty acid elongating multifunctional enzyme from *Mycobacterium tuberculosis var. bovis* bacillus Calmette-Guèrin. *J. Biol. Chem.* **267:**19388–19395.

McAdam, R. A., P. W. M. Hermans, D. van Soolingen, Z. F. Zainuddin, D. Catty, J. D. A. van Embden, and J. W. Dale. 1990. Characterization of a *Mycobacterium tuberculosis* insertion sequence belonging to the IS3 family. *Mol. Microbiol.* **4:**1607–1613.

Mintz, L., G. Gryan, and G. M. Church. 1993. Unpublished data.

Philipp, W., S. Poulet, L. Pascopella, K. Eiglmeier, B. Heym, W. R. Jacobs, Jr., and S. T. Cole. 1993. Genome organisation of *Mycobacterium tuberculosis*. Unpublished data.

Prober, J. M., G. L. Trainor, R. J. Dam, F. W. Hobbs, C. W. Robertson, R. J. Zagursky, A. J. Cocuzza, M. A. Jensen, and K. Baumeister. 1987. A system for rapid DNA sequencing with fluorescent chain-terminating dideoxynucleotides. *Science* **238:**336–341.

Ranes, M. G., J. Rauzier, M. Lagranderie, M. Gheor-giu, and B. Gicquel. 1990. Functional analysis of pAL5000, a plasmid from *Mycobacterium fortuitum*: construction of a "mini" mycobacterium-*Escherichia coli* shuttle vector. *J. Bacteriol.* **172:**2793–2797.

Rauzier, J., J. Moniz-Pereira, and B. Gicquel-Sanzey. 1988. Complete nucleotide sequence of pAL5000, a plasmid from *Mycobacterium fortuitum*. *Gene* **71:**315–321.

Richterich, P., and G. M. Church. 1993. DNA sequencing by direct transfer electrophoresis and nonradioactive detection. *Methods Enzymol.* **218:**187–222.

Robison, K., and G. M. Church. 1993. Unpublished data.

Roncero, C., and M. J. Casadaban. 1992. Genetic analysis of the genes involved in synthesis of the lipopolysaccharide core in *Escherichia coli* K-12: three operons in the *rfa* locus. *J. Bacteriol.* **174:**3250–3260.

Saiki, R. K., D. H. Gelfand, S. Stoffel, S. J. Scharf, R. Higuchi, G. T. Horn, K. B. Mullis, and H. A. Erlich. 1988. Primer-directed enzymatic amplification of DNA with a thermostable DNA polymerase. *Science* **239:**487–491.

Schwartz, D. C., and C. R. Cantor. 1984. Separation of yeast chromosome-sized DNAs by pulsed-field gel electrophoresis. *Cell* **37:**67–75.

Shine, J., and L. Dalgarno. 1975. Terminal-sequence analysis of bacterial ribosomal RNA: correlation between the 3'-terminal-polypyrimidine sequence of 16S RNA and translational specificity of the ribosome. *Eur. J. Biochem.* **57:**221–230.

Smith, C. L., P. E. Warburton, A. Gaal, and C. R. Cantor. 1986a. Analysis of genome organization and rearrangements by pulsed field gradient gel electrophoresis, p. 45–70. *In* J. K. Setlow and A. Hollaender (ed.), *Genetic Engineering*. Plenum Publishing Corp., New York.

Smith, D. R., T. Avruch, C. Butler, N. Capparell, S. Drill, K. Falls, H. Lee, M. Rubenfield, A. Smyth, D. Torrey, Q. Xu, and J. Mao. 1993. Unpublished data.

Smith, L. M., J. Z. Sanders, R. J. Kaiser, P. Hughes, C. Dodd, C. R. Connell, C. Heiner, S. B. H. Kent, and L. E. Hood. 1986b. Fluorescence detection in automated DNA sequence analysis. *Nature* (London) **321:**674–679.

Snapper, S. B., L. Lugosi, A. Jekkel, R. E. Melton, T. Kieser, B. R. Bloom, and W. R. Jacobs. 1988. Lysogeny and transformation in mycobacteria: stable expression of foreign genes. *Proc. Natl. Acad. Sci. USA* **85:**6987–6991.

Snapper, S. B., R. E. Melton, S. Mustafa, T. Kieser, and W. R. Jacobs. 1990. Isolation and characterization of efficient plasmid transformation mutants of *Mycobacterium smegmatis*. *Mol. Microbiol.* **4:**1911–1919.

Snider, D. E., Jr., and W. L. Roper. 1992. The new tuberculosis. *N. Engl. J. Med.* **326:**703–705.

Sulston, J., F. Mallett, R. Staden, R. Durbin, T. Horsnell, and A. Coulson. 1988. Software for genome mapping by fingerprinting techniques. *Comput. Appl. Biosci.* **4:**125–132.

Thierry, D., A. Brisson-Noël, V. Vincent-Lévy-Frébault, S. Nguyen, J. Guesdon, and B. Gicquel. 1990a. Characterization of a *Mycobacterium tuberculosis* insertion sequence, IS*6110*, and its application in diagnosis. *J. Clin. Microbiol.* **28:**2668–2673.

Thierry, D., M. D. Cave, K. D. Eisenach, J. T. Crawford, J. H. Bates, B. Gicquel, and J. L. Guesdon. 1990b. IS*6110*, an IS-like element of *Mycobacterium tuberculosis* complex. *Nucleic Acids Res.* **18:**188.

Varnerot, A., F. Clément, M. Gheorghiu, and V. Vincent-Lévy-Frébault. 1992. Pulsed field gel electrophoresis of representatives of *Mycobacterium tuberculosis* and *Mycobacterium bovis* BCG strains. *FEMS Microbiol. Lett.* **98:**155–160.

Winter, N., M. Lagranderie, J. Rauzier, J. Timm, C. Leclerc, B. Guy, M. P. Kieny, M. Gheorghiu, and B. Gicquel. 1991. Expression of heterologous genes in *Mycobacterium bovis* BCG: induction of a cellular response against HIV-1 Nef protein. *Gene* **109:**47–54.

Young, D., R. Lathigra, R. Hendrix, D. Sweetser, and R. A. Young. 1988. Stress proteins are immune targets in leprosy and tuberculosis. *Proc. Natl. Acad. Sci. USA* **85:**4267–4270.

Young, D. B., and S. T. Cole. 1993. Leprosy, tuberculosis, and the new genetics. *J. Bacteriol.* **175:**1–6.

Young, R. A., B. R. Bloom, C. Grosskinsky, J. Ivanyi, D. Thomas, and R. W. Davis. 1985a. Dissection of *Mycobacterium tuberculosis* antigens using recombinant DNA. *Proc. Natl. Acad. Sci. USA* **82:**2583–2587.

Young, R. A., V. Mehra, D. Sweetser, T. Buchanan, J. Clark-Curtiss, R. W. Davis, and B. R. Bloom. 1985b. Genes for the major protein antigens of the leprosy parasite *Mycobacterium leprae*. *Nature* (London) **316:**450–452.

Tuberculosis: Pathogenesis, Protection, and Control
Edited by Barry R. Bloom
© 1994 American Society for Microbiology, Washington, DC 20005

Chapter 17

Expression of Foreign Genes in Mycobacteria

Jeanne E. Burlein, C. Kendall Stover, Shawn Offutt, and Mark S. Hanson

The identification and characterization of mycobacteria as etiologic agents of leprosy and tuberculosis over 100 years ago constituted the origins of the study of bacterial pathogenesis. In the intervening time, substantial effort has resulted in the elucidation of much of the physiology, biochemistry, and immunology of the mycobacteria, but efforts at describing the genetics of mycobacteria have been rewarded only very recently. The first reports of characterization of cloned mycobacterial genes came in 1985 with the identification of protein antigens from *Mycobacterium leprae* (Young et al., 1985b; Clark-Curtiss et al., 1985), *M. tuberculosis* (Young et al., 1985a), and BCG (Thole et al., 1985) by their cloning and expression in *Escherichia coli*. These studies showed that while mycobacterial translational signals seemed to function in *E. coli*, transcription initiation signals functional in this heterologous background were isolated very infrequently. These findings underscored the need to develop systems for the expression of mycobacterial genes in a homologous background. Much of the impetus for the increased interest in the study of mycobacterial genetics stems from the increased incidence of tuberculosis worldwide. As the mechanisms of pathogenesis of many infectious agents (Finlay and Falkow, 1989) have been defined through the use of genetics, it is expected that the same will be true for tuberculosis. Also, genetic manipulation of the closely related BCG, an attenuated strain of the bovine tubercle bacillus *M. bovis*, may produce new recombinant vaccines that use this safe and immunogenic tuberculosis vaccine as a delivery vehicle. In this chapter, we review the development of genetic systems for the expression of foreign genes in mycobacteria.

INTRODUCTION AND MAINTENANCE OF FOREIGN DNA IN MYCOBACTERIA

Phage-Based Systems

Mycobacteriophage have been used for many years to type mycobacterial isolates and have more recently been modified as vectors for efficient delivery of foreign DNA into mycobacteria (see chapter 12 in this volume). These modified phage vectors, termed "shuttle phasmids," were constructed by insertion of a portion of an *E. coli* cosmid cloning vector into the mycobacteriophage genome (Jacobs et al., 1987). Use of DNA from a temperate phage allowed construction of a shuttle plasmid,

Jeanne E. Burlein, Shawn Offutt, and Mark S. Hanson • MedImmune, Inc., 35 West Watkins Mill Road, Gaithersburg, Maryland 20878.   *C. Kendall Stover* • PathoGenesis Corp., Department of Tuberculosis and Infectious Diseases, 201 Elliott Avenue, West, Seattle, Washington 98119.

phAE1, capable of integrating as a single copy into the mycobacterial genome while expressing a foreign antibiotic resistance gene and maintaining itself as a stable element replicating with the bacterial chromosome (Snapper et al., 1988). Further improvements in the versatility and capacity for foreign DNA of phage-based cloning systems were achieved when the minimal sequences necessary for site-specific integration into the chromosomal *attB* site were identified (Lee et al., 1991) and incorporated into plasmid vectors, for example, the integrating vector pMV361 (Stover et al., 1991) (Fig. 1).

Plasmid-Based Systems

Plasmid-based expression systems extend the capabilities of phage-based systems by providing increased cloning capacity, increased copy number in the mycobacterial host, and ease of manipulation. Although plasmids have been identified in several species of fast-growing mycobacteria (see chapter 13 in this volume),

plasmids native to or capable of replication in slow-growing mycobacteria were not known at the time the phage-based vectors were initially constructed. Subsequently, it was shown (Snapper et al., 1988) that a shuttle plasmid capable of extrachromosomal replication in both *E. coli* and slow-growing mycobacteria could be constructed using the 5.0-kb cryptic plasmid pAL5000 from fast-growing *M. fortuitum* (Labidi et al., 1985) in conjunction with an *E. coli* cloning vector. This mycobacterial replicon in pAL5000 was later localized to a segment spanning approximately half the plasmid (Ranes et al., 1990) and then further defined to a 1.8-kb segment of pAL5000 DNA (Stover et al., 1991), allowing construction of compact mycobacterium-*E. coli* shuttle vectors, e.g., pMV261 (Fig. 1).

Some promiscuous plasmid replicons of nonmycobacterial origin have also been shown to be functional in mycobacteria. The 10.2-kb cosmid pJRD215, derived from a broad-host-range IncQ plasmid, can replicate in the fast-growing *M. aurum* and *M.*

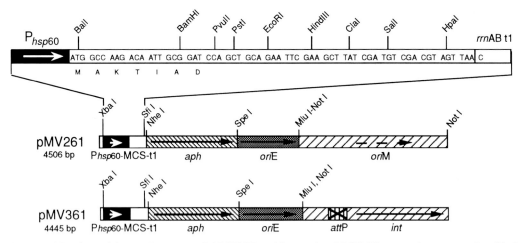

Figure 1. Mycobacterial extrachromosomal (pMV261) and integrative (pMV361) expression vectors (modified from Stover et al., 1991). Common elements in these two vectors include an expression cassette, the Tn*903*-derived *aph* gene (kanamycin resistance), and an origin of replication functional in *E. coli* (*ori*E) derived from pUC19. The expression cassette contains 0.4 kb of the 5′ end of the BCG *hsp-60* gene, including the promoter region, ribosome-binding site, and first six codons (MAKTIA) as well as a multiple cloning site and the *E. coli* *rrnAB*$_{t1}$ transcriptional terminator. The vectors differ by inclusion of either a mycobacterial plasmid replication origin (*ori*M) or the *attP* and *int* genes of mycobacteriophage L5.

smegmatis, but some transformants undergo deletion of some plasmid sequence (Hermans et al., 1991). The corynebacterial pNG2 plasmid replicon was also shown to function in *E. coli* as well as in *M. smegmatis* and BCG (Radford and Hodgson, 1991).

Introduction of DNA into Mycobacteria

Among the early impediments to working with mycobacteria was difficulty in transforming these cells relative to other bacteria such as *E. coli*. Transformation of mycobacterial protoplasts with phage DNA results in efficiencies of 10^3 to 10^4 PFU/μg (Jacobs et al., 1987), and plasmid transformations result in similar efficiencies. Electroporation is even more effective, with efficiencies of 10^6 transformants per μg of DNA (Jacobs et al., 1991). Introduction of foreign DNA by means of a recombinant mycobacteriophage can be even more efficient (see chapter 12) (Jacobs et al., 1993). Conjugative transfer of a shuttle plasmid from *E. coli* to *M. smegmatis* has also been reported (Lazraq et al., 1990).

FEATURES OF EXPRESSION VECTORS

Extrachromosomal and Integrating Modes of Replication

Various derivatives of the pAL5000 plasmid replicon have been combined with *E. coli* plasmid replication origins, such as ColE1 and p15A, by several groups to fashion *E. coli*-mycobacterium shuttle vectors. However, not all versions appear to be equally stable in mycobacteria (Lazraq et al., 1991). In one study, the vector containing the smallest replication origin derived from pAL5000, pMV261, replicated to approximately five copies per genome equivalent (Stover et al., 1991). These vectors have also proved to be remarkably stable. We have found that this vector can be maintained in BCG for over 18 serial passages (about 70 to 80 generations) in liquid

culture in the absence of any selection. Other antigen-expressing plasmids based on this replicon are much less stable in the absence of selection, although we have not yet determined whether this instability is due to loss of the replicon or of the antigen insert DNA. This replicon has also been shown to be stable in recombinant BCG (rBCG) during several months of persistence of the bacterium in vivo; BCG recovered from mice still express the foreign gene (Stover et al., 1991; Connell et al., 1993).

Shuttle vectors that circumvent the question of plasmid instability in mycobacteria have been constructed by utilizing integration functions of temperate mycobacteriophages (see chapter 12). As single-copy elements replicating with the bacterial chromosome, foreign genes from integrating vectors have had lower expression levels, in most cases, than the same genes expressed from multicopy plasmids. Some genes seem to be expressed in mycobacteria only in a single-copy format, an observation usually interpreted to indicate over-expression lethality. The full-length human immunodeficiency virus type 1 (HIV-1) gp120 gene can be expressed from the *hsp-60* promoter only when it is integrated (Stover et al., 1991), but expression from multicopy plasmid vectors is possible if weaker promoters are used (Galen, unpublished data). The integrating vectors also have the potential to be maintained in the same cell with the extrachromosomal plasmid vectors, therefore allowing the opportunity for further versatility of foreign gene expression.

Selectable Markers

Typically, genes encoding resistance to antibiotics are used to select for bacterial transformants receiving cloning vectors. For antibiotic selection of mycobacterial transformants, the choice of drugs is somewhat limited. The cell surface glycolipids of mycobacteria are thought to be responsible for the impermeability of mycobacteria to many commonly used antibiotics (see chapter 22 in this volume). β-Lactamases are common among most fast- and slow-growing mycobacteria. Antibiotics such as tetracycline that are unstable during the prolonged incubation periods required for selection of transformants are unsuitable for mycobacteria. Aminoglycoside antibiotics avoid the aforementioned problems of ampicillin and tetracycline. Although naturally occurring aminoglycoside resistance is known in fast-growing strains (Hull et al., 1984), no convenient plasmid-encoded drug markers have been identified. Fortunately, foreign kanamycin resistance markers derived from Tn5 and Tn903 were shown to be effective selectable markers for both phage-based and plasmid-based shuttle vectors in mycobacteria (Snapper et al., 1988). The aminoglycoside phosphotransferases, particularly APH(3')I of Tn903, which has a somewhat narrower substrate specificity, are currently the most widely used antibiotic resistance markers for mycobacterial gene manipulation. Other markers functional in mycobacteria are also known. Chloramphenicol resistance has been shown to be functional as a selectable marker in M. smegmatis (Snapper et al., 1988), although the spontaneous mutation rate to resistance makes use of chloramphenicol selection less attractive. Hygromycin resistance can be used as a selectable marker in both slow- and fast-growing mycobacteria (Radford and Hodgson, 1991), but the sensitivity of the drug to salts necessitates the use of synthetic media, which is suboptimal for growth. A sulfonamide resistance determinant identified on an M. fortuitum transposable element (Martin et al., 1990) should be effective as a selectable marker for plasmid maintenance. Mercuric reductase activity has been characterized on a plasmid from M. scrofulaceum (Meissner and Falkingham, 1984), but this activity has not yet been utilized as a selectable marker for foreign gene expression in mycobacteria.

A goal of foreign gene expression in mycobacteria is to achieve selection of transformants without the use of antibiotic resistance markers that might be transferred from the recombinant strain to other pathogenic mycobacterial strains. This is particularly important for recombinant BCG vaccines, which could achieve wide use in humans. One strategy to achieve this end is based on the mycobacteriophage L5 gene 71 repressor-like protein (see chapter 12). Expression of this gene on mycobacterial shuttle vectors allows selection of transformants of M. smegmatis in the presence of mycobacteriophages that would otherwise be lytic (Donnelly-Wu et al., 1993). We have successfully used this strategy to select for BCG recombinants expressing foreign genes from such phage resistance vectors.

Future goals for nondrug selection include the development of vectors containing genes capable of complementing mycobacterial auxotrophic mutations and of systems for generating these mutations (see chapters 14 and 18 in this volume). This selection strategy has proved to be effective for maintaining plasmids in Salmonella vaccine strains in vivo (Nakayama et al., 1988).

Transcription and Translation Initiation

The first foreign genes expressed in mycobacteria were the APH gene of Tn903 and the gene for M. leprae Hsp60 antigen, both expressed from their own promoters (Snapper et al., 1988). In the construction of expression vectors, promoters of mycobacterial stress-regulated genes (we will use the term "heat shock proteins") were chosen as the first candidates to drive expression of foreign genes in mycobacteria for several reasons: (i) expression of these genes is observed under all growth conditions; (ii) in other bacteria (Buchmeier and Heffron, 1990), their expression is induced upon infection of macrophages, the site of replication of infectious mycobacteria in vivo; and (iii) the sequences of these genes were among the first available (Young et al., 1985b; Mehra et al., 1986; Shinnick, 1987). Analysis of potential promoter sequences of mycobacterial genes by computer algorithms based on prokaryotic consensus sequences is only somewhat helpful in predicting the promoter sequences (Dale and Patki, 1990). In the instances where transcriptional start sites have been mapped, the promoters for the BCG *hsp-60* (Stover et al., 1991) and *hsp-70* (Lathigra et al., unpublished data) genes show, at best, weak homology to these consensus sequences. These promoters do appear to be stress regulated in vitro, but only when they are used in integrating vectors (Stover et al., 1991). These promoters can drive expression of foreign genes to 10% or more of total mycobacterial protein. Other promoters successfully used in mycobacterial expression vectors include those from genes encoding the *M. kansasii* alpha antigen (Matsuo et al., 1990a), the *M. paratuberculosis* IS*900* ORF2 (Murray et al., 1992), the *M. tuberculosis* 19-kDa antigen (Stover et al., 1993a, b) and 38-kDa antigen (unpublished data), the *Streptomyces albus* *groES/groEL1* (Winter et al., 1991) reading frames from various mycobacteriophages (Barletta et al., 1992), and the *E. coli lac* promoter (unpublished data). At this point, the in vivo expression levels of these promoters, for example, as resident in rBCG-infected macrophages, can only be inferred from the immunogenicity of the protein product of the gene in question, but methods to measure expression levels directly are under investigation.

PROTEIN EXPRESSION

Translational Efficiency

Expression of foreign proteins in recombinant organisms is influenced by many factors. At the translational level, accumulation of protein is dictated by the balance of peptide synthesis rate, posttranslational modification and protein folding, and degradation by endogenous proteases (Goldberg and Goff, 1986). At present, we cannot directly address the issue of proteolytic degradation of foreign gene products in mycobacteria by eliminating genes encoding endogenous proteases, and we are just beginning to be able to address some of the other factors affecting protein stability in mycobacteria.

One factor potentially influencing translation rate is the codon usage of foreign genes (de Boer and Kastelein, 1986). Several compilations of codon usages of genes of mycobacteria (Dale and Patki, 1990; Wada et al., 1992) and the mycobacteriophage L5 (Hatfull and Sarkis, 1993) have been published. The high G+C content of mycobacteria (around 65%) is reflected in a bias for codons with G or C at the third position. This is substantially different from the codon bias of most other organisms and might be expected to severely limit the translational efficiency of genes from most nonmycobacterial sources, but this is not necessarily the case. The *ospA* gene of *Borrelia burgdorferi*, an organism with a G+C content of about 30%, utilizes the Leu codon UUA with a frequency of approximately 38% (Bergstrom et al., 1989), while mycobacterial genes utilize this codon for Leu at a frequency of about 1%. Clearly, from the high expression levels of OspA in BCG in amino acid-rich medium (Stover et al., 1993a), codon bias is not the major factor influencing protein expression in this case. We have not yet determined whether the same expression levels are seen in amino-limiting conditions.

Although the codon bias of foreign genes expressed in mycobacteria may play a role in determining expression level, other factors affecting translation initiation are likely to be more important in influencing protein expression (Buell and Panayotatos, 1986).

These include the sequence around the ribosome-binding site, the structure of the 5' end of the mRNA, and the sequence around the initiation codon. These factors have not yet been examined systematically for mycobacteria, but two features of the sequences of the 5' ends of mycobacterial genes characterized to date can be noted (Dale and Patki, 1990; Hatfull and Sarkis, 1993). In general, the putative Shine-Dalgarno sequence preceding the initiator codon of mycobacterial genes appears similar in base content and position to the prokaryotic consensus sequence. Also, the nearly equal usage of AUG and GUG as potential initiator codons again reflects the high G+C content of mycobacterial DNA, but the effect of the choice of initiator codon on correct initiation or incorrect internal initiation of translation of foreign genes remains uncertain. For the most part, foreign proteins can be successfully expressed in mycobacteria as fusions with a small portion of the 5' end of an efficiently expressed mycobacteria gene, including the Shine-Dalgarno sequence, initiator codon, and several codons from the amino terminus of the fusion partner (Stover et al., 1991).

Posttranslational Modifications

Not only do posttranslational modifications affect the ultimate structure and function of proteins, but incorrect or inefficient modification can also influence protein stability and therefore expression level. Expression of foreign proteins with posttranslational modifications similar to those of the proteins in their native host may increase their stability in mycobacteria and aid in their adopting a more native conformation. For proteins from eukaryotes, not all possible modification are likely to occur, however. Along with inappropriate folding, lack of proper posttranslational modification is a factor thought to play a role in the formation of insoluble aggregates of foreign proteins expressed in recombinant organisms (Schein, 1989). Very few examples of posttranslationally modified gene products from mycobacteria have been described at the molecular level to date (see chapter 21 in this volume). Genes encoding three proteins appearing to be classic bacterial lipoproteins have been sequenced (Ashbridge et al., 1989; Andersen and Hansen, 1989; Nair et al., 1992), and their gene products have been partially characterized (Young and Garbe, 1991). Some recent evidence indicates that these products may undergo lipid acylation as well as glycosylation (Garbe et al., 1993), a form of posttranslational modification not previously observed in prokaryotes. It is thought that surface antigens of mycobacteria may be more accessible to immune processing in the macrophage and may therefore be more immunogenic than internal antigens. The leader sequences of the 19-kDa (Stover et al., 1993a, b) and 38-kDa (unpublished data) antigens have been used as fusion partners to direct the secretion and lipid acylation of several surface proteins to the membrane of rBCG. For most foreign proteins that are normally exported from their native host, this mycobacterial expression system has worked well. For the limited number of examples examined thus far, proteins successfully expressed as lipoprotein fusions in rBCG, even though expressed at lower levels, are more immunogenic than when they are expressed as cytoplasmic proteins (Stover et al., 1993a, b). However, as with attempts at secretion in other bacteria (Lee et al., 1989), fusion of a protein that is normally cytoplasmic to an export signal does not typically effect secretion. Expression of a given protein with a leader peptide, either with its natural leader or as a fusion with a mycobacterial leader, often results in lower expression levels than that achievable as a cytoplasmic protein (Stover et al., 1993a, b). In some cases, it has not yet been possible to express particular foreign proteins with their natural leader peptides or as fusions with mycobacterial leaders in BCG.

The mycobacterial alpha antigens (see chapter 21 in this volume), or antigen 85 complex, are another class of exported and therefore posttranslationally modified proteins. Homologous genes from several mycobacterial species have been sequenced (Borremans et al., 1989; Matsuo et al., 1990b; Content et al., 1991; Thole et al., 1992) and shown to encode unusually long leader peptides. These proteins have also been used as fusion partners to export epitopes (Matsuo et al., 1990a) or whole foreign proteins from rBCG (Stover et al., 1993a).

APPLICATIONS OF FOREIGN GENE EXPRESSION IN MYCOBACTERIA

Elucidation of Mycobacterial Virulence Determinants

A commonly used method of analyzing genes that might be involved in the virulence of a pathogen is to clone candidates for these genes in *E. coli*, mutate them in some manner, exchange the mutated allele back into the original genetic background by homologous recombination, and assess the effect on virulence phenotype. This approach is not yet tenable in the slow-growing mycobacteria, as they appear to be refractory to gene replacement (Kalpana et al., 1991). A recent report indicates that single recombination events between homologous sequences can occur at low frequency in BCG, raising the possibility of achieving targeted gene disruption in slow-growing mycobacteria by homologous recombination with cloned DNA (Aldovini et al., 1993). Alternate approaches include (i) reconstitution of a virulence phenotype in an avirulent strain by the expression of genes cloned from a virulent mycobacterium and (ii) insertional mutagenesis of virulent mycobacteria with transposons (see chapter 14 in this volume). Also, expres-

sion of genes as fusions with conveniently assayed enzymes such as β-galactosidase (Miller et al., 1989), alkaline phosphatase (Goldberg et al., 1990), and luciferase (Park et al., 1992) has been instrumental in the analysis of regulation of candidate virulence genes in other bacteria. Similar studies of transcriptional regulation of expression of these reporters in mycobacteria are in progress in several laboratories.

Understanding Drug Action and Resistance

Much of the increased interest in mycobacteria is a result of the emergence of multidrug-resistant *M. tuberculosis*. Expression of genes encoding targets of antibiotic action in a drug-resistant background is one strategy toward understanding mechanisms of drug action. *M. tuberculosis* is normally highly susceptible to isoniazid (INH), but strains resistant to this drug are becoming increasingly common. *M. smegmatis* is relatively resistant to INH, so that as a first step in understanding this phenotype at the genetic level, *M. smegmatis* was transformed to INH sensitivity with a shuttle cosmid containing *M. tuberculosis* DNA (Zhang et al., 1992). The INH sensitivity gene, *katG*, was found to be deleted in a proportion of INH-resistant *M. tuberculosis* isolates. More recently, an additional mechanism for INH resistance was revealed by expressing genes from spontaneous INH-resistant *M. smegmatis* and BCG mutants in INH-sensitive *M. smegmatis* (Banerjee et al., 1994). The candidate target of INH action common to these mutants, *inhA*, has similarity to *envM* of enteric bacteria, a gene thought to be involved in fatty acid biosynthesis. Thus, expression of the *katG* and *inhA* genes in heterologous mycobacterial species provided crucial insight into the potential mechanism of action of INH.

Expression of foreign reporter genes in virulent mycobacteria such as *M. tuberculosis* is obviously dependent on transcriptional and translational activities and can therefore be used to assess the metabolic health of the bacterial cell in response to antibiotics. Two recent reports demonstrate the effectiveness of this approach by showing that the activity of firefly luciferase either introduced on a plasmid vector (Jacobs et al., 1993) or expressed from a stable plasmid vector (Cooksey et al., 1993) can be used to reveal the susceptibility of *M. tuberculosis* to various drugs (see chapters 12 and 30 in this volume).

Expression of Complex Secondary Gene Products

Complex surface macromolecules, such as oligosaccharides and glycolipids, require the products of many genes and the correct cell envelope structure for proper assembly. The roles of many mycobacterial glycolipids as potential virulence factors and modulators of the immune response have been described elsewhere (see chapter 20 in this volume), and, as surface structures, they could potentially play a role in drug permeability. Attempts at expression of such macromolecules from mycobacteria in a cloning host such as *E. coli* are fraught with difficulties. When *M. smegmatis* was used as a cloning host, the genes required for the terminal sugar modifications of the serovar 2 glycopeptidolipid of *M. avium* were successfully identified (Belisle et al., 1991). This accomplishment would have undoubtedly been more difficult or impossible in a nonmycobacterial background.

Biochemical Transformations

Strains of fast-growing saprophytic mycobacteria can degrade toxic waste products such as alkenes and chlorinated alkenes. It has been suggested that strains of soil mycobacteria such as *M. aurum* may have utility as bioremediation agents (Hermans et al., 1991), and investigation of foreign gene expression in this species are in progress.

RECOMBINANT MYCOBACTERIAL VACCINES

Recombinant BCG Vaccines

One of the goals of the earlier work (Jacobs et al., 1987) on expression of foreign genes in mycobacteria was the development of an rBCG vaccine delivery system for heterologous antigens. It was hoped at the time that uncertainties about genetically manipulating the organism would be outweighed by several advantages: (i) BCG is one of the most effective adjuvants known, (ii) BCG has been used in approximately 3 billion people since 1948 with a very low incidence of serious complications, (iii) BCG immunizations elicit long-lasting immune responses, (iv) BCG can be administered at birth, and (v) the current BCG vaccines are inexpensive to produce (see chapter 31 in this volume). Apart from its effectiveness as a vaccine for tuberculosis, BCG is an effective adjuvant in both humans (Convit et al., 1982) and animals (Fortier et al., 1987; Pearce et al., 1988) when combined with other antigens. Believing in the promise of effective recombinant BCG vaccines, several groups endeavored to make this possibility a reality.

The first successes at foreign gene expression in BCG came with the demonstration of resistance to kanamycin after transformation with pAL5000-derived shuttle plasmids (Snapper et al., 1988; Ranes et al., 1990). It was then shown that an 8-amino-acid epitope of HIV-1 p17$_{gag}$ could be expressed in BCG as an insertion into the alpha-antigen reading frame (Matsuo et al., 1990a). In 1991, several groups reported expression of entire foreign protein antigens from HIV-1 (Stover et al., 1991; Aldovini and Young, 1991; Winter et al., 1991) and bacterial antigens (Stover et al., 1991). Most important, these studies demonstrated that foreign proteins delivered by rBCG to mice can elicit all three types of immune response necessary for protection against a variety of pathogens: B-cell production of immunoglobulin G antibodies; T-cell proliferation and lymphokine production, including gamma interferon; and major histocompatibility complex class I-restricted cytotoxic T lymphocytes. Cytotoxic lymphocyte responses to SIV_{mac} *gag* delivered by rBCG have also been demonstrated (Yasutomi et al., 1993). *Plasmodium falciparum* antigens have also been expressed in rBCG, but immune responses to these antigens have been disappointing (Haeseleer et al., 1993; Lanar, unpublished data).

Recent work has shown not only that proteins delivered by rBCG can be immunogenic but also that these immune responses can be protective in animal models of disease. Expression of a nontoxigenic fragment of tetanus toxin in rBCG elicits antibody responses that protect approximately half of mice challenged with 100 50% lethal dose units of toxin (Cassatt et al., 1993). Boosting with either rBCG-ToxC or a subimmunogenic dose of tetanus toxoid increased protection levels substantially. BCG expressing the gp63 protein of *Leishmania major* can elicit cell-mediated immune responses that protect mice from cutaneous leishmaniasis (Connell et al., 1993). BCG expressing the OspA protein of *B. burgdorferi* has been shown to elicit sterilizing immunity in mice to intradermal challenge with 100 50% infective doses of the virulent spirochete (Stover et al., 1993a). BCG-OspA has been demonstrated to elicit strong immunoglobulin G responses in guinea pigs and sheep as well, again demonstrating that the immunogenicity of rBCG is not restricted to mice. Similar levels of protection to a challenge with *Streptococcus pneumoniae* are seen in mice immunized with rBCG expressing the *S. pneumoniae* PspA antigen (Stover et al., 1993b). When antigens expressed in rBCG elicit very strong immune responses, e.g., serum antibody enzyme-linked immunosorbent assay titers in excess of 10^5, protection from challenge can be complete. Thus far,

not all antigens are expressed in rBCG at levels high enough or in the correct conformation to elicit the strong immune responses required for good protection. BCG recombinants in earlier stages of development include those expressing antigens from papillomavirus, influenza virus, measles virus, rotavirus, *Haemophilus influenzae*, *Corynebacterium diphtheriae*, *Schistosoma mansoni*, *Schistosoma japonicum*, and *Fasciola hepatica*.

Expression levels of a foreign gene often vary in different strains of a given prokaryotic host species. In recombinant *E. coli*, this variability is sometimes due to differences in endogenous proteases that degrade improperly folded proteins (Goldberg and Goff, 1986), but doubtless other factors are also influential. There are many different vaccine substrains of BCG that differ in several characteristics (Osborne, 1983; chapter 31 in this volume). With this in mind, we sought to determine whether expression of foreign genes would also differ among the BCG substrains. At a gross level, expression of most endogenous proteins is quite similar among BCG substrains, as expected, but some small differences can be discerned by Coomassie blue-stained sodium dodecyl sulfate-polyacrylamide gel electrophoresis (SDS-PAGE) (Fig. 2A). The same is not true for expression of foreign genes. The OspA gene of *B. burgdorferi*, minus its leader sequence, transcribed from the BCG *hsp-60* promoter on an extrachromosomal vector (pMV261-OspA) is expressed at relatively high levels by most but not all of the BCG substrains, as demonstrated by immunoblotting with a monoclonal antibody reactive with OspA (Fig. 2B). Expressing OspA from this same vector but as a fusion with the *M. tuberculosis* 19-kDa lipoprotein leader peptide (p2619s) alters this profile of expression (Fig. 2C). The HIV-1 gp120 protein has also been expressed successfully in several BCG substrains from the BCG *hsp-60* promoter on the integrating vector

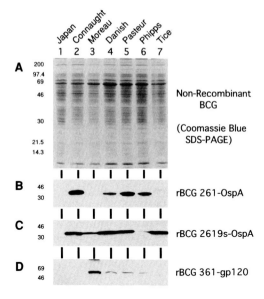

Figure 2. Expression of foreign antigens in different BCG substrains. BCG culture lysates equivalent to approximately 5×10^6 bacteria were analyzed by SDS-PAGE and Coomassie blue staining (A) or by immunoblotting with antibodies specific for foreign antigens *B. burgdorferi* OspA (B, C) or HIV-1 gp120 (D). Panel A shows the total proteins expressed by nonrecombinant BCG. Panels B through D show relevant portions of immunoblots of different BCG recombinants expressing the indicated foreign antigens.

the choice of substrain for expressing foreign antigens in BCG has to be determined empirically, with a final selection of the strain that imparts the best immune response.

One of the goals of development of rBCG vaccine vectors is the simultaneous expression and delivery of multiple foreign antigens. This goal has recently been achieved by the simultaneous expression of two foreign surface proteins from *S. pneumoniae* and *H. influenzae* in the same BCG recombinant (Hanson et al., in press). Similar results have been achieved for the simultaneous expression of two antigens from *P. falciparum* in rBCG (Haeseleer et al., 1993). The potential for these multivalent BCG vaccines to elicit a protective immune response to each of the foreign antigens is under investigation.

Recombinant Mycobacterial Vaccines for Tuberculosis

BCG, the current vaccine against tuberculosis, has provided variable protective efficacy against tuberculosis in different vaccine trials (see chapter 31 in this volume). The poor efficacy of BCG in some of these trials clearly indicates that a vaccine capable of eliciting less variable and more solid protection against tuberculosis is desirable. One possibility for an improved tuberculosis vaccine is to overexpress in rBCG the protective antigens of *M. tuberculosis* (see chapter 31). As there is very limited information as to which antigens individually or in combination would enhance protective immune responses (see chapters 24, 25, and 26), it is not yet clear which antigens should be chosen for expression in rBCG. To date, the *M. tuberculosis* 19- and 38-kDa lipoproteins have been expressed in rBCG, but these await testing in animal models for improved efficacy over nonrecombinant BCG. Several "atypical" mycobacteria, including *M. microti*, *M. vaccae*, and *M. habana*, have received at-

pMV361, albeit at low levels (Fig. 2D). This study has been expanded to include several additional foreign genes from both prokaryotic and eukaryotic sources and vectors utilizing several different mycobacterial promoters and translation initiation signals (over 230 total combinations of BCG substrain, expression vector, and foreign gene; data not shown). Unfortunately, few clear rules for choosing the optimal BCG substrain for expression of a given foreign protein emerge from the BCG recombinants examined to date. Some substrains seem to give uniformly poor levels of expression from these vectors, i.e., the Japan strain (Fig. 2, lane 1), while others are very frequently positive for expression of a wide variety of proteins, i.e., Pasteur 1173P2 (Fig. 2, lane 5). At this point, it appears that tention as potential vaccines against tuberculosis (see chapter 31). These species could also be considered as expression hosts for *M. tuberculosis* antigens.

Another intriguing possibility for creating an improved tuberculosis vaccine is to rationally attenuate the pathogen by introducing into the *M. tuberculosis* genome defined lesions that eliminate its ability to cause disease but not its ability to elicit a protective immune response (see chapter 31). Present strategies to accomplish this rely on the ability to deliver transposons capable of expressing transposition functions (see chapter 14) into *M. tuberculosis* through the use of phage or plasmid vectors with conditional replication functions (see chapters 12 and 18). It will take some time to reiterate in *M. tuberculosis*, even using the tools of modern molecular biology, the accomplishments of Calmette and Guérin with the attenuation of *M. bovis* achieved by more traditional means.

Other Recombinant Mycobacterial Vaccines

M. smegmatis offers advantages as a vaccine delivery vehicle for use in livestock animals when environmental stability of the vector is important, for example, in animal feed, and when consumer resistance to BCG-infected animals might be encountered. Immunization of chickens with recombinant *M. smegmatis* expressing an *Eimeria acervulina* surface antigen elicits partial protection against coccidiosis (Jenkins and Lillehoj, personal communication).

SUMMARY

Our ability to genetically manipulate the mycobacteria, some of the first microbial pathogens identified, is much less than a decade old. The new tools that make possible the expression of foreign genes in members of this genus will ultimately enhance our understanding of the molecular basis of the pathogenicity of *M. tuberculosis* and other infectious mycobacteria. We anticipate that this understanding will enable us to harness the unusual immunogenic properties of these bacilli and employ them to create novel recombinant vaccines effective against tuberculosis and other infectious diseases.

Acknowledgments. We thank Raju Lathigra and Jim F. Young for helpful discussions and for comments on the manuscript.

REFERENCES

Aldovini, A., R. N. Husson, and R. A. Young. 1993. The *uraA* locus and homologous recombination in *Mycobacterium bovis* BCG. *J. Bacteriol.* **175:**7282–7289.
Aldovini, A., and R. A. Young. 1991. Humoral and cell-mediated responses to live recombinant BCG-HIV vaccines. *Nature* (London) **351:**479–482.
Andersen, A. B., and E. B. Hansen. 1989. Structure and mapping of antigenic domains of protein antigen b, a 38,000-molecular weight protein of *Mycobacterium tuberculosis*. *Infect. Immun.* **57:**2481–2488.
Ashbridge, K. R., R. J. Booth, J. D. Watson, and R. Lathigra. 1989. Nucleotide sequence of the 19 kDa antigen gene from *Mycobacterium tuberculosis*. *Nucleic Acids Res.* **17:**1249.
Banerjee, A., E. Dubnau, A. Quemard, V. Balasubramanian, K. S. Um, T. Wilson, G. de Lisle, and W. R. Jacobs, Jr. 1994. inhA, a gene encoding a target for isoniazid and ethionamide in *Mycobacterium tuberculosis*. *Science* **263:**227–230.
Barletta, R. G., D. D. Kim, S. B. Snapper, B. R. Bloom, and W. R. Jacobs, Jr. 1992. Identification of expression signals of the mycobacteriophages Bxb1, L1, and TM4 using the *Escherichia*-mycobacterium shuttle plasmids pYUB75, and pYUB76 designed to create translational fusions to the *lacZ* gene. *J. Gen. Microbiol.* **138:**23–30.
Belisle, J. T., L. Pascopella, J. M. Inamine, P. J. Brennan, and W. R. Jacobs, Jr. 1991. Isolation and expression of a gene cluster responsible for biosynthesis of the glycopeptidolipid antigens of *Mycobacterium avium*. *J. Bacteriol.* **173:**6991–6997.
Bergstrom, S., V. G. Bundoc, and A. G. Barbour. 1989. Molecular analysis of linear plasmid-encoded major surface proteins, OspA and OspB, of the Lyme disease spirochaete *Borrelia burgdorferi*. *Mol. Microbiol.* **3:**479–486.
Borremans, M., L. de Wit, G. Volckaert, J. Ooms, J. de Bruyn, K. Huygen, J.-P. van Vooren, M. Stelan-

dre, R. Verhofstadt, and J. Content. 1989. Cloning, sequence determination, and expression of a 32-kilodalton-protein gene of *Mycobacterium tuberculosis. Infect. Immun.* **57**:3123–3130.

Buchmeier, N. A., and F. Heffron. 1990. Induction of *Salmonella* stress proteins upon infection of macrophages. *Science* **248**:730–732.

Buell, G., and N. Panayotatos. 1986. Mechanism and practice, p. 345–363. *In* W. Reznikoff and L. Gold (ed.), *Maximizing Gene Expression.* Butterworths, Boston.

Cassatt, D. R., V. F. de la Cruz, J. E. Burlein, J. Young, S. Koenig, and C. Kendall Stover. 1993. Protection of mice against tetanus challenge using an experimental tetanus vaccine based on recombinant BCG, p. 385–389. *In* H. S. Ginsberg, F. Brown, R. M. Channock, and R. A. Lerner (ed.), *Vaccines 93.* Cold Spring Harbor Laboratory Press, Plainview, N.Y.

Clark-Curtiss, J. E., W. R. Jacobs, M. A. Docherty, L. R. Ritchie, and R. Curtiss. 1985. Molecular analysis of DNA and construction of genomic libraries of *Mycobacterium leprae. J. Bacteriol.* **161**:1093–1102.

Connell, N. D., E. Medina-Acosta, W. R. McMaster, B. R. Bloom, and D. G. Russell. 1993. Effective immunization against cutaneous leishmaniasis with recombinant BCG expressing the *Leishmania* surface proteinase (gp63). *Proc. Natl. Acad. Sci. USA* **90**:11473–11477.

Content, J., A. de la Cuvellerie, L. de Wit, V. Vincent-Levy-Frebault, J. Ooms, and J. de Bruyn. 1991. The gene coding for the antigen 85 complexes of *Mycobacterium tuberculosis* and *Mycobacterium bovis* BCG are members of a gene family: cloning, sequence determination, and genomic organization of the gene coding for antigen 85-C of *M. tuberculosis. Infect. Immun.* **59**:3205–3212.

Convit, J., N. Aranzazu, M. Ulrich, M. E. Pinardi, O. Reyes, and J. Alvarado. 1982. Immunotherapy with a mixture of *Mycobacterium leprae* and BCG in different forms of leprosy and Matsuda negative contacts. *Int. J. Lepr.* **50**:415.

Cooksey, R. C., J. T. Crawford, W. R. Jacobs, and T. M. Shinnick. 1993. A rapid method for screening antimicrobial agents for activity against a strain of *Mycobacterium tuberculosis* expressing firefly luciferase. *Antimicrob. Agents Chemother.* **37**:1348–1352.

Dale, J. W., and A. Patki. 1990. Mycobacterial gene expression and regulation, p. 173–198. *In* J. McFadden (ed.), *Molecular Biology of the Mycobacteria.* Surrey University Press, London.

de Boer, H. A., and R. A. Kastelein. 1986. Biased codon usage: an exploration of its role in optimization of translation, p. 225–286. *In* W. Reznikoff and

L. Gold (ed.), *Maximizing Gene Expression.* Butterworths, Boston.

Donnelly-Wu, M. K., W. R. Jacobs, Jr., and G. F. Hatfull. 1993. Superinfection immunity of mycobacteriophage L5: applications for genetic transformation of mycobacteria. *Mol. Microbiol.* **7**:407–417.

Finlay, B. B., and S. Falkow. 1989. Common themes in microbial pathogenicity. *Microbiol. Rev.* **53**:210–230.

Fortier, A. H., B. A. Mock, M. S. Meltzer, and C. A. Nacy. 1987. *Mycobacterium bovis* BCG-induced protection against cutaneous and systemic *Leishmania major* infections of mice. *Infect. Immun.* **55**:1707–1714.

Galen, J. Unpublished data.

Garbe, T., D. Harris, M. Vordermeier, R. Lathigra, J. Ivanyi, and D. Young. 1993. Expression of the *Mycobacterium tuberculosis* 19-kilodalton antigen in *Mycobacterium smegmatis*: immunological analysis and evidence of glycosylation. *Infect. Immun.* **61**:260–267.

Goldberg, A. L., and S. A. Goff. 1986. The selective degradation of abnormal proteins in bacteria, p. 287–314. *In* W. Reznikoff and L. Gold (ed.), *Maximizing Gene Expression.* Butterworths, Boston.

Goldberg, M. B., S. A. Boyko, and S. B. Calderwood. 1990. Transcriptional regulation by iron of a *Vibrio cholerae* virulence gene and homology of the gene to the *Escherichia coli* Fur system. *J. Bacteriol.* **172**:6863–6870.

Haeseleer, F., J.-F. Pollet, M. Haumont, C. Dubeaux, A. Bollen, P. Jacobs, M. Modesti, and J. Cohen. 1993. Stable integration and expression of *Plasmodium falciparum* antigen coding sequences in mycobacteria, p. 413–417. *In* H. S. Ginsberg, F. Brown, R. M. Channock, and R. A. Lerner (ed.), *Vaccines 93.* Cold Spring Harbor Laboratory Press, Plainview, N.Y.

Hanson, M. S., C. V. Lapcevich, and S. L. Haun. Progress on development of the live BCG recombinant (rBCG) vaccine vehicle for combined delivery. *Ann. N.Y. Acad. Sci.*, in press.

Hatfull, G. F., and G. J. Sarkis. 1993. DNA sequence, structure, and gene expression of mycobacteriophage L5: a phage system for mycobacterial genetics. *Mol. Microbiol.* **7**:395–405.

Hermans, J., C. Martin, G. N. M. Huijberts, T. Goosen, and J. A. M. de Bont. 1991. Transformation of *Mycobacterium aurum* and *Mycobacterium smegmatis* with the broad host-range gram-negative cosmid vector pJRD215. *Mol. Microbiol.* **5**:1561–1566.

Hull, S. I., R. J. Wallace, Jr., D. G. Bobey, K. E. Price, R. A. Goodhines, J. M. Swenon, and V. A. Silcox. 1984. Presence of aminoglycoside acetyltransferase and plasmids in *Mycobacterium fortuitum. Am. Rev. Respir. Dis.* **129**:614–618.

Jacobs, W. R., Jr., R. G. Barletta, R. Udani, J. Chan, G. Kalkut, G. Sosne, T. Keiser, G. J. Sarkis, G. F. Hatfull, and B. R. Bloom. 1993. Rapid assessment of drug susceptibilities of *Mycobacterium tuberculosis* by means of luciferase reporter phages. *Science* **260**:819–822.

Jacobs, W. R., Jr., G. V. Kalpana, J. D. Cirillo, L. Pascopella, S. B. Snapper, R. A. Udani, W. Jones, R. G. Barletta, and B. R. Bloom. 1991. Genetic systems for mycobacteria. *Methods Enzymol.* **204**: 537–555.

Jacobs, W. R., Jr., M. Tuckman, and B. R. Bloom. 1987. Introduction of foreign DNA into mycobacteria using a shuttle phasmid. *Nature* (London) **327**: 532–535.

Jenkins, M. C., and H. S. Lillehoj. Personal communication.

Kalpana, G. V., B. R. Bloom, and W. R. Jacobs, Jr. 1991. Insertional mutagenesis and illegitimate recombination in mycobacteria. *Proc. Natl. Acad. Sci. USA* **88**:5433–5437.

Labidi, A., H. L. David, and D. Roulland-Dussoix. 1985. Cloning and expression of mycobacterial plasmid DNA in *Escherichia coli*. *FEMS Microbiol. Lett.* **30**:221–225.

Lanar, D. Unpublished data.

Lathigra, R., et al. Unpublished data.

Lazraq, R., S. Clavel-Seres, and H. L. David. 1991. Transformation of distinct mycobacterial species by shuttle vectors derived from the *Mycobacterium fortuitum* pAL5000 plasmid. *Curr. Microbiol.* **22**:9–13.

Lazraq, R., S. Clavel-Seres, H. L. David, and D. Roulland-Dussoix. 1990. Conjugative transfer of a shuttle plasmid for *Escherichia coli* to *Mycobacterium smegmatis*. *FEMS Microbiol. Lett.* **69**:135–138.

Lee, C., P. Li, H. Inouye, E. Brickman, and J. Beckwith. 1989. Genetic studies on the inability of β-galactosidase to be translocated across the *Escherichia coli* cytoplasmic membrane. *J. Bacteriol.* **171**:4609–4616.

Lee, M. H., L. Pascopella, W. R. Jacobs, Jr., and G. F. Hatfull. 1991. Site-specific integration of mycobacteriophage L5: integration-proficient vectors for *Mycobacterium smegmatis*, *Mycobacterium tuberculosis* and bacille Calmette-Guerin. *Proc. Natl. Acad. Sci. USA* **88**:3111–3115.

Martin, C., J. Timm, J. Rauzier, R. Gomez-Lus, J. Davies, and B. Gicquel. 1990. Transposition of an antibiotic resistance element in mycobacteria. *Nature* (London) **345**:739–743.

Matsuo, K., R. Yamaguchi, A. Yamazaki, H. Tasaka, K. Terasaka, M. Totsuka, K. Kobayashi, H. Yukitake, and T. Yamada. 1990a. Establishment of a foreign secretion system in mycobacteria. *Infect. Immun.* **58**:4049–4054.

Matsuo, K., R. Yamaguchi, A. Yamazaki, H. Tasaka, K. Terasaka, and T. Yamada. 1990b. Cloning and expression of the gene for the cross-reactive α antigen of *Mycobacterium kansasii*. *Infect. Immun.* **58**:550–556.

Mehra, V., D. Sweetser, and R. A. Young. 1986. Efficient mapping of protein antigen determinants. *Proc. Natl. Acad. Sci. USA* **83**:7013–7017.

Meissner, P. S., and J. O. Falkingham. 1984. Plasmid-encoded mercuric reductase in *Mycobacterium scrofulaceum*. *J. Bacteriol.* **157**:669–672.

Miller, J. F., C. R. Roy, and S. Falkow. 1989. Analysis of *Bordetella pertussis* virulence gene regulation by use of transcriptional fusions in *Escherichia coli*. *J. Bacteriol.* **171**:6345–6348.

Murray, A., N. Winter, M. Lagranderie, D. F. Hill, J. Rauzier, J. Timm, C. Leclerc, K. M. Moriarty, M. Gheorghiu, and B. Gicquel. 1992. Expression of *Escherichia coli* β-galactosidase in *Mycobacterium bovis* BCG using an expression system from *Mycobacterium paratuberculosis* which induced humoral and cellular immune responses. *Mol. Microbiol.* **6**:3331–3342.

Nair, J., D. A. Rouse, and S. L. Morris. 1992. Nucleotide sequence analysis and serologic characterization of the *Mycobacterium intracellulare* homologue of the *Mycobacterium tuberculosis* 19 kDa antigen. *Mol. Microbiol.* **6**:1431–1439.

Nakayama, K., S. M. Kelly, and R. Curtiss III. 1988. Construction of an Asd+ expression-cloning vector: stable maintenance and high level expression of cloned genes in a Salmonella vaccine vector strain. *Bio/Technology* **6**:693–697.

Osborne, T. W. 1983. Changes in BCG strains. *Tubercle* **64**:1–132.

Park, S. F., G. S. A. B. Stewart, and R. G. Kroll. 1992. The use of bacterial luciferase for monitoring the environmental regulation of expression of genes encoding virulence factors in Listeria monocytogenes. *J. Gen. Microbiol.* **138**:2619–2627.

Pearce, E. J., S. L. James, S. Hierny, D. E. Lanar, and A. Sher. 1988. Induction of protective immunity against *Schistosoma mansoni* by vaccination with schistosome paramyosin (Sm97), a nonsurface parasite antigen. *Proc. Natl. Acad. Sci. USA* **85**:5679–5682.

Radford, A. J., and A. L. M. Hodgson. 1991. Construction and characterization of a mycobacterium-*Escherichia coli* shuttle vector. *Plasmid* **25**:149–153.

Ranes, M. G., J. Rauzier, M. Lagranderie, M. Gheorghiu, and B. Gicquel. 1990. Functional analysis of pAL5000, a plasmid from *Mycobacterium fortuitum*: construction of a "mini" mycobacterium-*Escherichia coli* shuttle vector. *J. Bacteriol.* **172**:2793–2797.

Schein, C. 1989. Production of soluble recombinant proteins in bacteria. *Bio/Technology* **7**:1141–1149.

Shinnick, T. M. 1987. The 65-kilodalton antigen of *Mycobacterium tuberculosis*. *J. Bacteriol.* **169:** 1080–1088.

Snapper, S. B., L. Lugosi, A. Jekkel, R. Melton, T. Kieser, B. R. Bloom, and W. R. Jacobs, Jr. 1988. Lysogeny and transformation of mycobacteria: stable expression of foreign genes. *Proc. Natl. Acad. Sci. USA* **85:**6987–6991.

Stover, C. K., G. P. Bansal, M. S. Hanson, J. E. Burlein, S. R. Palaszynski, J. F. Young, S. Koenig, D. B. Young, A. Sadziene, and A. Barbour. 1993a. Protective immunity elicited by a recombinant bacille Calmette-Guerin (BCG) expressing outer surface protein A (OspA) lipoprotein: a candidate Lyme disease vaccine. *J. Exp. Med.* **178:**197–209.

Stover, C. K., V. F. de la Cruz, T. R. Fuerst, J. E. Burlein, L. A. Benson, L. T. Bennett, G. P. Bansal, J. F. Young, M. H. Lee, G. F. Hatfull, S. B. Snapper, R. G. Barletta, W. R. Jacobs, Jr., and B. R. Bloom. 1991. New use of BCG for recombinant vaccines. *Nature* (London) **351:**458–460.

Stover, C. K., S. Langermann, M. S. Hanson, J. E. Burlein, S. R. Palaszynski, S. Koenig, L. S. McDaniel, and D. E. Briles. 1993b. Candidate pneumococcal vaccines based on the recombinant BCG vaccine vehicle, abstr. E-79. *Abstr. 93rd Gen. Meet. Am. Soc. Microbiol. 1993.*

Thole, J. E., H. G. Dauwerse, P. K. Das, D. G. Groothuis, L. M. Schouls, and J. D. A. van Embden. 1985. Cloning of *Mycobacterium bovis* DNA and expression of antigens in *Escherichia coli*. *Infect. Immun.* **50:**800–806.

Thole, J. E. R., R. Schoningh, A. A. M. Janson, T. Garbe, Y. E. Cornelisse, J. E. Clark-Curtiss, A. H. J. Kolk, T. H. M. Ottenhoff, R. R. R. De Vries, and C. Abou-Zeid. 1992. Molecular and immunological analysis of a fibronectin-binding protein antigen secreted by *Mycobacterium leprae*. *Mol. Microbiol.* **6:**153–163.

Wada, K., Y. Wada, F. Ishibashi, T. Gojobori, and T. Ikemura. 1992. Codon usage tabulated from the GenBank genetic sequence data. *Nucleic Acids Res.* **20:**S2111–S2118.

Winter, N., M. Lagranderie, J. Rauzier, J. Timm, C. Leclerc, B. Guy, M. P. Kieny, M. Gheorghiu, and B. Gicquel. 1991. Expression of heterologous genes in *Mycobacterium bovis* BCG: induction of a cellular response against HIV-1 Nef protein. *Gene* **109:**47–54.

Yasutomi, Y., S. Koenig, S. S. Haun, C. K. Stover, R. K. Jackson, P. Conrad, A. J. Conley, E. A. Emini, T. R. Fuerst, and N. L. Letvin. 1993. Immunization with recombinant BCG-SIV elicits SIV-specific cytotoxic T lymphocytes in rhesus monkeys. *J. Immunol.* **150:**3101–3107.

Young, D. B., and T. R. Garbe. 1991. Lipoprotein antigens of *Mycobacterium tuberculosis*. *Res. Microbiol.* **142:**55–65.

Young, R. A., B. R. Bloom, C. M. Grosskinsky, J. Ivanyi, D. Thomas, and R. W. Davis. 1985a. Dissection of *Mycobacterium tuberculosis* antigens using recombinant DNA. *Proc. Natl. Acad. Sci. USA* **82:**2583–2587.

Young, R. A., V. Mehra, D. Sweetser, T. Buchanan, J. Clark-Curtiss, R. W. Davis, and B. R. Bloom. 1985b. Genes for the major protein antigens of the leprosy parasite, *Mycobacterium leprae*. *Nature* (London) **316:**450–452.

Zhang, Y., B. Heym, B. Allen, D. Young, and S. Cole. 1992. The catalase-peroxidase gene and isoniazid resistance of *Mycobacterium tuberculosis*. *Nature* (London) **358:**591–593.

Tuberculosis: Pathogenesis, Protection, and Control
Edited by Barry R. Bloom
© 1994 American Society for Microbiology, Washington, DC 20005

Chapter 18

Molecular Genetic Strategies for Identifying Virulence Determinants of *Mycobacterium tuberculosis*

William R. Jacobs, Jr., and Barry R. Bloom

THE GENOTYPE OF VIRULENCE

In 1881, the causes of tuberculosis were variously perceived to be (i) the wrath of God, (ii) bad air, (iii) a cancer, or (iv) microbes. Depending on which hypotheses were correct, the respective therapies that would have been advocated were radically different: (i) repentance, (ii) prayer, (iii) a change to a dry climate, or (iv) a psychiatrist. The knowledge of the true etiology of tuberculosis allowed new approaches to prevention, treatment, and ultimately cure of the disease. One can argue that a rational approach to understanding the unique characteristics of an infectious pathogen, its phenotype, is to define the genetic constitution, the genotype, that encodes and controls the particular phenotype. This chapter is concerned with how knowledge of other bacterial pathogens may provide insight into the pathogenesis of tuberculosis.

In 1882, Robert Koch's landmark paper demonstrated that tuberculosis was caused by *Mycobacterium tuberculosis* (Koch, 1882). Perhaps as important, Koch was able to generalize from his studies of anthrax and tuberculosis and develop a systematic approach to establishing whether a microorganism is the causative agent of a disease by experimentally fulfilling three conditions that have come to bear his name, i.e., Koch's postulates (Table 1). By analogy, "molecular Koch's postulates" (Falkow, 1988) or Koch's molecular postulates (Jacobs, 1992) (Table 1) define the comparable conditions that must be satisfied in order to establish whether a particular characteristic of a bacterium, i.e., its phenotype, results from the presence and expression of a specific gene. This postulate can be used to establish that any phenotype, such as virulence, antibiotic resistance, tissue tropism, or ability to grow on a particular carbon source, results from the presence and expression of a specific gene, i.e., the genotype. For example, to identify a gene required for virulence of *M. tuberculosis*, one would (i) identify or generate a mutant of *M. tuberculosis* that is avirulent because of a mutation in a specific gene, (ii) clone the putative virulence gene from the virulent *M. tuberculosis* strain, and (iii) introduce the cloned gene into the avirulent mutant and demonstrate that that gene restores

William R. Jacobs, Jr., and Barry R. Bloom • Howard Hughes Medical Institute, Albert Einstein College of Medicine, Bronx, New York 10461.

Table 1. Comparison of Koch's postulates and Koch's molecular postulates

Koch's postulates
"To prove that tuberculosis is caused by the invasion of bacilli and the growth and multiplication of bacilli, it was necessary

(1) to isolate the bacilli from the body;

(2) to grow them in pure culture. . . and;

(3) by administering the isolated bacilli to animals, reproduce the same morbid condition. . . ."
(Koch, 1882)

Koch's molecular postulates
To prove that a phenotype such as virulence is caused by the presence and expression of a specific gene, it is necessary

(1) to isolate a mutant bacterium with a phenotype that differs from the wild-type phenotype,

(2) to clone the wild-type gene, and

(3) by introducing the wild-type gene back into the mutant bacterium, to reproduce the wild-type phenotype.

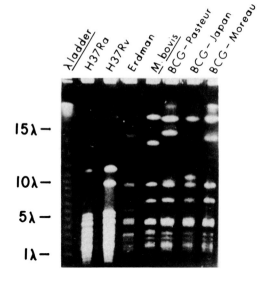

Figure 1. Macrorestriction analyses of *M. tuberculosis* genomes. The chromosomes of *M. tuberculosis* H37Ra and H37Rv and *M. bovis* and BCG strains were isolated and digested with *Dra*I. Following digestions, the DNA fragments were separated by pulsed-field gel electrophoresis. Note the 475-kb band present in the virulent H37Rv strain but absent in the avirulent H37Ra strain. Molecular weight markers are multimers of the bacteriophage λ genome.

virulence. One would infer from such an experiment that the cloned gene encodes a virulence factor or determinant. Indeed, biology was revolutionized earlier in this century with the discoveries of transformation, transduction, and conjugation, because these systems permitted the fulfillment of Koch's molecular postulates for bacteria. These gene transfer systems thus enabled researchers to know whether a genotype was responsible for a phenotype.

The necessity for defining virulence determinants stringently can readily be illustrated by the following example from our own studies of *M. tuberculosis*. When the genomes of the related *M. tuberculosis* strains H37Rv and H37Ra were analyzed by macrorestriction analysis (Jacobs et al., unpublished result) (Fig. 1), a prominent 475-kb band observed in the virulent strain of *M. tuberculosis* was absent in the avirulent strain. This macrorestriction analysis was performed by digesting the intact *M. tuberculosis* chromosomal DNAs with the restriction enzyme *Dra*I, an enzyme that cleaves the 6-bp sequence ATATAT. Since

M. tuberculosis has a high guanine-plus-cytosine content, *Dra*I cuts the genome only a limited number of times, resulting in the generation of large DNA fragments that can be resolved by pulsed-field gel electrophoresis. This simple physical analysis of the genome revealed one clear genetic difference between the virulent and the avirulent strain, but the question of whether this particular genetic difference is responsible for the loss of virulence in the avirulent H37Ra strain or is irrelevant cannot be resolved by mere physical or chemical analysis. Without fulfilling Koch's molecular postulates, we cannot know whether this particular genetic difference is related to virulence and attenuation. It is entirely possible that the loss of virulence results from some other genetic difference that is not visible by the relatively crude restriction analysis. For example, the presence or absence of the 475-kb *Dra*I fragment could have resulted simply from a point mutation or polymorphism that generated a novel *Dra*I site. Alternatively, the mutation could have arisen from the transposition of IS*6110*, which contains an internal *Dra*I site, into the 475-kb fragment, which may or may not affect virulence, since possibly hundreds of other mutations acquired by the H37Rv strain during and after its initial isolation could be responsible for the avirulence phenotype.

THE PHENOTYPE OF VIRULENCE

Webster's dictionary defines virulence as "the relative capacity of a pathogen to overcome body defenses." Virulence is a complex phenotype dependent not only on the genetic nature of the pathogen but also on the genetic and immunologic makeup of the host. To the extent it is understood in gram-negative bacterial pathogens, virulence is generally determined by a multiplicity of traits that endow the pathogen with its ability to exploit anatomical weaknesses and overcome the immune defenses of the host (Table 2). The usefulness of that definition of virulence is illustrated by the opportunistic pathogens, agents not normally pathogenic in immunocompetent hosts yet often highly virulent in immunocompromised individuals. Thus, even BCG and *M. avium* have virulence genes that

Table 2. Properties of a virulent organism

1. Infectious; capable of being spread from one individual to another
2. Capable of entering mammalian host cells
3. Capable of surviving or escaping phagocyte cellular defenses
4. Capable of multiplying in host cells, e.g., macrophages
5. Capable of spreading from one infected cell to another
6. Capable of causing cell injury that results in pathology
7. Capable of killing the host

can cause pathogenicity in immunocompromised hosts.

DEVELOPMENT OF GENETIC SYSTEMS FOR MYCOBACTERIA

Despite the fact that the first condition of Koch's molecular postulates, that requiring the isolation of virulence mutants, was first fulfilled with the isolation of BCG (bacillus Calmette-Guérin) by Calmette and Guérin in 1908 (Calmette and Guérin, 1909), methods for addressing the remaining postulates with *M. tuberculosis* or *M. bovis*, in contrast to many other bacterial pathogens, were not available until quite recently. The second condition, requiring the cloning of genes, was achieved with the development of recombinant DNA technologies that permitted efficient cloning of mycobacterial genes into cloning vectors in *Escherichia coli*. Numerous genes encoding protein antigens (Young et al., 1985a, b) and enzymes (Jacobs et al., 1986) have been cloned in recent years from the slow-growing, pathogenic mycobacteria. This approach has yielded considerable information about the nature of many important antigens found in mycobacterial infections. However, the testing of the function of genes requires that the third condition of Koch's molecular postulates be fulfilled and necessitates that ways be found to introduce recombinant DNA into mycobacteria.

The first vector that allowed the introduction of recombinant DNA into mycobacteria was a shuttle vector, a hybrid molecule that replicated as a plasmid in *E. coli* and as a phage in mycobacteria. These shuttle phasmids (Jacobs et al., 1987) (see chapter 12) could be introduced into *M. smegmatis* protoplasts as plasmid DNAs isolated from *E. coli*. The shuttle phasmid DNAs replicated as phages in *M. smegmatis*, where they could be packaged into the heads of mycobacteriophages. This permitted the introduction of genes into both

rapidly growing and slow-growing mycobacteria, including BCG and *M. tuberculosis*. This technology was extended with the
construction of temperate shuttle phasmids, vectors that retained their ability to
integrate site specifically into the chromosomes of mycobacteria (Snapper et al.,
1988). These shuttle phasmids were instrumental in demonstrating that kanamycin
and kanamycin resistance genes functioned
as selectable markers in mycobacteria. The
efficiency of introducing the DNA into mycobacteria, including *M. smegmatis*, BCG,
and *M. tuberculosis*, was greatly enhanced
by the use of electroporation of these vectors (Snapper et al., 1988). This technique
allowed the isolation of efficient plasmid
transformation mutants of *M. smegmatis*
(Snapper et al., 1990) which subsequently
enhanced the development of plasmid
transformation systems using multicopy
plasmids (Stover et al., 1991) and single-
copy integrating vectors (Lee et al., 1991)
(see chapter 17). These vector systems now
represent genetic tools by which cloned
DNA fragments can be efficiently introduced into the mycobacteria and provide a
definitive means of analyzing the genetic
basis for virtually any phenotype expressed
in the mycobacteria (see chapter 17). Although these systems now constitute a
powerful methodology for understanding
mycobacterial genes, there remain critical
limitations that restrict our ability to dissect
and define the genetic determinants of virulence, pathogenesis, and protection.

PROGRESS TOWARD FULFILLING KOCH'S MOLECULAR POSTULATES

Isolation of Avirulent Mutants of *M. bovis* and *M. tuberculosis* by Serial Passage

The first step in identifying virulence
genes is to isolate mutants that are avirulent. All of the early attenuated viral mutants and vaccine strains were generated by
serial passage of a virulent isolate in laboratory culture. Applying this approach to a
virulent *M. bovis* strain, Calmette and
Guérin in 1909 noted that after 208 passages
in vitro, a bacterium that had a distinctly
different colony morphology was isolated
(see chapter 2). Over a period of many
years, this strain, BCG, was shown to be
attenuated and unable to revert to virulence
in animal models, and it now represents the
most widely used vaccine in the world.
However, the critical point here is that to
this day, the precise nature of the mutations
that result in attenuation of the virulent *M.
bovis* strain remains a mystery. The identification of the precise mutations that cause
avirulence is further confounded by the
facts that since there were no freezers in
1908 or 1921, the original virulent and attenuated *M. bovis* strains from which BCG
was derived have been irretrievably lost.
Propagation of BCG vaccine strains has
occurred in many laboratories all over the
world and has most likely resulted in the
accumulation of large numbers of mutations, some of which may also contribute to
the attenuation of these strains (note the
*Dla*I polymorphisms in Fig. 1). Thus, the
introduction of a single specific DNA fragment from the virulent strain of *M. bovis*
back into BCG is not likely to restore
virulence. In an analogous manner, *M. tuberculosis* H37 lost its virulence following
prolonged passage on agar slants. A culture
of highly virulent organisms was obtained
following passage of the less virulent
strains in mice. Steenken and Petroff
cloned the virulent and avirulent variants of
isolate H37 and designated them H37Rv
and H37Ra, respectively (Steenken et al.,
1934). However, these strains were not
frozen until 1940, and thus the original
clones have been lost.

Complementation Analyses of the Avirulent *M. tuberculosis* H37Ra Strain

Avirulent mutants of *M. tuberculosis* or
M. bovis such as H37Ra and BCG can be

distinguished from virulent mutants by their growth in animals (Mackaness et al., 1954; Collins and Smith, 1969; North and Izzo, 1993). Virulent strains of *M. tuberculosis* multiply more rapidly in the mouse and in high challenge doses cause death, while avirulent mutants cause a self-limiting infection. One strategy for identifying genes that are necessary to restore a virulence phenotype to an avirulent mutant is to screen for restoration of virulence in an animal model (Fig. 2). In order to reduce the number of clones that need to be screened and to ensure that cloned genes are not lost during animal passage, we developed an integrating cosmid vector, pYUB178, for mycobacteria. This integrating vector, approximately 7 kb long, can accommodate 40 kb of DNA and uses the site-specific integration system of mycobacteriophage L5 (Lee et al., 1991) to integrate recombinant DNA into a unique *attB* site of the *M. tuberculosis* chromosome. This vector thus can represent 99% of the entire *M. tuberculosis* genome in as few as 300 clones. Another advantage of the system is that the recombinant DNA introduced in single copy is stably maintained in *M. tuberculosis* cells in the absence of antibiotic selection even when the strain is passed through animals.

To test the utility of this system, cosmid genomic libraries of *M. tuberculosis* H37Rv were constructed and introduced into the avirulent H37Ra strain (Pascopella et al., in press a, b). These integrated libraries were passaged through mice, and a number of clones that grew to greater numbers in the lungs or in spleens of infected animals than the *M. tuberculosis* H37Ra vector control were isolated. We have analyzed the *M. tuberculosis* H37Rv inserts from clones iso-

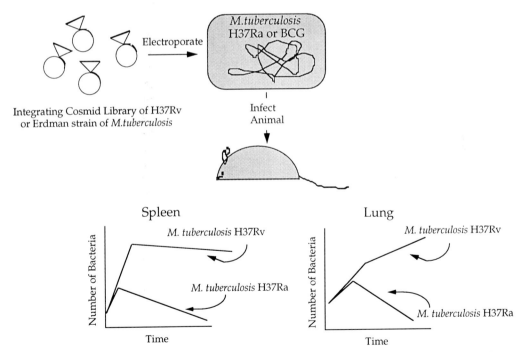

Figure 2. Virulence complementation assay. Cosmid genomic libraries of the virulent *M. tuberculosis* strain are constructed in an integrating cosmid vector and introduced into an avirulent mutant such as *M. tuberculosis* H37Ra or BCG. The resulting library of recombinant clones is injected into mice. Theoretically, clones that restore virulence will have a selective advantage and be enriched for in the mouse.

lated from different experiments that had the ability to preferentially localize in spleen and found several clones with overlapping DNA fragments (Fig. 3, lanes 2, 3, and 4). However, although this experiment has been repeated numerous times and in different ways, no clones capable of restoring full virulence to the *M. tuberculosis* H37Ra mutant were identified. This result suggests at least two quite different possibilities: (i) the H37Ra mutant has acquired a number of mutations on noncontiguous chromosomal locations that result in its avirulent phenotype, or alternatively, (ii) the H37Ra strain has a missense mutation in the putative virulence gene or a virulence regulatory gene such that when the wild-type gene is cloned into H37Ra in a merodiploid state, as we have done, it may exhibit an intermediate phenotype. This experiment points out the two significant needs for using this approach in identifying virulence

A. Growth of H37Ra recombinants containing H37Rv cosmids in spleen

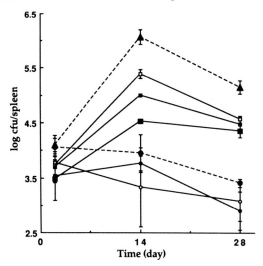

B. PstI digests of H37Rv cosmids

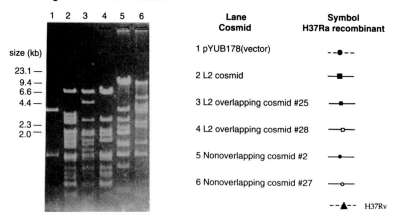

Lane Cosmid	Symbol H37Ra recombinant
1 pYUB178(vector)	--●--
2 L2 cosmid	—■—
3 L2 overlapping cosmid #25	—■—
4 L2 overlapping cosmid #28	—□—
5 Nonoverlapping cosmid #2	—◆—
6 Nonoverlapping cosmid #27	—○—
	--▲-- H37Rv

Figure 3. Characterization of *M. tuberculosis* H37Rv DNA fragments that confer an in vivo growth advantage in spleen on *M. tuberculosis* H37Ra. Several overlapping clones that confer a selective growth advantage upon transformation into *M. tuberculosis* H37Ra have been identified.

genes. First, methods of efficiently isolating mutants of *M. tuberculosis* that arise from single clones, such as a transposon mutagenesis system described below, are needed. Second, there is a crucial need for efficient methods of performing allele exchange or gene replacement experiments in *M. tuberculosis* and BCG to eliminate the need for a merodiploid state. Although numerous investigators have demonstrated that homologous recombination can be readily achieved in *M. smegmatis*, this has not yet been achieved for *M. tuberculosis* and has been achieved inefficiently for BCG (Aldovini et al., 1993). The introduction of linear DNA fragments into both *M. tuberculosis* and BCG results in their incorporation primarily in nonhomologous sites around the *M. tuberculosis* chromosome (Kalpana et al., 1991). The surprising discovery that the *M. tuberculosis recA* gene is expressed as a protein that undergoes protein splicing (Davis et al., 1991, 1992; see also chapter 15 in this volume) suggests that the recombination systems of *M. tuberculosis* might be unusual and that they may need to be characterized before we can achieve efficient homologous recombination.

Identification of Putative Virulence Genes: Use of *E. coli* as a Surrogate Host

One successful strategy has been to use *E. coli* as a surrogate host for the cloning and screening of virulence genes of pathogenic gram-negative bacteria. A classic experiment utilizing such an approach was the identification of the invasin gene of *Yersinia pseudotuberculosis* by Isberg and Falkow (1985; Isberg et al., 1987). In this experiment, a genomic library of *Y. pseudotuberculosis* was constructed and screened for recombinant clones that had the ability to adsorb to and enter eukaryotic epithelial cells in culture, which *E. coli* itself is unable to do. Recombinant clones with such a

phenotype were shown to possess a common DNA fragment encoding a gene, named *invA*, that produced an 86-kDa protein that mediates the efficient uptake of *E. coli* into HeLa cells. It is worth noting that insertional mutation of the *invA* gene into *Yersinia* sp. did not abolish the ability to enter epithelial cells or virulence in vivo, nor is *invA* protective by itself. Thus, since their very survival depends on overcoming host defenses, most pathogens will likely have multiple genes responsible for entering or surviving within the host, and that multiplicity represents the challenge to our understanding.

Recently, this same approach was successfully utilized by Arruda et al. (1993) to screen a genomic library of *M. tuberculosis* in *E. coli* for the ability to efficiently invade or be taken up by mouse macrophages. The DNA sequence of the clone showed 27% homology with the internalin gene of *Listeria monocytogenes* and 19% homology with *invA*; both of these genes are associated with mammalian cell entry in their respective pathogens. Of particular interest was the finding that *E. coli* expressing InvA also survived longer within the macrophage. This is an exciting development and represents the identification of the first putative invasin gene described for any mycobacterial pathogen.

Recent reports have described the use of subtractive mRNA library approaches for the identification of genes that are made specifically in either virulent mycobacteria (Kinger and Tyagi, 1993) or genes that are induced when the mycobacteria are grown in macrophages (Plum and Clark-Curtiss, 1994). These are very promising approaches that should lead to the identification of many of the genes involved in intracellular growth and virulence.

Finally, it has long been appreciated that there are significant homologs of many virulence genes of gram-negative pathogens, even in different genera. For example, in *Salmonella*, *Yersinia*, *Vibrio*, and *Shigella* spp. as well as *Bordetella* spp., there are key regulatory genes that control virulence. One set is a series of molecular sensors and signal transducers that respond to the environment in which the organism is found (Miller et al., 1989). These regulatory genes can control expression of a whole series of virulence genes. For example, a mutation in the *bvgAS* gene in *Bordetella pertussis* results in the failure to express pertussis toxin, an adenosyl cyclase, a filamentous hemagglutinin, and a hemolysin. While the G+C content of *M. tuberculosis* is higher than that of most gram-negative bacteria, since it has been possible to identify some mycobacterial antigen and enzyme genes by hybridization with degenerate oligonucleotides on the basis of coding sequences of genes of interest from *E. coli*, it may be possible to identify homologs of virulence genes by a similar strategy. In this context, Gupta and Tyagi (1993) have reported the cloning of a mycobacterial homolog of the *virF* gene of *Shigella* spp. Clearly, the demonstration that such homologs are involved in mycobacterial virulence will depend on fulfillment of Koch's molecular postulates, namely, mutation and transfer to avirulent strains.

FUTURE STRATEGIES

A number of general approaches to delineating molecular mechanisms of microbial pathogenesis are being developed. Some of those that we believe may be particularly relevant to understanding mycobacterial pathogenesis are outlined in Table 3 and summarized briefly here.

The Power of Transposon Mutagenesis for Identifying Virulence Genes

While there are multiple ways of inducing mutations in bacteria, including use of chemical mutagens and irradiation, insertional mutagenesis has unique advantages

Table 3. Strategies successfully used to identify virulence genes

Experiment	Example
Transfer of virulence genes to avirulent strains	Isberg and Falkow, 1985
Screening libraries of transposon mutants for avirulent phenotypes	Fields et al., 1986
Screening reporter transposon libraries for virulence-associated phenotypes	Maurelli and Curtiss, 1984
Screening for cell surface or secreted proteins by using a *phoA* reporter	Taylor et al., 1989
In vivo expression technology	Mahan et al., 1993

(Table 4). Insertional mutagenesis is usually achieved by using a transposon, a DNA element that can move from its original site on a DNA molecule to a random site in the same or a different DNA molecule (chapter 14). The transposition event, i.e., the transfer of the transposon from one site to another, is mediated by a gene encoding a transposase. In addition to carrying the transposase, the transposon carries a selectable marker gene, such as an antibiotic resistance gene, that usually confers a selective advantage on a bacterium under certain growth conditions. Thus, to generate a library of insertional mutants, the transposon is introduced into the host bac-

Table 4. Why insertional mutagenesis?

Parameter	Physical or chemical DNA-damaging agent	Insertional mutagen
Direct selection for mutants (even in clumps)	No	Yes
Frequency of mutants/treatment	10^{-4}	100%
No. of mutations/cell	>1	1
Reporter screens	No	Yes
Random mutations	Yes	Yes and No

terium by means of a transposon delivery vector that cannot replicate in that organism. In a small fraction of the cells (usually between 10^{-3} and 10^{-5}), the transposon will hop from the delivery vector to the chromosome of the bacterium of interest. The cells to which the delivery vector containing the transposon has been introduced are plated on medium containing the selective agent. Only the cells in which the transposon has hopped from the delivery vector to its chromosome will stably express the selectable marker gene and thus give rise to a colony of cells arising from a single mutated cell in the presence of the antibiotic. By collecting a large set of colonies from such an experiment, a library of insertion mutants can be assembled. The generation of such a library of mutants for the identification of virulence mutants is particularly well suited for *M. tuberculosis* and BCG for several reasons. First, since *M. tuberculosis*, like other mycobacteria, grows in clumps of 10 to 20 bacterial cells even when grown in detergent, the introduction of a selectable marker gene and the growth of cells in the presence of the selecting agent allow cells that did not receive the transposon to be selected against and killed. This selection ensures that the colony that arises on a selection plate is clonal, i.e., derived from a single cell containing the transposon. Second, since selection will enrich for cells in which a transposon has hopped into a cell's chromosome, transposon mutagenesis generates a set of colonies in which every colony has arisen from a single mutated cell. In contrast, procedures using mutagenic agents such as irradiation or chemicals generally yield one mutant colony for every 1,000 to 10,000 nonmutated colonies, and there is always a possibility that the mutated cell contains more than one lesion caused by the DNA-damaging agent. Transposon mutagenesis is thus highly desirable for the identification of mutations in virulence genes, since such mutations cannot be directly selected for

but rather must be screened for. If one considers that each assay for virulence involves growth in an animal or in a cultured cell line, there is a need for a method that requires screening as few candidate clones as possible. For *M. tuberculosis*, there is an additional advantage to transposon mutagenesis, since the generation time of *M. tuberculosis* cells is 20 to 24 h, and thus at least 2 to 4 weeks are required to yield colonies on plates and much longer times are needed to perform in vivo virulence assays.

If one assumes that a bacterium contains over 3,000 genes and that it could tolerate insertion mutants in each of them, a minimum of 3,000 mutants would be required to screen a complete mutant library. However, even if a transposon hops in a purely random fashion, producing random mutations, approximately three times as many mutants would have to be screened to ensure that a mutation has been generated in the majority of genes. Such an approach was utilized by Heffron and colleagues to identify genes important for the growth and survival of *Salmonella typhimurium* in mouse macrophages (Fields et al., 1986). A library of 9,516 *S. typhimurium* transformants generated with Tn*10* were screened for their abilities to grow in macrophages in tissue culture. This approach led to the identification of 83 mutants that had diminished capacity for intracellular survival. All of the mutants were less virulent than the parent in 50% lethal dose assays in mice, suggesting that for *S. typhimurium*, survival within macrophages is essential for virulence. The range of mutations included a variety of amino acid auxotrophies as well as mutations that confer sensitivities to a several of microbicidal mechanisms, including defensins. This approach was quite productive but very labor intensive, even though the transposon mutagenesis reduced the number of mutants that had to be screened to a manageable number.

Generation of Insertion Mutations in BCG and *M. tuberculosis*

Mutagenesis of a slow-growing mycobacterium that requires 3 to 4 weeks to yield colonies on a plate, such as BCG or *M. tuberculosis*, would be greatly facilitated by insertional mutation approaches that permit direct selection for mutants (Fig. 4). Several transposons have been identified, and progress in trying to develop such a strategy has been made in several laboratories (see chapter 14). When studies were initiated in our laboratory, no transposons had

yet been described for the mycobacteria. Consequently, we sought to develop a shuttle mutagenesis strategy in which mycobacterial DNA was cloned onto shuttle plasmids that were insertionally mutagenized by passage in *E. coli* containing Tn5 derivatives. When the mutagenized DNA was shuttled into *M. smegmatis*, we were successful in generating auxotrophic mutants by homologous recombination and allelic exchange. However, we were surprised to find that when similar allele exchanges were attempted in BCG and *M. tuberculo-*

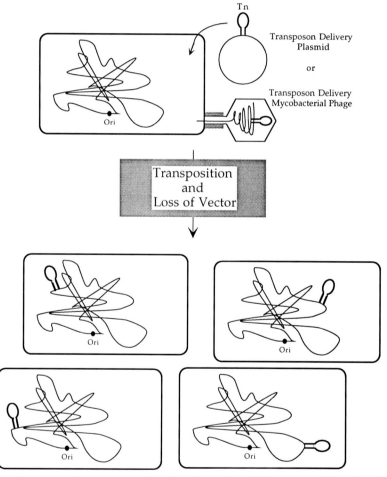

Figure 4. Strategy for constructing transposon libraries. A mycobacterial transposon is introduced on a suicide delivery vector, and clones that have obtained the transposon containing a selectable marker gene randomly inserted in the genome are selected for.

sis, no recombination was obtained with circular plasmids, and linear DNA fragments inserted randomly into the genome of these slow-growing mycobacteria (Kalpana et al., 1991). Although we have even been able to isolate auxotrophic mutants of BCG by taking advantage of this illegitimate recombination mechanism, the frequency is too low to generate useful libraries of mutants.

In independent experiments aimed at generating auxotrophic mutants in the diaminopimelic acid biosynthetic pathway essential for cell wall production, we inadvertently found that the construction used served as a transposon trap that allowed us to discover the insertion element IS*1096* of *M. smegmatis* (Cirillo et al., 1991), which appears to transpose in a random fashion into target DNA. Sequencing of this 2.2-kb DNA element identified two open reading frames. We have subsequently engineered transposon derivatives of this insertion element by placing a kanamycin resistance gene at various locations throughout IS*1096*. Libraries of insertional mutants of BCG using these transposon derivatives have been generated, and detailed analysis of 30 insertional mutants established that the IS*1096*-derived transpositions all inserted into different sites of the chromosome (McAdam et al., in press). These experiments thus suggest that this insertion element can transpose in a random fashion in BCG and possibly in *M. tuberculosis*. To date, three auxotrophic mutants have been characterized: two with mutations in leucine and one with mutations in methionine biosynthesis (McAdam et al., unpublished results). Initial characterization of the growth of the auxotrophs in mice has revealed interesting findings. The methionine auxotroph mimics the parent BCG strain, showing modest increases of growth in the mice. In contrast, both leucine auxotrophs show no growth and are cleared from the mice in 3 to 4 weeks.

Since phages at an appropriate multiplic-ity of infection can infect every cell in a mycobacterial population, whereas the frequency of transformation is only on the order of 10^{-5}, the next methodological advance required will be to develop a suicide phage delivery system to increase the frequency of transpositions.

Potential Uses of Reporter Screens for Identification of Genes with Virulence-Associated Phenotypes

Another useful property of transposons is that they can be engineered to contain promoterless reporter genes such as the *lacZ* gene that encodes β-galactosidase or the firefly luciferase gene. Expression of β-galactosidase can be readily detected by using a variety of substrate analogs such as 5-bromo-4-chloro-3-indolyl-β-D-galactopyranoside (X-Gal) or *o*-nitrophenyl-β-D-galactopyranoside (ONPG) that can be easily detected in media or by using spectrophotometric assays, and luciferase can be detected by measuring luminescence. The utility of a promoter probe transposon lies in the abilities of these constructs to transpose downstream of promoters of random genes, thereby placing the reporter gene under the regulatory control of a chromosomally encoded gene. Since the gene products of many genes will not be easily assayable, this process provides a powerful method for assaying the activities of interesting genes under a variety of culture or in vivo conditions. Reporter transposons provide a powerful method for identifying novel genes that share a common mode of regulation. For example, this method was first used to identify a novel virulence gene of *Shigella flexneri* on the basis of the observation that the virulence phenotype of *Shigella* spp. is regulated by temperature (Maurelli and Curtiss, 1984). Specifically, *Shigella flexneri* grown at 37°C was fully virulent and capable of invading HeLa cell monolayers; however, if grown at 30°C, the *Shigella flexneri* was noninvasive of the

HeLa cell monolayer. It appeared as if the genes required for invasion of HeLa cells were turned on at 37°C but turned off at 30°C. A library of reporter transposon insertions was constructed in *Shigella flexneri* by using a Mud *lac* phage, in which the phage Mu functions like a transposon. Mutants that made β-galactosidase at 37°C but not at 30°C were identified. This family of mutants was screened for loss of virulence at 37°C, and mutants that were completely avirulent were found. One such mutant had acquired a Mud *lac* insertion in a previously unidentified gene that is essential for the virulence of *Shigella flexneri*. The advantage of this method is that it reduced the number of transposon mutants that had to be screened in a time-consuming virulence assay by identifying a set of genes that shared an expression pattern with the phenotype of virulence.

In analogous reasoning, several investigators made the assumption that a number of proteins associated with virulence would be secreted or associated with the cell wall of the pathogen. They used a secretion reporter transposon, Tn*phoA*, a transposon containing a promotorless alkaline phosphatase gene, to generate libraries of mutants in *Vibrio cholerae* (Taylor et al., 1989), *B. pertussis* (Finn et al., 1991), or *Shigella flexneri* (Allaoui et al., 1992) to identify novel genes associated with virulence. In the presence of substrate, Tn*phoA* produces a color when the molecule is expressed extracellularly or in the periplasm. By linking the Tn*phoA* strategy with imaginative screens, it has been possible even to identify sets of genes required to permit *Salmonella* spp. to transcytose polarized cells (Finlay et al., 1988).

Reporter Genes That Should Be Useful for Mycobacteria

The use of reporter genes offers tremendous advantages for screening for novel genes with phenotypes that are not easily assayable. For mycobacteria, a number of reporter genes have been demonstrated to function. The *E. coli lacZ* gene, encoding β-galactosidase, is expressed when fused to mycobacterial promoters and can easily be assayed for in mycobacteria by using X-Gal (Stover et al., 1991; Barletta et al., 1991). The gene is useful for screening for promoter activities on agar media, but accurate activity analyses require that the cells be sonicated prior to assay (Levin and Hatfull, 1993), a major hazard for its use with virulent *M. tuberculosis* strains. In contrast, the firefly luciferase gene has been demonstrated to be assayable in intact *M. smegmatis*, BCG, and *M. tuberculosis* cells simply by adding the substrate luciferin, which readily enters mycobacterial cells (Jacobs et al., 1993). Moreover, the expression of the luciferase gene provides a novel assay for assessing viability and thus can be used in a variety of drug-screening or possible cell-killing assays (Jacobs et al., 1993; Cooksey et al., 1993).

The enzyme alkaline phosphatase is extremely useful as a secreted reporter gene, as its activity is seen only when the protein is secreted and not when the protein is present in the cytoplasm. To date, attempts to express an active alkaline phosphatase enzyme in mycobacteria have not been successful (Connell, unpublished results). As an alternative enzyme for studying secretion, we have cloned several genes that are secreted from *Streptomyces coelicolor* as potential secretion reporter probes. We have found that the secreted streptomyces β-galactosidase can be expressed in *M. smegmatis* (Connell et al., unpublished results). In addition, we have observed that the plasmid-encoded agarase gene (*dagA*) can be expressed in both *M. smegmatis* and BCG, where it causes colonies to sink into the agar plate. Experiments are under way to test the usefulness of these genes in identifying secreted genes of *M. tuberculosis*.

In Vivo Gene Expression Assays Using Auxotrophs of BCG and *M. tuberculosis*

Mekalanos and his coworkers have recently described a very appealing system for identifying genes that are expressed exclusively when *Salmonella typhimurium* is grown in vivo (Mahan et al., 1993). The method requires an auxotrophic host strain that can be converted to a prototroph by a plasmid containing the complementing gene required for growth linked to a reporter gene, such as that for β-galactosidase. They utilized a *purA* auxotroph created by deletion of the chromosomal *purA* gene in *S. typhimurium*. They then generated a vector that had a unique cloning site located at the 5′ end of the promoterless *purA* gene, which had a β-galactosidase gene situated downstream in an operon with the *purA* gene. A genomic library of random sequences of *Salmonella* DNA was introduced into the unique cloning site in front of the biosynthetic gene, and this library was introduced in single copy into the bacterial pathogen. The auxotroph is unable to grow unless a promoter sequence is cloned in the unique cloning site situated proximal to the truncated biosynthetic gene. Any bacteria constitutively expressing the reporter in vitro, presumably reflecting insertion of a constitutive promoter sequence, are excluded, and the remainder are used to infect

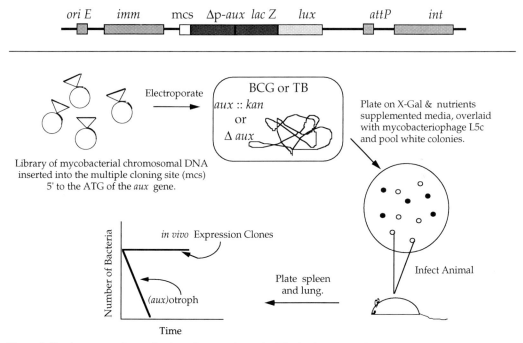

Figure 5. In vivo expression technology for mycobacteria. The basic strategy has been described by Mekalanos and colleagues (Mahan et al., 1993) for *Salmonella* spp. An appropriate auxotroph is identified and found not to grow in an animal host. A genomic library from the virulent organism is constructed in a vector in a unique restriction site present immediately upstream of the complementing gene. The reporter operon is used to identify genes that are turned on constitutively that are then removed from the library. The remaining library is passed through animals, and only those recombinant clones that are expressed in vivo will grow in the selective environment of the mouse.

animals. The organisms surviving in any tissue are then plated, and colonies not expressing the reporter must reflect a fusion of the biosynthetic and reporter genes with a promoter that was activated only in vivo. That sequence is then used to isolate the gene controlled by that promoter. In *Salmonella* spp., about 100 in vivo-expressed genes, many of them known virulence factors, have been identified (Mekalanos, in press). This is a general strategy that can be applied, in principle, to any pathogen.

We have been successful in using insertional mutagenesis to generate several auxotrophic mutations for leucine, isoleucine-valine, and methionine genes in BCG (Kalpana et al., unpublished results; McAdam et al., unpublished results). It has been gratifying to note that the *leu* and *ile* mutants fail to grow in mice and thus might be promising candidates for adapting the in vivo expression technology to pathogenic mycobacteria. One possible strategy for detecting genes expressed in vivo from mycobacteria is illustrated in Fig. 5.

ACQUISITION OF NEW KNOWLEDGE THROUGH GENETIC STUDIES

Koch's postulates set out both criteria and a methodology for understanding, at the level of causation, the pathogenesis of a whole new category of human and animal diseases. Through application of those principles and epidemiological studies, the etiologies of hundreds of human diseases have been established as attributable to infectious viral, bacterial, or parasitic pathogens. In every case, production of disease requires unique adaptations of the pathogenic agent to overcome defenses of the host or modifications of host responses, as in immunodeficiency, becoming susceptible to pathogenesis by opportunistic agents.

The advances in molecular biology and immunology in recent years now provide the tools for understanding the pathogenesis of disease at a molecular level. Yet fundamentally those advances depend on understanding of genetics. By the analogous Koch's molecular postulates, it is now possible, through the study of mutants, to identify regulatory and functional genes contributing to virulence of bacterial pathogens such as *M. tuberculosis* and by means of gene transfer techniques to formally establish their role in pathogenesis. By extending the Human Genome Project to these major pathogens, within but a few years the entire DNA sequences of *M. tuberculosis*, *M. leprae*, and attenuated tuberculosis strains will be known, and that knowledge will enable us to predict the amino acid sequence of every enzyme, every protein, and every antigen. The application of these molecular genetic approaches to tuberculosis will yield a vast amount of knowledge at a molecular level of the mechanisms of pathogenesis and protection. We hope it will also provide previously unimagined opportunities for developing new and effective drugs, diagnostics, and vaccines that will ensure the effective control of tuberculosis globally.

Acknowledgment. We thank V. Balasubramanian for excellent help in preparing the drawings.

REFERENCES

Aldovini, A., R. N. Husson, and R. A. Young. 1993. The *uraA* locus and homologous recombination in *Mycobacterium bovis* BCG. *J. Bacteriol.* **175:**7282–7289.

Allaoui, A., P. J. Sansonetti, and C. Parsot. 1992. MxiJ, a lipoprotein involved in secretion of *Shigella* Ipa invasins, is homologous to YacJ, a secretion factor of the *Yersinia* Yop proteins. *J. Bacteriol.* **174:**7661–7669.

Arruda, S., G. Bomfim, R. Knights, T. Huima-Byron, and L. W. Riley. 1993. Cloning of an *M. tuberculosis* DNA fragment associated with entry and survival inside cells. *Science* **261:**1454–1457.

Barletta, R. G., D. D. Kim, S. B. Snapper, B. R. Bloom, and W. R. Jacobs, Jr. 1991. Identification of expression signals of the mycobacteriophages Bxb1, L1, and TM4 using the *Escherichia-Mycobacterium* shuttle plasmids. *J. Gen. Microbiol.* **138:**23–30.

Calmette, A., and C. Guérin. 1909. Sur quelques propriétés du bacille tuberculeux d'origine bovine, cultivé sur la bile de boeuf glycérinée. *C. R. Acad. Sci.* **149:**716.

Cirillo, J. D., R. G. Barletta, B. R. Bloom, and W. R. Jacobs, Jr. 1991. A novel transposon trap for mycobacteria: isolation and characterization of IS*1096*. *J. Bacteriol.* **173:**7772–7780.

Collins, F. M., and M. M. Smith. 1969. A comparative study of the virulence of *Mycobacterium tuberculosis* measured in mice and guinea pigs. *Am. Rev. Respir. Dis.* **100:**631–639.

Connell, N. Unpublished results.

Connell, N., B. R. Bloom, and W. R. Jacobs, Jr. Unpublished results.

Cooksey, R. C., J. T. Crawford, W. R. Jacobs, Jr., and T. M. Shinnick. 1993. A rapid method for screening antimicrobial agents for activities against a strain of *Mycobacterium tuberculosis* expressing firefly luciferase. *Antimicrob. Agents Chemother.* **37:**1348–1352.

Davis, E. O., P. J. Jenner, P. C. Brooks, M. J. Colston, and S. G. Sedgwick. 1992. Protein splicing in the maturation of *M. tuberculosis* RecA protein: a mechanism for tolerating a novel class of intervening sequence. *Cell* **71:**201–210.

Davis, E. O., S. G. Sedgwick, and M. J. Colston. 1991. Novel structure of the *recA* locus of *Mycobacterium tuberculosis* implies processing of the gene product. *J. Bacteriol.* **173:**5653–5662.

Falkow, S. 1988. Molecular Koch's postulates applied to microbial pathogenicity. *Rev. Infect. Dis.* **10:**S274–S276.

Fields, P. I., R. V. Swanson, C. G. Haidaris, and F. Heffron. 1986. Mutants of *Salmonella typhimurium* that cannot survive within the macrophage are avirulent. *Proc. Natl. Acad. Sci. USA* **83:**5189–5193.

Finlay, B. B., M. N. Starnbach, C. L. Francis, B. A. Stocker, and S. Falkow. 1988. Identification and characterization of Tn*phoA* mutants of *Salmonella* that are unable to pass through a polarized MDCK epithelial cell monolayer. *Mol. Microbiol.* **2:**757–766.

Finn, T. M., R. Shahin, and J. J. Mekalanos. 1991. Characterization of *vir*-activated Tn*phoA* gene fusions in *Bordetella pertussis*. *Infect. Immun.* **59:**3273–3279.

Gupta, S., and A. K. Tyagi. 1993. Sequence of a newly identified *Mycobacterium tuberculosis* gene encoding a protein with a sequence homology to virulence-regulating proteins. *Gene* **126:**157–158.

Isberg, R. R., and S. Falkow. 1985. A single genetic locus encoded by *Yersinia pseudotuberculosis* permits invasion of cultured animal cells by *Escherichia coli* K-12. *Nature* (London) **317:**262–265.

Isberg, R. R., D. L. Voorhis, and S. Falkow. 1987.

Identification of invasin: a protein that allows enteric bacteria to penetrate cultured mammalian cells. *Cell* **50:**769–778.

Jacobs, W. R., Jr. 1992. Advances in mycobacterial genetics: new promises for old diseases. *Immunobiology* **184:**147–156.

Jacobs, W. R., Jr., R. Barletta, R. Udani, J. Chan, G. Kalkut, G. Sarkis, G. F. Hatfull, and B. R. Bloom. 1993. Rapid assessment of drug susceptibilities of *Mycobacterium tuberculosis* by means of luciferase reporter phages. *Science* **260:**819–822.

Jacobs, W. R., M. A. Docherty, R. Curtiss III, and J. E. Clark-Curtiss. 1986. Expression of *Mycobacterium leprae* genes from a *Streptococcus mutans* promoter in *Escherichia coli* K-12. *Proc. Natl. Acad. Sci. USA* **83:**1926–1930.

Jacobs, W. R., Jr., M. Tuckman, and C. Smith. Unpublished result.

Jacobs, W. R., Jr., M. Tuckman, and B. R. Bloom. 1987. Introduction of foreign DNA into mycobacteria using a shuttle phasmid. *Nature* (London) **327:**532–536.

Kalpana, V. G., B. R. Bloom, and W. R. Jacobs, Jr. 1991. Insertional mutagenesis and illegitimate recombination in mycobacteria. *Proc. Natl. Acad. Sci. USA* **88:**5433–5437.

Kalpana, G., W. R. Jacobs, Jr., and B. R. Bloom. Unpublished results.

Kinger, A. K., and J. S. Tyagi. 1993. Identification and cloning of genes differentially expressed in the virulent strain of *Mycobacterium tuberculosis*. *Gene* **131:**113–117.

Koch, R. 1882. Die Aetiologie der Tuberculos. *Ber. Klin. Wochenschr.* **19:**221. (Reprinted as a translation by Berna Pinner and Max Pinner, *Am. Rev. Tuberc.* **25:**285–323, 1932.)

Lee, M. H., L. Pascopella, W. R. Jacobs, Jr., and G. F. Hatfull. 1991. Site-specific integration of mycobacteriophage L5: integration-proficient vectors for *Mycobacterium smegmatis*, BCG, and *M. tuberculosis*. *Proc. Natl. Acad. Sci. USA* **88:**3111–3115.

Levin, M., and G. F. Hatfull. 1993. Mycobacterium smegmatis RNA polymerase, DNA supercoiling, action of rifampicin and the mechanism of rifampicin resistance. *Mol. Microbiol.* **8:**277–285.

Mackaness, G. B., N. Smith, and A. Q. Wells. 1954. The growth of intracellular tubercle bacilli in relation to their virulence. *Am. Rev. Tuberc.* **69:**479–494.

Mahan, M. J., J. M. Slauch, and J. J. Mekalanos. 1993. Selection of bacterial virulence genes that are specifically induced in host tissues. *Science* **259:**686–688.

Maurelli, A. T., and R. Curtiss III. 1984. Bacteriophage Mu d1(Apʳ *lac*) generates *vir-lac* operon fusions in *Shigella flexneri* 2a. *Infect. Immun.* **45:**642–648.

McAdam, R., J. D. Cirillo, T. Weisbrod, and W. R. Jacobs, Jr. Genetic analysis of IS*1096*: transposition in *M. bovis* BCG. *J. Bacteriol.*, in press.

McAdam, R. A., J. Martin, T. Weisbrod, J. Scuderi, and W. R. Jacobs, Jr. Unpublished results.

Mekalanos, J. J. Bacterial response to host signals. *Harvey Soc.*, in press.

Miller, J. F., J. J. Mekalanos, and S. Falkow. 1989. Coordinate regulation and sensory transduction in the control of bacterial virulence. *Science* **243:**916–922.

North, R. J., and A. A. Izzo. 1993. Mycobacterial virulence: virulent strains of *Mycobacterium tuberculosis* have faster *in vivo* doubling times and are better equipped to resist growth-inhibiting functions of macrophages in the presence and absence of specific immunity. *J. Exp. Med.* **177:**1723–1734.

Pascopella, L., F. M. Collins, J. M. Martin, W. R. Jacobs, Jr., and B. R. Bloom. Identification of a genomic fragment of *Mycobacterium tuberculosis* responsible for in vivo growth advantage. *Infect. Agents Dis.*, in press a.

Pascopella, L., F. M. Collins, J. M. Martin, M. H. Lee, G. F. Hatfull, C. K. Stover, B. R. Bloom, and W. R. Jacobs, Jr. Use of in vivo complementation in *Mycobacterium tuberculosis* to identify a genomic fragment associated with virulence. *Infect. Immun.*, in press b.

Plum, G., and J. E. Clark-Curtiss. 1994. Induction of *Mycobacterium avium* gene expression following phagocytosis by human macrophages. *Infect. Immun.* **62:**476–483.

Snapper, S. B., L. Lugosi, A. Jekkel, R. Melton, T. Kieser, B. R. Bloom, and W. R. Jacobs, Jr. 1988. Lysogeny and transformation of mycobacteria: stable expression of foreign genes. *Proc. Natl. Acad. Sci. USA* **85:**6987–6991.

Snapper, S. B., R. E. Melton, S. Mustafa, T. Kieser, and W. R. Jacobs, Jr. 1990. Isolation and characterization of efficient plasmid transformation mutants of *Mycobacterium smegmatis*. *Mol. Microbiol.* **4:**1911–1919.

Steenken, Jr., W., W. H. Oatway, Jr., and S. A. Petroff. 1934. Biological studies of the tubercle bacillus. III. Dissociation and pathogenicity of the R and S variants of the human tubercle bacillus (H_{37}). *J. Exp. Med.* **60:**515–540.

Stover, C. K., V. F. de la Cruz, T. R. Fuerst, J. E. Burlein, L. A. Benson, L. T. Bennett, G. P. Bansal, J. F. Young, M. H. Lee, G. F. Hatfull, S. B. Snapper, R. G. Barletta, W. R. Jacobs, Jr., and B. R. Bloom. 1991. New use of BCG for recombinant vaccines. *Nature* (London) **351:**456–460.

Taylor, R. K., C. Manoil, and J. J. Mekalanos. 1989. Broad-host-range vectors for the delivery of Tn*phoA*: use in genetic analysis of secreted virulence determinants of *Vibrio cholerae*. *J. Bacteriol.* **171:**1870–1878.

Young, R. A., B. R. Bloom, C. M. Grosskinsky, J. Ivanyi, D. Thomas, and R. W. Davis. 1985a. Dissection of *Mycobacterium tuberculosis* antigens using recombinant DNA. *Proc. Natl. Acad. Sci. USA* **82:**2583–2587.

Young, R. A., V. Mehra, D. Sweetzer, T. Buchanan, J. E. Clark-Curtiss, R. W. Davis, and B. R. Bloom. 1985b. Genes for the major protein antigens of the leprosy parasite, *Mycobacterium leprae*. *Nature* (London) **316:**450–452.

IV. PHYSIOLOGY OF *MYCOBACTERIUM TUBERCULOSIS*

Tuberculosis: Pathogenesis, Protection, and Control
Edited by Barry R. Bloom
© 1994 American Society for Microbiology, Washington, DC 20005

Chapter 19

Ultrastructure of *Mycobacterium tuberculosis*

Patrick J. Brennan and Philip Draper

Mycobacterium tuberculosis was an early object of study by electron microscopy (Rosenblatt et al., 1942), consonant with its importance as a human pathogen. This species and other fast- and slow-growing mycobacterial species have subsequently been studied by a variety of electron microscopical techniques, so a considerable body of ultrastructural data exists. This chapter attempts to describe what is understood of the ultrastructure of *M. tuberculosis* and to point out problems of interpretation and areas where further investigation, probably involving the development of new techniques, is needed. Several reviews discussing the ultrastructure of mycobacteria have been published (Imaeda et al., 1968; Draper, 1982; McNeil and Brennan, 1991).

Most bacteria do not possess the elaborate system of internal compartments found in eukaryotic cells, and the information obtained about mycobacteria by electron microscopy is primarily information about the envelope layers, a discussion of which forms the major part of this chapter. A few ultrastructurally significant objects do occur within the mycobacterial cell, however; these will be discussed briefly. *M. tuberculosis* differs from the majority of bacteria, and from most mycobacteria, in being a pathogen that can multiply within the phagocytic cells of its host. The interaction between bacterium and host cells is clearly important, and some aspects of the ultrastructure of this interaction, which has been considerably studied, will also be described in this chapter.

LIMITATIONS OF ULTRASTRUCTURAL STUDIES OF MYCOBACTERIA

Most electron microscopical techniques available have been applied to mycobacterial cells, yet progress in understanding the ultrastructure of these cells has been less dramatic than for some other bacteria, a fact not entirely explained by the small number of researchers investigating mycobacteria. Some likely reasons for this are worth noting. Mycobacteria are distinctly smaller than most "laboratory" bacteria, so problems of resolution of their structures are greater. For reasons not entirely clear but probably associated with the massive amounts of complex lipid present, the cells are difficult to embed and to section optimally. Fixatives that reliably stabilize neutral carbohydrates and lipids are not available, and stains supplying electron density to such structures are few, and their speci-

Patrick J. Brennan • Department of Microbiology, Colorado State University, Fort Collins, Colorado 80523.   *Philip Draper* • National Institute for Medical Research, Mill Hill, London NW7 1AA, England.

ficities are uncertain. Immunostaining does not at present have the resolution needed to localize molecules within structures as small as mycobacterial cells. It is clear that new techniques are needed if the various ultrastructural problems mentioned in this chapter are to be resolved.

NATURE OF THE ENVELOPE OF *M. TUBERCULOSIS*

Bacterial envelopes provide protection and support for the bacterial cell and also contain the mechanisms that allow (or prevent) traffic of substances between the bacterial cell and its environment. There are remarkable similarities, both chemical and ultrastructural, among the envelopes of most bacteria. A major structural division is between gram-positive and gram-negative species: the structural distinction is believed to be mainly responsible for and corresponds broadly to the behavior of the organisms in the classical Gram stain. *M. tuberculosis* and other mycobacteria are biologically part of the gram-positive group (though they behave anomalously with the Gram stain), but they have some distinctive features. In particular, although all gram-positive bacteria possess peptidoglycan (a cross-linked polymer of amino sugars and amino acids that determines the shape of the bacterial cell), the molecules attached to or associated with this polymer are predominantly lipids in mycobacteria rather than the proteins and polysaccharides found in other bacteria (Lederer et al., 1975). However, mycobacteria possess a wall polysaccharide that resembles that of other gram-positive bacteria in having a disaccharide-phosphoryl linker between the peptidoglycan and the polysaccharide (McNeil et al., 1990).

Since *M. tuberculosis* is one of a small group of species able to survive inside the phagocytic cells of a animal host, it is likely that its envelope has special properties defending the bacterium against host microbicidal processes. However, though attempts have been made to associate ultrastructural features with resistance to phagocytes, no special feature has yet been conclusively identified: the envelopes of *M. tuberculosis* do not differ visibly from those of non-pathogenic mycobacteria. Because other, nonpathogenic and faster-growing mycobacterial species are easier and safer to handle than *M. tuberculosis*, many ultrastructural studies have been made with them rather than with *M. tuberculosis* itself. Thus, much of the information presented in this chapter has been obtained from other species but is believed to be applicable to the pathogen. Ultrastructural features that are found in other species or groups of species but that do not occur in *M. tuberculosis* itself will not be discussed. However, it will be assumed that the ultrastructure of the various members of the "*M. tuberculosis* complex," including pathogenic *M. bovis* and its attenuated vaccine strain BCG (bacille Calmette-Guérin), is similar. The various members of the complex are generally very similar except as concerns pathogenicity.

The envelope consists of two distinct parts: the plasma membrane and, around it, the wall. These parts provide osmotic protection plus transport of ions and molecules and mechanical support plus protection, respectively. The parts may be mechanically separated and studied independently, which is especially convenient for chemical and biochemical investigations, but have often been examined together for ultrastructural purposes. An important theme of ultrastructural investigation has been the attempt to relate chemical identity to visible structure and to relate both to biological function, so subcellular fractionation, chemical investigation, and ultrastructural study have often been linked. As discussed below, these attempts have been partially successful as far as the major components of the envelope are concerned, but the distribution and arrangement of the numerous minor (though potentially important) envelope-associated molecules found in *M. tuberculosis* are still poorly understood.

FRACTIONATION OF THE MYCOBACTERIAL ENVELOPE

Although the ultrastructure of the envelope may be studied in intact bacteria, it is necessary to fractionate the cells in order to study the chemistry of the various parts and to correlate knowledge of the chemical composition with ultrastructural appearance. Mycobacteria present various problems to the would-be fractionator: they are mechanically tough, the various fractions tend to adhere to one another, and some of the associated molecules appear to redistribute themselves during fractionation. Typically, the cells have been broken by mechanical stress (sonication, grinding with abrasives, or shearing in the French pressure cell) and then fractionated by differential centrifugation or density gradients. Electron microscopy and chemical and biochemical analyses of the fractions are essential to ensure their purity. Techniques for isolating mycobacterial plasma membranes were worked out by Brodie and his group (Brodie et al., 1979). Although most of this work was done with rapid-growing species, it seems likely that all mycobacterial plasma membranes are similar.

THE PLASMA MEMBRANE OF MYCOBACTERIA

Membranes of mycobacteria, including *M. tuberculosis*, appear in ultrathin sections as classic bilayers, with two electron-dense layers separated by a transparent layer (Silva and Macedo, 1983a). This appearance, coupled with their known chemical composition (Kumar et al., 1979), indicates that these are "normal" biological membranes. (Extensive research by Brodie's group showed that membranes of the rapid-growing species *M. phlei* have the characteristic metabolic functions of bacterial membranes [Brodie et al., 1979].) Mycobacterial membranes do, however, have some distinctive components, notably the lipopolysaccharides lipoarabinomannan (LAM) and lipomannan and the phosphatidylinositol mannosides. Freeze fracture confirms their normal nature and shows a fracture plane between the electron-dense layers and typical images of integral membrane proteins embedded in the layers (Nguyen et al., 1979). It should be noted that thin sections of specimens prepared by several techniques show no indication of an additional, outer membrane (such as is found in gram-negative bacteria), although there is an additional plane of fracture in the envelope, and this feature has been important in the development of theoretical models of the envelope (see below).

The appearance of the mycobacterial plasma membrane is not symmetrical in bacteria cells carefully fixed from a viable state: the outer, electron-dense layer is thicker (measured in thin sections) than the inner layer (Fig. 1). The asymmetry is lost when the cells are killed before fixation for microscopy or when fixation is inadequate. The asymmetrical appearance is also preserved when mycobacterial cells (at least those of rapid-growing species) are subjected to the process of freeze-substitution as an alternative to conventional fixation and embedding (Paul and Beveridge, 1992). There is electron-cytochemical evidence that the "extra" thickness is associated with carbohydrate (Silva and Macedo, 1983b), and possible candidate molecules are phosphatidylinositol mannosides or LAM, though why and how these should be redistributed (or removed) in dead cells is not clear.

In killed or degenerated mycobacterial cells, the plasma membrane is seen clearly separated from the other layers of the en-

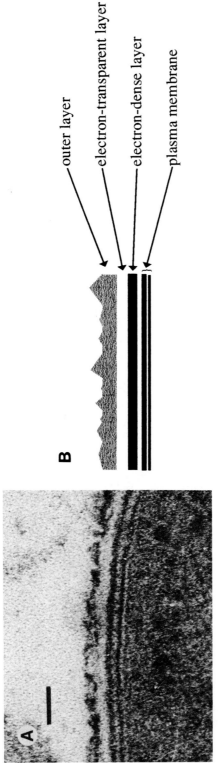

Figure 1. Appearance of mycobacterial envelope in thin sections. (A) Electron micrograph of envelope and part of cell contents of *M. phlei* 425. Cells were fixed by freeze-substitution (Paul and Beveridge, 1992) to optimize preservation of structure and to reduce extraction of lipid components by solvents used in processing. (Photograph kindly supplied by Terry Paul, University of Guelph, Guelph, Ontario, Canada.) Bar indicates 30 nm. (B) Interpretation of image shown in panel A in terms of layer structure described in text. Thickness of layers is enlarged about twofold compared with thickness in the micrograph. Modified from Fig. 15 of Paul and Beveridge (1992).

velope, but in bacteria that were viable before fixation, the outer layer of the membrane is more or less closely apposed to the inner layer of the wall (Silva and Macedo, 1983a; Paul and Beveridge, 1992), which has sometimes caused some confusion in interpretation of images of sections (Daffé et al., 1989). The spacing of the outer layer of the membrane and the inner layer of the wall appears to depend on the fixation, staining, and embedding protocols used in preparing the cells for microscopy. In some cases, a distinct gap with moderate electron density is observed. Experiments (using plasmolysis, for example) to test whether there is any physical attachment between wall and membrane have not been made, but any attachment is clearly broken in degenerating cells.

If the hypothesis is that the walls of *M. tuberculosis* and other mycobacteria form permeability barriers somewhat analogous to the outer membranes of gram-negative bacteria (see below), then the space between the outer leaflet of the membrane and the wall forms a compartment analogous to the periplasmic space of gram-negative bacteria. As such, it merits further study to identify molecules trapped or stored in this compartment.

APPEARANCE OF THE WALL OF *M. TUBERCULOSIS*

Isolated walls of bacteria, including mycobacteria, retain the shape of the intact bacteria, so the wall determines the size and shape of the bacterial cell. In the case of mycobacteria, it seems that this basic function is accompanied by important activities that control access to the plasma membrane of molecules in the environment of the cell. The study of ultrastructure attempts to clarify how the arrangement of chemical components of the wall achieves this double function. Unfortunately, the various ultrastructural techniques applied

to mycobacterial walls give inconsistent or even, apparently, contradictory data, and the reconciliation of these data has yet to be completed.

The chemistry of the mycobacterial wall is discussed in detail elsewhere (see, for example, Lederer et al. [1975] and McNeil and Brennan [1991]), but a brief summary will simplify discussion of the observed ultrastructure. The shape-forming properties of the wall are attributable to the peptidoglycan, whose chemical structure in *M. tuberculosis* closely resembles that found in other bacteria. Attached to this by phosphodiester bonds is a branched-chain polysaccharide, the arabinogalactan, whose distal ends are esterified with high-molecular-weight fatty acids (mycolic acids) of sizes and structures unique to mycobacteria. Mycolic acids are 1-alkyl branched 2-hydroxy fatty acids, typically with 70 to 90 carbon atoms. The branch is commonly about 24 carbon atoms long and is a simple alkyl chain, but the main chain contains (in *M. tuberculosis*) cyclopropyl, methoxyl or keto, and methyl groups. This asymmetry between the two alkyl chains is important in the construction of models of the mycobacterial envelope (see below). Peptidoglycan-arabinogalactan mycolate forms the so-called cell wall skeleton, which is readily isolated and studied. Associated with the skeleton is a large variety of lipids and glycolipids (and possibly some proteins). These differ considerably among mycobacterial species or groups of species, and a few have highly distinctive ultrastructural appearances, but those associated with *M. tuberculosis* (many of which are well studied and well understood from a chemical point of view) are not among the ultrastructurally recognizable types. For none of these associated molecules is the anatomical situation in *M. tuberculosis* known, and their connections with ultrastructure (if any) are not definitely known. New wall-associated molecules continue to be described, and it seems certain that some remain to be isolated and identified. Consequently, one must admit the possibility that some features of the appearance of the wall are caused by substances still unknown.

The simplest images of the wall of *M. tuberculosis* are obtained from ultrathin sections of embedded bacteria. A recent publication (though dealing with fast-growing mycobacteria) describes the use of freeze-substitution to minimize extraction of associated lipids from the wall, a procedure whose efficacy was confirmed by measuring extraction of radiolabeled lipids from the mycobacteria during processing for microscopy (Paul and Beveridge, 1992). Among those so far published, these images seem likely to be the least affected by processing artifacts, but they differ only quantitatively (thicknesses and densities of the layers, improved technical quality) from images obtained by earlier techniques (Imaeda et al., 1968), including images of *M. tuberculosis* itself. The wall is constructed of three layers (Fig. 1). With conventional staining, their appearance is as follows: an inner layer of moderate electron density, a wider electron-transparent layer, and an outer electron-opaque layer of extremely variable appearance and thickness. The inner layer probably contains the peptidoglycan; its moderate electron density is consistent with the known staining properties of this molecule, which contains carboxyl groups (of diaminopimelic acid) that bind metal ions (Beveridge and Murray, 1980). Binding of uranium by mycobacterial walls has been described elsewhere (Andres et al., 1993). The electron-transparent layer appears to be the arabinogalactan mycolate, the lipopolysaccharide that forms a large part of the wall. Its transparency to electrons is probably explained by its extremely hydrophobic nature (so that water-soluble stains fail to penetrate) together with a lack of reactive chemical groups that might bind commonly used electron microscopical stains. In isolated walls, removal of the mycolate by gentle saponification

followed by solvent extraction removes the electron-transparent layer, implying that the inner layer contains both peptidoglycan and arabinogalactan (Draper, 1971). However, this residual material also loses much of its structural rigidity, implying that there has been some rearrangement of the molecules following the loss of the lipid. The peptidoglycan-arabinogalactan may be stained with silver, indicating the presence of carbohydrate, but the stain is not successful with intact cells or undegraded walls (Rastogi et al., 1984), indicating that the mycolic acids prevent access to the arabinogalactan.

The outermost layer of the wall as seen in thin sections has been clearly identified as a distinct entity only recently. The layer has been detected in at least 18 mycobacterial species, including *M. tuberculosis* and *M. bovis*, where it could be seen in 50 to 80% of individual mycobacterial cells (Rastogi et al., 1986). Without special staining, the layer (which can be observed in many published electron micrographs of mycobacteria) varies in thickness (from negligible to massive), electron density, and appearance (fibrillar, granular, or homogeneous). Part of this variability seems to be attributable to preparation methods for microscopy; other variables may be methods of growing the bacteria and differences between mycobacterial species. The use of the dye ruthenium red allowed the layer to be clearly and consistently visualized. While the interpretation of cytochemical methods usable for electron microscopy is difficult and often uncertain, it seems clear that (i) the layer is real and may be interpreted as a capsule of the mycobacterial cell and (ii) it contains charged groups. The latter conclusion is indicated by the intense staining of the layer by ruthenium red. This dye is used in electron microscopy as a basic stain that does not penetrate membranes; it confers excellent contrast to the glycocalyx of eukaryotic cells, apparently by binding to acidic polysaccharides (Hayat, 1989). It is not clear what component of the mycobacterial envelope binds to ruthenium red. The lipopolysaccharide LAM, which contains succinate and phosphate groups, is a possibility (Hunter et al., 1986). Tannic acid also emphasizes the outer layer in the case of *M. vaccae* (Takade et al., 1983); those authors discuss what information this fact gives about the layer and suggest that it may indicate the presence of a polysaccharide. Since the outer layer survives the treatment with organic solvents used in conventional electron microscopic embedding, it is unlikely to consist of lipid or glycolipid; for example, its appearance was not much affected whether mycobacterial cells were processed by conventional techniques or by freeze-substitution (Paul and Beveridge, 1992), although massive losses of extractable lipid occurred in the former process.

An alternative interpretation of the layers of the mycobacterial envelope (specifically, those of the rapid-growing *M. smegmatis*) has been made elsewhere (Daffé et al., 1989). Though various special staining methods were used, the images obtained were not fundamentally different from those seen by other workers. The interpretation differs because the "periplasmic layer" between the membrane and the peptidoglycan (in the terms used above) is considered to be peptidoglycan, while the outer layer is ignored. This alternative interpretation does not seem to accord with the known properties of the chemically identified layers, nor does it take into account the appearance of sectioned isolated walls or of degenerating, and so plasmolyzed, whole mycobacteria.

The relatively recent techniques of freeze fracture and freeze-etching have been applied to mycobacterial walls. The techniques have the advantage that they involve minimal processing of the material to be examined prior to freezing to liquid nitrogen temperatures, so that labile structures are likely to be well preserved. Further, no organic solvents at room temperature are employed, so that lipid components are not extracted as they are during conventional embedding procedures. It should be noted, however, that considerations of safety demand that fixed cells of mycobacterial pathogens be used, so the bacteria are not, strictly, in their native form.

The most striking feature of freeze fractured mycobacteria is the presence of a plane of fracture within the wall (in addition to the plane within the plasma membrane, discussed above) (Nguyen et al., 1979). This publication by Nguyen et al. (1979) dealt with *M. leprae* and *M. lepraemurium* only, but similar images were obtained with BCG (Binkhuysen and Das, 1982), so the phenomenon may be taken to occur in *M. tuberculosis* also. Fracture planes are believed to arise within hydrophobic areas of specimens, for example, between the paired layers of alkyl chains in biological membranes, so the existence of such a hydrophobic layer in the wall is implied. It is unlikely that the fracture corresponds to the interface between inner electron-dense and intermediate electron-transparent layers seen in thin sections, assuming that the interpretation of these layers given above is correct, since the inner layer is hydrophilic and a fracture would involve breakage of a large number of covalent bonds. It is more likely that the fracture occurs within the hydrophobic part of the wall, and considerable ingenuity has been exercised in devising models that include a suitable hydrophobic interface.

MODELS OF THE STRUCTURE OF THE MYCOBACTERIAL ENVELOPE

Two main models of the arrangement of the mycoloyl residues and the accessory lipids and glycolipids in the wall have been discussed; both assume that the mycolic acids of the mycoloyl arabinogalactan are arranged with their hydrocarbon chains parallel and their methyl ends pointing to the outside of the mycobacterial cell. Such an arrangement would be consistent with the hydrophobic properties of intact cells of many species of mycobacteria and their tendency to adhere to one another in an aqueous environment in the absence of stabilizing agents. There is also evidence from X-ray diffraction that indicates that the walls of at least one mycobacterial species contain parallel, close-packed alkyl chains (Nikaido et al., 1993). In the model proposed by Minnikin (1982) and elaborated, notably by the inclusion in the proposed structure of wall-associated proteins and LAM, by Brennan and coworkers (McNeil and Brennan, 1991), the hydrocarbon chains of mycolic acids are intercalated with the hydrocarbon chains of the numerous wall-associated lipids and glycolipids. The branched nature of the mycolic acids, with a longer and a shorter hydrocarbon chain, makes such intercalation structurally plausible. It is possible that methyl branches and other side groups on the alkyl chains of the lipids control the depth to which the intercalation can occur. Further, the particular (and unusual) structures of the alkyl chains both of mycolic acids and of the various fatty acids found in wall-associated mycobacterial lipids and glycolipids are consistent with an intercalation model (and were, in fact, the basis for the original proposal). It is supposed that the intercalated alkyl chains are pulled apart in freeze fracture; this would involve overcoming only weak hydrophobic interactions rather than covalent chemical bonds.

The model receives some support from the immunological properties of intact cells of *M. leprae* and most members of the *M. avium-M. intracellulare* group. Of 24 mouse monoclonal antibodies against *M. leprae*, 7 reacted with unsonicated whole bacteria in an indirect fluorescence test. Five of these recognized either phenolic glycolipid I, a well-characterized wall-associated lipid, or unidentified lipid or carbohydrate antigens (Engers et al., 1985). In the case of *M.*

avium, the bacteria are agglutinated by the antibodies to oligosaccharide moieties of wall-associated glycopeptidolipids (Good and Beam, 1984). This indicates that the hydrophilic ends of the glycolipids protrude from the surface, while their lipid parts are attached to the mycobacterial envelope.

An alternative model has been developed by Rastogi (1991), who suggests that the amphipathic, wall-associated lipids form a superficial layer on the wall, with their hydrocarbon chains forming a packed monolayer on the inner side. This arrangement would form a bilayer structure with the outward-pointing hydrocarbon chains of the mycolic acids, exactly analogous to the structure of a normal biological membrane. In addition to the recognized wall-associated lipids, this model supposes that phospholipids (particularly phosphatidylinositol mannosides) form part of the outer layer. Phospholipids are usually associated with membranes rather than walls, but the mannosides apparently have a dual distribution, being found associated with isolated walls as well as with membranes (Goren and Brennan, 1979). It is not clear whether this represents their natural position or occurs as a result of redistribution of suspended lipids during the rather violent mechanical stresses needed to prepare mycobacterial walls.

Figure 2 shows a model of the wall incorporating features of both earlier models and including both intercalated and "bilayer-type" arrangements of alkyl chains, which allows for the fact that wall-associated lipids include those with medium-length (C_{24} to C_{36}) and short (C_{12} to C_{20}) fatty acyl groups.

In principle, the models might be differentiated by ultrastructural appearance, since the bilayer-type arrangement could lead to a sharply layered structure on the outside of the walls. As discussed above, a layer of polar material is commonly seen on the outer surface of mycobacterial walls, but its highly variable nature seems incon-

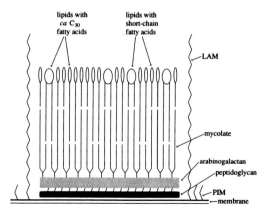

Figure 2. Model of the structure of the mycobacterial cell envelope. Positions of the asymmetric plasma membrane, peptidoglycan, and covalently attached arabinogalactan are indicated, together with LAM and phosphatidylinositol mannosides (PIM), at least some of which are known to be associated with the plasma membrane. A possible arrangement of the wall-associated lipids is also shown. Mycolic acids residues are known to be attached to the majority of the terminal and penultimate arabinose residues of the arabinogalactan. Since the mycolates possess two hydrocarbon chains of unequal lengths that would form an irregular monolayer, it is proposed that these are complemented by two classes of polar lipids with medium-chain (e.g., mycocerosates) and short-chain (e.g., acylglycerols) fatty acyl chains, respectively. There is evidence for a small number of porins in the envelope, presumably within the outer hydrophobic bilayer. Adapted from Minnikin (1982), McNeil and Brennan (1991), and Nikaido et al. (1993).

ENVELOPE ULTRASTRUCTURE AS SEEN BY OTHER ELECTRON MICROSCOPICAL TECHNIQUES

Extensive studies of mycobacteria were made by using the technique of negative staining, which offers greater resolution than sectioning but is more problematic to interpret. Mycobacterial cells (and isolated walls) exhibit a remarkable variety of structures when treated with negative stains, and an elaborate model of the wall was developed by Imaeda et al. (1968) and subsequently modified by Barksdale and Kim (1977), who took account of freeze fracture images as well. Unfortunately, it is not easy to reconcile every feature seen when negative stains are used with what is seen in thin sections. The situation is further confused by the appearance of features that are probably specific to individual species or groups of species of mycobacterium (connected with the possession of particular wall-associated molecules, for example, quasicrystalline arrays of glycopeptidolipid in *M. avium* complex [Draper, 1974; Barrow and Brennan, 1982]); this variability was apparently not appreciated in the original publications on the appearance of mycobacteria. It may be noted that *M. tuberculosis* does not possess "crystalline" glycolipids of this type.

A consistent feature are the "paired fibrous structures," which are ridges (or possibly grooves) forming a network over the mycobacterial wall that were originally described by Takeya et al. (1958) but have been observed repeatedly since then. With optimal resolution, these structures appear as pairs of parallel lines. Interestingly, on negatively stained specimens, they are visible only on damaged cells or isolated walls (Takeya et al., 1961), indicating that they are internal structures that are inaccessible to the stain in intact cells. However, they are also seen in cells shadowed with heavy metals, which seems to contradict this simple interpretation. Their nature is un-

sistent with a structure universal among mycobacterial species, and its thickness is frequently much greater than would be expected from a lipid monolayer. Further, it survives conditions known to extract significant amounts of lipids from the wall. Quantitative studies might also be helpful, answering the question of whether sufficient suitable amphipathic substances are present to form a monolayer on the wall. The intercalation model could allow any quantity of associated lipid from none to complete saturation (all possible intercalation sites occupied). However, either approach requires the exact anatomical site of the molecules involved to be determined.

known. A possible interpretation is that they are simple folds in the wall that occur when the internal contents of the mycobacterial cell collapse, but this does not explain their "paired" appearance. Also seen on negatively stained and metal-shadowed mycobacteria (including *M. tuberculosis*) are radial bands, usually near the end of the cell (Nishiura et al., 1969). These appear to be scars remaining from cell division; similar structures have been noted on other microorganisms, and what is known of the process of cell division in mycobacteria (see below) would lead one to expect a discontinuity in the surface of the wall at the site of separation of the daughter cells.

PROTEINS IN THE MYCOBACTERIAL WALL

It is certain that the mycobacterial wall contains proteins. First, proteins in the process of being exported from the cell must pass through the wall. Second, enzymes needed for construction and reconstruction of the wall polymers during growth and division must occur within the structure of the wall. Such proteins are well known in more fully investigated bacterial species. Third, and most interesting, is the recently discovered occurrence of porins in the envelope of one mycobacterial species, *M. chelonae* (Trias et al., 1992). Porins are special proteins that form hydrophilic channels through the outer membrane of gram-negative bacteria so that small aqueous solutes can pass this barrier. They were originally sought in mycobacteria as part of an investigation of the extreme general resistance to antibiotics found in some mycobacteria, notably *M. avium* and its relatives; *M. chelonae* is a rapid-growing species with similar general resistance. Porin-type proteins were found in carefully prepared walls of *M. chelonae* shown to be free of residual plasma membrane by the absence of characteristic enzymes. The

amount of these proteins is quite small, consistent with the very low measured permeability of the wall to hydrophilic molecules, but the proteins have the characteristic properties of a porin (Trias and Benz, 1993).

M. tuberculosis is much less generally resistant to drugs than *M. avium*, which implies either that the wall structure is different and does not contain the outer lipid layer discussed above or, alternatively, that porins and similar hydrophilic channels are more abundant in *M. tuberculosis* than in *M. chelonae*. All the ultrastructural and chemical evidence suggests that *M. avium* and *M. tuberculosis* have rather similar envelope structures, which makes the first alternative unattractive. There is some evidence for a porin-type protein in *M. tuberculosis*. A 23-kDa polypeptide that had amino acid homology with the protein OmpF of *Escherichia coli* was released by trifluoromethanesulfonic acid from purified walls of *M. tuberculosis* H37Ra (Hirschfield et al., 1990). This was the only insoluble wall-associated protein found. Small amounts of the same protein were detected in virulent strains (Erdman and H37Rv), but massive amounts of polyglutamic acid in these walls made further investigation difficult.

No ultrastructural visualization of the porins or of any other protein within the structure of the wall has yet been achieved. However, mention should be made of a report that BCG possesses a superficial layer of particles (presumably protein) forming an ordered array (Lounatmaa and Brander, 1989). Such layers, the so-called S-layer glycoproteins (Messner and Sleytr, 1992), are well known in some gram-positive bacteria but have not been reported by other workers in any mycobacterial cells. On the other hand, it is well known that mycobacteria secrete a variety of proteins (Wiker et al., 1991). For the present, the status of the layer in mycobacteria must be considered uncertain, and the possibility that the observed cells were contaminants of the culture of BCG must be borne in mind.

CELL DIVISION IN MYCOBACTERIA

Images of cell division in mycobacteria are readily observed in ultrathin sections, but descriptions of the process have been published only for three slow-growing species, not including *M. tuberculosis*: *M. leprae* (Edwards, 1970), *M. lepraemurium* (Hirata, 1979), and *M. avium* (Rastogi and David, 1981). The material used in these studies was not entirely technically satisfactory: the *M. leprae* cells included many partly degenerated cells, the *M. lepraemurium* cells were visibly distorted by the processing for electron microscopy, and the *M. avium* cells were physiologically abnormal and filamentous. However, the process of division seemed to be similar in each case. An elegant set of pictures that illustrates the process has been made by using the fast-growing *M. vaccae* (Takade et al., 1983) and may be taken as a definitive description. A notable feature is the behavior of the layers (inner electron dense, electron transparent, and outer electron dense) of the wall, since the formation of the daughter cells involves the breaking of the inner layer, (presumably) the spreading of the outer layer across the break, and the formation of the outer layer outside the new sections of wall. Formation of the new plasma membrane in an annular fashion beginning at the periphery and spreading toward the center is the first step in division. New wall, in two layers, is laid down on the external faces of the new membranes as they develop, but the original wall remains intact at this stage. The final stage is the splitting of the old wall at the periphery of the new septum and the formation of a complete electron-transparent layer over the broken end of the peptidoglycan layer. It is clear that the radial bands mentioned

above are scars left at the site of the break, and the deformation of the newly cleaved cells at this point is clearly seen in the sections of *M. vaccae*. In the case of *M. vaccae*, at least some of the daughter cells failed to separate completely, but this phenomenon has not been noted in cultures of *M. tuberculosis*.

Understanding of cell division in mycobacteria is incomplete: it is not known whether the outer layer is present but unstained in the new septum or whether it forms after the daughter cells split or how the electron-transparent layer spreads across the cleaved ends of the inner, electron-dense layer, though the images of *M. vaccae* suggest that this process is rapid. A problem is that all mycobacteria grow relatively slowly, and the slow-growing species, including *M. tuberculosis*, are particularly sluggish. Consequently, only a small proportion of cells observed at any given time are in any stage of division. Electron microscopical experiments using synchronized cultures might give the required information, since suitable choice of the moment of fixation would yield a high proportion of cells in the process of division. A system for synchronizing *M. tuberculosis* for at least a few generations has been described elsewhere (Wayne, 1977).

ULTRASTRUCTURE OF INTRACELLULAR *M. TUBERCULOSIS*

Though *M. tuberculosis* grows readily (but slowly) in vitro, it is also able to survive and multiply inside phagocytic cells of humans and animals, an ability of importance in the pathogenesis of tuberculosis. The commonest type of host cell is the macrophage; inside this cell, the bacteria occur within vacuoles, apparently the phagosomes formed as the bacteria are engulfed by the cells. However, living mycobacteria are not usually found in direct contact with the other contents of the vacuole but are separated from them by a distinct "electron-transparent zone" (Armstrong and Hart, 1971). It should be noted that this structure is quite different from the electron-transparent layer of the wall; some confusion has occurred because of the similar names of these structures, but they are distinct, and the boundary between them can usually be seen. The boundary occurs in the position of the outer layer seen on cells grown in vitro. Despite considerable effort, the nature of the electron-transparent zone is not clear. Its contents are unknown, and it is not certain whether it is of mycobacterial or host cell origin. Nor is it clear in general whether it forms only around viable bacteria, though there is some evidence that this is not the case for *M. avium* (Frehel et al., 1986). In some pathogenic mycobacteria (*M. leprae* and *M. lepraemurium*), structures that are clearly mycobacterial and that occur in the position occupied by the electron-transparent zone in thin sections have been observed by freeze fracture (Nishiura et al., 1977). The structures can be identified with known lipid and glycolipid products that are produced on a massive scale by these species. Intracellular *M. tuberculosis* seems not to have been studied by freeze fracture, but in any case, it produces none or very little of the glycolipids thought to be involved. On the other hand, mycobacteria secrete protein (Wiker et al., 1991) and possibly carbohydrate (carbohydrate was present in "old tuberculin"), and these may occupy the electron-transparent zone.

In fact, it is not entirely clear that *M. tuberculosis* invariably possesses an electron-transparent zone. Though the structure has been described and illustrated (Armstrong and Hart, 1971), it is scarcely evident in a more recent set of images of essentially the same system (mouse peritoneal macrophages) fixed in a similar way (McDonough et al., 1993), while quantitative measurements indicated that the percentage of *M. tuberculosis* cells with an electron-transparent zone was low (unlike the situation with *M. avium*) (Frehel et al., 1986). The matter is of some importance, because the zone separates the pathogen from the host and is a putative part of the mechanisms that permit intracellular growth; further investigation of the intracellular situation of *M. tuberculosis* seems warranted.

CONCLUSIONS

M. tuberculosis shares many ultrastructural features with other mycobacteria, including nonpathogens. Based on thin sections and images of the wall obtained by freeze fracture plus chemical considerations, a plausible model of the arrangement of the mycobacterial wall may be constructed. However, it is not yet possible to reconcile this model with detail seen by earlier workers in negatively stained or metal-shadowed preparations. Some aspects of mycobacterial ultrastructure are not yet fully understood, for example, the exact localization and arrangement of the many wall-associated substances already identified by chemists. Also, the spectrum of wall-associated molecules present differs among mycobacterial species, so there may be important differences in wall structure and properties. Some of these problems may be solved by application of existing techniques, but others await the development of new methods, particularly the ability to identify and localize lipids and carbohydrates with high resolution. Eventual solutions to the problems are likely to be applicable to all or most mycobacteria, and the use of rapidly growing, nonpathogenic species seems sensible. In addition, the special ability of *M. tuberculosis* to survive in a mammalian host and to cause a potentially fatal disease presumably derives at least in part from the nature and arrangement of particular chemicals in the bacterial cell. Further study of the ultrastructure of this particular species is needed to understand its pathogenic properties.

REFERENCES

Andres, Y., H. J. MacCordick, and J. C. Hubert. 1993. Adsorption of several actinide (Th, U) and lanthanide (La, Eu, Yb) ions by *Mycobacterium smegmatis. Appl. Microbiol. Biotechnol.* **39:**413–417.

Armstrong, J. A., and P. D. Hart. 1971. Response of cultured macrophages to *Mycobacterium tuberculosis*, with observations on fusion of lysosomes with phagosomes. *J. Exp. Med.* **134:**713–740.

Barksdale, L., and K. S. Kim. 1977. *Mycobacterium. Bacteriol. Rev.* **41:**217–372.

Barrow, W. W., and P. J. Brennan. 1982. Isolation in high frequency of rough variants of *Mycobacterium intracellulare* lacking C-mycoside glycopeptidolipid antigens. *J. Bacteriol.* **150:**381–384.

Beveridge, T. J., and R. G. E. Murray. 1980. Sites of metal deposition in the cell wall of *Bacillus subtilis. J. Bacteriol.* **141:**876–887.

Binkhuysen, F., and P. K. Das. 1982. Ultrastructural characteristics of *Mycobacterium bovis* BCG and *Mycobacterium leprae. Int. J. Lepr.* **50:**76–82.

Brodie, A. F., V. K. Kalra, S. H. Lee, and N. S. Cohen. 1979. Properties of energy-transducing systems in different types of membrane preparations from *Mycobacterium phlei*—preparation, resolution, and reconstitution. *Methods Enzymol.* **55:**175–200.

Daffé, M., M. A. Dupont, and N. Gas. 1989. The cell envelope of *Mycobacterium smegmatis*: cytochemistry and architectural implications. *FEMS Microbiol. Lett.* **61:**89–94.

Draper, P. 1971. The walls of *Mycobacterium lepraemurium*: chemistry and ultrastructure. *J. Gen. Microbiol.* **69:**313–324.

Draper, P. 1974. The mycoside capsule of *Mycobacterium avium* 357. *J. Gen. Microbiol.* **83:**431–433.

Draper, P. 1982. The anatomy of mycobacteria, p. 9–52. *In* C. Ratledge and J. Stanford (ed.), *The Biology of the Mycobacteria*, vol. 1. *Physiology, Identification and Classification*. Academic Press, Inc., London.

Edwards, R. P. 1970. Electron-microscope illustrations of division in *Mycobacterium leprae. J. Med. Microbiol.* **3:**493–499.

Engers, H. D., M. Abe, B. R. Bloom, V. Mehra, W. Britton, T. M. Buchanan, S. K. Khanolkar, D. B. Young, O. Closs, T. Gillis, M. Harboe, J. Ivanyi, A. H. J. Kolk, and C. C. Shepard. 1985. Results of a World Health Organization-sponsored workshop on monoclonal antibodies to *Mycobacterium leprae. Infect. Immun.* **48:**603–605.

Frehel, C., A. Ryter, N. Rastogi, and H. David. 1986. The electron-transparent zone in phagocytosed *Mycobacterium avium* and other mycobacteria: formation, persistence and role in bacterial survival. *Ann. Inst. Pasteur/Microbiol.* **137B:**239–257.

Good, R. C., and R. E. Beam. 1984. Seroagglutination, p. 105–122. *In* G. P. Kubica and L. G. Wayne (ed.), *The Mycobacteria—a Sourcebook*, part A. Marcel Dekker, Inc., New York.

Goren, M. B., and P. J. Brennan. 1979. Mycobacterial lipids: chemistry and biologic activities, p. 63–193. *In* G. P. Youmans (ed.), *Tuberculosis*. The W.B. Saunders Co., Philadelphia.

Hayat, M. A. 1989. *Principles and Techniques of Electron Microscopy*, 3rd ed. Macmillan, Basingstoke.

Hirata, T. 1979. Electron microscopic observations of intracytoplasmic membrane systems and cell division in *Mycobacterium lepraemurium. Int. J. Lepr.* **47:**585–596.

Hirschfield, G. R., M. McNeil, and P. J. Brennan. 1990. Peptidoglycan-associated polypeptides of *Mycobacterium tuberculosis. J. Bacteriol.* **172:**1005–1013.

Hunter, S. W., H. Gaylord, and P. J. Brennan. 1986. Structure and antigenicity of the phosphorylated lipopolysaccharide antigens from the leprosy and tubercle bacilli. *J. Biol. Chem.* **261:**12345–12351.

Imaeda, T., F. Kanetsuna, and B. Galindo. 1968. Ultrastructure of cell walls of genus *Mycobacterium. J. Ultrastruct. Res.* **25:**46–63.

Kumar, G., V. K. Kalra, and A. F. Brodie. 1979. Asymmetric distribution of phospholipids in membranes from *Mycobacterium phlei. Arch. Biochem. Biophys.* **198:**22–30.

Lederer, E., A. Adam, R. Ciorbaru, J. F. Petit, and J. Wietzerbin. 1975. Cell walls of mycobacteria and related organisms; chemistry and immunostimulant properties. *Mol. Cell. Biochem.* **7:**87–104.

Lounatmaa, K., and E. Brander. 1989. Crystalline surface layer of *Mycobacterium bovis* BCG. *J. Bacteriol.* **171:**5756–5758.

McDonough, K. A., Y. Kress, and B. R. Bloom. 1993. Pathogenesis of tuberculosis: interaction of *Mycobacterium tuberculosis* with macrophages. *Infect. Immun.* **61:**2763–2773.

McNeil, M., M. Daffé, and P. J. Brennan. 1990. Evidence for the nature of the link between the arabinogalactan and peptidoglycan of mycobacterial cell walls. *J. Biol. Chem.* **265:**18200–18206.

McNeil, M. R., and P. J. Brennan. 1991. Structure, function and biogenesis of the cell envelope of mycobacteria in relation to bacterial physiology, pathogenesis and drug resistance; some thoughts and possibilities arising from recent structural information. *Res. Microbiol.* **142:**451–463.

Messner, P., and U. B. Sleytr. 1992. Crystalline bacterial cell-surface layers. *Adv. Microb. Physiol.* **33:**213–275.

Minnikin, D. E. 1982. Lipids: complex lipids, their chemistry, biosynthesis and roles, p. 95–184. *In* C. Ratledge and J. Stanford (ed.), *The Biology of the Mycobacteria*, vol. 1. *Physiology, Identification and Classification*. Academic Press, Inc., London.

Nguyen, H. T., D. D. Trach, N. V. Man, T. H. Ngoan, I. Dunia, M. A. Ludosky-Diawara, and E. L. Benedetti. 1979. Comparative ultrastructure of *Mycobacterium leprae* and *Mycobacterium lepraemurium* cell envelopes. *J. Bacteriol.* **138:**552–558.

Nikaido, H., S. H. Kim, and E. Y. Rosenberg. 1993. Physical organization of lipids in the cell wall of *Mycobacterium chelonae*. *Mol. Microbiol.* **8:**1025–1030.

Nishiura, M., S. Izumi, T. Mori, K. Takeo, and T. Nonaka. 1977. Freeze-etching study of human and murine leprosy bacilli. *Int. J. Lepr.* **45:**248–254.

Nishiura, M., S. Okada, S. Izumi, and H. Takizawa. 1969. An electron microscope study of the band structure of the leprosy bacillus and other mycobacteria. *Int. J. Lepr.* **37:**225–238.

Paul, T. R., and T. J. Beveridge. 1992. Reevaluation of envelope profiles and cytoplasmic ultrastructure of mycobacteria processed by conventional embedding and freeze-substitution protocols. *J. Bacteriol.* **174:**6508–6517.

Rastogi, N. 1991. Recent observations concerning structure and function relationships in the mycobacterial cell envelope: elaboration of a model in terms of mycobacterial pathogenicity, virulence and drug-resistance. *Res. Microbiol.* **142:**464–476.

Rastogi, N., and H. L. David. 1981. Growth and cell division of *Mycobacterium avium*. *J. Gen. Microbiol.* **126:**77–84.

Rastogi, N., C. Frehel, and H. L. David. 1984. Evidence for taxonomic utility of periodic acid-thiocarbohydrazide-silver proteinate cytochemical staining for electron microscopy. *Int. J. Syst. Bacteriol.* **34:**293–299.

Rastogi, N., C. Frehel, and H. L. David. 1986. Triple-layered structure of mycobacterial cell wall: evidence for the existence of a polysaccharide-rich outer layer in 18 mycobacterial species. *Curr. Microbiol.* **13:**237–242.

Rosenblatt, M. B., E. F. Fullam, and A. E. Gessler. 1942. Studies of mycobacteria with the electron microscope. *Am. Rev. Tuberc.* **46:**587–599.

Silva, M. T., and P. M. Macedo. 1983a. The interpretation of the ultrastructure of mycobacterial cells in transmission electron microscopy of ultrathin sections. *Int. J. Lepr.* **51:**225–234.

Silva, M. T., and P. M. Macedo. 1983b. A comparative ultrastructural study of the membranes of *Mycobacterium leprae* and of cultivable mycobacteria. *Biol. Cell.* **47:**383–386.

Takade, A., K. Takeya, H. Taniguchi, and Y. Mizuguchi. 1983. Electron microscopic observations of cell division in *Mycobacterium vaccae* V1. *J. Gen. Microbiol.* **129:**2315–2320.

Takeya, K., R. Mori, M. Koike, and T. Toda. 1958. Paired fibrous structures in mycobacteria. *Biochim. Biophys. Acta* **30:**197–198.

Takeya, K., R. Mori, T. Tokunaga, M. Koike, and K. Hisatsune. 1961. Further studies on the paired fibrous structures of mycobacterial cell wall. *J. Biophys. Biochem. Cytol.* **9:**496–501.

Trias, J., and R. Benz. 1993. Characterization of the channel formed by the mycobacterial porin in lipid bilayer membranes. Demonstration of voltage gating and of negative point charges at the channel mouth. *J. Biol. Chem.* **268:**6234–6240.

Trias, J., V. Jarlier, and R. Benz. 1992. Porins in the cell wall of mycobacteria. *Science* **258:**1479–1481.

Wayne, L. G. 1977. Synchronized replication of *Mycobacterium tuberculosis*. *Infect. Immun.* **17:**528–530.

Wiker, H. G., M. Harboe, and S. Nagai. 1991. A localization index for distinction between extracellular and intracellular antigens of *Mycobacterium tuberculosis*. *J. Gen. Microbiol.* **137:**875–884.

Tuberculosis: Pathogenesis, Protection, and Control
Edited by Barry R. Bloom
© 1994 American Society for Microbiology, Washington, DC 20005

Chapter 20

Lipids and Carbohydrates of *Mycobacterium tuberculosis*

Gurdyal S. Besra and Delphi Chatterjee

The mycobacterial cellular envelope contains a high proportion of lipids whose diverse structures have obvious chemosystematic potential. Research extending back over the last 50 years has implicated various components of the mycobacterial cell wall matrix in many host responses associated with tuberculosis and other mycobacterioses (Goren and Brennan, 1979). However, current chemical knowledge of the mycobacterial cellular envelope greatly outweighs our understanding of the disease process (Brennan, 1989). The elaborate and distinctive features of many of the cell wall moieties has led us to speculate that these are involved in the virulence and pathogenesis of *Mycobacterium tuberculosis*. These structures include mAGP, LAM, LM, PIM, SL, trehalose 6,6'-dimycolate (cord factor), other acylated trehaloses, phenolic glycolipid, lipooligosaccharides, and attenuation indicator lipid. While some of these molecules, such as SL and cord factor, have previously been implicated in host-pathogen interactions (Goren and Brennan, 1979), proof of their involvement in pathogenesis is far from conclusive.

In the context of this review, a broad structural definition of these complex mycobacterial lipids will be presented along with a discussion of the possible roles of these lipids found within *M. tuberculosis*.

ABBREVIATIONS AND TERMS USED

Ara*f*, arabinofuranose; Fuc*p*, fucopyranose; Gal*f*, galactofuranose; GC, gas chromatography; GlcNac, *N*-acetylglucosamine; HPLC, high-performance liquid chromatography; IL-1, interleukin-1; Ins, inositol; IR, infrared; LAM, lipoarabinomannan; LM, lipomannan; mAGP, mycolyl-arabinogalactan-peptidoglycan complex; Man*p*, mannopyranose; MS, mass spectrometry; NMR, nuclear magnetic resonance; P, phosphate; PDIM, phthiocerol dimycocerosate; PIM, phosphatidyl-*myo*-inositol mannoside; Rha*p*, rhamnopyranose; SL, sulfatide; TNF, tumor necrosis factor; Phe Gl, phenolic glycolipid

cis and *trans*: geometrical isomers resulting from a double bond

D and L: When two enantiomorphs differ only in their abilities to rotate the plane of polarized light by equal amounts in opposite directions, the plane to the right is called *dextro* (D), and the one to the left is called *levo* (L). The enantiomorphs are also

Gurdyal S. Besra and Delphi Chatterjee • Department of Microbiology, Colorado State University, Fort Collins, Colorado 80523.

referred to as optical isomers and occur when four different atoms or groups are attached to a carbon atom. The D or L rotation is also used in assigning the absolute configuration of glycosyl residues. For instance, any hexose in which the configuration at C-5 is the same as that in (+)-glyceraldehyde is a D-hexose.

erythro: refers to the relative stereochemistry between two centers

R or *S*: the absolute stereochemistry at a carbon atom carrying four different groups as specified by the Cahn-Ingold-Prelog sequence rule

WAXES

A lipid apparently not present in other actinomycetes was isolated from *M. tuberculosis* by Noll (1957) and was degraded by lithium aluminum hydride to yield two products. The spectroscopic data for these products were consistent with those for phthiocerol A and reduced mycocerosic acids (also known as mycosanoic/mycoceranoic acids) (Table 1). It was concluded that the lipid had a PDIM structure in which

the mycocerosic acids were esterified to both hydroxyls of phthiocerol A.

Noll (1957) reviewed studies establishing the structures of phthiocerol A as 3-methoxy-4-methyl do-(and tetra)-triacontane-9,11-diol. Compounds related to phthiocerol A have the terminal ethyl group replaced by a terminal methyl group (phthiocerol B), the methoxy group replaced by a keto group (phthiodiolone A), and the methoxy group replaced by a hydroxyl group (phthiotriol A) (Table 1). Minnikin and Polgar (1967a) confirmed the structures of phthiodiolone A from *M. tuberculosis* on the basis of MS, ^{1}H NMR, and IR of phthiodiolone A and its ethylidene acetal derivative. Minnikin and Polgar (1966) applied similar studies to confirm the structures of phthiocerol A and also presented evidence for phthiocerol B.

The mycocerosic acids were first isolated from the waxes of *M. tuberculosis* (Ginger and Anderson, 1945). The mycocerosic acids were also studied by Asselineau et al. (1959) and by Polgar's group (Marks and Polgar, 1955; Polgar and Smith, 1963). A brief review of the studies leading to their structural elucidation is given by Goren and Brennan (1979) and Cason et al. (1964). In summary, GC, MS, and stepwise degradation experiments established that the mycocerosic acids were composed of a complex mixture of multi-methyl-branched acids with a major C_{32} component, 2,4,6,8-tetramethyloctacosanoate. Minor components; C_{30} and probably C_{31} and C_{34} tetramethyl acids; and C_{25}, C_{27}, C_{29}, and possibly C_{26} trimethyl branched acids were also present. Related to the PDIM family of waxes are the phenolphthiocerols (Table 1), which form the basic lipid core of the phenolic glycolipids isolated from *M. tuberculosis* Canetti (Daffe et al., 1987) and also the so-called "attenuation indicator" lipid of attenuated strains of *M. tuberculosis*.

The proposed biosynthetic route leading to phthiocerol A is outlined in Fig. 1; for phthiocerol B, Minnikin and Polgar (1965)

Table 1. Long-chain diols and fatty acids

Phthiocerol A	$CH_3(CH_2)_{20,22}$ ... OH OH ... OCH$_3$, CH$_3$
Phthiocerol B	$CH_3(CH_2)_{20,22}$ ... OH OH ... OCH$_3$, CH$_3$
Phthiodiolone A	$CH_3(CH_2)_{20,22}$ ... OH OH ... O, CH$_3$
Phthiotriol A	$CH_3(CH_2)_{20,22}$ ... OH OH ... OH, CH$_3$
Phenolphthiocerol A	HO—⟨ ⟩—(CH$_2$)$_{14-18}$ ... OX OX ... OCH$_3$, CH$_3$ x = Mycocerosic Acid
Mycocerosic Acid	$CH_3(CH_2)_{20}$ ... CH$_3$ CH$_3$ CH$_3$ CH$_3$ ... COOH

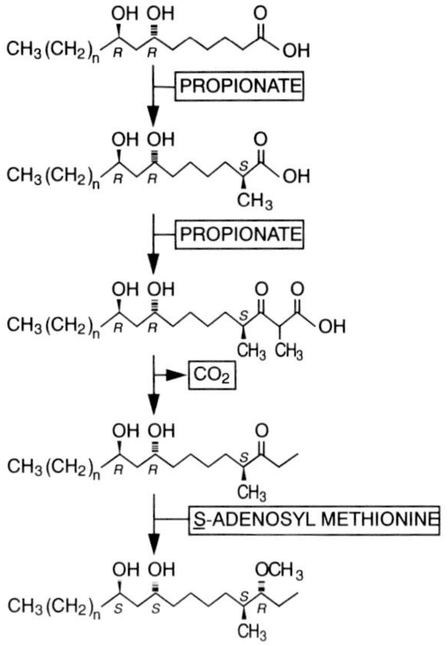

Figure 1. Final stages of phthiocerol A biosynthesis. n = 20 or 22.

suggested that acetate rather than propionate may be incorporated in the final stage. Studies carried out by Gastambide-Odier and Sarda (1970) suggested that the biosynthesis of the phenolphthiocerols may arise from *p*-hydroxybenzoate, formed via shikimic and chorismic acids, which is then elongated to give the long-chain diol.

Early studies demonstrated the incorporation of propionate into mycocerosic acids, which gave rise to methyl branches (Gastambide-Odier et al., 1963). A cell extract of *M. bovis* BCG was used to show that 18- and 20-carbon primers were elongated to give mycocerosates (Rainwater and Kolattukudy, 1983, 1985) and later were used to identify the fatty acyl synthetase complex associated with mycocerosic acid biosynthesis (Kikuchi et al., 1992; Manjula and Kolattukudy, 1992).

The biosynthetic systems leading to the glycosidation of phenolphthiocerol A dimycocerosate have recently been investigated by Thurman et al. (1993), who used *M. microti*. However, the acylation of glycosylphenolphthiocerol A with mycocerosates has not been studied.

In addition to discussing the PDIM waxes, the older literature discusses in considerable detail the waxes A, B, C, and D, isolated from various mycobacterial species (Anderson, 1941). Wax A was shown to be characteristic triacylglycerol (Brennan et al., 1970b), and a study conducted by Walker et al. (1970) demonstrated that fatty acids longer than C_{20} occupied position *sn*-3, C_{16} fatty acids occupied position 2, and either octadecanoate or 10-methyloctadecanoate occupied position 1. Interestingly, triacylglycerols are virtually absent in mycobacteria grown in glucose-containing media. However, Tween 80, a common constituent of growth medium that provides metabolizable oleic acid (Weir et al., 1972), and nitrogen starvation (Antoine and Tepper, 1969) both enhance triglycerol production. Few insights can be gleaned from these unusual observations, but they demonstrate that the polyol components of neutral acyl glycerols exhibit wide differences depending on the major carbon source in the medium (Brennan et al., 1970a, b). Wax D was characterized as an autolytic product of the cell wall's mAGP (Goren and Brennan, 1979). However, waxes B and C have never been structurally defined.

PHOSPHOLIPIDS

The phospholipids found within mycobacterial species are almost invariably phosphodiacylglycerols based on phosphatidic acid. The most common of the phosphodiacylglycerols are phosphatidylglycerol, diphosphatidylglycerol, phosphatidylethanolamine, and the mannosides of phosphatidylinositol.

Among the phospholipids found in mycobacteria, the most unusual and highly characteristic members are the phosphatidylinositols. In 1939, Anderson isolated from virulent *M. tuberculosis* a phospholipid that upon alkaline saponification and dephosphorylation, produced a "mannoinositide"

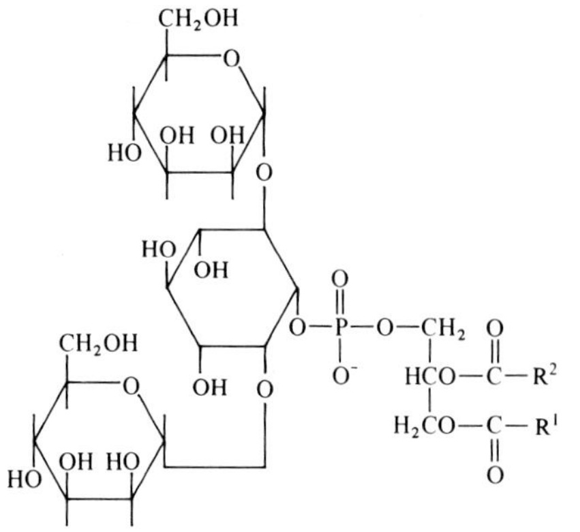

R^1C and R^2C = mixture of palmitoyl and tuberculostearoyl groups
$\parallel$ $\parallel$
O   O

Figure 2. Phosphatidylinositol dimannoside.

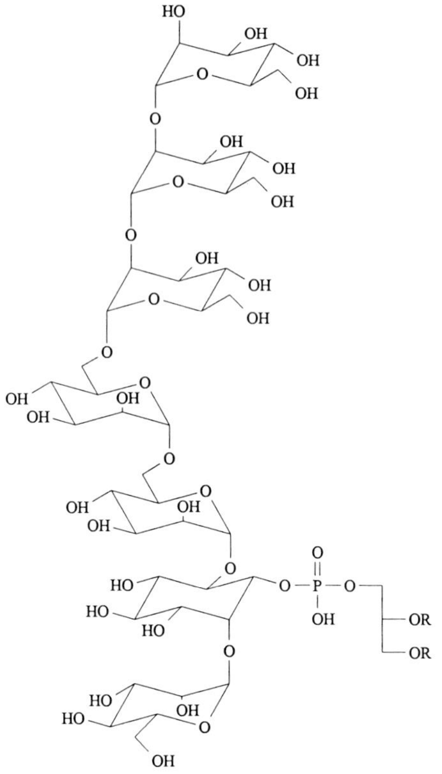

Figure 3. Phosphatidyl-*myo*-inositol hexamannoside. R, palmitic acid or tuberculostearic acid.

containing mannose and inositol in a ratio of 2:1 (Anderson, 1939). Some 25 years later, Lee and Ballou (1964) arrived at the complete structure of phosphatidylinositol dimannoside (PIM$_2$) (Fig. 2) from *M. tuberculosis* and *M. phlei*. Earlier studies (Ballou et al., 1963) and the use of ^{1}H NMR (Lee and Ballou, 1964) clearly established that the glycerol phosphate moiety was attached to the L-1 position of the *myo*-inositol ring and the mannose residues were glycosidically linked to the 2 and 6 positions of the *myo*-inositol ring. More recently, Chatterjee et al. (1992a) have described the presence of a phosphatidyl-*myo*-inositol hexamannoside (PIM$_6$) (Fig. 3) isolated from *M. tuberculosis* that contains an $\alpha1\rightarrow2$-linked mannose at the end of the tetrasaccharide backbone. Evidence for the existence of a phosphatidyl-*myo*-inositol pentamannoside (PIM$_5$) had been reported by Ballou et al. (1963), and the molecule was later structurally defined by Lee and Ballou (1965).

Early investigations conducted by Ballou and colleagues used deacylated glycophospholipids, and it was assumed that the parent lipids contained no additional fatty acyl groups except those on the glycerol moiety. However, Pangborn and McKinney (1966) isolated from *M. tuberculosis* a series of phosphatidyl-*myo*-inositol diman-

nosides containing two, three, and four acyl residues. The positions of these extra acyl groups are not known with certainty. It is also assumed that mono- and diacylphosphatidyl-*myo*-inositol pentamannosides are present in *M. tuberculosis* (Pangborn and McKinney, 1966). Biosynthesis of the phosphatidyl-*myo*-inositol mannosides still raises several unanswered questions. Brennan and Ballou (1968), Goren and Brennan (1979), and Minnikin (1982) have reviewed this area.

The cytoplasmic membranes of all actinomycetes and related bacteria contain small quantities of glycosylphosphopolyisoprenols involved in the synthesis of peptidoglycan and cell wall polysaccharides. In *M. tuberculosis* H37Ra, 60% of the lipid-bound [^{14}C]mannose from a cell-free system was found to be incorporated into two

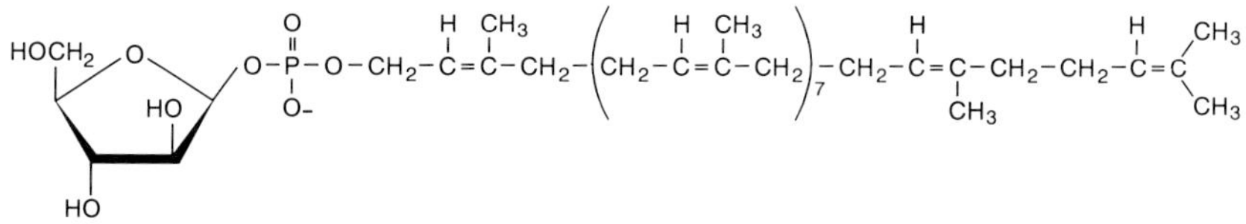

Figure 4. β-ᴅ-Arabinofuranosyl-1-phosphodecaprenol.

mannosylphosphopolyprenols (Takayama and Goldman, 1970). Incidentally, similar products were also found in *M. smegmatis* and were later characterized as mannosyl-1-phosphodecaprenol (Takayama and Armstrong, 1971; Takayama et al., 1973). More recently, the carrier lipid β-ᴅ-arabinofuranosyl-1-phosphodecaprenol (Fig. 4) was isolated and characterized by Wolucka et al. (submitted) and implicated in arabinogalactan and LAM biosynthesis.

ACYLATED TREHALOSES

Cord Factor

Middlebrook et al. (1947) observed that *M. tuberculosis* grows in the form of serpentine cords and also that avirulent and saprophytic species could be distinguished by an ability to absorb the cationic phenazine dye natural red. These two observations led to the early hypothesis that cell wall components are implicated in this phenomenon and are therefore related to virulence. A search for these components uncovered two families of trehalose-based lipids: cord factor (Fig. 5) and the SLs (Fig. 6). Even though there is little supporting evidence that the cord factors or the SLs

contribute to cord formation, these families of lipids are known to be implicated in several key disease-related events. Bloch's initial identification of cord factor, trehalose 6,6′-dimycolate, in virulent *M. tuberculosis* led to speculation concerning its role in virulence and cord formation (Bloch, 1950). However, later studies failed to show that this material had a role in the cord-forming ability of virulent *M. tuberculosis*; similarly, cord factors were also found in other noncording mycobacterial species and other mycolic acid-containing bacterial species (Goren, 1972).

The structural elucidation of the cord factors from *M. tuberculosis* were established through a series of classic studies conducted by Bloch, Noll, Asselineau, and Lederer (for a review of earlier structural work, see Noll [1956]). More recent studies using ^{13}C NMR (Polansky et al., 1977), MS (Adam et al., 1967), and field desorption MS (Puzo et al., 1978; Puzo and Prome, 1978) have been used to elucidate the finite structure of cord factor. The separation of individual cord factors on the basis of heterogeneity in mycolic acid composition was achieved by the use of thin-layer chromatography of trimethylsilyl ether derivatives (Prome et al., 1976). Studies conducted by Strain and colleagues (1977) resolved six separable mycolate-containing components: symmetrical α-α, methoxy-methoxy, and keto-keto and the unsymmetrical combinations of α-methoxy, methoxy-keto, and α-keto. Interestingly, the cord factors isolated from *M. bovis* were found to lack the methoxy-substituted class of cord factor (Strain et al., 1977). The authors of that study argued that virulence may be

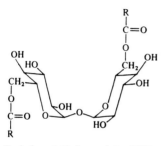

Figure 5. Trehalose 6,6′-dimycolate. RCO = mycolyl.

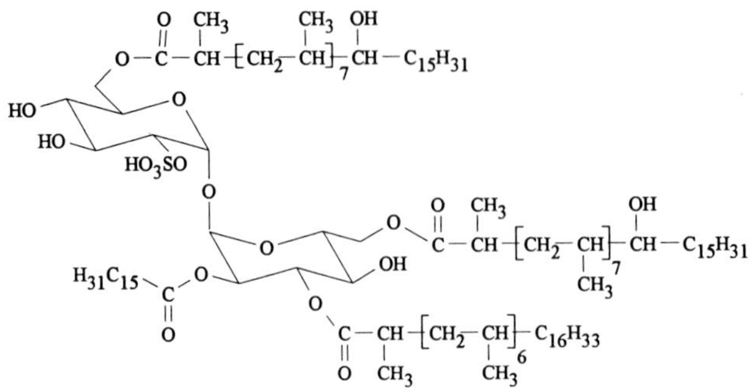

Figure 6. 2,3,6,6′-Tetra-*O*-acyltrehalose 2′-sulfate.

related to the presence or absence of a given mycolate component of cord factor.

Various biological activities for the cord factors have been described (Goren and Brennan, 1979; Goren, 1982), most of them seemingly related to the ability of cord factors to induce cytokine-mediated events such as systemic toxicity (Kato, 1973), antitumor activity (Lepoivre et al., 1982), granulomagenic activity, and macrophage release of chemotactic factors (Matsunaga et al., 1990). Cord factors were also noted to inhibit Ca^{2+}-induced fusion between phospholipid vesicles (Spargo et al., 1991) and migration of leukocytes (Goren and Brennan, 1979).

SLs

Investigations by Goren (1970a, b) recognized that the SLs (Fig. 6) of *M. tuberculosis* H37Rv were based on trehalose 2′-sulfate acylated with hydroxyphthioceranic, phthioceranic, and saturated straight-chain fatty acids. Chromatographic resolution of the natural mixture of SLs by using DEAE-cellulose gave rise to five components (Table 2).

In a series of experiments using per-*O*-methylated SL-I under nonisomerizing conditions, Goren et al. (1976a) established that SL-I is a 2,3,6,6′-tetra-*O*-acyltrehalose 2′-sulfate and SL-III is a 2,3,6-tri-*O*-acyl-

Table 2. SLs of *M. tuberculosis*

Sulfolipid	Acylation	No. of acyl residues		
		Palmitate/ stearate	Phthioceranate[a]	Hydroxyphthioceranate[b]
SL-I	2,4,6,6′	1	0	3
SL-I′	2,3,6,6′	1	0	3
SL-II	2,3,6,6′	1	1	2
SL-II′	2,3,6,6′	1	2	1
SL-III	2,3,6	1	0	2

[a] Phthioceranate: $C_{16}H_{33}$ $\left[-CH-CH_2 \right]_n CH-COOH$ $n = 2\text{-}9$ (with CH_3 substituents)

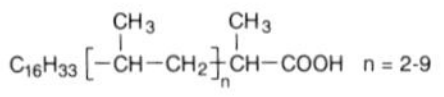

[b] Hydroxyphthioceranate: $C_{15}H_{31}$ $-CH\left[CH-CH_2 \right]_n CH-COOH$ $n = 2\text{-}10$ (with OH and CH_3 substituents)

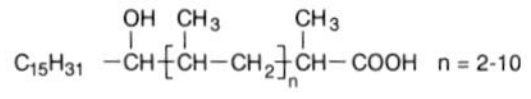

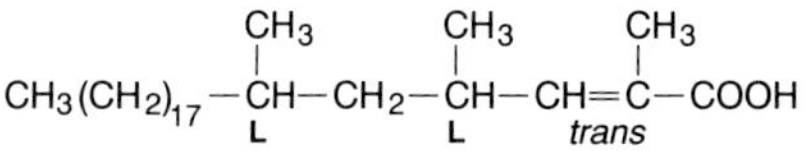

CH$_3$ CH$_3$ CH$_3$
| | |
CH$_3$(CH$_2$)$_{17}$—CH—CH$_2$—CH—CH=C—COOH
             L   L   *trans*

Figure 7. Mycolipenic acids.

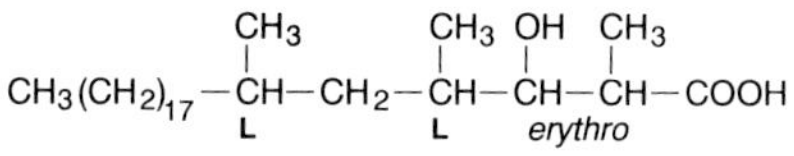

CH$_3$ CH$_3$ OH CH$_3$
| | | |
CH$_3$(CH$_2$)$_{17}$—CH—CH$_2$—CH—CH—CH—COOH
             L   L   *erythro*

Figure 9. Mycolipanolic acids.

trehalose 2′-sulfate. Also, through the use of partial methanolysis, a complete assignment of the acyl residues palmitate/stearate, phthioceranate, and hydroxyphthioceranate to a specific location on the trehalose moiety was established.

A later study by Goren et al. (1982) established a significant contribution between the SLs and the degree of virulence in the guinea pig among a broad span of *M. tuberculosis* isolates. Most of the virulent strains were prolific in elaborating the strongly acidic SLs, whereas the attenuated strains were notably deficient in these entities and were characterized by the presence of the attenuation indicator lipid (Goren et al., 1974, 1982). Subsequently, the biological activity of the SLs was proposed as an antagonist of the fusion of secondary lysosomes with phagosomes (Goren et al., 1976b; Goren, 1977). This original hypothesis has since been revised, and current evidence indicates that the SLs inhibit phagosome activation (Goren, 1987), thus promoting intracellular survival of the pathogen.

Other Trehalose Esters

Minnikin et al. (1985) and Besra et al. (1992) have recently added a new dimension to the chemistry of acylated trehaloses in describing two new families of widely differing polarities from *M. tuberculosis* H37Rv. The nonpolar classes are heavily acylated with saturated straight-chain C$_{16}$, C$_{18}$, and 2,4,6-trimethyltetracos-2-enoic acids (C$_{27}$ mycolipenic acids [Fig. 7]). It is tempting to postulate a role in virulence for these glycolipids (Daffe et al., 1988; Kataoka et al., 1986). First, mycolipenic acids are produced only by virulent strains (Daffe et al., 1988), and second, these acids have a dramatic influence on leukocyte migration (Goren and Brennan, 1979). It has been proposed that the highly branched structure of the mycolipenic acids renders their esters very difficult to hydrolyze and their free form barely sensitive to catabolism by the host organism.

The second class of relatively polar glycolipids were recently shown to be 2,3-di-*O*-acyltrehaloses (Fig. 8). They contain a combination of saturated straight-chain C$_{16}$-C$_{19}$, C$_{21}$-C$_{25}$ mycocerosate, C$_{24}$-C$_{28}$ mycolipanolic (Fig. 9) fatty acids and minor amounts of C$_{25}$-C$_{27}$ mycolipenic fatty acids (Besra et al., 1992). Interestingly, these simple acylated trehaloses appear to be restricted to virulent strains of *M. tuberculosis*. Also, they appear to be very reminiscent of the "core" acyltrehaloses of many of the multiglycosylated trehalose-containing lipooligosaccharides (Brennan, 1988).

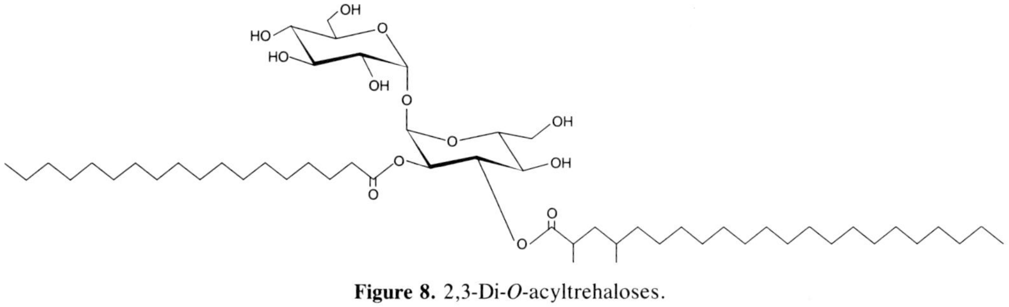

Figure 8. 2,3-Di-*O*-acyltrehaloses.

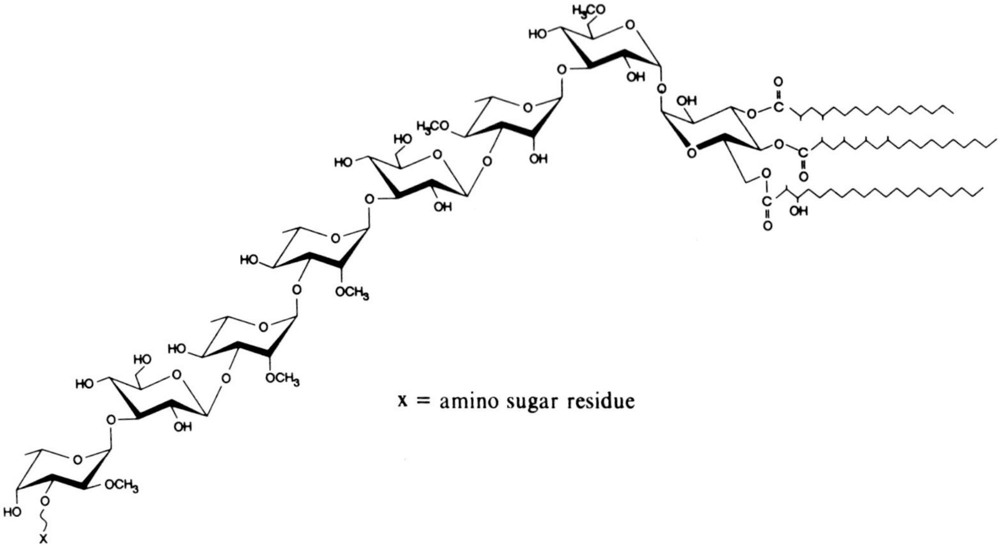

Figure 10. Lipooligosaccharide (LOS-I) isolated from *M. tuberculosis* Canetti.

However, the avirulent and atypical Canetti strain of *M. tuberculosis* appears to be the only *M. tuberculosis* strain to date that produces a highly glycosylated, acylated trehalose glycolipid (Fig. 10) (Daffe et al., 1991b).

The search for a phenolic glycolipid has proved to be unsuccessful with the majority of *M. tuberculosis* strains examined thus far (Goren et al., 1974; Koul and Gastambide-Odier, 1977; Minnikin et al., 1985; Daffe et al., 1991a). However, Daffe et al. (1987) identified a phenolic glycolipid from *M. tuberculosis* Canetti. The trisaccharide was found to consist of 2,3,4-tri-*O*-methyl-

α-L-Fuc*p*(1→3)-α-L-Rha*p*-(1→3)-2-*O*-methyl-α-L-Rha*p* (Fig. 11), and the aglycon moiety corresponded to the well-known phenolphthiocerol dimycocerosate. The phenolic glycolipids of *M. tuberculosis* Canetti and *M. bovis* appear to share some structural analogy. Indeed, both species contain Phe Gl B-1 (mycoside B), Phe Gl B-2, and PGT-1 but differ from Phe Gl B-3 by the distal tri-*O*-methyl-α-L-Fuc*p*.

MYCOLIC ACIDS

Mycolic acids were first identified in an unsaponifiable lipid extract isolated from

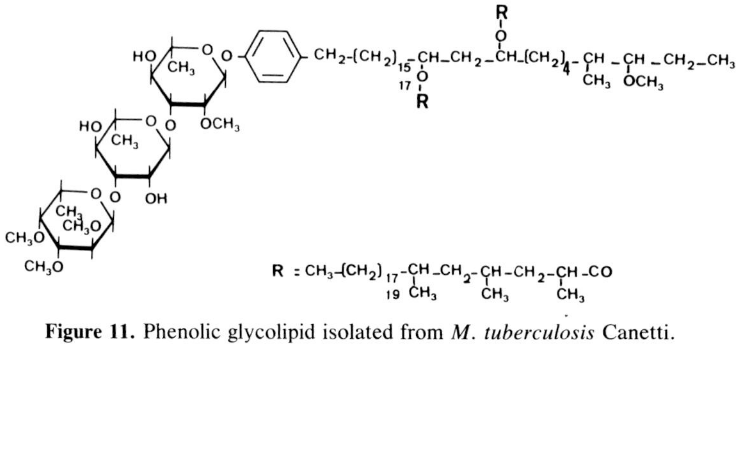

Figure 11. Phenolic glycolipid isolated from *M. tuberculosis* Canetti.

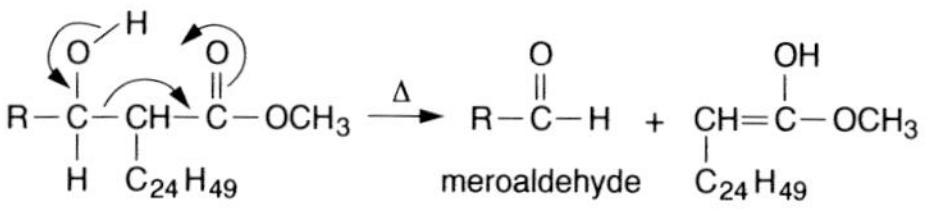

Figure 12. Reverse Claisen condensation reaction.

M. tuberculosis by Stodola et al. (1938). A typical characteristic of the mycolic acids is that they undergo a reverse Claisen-type condensation reaction (Etemadi, 1967a). For example, a methyl mycolate from *M. tuberculosis* will give a nonvolatile "meroaldehyde" and hexacosanoic acid methyl ester (Fig. 12).

Mycolic acids are high-molecular-weight, α-alkyl, β-hydroxy fatty acids. In the bacterial cell, they are present either in lipids, extractable by organic solvents mainly in the form of trehalose 6,6′-dimycolate, or, for the most part, as bound esters of arabinogalactan, a peptidoglycan-linked polysaccharide (Lechevalier, 1977; Minnikin and Goodfellow, 1980).

Mycobacterial mycolic acids are distinguished from those of other genera (such as *Corynebacterium*, *Nocardia*, and *Rhodococcus*) by the following features (Minnikin and Goodfellow, 1980): (i) they are the largest mycolic acids (C_{70} to C_{90}); (ii) they have the largest side chain (C_{20} to C_{24}); (iii) they contain one or two unsaturations, which may be double bonds or cyclopropane rings; (iv) they contain oxygen functions additional to the β-hydroxy group; and (v) they have methyl branches in the main carbon backbone.

The entire structural spectrum of mycolic acids was resolved in a series of elegant investigations carried out by Asselineau (1969), Etemadi (1967a, b, c), and Minnikin and Polgar (1967b, c) through the use of MS, NMR, and IR. As a consequence, the α branch, except for chain length, was found to be consistently conserved among the family of mycolic acids. The key structural changes, such as methoxy, keto, and methyl branches, double bonds, and cyclopropane rings, were always found in the *mero*-aldehyde portion.

Table 3. Structures of some mycobacterial mycolic acids

α-Mycolates[a]

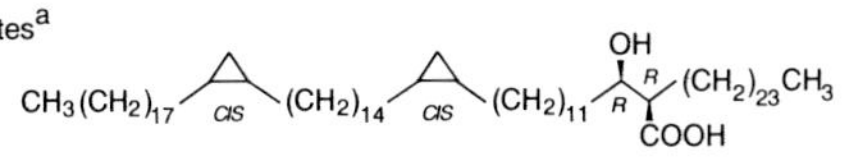

Ketomycolates

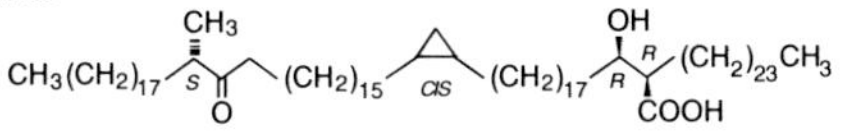

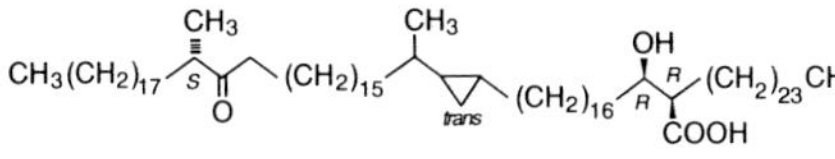

Methoxymycolates

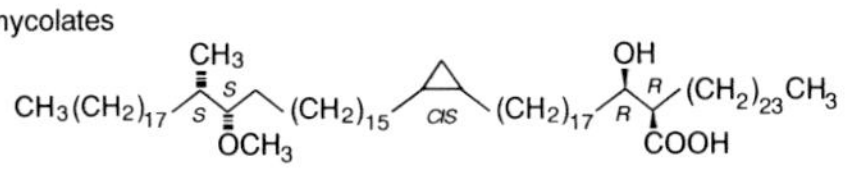

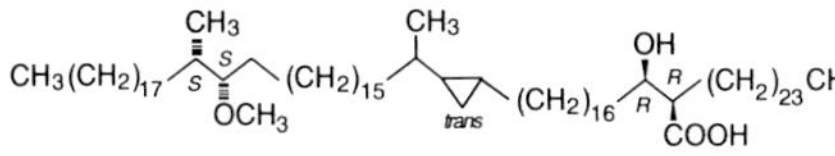

α′-Mycolates

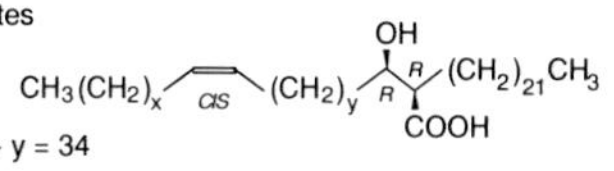

Where x + y = 34

Epoxymycolates

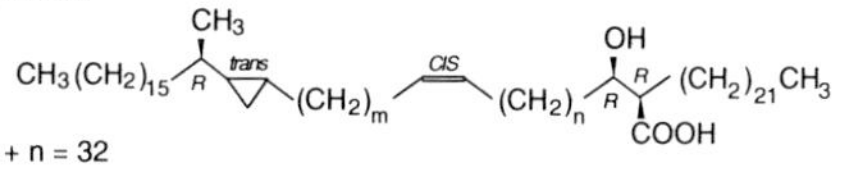

Where m + n = 32

Wax-ester Mycolates

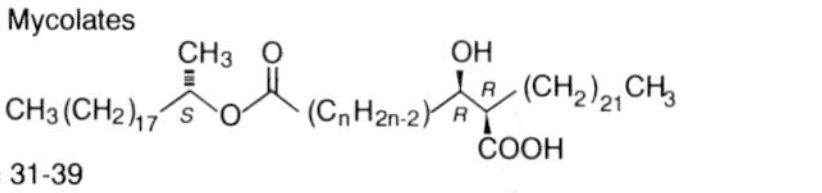

Where n = 31-39

[a] In addition to producing α-mycolates, certain mycobacteria produce similar diunsaturated mycolates.

Mycolic acids that lack extra oxygen functions in addition to the β-hydroxy group are termed α-mycolates (Table 3). The α-mycolates isolated from virulent *M. tuberculosis* have been studied in great detail and contain one major series containing two *cis*-cyclopropane rings (Etemadi, 1967b, c; Minnikin and Polgar, 1967b; Asselineau et al., 1969) (Table 3). In addition, keto- and methoxymycolates from virulent *M. tuberculosis* have been characterized

(Minnikin and Polgar, 1967c). They are composed of a series containing *cis*- and *trans*-cyclopropane rings (Table 3). The former was the major series for the methoxymycolates, and the latter was the major series for the ketomycolates.

The development of thin-layer chromatographic systems has proved invaluable for the assignment of superficial mycolate patterns. Mycolates could be separated by their polar functions, giving rise to multispot thin-layer chromatograms. Minnikin and coworkers have utilized this technique in the development of two-dimensional thin-layer chromatographic systems to analyze mycobacterial mycolates released by alkaline (Minnikin et al., 1984a) and acid methanolysis procedures (Wong and Gray, 1979; Minnikin et al., 1984b).

Goren and Brennan (1979) have reviewed the use of NMR, IR, and MS as aids to the resolution of the mycolic acids. MS permitted inferences about the degrees of unsaturation, chain lengths, and sizes of the mycolic acids (Etemadi, 1967b; Alshamaony et al., 1976a, b; Minnikin et al., 1974). Also, GC-MS of trimethylsilyl ethers of mycolic acids allowed the separation of individual mycolate components (Yano et al., 1978). The advent of HPLC proved to be a very valuable tool in the resolution of mycolic acids into individual mycolate populations and finally into a homologous series by reverse-phase HPLC by the use of *para*-bromophenacyl esters (Steck et al., 1978).

The biosynthesis of mycolic acids has been the subject of much discussion, but only recently has detailed evidence become available. Early studies showed that in *Corynebacterium diphtheriae*, C_{32} mycolic acids were formed by condensation and reduction of C_{16} fatty acids (Gastambide-Odier and Lederer, 1960), and similar condensations were established for the mycolic acids of *Nocardia asteroides* and *M. smegmatis* (Etemadi, 1967b). A detailed investigation into mycobacterial mycolic acid biosynthesis was carried out by Takayama and coworkers for *M. tuberculosis* H37Ra, as reviewed by Minnikin (1982) and Takayama and Davidson (1979a, b). The suggested pathway for the biosynthesis of the α-mycolic acids in *M. tuberculosis* H37Ra is outlined in Fig. 13. The *cis*-tetracos-5-enoic desaturase reaction was considered to be a step that was sensitive to the antitubercular drug isoniazid (Takayama and Davidson, 1979a, b; Winder, 1982), but a detailed mechanism for the inhibition and resistance of certain mycobacterial pathogens to this drug has not been proposed. Isoniazid also appears to inhibit the elongation of fatty acids having more than 30 carbons. Winder (1982) has reviewed the modes of action of several antimycobacterial agents that are

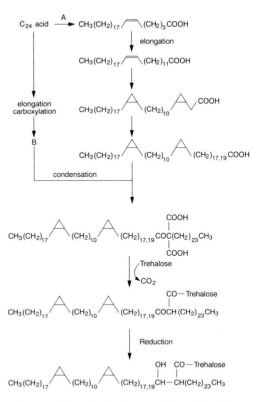

Figure 13. Biosynthesis of α-mycolic acids in *M. tuberculosis* H37Ra. A, Δ^5 desaturase; B, tetracosanyl malonate $CH_3(CH_2)_{23}$ $CH(COOH)_2$.

thought to be involved in inhibition of mycolic acid biosynthesis.

Fatty acyl-elongating enzymes are present in cell extracts from *M. tuberculosis* H37Ra, resulting in the incorporation of [^{14}C]malonyl coenzyme A into saturated and unsaturated fatty acids up to C_{56} (Qureshi et al., 1984). Incorporation of (*S*)-methyl-[^{14}C]adenosylmethionine and unlabeled malonyl coenzyme A gave mainly C_{48} to C_{56} acids, indicating that the introduction of cyclopropane rings or methyl groups into meromycolic acids occurs late in the pathway (Qureshi et al., 1984). When [^{14}C]oleate and labeled monounsaturates were used, only acids up to C_{32} were produced, suggesting that the correct double-bond position was essential for effective elongation.

This cell-free system (Qureshi et al., 1984), however, did not produce complete mycolic acids, though it did provide evidence for an elongation system leading to meromycolates. Lacave et al. (1990a, b) have utilized a cell-free system that is able to synthesize whole "true" mycolic acids from [1-^{14}C]acetate as a labeled precursor. Biosynthetic activity for mycolic acids occurred in an insoluble fraction from disrupted cells of *M. aurum* and produced unsaturated mycolic acids, while keto and wax-ester mycolic acids were synthesized to a lesser extent. Recent studies (Lacave et al., 1987, 1989) have also indicated that two parallel pathways must operate. The methyl branch adjacent to the epoxide group in epoxymycolates has an (*R*) absolute configuration in contrast to the (*S*)-methyl group next to the keto, methoxy, and wax-ester functions. This rules out a common epoxide intermediate in the biosynthetic pathway leading to all oxygenated mycolates. Metabolic studies and different chain lengths indicate that α-mycolates are not precursors of oxygenated mycolates (Minnikin, 1982). Instead, the pathways for α-mycolates and oxygenated mycolates appear to diverge from common intermedi-

ates. Lacave and coworkers (1990a, b) concluded that the biosynthesis of mycolic acids must involve a complex multienzyme system. More recently, Wheeler et al. (1993a) developed a low-water assay to investigate the incorporation of radioactive [1-^{14}C]acetate into α-, α'-, and epoxymycolates from *M. smegmatis* by using *cis*-tetracos-5-enoic acid, a key intermediate in mycolic acid biosynthesis. The results of this study positively identify for the first time a putative precursor in mycolic acid biosynthesis. Related studies demonstrated that methyl 4-(2-octadecylcyclopropen-1-yl) butanoate, a structural analog of *cis*-tetracos-5-cnoic acid, inhibited mycolic acid biosynthesis (Wheeler et al., 1993b).

Besides placing emphasis on structural deviation and biogenetic implications, the sections on mycolic acids from Goren and Brennan (1979), Minnikin (1982), and Brennan (1988) also deal with the effects of isoniazid and other antimycobacterial agents on the biosynthesis of mycolic acids.

MYCOBACTINS

All mycobacteria, with the notable exception of *M. paratuberculosis*, contain an iron-chelating component known as mycobactin. The structure of mycobactin T (Fig. 14) isolated from *M. tuberculosis* is similar to that of mycobactins isolated from other species. Ratledge (1987) has recently reviewed the isolation, purification, biosyn-

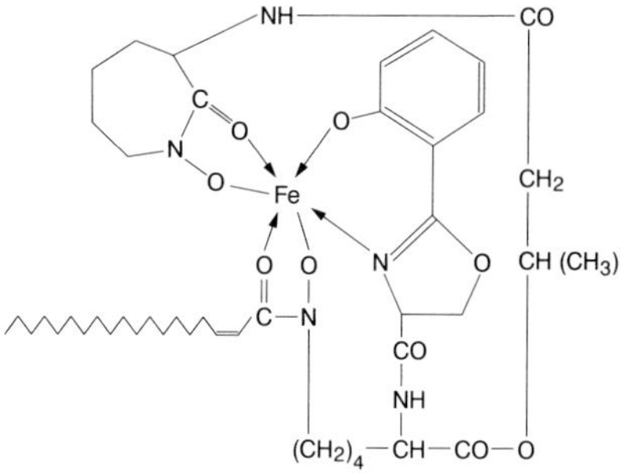

Figure 14. Mycobactin T.

thesis, and characterization of mycobactins.

LIPOGLYCANS OF *M. TUBERCULOSIS*

The structures of methylglucolipopolysaccharide and methylmannopolysaccharide have been pursued by Ballou for over 20 years (Dell and Ballou, 1983). These polysaccharides are truly cytosolic and have in common the role of generating complexes with long-chain fatty acids in which the fatty acid is included in the interior of the helically coiled polysaccharide. Ballou has suggested that the role of methylmannopolysaccharide may be to serve as a lipid carrier in the cell and to allow the synthesis of characteristically long-chain fatty acids.

mAGP Complex

The most characteristic feature of the mycobacterial cell wall is the chemotype IV peptidoglycan, which is composed of substantial quantities of *meso*-diaminopimelic acid (Lechevalier and Lechevalier, 1970). The tripartite structure of the mycobacterial cell wall was first suggested by Imaeda et al. (1968), who used negative staining and electron microscopy. Later, Barksdale and Kim (1977) labeled the layers of the trilaminar structure L1, L2, and L3, with the innermost layer being L3. Draper (1982) further concluded that the L3 layer corresponded to a true cell wall. The two outermost layers, L1 and L2, corresponded to capsule-like structures that were not covalently linked to the cell wall. Further electron microscopy studies defined the ultrastructure of the mycobacterial cell envelope (Draper, 1982). It is clear that the envelope possesses an electron-dense layer of peptidoglycan that is surrounded by an electron-transparent layer of arabinogalactan and mycolic acids. Basically, peptidoglycan is a highly cross-linked polymer of amino sugars and amino acids [repeating units of GlcNAc-(β1→4)-*N*-glycolylmuramic acid (Goodfellow and Cross, 1984)]. In addition, peptidoglycan is covalently linked to arabinogalactan via a phosphodiester bond, and mycolic acids are in turn attached to the arabinogalactan. A schematic representation of this cellular envelope of *M. tuberculosis* is depicted in Fig. 15.

During 50 years of intensive studies (Misaki et al., 1970, 1974, 1977; Azuma et al., 1968; Vilkas et al., 1973; Lederer et al., 1975), the arabinogalactan polymer was shown to consist exclusively of D-arabinose and D-galactose residues. Misaki et al. (1974) further demonstrated that the arabinosyl residues are 5-linked Ara*f* and the galactosyl residues are either 4-linked galactopyranoses or 5-linked Gal*f*. Following this study, Vilkas et al. (1973), by using partial acid hydrolysis, isolated Gal*f*-(1→6)-Gal, which established that some of the galactosyl residues were in fact linked to furanose and C-6.

The polymer is unusual in that, unlike most bacterial polysaccharides (Anderson and Unger, 1983), it lacks any repeating units of oligosaccharides but is composed of a few distinct, defined structural motifs. The use of partial depolymerization of per-*O*-alkylated polysaccharides (Daffe et al., 1990) and subsequent analyses of the generated oligomers by GC-MS and fast atom bombardment-MS established that (i) within the arabinogalactan, all arabinosyl and galactosyl residues are in the furanose form; (ii) the nonreducing terminal arrangements of arabinan consist of a hexaarabinofuranosyl structure [β-D-Ara*f*-(1→2)-α-D-Ara*f*]$_2$-3,5-α-D-Ara*f*-(1→5)-α-D-Ara*f*; (iii) the majority of the arabinan chain consists of 5-linked α-D-Ara*f* residues with branching introduced by 3,5-α-D-Ara*f* residues replaced at both branch positions with 5-α-D-Ara*f*; (iv) the arabinan chains are attached through the C-5 of some of the 6-linked Gal*f* units, and approximately two arabinan chains are attached to the galactan core; (v)

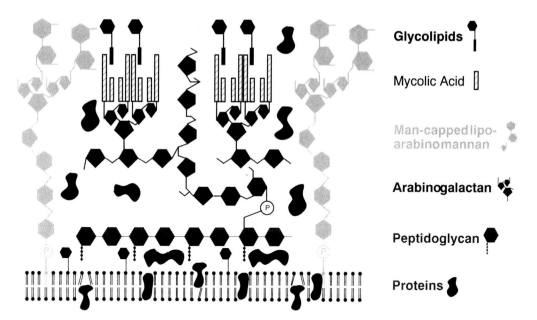

Glycolipids

Mycolic Acid

Man-capped lipo-
arabinomannan

Arabinogalactan

Peptidoglycan

Proteins

Figure 15. Schematic representation of the cell wall of *M. tuberculosis*.

the galactan region consists of linear alternating 5- and 6-linked β-D-Gal*f* residues; (vi) the galactan region of the arabinogalactan is linked to the C-6 of some muramyl residues of peptidoglycan via a unique diglycosylphosphoryl bridge, L-Rha*p*-(1→3)-D-GlcNAc-(1→P) (McNeil et al., 1990); and (vii) the mycolic acids are located in clusters of four on the terminal hexaarabinofuranosyl, but only two-thirds of these arrangements are mycolated (McNeil et al., 1991).

Recently, a novel family of arabinases and galactanases secreted by a *Cellulomonas* species was used to degrade base-solubilized arabinogalactan from virulent *M. tuberculosis*. The major degradation product was a hexaarabinofuranoside, [β-D-Ara*f*-(1→2)-α-D-Ara*f*-(1→]$_2$-3,5-α-D-Ara*f*-(1→5)-α-D-Ara*f*, and a linear disaccharide, α-D-Ara*f*-(1→5)-α-D-Ara*f*. Interestingly, the linear galactan backbone was degraded into cyclic oligosaccharides of the structure [-5-β-D-Gal*f*-(1→6)-β-D-Gal*f*-(1→]$_n$ (McNeil et al., in press). According to this observation, the galactan forms a short helical chain in

which four Gal*f* residues represent one turn of the helix.

The mAGP is known to be a strong immunogen, but very little is known about its interactions with host cells. It has been speculated that it provides a protective barrier and intransigence to drug permeation (McNeil and Brennan, 1991; Nikaido and Jarlier, 1991).

LAM

A second molecule that dominates the mycobacterial cell envelope is LAM. Earlier studies conducted by Menzel and Heidelberger (1939), Chargaff and Schaefer (1935), and Seibert and Watson (1941) all pointed toward the presence of a serologically active polysaccharide isolated from *M. tuberculosis*.

Misaki et al. (1977) and Azuma et al. (1968) established that the polysaccharide consisted of an α(1→6)-linked D-Man*p* backbone to which were attached short side chains of α(1→2)-linked D-Man*p* residues and α(1→5)-linked D-Ara*f* residues. Initial studies were conducted with a polysaccharide that was isolated after strong alkaline hydrolysis, which pointed to the conclusion that LAM was a neutral polysaccharide, although earlier studies by Ohashi (1970), Ohashi and Tsumita (1964), and Tsumita et al. (1959, 1960) described two classes of arabinomannan isolated from *M. tuberculosis*, i.e., acylated and nonacylated. The acylated version was shown to contain palmitic and tuberculostearic acids. Weber and Gray (1979) indicated that native arabinomannan isolated from *M. smegmatis* is phosphorylated and contains both succinyl and lactyl residues in addition to palmitic and tuberculostearic acids. They also corroborated the earlier observation of Misaki et al. (1977) and Ohashi (1970) that most of the Manp residues belong to a core region, with the main structural feature being α(1→5)-linked D-Araf units.

Hunter et al. (1986) isolated highly purified LAM by using anion-exchange and gel filtration chromatography; by polyacrylamide gel electrophoresis, this LAM yielded a broad, diffuse band with a mass of 30 to 35 kDa. Subsequent analyses of LAM showed that in addition to arabinose and mannose, it contained glycerol, inositol, phosphate, lactate, succinate, palmitate, and tuberculostearate, as suggested earlier. The phosphate was shown to occur in the form of an alkali-labile phosphatidyl-*myo*-inositol unit, and the two long-chain fatty acids occurred in the form of a diacylglycerol. Interestingly, both LAM and LM are considered prokaryotic versions of a growing body of biologically important phosphatidylinositol "membrane anchors" (Hunter and Brennan, 1990). The structure of LAM is summarized in Fig. 16.

LAM exhibits a wide spectrum of immunoregulatory functions such as abrogation of T-cell activation (Kaplan et al., 1987), inhibition of gamma interferon-mediated activation of murine macrophages (Sibley et al., 1988), scavenging of potentially cytotoxic oxygen-free radicals (Chan et al.,

1991), inhibition of protein kinase C activity (Chan et al., 1991), and evocation of a large array of cytokines associated with macrophages, such as TNF (Moreno et al., 1988, 1989; Chatterjee et al., 1992c; Roach et al., 1993), granulocyte macrophage colony-stimulating factor, IL-1a, IL-1b, IL-6, and IL-10 (Barnes et al., 1992; Orme et al., 1993). Thus, it has been speculated that LAM mediates the production of macrophage-derived cytokines that may give rise to many of the clinical manifestations of tuberculosis and leprosy (Wallis et al., 1990).

The structural definition of LAM has resulted in two distinct arrangements occupying the terminal end: branched hexaarabinofuranosides with the structure [β-D-Araf-(1→2)-α-D-Araf]₂-3,5-α-D-Araf-(1→5)-α-D-Araf and linear tetraarabinofuranosides of the structure β-D-Araf-(1→2)-α-D-Araf-(1→5)-α-D-Araf-(1→5)-α-D-Araf (Chatterjee et al., 1991). However, in the case of LAM isolated from the virulent Erdman strain of *M. tuberculosis*, these two types of arabinose termini are extensively capped with Manp residues, a product now termed ManLAM (Chatterjee et al., 1992b) (Fig. 16). It has also been shown that the ability to stimulate TNF of AraLAM is abrogated by mannose capping (Chatterjee et al., 1992c). Recently, studies conducted by Roach et al. (1993) have confirmed these observations and have shown further that the early response genes (including c-*fos* and the genes for JE as well as TNF) in macrophages exposed to LAMs are turned on or off depending on the structural differences discussed above.

The biological properties of LAM are also dependent on the native structure of LAM at the reducing end. Upon treatment of LAM with mild alkali to remove acyl functions, the capacity of the molecule to induce cytokine production and the suppression of antigen-induced proliferation are removed. This confirms that the phosphatidylinositol anchor is also crucial to

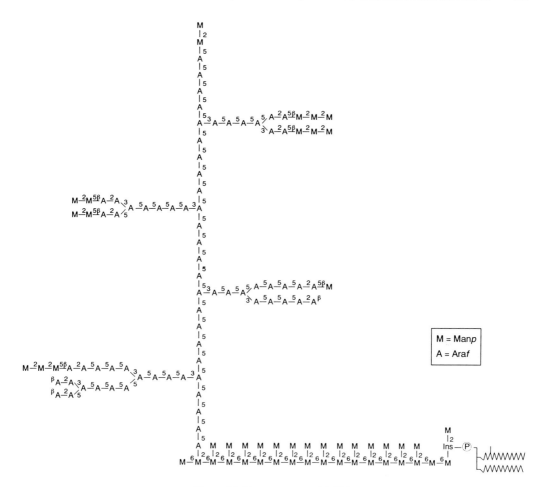

Figure 16. Mannose-capped LAM.

some of the biological functions of LAM. Recent studies have shown that *M. bovis* BCG and *M. tuberculosis* H37Rv also contain ManLAM with a molecular mass of 17,250 kDa, estimated by using laser desorption MS (Venisse et al., 1993). In addition, several investigators have suggested that the broadness of the band on a polyacrylamide gel is perhaps due to the presence of microheterogeneity within the molecule, analogous to the lipopolysaccharides of gram-negative bacteria. Structurally, it also appears that the arabinan portion of LAM is critical to its biological properties. In fact, LM, which is devoid of the arabinan portion of LAM but has a structure somewhat similar to the mannan backbone of LAM, is biologically inactive.

There has been considerable development in the structural definition of LAM, LM, and the PIMs, notably, confirmation that LAM and LM are essentially the multiglycosylated versions of the PIMs, which were described over 30 years ago; however, the biosyntheses of these unusual molecules are still unexplored. It is thought that a multifaceted enzyme complex will be involved in the formation of the complete molecule. Indeed, Yokoyama and Ballou (1989) have demonstrated the presence of a decaprenyl-P-Man carrier lipid involved in the biosynthesis of mannans, and a more recent study by Wolucka et al. (in press) has resulted in the isolation of a lipid that may be implicated in arabinan biosynthesis.

The location of LAM in the cell wall has been a topic of much controversy. The surface location of LAM has been demonstrated with the aid of electron microscopy (Hunter and Brennan, 1990), and because of the presence of its phosphatidylinositol lipid anchor, LAM is believed to be anchored in the plasma membrane of the mycobacterial cell envelope (Fig. 15). Therefore, it is envisaged that LAM traverses the entire cell wall of a mycobacterium (Fig. 15).

Although LAM may not be a virulence factor for tuberculosis, it is clear from the studies discussed above that with its unique structural features, it is a key molecule with an important role in the interaction of the pathogen with the host and may be a factor contributing to the survival of *M. tuberculosis* within host macrophages.

COMPREHENSIVE VIEW OF CARBOHYDRATES AND LIPIDS

An important feature of the mycobacterial cell wall is the integrity of the capsular lipids and the outer lipid matrix, mycolylarabinogalactan. Indeed, several models that accommodate various features of the cell wall have been suggested (Minnikin, 1991). The model presented by Minnikin (1982, 1991) suggests that the arabinogalactan chains would have an ordered arrangement due to the constraints placed on them by the mycolic acids packing tightly together. Therefore, any degree of disruption to the capsular lipids or the mycolylarabinogalactan complex would lead to a very disordered arrangement.

In addition, there are many plausible reasons given for the complexity of the cell wall entities produced by *M. tuberculosis*. The effort expended by the bacilli in their production of these entities alone suggests

that they are important in survival and proliferation; we do know from our experience with tissue-derived *M. leprae* that these constituents are produced in vivo. Universally, the modes for effecting bacterial survival include modulation of the bacterial interaction with the host immune response (i.e., evasion of complement-mediated lysis); the bacterium's influence on the macrophage (i.e., directing phagocytosis via nonactivating receptors or nonstimulation of inflammatory cytokines); and downregulation of the immune activation of mononuclear cells and moderation of the stimulation of the cellular response (i.e., reducing antigen-presenting activity). Several of these effects have been noted for the cell wall entities described earlier; however, the link between the expression of these molecules and virulence is still rather tenuous.

This lack of biological definition and the poor understanding of the overall physical characteristics of the mycobacterial cell wall were probably due to the inadequacy of the experimental systems of the time. As a consequence, there is an urgent need within the discipline to isolate or derive specific mutants with altered syntheses of defined cell wall products and to use these mutants in assessing the biological importance of individual molecules. Also, the use of sophisticated physical techniques, such as solid-state NMR or X-ray powder diffraction, may hold the key to unraveling the complex ultrastructure of the mycobacterial cell wall. Finally, a more comprehensive study of the L forms of mycobacteria (Barksdale and Kim, 1977) may provide additional information concerning both the physical characterization and the biological functions of the complex carbohydrates and lipids of *M. tuberculosis*.

Acknowledgments. We express our deepest gratitude to Patrick J. Brennan and David E. Minnikin for their introduction, direction, and continuous support in our endeavors. As a consequence, this chapter is dedicated to these two eminent scientists who have contributed to the structural elucidation of the myco-bacterial cell wall of *M. tuberculosis* over the past 25 years.

We also thank Michael R. McNeil for valuable assistance in the completion of this chapter, Marilyn K. Hein for preparation of the manuscript, and Carol Marander for the graphics.

We duly acknowledge the support of the National Institute of Allergy and Infectious Diseases, National Institutes of Health, for grant AI-18357 and contract AI-05074; and the Heiser Program for Research in Leprosy and Tuberculosis for a postdoctoral fellow-ship to G. S. Besra.

REFERENCES

Adam, A., M. Senn, E. Vilkas, and E. Lederer. 1967. Spectrometrie de masse de glycolipides. 2. Diesters de trehalose naturels et synthetiques. *Eur. J. Bio-chem.* **2**:460–468.

Alshamaony, L., M. Goodfellow, and D. E. Minnikin. 1976a. Free mycolic acids as criteria in the classifi-cation of *Nocardia* and the "*rhodochrous*" com-plex. *J. Gen. Microbiol.* **92**:188–199.

Alshamaony, L., M. Goodfellow, D. E. Minnikin, and H. Mordarska. 1976b. Free mycolic acids as criteria in the classification of *Gordona* and the "*rhodo-chrous*" complex. *J. Gen. Microbiol.* **92**:183–187.

Anderson, L., and F. M. Unger (ed.). 1983. *Bacterial Lipopolysaccharides.* ACS Symposium Series 231. American Chemical Society, Washington, D.C.

Anderson, R. J. 1939. The chemistry of the lipids of the tubercle bacillus and certain other microorganisms. *Prog. Chem. Org. Nat. Prod.* **3**:145–202.

Anderson, R. J. 1941. Structural peculiarities of acid-fast bacterial lipids. *Chem. Rev.* **29**:225–243.

Antoine, A. D., and B. S. Tepper. 1969. Environmental control of glycogen and lipid content of *Mycobacte-rium phlei. J. Gen. Microbiol.* **55**:217–226.

Asselineau, C., J. Asselineau, R. Ryhage, S. Stallberg-Stenhagen, and E. Stenhagen. 1959. Synthesis of (−)-methyl 2D, 4D, 6D-trimethylnonacosanoate and identification of C$_{32}$-mycocerosic acid as 2,4,6,8-tetramethyloctacosanoic acid. *Acta Chem. Scand.* **13**:822–824.

Asselineau, C., H. Montrozier, and J. C. Prome. 1969. Structure des acides α-mycoliques isoles de la souche Canetti de *Mycobacterium tuberculosis. Bull. Soc. Chim. Fr.* **51**:592–596.

Azuma, I., H. Kimura, T. Niinaka, I. Aoki, and Y. Yamamura. 1968. Chemical and immunological studies on mycobacterial polysaccharides. I. Purifi-cation and properties of polysaccharides from hu-man tubercle bacilli. *J. Bacteriol.* **95**:263–271.

Ballou, C. E., E. Vilkas, and E. Lederer. 1963. Struc-tural studies on the myo-inositol phospholipids of

Mycobacterium tuberculosis. J. Biol. Chem. **238**:69–76.

Barksdale, L., and K.-S. Kim. 1977. *Mycobacterium. Bacteriol. Rev.* **41**:217–372.

Barnes, P. F., D. Chatterjee, J. S. Abrams, S. Lu, E. Wang, M. Yamamura, P. J. Brennan, and R. L. Modlin. 1992. Cytokine production induced by *My-cobacterium tuberculosis* lipoarabinomannan: rela-tionship to chemical structure. *J. Immunol.* **149**:541–547.

Besra, G. S., R. C. Bolton, M. R. McNeil, M. Ridell, K. E. Simpson, J. Glushka, H. van Halbeek, P. J. Brennan, and D. E. Minnikin. 1992. Structural elu-cidation of a novel family of acyltrehaloses from *Mycobacterium tuberculosis. Biochemistry* **31**:9832–9837.

Bloch, H. 1950. Studies on the virulence of tubercle bacilli. Isolation and biological properties of a con-stituent of virulent organisms. *J. Exp. Med.* **91**:197–218.

Brennan, P. J. 1988. *Mycobacterium* and other actino-mycetes, p. 203–298. *In* C. Ratledge and S. G. Wilkinson (ed.), *Microbial Lipids*, vol. I. Academic Press, London.

Brennan, P. J. 1989. Structures of mycobacteria: re-cent developments in defining cell wall carbohy-drates and proteins. *Rev. Infect. Dis.* **11**(Suppl. 2):S420–S430.

Brennan, P. J., and C. E. Ballou. 1968. Biosynthesis of mannophosphoinositides of *Mycobacterium phlei. J. Biol. Chem.* **243**:2975–2984.

Brennan, P. J., D. P. Lehane, and D. W. Thomas. 1970a. Acylglucoses of the corynebacteria and my-cobacteria. *Eur. J. Biochem.* **13**:117–123.

Brennan, P. J., S. A. Rooney, and F. G. Winder. 1970b. The lipids of *Mycobacterium tuberculosis* BCG: fractionation, composition, turnover, and the effects of isoniazid. *Ir. J. Med. Sci.* **3**:371–390.

Cason, J., G. L. Lange, W. T. Miller, and A. Weiss. 1964. The multibranched higher saturated acids from tubercle bacillus. *Tetrahedron* **20**:91–106.

Chan, J., X. Fan, S. W. Hunter, P. J. Brennan, and B. R. Bloom. 1991. Lipoarabinomannan, a possible virulence factor involved in persistence of *Myco-bacterium tuberculosis* within macrophages. *Infect. Immun.* **59**:1755–1761.

Chargaff, E., and W. Schaefer. 1935. A specific poly-saccharide from the bacillus Calmette Guerin. *J. Biol. Chem.* **112**:393–405.

Chatterjee, D., C. M. Bozic, M. McNeil, and P. J. Brennan. 1991. Structural features of the arabinan component of the lipoarabinomannan of *Mycobac-terium tuberculosis. J. Biol. Chem.* **266**:9652–9660.

Chatterjee, D., S. W. Hunter, M. McNeil, and P. J. Brennan. 1992a. Lipoarabinomannan: multiglycosy-lated form of the mycobacterial mannosylphosphati-dylinositols. *J. Biol. Chem.* **267**:6228–6233.

Chatterjee, D., K. Lowell, B. Rivoire, M. R. McNeil, and P. J. Brennan. 1992b. Lipoarabinomannan of *Mycobacterium tuberculosis*: capping with mannosyl residue in some strains. *J. Biol. Chem.* **267**:6234–6239.

Chatterjee, D., A. D. Roberts, K. Lowell, P. J. Brennan, and I. M. Orme. 1992c. Structural basis of capacity of lipoarabinomannan to induce secretion of tumor necrosis factor. *Infect. Immun.* **60**:1249–1253.

Daffe, M., P. J. Brennan, and M. McNeil. 1990. Predominant structural features of the cell wall arabinogalactan of *Mycobacterium tuberculosis* as revealed through characterization of oligoglycosyl alditol fragments by gas chromatography/mass spectrometry and by ^{1}H and ^{13}C-NMR analyses. *J. Biol. Chem.* **265**:6734–6743.

Daffe, M., S.-N. Cho, D. Chatterjee, and P. J. Brennan. 1991a. Chemical synthesis and seroreactivity of a neoantigen containing the oligosaccharide hapten of the *Mycobacterium tuberculosis*-specific phenolic glycolipid. *J. Infect. Dis.* **163**:161–168.

Daffe, M., C. Lacave, M. A. Laneelle, M. Gillois, and G. Laneelle. 1988. Polyphthienoyl trehalose, glycolipids specific for virulent strains of the tubercle bacillus. *Eur. J. Biochem.* **172**:579–584.

Daffe, M., C. Lacave, M.-A. Laneelle, and G. Laneelle. 1987. Structure of the major triglycosylphenolphthiocerol of *Mycobacterium tuberculosis* strain Canetti. *Eur. J. Biochem.* **167**:155–160.

Daffe, M., M. R. McNeil, and P. J. Brennan. 1991b. Novel type-specific lipooligosaccharides from *Mycobacterium tuberculosis*. *Biochemistry* **30**:378–388.

Dell, A., and C. E. Ballou. 1983. Fast-atom-bombardment, negative ion mass spectrometry of the mycobacterial *O*-methyl-deuterium glucose polysaccharides and lipopolysaccharides. *Carbohydr. Res.* **120**:95–111.

Draper, P. 1982. The anatomy of mycobacteria, p. 9–52. *In* C. Ratledge and J. Sanford (ed.), *The Biology of Mycobacteria*, vol. 1. Academic Press, London.

Etemadi, A.-H. 1967a. The use of pyrolysis gas chromatography and mass spectrometry in the study of the structure of mycolic acids. *J. Gas Chromatogr.* **5**:447–456.

Etemadi, A.-H. 1967b. Correlations structurales et biogenetiques des acides mycoliques en rapport avec la phylogenese de quelques genres d'actinomycetales. *Bull. Soc. Chim. Biol.* **49**:695–706.

Etemadi, A.-H. 1967c. Les acides mycoliques structure, biogenese et interet phylogenetique. *Expo. Annu. Biochim. Med.* **28**:77–109.

Gastambide-Odier, M., J. M. Delaumeny, and E. Lederer. 1963. Biosynthesis of phthiocerol: incorporation of methionine and propionic acid. *Chem. Ind.* **1963**:1285–1286.

Gastambide-Odier, M., and E. Lederer. 1960. Biosynthese de l'acide corynomycolique a partir de deux molecules d'acide palmitique. *Biochem. Z.* **333**:285–295.

Gastambide-Odier, M., and P. Sarda. 1970. Contribution a etude de la structure et de la biosynthese de glycolipides specifiques isoles de mycobacterias: les mycosides A et B. *Pneumologie* **42**:241–255.

Ginger, L. G., and R. J. Anderson. 1945. The chemistry of the lipids of tubercle bacilli. LXXII. Fatty acids occurring in the wax prepared from tuberculin residues concerning mycocerosic acid. *J. Biol. Chem.* **157**:203–211.

Goodfellow, M., and T. Cross. 1984. Classification, p. 7–164. *In* M. Goodfellow, M. Mordorski, and S. T. Williams (ed.), *The Biology of the Actinomycetes*. Academic Press, London.

Goren, M. B. 1970a. Sulfolipid I of *Mycobacterium tuberculosis* strain H37Rv. I. Purification and properties. *Biochim. Biophys. Acta* **210**:116–126.

Goren, M. B. 1970b. Sulfolipid I of *Mycobacterium tuberculosis* strain H37Rv. II. Structural studies. *Biochim. Biophys. Acta* **210**:127–138.

Goren, M. B. 1972. Mycobacterial lipids: selected topics. *Bacteriol. Rev.* **36**:33–64.

Goren, M. B. 1977. Phagocyte lysosomes: interactions with infectious agents, phagosomes, and experimental perturbations in function. *Annu. Rev. Microbiol.* **31**:507–533.

Goren, M. B. 1982. Immunoreactive substances of mycobacteria. *Am. Rev. Respir. Dis.* **125**(Part 2):50–69.

Goren, M. B. 1987. Polyanionic agents do not inhibit phagosome-lysosome fusion in cultured macrophages. *J. Leukocyte Biol.* **41**:122–129.

Goren, M. B., and P. J. Brennan. 1979. Mycobacterial lipids: chemistry and biologic activities, p. 69–193. *In* G. P. Youmans (ed.), *Tuberculosis*. The W.B. Saunders Co., Philadelphia.

Goren, M. B., O. Brokl, P. Roller, H. M. Fales, and B. C. Das. 1976a. Sulfatides of *Mycobacterium tuberculosis*: the structure of the principle sulfatide (SL-I). *Biochemistry* **15**:2728–2735.

Goren, M. B., O. Brokl, and W. B. Schaefer. 1974. Lipids of putative relevance to virulence in *Mycobacterium tuberculosis*: correlation of virulence and elaboration of sulfatides and strongly acidic lipids. *Infect. Immun.* **9**:150–158.

Goren, M. B., J. M. Grange, V. R. Aber, B. W. Allen, and D. A. Mitchinson. 1982. Role of lipid content and hydrogen peroxide susceptibility in determining the guinea-pig virulence of *Mycobacterium tuberculosis*. *Br. J. Exp. Pathol.* **63**:693–700.

Goren, M. B., P. D. Hart, M. R. Young, J. A. Armstrong. 1976b. Prevention of phagosome-lysosome fusion in cultured macrophages by sulfatides of *Mycobacterium tuberculosis*. *Proc. Natl. Acad.*

Sci. USA **73:**2510–2514.

Hunter, S. W., and P. J. Brennan. 1990. Evidence for the presence of a phosphatidylinositol anchor on the lipoarabinomannan and lipomannan of *Mycobacterium tuberculosis. J. Biol. Chem.* **265:**9272–9279.

Hunter, S. W., H. Gaylord, and P. J. Brennan. 1986. Structure and antigenicity of the phosphorylated lipopolysaccharide antigens from the leprosy and tubercle bacilli. *J. Biol. Chem.* **261:**12345–12351.

Imaeda, T., F. Kanetsuna, and B. Galindo. 1968. Ultrastructure of cell walls of genus *Mycobacterium. J. Ultrastruct. Res.* **25:**46–63.

Kaplan, G., R. R. Gandhi, D. E. Weinstein, W. R. Levis, M. E. Patarroyo, P. J. Brennan, and Z. A. Cohn. 1987. *Mycobacterium leprae* antigen-induced suppression of T cell proliferation *in vitro. J. Immunol.* **138:**3028–3034.

Kataoka, N., I. Toida, I. Yano, and A. Misaki. 1986. Isolation and characterization of new glycolipids from *Mycobacterium tuberculosis* H37Rv. *Osaka City Med. J.* **32:**1–15.

Kato, M. 1973. Effect of anti-cord factor antibody on experimental tuberculosis in mice. *Infect. Immun.* **7:**14–21.

Kikuchi, S., D. L. Rainwater, and P. E. Kolattukudy. 1992. Purification and characterization of an unusually large fatty acid synthase from *Mycobacterium tuberculosis* var. bovis BCG. *Arch. Biochem. Biophys.* **295:**318–326.

Koul, A. K., and M. Gastambide-Odier. 1977. Microanalyse rapide de dimycocerosate de phthiocerol de mycoside et de glycerides dans les extraits a l'ether de petrole de *Mycobacterium kansasii* et du BCG, souchi Pasteur. *Biochimie* **59:**535–538.

Lacave, C., M. A. Laneelle, M. Daffe, H. Montrozier, M. P. Rols, and C. Asselineau. 1987. Etude structurale et metabolique des acides mycoliques de *Mycobacterium fortuitum. Eur. J. Biochem.* **163:**369–378.

Lacave, C., M. A. Laneelle, and G. Laneelle. 1990a. Mycolic acid synthesis by *Mycobacterium aurum* cell-free extracts. *Biochim. Biophys. Acta* **1042:**315–323.

Lacave, C., M. A. Laneelle, H. Montrozier, and G. Laneelle. 1989. Mycolic acid metabolic filiation and location in *Mycobacterium aurum* and *Mycobacterium phlei. Eur. J. Biochem.* **181:**459–466.

Lacave, C., A. Quemard, and G. Laneelle. 1990b. Cell-free synthesis of mycolic acids in *Mycobacterium aurum*: radioactivity distribution in newly synthesized acids and presence of cell wall in the system. *Biochim. Biophys. Acta* **1045:**58–65.

Lechevalier, M. P. 1977. Lipids in bacterial taxonomy—a taxonomist's view. *Crit. Rev. Microbiol.* **1977:**109–210.

Lechevalier, M. P., and H. Lechevalier. 1970. Chemical composition as a criterion in the classification of

aerobic actinomycetes. *Int. J. Syst. Bacteriol.* **20:**435–444.

Lederer, E., A. Adam, R. Ciorbaru, J.-F. Petit, and J. Wietzerbin. 1975. Cell walls of mycobacteria and related organisms; chemistry and immunostimulant properties. *Mol. Cell. Biochem.* **7:**87–104.

Lee, Y. C., and C. E. Ballou. 1964. Structural studies on the myo-inositol mannosides from the glycolipids of *Mycobacterium tuberculosis* and *Mycobacterium phlei. J. Biol. Chem.* **239:**1316–1327.

Lee, Y. C., and C. E. Ballou. 1965. Complete structures of the glycophospholipids of mycobacteria. *Biochemistry* **4:**1395–1404.

Lepoivre, M., J. P. Tenu, G. Lemaire, and J. F. Petit. 1982. Anti-tumor activity and hydrogen peroxide release by macrophages elicted by trehalose clusters. *J. Immunol.* **129:**860–866.

Manjula, M., and P. E. Kolattukudy. 1992. Molecular cloning and sequencing of the gene for mycocerosic acid synthase, a novel fatty acid elongating multifunctional enzyme from *Mycobacterium tuberculosis* var. *bovis* Bacillus Calmette-Guerin. *J. Biol. Chem.* **267:**19388–19395.

Marks, G. S., and N. Polgar. 1955. Mycoceranic acid. II. *J. Chem. Soc.* **1955**(Part IV):3851–3857.

Matsunaga, I., S. Oka, T. Inove, and I. Yano. 1990. Mycolyl glycolipids stimulate macrophages to release chemotactic factors. *FEMS Microbiol. Lett.* **67:**49–54.

McNeil, M., and P. J. Brennan. 1991. Structure, function, and biogenesis of the cell envelope of mycobacteria in relation to bacterial physiology, pathogenesis, and drug resistance; some thoughts and possibilities arising from recent structural information. *Res. Microbiol.* **142:**451–463.

McNeil, M., M. Daffe, and P. J. Brennan. 1990. Evidence for the nature of the link between the arabinogalactan and peptidoglycan components of mycobacterial cell walls. *J. Biol. Chem.* **265:**18200–18206.

McNeil, M., M. Daffe, and P. J. Brennan. 1991. Location of the mycolyl ester substituent in the cell walls of mycobacteria. *J. Biol. Chem.* **266:**13217–13223.

McNeil, M. R., K. G. Robuck, M. Harter, and P. J. Brennan. Enzymatic evidence for the presence of a critical terminal hexaarabinoside in the cell walls of *Mycobacterium tuberculosis. Glycobiology*, in press.

Menzel, A. E. O., and M. Heidelberger. 1939. Specific and nonspecific cell polysaccharides of bovine strain of tubercle bacillus. *J. Biol. Chem.* **127:**221–236.

Middlebrook, G., R. J. Dobos, and C. Pierce. 1947. Virulence and morphological characteristics of mammalian tubercle bacilli. *J. Exp. Med.* **86:**175–184.

Minnikin, D. E. 1982. Lipids: complex lipids, their chemistry, biosynthesis and roles, p. 95–184. *In* C. Ratledge and J. L. Stanford (ed.), *The Biology of the*

Mycobacteria, vol. I. Academic Press, London.

Minnikin, D. E. 1991. Chemical principles in the organization of lipid components in the mycobacterial cell envelope. *Res. Microbiol.* **142**:423–427.

Minnikin, D. E., G. Dobson, D. Sesardie, and M. Ridell. 1985. Mycolipenates and mycolipanolates of trehalose from *Mycobacterium tuberculosis*. *J. Gen. Microbiol.* **131**:1369–1374.

Minnikin, D. E., and M. Goodfellow. 1980. Lipid composition in the classification and identification of acid-fast bacteria, p. 189–256. *In* M. Goodfellow and R. G. Board (ed.), *Microbiological Classification and Identification*. Academic Press, London.

Minnikin, D. E., S. M. Minnikin, I. G. Hutchinson, M. Goodfellow, and J. M. Grange. 1984a. Mycolic acid patterns of representative strains of *Mycobacterium fortuitum*, *Mycobacterium peregrinum*, and *Mycobacterium smegmatis*. *J. Gen. Microbiol.* **130**:363–367.

Minnikin, D. E., S. M. Minnikin, J. H. Parlett, M. Goodfellow, and M. Magnusson. 1984b. Mycolic acid patterns of some species of *Mycobacterium*. *Arch. Microbiol.* **139**:225–231.

Minnikin, D. E., P. V. Patel, and M. Goodfellow. 1974. Mycolic acids of representative strains of *Nocardia* and ''*rhodochrous*'' complex. *FEBS Lett.* **39**:322–324.

Minnikin, D. E., and N. Polgar. 1965. Phthiocerol B, a constituent of the lipids of the tubercle bacilli. *Chem. Commun.* **20**:495.

Minnikin, D. E., and N. Polgar. 1966. Studies relating to phthiocerol. V. Phthiocerol A and B. *J. Chem. Soc.* (C) **1966**:2107–2112.

Minnikin, D. E., and N. Polgar. 1967a. Studies relating to phthiocerol. VII. Phthiodiolone A. J. Chem. Soc. (C) **1967**:803–807.

Minnikin, D. E., and N. Polgar. 1967b. The mycolic acids from human and avian tubercle bacilli. *Chem. Commun.* **18**:916–918.

Minnikin, D. E., and N. Polgar. 1967c. The methoxymycolic and ketomycolic acids from human tubercle bacilli. *Chem. Commun.* **22**:1172–1174.

Misaki, A., I. Azuma, and Y. Yamamura. 1977. Structural and immunochemical studies on D-arabino-D-mannans and D-mannans of *Mycobacterium tuberculosis* and other *Mycobacterium* species. *J. Biochem.* **82**:1759–1770.

Misaki, A., N. Ikawa, T. Kato, and S. Kotani. 1970. Cell wall arabinogalactan of *Mycobacterium phlei*. *Biochim. Biophys. Acta* **215**:405–408.

Misaki, A., N. Seto, and I. Azuma. 1974. Structure and immunological properties of D-arabino-D-galactan isolated from cell walls of *Mycobacterium* species. *J. Biochem.* **76**:15–22.

Moreno, C., A. Mehlert, and J. Lamb. 1988. The inhibitory effects of mycobacterial lipoarabinomannan and polysaccharides upon polyclonal human T-cell proliferation. *Clin. Exp. Immunol.* **74**:206–210.

Moreno, C., J. Taverne, A. Mehlert, C. A. W. Bate, R. J. Brealey, A. Meager, G. A. W. Rook, and J. H. L. Playfair. 1989. Lipoarabinomannan from *Mycobacterium tuberculosis* induces the production of tumor necrosis factor from human and murine macrophages. *Clin. Exp. Immunol.* **76**:240–245.

Nikaido, H., and V. Jarlier. 1991. Permeability of the mycobacterial cell wall. *Res. Microbiol.* **142**:437–443.

Noll, H. 1956. The chemistry of cord-factor, a toxic glycolipid of *M. tuberculosis*. *Adv. Tuberc. Res.* **7**:149–183.

Noll, H. 1957. The chemistry of some native constituents of the purified wax of *Mycobacterium tuberculosis*. *J. Biol. Chem.* **224**:149–164.

Ohashi, M. 1970. Studies on the chemical structure of serologically active arabinomannan from mycobacteria. *Jpn. J. Exp. Med.* **40**:1–14.

Ohashi, M., and J. Tsumita. 1964. The fatty acid composition of the lipopolysaccharide of *Mycobacterium tuberculosis*, the hemagglutination antigen. *Jpn. J. Exp. Med.* **34**:323–328.

Orme, I. M., A. D. Roberts, J. P. Griffin, and J. S. Abrams. 1993. Cytokine secretion by CD4 T lymphocytes acquired in response to *Mycobacterium tuberculosis* infection. *J. Immunol.* **151**:518–525.

Pangborn, M. C., and J. A. McKinney. 1966. Purification of serologically active phosphoinositides of *Mycobacterium tuberculosis*. *J. Lipid Res.* **7**:627–637.

Polansky, J., E. Solar, R. F. Toubiana, K. Takayama, M. S. Raju, and E. Wankert. 1977. A carbon-13 nuclear magnetic resonance spectral analysis of cord-factors and related substances. *Nouv. J. Chim.* **2**:317–320.

Polgar, N., and W. Smith. 1963. Mycoceranic acid. III. *J. Chem. Soc.* (Part III) **1963**:3081–3085.

Prome, J. C., C. Lacave, A. Ahibo-Coffy, and A. Savagnac. 1976. Separation et etude structurale des especes moleculaires de monomycolates et de dimycolates de α-D-trehalose presents chez *Mycobacterium phlei*. *Eur. J. Biochem.* **63**:543–552.

Puzo, G., and J. C. Prome. 1978. Field desorption mass spectrometry of oligosaccharides and glycolipids in presence of metal salts. *Adv. Mass Spectrom.* **7**:1596–1602.

Puzo, G., G. Tissie, C. Lacave, H. Aurelle, and J. C. Prome. 1978. Structural determination of 'cord-factor' from a *Cornybacterium diphtheriae* strain by the use of combined ionization methods in mass spectrometry: field desorption cesium cationization and electron impact mass spectrometry. *Biomed. Mass Spectrom.* **5**:699–703.

Qureshi, N., N. Sathyamoorthy, and K. Takayama. 1984. Biosynthesis of C_{30} to C_{56} fatty acids by an extract of *Mycobacterium tuberculosis* H37Ra. *J. Bacteriol.* **157**:46–52.

Rainwater, D. L., and P. E. Kolattukudy. 1983. Synthesis of mycocerosic acids from methylmalonyl coenzyme A by cell-free extracts of *Mycobacterium tuberculosis* var. *bovis* BCG. *J. Biol. Chem.* **258**: 2979–2985.

Rainwater, D. L., and P. E. Kolattukudy. 1985. Fatty acid biosynthesis in *Mycobacterium tuberculosis* var. *bovis Bacillus Calmette-Guerin*. *J. Biol. Chem.* **260**:616–623.

Ratledge, C. 1987. Iron metabolism in mycobacteria, p. 207–221. *In* G. Winkleman, D. van der Jalm, and J. Weilands (ed.), *Iron Transport in Microbes, Plants, and Animals*. VCH, Weinheim, Germany.

Roach, T. I. A., C. H. Barton, D. Chatterjee, and J. M. Blackwell. 1993. Macrophage activation: lipoarabinomannan from avirulent and virulent strains of *Mycobacterium tuberculosis* differentially induces the early genes c-fos, KC, JE, and tumor necrosis factor-α. *J. Immunol.* **150**:1886–1896.

Seibert, F. B., and D. W. Watson. 1941. Isolation of the polysaccharides and nucleic acid of tuberculin by electrophoresis. *J. Biol. Chem.* **140**:55–69.

Sibley, L. D., S. W. Hunter, P. J. Brennan, and J. L. Krahenbuhl. 1988. Mycobacterial lipoarabinomannan inhibits gamma interferon-mediated activation of macrophages. *Infect. Immun.* **56**:1232–1236.

Spargo, B. J., L. M. Crowe, T. Ioneda, B. L. Beaman, and J. H. Crowe. 1991. Cord-factor (α-α′-trehalose 6,6′ dimycolate) inhibits fusion between phospholipid vesicles. *Proc. Natl. Acad. Sci. USA* **88**:737–740.

Steck, P. A., B. A. Schwartz, M. S. Rosendahl, and G. R. Gray. 1978. Mycolic acids: a reinvestigation. *J. Biol. Chem.* **253**:5625–5709.

Stodola, F. H., A. Lesuk, and R. J. Anderson. 1938. The chemistry of lipids of tubercle bacilli. LIV. The isolation and properties of mycolic acids. *J. Biol. Chem.* **126**:505–513.

Strain, S. M., R. Toubiana, E. Ribi, and R. Parker. 1977. Separation of the mixture of trehalose 6,6′-dimycolates comprising the mycobacterial glycolipid fraction. *Biochem. Biophys. Res. Commun.* **77**:449–456.

Takayama, K., and E. L. Armstrong. 1971. Mannolipid synthesis in a cell-free system of *Mycobacterium smegmatis*. *FEBS Lett.* **18**:67–69.

Takayama, K., and L. A. Davidson. 1979a. Antimycobacterial drugs that inhibit mycolic acid synthesis. *Trends Biochem. Sci.* **4**:280–282.

Takayama, K., and L. A. Davidson. 1979b. Isonicotinic acid hydrazide, p. 98–119. *In* F. E. Hahn (ed.), *Antibiotics VI, Mechanism of Action of Antibacterial Agents*. Springer Verlag, Berlin.

Takayama, K., and D. S. Goldman. 1970. Enzymatic synthesis of mannosyl-1-phosphoryldecaprenol by a cell-free system of *Mycobacterium tuberculosis*. *J. Biol. Chem.* **245**:6251–6257.

Takayama, K., H. K. Schnoes, and E. J. Semmlier. 1973. Characterization of the alkali-stable mannophospholipids of *Mycobacterium smegmatis*. *Biochim. Biophys. Acta* **136**:212–221.

Thurman, P. F., W. Chai, J. R. Rosankiewicz, H. J. Rogers, A. M. Lawson, and P. Draper. 1993. Possible intermediates in the biosynthesis of mycoside B by *Mycobacterium microti*. *Eur. J. Biochem.* **212**: 705–711.

Tsumita, T., R. Matsumoto, and D. Mizuno. 1959. The nature of the Middlebrook-Dubos haemagglutination antigen of *Mycobacterium tuberculosis*. *Jpn. J. Med. Sci.* **12**:167–170.

Tsumita, T., R. Matsumoto, and D. Mizuno. 1960. Chemical and biological properties of the haemagglutination antigen, a lipopolysaccharide of *Mycobacterium tuberculosis*. *Jpn. J. Med. Sci.* **13**:131–138.

Venisse, A., J.-H. Berjeaud, P. Chaurand, P. Gilleron, and G. Puzo. 1993. Structural features of lipoarabinomannan from *Mycobacterium bovis* BCG. Determination of molecular mass by laser desorption mass spectrometry. *J. Biol. Chem.* **268**:12401–12411.

Vilkas, E., C. Amar, J. Markovits, J. G. F. Vliegenthart, and J. P. Kamerling. 1973. Occurrence of a galactofuranose disaccharide in immunoadjuvant fractions of *Mycobacterium tuberculosis* (cell walls and wax D). *Biochim. Biophys. Acta* **297**:423–435.

Walker, R. W., H. Barakat, and J. G. C. Hung. 1970. The positional distribution of fatty acids in the phospholipids and triglycerides of *Mycobacterium smegmatis* and *M. bovis* BCG. *Lipids* **5**:684–691.

Wallis, R. S., M. Amir-Tahmasseb, and J. J. Ellner. 1990. Induction of interleukin 1 and tumor necrosis factor by mycobacterial proteins: the monocyte Western blot. *Proc. Natl. Acad. Sci. USA* **87**:3348–3352.

Weber, P. L., and G. L. Gray. 1979. Structural and immunochemical characterization of the acidic arabinomannan of *Mycobacterium smegmatis*. *Carbohydr. Res.* **74**:259–278.

Weir, M. P., W. H. R. Langridge, and R. H. Walker. 1972. Relationships between oleic acid uptake and lipid metabolism in *Mycobacterium smegmatis*. *Am. Rev. Respir. Dis.* **106**:450–457.

Wheeler, P. R., G. S. Besra, D. E. Minnikin, and C. Ratledge. 1993a. Stimulation of mycolic acid biosynthesis by incorporation of *cis*-tetracos-5-enoic acid in a cell wall preparation from *Mycobacterium smegmatis*. *Biochim. Biophys. Acta* **1167**:182–188.

Wheeler, P. R., G. S. Besra, D. E. Minnikin, and C. Ratledge. 1993b. Inhibition of mycolic acid biosynthesis in a cell wall preparation from *Mycobacterium smegmatis* by methyl 4-(2-octadecylcyclpropen-1-yl) butanoate, a structural analogue of a key precursor. *Lett. Appl. Microbiol.* **17**:33–36.

Winder, F. G. 1982. Mode of action of the antimyco-bacterial agents and associated aspects of the molecular biology of the mycobacterias, p. 354–438. *In* C. Ratledge and J. L. Stanford (ed.), *The Biology of the Mycobacteria*, vol. 1. Academic Press, London.

Wolucka, B. A., M. R. McNeil, E. Hoffmann, T. Chojnacki, C. Cocito, R. Comber, and P. J. Brennan. Recognition of the likely carrier lipid for arabinan biosynthesis and its relation to the mode of action of ethambutol in mycobacteria. Submitted for publication.

Wong, M. Y. H., and G. R. Gray. 1979. Structures of the homologous series of mono-alkene mycolic acids from *Mycobacterium smegmatis*. *J. Biol. Chem.* **254:**5741–5744.

Yano, I., K. Kageyama, Y. Ohno, M. Masui, E. Kusunose, and M. Kusunose. 1978. Separation and analysis of molecular species of mycolic acids in *Nocardia* and related taxa by gas chromatography mass spectrometry. *Biomed. Mass Spectrom.* **5:**14–24.

Yokoyama, K., and C. E. Ballou. 1989. Synthesis of alpha 1→6 mannooligosaccharides in *Mycobacterium smegmatis*. Function of beta-mannosylphosphoryldecaprenol as the mannosyl donor. *J. Biol. Chem.* **264:**21621–21628.

Tuberculosis: Pathogenesis, Protection, and Control
Edited by Barry R. Bloom
© 1994 American Society for Microbiology, Washington, DC 20005

Chapter 21

Proteins and Antigens of *Mycobacterium tuberculosis*

Åse Bengård Andersen and Patrick Brennan

The proteins of the causative agent of tuberculosis, *Mycobacterium tuberculosis*, have been a major research topic almost since the days of the discovery of the organism by Robert Koch in 1882 (Koch, 1882). Looking back, it appears that there was, and still is, a general tendency to approach the topic from at least two angles: (i) basic research aimed at improving knowledge of the physiology of the bacteria, identifying metabolic pathways and enzyme systems, etc., and (ii) research aimed at understanding the interaction of the individual mycobacterial components with the immune systems of human beings or animal models. The goals of these latter efforts are to identify antigens that may be important in conferring protection against tuberculosis. The search for improved diagnostic reagents such as improved skin test reagents and/or serological markers is another aspect of such studies.

Obviously, each protein of *M. tuberculosis*, like proteins of any other organism, serves different functions. Regardless of whether a given protein is looked upon as a more or less potent antigen by the immunologist, in every case it serves a distinct and sometimes indispensable function in the bacterium.

The reasons for the division in approach are diverse: one is that laboratory techniques are subject to influence by the "trends of the time." Clearly, classic biochemistry and physiology were put somewhat in the background when molecular biology and modern immunology made their entry into mycobacteriology in the mid-1980s. The possibilities and achievements already attained with recombinant DNA techniques are astonishing and provide tools that are indispensable in modern research. However, it is important for the two lines of research to meet and, one hopes, to merge. Much effort has been devoted to the study of the nutritional requirements of mycobacteria in order to provide better support of bacteria in clinical specimens. Many of the important and fundamental biochemical studies on the growth and metabolism of mycobacteria date from several decades ago, and a good deal of information is available. However, in comparison to what is known about the physiology of and gene expression in *Escherichia coli*, the data concerning mycobacteria seem scarce. The slow generation time

Åse Bengård Andersen • Mycobacteria Department, Sector for Biotechnology, Statens Seruminstitut, DK 2300 Copenhagen, Denmark. *Patrick Brennan* • Department of Microbiology, Colorado State University, Fort Collins, Colorado 80523.

of *M. tuberculosis* combined with the tendency of the bacteria to aggregate when cultured in liquid medium and the safety precautions needed to work with it have discouraged the application of modern microbiological methods such as chemostats or fermentors in experiments designed to add to our understanding of the physiology and metabolism of *M. tuberculosis*. As will be discussed in more detail later in this chapter, it is extremely important for a number of reasons to know how the expression of various genes is regulated: from a vaccine-oriented and diagnostic point of view, it is important to know at what stage during infection certain proteins (antigens) are being expressed. It is important to know which in vitro conditions mimic in vivo situations, and this knowledge will also be important in the search for better antituberculosis drugs.

TUBERCULIN: A FAMOUS MYCOBACTERIAL ANTIGEN

Less than 10 years after the discovery of *M. tuberculosis* was published (Koch, 1882), Koch reported on his attempts to purify the components released to the culture medium by *M. tuberculosis* (Koch, 1891). He prepared a product later known as "Koch's old tuberculin." This product is a heat-inactivated concentrate of the constituents present in a glycerol-containing broth that has supported growth of *M. tuberculosis* for 8 weeks. Koch initially believed that this product might be useful in the treatment of tuberculosis (Koch, 1897). This theory was later abandoned, but Koch also made the important observation that the product was able to elicit a characteristic reaction 24 to 48 h after subcutaneous injection in tuberculous animals and humans. He suggested that the product, which he termed "tuberculin," could be used in the diagnosis of tuberculous infection (Koch, 1891, 1897). The reaction elic-

ited in the skin by tuberculin was referred to as "Koch's phenomenon" and is largely synonymous with what is today designated a delayed-type hypersensitivity (DTH) reaction. Tuberculin skin testing soon became accepted by clinicians and epidemiologists, and the impact of Koch's initial observation on tuberculosis control and surveillance cannot be overemphasized. There were, however, problems that were related to the crude nature of the product and the fact that a lot of components originating from the broth itself were concentrated with the mycobacterial proteins. Later, it became possible to use synthetic, protein-free media to support growth for tuberculin production. A much cleaner product was thus obtained, and F. Seibert and B. Munday were able to demonstrate that the active principle of tuberculin is present in the ammonium sulfate-precipitable protein fraction of the culture filtrate (Seibert and Munday, 1932). The material was termed "tuberculin purified protein derivative" (PPD). PPD has been and still is an extremely useful diagnostic and epidemiological tool. The production methods may vary from one producer to another, but essentially the products consist of proteins, released to the growth medium from stationary cultures of *M. tuberculosis*, that are recovered by precipitation with ammonium sulfate or trichloric acetic acid after heat inactivation, filtration, and concentration of the culture. The complexity of constituents of the product and the lack of knowledge at the molecular level as to which of the many components the major biological activity could be attributed made standardization of the product difficult. The need for international standards and master batches of the product became obvious. In 1941, Seibert produced PPD-S (Seibert and Glenn, 1941), which was later chosen to be the international standard of tuberculin intended to be used in comparative potency assays. The World Health Organization (WHO) and United Nations Children's

Fund (UNICEF) sponsored production of the master batch of PPD, termed RT23, at Statens Seruminstitut in Denmark, and it was agreed that UNICEF would make this preparation available for general use (Magnusson and Bentzon, 1958; Guld et al., 1958). It has been estimated that some 2 billion doses of RT23 have been administered to humans, and the product is still being widely used.

As will be discussed later, many bacterial proteins are highly conserved, not only within the genus *Mycobacterium* but also in a broad range of other bacterial species. One example is the group of stress or heat shock proteins that are produced in abundant quantities by *M. tuberculosis* and that exhibit at least 50% homology at the amino acid level with stress proteins from other bacterial species. It is therefore not surprising that PPD is not a fully species-specific reagent but is widely cross-reacting. It is still a prominent challenge for future research to apply modern biotechnology to the task of improving or finding candidates to replace a product that was developed in the period 1890 to 1932. Readers interested in details of the history of tuberculin should consult reviews by Magnusson (1967) and Landi (1984).

IDENTIFICATION AND ISOLATION OF ANTIGENS FROM *M. TUBERCULOSIS*

Classic Methods

The search for improved diagnostic reagents, such as more species-specific skin test antigens and serological markers, has been a driving force in many of the efforts devoted to the fractionation and identification of mycobacterial protein antigens. A comprehensive overview of the early attempts in this field may be found in, e.g., a review by Daniel and Janicki (1978).

The use of polyclonal antibodies raised in rabbits or goats hyperimmunized with sonicates or culture filtrates from unheated cultures of *M. tuberculosis* was at an early stage implemented in an immunoelectrophoresis system, and 11 major precipitates were thereby identified. The system was standardized with respect to reagents and nomenclature under the sponsorship of the United States-Japan Cooperative Medical Sciences Program and is referred to as the US-Japan reference system. However, the technique did not have enough resolving power to illustrate the complexity of the protein composition of the bacteria. This became evident when the two-dimensional technique, the so-called crossed-immunoelectrophoresis (CIE) technique, appeared (Wright and Roberts, 1974), and the number of observed precipitates was increased to 36.

The CIE method was introduced as a reference system for soluble antigens from BCG (Closs et al., 1980) and *M. tuberculosis* (Wright and Roberts, 1974; Wiker et al., 1988) (Fig. 1). However, the method has never been widely used despite the fact that it has analytical advantages that are not offered by other electrophoretic methods. The proteins are analyzed in their native configuration, and it is possible to study the antigenic relatedness of groups or families of proteins. As an example, the CIE method demonstrated the partial identity of the three members of the so-called 85 complex (Wiker et al., 1986a), which will be covered in more detail later in this chapter. The native status of the proteins in the precipitates has in some cases allowed direct demonstration of enzyme activity and thereby provided a method of identifying the function of the antigens (Ridell et al., 1987; Wiker et al., 1988).

The conventional biochemical tools for fractionating and analyzing mycobacterial proteins, as mentioned above, have not been in common use during recent years. Only a few groups have mastered the discipline and succeeded in purifying preparative quantities of single proteins. An outstanding exception should be mentioned: S.

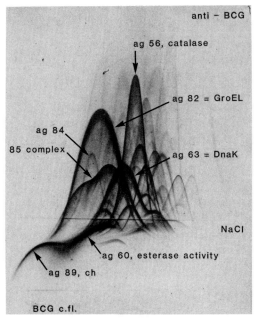

anti – BCG

ag 56, catalase

ag 82 = GroEL

ag 84

85 complex

ag 63 = DnaK

NaCl

ag 60, esterase activity

ag 89, ch

BCG c.fl.

Figure 1. Example of CIE of BCG culture fluid (BCG c.fl.). The second-dimension gel contained rabbit anti-BCG immunoglobulins (anti-BCG), and the intermediate gel contained 100 μl of 0.1 M NaCl. Numbers refer to the CIE reference system introduced by Closs et al. (1980). Staining for the esterase activity was performed prior to Coomassie staining of the CIE plate. The figure was kindly provided by Morten Harboe, Oslo, Norway. ag, antigen.

Nagai and coworkers, who have purified a large panel of mycobacterial proteins, of which several have been shown to be proteins actively secreted by the growing bacteria (Harboe et al., 1986; Wiker et al., 1986a, b; Nagai et al., 1991). This group of proteins will also be dealt with in more detail later. The laboratory of P. Brennan is also taking this approach (e.g., Lee et al., 1992). Recent reports on posttranslational modifications of several mycobacterial antigens such as acylations (Young and Garbe, 1991b) and maybe even glycosylations (Garbe et al., 1993) stress the importance of obtaining native bacterial products. It will be of utmost importance to compare the biological potency of immunologically interesting proteins in both native and recombinant, and therefore possibly

nonmodified or differently modified, versions.

MAbs and Recombinant DNA Techniques

The application of modern biotechnology to the study of the causative agent of tuberculosis was effectively stimulated by the WHO after the presentation of a comprehensive research plan in 1983 (Bulletin of the World Health Organization, 1983). A new group of researchers were thereby recruited to the field from other disciplines, and the microorganism was soon approached at both the DNA level and the protein level by the development of monoclonal antibodies (MAbs) raised against *M. tuberculosis*. The MAbs offered the unique possibility of tagging individual proteins by the recognition and binding of single epitopes. This property makes MAbs extremely useful reagents for a number of purposes in this context, most importantly for the affinity purification of the protein bound by the MAb and for the detection of mycobacterial proteins expressed by other microorganisms carrying and expressing recombinant mycobacterial DNA. The WHO has supported three international workshops, which aimed at reaching a consensus regarding the reactivity patterns of antimycobacterial MAbs submitted to the workshops. The results have been published, and samples of the MAbs are available on request from interested researchers (Engers et al., 1985, 1986; Khanolkar-Young et al., 1992). This initiative has been extremely useful, and much confusion and duplicate work have been avoided. The cloning of DNA from *M. tuberculosis* in fast-growing hosts like *E. coli* was initially and very successfully accomplished by R. Young, who constructed DNA expression libraries of both *M. tuberculosis* and *M. leprae* in the lambda gt11 vector (Young et al., 1985a, b), and by J. Thole and J. van Embden, who made the first BCG DNA bank in the EMBL3 phage lambda derivative (Thole et al., 1985). After encouragement by the WHO, the lambda gt11 gene libraries were made available to the scientific community. The speed with which a large number of laboratories became involved in the study of mycobacterial genes and their gene products was thereby greatly enhanced.

Five recombinant antigens have been produced in large enough quantities to be distributed to interested researchers through a WHO-organized "antigen bank." Obviously, the body of immunological data on these antigens by far exceeds what is known about other antigens. This does not necessarily mean that these antigens are more "interesting" than others, but they certainly have provided us with a baseline against which other antigens can be measured.

In a recent review, about 50 mycobacterial protein antigens were listed; the nucleotide sequences were known for about 20 of them (Young et al., 1992). A great many but not all of these antigens have been characterized in *M. tuberculosis*, *M. bovis*, and *M. leprae*. The organization and physical mapping of the *M. tuberculosis* genome is currently in progress (Cole, personal communication), and the eventual sequencing of the entire genome is now an attainable goal.

STRATEGIES FOR SELECTION OF ANTIGENS: WHAT DO WE FIND AND WHAT IS MISSED?

The mass of the genome of *M. tuberculosis* (3×10^9 Da [Baess and Mansa, 1978]) is comparable to that of the *E. coli* genome, in which more than 1,000 genes have been identified (Bachmann, 1990). In what order of priority should all these genes and gene products be studied? In the following, we will discuss some of the biases and limitations of the experimental conditions that are often encountered when working with mycobacteria.

As mentioned above, the goal for many of the projects dealing with characterization of mycobacterial proteins is the eventual identification of candidates that are important in eliciting a protective immune response in humans. Without devaluing all the unique properties of murine MAbs, it has been frustrating and a matter of much discussion as to what relevance antigens selected by virtue of their B-cell immunogenicity would have in a situation where T lymphocytes are known to play the major part. Obviously, the results and information obtained by means of MAbs have proved important and have led, for example, to the opening of a whole new field of research in stress and heat shock responses in mycobacteria and the role of these antigens in autoimmunity. However, this discussion has prompted several initiatives in which the bias of antibody selection has been bypassed. A relevant parameter to screen for is the ability of a protein to induce in vitro proliferation of T lymphocytes from diseased or vaccinated humans or animals. Direct screening of lysates of *E. coli* harboring recombinant phage clones from the lambda gt11 *M. tuberculosis* gene library (Young et al., 1985a) was therefore attempted by Mustafa et al. (1988), but the method is cumbersome, and because of the crude nature of the material, background proliferation is a problem unless T-cell clones are used. Another approach is the transfer of antigens separated by one-dimensional gel electrophoresis to nitrocellulose, which subsequently is cut into strips and presented to the cell culture (Young and Lamb, 1986; Abou-Zeid et al., 1987). This method suffers from the drawback that it is difficult to quantitate the proteins, and therefore it is difficult to rank one antigen as better than another. Gulle and colleagues refined the method by separating the antigens by isoelectric focusing in the first dimension followed by native polyacrylamide gel electrophoresis (PAGE) in the second dimension. The proteins were thereafter electroeluted to a soluble phase in a specially designed device containing 480 wells and were then presented to the cell cultures (Gulle et al., 1990; Daugelat et al., 1992). This appears to be a very attractive method. However, the yield of material that can be collected by this method may be a problem. A similar approach was taken by Andersen and Heron (1993a, b), who described a semipreparative method of electroeluting proteins after conventional sodium dodecyl sulfate (SDS)-PAGE. By this method, it was possible to fractionate a pool of secreted protein antigens into distinct fractions devoid of SDS in a cell-compatible buffer in quantities that allowed dose-response assays (Fig. 2).

The ability to induce proliferation of immune T lymphocytes is clearly important, but monitoring the release of specific cytokines may give a more detailed picture. Already in 1986, it was observed that mycobacterial antigens directly stimulated human monocytes to release interleukin-1 (Wallis et al., 1986). The use of SDS-PAGE-separated proteins transferred to nitrocellulose made it possible to relate the

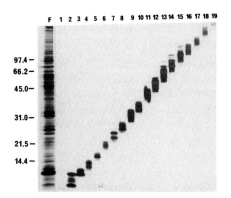

Figure 2. Example of SDS-PAGE of fractions of secreted proteins of *M. tuberculosis*. Lane F contains the starting material: secreted proteins from *M. tuberculosis* devoid of autolytic products. Lanes 1 to 19 contain different fractions obtained after preparative SDS-PAGE and subsequent electroelution (Andersen and Heron, 1993b). The figure was kindly provided by Peter Andersen, Copenhagen, Denmark.

release of both interleukin-1 and tumor necrosis factor (TNF) to two fractions representing molecular weights of 46,000 and 20,000 (Wallis et al., 1990). Recently, by use of two-dimensional gel electrophoresis, a 58-kDa protein inducing significant release of TNF-α from human macrophages was identified (Wallis et al., 1993). The N-terminal amino acid sequence of the protein revealed that this approach had identified a novel protein. TNF-α is a potent macrophage-activating cytokine, and these proteins may therefore be important in mycobacterial immunity and pathogenesis.

It is almost a dogma that protection against tuberculosis can be achieved only by vaccination with a live vaccine. G. Rook and colleagues observed that human T-cell lines reactive to sonicates of *M. tuberculosis* responded very poorly under similar conditions to live bacteria (Rook et al., 1986). It was proposed that an explanation might be sought in "important protective antigens released by live bacilli, which are not present in any significant quantity in dead ones. Conversely, internal mycobacterial antigens may be irrelevant to protection if not released by live bacilli." This hypothesis was supported by others on the basis of experiments, mainly in the murine system, that pointed in the direction of secreted or at least surface-exposed antigens being of major importance in the immune response to mycobacteria (Orme, 1988a, b; Andersen et al., 1991c, 1992b; Andersen and Heron, 1993a; Orme et al., 1992) (for a review, see Orme et al. [1993]). The proteins secreted to the culture medium were recovered and used as vaccines in protection experiments in mice (Hubbard et al., 1992) and guinea pigs (Pal and Horwitz, 1992), and in both cases significant reductions in the numbers of CFU recovered from spleen or lungs were observed. However, the potency of the experimental vaccine was not compared with that of the existing vaccine, BCG. Study of the composition of secreted proteins has been pursued by several groups and will be covered in more detail below.

Gamma interferon is another cytokine that is extremely potent in triggering macrophages to express enhanced antimicrobial activity (Kawamura et al., 1992). Two molecular mass regions of secreted proteins (from 4 to 11 and 26 to 35 kDa) purified by preparative SDS-PAGE exhibited a marked stimulatory capacity on T lymphocytes isolated from mice infected intravenously with live *M. tuberculosis*, and this profile was even more clearly observed when the supernatants of the cultures were assayed for their contents of gamma interferon (Andersen et al., 1992b). It was thereafter shown that the specificity of the T lymphocytes of memory immune mice (that is, mice that have been cured from infection with *M. tuberculosis* and have thereby acquired resistance to a secondary infection) was specifically directed towards these two molecular weight fractions, and it was also observed that T cells directed against the low-molecular-weight fractions were responsible for the recall of protective immunity (Andersen and Heron, 1993a).

Another example of alternative screening procedures was reported by the group of G. Marchal. They looked for diagnostic reagents that would be able to differentiate between infection with live, actively replicating mycobacteria and mere sensitization with killed or dormant mycobacteria. The culture filtrate proteins of young BCG cultures were fractionated by three chromatographic principles (size, charge, and hydrophobicity), and the screening of the fractions was based on comparative analyses of either the serological responses or the DTH responses of two groups of guinea pigs immunized with either live or killed BCG. By this method, two new antigens were identified, both with a very unusual amino acid composition. A 45/47-kDa protein was identified as a serological marker for replicating mycobacteria (Romain et al., 1993b), and another protein with a proline

content of 40% was identified as having the ability to differentiate infection from sensitization in DTH reactions (Romain et al., 1993a, b).

The choice of bacterial strain is another matter of controversy. In most cases, laboratory strains like *M. tuberculosis* H37Rv or Erdman are used, but expression of the antigens in virulent strains isolated from clinical specimens is important to confirm. Along with considerations concerning which strain to choose, it should be remembered that gene expression, as in other systems, varies according to culture conditions. A shift in temperature or the addition of a physiological stress stimulus like ethanol will increase the synthesis of a certain set of stress proteins (Young and Garbe, 1991a). The cultivation of *M. tuberculosis* in medium deficient of zinc or phosphate will induce the synthesis of yet another set of proteins (e.g., De Bruyn et al., 1989; Andersen et al., 1990; Espitia et al., 1992). *M. tuberculosis* has all the metabolic pathways needed for the de novo synthesis of all amino acids if needed. In other systems, the deprivation of any nutritional component will lead to compensatory synthesis of the enzymes required for the supply of the needed component, and there is no reason to believe that this is any different in mycobacteria. In other words, the protein profile of the mycobacterial sonicate or culture filtrate will expectedly vary in composition according to the conditions in the culture vessel. We do not know as yet the details of the metabolic conditions within an activated macrophage and what consequences these may have on the phenotypic appearance of *M. tuberculosis*.

Salmonella is another bacterial genus that is able to survive and replicate within macrophages. Increased synthesis of a distinct subset of at least 30 different *Salmonella* proteins was demonstrated when the bacteria were cultured in macrophages rather than in medium alone (Buchmeier and Heffron, 1990). Some of the induced proteins belonged to the stress protein family, but clearly, a large group of proteins contribute to bacterial survival in the macrophage. A similar study involving *M. tuberculosis* would be most relevant.

Finally, once an interesting antigen is identified, there is a wish to identify the biological function of the protein. The traditional way to do this is to search existing databases for sequence homology to other proteins and then demonstrate the function. However, this method inherently picks up only homologies to very conserved structures. Even so, we know the biological function of only a fraction of the antigens hitherto identified, and as will be discussed below, the function of a large group of mainly secreted proteins produced in substantial amounts by the organism is completely unknown. Information on the importance and function of single genes and their gene products has in other systems been greatly facilitated by gene inactivation by, e.g., site-directed mutagenesis. This approach has not been an easy task in mycobacteria, as is described in the section covering the genetics of *M. tuberculosis*.

STRUCTURE AND FUNCTION OF *M. TUBERCULOSIS* PROTEINS

In the following, a panel of *M. tuberculosis* proteins will be described according to their subcellular location. They may be cytoplasmic, cell membrane or cell wall associated, or secreted to the surrounding medium. This review is not intended to be exhaustive but rather is an introduction to some of the major groups of mycobacterial proteins. Recently, a compilation of mycobacterial protein antigens was published (Young et al., 1992), and two tables from that paper are reproduced in this chapter (Tables 1 and 2). Each antigen was assigned a code consisting of a number followed by a letter that indicates whether the gene is from *M. tuberculosis* (T), *M. bovis* (B), or

M. leprae (L). This code is appended in square brackets to the protein names in this chapter whenever applicable.

CYTOPLASMIC PROTEINS

Enzymes Involved in Amino Acid and Protein Biosynthesis

The mycobacteria constitute the members of the separate genus *Mycobacterium*, which belongs to the family *Mycobacteriaceae*. Despite their isolated position in the family tree, it appears that mycobacteria behave metabolically like most other bacteria. For a detailed review of this topic, consult chapter 22 of this book. A renewed interest in the metabolic pathways of mycobacteria has arisen in recent years. The idea of improving the existing BCG vaccine by genetic manipulation has prompted a demand for selectable cloning markers, which do not imply the biohazard problems of antibiotic resistance genes. Inactivation of genes involved in the synthesis of aromatic amino acids has in *Salmonella* spp. proved to be a successful way to obtain an attenuated vaccine strain (Hoiseth and Stocker, 1981), and an analogous approach might work in mycobacteria. The search for new drug targets is another reason to be interested in vital metabolic pathways, and finally, the enzymes of the cytosol may be as antigenic as any other proteins.

The *aroA* gene from *M. tuberculosis* encoding the 5-enolpyruvylshikimate-3-phosphate synthetase, which is involved in the synthesis of aromatic amino acids, was cloned by complementation of an *aroA E. coli* mutant with phages from a lambda gt11 *M. tuberculosis* DNA library (Garbe et al., 1990). The expression and antigenic cross-reactivity of the *M. tuberculosis aroA* gene product and the *aroA* product from *E. coli* were demonstrated by the Western blot (immunoblot) technique. By similar complementation studies, the *lysA* gene from *M. tuberculosis* was cloned (Andersen and

Hansen, 1993). The *lysA* gene encodes the diaminopimelic acid decarboxylase, which catalyzes the conversion of diaminopimelic acid to lysine. The expression of the gene product was verified in so-called maxicell experiments, but the enzyme is not believed to be of immunological importance. The deduced amino acid sequences of both the *aroA* and the *lysA* genes exhibited significant homology (from 27 to 53% identity) to similar sequences isolated from other bacterial species.

Recently, a 40-kDa protein antigen of *M. tuberculosis* [6T] was identified by sequence homology and functional analyses to be an L-alanine dehydrogenase. This enzyme catalyzes the reversible conversion of pyruvate to L-alanine in an NAD/NADH-dependent process. The protein was initially identified by MAb HBT10, which binds to *M. tuberculosis* strains and *M. marinum* but not to BCG (Ljungqvist et al., 1988; Worsaae et al., 1988; Andersen et al., 1992a). It was possible to demonstrate enzyme activity only in the HBT10-reactive strains, and only very low activity occurred in the attenuated strain *M. tuberculosis* H37Ra. In a study from 1970, growth responses to various sources of nitrogen were compared (it is well known that asparagine is a source for nitrogen that is usually added to synthetic media to enhance growth rate), and alanine was shown to be superior to glutamate and asparagine when H37Ra was cultured (Lyon et al., 1970). In *E. coli*, at least two but maybe four different pathways leading to L-alanine synthesis have been described (Reitzer and Magasanik, 1987). It is not known how many routes mycobacteria possess, but these data indicate that L-alanine dehydrogenases play a quantitatively larger role in *M. tuberculosis* than in, e.g., BCG. It might be that one aspect of attenuation of virulent mycobacteria relies on altered expression or deletion of probably several genes that are not vital but certainly make survival of the strain more difficult.

A strong homology between L-alanine dehydrogenases from *Bacillus* spp. and *M. tuberculosis* was recently extended to the pyridine nucleotide transhydrogenase of *E. coli* (Delforge et al., 1993). Pyridine nucleotide transhydrogenases are found in the plasma membranes of prokaryotes and the inner membranes of mitochondria and are involved in the regeneration of NADPH for amino acid synthesis, the concomitant oxidation of NADH to NAD^+, and the translocation of protons across the membrane. It was suggested that the MAb HBT10 cross-reacted with the *M. tuberculosis* pyridine nucleotide transhydrogenase and that virulence could be linked to the level of membrane-bound pyridine nucleotide transhydrogenase available for anabolic metabolism. In fact, HBT10 reactive protein was found to be secreted by *M. tuberculosis* despite the fact that no signal peptide was identified (Andersen et al., 1992a). It was hypothesized that extracellular L-alanine dehydrogenase might be involved in cell wall synthesis, because L-alanine is one of the four amino acids constituting the peptide moiety of the peptidoglycan layer.

A very important part of the protein synthesis machinery is the group of so-called elongation factors, EF-Tu. The *tuf* gene encoding EF-Tu of *M. tuberculosis* (Carlin et al., 1992) and that from *M. leprae* (Honoré et al., 1993) were recently cloned. In *E. coli*, the gene is present in two copies (Furano, 1978), but *M. tuberculosis* holds only one copy. The MAbs used to isolate the gene from *M. tuberculosis* were generated from LOU/C rats immunized with live BCG. In *E. coli*, EF-Tu is one of the most abundant proteins in the cell. EF-Tu is apparently also represented in PPD, because MAb 76-3, raised against PPD, recognized the *tuf* gene product (Klausen, unpublished data). EF-Tu may be a potential drug target, as the activity of EF-Tu in other systems has been shown to be sensi-

Table 1. Antigens with identified functions[a]

Code no.[b]	Name	Organism	Subunit size (kDa)[c]	Alternative name(s)[d]	MAbs[e]	Function[f]	Immunological characteristics
1T	DnaK	*M. tuberculosis*	71	CIE Ag63	51A, HAT1, HAT3	Heat shock protein; role in protein folding and translocation; >50% sequence identity with *E. coli* DnaK and human *hsp-70*	Antibody response in mouse and humans; proliferative T-cell response in patients and controls; potential target of autoreactivity?
1B	DnaK	BCG	70				
1L	DnaK	*M. leprae*	70				
2T	GroEL	*M. tuberculosis*	65	CIE Ag82	HAT5, CBA1, H2.16, TB78*	Heat shock protein; role in protein folding and translocation; >50% sequence identity with *E. coli* GroEL and human *hsp-60*; functions with GroES	Antibody response in mouse and humans; proliferative and cytotoxic T-cell responses in patients and controls; recognized by some γδ T cells; multiple peptide epitopes mapped; autoreactive responses in rodents and humans
2B	GroEL	BCG	65	64-kDa antigen, MbaA, CIE Ag82			
2L	GroEL	*M. leprae*	65		IIIE9,* IVD8,* IIH9, D5H, IIC8, Y1.2, ML30, CW1F2E8		

						Proposed function	Comments
3T	PhoS	*M. tuberculosis*	38	CIE Ag78, Pab, US Japan Ag5	TB71,* TB72,* HYT28,* HBT12,* C38.D1,* F67.19,* HAT2	Role as "binding protein" in phosphate transport potential; signal peptide and lipoprotein consensus; carbohydrate associated with purified protein	*M. tuberculosis* complex-specific antibody response in smear-positive patients; proliferative T-cell response in patients and after BCG vaccination
4T	SodA	*M. tuberculosis*	23	CIE Ag62		Superoxide dismutase; >50% sequence identity with *E. coli*	Recognized by MAbs
4L	SodA	*M. leprae*	28		F116.5, D2D	SodA and MnSod from human mitochondria	
5T	GroES	*M. tuberculosis*	12			Heat shock protein; role in protein folding and translocation; functions with GroEL; extensive sequence identity with *E. coli* GroES	Recognized by MAbs; induces strong proliferative T-cell response
5B	GroES	BCG	12	MPB57, BCG-a, MCP-I	SA12		
5L	GroES	*M. leprae*	14		CS-01		Response in tuberculoid leprosy and lepromin tests
6T		*M. tuberculosis*	40		HBT10*	L-Alanine dehydrogenase	Antibody HBT10 distinguishes BCG and *M. tuberculosis*

[a] Modified from Young et al., 1992.

[b] An antigen is assigned a code number if (i) its subunit molecular mass is known and (ii) either the complete gene has been cloned or the N-terminal sequence has been established. A letter added after the code number designates *M. tuberculosis* (T), *M. bovis* (B), or *M. leprae* (L).

[c] Estimates of subunit molecular mass are based on those observed during SDS-PAGE, which often differ from those derived by sequence analysis.

[d] CIE numbers refer to the system based on analysis of mycobacterial extracts by CIE.

[e] Only MAbs included in WHO workshops are listed. In addition to the workshops already published (Engers et al., 1985, 1986), this includes results of a third workshop completed in May 1991 (Khanolkar-Young et al., 1992). Asterisks denote antibodies reported to show species specificity.

[f] In most cases, the proposed function is based on sequence comparison rather than on direct experiments with the mycobacterial proteins.

Table 2. Antigens with known sequences but without identified function[a]

Code no.[b]	Organism	Subunit size (kDa)[c]	Alternative name(s)[d]	MAbs[e]	Structural features	Immunological characteristics
7I	M. intracellulare	43	MI43			Serologically active, recognized by T cells
8L	M. leprae	36	Proline rich	F47.9*	Proline-rich repeated motif in amino-terminal region	Specific antibody response in leprosy patients; proliferative and suppressive T-cell responses
9T	M. tuberculosis	35			Membrane associated	
10T(a)	M. tuberculosis	30/31	CIE Ag85 antigen, P32, MPT44	HYT27	Multigene family encoding three or more closely related major secreted proteins; signal peptide cleaved in mature proteins; fibronectin-binding proteins	Recognized by MAbs; cross-reactive antibody response in leprosy and tuberculosis patients; proliferative T-cell response in mouse and humans; recognized by T cells from synovial fluid of rheumatoid arthritis patients
10B(a)	BCG	30/31	CIE Ag85A, MPB44	HYT27		
10B(b)	BCG	30/31	CIE Ag85B, MPB59, α antigen, US Japan Ag6	HYT27		
10K(b)	M. kansasii	30/31	α Antigen, antigen a2	HYT27		
10L(b)	M. leprae	30/31				
11L	M. leprae	28			Possible iron-regulated protein; potential signal sequence	Antibody response in lepromatous leprosy patients

Code	Species	Mass (kDa)	Antigen	Additional designation	Properties	Immune response
12B	BCG	23	MPB64	L24.b4, C24.b1	Major secreted protein specific to *M. tuberculosis* complex	
13T	*M. tuberculosis*	19		TB23, HYT6, F29.47, 21-2H3	Potential signal peptide and lipoprotein consensus sequence; carbohydrate associated with purified protein	Antibody response in mouse and humans; proliferative T-cell response in patients and controls
13B	*M. bovis*	19				
14L	*M. leprae*	18	L5*		Member of low-molecular-weight heat shock protein family	Antibody response in mouse and humans; proliferative T-cell responses in patients and contacts
15B	BCG	18	MPB70		Major secreted protein of *M. bovis*	Specific antibody response in *M. bovis* infection
			MPB80		Signal peptide; variant forms found with masses of 22–25 kDa; carbohydrate associated with purified protein	
16L	*M. leprae*	15			Expressed as free protein; sequenced	Antibody and T-cell responses in leprosy patients and healthy contacts
17T	*M. tuberculosis*	14	MPT40			Antibody and proliferative T-cell responses in patients; species-specific antigen
18L	*M. leprae*	12	MLA12A			Recognized by MAbs
19T	*M. tuberculosis*	10			Sequenced from purified protein	DTH response in guinea pigs

[a] Modified from Young et al., 1992.

[b] An additional designation in parenthesis (a, b, c) has been included in order to refer to the original CIE reference system describing related antigens as 85A, 85B, and 85C. A letter added after the code number designates *M. tuberculosis* (T), *M. bovis* (B), *M. leprae* (L), *M. kansasii* (K), or *M. intracellulare* (I).

[c] Estimates of subunit molecular mass are based on those observed during SDS-PAGE, which often differ from those derived by sequence analysis.

[d] CIE numbers refer to the system based on analysis of mycobacterial extracts by CIE.

[e] Only MAbs included in WHO workshops are listed. In addition to the workshops already published (Engers et al., 1985, 1986), this includes results of a third workshop completed in May 1991 (Khanolkar-Young et al., 1992). Asterisks denote antibodies reported to show species specificity.

tive to tetracycline derivatives (Van de Klundert et al., 1978).

Stress Proteins

Among the first proteins to be identified by the use of MAbs was a group of proteins that later were shown to be significantly homologous to the widely conserved protein family of so-called heat shock proteins (hsp) or stress proteins (Young et al., 1988). This family of proteins has been found in eukaryotic cells, even in plants, and in prokaryotic bacteria (reviewed by Neidhardt and VanBogelen [1987] and Ang et al. [1991]). The stress proteins apparently serve multiple functions. An important role is to assist the microorganism in adaptation to environmental changes. Stress proteins are synthesized in considerable amounts in unstressed cells, but the transcription and translation levels increase markedly when the cell is exposed to elevated temperature or to other stress factors like oxygen radicals, metal ions, or ethanol. Members of the stress protein family act as "molecular chaperones" by mediating protein folding and assembly and maybe membrane translocation.

Three members of the stress protein family have been studied extensively in both prokaryotes and eukaryotes: hsp70/DnaK, hsp60/GroEL, and GroES. A 71-kDa protein of *M. tuberculosis* [1T] appeared homologous to DnaK of *E. coli* (Young et al., 1988) and hsp70 in eukaryotes (Garsia et al., 1989). The gene was isolated from *M. tuberculosis* by several researchers (Husson and Young, 1987; Shinnick et al., 1987a; Andersen et al., 1988a), and the nucleotide sequence was determined by Lathigra et al. (in press). The *dnaK* gene from *E. coli* is located just upstream of the *dnaJ* gene, and the two genes form an operon. Sequence analyses revealed a similar gene structure in *M. tuberculosis*, as an open reading frame identified downstream of the *dnaK* gene shared significant se-

quence homology with *dnaJ* from *E. coli* (Lathigra et al., 1988). By analogy with the function of DnaK from *E. coli*, DnaK from *M. bovis* has been demonstrated to possess ATPase and autophosphorylating activities that could be modulated by its binding to proteins and peptides (Peake et al., 1991).

A 65-kDa protein of *M. tuberculosis* [2T] appeared to be homologous to GroEL of *E. coli* (Young et al., 1988). The gene was isolated from *M. tuberculosis* in several laboratories (Young et al., 1985a; Shinnick et al., 1987a; Andersen et al., 1988a), and the nucleotide sequence was established from *M. tuberculosis* (Shinnick, 1987), BCG (Thole et al., 1987), and *M. leprae* (Mehra et al., 1986). The amino acid sequences of the GroEL analogs of *M. leprae*, BCG, and *M. tuberculosis* displayed more than 95% homology (Shinnick et al., 1987b). These proteins are at present the most extensively studied proteins of all mycobacterial proteins, and the literature on this topic has recently been reviewed by Thole and van der Zee (1990). In *E. coli*, the *groEL* gene is located in an operon with *groES*. *groES* and GroES form a complex that ensures proper folding and assembling of newly synthesized polypeptides in the cell. A *groES* homolog was also identified in *M. tuberculosis* [5T], but it was located separately from the 65-kDa gene (Baird et al., 1989). Subsequent studies have demonstrated a second version of a gene with very strong homology to the *groEL* gene (Kong et al., 1993; De Wit et al., 1992). This gene is located less than 100 bp downstream of the *groES* gene of *M. tuberculosis*. The in vivo consequences of two *groEL* genes are not yet clear. The chaperone proteins direct the precursor versions of the secreted proteins to the cell membrane. It has been suggested that antigens translocated across the cell membrane need another chaperone to assist them in traversing of the cell wall, and the GroES protein might be involved in this process. This would explain why the 10-kDa GroES homolog is in fact found at a very early stage in culture filtrates (Andersen et al., 1992b). The GroES protein of *M. tuberculosis* proved to be a major T-cell immunogen in human and murine studies (Barnes et al., 1992; Mehra et al., 1992; Orme et al., 1992).

The proteins encoded by the *hsp* genes have all been shown to interact with the immune systems of animals and humans (reviewed by Murray and Young [1992] and Polla [1988]). The 65-kDa protein has been mapped at the epitope level with respect to both B- and T-lymphocyte recognition (Mehra et al., 1986; Lamb et al., 1987; Anderson et al., 1988b; Kale et al., 1990; Munk et al., 1990). However, an association between autoimmune disorders and stress proteins has also been indicated (reviewed by Cohen and Young [1991] and Harboe and Quayle [1991]), and this association has reduced interest in these antigens from the vaccine point of view. The possible influence on antigen processing and presentation of these proteins as a consequence of the chaperone function involving direct interaction with antigens was recently reviewed by Young et al. (1993). Indeed, the study of this group of proteins in relation to pathogenesis and in improving our understanding of the physiology of mycobacteria has been and still is of great importance.

PROTEINS SECRETED ACROSS THE CELL BOUNDARY

Prokaryotic Transport across Cell Membranes

The bacterial cytoplasm is bounded by a bilaminar lipid membrane that is impermeable to solutes, nutrients, and macromolecules unless a specific transport system is available. In gram-negative bacteria, the cell wall consists of three layers: the cytoplasmic membrane, the peptidoglycan layer, and an outer lipopolysaccharide-containing cell membrane. A periplasmic space has been defined between the cytoplasmic membrane and the peptidoglycan layer. The outer membrane of a gram-negative bacterium is to some degree permeable to solutes through nonspecific pores. The peptidoglycan layer is considered freely permeable and is thought to function mainly as a skeleton for the organism. Gram-positive bacteria do not have outer membranes or periplasmic spaces. The composition of the cell walls of mycobacteria resembles that of gram-positive bacteria, although the Gram classification is not usually applied to this genus.

Proteins synthesized in the cytoplasm may be destined to function outside the cytoplasmic membrane, either in association with the cytoplasmic membrane or cell wall or exported all the way to the surrounding medium. The first critical event in this process is translocation across the cytoplasmic membrane. Several studies, mostly with gram-negative organisms, have shown that secreted proteins are synthesized in a precursor form that is processed to a mature version during translocation (reviewed by, e.g., Oliver [1985] and Pugsley et al. [1990]). The precursor versions of the proteins are usually synthesized with an N-terminal sequence of 20 to 40 amino acids, i.e., the signal peptide (or leader sequence), which is required for transport across membranes and is later cleaved off. The N-terminal two or three amino acids are positively charged and are followed by a stretch of nonpolar amino acids. The mature protein is demarcated by a conserved sequence that is recognized and cleaved by specific signal peptidases. However, signal peptide-independent extracellular secretion, for example, the α-hemolysin secretion pathway of *E. coli* and the adenylate/hemolysin secretion pathway of *Bordetella pertussis*, has also been described (Pugsley et al., 1990). The secretion of these proteins is dependent on the expression of secretion factors, which are encoded on distinct structural genes. The secretion signals of the α-hemolysin are

believed to be located in the carboxy-terminal part of the protein, but no common
denominator has been identified for this
secretion pathway. As described below,
both signal peptide-mediated and signal
peptide-independent secretion pathways
are represented in mycobacteria.

Proteins Secreted by *M. tuberculosis*

Human pathogenic bacteria interact with
their hosts in different ways. Each bacterial
species has evolved a unique way of either
attacking the host or evading host defense
mechanisms. Mycobacteria make use of
subtle but efficient means of surviving
within the host. No true exotoxins have
ever been described, and much of the tissue
damage that occurs in relation to a tuberculous infection is a result of the host
immune response attempting to combat the
infection. Mycobacteria secrete a number
of proteins to the surrounding medium
(Harboe and Nagai, 1984; Harboe et al.,
1986; Wiker et al., 1986a, b, 1991; Abou-
Zeid et al., 1988a, b; Andersen et al.,
1991b), and these proteins are extremely
potent in generating a cellular immune response in mice infected with live *M. tuberculosis* (Andersen et al., 1991c). It has been
observed in animal models that specific
protection against disease may be conferred only by the administration of live
BCG vaccine. One explanation for this may
be sought in the secreted proteins. After
administration of a live vaccine strain, the
protein synthesis machinery of the bacteria
is still working, and proteins are continuously being secreted into the surroundings.
T lymphocytes directed toward these proteins may be responsible for the initial
recognition of the infected macrophage
leading to efficient control of the infection
at a very early stage (Rook et al., 1986;
Orme, 1988a; Andersen et al., 1991c; Hubbard et al., 1992; Orme et al., 1992).

To determine whether a given protein is
actively secreted by an organism like *M.*

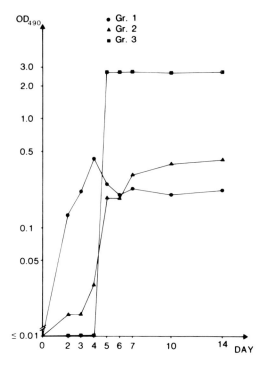

Figure 3. Kinetics of release of *M. tuberculosis* antigens into culture filtrates. Group 1 represents antigens
rapidly secreted or excreted into the medium. Group 2
contains antigens secreted or released gradually
throughout the culture period. Group 3 contains antigens present in SDS cell extracts that represent release
of cytoplasmic constituents rather than secreted proteins. OD_{490}, optical density at 490 nm.

tuberculosis is not trivial. The emergence
of ^{35}S-labeled proteins in the culture medium at very early times was studied by
SDS-PAGE (Abou-Zeid et al., 1988b). In
another study, a formula for a so-called
localization index was described (Wiker et
al., 1991). The method is based on the
quantitation of different antigens in the culture fluid relative to the amount found in the
bacterial sonicate. Others have monitored
the release of the GroEL/65-kDa protein
and the activity of isocitrate dehydrogenase
as markers for autolysis, and thus only
proteins appearing in the culture medium
before the emergence of these two markers
were considered true secreted proteins
(Fig. 3) (Andersen et al., 1991c). As judged

by the appearance after SDS-PAGE of a culture filtrate preparation consisting predominantly of secreted proteins, at least 33 individual protein bands may be identified (Andersen et al., 1991b). The functions of only a few of these proteins are known.

Proteins associated with the cell membrane or cell wall

A direct approach to the study of membrane-integrated proteins was made by the isolation of a 19-kDa protein from enriched membrane fractions of *M. tuberculosis* (Lee et al., 1992). The amino acid sequence was determined by direct sequencing of the purified protein or the peptides thereof. The sequence appeared to be unique, and immunoblotting results showed that the protein is immunogenic and is present in substantial quantities in virulent strains of *M. tuberculosis*.

Lipoproteins are generally associated with cell surfaces and are well known, especially in gram-negative bacteria (e.g., Pugsley et al., 1990) but also in gram-positive bacteria. It has been suggested that lipoproteins of gram-positive organisms might be functional equivalents of the periplasmic protein of gram-negative bacteria (Nielsen and Lampen, 1982). It is envisaged that the lipid moieties of these proteins are integrated into the cell surface and the protein part is exposed on the exterior, thereby allowing the proteins to carry out functions like binding of certain nutrients, etc. Young and Garbe (1991b) demonstrated [3H]palmitate incorporation in four *M. tuberculosis* proteins of molecular masses 19, 26, 27, and 38 kDa, indicating that these proteins are posttranslationally modified by acylation. The 26- and 27-kDa proteins have not been characterized in detail as yet, as opposed to the 19- and 38-kDa proteins. The amino acid sequence deduced from the nucleotide sequence of the gene encoding the 38-kDa protein [3T] exhibited 30% homology to the amino acid

sequence of the periplasmic protein PstS (=PhoS) from *E. coli*. PstS is part of the phosphate regulon of *E. coli* that is activated during phosphate starvation (reviewed by Torriani [1990]). Phosphate is an essential nutrient for all living organisms, and the phosphate uptake system utilized by *E. coli* has been studied extensively (reviewed by Torriani-Gorini et al. [1987]). Two different systems have been described: the constitutively expressed low-affinity system, designated the phosphate inorganic transport system, and the tightly regulated high-affinity phosphate-specific transport system. In *E. coli*, phosphate is transported through the outer membrane by a phosphate-specific porin and is captured in the periplasmic space by PstS. PstS releases the phosphate to the cytoplasm via a phosphate-specific channel spanning the cytoplasmic membrane. Recently, the synthesis of the 38-kDa protein of *M. tuberculosis* was shown to be enhanced during phosphate starvation, thus strengthening the evidence that the protein is involved in phosphate metabolism (Andersen et al., 1990; Espitia et al., 1992).

The deduced amino acid sequence of the *M. tuberculosis* PstS homolog does possess a consensus signal sequence, which allows the protein to be transported across the cytoplasmic membrane (Andersen and Hansen, 1989; Andersen et al., 1990). Given that the function of the 38-kDa protein in *M. tuberculosis* is to bind and make phosphate available to the bacterium, it needs to remain attached in some way to the cell wall. The data indicating that the protein is a lipoprotein and anchored in the cell wall by the lipid moiety (Young and Garbe, 1991b) fit nicely into the theory of Nielsen and Lampen (1982). An amino acid sequence similar to that of a lipoprotein consensus element was identified at the carboxy-terminal part of the signal sequence of the 38-kDa protein, and data obtained by immunodetection of the 38-kDa protein by electron microscopy confirmed the ultrastructural location of the protein on the surface of *M. tuberculosis* (Espitia et al., 1992). PstS from *E. coli* has been crystallized, and the X-ray structure of the liganded form of the protein has been described (Luecke and Quiocho, 1990). The structural analyses revealed that phosphate (monobasic or dibasic) is bound by 12 strong hydrogen bonds formed by seven amino acids. Six of these amino acids are conserved in the *M. tuberculosis* version of PstS. Very little is known about the mechanisms utilized by mycobacteria for assimilation of nutrients (although recently, a porin from *M. chelonae* was described [Trias et al., 1992]). The study of the phosphate uptake system may shed some light on one aspect of this question.

Another protein identified as a lipoprotein (Young and Garbe, 1991b) is the 19-kDa protein [13T]. It has been suggested that this protein is also involved in phosphate uptake. In fact, the synthesis of this protein is enhanced during phosphate starvation (Andersen, unpublished data). This protein appears to be structurally much more conserved within the mycobacterial species as judged by the cross-reactivity of the MAbs (Andersen et al., 1986; Engers et al., 1985).

Besides the functional aspects, lipoproteins from other species have in several cases proved to be highly immunogenic (e.g., Deres et al., 1989; Chamberlain et al., 1989). The immunological and immunochemical information on the 38-kDa protein [3T] is quite extensive, and the entire "history" of the protein has recently been thoroughly reviewed by Harboe and Wiker (1992). In 1981, the first publication describing results on the production of MAbs reactive to mycobacteria appeared (Coates et al., 1981). Two of these MAbs, TB71 and TB72, were reported to be able to discriminate between *M. tuberculosis*, BCG, and other mycobacterial species in radioimmunoassays. These MAbs therefore seemed to be very promising tools in mycobacterial taxonomy, and the target was later known to be the 38-kDa protein (Engers et al., 1986). However, the initial assumption that the 38-kDa protein was not present in BCG was contradicted by Andersen et al. (1986) and Wiker et al. (1990), who demonstrated that the protein is present in BCG, although in smaller quantities. Recently, a 38-kDa reactive MAb, HAT2, was shown to bind to *M. intracellulare* (Khanolkar-Young et al., 1992). In light of the important biological function of the protein, it may not be surprising that analogous proteins are also present in other mycobacteria. However, the *M. tuberculosis* version of the protein predominantly possesses species-specific B-cell epitopes, because hyperimmune sera from rabbits immunized with mycobacteria other than *M. tuberculosis* do not react with affinity-purified 38-kDa protein from *M. tuberculosis* (Kadival et al., 1987).

The 38-kDa protein stimulates T-lymphocytes from immunized mice, guinea pigs, and humans (Young et al., 1986; Worsaae et al., 1987; Kadival et al., 1987; Hasløv et al., 1990; Vordermeier et al., 1991, 1992a, b). Peptides derived from this molecule have in preliminary studies shown some potential as alternatives for PPD (Vordermeier et al., 1991, 1992b), although tuberculosis patients with active disease appeared to be selectively unresponsive to one particular epitope (designated 38.G) on the protein (Vordermeier et al., 1992a).

Serology has never gained a footing as a diagnostic alternative in tuberculosis. The inherent problems within this field will be covered in another chapter, but one of the few antigens that has showed some potential is in fact the 38-kDa protein (reviewed by Harboe and Wiker [1992]).

Proteins exported to the exterior

Superoxide dismutase (SOD) is an example of an enzyme that serves a very distinct function, namely, paralyzing a host defense mechanism by inactivating the toxic superoxide radicals generated by the activated macrophage (Fridovic, 1978). The gene was isolated from *M. tuberculosis* by means of a MAb, and the amino acid sequence was deduced from the nucleotide sequence [4T] (Zhang et al., 1991). SOD is an example of a protein exported to the surrounding medium by a mechanism that is not dependent on a consensus signal sequence. The mechanism by which the enzyme reaches the extracellular environment is as yet unknown. Interestingly, a mutation in the SOD gene was found to correlate with resistance to isoniazid (Zhang et al., 1991, 1992).

One of the prominent bands observed among the secreted proteins is a double band of molecular weights 30/31.000 (Abou-Zeid et al., 1988a; Andersen et al., 1991b; Nagai et al., 1991; Wiker et al., 1986a, b). This protein complex consists of at least three distinct proteins, with partial identities as shown by CIE. In CIE, the proteins precipitate in fusing lines and are designated the 85-complex (Closs et al., 1980; Wiker et al., 1988). The data available on this protein complex were thoroughly reviewed by Wiker and Harboe (1992). The three proteins [1O], also termed 85A or MP44 (31 kDa), 85B or MP59 (30 kDa), and 85C or MP45 (31.5 kDa), have been purified from BCG culture fluid (Wiker et al., 1986a, b; De Bruyn et al., 1987; Nagai et al., 1991). The complex is encoded by three homologous but distinct structural genes (Wiker et al., 1990; Content et al., 1991). The genes encoding the 85A component from *M. tuberculosis* and the 85B component from BCG have been isolated and sequenced (Borremans et al., 1989; Matsuo et al., 1988; De Wit, 1990). The gene encoding the 85C component has been isolated (Abou-Zeid et al., 1991) and sequenced (Content et al., 1991). Recently, antigenic cross-reactivity between the 85B component and a 27-kDa protein designated MPT51 was demonstrated, and by comparing the N-terminal amino acid sequences, 60% homology was observed (Nagai et al., 1991). This observation led those authors to suggest that there may exist a whole family of structurally closely related secreted proteins in mycobacteria.

All three members of the 85 complex are recognized by MAb HYT27 (Abou-Zeid et al., 1988a), and homologous proteins may be found in a wide range of mycobacterial species, as judged by the interspecies reactivity of this MAb (Andersen et al., 1986). Structural genes encoding homologous proteins displaying from 75 to 85% sequence identity have also been isolated from *M. leprae* (Thole et al., 1992) and *M. kansasii* (Matsuo et al., 1990).

It was shown by Ratliff et al. (1987) that mycobacteria bind to fibronectin-coated surfaces. This property was later ascribed to the 30/31-kDa protein complex (Abou-Zeid et al., 1988a). Although the 30/31-kDa proteins do possess true signal sequences that are cleaved off before release of the proteins to the exterior, a fraction of the proteins remains attached, at least temporarily, to the bacterial cell surface (Rambukkana et al., 1991). This fraction is believed to be of importance for the adhesion of the bacteria to and subsequent infection of eukaryotic cells. BCG has proved useful in the therapy of carcinoma in situ malignancies in the urinary bladder. The initial attachment of the bacteria to the epithelium of the bladder is assumed to be mediated by fibronectin (Ratliff et al., 1987).

The diagnostic potential of the protein complex has been assessed by several researchers. Some of the studies have been conducted with affinity-purified material consisting of all three components, and in other studies, there has been access to the individual components. The 85 complex elicited a medium-sized DTH response in guinea pigs (Hasløv et al., 1990). However, further studies using the purified components showed that there may be differences in the T-cell-stimulating capacities of the individual components, which is surprising considering the high level of homology between these proteins. Godfrey and colleagues showed that an 85A-enriched antigen preparation was able to markedly reduce the DTH response to PPD and also that T-cell-derived fibronectin is bound by these molecules (Godfrey et al., 1992). T-cell fibronectin is involved in the initiation of DTH reactions, and the specific adsorption of this lymphokine by the 85 complex is therefore thought to depress the cellular immune response.

The 85A component induced T-lymphocyte proliferation and gamma interferon release in the murine system when peripheral blood lymphocytes from human tuberculin-positive healthy controls and tuberculosis patients were assayed (Huygen et al., 1988a, b).

Another major component of the secreted products of *M. tuberculosis* is a protein with a molecular weight of 24,000. The protein was initially isolated from culture fluid preparations from *M. bovis* BCG Tokyo and was designated MPB64 [12B] (Harboe et al., 1986). MPB64 attracted attention because it was able to elicit a strong DTH reaction in guinea pigs immunized with mycobacteria belonging to the tuberculosis complex but not in animals immunized with other mycobacteria (Harboe et al., 1986; Andersen et al., 1991a). The species specificity in the DTH response pattern is somewhat surprising, because the protein was detected in a serologically cross-reactive form in *M. kansasii* (Andersen et al., 1991a). The gene has been cloned and sequenced from BCG Tokyo (Yamaguchi et al., 1989) and from *M. tuberculosis* (Oettinger and Andersen, unpublished data). Analyses of the protein profiles of a panel of different substrains of BCG revealed marked differences in the level of expression of MPB64 (Harboe et al., 1986). In fact, the MPB64-encoding gene appeared to be absent from four of the BCG substrains (Li et al., 1993). The function of MPB/T 64 is as yet unknown.

CONCLUDING REMARKS

The application of molecular biological methods to slow-growing, pathogenic mycobacteria was somewhat delayed compared to their use with other microorganisms. However, the technical progress made over the last decade is impressive. More genes and proteins are constantly added to the list of those investigated. The ultimate determination of the structure of the genomes of both *M. tuberculosis* and *M. leprae*, which will be completed in the years to come, will supply mycobacteriologists with enormous amounts of data. All the genes and gene products with structural homologies to genes and enzymes with known functions will be mapped. The remaining challenges will be to analyze this information and to identify and characterize the proteins that may be unique to mycobacteria and that may be responsible for pathogenicity. For this purpose, a reliable, site-specific gene inactivation system is most urgently needed, and collaboration between the disciplines of genetics, physiology, and immunology is important in an attempt to explain the abilities of mycobacteria to survive within macrophages, evade the immune system, and resist the effects of so many drugs.

Acknowledgments. We cordially thank Peter Andersen, Morten Harboe, and Kaare Hasløv for helpful discussions. Thomas Oettinger is thanked for sharing unpublished results.

REFERENCES

Abou-Zeid, C., E. Filley, J. Steele, and G. A. W. Rook. 1987. A simple new method for using antigens separated by polyacrylamide gel electrophoresis to stimulate lymphocytes in vitro after converting bands cut from Western blots into antigen-bearing particles. *J. Immunol. Methods* **98:**5–10.

Abou-Zeid, C., T. Garbe, R. Lathigra, H. Wiker, M. Harboe, G. A. W. Rook, and D. B. Young. 1991. Genetic and immunological analysis of *Mycobacterium tuberculosis* fibronectin-binding proteins. *Infect. Immun.* **59:**2712–2718.

Abou-Zeid, C., T. L. Ratliff, H. G. Wiker, M. Harboe,

J. Bennedsen, and G. A. W. Rook. 1988a. Characterization of fibronectin-binding antigens released by *Mycobacterium tuberculosis* and *Mycobacterium bovis* BCG. *Infect. Immun.* **56:**3046–3051.

Abou-Zeid, C., I. Smith, J. M. Grange, T. L. Ratliff, J. Steele, and G. A. W. Rook. 1988b. The secreted antigens of *Mycobacterium tuberculosis* and their relationship to those recognized by the available antibodies. *J. Gen. Microbiol.* **134:**531–538.

Andersen, Å. B. Unpublished data.

Andersen, Å. B., P. Andersen, and L. Ljungqvist. 1992a. Structure and function of a 40,000-molecular-weight protein antigen of *Mycobacterium tuberculosis. Infect. Immun.* **60:**2317–2323.

Andersen, Å. B., and E. B. Hansen. 1989. Structure and mapping of antigenic domains of protein antigen b, a 38,000-molecular-weight protein of *Mycobacterium tuberculosis. Infect. Immun.* **57:**2481–2488.

Andersen, Å. B., and E. B. Hansen. 1993. Cloning of the *lysA* gene from *Mycobacterium tuberculosis. Gene* **124:**105–109.

Andersen, Å. B., L. Ljungqvist, K. Hasløv, and M. W. Bentzon. 1991a. MPB64 possesses 'tuberculosis-complex'-specific B- and T-cell epitopes. *Scand. J. Immunol.* **34:**365–372.

Andersen, Å. B., L. Ljungqvist, and M. Olsen. 1990. Evidence that protein antigen b of *Mycobacterium tuberculosis* is involved in phosphate metabolism. *J. Gen. Microbiol.* **136:**477–480.

Andersen, Å. B., A. Worsaae, and S. D. Chaparas. 1988a. Isolation and characterization of recombinant lambda gt11 bacteriophages expressing eight different mycobacterial antigens of potential immunological relevance. *Infect. Immun.* **56:**1344–1351.

Andersen, Å. B., Z. L. Yuan, K. Hasløv, B. Vergmann, and J. Bennedsen. 1986. Interspecies reactivity of five monoclonal antibodies to *Mycobacterium tuberculosis* as examined by immunoblotting and enzyme-linked immunosorbent assay. *J. Clin. Microbiol.* **23:**446–451.

Andersen, P., D. Askgaard, A. Gottshau, J. Bennedsen, S. Nagai, and I. Heron. 1992b. Identification of immunodominant antigens during infection with *Mycobacterium tuberculosis. Scand. J. Immunol.* **36:**823–831.

Andersen, P., D. Askgaard, L. Ljungqvist, J. Bennedsen, and I. Heron. 1991b. Proteins released from *Mycobacterium tuberculosis* during growth. *Infect. Immun.* **59:**1905–1910.

Andersen, P., D. Askgaard, L. Ljungqvist, M. W. Bentzon, and I. Heron. 1991c. T-cell proliferative response to antigens secreted by *Mycobacterium tuberculosis. Infect. Immun.* **59:**1558–1563.

Andersen, P., and I. Heron. 1993a. Specificity of a protective memory immune response against *Mycobacterium tuberculosis. Infect. Immun.* **61:**844–851.

Andersen, P., and I. Heron. 1993b. Simultaneous elec-troelution of whole SDS-polyacrylamide gels for the direct cellular analysis of complex protein mixtures. *J. Immunol. Methods* **161:**29–39.

Anderson, D. C., M. E. Barry, and T. M. Buchanan. 1988b. Exact definition of species-specific and cross-reactive epitopes of the 65-kilodalton protein of *Mycobacterium leprae* using synthetic peptides. *J. Immunol.* **141:**607–613.

Ang, D., K. Liberek, D. Skowyra, M. Zylicz, and C. Georgeopolous. 1991. Biological role and regulation of the universally conserved heat shock proteins. *J. Biol. Chem.* **266:**24233–24236.

Bachmann, B. J. 1990. Linkage map of *Escherichia coli* K-12, edition 8. *Microbiol. Rev.* **54:**130–197.

Baess, I., and B. Mansa. 1978. Determination of genome size and base ratio on deoxyribonucleic acid from mycobacteria. *Acta Pathol. Microbiol. Scand. Sect. B* **86:**309–312.

Baird, P. N., L. M. C. Hall, and A. R. M. Coates. 1989. Cloning and sequence analysis of the 10 kDa antigen gene of *Mycobacterium tuberculosis. J. Gen. Microbiol.* **135:**931–939.

Barnes, P. F., V. Mehra, G. R. Hirchfield, S. J. Fong, C. Abou-Zeid, G. Rook, G. A. W. Hunter, P. J. Brennan, and R. Modlin. 1989. Characterization of T cell antigens associated with the cell wall protein-peptidoglycan complex of *Mycobacterium tuberculosis. J. Immunol.* **143:**2656.

Barnes, P. F., V. Mehra, B. Rivoire, S.-J. Fong, P. J. Brennan, M. S. Voegtline, P. Minden, R. A. Houghten, B. R. Bloom, and R. L. Modlin. 1992. Immunoreactivity of a 10-kDa antigen of *Mycobacterium tuberculosis. J. Immunol.* **148:**1835–1840.

Borremans, M., L. De Wit, G. Volkaert, J. Ooms, J. De Bruyn, K. Huygen, J. P. Van Vooren, M. Stelandre, R. Verhofstadt, and J. Content. 1989. Cloning, sequence determination, and expression of a 32 kilodalton-protein gene of *Mycobacterium tuberculosis. Infect. Immun.* **57:**3123–3130.

Buchmeier, N. A., and F. Heffron. 1990. Induction of *Salmonella* stress proteins upon infection of macrophages. *Science* **248:**730–732.

Bulletin of the World Health Organization. 1983. Memorandum from a WHO meeting: plan of action for research in the immunology of tuberculosis. *Bull. W.H.O.* **61:**779–785.

Carlin, N. I. A., S. Löfdahl, and M. Magnusson. 1992. Monoclonal antibodies specific for elongation factor Tu and complete nucleotide sequence of the *tuf* gene in *Mycobacterium tuberculosis. Infect. Immun.* **60:**3136–3142.

Chamberlain, N. R., M. E. Brandt, A. L. Erwin, J. D. Radolf, and M. V. Norgard. 1989. Major integral membrane protein immunogens of *Treponema pallidum* are proteolipids. *Infect. Immun.* **57:**2872–2877.

Closs, O., M. Harboe, N. H. Axelsen, K. Bunch-

Christensen, and M. Magnusson. 1980. The antigens of *Mycobacterium bovis*, strain BCG, studied by crossed immunoelectrophoresis: a reference system. *Scand. J. Immunol.* **12**:249–263.

Coates, A. R. M., J. Hewitt, B. W. Allen, J. Ivanyi, and D. A. Mitchison. 1981. Antigenic diversity of *Mycobacterium tuberculosis* and *Mycobacterium bovis* detected by means of monoclonal antibodies. *Lancet* ii:167–169.

Cohen, I. R., and D. B. Young. 1991. Autoimmunity, microbial immunity and the immunological homonculus. *Immunol. Today* **12**:105–110.

Cole, S. Personal communication.

Content, J., A. de la Cuvellerie, L. de Wit, V. Vincent-Levy-Frébault, J. Ooms, and J. de Bruyn. 1991. The genes coding for the antigen 85 complexes of *Mycobacterium tuberculosis* and *Mycobacterium bovis* BCG are members of a gene family: cloning, sequence determination, and genomic organization of the gene coding for antigen 85-C of *M. tuberculosis*. *Infect. Immun.* **59**:3205–3212.

Daniel, T. M., and B. W. Janicki. 1978. Mycobacterial antigens: a review of their isolation, chemistry, and immunological properties. *Microbiol. Rev.* **42**:84–113.

Daugelat, S., H. Gulle, B. Schoel, and S. H. E. Kaufman. 1992. Secreted antigens of *Mycobacterium tuberculosis*: characterization with T lymphocytes from patients and contacts after two-dimensional separation. *J. Infect. Dis.* **166**:186–190.

De Bruyn, J., R. Bosmans, J. Nyabenda, and J. P. Van Vooren. 1989. Effect of zinc deficiency on the appearance of two immunodominant protein antigens (32kDa and 65kDa) in culture filtrates of mycobacteria. *J. Gen. Microbiol.* **135**:79–84.

De Bruyn, J., J. Huygen, R. Bosmans, M. Fauville, R. Lippens, J. P. Van Vooren, P. Falmagne, M. Weckx, H. G. Wiker, M. Harboe, and M. Turneer. 1987. Purification, characterization and identification of a 32 kDa protein antigen of *Mycobacterium bovis* BCG. *Microb. Pathog.* **2**:351–366.

Delforge, D., E. Depiereux, X. de Bolle, E. Feytmans, and J. Remacle. 1993. Similarities between alanine dehydrogenase and the N-terminal part of pyridine nucleotide transhydrogenase and their possible implication in the virulence mechanism of *Mycobacterium tuberculosis*. *Biochem. Biophys. Res. Commun.* **190**:1073–1079.

Deres, K., H. Schild, K. H. Wiesmuller, G. Jung, and H. G. Ramensee. 1989. *In vivo* priming of virus-specific cytotoxic T lymphocytes with synthetic lipopeptide vaccine. *Nature* (London) **342**:561–564.

De Wit, L., A. de la Cuvellerie, J. Ooms, and J. Content. 1990. Nucleotide sequence of the 32 kDa-protein gene (antigen 85A) of *Mycobacterium bovis* BCG. *Nucleic Acids Res.* **18**:3995.

De Wit, T. F. R., S. Bekelie, A. Osland, T. L. Miko,

P. W. M. Hermans, D. van Soolingen, J.-W. Drijfhout, R. Schöningh, A. A. M. Janson, and J. E. R. Thole. 1992. Mycobacteria contain two *groEL* genes: the second *Mycobacterium leprae groEL* gene is arranged in an operon with *groES*. *Mol. Microbiol.* **6**:1995–2007.

Engers, H. D., and Workshop Participants. 1985. Results of a World Health Organization-sponsored workshop on monoclonal antibodies to *Mycobacterium leprae*. *Infect. Immun.* **48**:603–605. (Letter to the editor.)

Engers, H. D., and Workshop Participants. 1986. Results of a World Health Organization-sponsored workshop to characterize antigens recognized by mycobacterium-specific monoclonal antibodies. *Infect. Immun.* **51**:718–720. (Letter to the editor.)

Espitia, C., M. Elinos, R. Hernández-Pando, and R. Mancilla. 1992. Phosphate starvation enhances expression of the immunodominant 38-kilodalton protein antigen of *Mycobacterium tuberculosis*: demonstration by immunogold electron microscopy. *Infect. Immun.* **60**:2998–3001.

Fridovic, I. 1978. The biology of oxygen radicals. *Science* **201**:875–880.

Furano, A. V. 1978. Direct demonstration of duplicate *tuf* genes in enteric bacteria. *Proc. Natl. Acad. Sci. USA* **75**:3104–3108.

Garbe, T., D. Harris, M. Vordermeier, R. Lathigra, J. Ivanyi, and D. Young. 1993. Expression of the *Mycobacterium tuberculosis* 19-kilodalton antigen in *Mycobacterium smegmatis*: immunological analysis and evidence of glycosylation. *Infect. Immun.* **61**:260–267.

Garbe, T., C. Jones, I. Charles, G. Dougan, and D. Young. 1990. Cloning and characterization of the *aroA* gene from *Mycobacterium tuberculosis*. *J. Bacteriol.* **172**:6774–6782.

Garsia, R. J., L. Hellqvist, R. J. Booth, A. J. Radford, W. J. Britton, L. Astbury, R. J. Trent, and A. Basten. 1989. Homology of the 70-kilodalton antigens from *Mycobacterium leprae* and *Mycobacterium bovis* with the *Mycobacterium tuberculosis* 71-kilodalton antigen and with the conserved heat shock protein 70 of eucaryotes. *Infect. Immun.* **57**:204–212.

Godfrey, H. P., Z. Feng, S. Mandy, K. Mandy, K. Huygen, J. De Bruyn, C. Abou-Zeid, H. G. Wiker, S. Nagai, and H. Tasaka. 1992. Modulation of expression of delayed hypersensitivity by mycobacterial antigen 85 fibronectin-binding proteins. *Infect. Immun.* **60**:2522–2528.

Guld, J., W. W. Bentzon, M. A. Bleiker, W. A. Griep, M. Magnusson, and H. Waaler. 1958. Standardization of a new batch of purified tuberculin (PPD) intended for international use. *Bull. Org. Mond. Sante* **19**:845–951.

Gulle, H., B. Schoel, and S. H. Kaufmann. 1990. Direct

blotting with viable cells of protein mixtures separated by two-dimensional gel electrophoresis. *J. Immunol. Methods* **133**:253–261.

Harboe, M., and S. Nagai. 1984. MPB70, a unique antigen of *Mycobacterium bovis* BCG[1–3]. *Am. Rev. Respir. Dis.* **129**:444–452.

Harboe, M., S. Nagai, M. E. Patarroyo, M. L. Torres, C. Ramirez, and N. Cruz. 1986. Properties of proteins MPB64, MPB70, and MPB80 of *Mycobacterium bovis* BCG. *Infect. Immun.* **52**:293–302.

Harboe, M., and A. J. Quayle. 1991. Heat shock proteins: friend and foe? *Clin. Exp. Immunol.* **86**: 2–5.

Harboe, M., and H. G. Wiker. 1992. The 38-kDa protein of *Mycobacterium tuberculosis*: a review. *J. Infect. Dis.* **166**:874–884.

Hasløv, K., Å. B. Andersen, L. Ljungqvist, and M. W. Bentzon. 1990. Comparison of the immunological activity of five defined antigens from *Mycobacterium tuberculosis* in seven inbred guinea pig strains. The 38-kDa antigen is immunodominant. *Scand. J. Immunol.* **31**:503–514.

Hoiseth, S. K., and B. A. D. Stocker. 1981. Aromatic-dependent *Salmonella typhimurium* are nonvirulent and effective as live vaccines. *Nature* (London) **291**:238–239.

Honoré, N., S. Bergh, S. Chanteau, F. Doucet-Populaire, K. Eiglmeier, T. Garnier, C. Georges, P. Launois, T. Limpaiboon, S. Newton, K. Niang, P. del Portillo, G. R. Ramesh, P. Reddi, P. R. Ridel, N. Sittisombut, S. Wu-Hunter, and S. T. Cole. 1993. Nucleotide sequence of the first cosmid from the *Mycobacterium leprae* genome project: structure and function of the Rif-Str regions. *Mol. Microbiol.* **7**:207–214.

Hubbard, R. D., C. M. Flory, and F. M. Collins. 1992. Immunization of mice with mycobacterial culture filtrate proteins. *Clin. Exp. Immunol.* **87**:94–98.

Husson, R. N., and R. A. Young. 1987. Genes for the major protein antigens of *Mycobacterium tuberculosis*: the etiologic agent of tuberculosis and leprosy share an immunodominant antigen. *Proc. Natl. Acad. Sci. USA* **84**:1679–1683.

Huygen, K., K. Palfliet, F. Jurion, J. Hilgers, R. ten Berg, J.-P. van Vooren, and J. de Bruyn. 1988a. *H-2*-linked control of in vitro gamma interferon production in response to a 32-kilodalton antigen (P32) of *Mycobacterium bovis* bacillus Calmette-Guérin. *Infect. Immun.* **56**:3196–3200.

Huygen, K., J.-P. van Vooren, M. Turneer, R. Bosmans, P. Dierckx, and J. de Bruyn. 1988b. Specific lymphoproliferation, gamma interferon production, and serum immunoglobulin G directed against a purified 32 kDa mycobacterial protein antigen (P32) in patients with active tuberculosis. *Scand. J. Immunol.* **27**:187–194.

Kadival, G. V., S. D. Chaparas, and D. Hussong. 1987.

Characterization of serologic and cell-mediated reactivity of a 38-kDa antigen isolated from *Mycobacterium tuberculosis*. *J. Immunol.* **139**:2447–2451.

Kale, Ab, B., R. Kiessling, J. D. A. van Embden, J. E. R. Thole, D. S. Kumararatne, P. Pisa, A. Wondimu, and T. H. M. Ottenhoff. 1990. Induction of antigen-specific CD4[+] HLA-DR-restricted cytotoxic T lymphocytes as well as nonspecific nonrestricted killer cells by the recombinant mycobacterial 65-kDa heat-shock protein. *Eur. J. Immunol.* **20**:369–377.

Kawamura, I., H. Tsukada, H. Yoshikawa, M. Fujita, K. Nomoto, and M. Mitsuyama. 1992. IFN-γ-producing ability as a possible marker for the protective T cells against *Mycobacterium bovis* BCG in mice. *J. Immunol.* **148**:2887–2893.

Khanolkar-Young, S., A. H. J. Kolk, Å. B. Andersen, J. Bennedsen, P. J. Brennan, S. Rivoire, S. Kuijper, K. P. W. J. McAdam, C. Abe, H. V. Batra, S. D. Chaparas, G. Damiani, M. Singh, and H. D. Engers. 1992. Results of the Third Immunology of Leprosy/ Immunology of Tuberculosis Antimycobacterial Monoclonal Antibody Workshop. *Infect. Immun.* **60**:3925–3927.

Klausen, J. Unpublished data.

Koch, R. 1882. Die Ätiologie der Tuberkulose. *Berliner Klin. Wochenschr.* **15**:221–230.

Koch, R. 1891. Weitere Mitteilung über das Tuberkulin. *Dtsch. Med. Wochenschr.* **43**:1189–1192.

Koch, R. 1897. Über neue Tuberkulinpräparate. *Dtsch. Med. Wochenschr.* **14**:209–213.

Kong, T. H., A. R. M. Coates, P. D. Butcher, C. J. Hickman, and T. M. Shinnick. 1993. *Mycobacterium tuberculosis* expresses two chaperonin-60 homologs. *Proc. Natl. Acad. Sci. USA* **90**:2608–2612.

Lamb, J. R., J. Ivanyi, A. D. M. Rees, J. B. Rothbard, K. Howland, R. A. Young, and D. B. Young. 1987. Mapping of T cell epitopes using recombinant antigens and synthetic peptides. *EMBO J.* **6**:1245–1249.

Landi, S. 1984. Production and standardization of tuberculin, p. 505–535. *In* G. P. Kubica and L. G. Wayne (ed.), *The Mycobacteria—a Sourcebook*, part A. Marcel Dekker, Inc., New York.

Lathigra, R., W. Alexander, K. Stover, J. Coadwell, R. Young, and D. Young. *J. Biol. Chem.*, in press.

Lathigra, R. B., D. B. Young, D. Sweetser, and R. A. Young. 1988. A gene from *Mycobacterium tuberculosis* which is homologous to the DnaJ heat shock protein of *E. coli*. *Nucleic Acids Res.* **16**:1636.

Lee, B.-Y., S. A. Hefta, and P. J. Brennan. 1992. Characterization of the major membrane protein of virulent *Mycobacterium tuberculosis*. *Infect. Immun.* **60**:2066–2074.

Li, H., J. C. Ulstrup, T. Ø. Jonassen, K. Melby, S. Nagai, and M. Harboe. 1993. Evidence for absence of the MPB64 gene in some substrains of *Mycobacterium bovis* BCG. *Infect. Immun.* **61**:1730–1734.

Ljungqvist, L., A. Worsaae, and I. Heron. 1988. Antibody responses against *Mycobacterium tuberculosis* in 11 strains of inbred mice: novel monoclonal antibody specificities generated by fusions, using spleens from BALB.B10 and CBA/J mice. *Infect. Immun.* **56**:1994–1998.

Luecke, H., and F. A. Quiocho. 1990. High specificity of a phosphate transport protein determined by hydrogen bonds. *Nature* (London) **347**:402–406.

Lyon, R. H., H. H. Wendell, and C. Costas-Martinez. 1970. Utilization of amino acids during growth of *Mycobacterium tuberculosis* in rotary cultures. *Infect. Immun.* **1**:513–520.

Magnusson, M. 1967. Das Tuberkulin. Herstellung, Reinigung, Standardiserung und chemischer Aufbau, p. 191–237. *In* G. Meissner and A. Schmiedel (ed.), *Mykobakterien und Mykobakterielle Krankheiten*, teil II. VEB Gustav Fischer Verlag Jena, Munich.

Magnusson, M., and M. W. Bentzon. 1958. Preparation of purified tuberculin RT 23. *Bull. Org. Mond. Sante* **19**:829–843.

Matsuo, K., R. Yamaguchi, A. Yamazaki, H. Tasaka, K. Teresaka, and T. Yamada. 1990. Cloning and expression of the gene for the cross-reactive α antigen of *Mycobacterium kansasii. Infect. Immun.* **58**:550–556.

Matsuo, K., R. Yamaguchi, A. Yamazaki, H. Tasaka, and T. Yamada. 1988. Cloning and expression of the *Mycobacterium bovis* BCG gene for extracellular α antigen. *J. Bacteriol.* **170**:3847–3854.

Mehra, V., B. R. Bloom, A. C. Bajardi, C. L. Grisso, P. A. Sieling, D. Alland, J. Convit, X. Fan, S. W. Hunter, P. J. Brennan, T. H. Rea, and R. L. Modlin. 1992. A major T cell antigen of *Mycobacterium leprae* is a 10-kD heat-shock cognate protein. *J. Exp. Med.* **175**:275–284.

Mehra, V., D. Sweetser, and R. A. Young. 1986. Efficient mapping of protein antigenic determinants. *Proc. Natl. Acad. Sci. USA* **83**:7013–7017.

Munk, M. E., T. M. Shinnick, and S. H. E. Kaufmann. 1990. Epitopes of the mycobacterial heat shock protein 65 for human T cells comprise different structures. *Immunobiology* **180**:272–277.

Murray, P. J., and R. A. Young. 1992. Stress and immunological recognition in host-pathogen interactions. *J. Bacteriol.* **174**:4193–4196.

Mustafa, A. S., F. Oftung, A. Deggerdal, H. K. Gill, R. A. Young, and T. Godal. 1988. Gene isolation with human T lymphocyte probes. Isolation of a gene that expresses an epitope recognized by T cells specific for *Mycobacterium bovis* BCG and pathogenic mycobacteria. *J. Immunol.* **141**:2729–2733.

Nagai, S., H. G. Wiker, M. Harboe, and M. Kinomoto. 1991. Isolation and partial characterization of major protein antigens in the culture fluid of *Mycobacterium tuberculosis. Infect. Immun.* **59**:372–382.

Neidhardt, F. C., and R. A. VanBogelen. 1987. Heat shock response, p. 1334–1345. *In* F. C. Neidhardt, J. L. Ingraham, K. B. Low, B. Magasanik, M. Schaechter, and H. E. Umbarger (ed.), *Escherichia coli and Salmonella typhimurium: Cellular and Molecular Biology*, vol. 2. American Society for Microbiology, Washington, D.C.

Nielsen, J. B. K., and J. O. Lampen. 1982. Glyceride-cysteine lipoproteins and secretion by gram-positive bacteria. *J. Bacteriol.* **152**:315–322.

Oettinger, T., and Å. B. Andersen. Unpublished data.

Oliver, D. 1985. Protein secretion in *Escherichia coli. Annu. Rev. Microbiol.* **39**:615–648.

Orme, I. M. 1988a. Characteristics and specificity of acquired immunologic memory to *Mycobacterium tuberculosis* infection. *J. Immunol.* **140**:3589–3593.

Orme, I. M. 1988b. Induction of nonspecific acquired resistance and delayed-type hypersensitivity, but not specific acquired resistance, in mice inoculated with killed mycobacterial vaccines. *Infect. Immun.* **56**:3310–3312.

Orme, I. M., P. Andersen, and W. H. Boom. 1993. The T cell response to *Mycobacterium tuberculosis. J. Infect. Dis.* **167**:1481–1497.

Orme, I. M., E. S. Miller, A. D. Roberts, S. K. Furney, J. P. Griffin, K. M. Dobos, D. Chi, B. Rivoire, and P. J. Brennan. 1992. T lymphocytes mediating protection and cellular cytolysis during the course of *Mycobacterium tuberculosis* infection. *J. Immunol.* **148**:189–196.

Pal, P. G., and M. A. Horwitz. 1992. Immunization with extracellular proteins of *Mycobacterium tuberculosis* induces cell-mediated immune responses and substantial protective immunity in a guinea pig model of pulmonary tuberculosis. *Infect. Immun.* **60**:4781–4792.

Peake, P., A. Basten, and W. J. Britton. 1991. Characterization and functional properties of the 70-kDa protein of *Mycobacterium bovis. J. Biol. Chem.* **266**:20828–20832.

Polla, B. S. 1988. A role for heat shock proteins in inflammation? *Immunol. Today* **9**:134–137.

Pugsley, A. P., D. d'Enfert, I. Reyss, and M. G. Kornacker. 1990. Genetics of extracellular protein secretion by gram-negative bacteria. *Annu. Rev. Genet.* **24**:67–90.

Rambukkana, A., P. K. Das, A. Chand, J. G. Baas, D. G. Groothuis, and A. H. J. Kolk. 1991. Subcellular distribution of monoclonal antibody defined epitopes on immunodominant *Mycobacterium tuberculosis* proteins in the 30-kDa region: identification and localization of 29/33-kDa doublet proteins on mycobacterial cell wall. *Scand. J. Immunol.* **33**:763–775.

Ratliff, T. L., J. O. Palmer, J. McGarr, and E. J. Brown. 1987. Intravesical bacillus Calmette-Guérin therapy for murine bladder tumors: initiation of the response by fibronectin-mediated attachment of bacillus Calmette-Guérin. *Cancer Res.* **47**:1762–1766.

Reitzer, L. J., and B. Magasanik. 1987. Ammonia assimilation and the biosynthesis of glutamine, glutamate, aspartate, asparagine, L-alanine, and D-alanine, p. 302–320. *In* F. C. Neidhardt, J. L. Ingraham, K. B. Low, B. Magasanik, M. Schaechter, and H. E. Umbarger (ed.), *Escherichia coli and Salmonella typhimurium: Cellular and Molecular Biology*, vol. 1. American Society for Microbiology, Washington, D.C.

Ridell, M., R. Öhman, and G. Wallerström. 1987. Characterization of mycobacterial immunoprecipitates by selective staining of enzymes. *J. Gen. Microbiol.* **133**:1983–1986.

Romain, F., J. Augier, P. Pescher, and G. Marchal. 1993a. Isolation of a proline-rich mycobacterial protein eliciting delayed-type hypersensitivity reactions only in guinea pigs immunized with living mycobacteria. *Proc. Natl. Acad. Sci. USA* **90**:5322–5326.

Romain, F., A. Laqueyrerie, P. Militzer, P. Pescher, P. Chavarot, M. Lagranderie, G. Auregan, M. Gheorghiu, and G. Marchal. 1993b. Identification of a *Mycobacterium bovis* BCG 45/47-kilodalton antigen complex, an immunodominant target for antibody response after immunization with living bacteria. *Infect. Immun.* **61**:742–750.

Rook, G. A. W., J. Steele, S. Barnass, J. Mace, and J. L. Stanford. 1986. Responsiveness to live *M. tuberculosis*, and common antigens, of sonicate-stimulated T cell lines from normal donors. *Clin. Exp. Immunol.* **63**:105–110.

Seibert, F. B., and J. T. Glenn. 1941. Tuberculin purified protein derivative. Preparation and analyses of a large quantity for standard. *Am. Rev. Tuberc.* **44**:9–25.

Seibert, F. B., and B. Munday. 1932. The chemical compositions of the active principles of tuberculin. XV. A precipitated purified tuberculin protein suitable for the preparation of a standard tuberculin. *Am. Rev. Tuberc.* **25**:724–737.

Shinnick, T. M. 1987. The 65-kilodalton antigen of *Mycobacterium tuberculosis*. *J. Bacteriol.* **169**:1080–1088.

Shinnick, T. M., C. Krat, and S. Schadow. 1987a. Isolation and restriction site maps of the genes encoding five *Mycobacterium tuberculosis* proteins. *Infect. Immun.* **55**:1718–1721.

Shinnick, T. M., D. Sweetser, J. Thole, J. van Embden, and R. A. Young. 1987b. The etiologic agents of leprosy and tuberculosis share an immunoreactive protein antigen with the vaccine strain *Mycobacterium bovis* BCG. *Infect. Immun.* **55**:1932–1935.

Thole, J. E. R., H. G. Dauwerse, P. K. Das, D. G. Groothuis, L. M. Schouls, and J. D. A. van Embden. 1985. Cloning of *Mycobacterium bovis* BCG DNA and expression of antigens in *Escherichia coli*. *Infect. Immun.* **50**:800–806.

Thole, J. E. R., W. J. Keulen, A. H. J. Kolk, D. G. Groothuis, L. G. Berwald, R. H. Tiesjema, and J. D. A. van Embden. 1987. Characterization, sequence determination, and immunogenicity of a 64-kilodalton protein of *Mycobacterium bovis* BCG expressed in *Escherichia coli* K-12. *Infect. Immun.* **55**:1466–1475.

Thole, J. E. R., R. Schöningh, A. A. M. Janson, T. Garbe, Y. E. Cornelisse, J. E. Clark-Curtiss, A. H. J. Kolk, T. H. M. Ottenhoff, R. R. P. De Vries, and C. Abou-Zeid. 1992. Molecular and immunological analysis of a fibronectin-binding protein antigen secreted by *Mycobacterium leprae*. *Mol. Microbiol.* **6**:153–163.

Thole, J. E. R., and R. van der Zee. 1990. The 65kD antigen: molecular studies on a ubiquitous antigen, p. 37–67. *In* J. McFadden (ed.), *Molecular Biology of the Mycobacteria*. Academic Press Ltd., London.

Torriani, A. 1990. From cell membrane to nucleotides: the phosphate regulon in *Escherichia coli*. Bioessays **12**:371–376.

Torriani-Gorini, A., F. G. Rothman, S. Silver, A. Wright, and E. Yagil (ed.). 1987. *Phosphate Metabolism and Cellular Regulation in Microorganisms*. American Society for Microbiology, Washington, D.C.

Trias, J., V. Jarlier, and R. Benz. 1992. Porins in the cell wall of mycobacteria. *Science* **258**:1479–1481.

Van de Klundert, J. A. M., P. Van der Meide, P. Van de Putte, and L. Bosch. 1978. Mutants of *Escherichia coli* altered in both genes coding for the elongation factor Tu. *Proc. Natl. Acad. Sci. USA* **75**:4470–4473.

Vordermeier, H. M., D. P. Harris, G. Friscia, E. Román, H. M. Surcel, C. Moreno, G. Pasvol, and J. Ivanyi. 1992a. T cell repertoire in tuberculosis: selective anergy to an immunodominant epitope of the 38-kDa antigen in patients with active disease. *Eur. J. Immunol.* **22**:2631–2637.

Vordermeier, H. M., D. P. Harris, P. K. Mehrotra, E. Roman, A. Elsaghier, C. Moreno, and J. Ivanyi. 1992b. *M. tuberculosis*-complex specific T-cell stimulation and DTH reactions induced with a peptide from the 38-kDa protein. *Scand. J. Immunol.* **35**:711–718.

Vordermeier, H. M., D. P. Harris, E. Roman, R. Lathigra, C. Moreno, and J. Ivanyi. 1991. Identification of T-cell stimulatory peptides from the 38-kDa protein of *Mycobacterium tuberculosis*. *J. Immunol.* **147**:1023–1029.

Wallis, R. S., M. Amir-Tahmasseb, and J. J. Ellner. 1990. Induction of interleukin 1 and tumor necrosis factor by mycobacterial proteins: the monocyte Western blot. *Proc. Natl. Acad. Sci. USA* **87**:3348–3352.

Wallis, R. S., H. Fujiwara, and J. J. Ellner. 1986. Direct stimulation of monocyte release of interleukin 1 by mycobacterial protein antigens. *J. Immunol.* **136**:193–196.

Wallis, R. S., R. Paranjape, and M. Phillips. 1993. Identification by two-dimensional gel electrophoresis of a 58-kilodalton tumor necrosis factor-inducing protein of *Mycobacterium tuberculosis*. *Infect. Immun.* **61**:627–632.

Wiker, H. G., and M. Harboe. 1992. The antigen 85 complex: a major secretion product of *Mycobacterium tuberculosis*. *Microbiol. Rev.* **56**:648–661.

Wiker, H. G., M. Harboe, J. Bennedsen, and O. Closs. 1988. The antigens of *Mycobacterium tuberculosis*, H37Rv, studied by crossed immunoelectrophoresis. Comparison with a reference system for *Mycobacterium bovis*, BCG. *Scand. J. Immunol.* **27**:223–239.

Wiker, H. G., M. Harboe, and T. E. Lea. 1986a. Purification and characterization of two protein antigens from the heterogenous BCG85 complex in *Mycobacterium bovis* BCG. *Int. Arch. Allergy Appl. Immun.* **81**:298–306.

Wiker, H. G., M. Harboe, and S. Nagai. 1991. A localization index for distinction between extracellular and intracellular antigens of *Mycobacterium tuberculosis*. *J. Gen. Microbiol.* **137**:875–884.

Wiker, H. G., M. Harboe, S. Nagai, M. E. Patarroyo, C. Ramirez, and N. Cruz. 1986b. MPB59, a widely cross-reacting protein of *Mycobacterium bovis* BCG. *Int. Arch. Allergy Appl. Immun.* **81**:307–314.

Wiker, H. G., K. Sletten, S. Nagai, and M. Harboe. 1990. Evidence for three separate genes encoding the proteins of the mycobacterial antigen 85 complex. *Infect. Immun.* **58**:272–274.

Worsaae, A., L. Ljungqvist, K. Hasløv, I. Heron, and J. Bennedsen. 1987. Allergenic and blastogenic reactivity of three antigens from *Mycobacterium tuberculosis* in sensitized guinea pigs. *Infect. Immun.* **55**:2922–2927.

Worsaae, A., L. Ljungqvist, and I. Heron. 1988. Monoclonal antibodies produced in BALB.B10 mice define new antigenic determinants in culture filtrate preparations of *Mycobacterium tuberculosis*. *J. Clin. Microbiol.* **26**:2608–2614.

Wright, G. L., and D. B. Roberts. 1974. Two-dimensional immunoelectrophoresis of mycobacterial antigens. Comparison with a reference system. *Am. Rev. Respir. Dis.* **109**:306–310.

Yamaguchi, R., K. Matsuo, A. Yamazaki, C. Abe, S. Nagai, K. Terasaka, and T. Yamada. 1989. Cloning and characterization of the gene for immunogenic protein MPB64 of *Mycobacterium bovis* BCG. *Infect. Immun.* **57**:283–288.

Young, D., L. Kent, A. Rees, J. Lamb, and J. Ivanyi. 1986. Immunological activity of a 38-kilodalton protein purified from *Mycobacterium tuberculosis*. *Infect. Immun.* **54**:177–183.

Young, D., R. Lathigra, R. Hendrix, D. Sweetser, and R. A. Young. 1988. Stress proteins are immune targets in leprosy and tuberculosis. *Proc. Natl. Acad. Sci. USA* **85**:4267–4270.

Young, D., E. Roman, C. Moreno, R. O'Brien, and W. Born. 1993. Molecular chaperones and the immune response. *Phil. Trans. R. Soc. London Ser. B* **339**:363–368.

Young, D. B., and T. R. Garbe. 1991a. Heat shock proteins and antigens of *Mycobacterium tuberculosis*. *Infect. Immun.* **59**:3086–3093.

Young, D. B., and T. R. Garbe. 1991b. Lipoprotein antigens of *Mycobacterium tuberculosis*. *Res. Microbiol.* **142**:55–65.

Young, D. B., S. H. E. Kaufmann, P. W. M. Hermans, and J. E. R. Thole. 1992. Mycobacterial protein antigens: a compilation. *Mol. Microbiol.* **6**:133–145.

Young, D. B., and J. R. Lamb. 1986. T lymphocytes respond to solid-phase antigen: a novel approach to the molecular analysis of cellular immunity. *Immunology* **59**:167–171.

Young, R. A., B. R. Bloom, C. M. Grossinsky, J. Ivany, D. Thomas, and R. W. Davis. 1985a. Dissection of *Mycobacterium tuberculosis* antigens using recombinant DNA. *Proc. Natl. Acad. Sci. USA* **82**:2583–2587.

Young, R. A., V. Mehra, D. Sweetser, T. Buchanan, J. Clark-Curtiss, R. W. Davis, and B. R. Bloom. 1985b. Genes for the major protein antigens of the leprosy parasite *Mycobacterium leprae*. *Nature* (London) **316**:450–452.

Zhang, Y., B. Heym, B. Allen, D. Young, and S. Cole. 1992. The catalase-peroxidase gene and isoniazide resistance of *Mycobacterium tuberculosis*. *Nature* (London) **358**:591–593.

Zhang, Y., R. Lathigra, T. Garbe, D. Catty, and D. Young. 1991. Genetic analysis of superoxide dismutase, the 23 kilodalton antigen of *Mycobacterium tuberculosis*. *Mol. Microbiol.* **5**:381–391.

Tuberculosis: Pathogenesis, Protection, and Control
Edited by Barry R. Bloom
© 1994 American Society for Microbiology, Washington, DC 20005

Chapter 22

Membrane Permeability and Transport in *Mycobacterium tuberculosis*

Nancy D. Connell and Hiroshi Nikaido

STRUCTURE OF CELL WALL AND CELL MEMBRANE

As in other mycobacterial species, cells of *Mycobacterium tuberculosis* are covered by a lipid-rich cell wall. This structure has been examined in previous chapters, but here we want to draw attention to its functional implications. Much of our knowledge in this area comes from studies of mycobacteria other than *M. tuberculosis*, yet in view of the similarity of chemical composition of the cell walls from various organisms, we believe that all mycobacteria have the same basic features in the construction of cell wall.

What is most striking in the cell wall is the presence of a large amount of mycolic acids, most of which are covalently linked to the underlying arabinogalactan, which in turn is covalently linked to the peptidoglycan. Minnikin proposed in 1982 that the mycolic acid chains are arranged perpen-

Nancy D. Connell • Department of Microbiology and Molecular Genetics, University of Medicine and Dentistry of New Jersey, New Jersey Medical School, 185 South Orange Avenue, Newark, New Jersey 07103. *Hiroshi Nikaido* • Department of Molecular and Cell Biology, c/o Stanley/Donner Administrative Services Unit, 229 Stanley Hall, Berkeley, California 94720.

dicularly to the cell surface, forming an inner leaflet of an asymmetric bilayer structure (Minnikin, 1982). The outer leaflet of this bilayer structure was assumed to be made up of polar lipids containing short-chain ($<C_{20}$) or intermediate-chain hydrocarbons (Fig. 1). Head groups of some of these lipids were indeed shown to be exposed on the cell surface, i.e., the outer surface of the cell wall, in various mycobacterial species, as described in the earlier chapters of this book.

There were two major lines of criticism of this model. First, the fact that mycolic acid residues are covalently linked to a macromolecule, arabinogalactan, was thought to make it difficult for the mycolic acid chains to undergo lateral movements to produce the tight, parallel packing needed for the proposed structure. However, the structure of the arabinogalactan (Daffe et al., 1990; McNeil et al., 1991) appears to provide an answer to this problem. The backbone of this polysaccharide is made up of galactofuranose units, linked mostly via 1,6 linkages, and its side chains are made up of arabinofuranose units, linked via 1,5 linkages. Both linkages allow maximum flexibility (Fig. 2), and this flexibility facilitates the lateral movement of mycolic acid chains even though the head

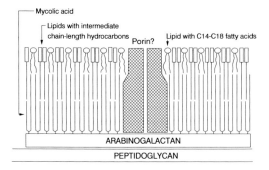

Figure 1. Modified Minnikin model of the mycobacterial cell wall.

group is nominally a macromolecule. Moreover, mycolic acid residues are always linked to nonreducing terminal arabinose residues, further enhancing the flexibility of the entire structure.

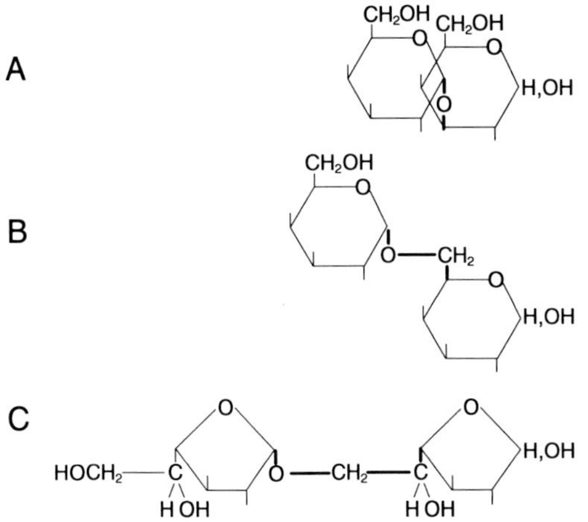

A

B

C

Figure 2. Flexibility of linkages between sugars, with galactosyl-galactose linkages shown as examples. In all formulae, bonds separating the two sugar rings are shown as thick lines. (A) The glycosidic linkage in α-galactopyranosyl-(1-3)-galactopyranose allows only very limited flexibility because of steric hindrance between the rigid, large pyranose rings. (B) The linkage in α-galactopyranosyl-(1-6)-galactopyranose has more flexibility because the two pyranose rings are one bond length farther away from each other. (C) Flexibility is maximized in α-galactofuranosyl-(1-6)-galactofuranose because separation between the sugar rings has been increased by one more bond length. The galactose residues in the main chain of mycobacterial arabinogalactan are connected in this manner (McNeil et al., 1991).

The Minnikin model demands that the cell wall contain the right amount of the other lipids that are assumed to make up the outer leaflet. The second objection to this model came from the observation that, in contrast to *M. tuberculosis*, saprophytic mycobacterial species were not known to contain many of these lipid species, except C-mycosides. However, our recent quantitative analysis of the cell wall isolated from a saprophytic species, *M. chelonae*, showed clearly that there are enough lipids containing short and intermediate-length hydrocarbon chains in this structure to make the Minnikin model plausible even in these organisms (Rosenberg and Nikaido, unpublished data).

These considerations show that the model is not unreasonable, but it was not tested experimentally until quite recently. An X-ray diffraction study (Nikaido et al., 1993), however, has now shown that many of the hydrocarbon chains, presumably the mycolic acid chains, are arranged as paracrystalline arrays perpendicular to the cell surface in the isolated cell wall of *M. chelonae*.

Thus, a large portion of the cell wall of *M. chelonae* appears to be an asymmetric bilayer. This structure reminds us of the bilayer in the outer membranes of gram-negative bacteria (Nikaido and Vaara, 1985). Here, too, the bilayer is highly asymmetric, and one of the leaflets (in this case, the outer leaflet) is exclusively composed of lipopolysaccharide (LPS). Six to seven fatty acid chains are connected to a common head group in LPS, making the lateral interaction between neighboring LPS molecules much stronger than that between neighboring glycerophospholipid molecules. Furthermore, there are no double bonds in the fatty acid chains, decreasing the mobility of the chains and the fluidity of the lipid interior (Fig. 3). These factors doubtless contribute to the lower permeability of the outer membrane bilayer to lipophilic molecules, estimated to be about

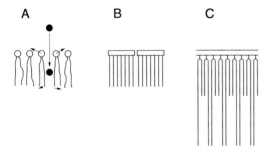

A   B   C

Figure 3. Comparison of bilayer leaflets composed of various lipids. (A) Glycerophospholipid leaflets allow easy entry of lipophilic solutes from the medium because transient lacunae can be created readily by lipid molecules moving away from each other (arrows on top) and by hydrocarbon chains bending in a fluid environment (arrows at bottom). (B) Creation of such lacunae becomes more difficult in LPS leaflet, because neighboring LPS molecules interact more strongly with each other and because there is less bending of the hydrocarbon chains, as these chains are saturated and therefore produce a tightly packed, nearly crystalline domain. (C) In a leaflet composed of arabinogalactan mycolate, the principles seen with the LPS leaflet have been pushed to their extreme, and it becomes extremely difficult for any solute to gain entry into the hydrocarbon domain in this structure.

50- to 100-fold lower than in the "typical" glycerophospholipid bilayer (Plesiat and Nikaido, 1992). We can see that in the mycobacterial cell wall, the principles used in the construction of the low-permeability barrier in the gram-negative outer membrane were utilized to an even higher extent. The hydrocarbon chains of mycolic acid are much longer (>40 and 22 carbon atoms) than those that are present in LPS (usually 12 and 14 carbon atoms) and contain few or no double bonds. The lengths of the chains increase lateral interaction between the hydrocarbon chains. Thus, mycolic acid chains are expected to produce an exceptionally tightly packed array with a very rigid interior (Fig. 3). Furthermore, instead of six or seven fatty acid residues, thousands of mycolic acid residues are linked to a single, albeit somewhat flexible, macromolecular head group. Both of these factors hinder, with an exceptional effi-

ciency, the entry of lipophilic molecules such as drugs into the lipid interior and hence the diffusion of these molecules across the bilayer. We will come back to this point later in this chapter.

One important question is whether the structure observed experimentally in a saprophytic species, *M. chelonae*, also applies to pathogenic organisms such as *M. tuberculosis*. It is difficult to answer this question experimentally. The lipophilicity of the cell surface in the latter organism and the consequent spontaneous aggregation of cells and cell envelope fractions make the purification of cell wall difficult. If one uses surfactants to prevent the aggregation of cells and cell walls, there is no guarantee that they will not affect the packing of lipids. Treatments necessary to kill the organism may alter the organization of the cell wall. Thus, at least for the time being, we can only speculate on some aspects of the structure of *M. tuberculosis* cell wall. We believe, however, that there is no fundamental difference in cell wall structure between saprophytic and pathogenic mycobacteria. First, the 16S rRNA sequence shows that *Mycobacterium* spp. are a tightly knit group, and the diversity among mycobacterial species is comparable approximately to that among members of the family *Enterobacteriaceae*, another tightly clustered group (Stahl and Urbance, 1990). Second, cell surfaces that appear quite hydrophobic are produced, for example, by rough mutants of *Enterobacteriaceae*, although these cells are still covered by carbohydrate head groups of LPS. This suggests that the exposure of hydrocarbons on the cell surface is not necessary to produce a rough surface. Third, the amount of mycolic acid present in *M. tuberculosis* is just enough to cover the cell surface as a monolayer, as predicted by the model (Nikaido et al., 1993). We have already mentioned that pathogenic species contain several candidate lipids that could form the outer leaflet and that the head groups of some of them are indeed exposed on the cell surface.

The presence of this efficient permeability barrier would, however, prevent the entry of nutrients and the exit of waste products. Gram-negative bacteria solve this problem by incorporating into the outer membrane bilayer porins, which are proteins that produce nonspecific, open, water-filled channels allowing the diffusion of small molecules across the membrane (Nikaido and Vaara, 1985; Nikaido, 1992). Interestingly, a cell wall protein forming a water-filled channel was recently identified in *M. chelonae* (Trias et al., 1992). This porin is a minor protein of 59,000 Da that allows the nonspecific diffusion of small molecules when it is reconstituted into liposomes composed of egg phosphatidylcholine. The dependence of penetration rates on the size of the solute suggests a pore diameter of 2.2 nm. It should be noted that this method gave a reasonably close estimate (1.0-nm diameter) of the size of *Escherichia coli* OmpF porin (Nikaido and Rosenberg, 1983) in comparison with the size determined by X-ray crystallography (Cowan et al., 1992). The mycobacterial porin had a specific activity at least 20-fold less than that of *E. coli* porin. This low activity may be due to reconstitution with lipids that may not exist in the mycobacterial cell wall. However, if the low activity is indeed an intrinsic property of this porin, this property and the low abundance of this protein in the cell wall would explain the low permeation rates of hydrophilic solutes measured in intact cells of *M. chelonae* (Jarlier and Nikaido, 1990) (see below). When a membrane protein shows a marginal activity in increasing the nonspecific permeability of liposomes, there is always a possibility that this activity is due to the creation of bilayer instability, i.e., the generation of transient leakage pathways between the protein and the surrounding lipids. Thus, it is important that Trias et al. (1992) showed that upon incorporation into

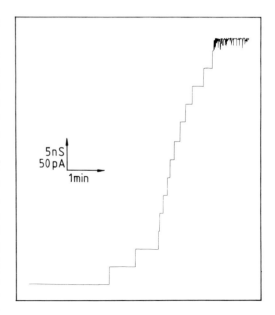

Figure 4. Insertion of "single channels" of 59-kDa protein into a black lipid film. From Trias et al. (1992) with permission.

a black lipid film, the protein produced "single-channel conductances" of a finite size (Fig. 4), a result conclusively showing that the protein is a bona fide pore-forming protein.

Finally, the mycobacterial porin channel tends to exclude anionic solutes, presumably because of the presence of several positively charged amino acid residues at the entrance of the channel (Trias et al., 1992; Trias and Benz, 1993).

It should be emphasized that low permeation rates through the porin pathway would lose their physiological significance without the exceptional barrier property of the bilayer continuum. This is so because even fairly hydrophilic compounds can dissolve into the lipid interior if the lipid shows a high degree of fluidity. In fact, calculations show that monoanionic cephalosporins used in the work of Jarlier and Nikaido (1990) would have diffused at more than 10 times higher rates through the lipid domain of the *M. chelonae* cell wall (Nikaido et al., 1993) if the cell wall lipids were not organized into the unusual structure described above.

There is very little information on the lipid constituents of the cytoplasmic membrane. It has been reported that *M. smegmatis* and *M. phlei* contain, as extractable lipids, cardiolipin and phosphatidylethanolamine as well as tri-, tetra-, and penta-acylated mannophosphoinositides (Dhariwal et al., 1976). The last group of compounds is interesting if these compounds indeed came from the cytoplasmic membrane, because it is known that the presence of a triacylated glycolipid produces the striking thermal stability of *Thermus aquaticus* cell membrane (Nikaido, 1990). However, now that we know about the existence of lipids containing fatty acids of less than 20 carbon atoms in the cell wall of fast-growing mycobacteria (see above), it seems possible that these lipids were derived from the cell wall. More detailed knowledge of the lipid composition of the cytoplasmic membrane will be indispensable for future studies of active transport in mycobacteria at the molecular level.

PERMEABILITY OF THE MYCOBACTERIAL CELL WALL

β-Lactams

Precise measurement of the permeability of mycobacterial cell wall to drugs is not easy. In the past, this was often attempted by measuring cell uptake of radioactively labeled drugs. However, most drugs bind to their target (and sometimes to other macromolecular structures), and it is difficult to distinguish binding from entry into the cells. Many of the antimycobacterial agents are quite hydrophobic, and with these compounds it is impossible to distinguish partition into the lipid interior of the walls and membranes from true entry across these barriers. When the agents have sites of protonation, they show unequal distribution across the cytoplasmic membrane because of the proton motive force across this membrane (Nikaido and Thanassi, 1993). Finally, some drugs are modified or degraded, as exemplified by the hydrolysis of penicillins and cephalosporins by β-lactamases.

Jarlier and Nikaido (1990) circumvented these difficulties by utilizing the Zimmermann-Rosselet method (Zimmermann and Rosselet, 1977). They first selected mycobacterial strains that produced sufficient levels of β-lactamase but did not leak any measurable amount of this enzyme into the medium. The enzyme molecules were presumably retained in the space between the cell wall and the cytoplasmic membrane, i.e., in the space corresponding to the periplasmic space of the gram-negative bacteria. Then a strain was selected that did not aggregate even in the absence of surfactants, which could affect the organization of lipids and thereby the permeability of the cell wall. Intact cells of a strain of *M. chelonae* selected in this way were incubated with cephalosporins, and their rates of hydrolysis were determined spectrophotometrically. Maximum rate of metabolism (V_{max}) and K_m of the β-lactamase were also determined after disruption of the cells. Diffusion across the cell wall should occur according to Fick's first law of diffusion, and hydrolysis in the "periplasmic space" should occur according to Michaelis-Menten kinetics. Also, at steady state, the net rate of drug influx should be equal to the rate of drug degradation, which is measured (Fig. 5). Calculations then yield the permeability coefficients, which show the rates of diffusion of cephalosporins across the cell wall in the presence of unit driving force to be nearly 4 orders of magnitude lower than those in the outer membrane of *E. coli* (Fig. 6). In fact, the permeability of *M. chelonae* cell wall is lower than permeability across the notoriously impermeable outer membrane of *Pseudomonas aeruginosa* (Fig. 6).

If the cephalosporins diffuse mainly through the lipid domains of the cell wall,

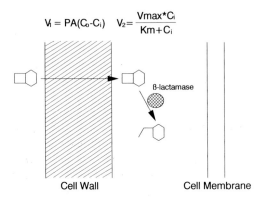

Figure 5. Measurement of cell wall permeability by the Zimmermann-Rosselet method. The net entry rate of cephalosporins across cell wall (V_1) is defined by Fick's first law of diffusion and is equal to the product of permeability coefficient (P), area of the cell surface per unit weight of cells (A), and the difference between outside (C_o) and inside (C_i) concentrations of the drug. The rate of hydrolysis of the cephalosporin in the space between the cell wall and cell membrane ("periplasm" in gram-negative bacteria) (V_2) is determined by the kinetic constants, V_{max} and K_m, of the β-lactamase as well as by the concentration of the cephalosporin in this space (C_i). Since at steady state $V_1 = V_2$, these equations can be combined and solved to determine the value of P.

their permeability coefficients should have a strong correlation with the lipophilicity of the agents (Stein, 1967). However, comparison among several agents of widely different lipophilicities showed little correlation

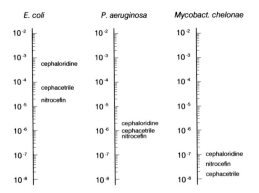

Figure 6. Permeability of *M. chelonae* cell wall in comparison to that of *E. coli* and *P. aeruginosa* outer membranes. Modified from Jarlier and Nikaido (1990).

with this parameter (Jarlier and Nikaido, 1990), a result consistent with diffusion of the agents mainly through the aqueous channels of the porin mentioned above. Another piece of evidence consistent with this idea is the rather low temperature coefficient of the diffusion rate (Jarlier and Nikaido, 1990); a much higher dependence on temperature would be expected if the diffusion occurred mainly through the lipid domain.

Among cephalosporins, cephaloridine, which carries no net charge, diffused much more rapidly than monoanionic cephalosporins (Jarlier and Nikaido, 1990). This observation is also consistent with the influx of cephalsosporins through the porin channels, because these channels tend to exclude anionic solutes, as mentioned above.

The low permeability of *M. chelonae* cell wall completely explains the level of resistance of this organism to cephalosporins. We can "predict" theoretically the MICs for cephalosporins from the values of the permeability coefficients, kinetic constants of the enzyme, and affinities of the drugs for the targets (Nikaido and Normark, 1987). Essentially, we assume that the influx of the antibiotics across the cell envelope occurs by the simple diffusion process with the permeability coefficient determined earlier and that the drug then has to survive the attack of the periplasmic β-lactamase before reaching the target, the penicillin-binding proteins (PBPs). The MIC is then the external drug concentration that will produce, at the target, the concentration just sufficient to cause significant inhibition of growth. The latter concentration, called c_{inh} by Nikaido and Normark (1987), is difficult to evaluate with precision, but it was shown that the use, as a surrogate for c_{inh}, of the I_{50}, i.e., the β-lactam concentration inhibiting by 50% the binding of benzylpenicillin to the PBPs, resulted in a good fit between predicted and experimentally determined

MICs for *E. coli* (Nikaido and Normark, 1987).

The I_{50}s were therefore determined, using the PBPs of *M. chelonae*, for three cephalosporins: cephacetrile, cephaloridine, and cefazolin (Jarlier et al., 1991). We found two prominent PBPs in this organism, with apparent molecular weights and I_{50}s similar to those reported for PBPs in *M. avium-M. intracellulare* (Mizuguchi et al., 1985). When the expected MICs were calculated by using these I_{50}s as well as the previously determined permeability coefficients and kinetic constants of the β-lactamase (Jarlier and Nikaido, 1990), we found them to be within 1 to 2 twofold dilutions from the experimentally determined values (Jarlier et al., 1991). The Zimmermann-Rosselet assay is based on several rather uncertain assumptions. These include the assumptions that there are no β-lactamase molecules either on the surface of the cells or in the cytoplasm, that the kinetic parameters of the enzyme in the "periplasmic space" are the same as those determined under laboratory conditions, and that the value of the cell surface per weight ratio used is reasonably correct. However, the fit between the theoretically predicted and experimentally determined MICs shows that these assumptions were probably correct and that the permeability coefficients obtained were not far off.

We can see from these data that because of low cell wall permeability, mycobacteria can develop very strong resistance to β-lactams in spite of relatively low levels of β-lactamase inside the cell wall barrier. In terms of V_{max}, the enzyme in *M. chelonae* hydrolyzes cephaloridine at a rate lower than 20% of that of the enzyme found in TEM plasmid-containing *E. coli*. Yet when we challenge these bacteria with 1 mM cephaloridine, the cell wall and the weak enzyme of *M. chelonae* are able to decrease the drug concentration by 99.8% (that is, the "periplasmic" concentration becomes about 0.2% of the external concentration).

In *E. coli*, in contrast, the local drug concentration can be decreased only by about 20% by the two "barriers," although one of the barriers, β-lactamase, is much more active than in *M. chelonae*.

More recently, permeability of cell wall to β-lactam compounds was determined in two other species of mycobacteria. Trias and Benz (in press) showed that *M. smegmatis* allows an approximately 10-fold-faster influx of cephalosporins than *M. chelonae*. Rosenberg and Nikaido (unpublished data) succeeded in measuring the permeability of the cell wall of *M. tuberculosis* H37Ra by a further modification of the Zimmermann-Rosselet method, and preliminary data show that *M. tuberculosis* is several times more permeable than *M. chelonae* to several cephalosporin compounds.

Other Agents

The extremely low permeability of the mycobacterial cell wall to β-lactams undoubtedly applies to other antimicrobial agents and most probably is the main reason that many agents are ineffective against mycobacteria. However, to our knowledge, direct measurement of permeability has not been carried out properly with any other agent. Furthermore, the simplistic assumption that slower penetration always produces higher resistance may not be valid in many cases, because if the drug is not inactivated, degraded, or pumped out, its intracellular concentration will eventually reach a value that is in equilibrium with the external concentration. All that is required for the activity of the drug is that the equilibrium be attained relatively rapidly in relation to the generation time of the organism. On the other hand, we must note that the extremely low permeability of the cell wall means that even very slow inactivation processes, which would be impossible to detect with the existing techniques, would still be sufficient to create significant levels of resistance. Thus, the fact that an agent is not known to be detectably inactivated by mycobacteria may not mean much.

Our knowledge that the aqueous porin channel has a rather large diameter (see above) makes it likely that many of the small, hydrophilic antimycobacterial agents diffuse predominantly through this pathway. These agents include isoniazid, pyrazinamide, *p*-aminosalicylic acid, cycloserine, and perhaps dapsone (Nikaido and Jarlier, 1991).

An alternative pathway of diffusion across the cell wall is through the lipid domain. The contribution of the lipid domain is rather minor in the outer membrane of enteric bacteria, because rapid penetration through the porin pathway is usually predominant (Nikaido and Vaara, 1985). However, the lipid pathway may be expected to play a more significant role in the mycobacterial cell wall, because the hydrophilic pathway is so inefficient. Indeed, many of the antimycobacterial agents, for example, rifamycins and clofazimine, show significant lipophilicity. Even those agents with potential protonation sites exist in uncharged forms much more frequently than usually anticipated (Nikaido and Thanassi, 1993) and thus have a possibility of utilizing the lipid pathway.

The diffusion rate of a lipophilic molecule through a given lipid domain is nearly proportional to the oil-water partition coefficient of that molecule (Stein, 1967), at least within a certain range. Thus, increasing the lipophilicity of an antibacterial agent should increase its efficacy. However, this does not always occur, because even the least lipophilic member of a homologous series may diffuse through the lipid domains of the usual phospholipid bilayer sufficiently rapidly, and thus, increasing the permeation rate further may not increase the efficacy. In mycobacteria, however, the intrinsic permeability of the lipid domain of the cell wall is so low that increases in the lipophilicities of the agents are expected to increase the penetration rate from an unac-

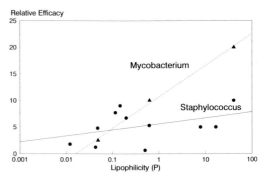

Figure 7. Efficacy of various tetracycline derivatives in *S. aureus* and *M. fortuitum*. Hydrophobicity values are the logarithms of the apparent octanol-water coefficients. *S. aureus* data are from Blackwood and English (1970). *M. fortuitum* data points show MICs for 30% of strains as determined with 59 strains (Wallace et al., 1979); this unusual choice of endpoint was dictated by the fact that the collection included many strains that were very highly resistant. The original publication gives the actual population distribution, and it is clearly seen that minocycline is more effective than doxycycline, which in turn is much more effective than tetracycline. The three drugs used with *M. fortuitum*, represented by triangles from left to right, are tetracycline, doxycycline, and minocycline.

ceptably low one to a reasonable one (in comparison with the rates of degradation, efflux, etc., or with the generation time) and will thus increase the efficacy (Nikaido and Thanassi, 1993). This was found to be true in several cases. Many derivatives of tetracycline that differ as much as 1,000-fold in terms of lipophilicity, as measured by the octanol-water partition coefficient, have been synthesized. If their efficacy is measured with *Staphylococcus aureus*, then there is no correlation with lipophilicity (Fig. 7). This is as expected, because even the least lipophilic of these compounds is expected to equilibrate across the cytoplasmic membrane bilayer within a few seconds (Nikaido and Thanassi, 1993). However, against mycobacteria, the more hydrophobic derivatives (minocycline and doxycycline) were found to show higher activity than the hydrophilic tetracycline (Fig. 7) (Wallace et al., 1979; Gelber, 1987; Franzblau, 1989). Another example involves the

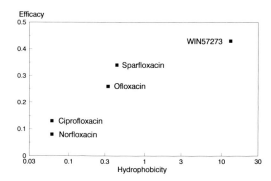

Efficacy

WIN57273

Sparfloxacin

Ofloxacin

Ciprofloxacin

Norfloxacin

Hydrophobicity

Figure 8. Lipophilicity and efficacy of fluoroquinolones. Hydrophobicity values are the logarithms of apparent octanol-water coefficients determined at pH 7.4 by Furet et al. (1992). Thus, WIN57273 partitions into the organic phase more than 100-fold better than norfloxacin or ciprofloxacin. Efficacies against *M. leprae* are the extent of growth inhibition at 1.25 µg/ml determined by Franzblau and White (1990) using the BACTEC 460 system.

fluoroquinolones. These compounds equilibrate across the usual cytoplasmic membrane bilayer within a few seconds, and thus there is no correlation between lipophilicity and efficacy against *S. aureus* (Nikaido and Thanassi, 1993). In contrast, there is a clear positive correlation between their lipophilicity and their efficacy against *M. leprae* (Fig. 8) (Gelber et al., 1992). In another interesting study, the addition of long, alkyl substituents to the 1 position of ciprofloxacin, which made the compound more hydrophobic, was shown to produce agents more active against *M. tuberculosis* and *M. avium* (but curiously, not against *M. chelonae*), although these hydrophobic derivatives were less active than ciprofloxacin against most other bacteria (Haemers et al., 1990). Still another example of the effect of hydrophobicity involves macrolides. Making the erythromycin structure more hydrophobic, as in clarithromycin or roxithromycin, produces agents significantly more active against *M. tuberculosis* (Gorzynski et al., 1989), *M. avium-M. intracellulare-M. scrofulaceum* (MAIS) complex (Fernandes et al., 1989; Naik and Ruck, 1989), and *M. leprae* (Franzblau and

Hastings, 1988; Franzblau, 1989; Ramasesh et al., 1989). With rifamycins, again, the semisynthetic derivatives that showed higher activities against mycobacteria, especially *M. avium*, were those, such as rifabutin, rifapentine, CGP-7040, and KRM-1648, that appeared to have more hydrophobic structures (Heifets et al., 1990; Tomioka et al., 1993). Finally, even with a small, hydrophilic agent, isoniazid, which is expected to use predominantly the porin pathway, Rastogi et al. (1988) showed that its activity can be enhanced against MAIS complex as well as against *M. tuberculosis* by the addition of long hydrocarbon chains, a result emphasizing the relative importance of the lipid pathway in mycobacteria (Nikaido and Jarlier, 1991).

Among antibiotics showing significant antimycobacterial activity, aminoglycosides, which are fairly large and very hydrophilic, appear to be exceptional. How do the aminoglycosides overcome the permeability barrier of the mycobacterial cell wall? We believe that the most likely mechanism is the one previously proposed by Hancock (1984) in order to explain why *P. aeruginosa*, another organism producing a very low permeability cell envelope, is quite susceptible to aminoglycosides. Hancock believes that aminoglycosides, being polycations, bind tightly to the negatively charged components on the external surface of the outer membrane, i.e., LPS, and thereby disorganize this membrane, eventually leading to penetration across this barrier. This hypothesis of "self-promoted uptake" is indeed supported by the experimental demonstration that the addition of low concentrations of aminoglycosides produces perturbation of the outer membrane barrier (although so far, the experimental conditions required unreasonably low ionic strength). The surface of the mycobacterial cell wall is similar to the surface of the gram-negative outer membrane in containing high concentrations of lipids with negatively charged head groups, for example, cardiolipin, phosphoinositides, and, in some species, sulfolipids and acidic glycolipids. Thus, we can imagine that aminoglycosides bind to the negatively charged surface of the mycobacterial cell wall and essentially traverse this barrier by disorganizing it. This notion is supported by the observation that another polycationic antibiotic, polymyxin, which is known to traverse the gram-negative outer membrane by a similar mechanism, inhibits at least some species of mycobacteria (David and Rastogi, 1985).

If the tight organization of the lipid hydrocarbons is important in the barrier property of the intact mycobacterial cell wall, agents that inhibit the biosynthesis of its components are expected to increase the permeability of the traditional antimicrobial drugs and thus their efficacy in a synergistic manner. Such results were indeed obtained by adding 2-deoxyglucose, ethambutol, and cerulenin, which are thought to inhibit the synthesis of polysaccharides, arabinogalactan, and fatty acids, respectively (Rastogi et al., 1990, 1992; Barrow et al., 1993). The specificity of action of some of the agents has not been established rigorously, and it is not clear whether permeation through the cell wall was truly affected. Nevertheless, these results are interesting and suggest a potentially fruitful direction for future research.

Possible Differences among Different Species of Mycobacteria

There are significant differences in drug susceptibility among mycobacteria, and some mycobacterial species other than *M. tuberculosis* are more resistant to some of the traditional antimycobacterial agents. In some ways, the situation seems similar to what we find in other groups of bacteria. For example, among the enteric/pseudomonad group (the γ-purple division of the phylogenetic tree of eubacteria), many of the saprophytic organisms living in soil and water (e.g., *P. aeruginosa*) must defend themselves against antibiotics present in their natural habitat, and thus they tend to produce less permeable outer membrane and to be intrinsically more resistant to antibiotics than are the obligate pathogens such as *Shigella* or *Salmonella* spp. Similarly, saprophytic, fast-growing, soil-dwelling mycobacteria such as *M. fortuitum* and *M. chelonae* are quite resistant to most of the antimycobacterial drugs, possibly because their cell walls have very low permeability. Among slow-growing mycobacteria, organisms of the *M. avium* complex, also thought to be inhabitants of soil, are resistant to most agents, presumably because both their porin and their lipid pathways have very low permeability. This assumption was indeed proven to be correct, as permeability to cephalosporins entering through the porin channels was shown to be significantly higher in *M. tuberculosis* than in *M. chelonae* (see above). The higher porin-mediated permeability in *M. tuberculosis* is consistent with much higher susceptibility of this organism to small, hydrophilic reagents such as ticarcillin and ciprofloxacin in comparison with *M. chelonae* (Casal et al., 1987; Collins and Hutley, 1988).

Some organisms (the more susceptible pathogens such as *M. tuberculosis* and the generally resistant organisms such as *M. avium* and *M. fortuitum*) are intermediate between these two extremes, and sometimes one can discern a pattern. For example, *M. marinum* is reported to be resistant to small, hydrophilic compounds such as isoniazid and *p*-aminosalicylic acid but susceptible to more hydrophobic compounds such as rifamycins and ethambutol. Thus, in this case, we can at least assume as a starting point that in this organism, the porin pathway has an exceptionally low permeability. Similarly, according to the self-promoted aminoglycoside uptake hypothesis, we can predict that some mycobacteria that are resistant to these agents

Table 1. Estimated permeability coefficients of mycobacterial cell wall to nutrients

Organism	Compound	$V_{max}{}^{a}$ (nmol/ mg/min)	K_m (μM)	Estimated P^b (nm/s)	Reference[c]
M. chelonae	Glucose	3.6	810	2.8	JN
	Glycerol	0.6	230	1.5	JN
	L-Leucine	0.3	25	1.7	JN
	Glycine	2.0	25	50	JN
M. smegmatis	Glucose	5	100	60	JB
	L-Glutamate	5	240	2.6	Yabu
M. phlei	L-Proline	0.6	4	400	Israeli
	L-Glutamate	5	8	800	Israeli

[a] When V_{max} was reported per milligram of protein, it was assumed that the protein content was about 50% of the dry weight of the cells.

[b] These values are minimal estimates, and the actual permeability coefficients may be higher.

[c] JN, Jarlier and Nikaido (1990); JB, Jayantha Bai et al. (1978); Yabu, Yabu (1967); Israeli, Israeli et al. (1977).

must have fewer of the acidic lipids on the surface, a notion that can be readily tested.

Permeability of Cell Wall to Nutrients

By using the Zimmermann-Rosselet procedure, the permeability of *M. chelonae* cell wall to small nutrient molecules was estimated (Jarlier and Nikaido, 1990). It was assumed that the nutrients cross the cell wall by a simple diffusion process and then are taken up by the active transport systems located in the cytoplasmic membrane. The latter system is equivalent to the periplasmic β-lactamase in the original Zimmermann-Rosselet assay and serves as the "sink" for removing nutrient molecules. We do not know the precise kinetic constants of the active transporters, and thus the permeability coefficients obtained correspond to minimal estimates. With this approach, the estimated permeability coefficients of *M. chelonae* cell wall toward D-glucose, L-leucine, and glycerol were in the range of 1.5 to 3 nm/s (Table 1). These values are about an order of magnitude higher than the permeability coefficients for most of the cephalosporins tested, an expected finding, because smaller solutes penetrate much faster through water-filled channels of a limited diameter (Nikaido and Vaara, 1985). These coefficients are still about 5 orders of magnitude lower than the

permeability coefficient of *E. coli* outer membrane toward glucose, which is 1.4×10^{-2} cm/s (Bavoil et al., 1977).

We can treat the published kinetic parameters for the active transport of several nutrients, which are discussed in the next section (Table 1), in the same way. Interestingly, many of the published data obtained with *M. phlei* and *M. smegmatis* suggest much higher cell wall permeability than that obtained by Jarlier and Nikaido with *M. chelonae*. This observation is consistent with the higher permeability of *M. smegmatis* cell wall reported by Trias and Benz (1993). It is also consistent with the generally higher drug susceptibility of *M. smegmatis* (and probably *M. phlei*) in comparison with *M. chelonae*.

PERMEABILITY OF THE MYCOBACTERIAL MEMBRANE: CARRIER-MEDIATED TRANSPORT

Like most areas of mycobacterial basic physiology and genetics, nutrient transport in mycobacteria is little known. The extensive studies of Brodie and colleagues detailing the transport characteristics of a single amino acid, proline, in a single organism, *M. phlei*, will be described below; other amino acids, sugars, and ions have been subjects of isolated publications. In addition, there is a notable dearth in genetic approaches to the question of membrane transport; no transport mutants have been described in the literature, nor have any of the genes encoding carrier proteins been cloned or sequenced. There follows a summary of information relating to transport in mycobacteria in general, with most of the research being directed to nonpathogenic strains such as *M. smegmatis* and *M. phlei*.

Small molecules traverse the cell membrane and enter the cell by a number of protein-mediated processes, each of which is characterized by a set of kinetic parameters. Permeases, which often represent the rate-limiting step in the conversion of small molecule to cellular products, have enzyme-like properties such as stereospecificity, saturation kinetics, and sensitivity to various kinds of inhibition. The basic types of carrier-mediated transport processes have been extensively reviewed (Saier, 1985; Romano, 1986) and are briefly introduced below.

Types of Carrier-Mediated Membrane Transport Processes

Facilitated diffusion

Molecules can be conducted down their concentration gradient by stereospecific carriers situated in the cytoplasmic membrane. There is no energy requirement for facilitated diffusion, so the substrate is not concentrated within the cell. However, facilitated diffusion is mediated by a finite number of carriers, and this fact is reflected in saturation kinetics. In addition, such transport is subject to competitive inhibition by structural analogs. Glycerol appears to be universally transported by a facilitated-diffusion mechanism that is well characterized in *E. coli* (Lin, 1976); monosaccharides are similarly transported in *Saccharomyces cerevisiae* (Bisson and Fraenkel, 1983). The glycerol transporter of *E. coli* is encoded by the *glpF* gene, which has been cloned (Sweet et al., 1990) and

sequenced (Truniger et al., 1992) and shows homology to members of the major intrinsic protein family of bacteria, plants, and animals (Pao et al., 1991). In low concentrations of glycerol, $glpF^+$ strains have a definite growth advantage over $glpF$ mutants (Richey and Lin, 1972). Once inside the cell, glycerol is trapped by ATP-dependent phosphorylation.

However, bacterial membranes are intrinsically permeable to glycerol as a consequence of its small size and neutral charge, so both passive diffusion and facilitated diffusion are involved in glycerol entry into bacterial cells, the former playing a lesser role when concentrations of glycerol are low. As mentioned above, the precise kinetic constants of glycerol transport have not been measured in mycobacteria, although preliminary kinetic evidence (Tuckman and Connell, unpublished data) suggests that the mycobacteria are not exceptional in this regard.

Active transport

Stereospecific carriers are also involved in active transport of substrates, but the concentrative effect of active transport is often as high as 100-fold over external levels. An expenditure of energy is required to concentrate against a gradient. Thus, in addition to exhibiting the characteristics of stereospecificity, saturation kinetics, and inhibition by analogs, active transport is sensitive to metabolic inhibitors. A number of energy-coupling mechanisms are found in bacterial cells. They fall into three distinct classes.

(i) Chemiosmotic coupling is the harnessing of the proton motive force resulting from the chemical (hydrogen ion) and electrical gradient established across active cellular membranes. The process is also known as "symport" when a proton moves across the membrane simultaneously with the substrate. "Antiport" is the energy-dependent exchange of one ion for another.

Many sugars, amino acids, and other metabolites are transported by chemiosmotic coupling.

(ii) Direct chemical-energy coupling is the direct use of a high-energy phosphate bond during transport. In these multicomponent transport systems, described in greatest detail for gram-negative organisms (Higgins, 1992), the actions of a number of proteins (up to five) contribute to the process: extracytoplasmic binding of the substrate, transfer to one or two membrane-bound permeases for translocation across the cytoplasmic membrane, and ATP hydrolysis by one or two proteins located on the cytoplasmic side of the membrane (Tam and Saier, 1993). Binding-protein-dependent transport systems are immediately distinguishable from other bacterial transporters on the basis of their sensitivity to (i) cold osmotic shock and (ii) metabolic inhibitors that interfere with ATP hydrolysis (i.e., nonmetabolizable analogs of ATP or agents that deplete the intracellular stores of ATP). The energy-requiring step is the hydrolysis of ATP by the ATP-binding subunit: a conformational change is then transmitted to the membrane-bound components that mediate passage through the membrane.

Many binding-protein-dependent transport systems for sugars, amino acids, and inorganic ions have been defined for gram-negative organisms. The components of these systems are closely related members of the larger structural superfamily called the ''ABC (ATP-binding cassette) transporters'' (Higgins et al., 1990). Such transport systems were initially not thought to be necessary and therefore not found in gram-positive organisms in the absence of a defined periplasmic space bounded by two separate membranes. However, proteins with sequences highly homologous to the periplasmic binding protein components of the ABC transporter systems of gram-negative organisms have been found in *Streptococcus pneumoniae* (Gilson et al., 1988),

Bacillus subtilis (Perego et al., 1991), and the mycobacteria (Young et al., 1992). The sequences suggest additional homology to lipoproteins, which are anchored to the cell membrane. It is thought, then, that such binding proteins may be instrumental in securing substrate within the region outside the cytoplasmic membrane of gram-positive bacteria and, in the case of mycobacteria, inside the lipid-rich cell wall (Higgins et al., 1990). Further characterization of such transporters in mycobacteria awaits a genetic approach by cloning such genes by homology with known proteins or by complementation of transport mutants.

(iii) Group translocation involves the chemical modification of the substrate during translocation. The best-described example of group translocation is the phosphoenolpyruvate:sugar phosphotransferase system (PTS) that is widely distributed among facultatively anaerobic bacteria. However, the PTS is most likely not utilized by mycobacteria, which are strict aerobes, as indicated by the absence of the phosphocarrier protein HPr in cell extracts of *M. smegmatis* (Romano et al., 1970; Jayanthai Bai et al., 1978).

Regulation of Transport

There are several levels of regulation of nutrient transport in bacteria. The simplest is competition among structurally related substrates for binding to permeases with overlapping specificities. Of crucial importance is the influence of cellular metabolism, resulting in induction and/or repression of transport activity and exerted at the level of transcription of the permease genes. Unfortunately, no formal descriptions of regulated transport in mycobacteria exist, although induced metabolism of several nutrients has been cursorily described and will be discussed below.

The mechanisms of inducer exclusion and inducer expulsion are found in organisms that use PTS transport and demonstrate an ordered hierarchy of carbon source utilization, usually headed by glucose (Meadow et al., 1990). These regulatory mechanisms are based on protein interactions between the PTS components (De Reuse et al., 1992). There remains the problem of regulation in non-PTS organisms, many of which do not use sugars as a preferred carbon source. The mycobacteria fall into this class because of their efficient use of glycerol instead of glucose or fructose (Edson, 1951). There is mounting evidence for regulation of permease activity by hexokinase itself in non-PTS organisms; in *E. coli*, glycerol uptake and utilization rely on the interaction between the glycerol facilitator and glycerol kinase, the first step in glycerol catabolism (Voegele et al., 1993). In addition, there are two cases of regulation of bacterial transport systems mediated by external inducer via a two-component signal transduction system: the sugar-phosphate transport system of *E. coli* (Weston and Kadner, 1988) and the phosphoglycerate transport system of *Salmonella typhimurium* (Yang et al., 1988). The proteins in these two regulatory systems are homologous to the larger family of sensor and regulator proteins that are involved in response to environmental signals (Stock et al., 1989).

SPECIFIC SYSTEMS FOR NUTRIENT TRANSPORT IN MYCOBACTERIA

Amino Acids

Very early studies of mycobacterial amino acid transport were not confined to fast-growing species. In an extensive analysis of nutrient utilization by logarithmic-phase *M. tuberculosis* H37Ra, Lyon and colleagues observed a time lag only in glutamate oxidation. They proceeded to examine glutamate transport in both *M. tuberculosis* H37Ra and *M. smegmatis* and found that uptake rates were higher in cells pregrown in glutamate, whereas enzyme activ-

ities in extracts from induced and uninduced cultures were the same (Lyon et al., 1970). Scrutiny of the data reveals nonlinear Lineweaver-Burk kinetics, as Yabu later observed for accumulation of a number of amino acids (Yabu, 1967, 1970, 1971). In careful kinetic studies, Yabu showed two-component accumulation of L-glutamic acid, L-alanine, L-aspartic acid, and L-valine. The kinetic analyses are consistent with both active (metabolic-inhibitor-sensitive, permease-mediated) transport and facilitated diffusion (at higher substrate concentrations and after saturation of the permease). Attempts to distinguish between these two processes by isolation of a permeaseless mutant of *M. smegmatis* were "numerous but unsuccessful" (Yabu, 1970) and not further discussed. A possible approach would entail the selection of mutants resistant to a toxic analog of the amino acid that enters only by the permease pathway. This would leave the diffusion component free to be studied without interference from permease activity. In lieu of such mutants, Yabu distinguished between the two processes by measuring temperature dependence, metabolic inhibitors, and competition by other amino acids (Yabu, 1970).

The D isomers of three amino acids show different entry processes in *M. smegmatis*: D-glutamic acid and D-aspartic acid appear to enter the cell only by diffusion; D-alanine appears to require a permease and enter only by active transport; and the kinetics of D-valine accumulation indicate both transport processes, as with its L isomer. Two of these D-amino acids, alanine and glutamic acid, are found in high abundance in the cell wall despite their slow rates of accumulation.

Brodie and colleagues gave extensive attention to the transport of amino acids by mycobacteria, specifically *M. phlei*, particularly in the context of a broader approach to understanding energy coupling and membrane processes in bacteria. Most of the publications from this prolific group focused on proline transport (Hirata and Brodie, 1972; Lee and Brodie, 1978). By using then-novel techniques of measuring transport in isolated membrane vesicles, Brodie et al. showed that proline is accumulated by active transport, which depends on oxidation of substrate (oxidative phosphorylation), and requires Li^+ or Na^+ ion (Hirata et al., 1974). Curiously, Na^+ ion appears to change the V_{max} of the transporter but not the K_m; in other words, the activity but not the specificity of the enzyme is altered. This is not the case with proline transport in either *S. typhimurium* or animal systems.

Other differences in the modes of energy transduction in *E. coli* and *M. phlei* were also found. Using whole cells of *M. phlei*, Prasad et al. contrasted transport of proline with that of lysine, leucine, glutamine, glutamate, tryptophan, and histidine (Prasad et al., 1976). Proline uptake, unlike uptake of the other amino acids, was insensitive to respiratory inhibitors (such as cyanide, arsenate, and azide) that block the respiratory chain; no amino acid tested was accumulated under anaerobic conditions. In view of the ability of O_2 to rescue proline transport in the presence of these inhibitors, it was proposed that a bypass of the respiratory chain is possible for proline transport energization, with molecular oxygen as the terminal electron acceptor.

It is possible to measure the relative contributions of the proton and electrochemical gradients to the activated membrane state. Proline transport seems to be driven by electrochemical gradient alone, since it is insensitive to ionophores (which change the permeability of the membrane to ions) and not to uncouplers (which change the pH gradient). Other amino acids in this study were sensitive to both classes of inhibitors.

The proline carrier was solubilized from membrane vesicles by Lee and coworkers (Lee et al., 1979) and shown to be a monomeric 20,000-Da protein. The purified protein was reconstituted into detergent-extracted membrane vesicles as well as liposomes, which restored specific proline transport requiring Na^+ and substrate oxidation.

Berger and Heppel (1975) proposed that in *E. coli*, various sensitivities of transport mechanisms to osmotic shock reflect underlying differences in energy coupling. We now know that one result of osmotic shock is the release of the soluble components of binding-protein-dependent transport systems necessary for uptake, as described earlier. Brodie and coworkers showed that in *M. phlei*, osmotic shock results in the production of protoplast ghosts (Asano et al., 1973) and amino acid uptake is unaffected; they concluded that the permeases are tightly associated with the membrane. Whether or not this is true for other mycobacteria remains to be tested; some transport systems in other gram-positive organisms appear to utilize "binding proteins" that have regions of homology with lipoprotein anchors and may indeed be tightly associated with the cell membrane.

Sugars and Other Carbohydrates

Few publications addressing the transport of specific sugars are to be found. The mycobacteria utilize a wide variety of sugars as sole carbon source, yet the transport of only a few has been evaluated. Ellard and Clarke (1959) presented initial evidence of inducible transport of fumarate and perhaps acetate but were unable with existing techniques to confirm their observations. As mentioned above, Romano et al. (1970) showed that enzyme I of the PTS system is not found in *M. smegmatis*, and this was confirmed by Jayanthai Bai et al. (1978). These latter workers also measured the K_m for glucose transport (100 μM) by *M. smegmatis* and found that the system was constitutive. Fructose, on the other hand, was actively transported by an inducible system. However, as these workers correctly point out, it is difficult to separate transport from phosphorylation and subsequent steps in sugar metabolism. Studies with nonmetabolizable analogs of these sugars as well as the isolation of metabolic mutants will be required for the biochemical characterization of sugar transport.

Other Nutrients

Iron acquisition has been extensively studied by Ratledge and colleagues, and several reviews have been published (Snow, 1970; Ratledge, 1982). Nevertheless, the precise details of the actual movement of iron molecules across the mycobacterial cytoplasmic membrane remain undescribed. In the presence of oxygen, iron is found in the form of ferric iron (Fe^{3+}). However, iron is scarce in the microbial environment because (i) $Fe(OH)_3$ is highly insoluble in aqueous solution, and (ii) in animal tissues, most iron is chelated by host molecules such as lactoferrin and transferrin. Microorganisms, including the mycobacteria, have high-affinity iron-binding compounds called siderophores; mycobacteria synthesize a number of small, water-soluble, iron-binding peptides that are called exochelins (Macham et al., 1975). Exochelins are excreted into the extracellular environment, where they chelate with iron and are returned into the cell. The iron molecule is then transferred to another class of molecules, the mycobactins, which are water-insoluble iron-binding proteins associated with the cytoplasmic membrane. The synthesis of both classes of compound is derepressed under iron-deficient conditions.

The actual uptake process depends on the type of exochelin involved. MB-type exochelins, found in BCG, M. avium, M. intracellulare, and M. tuberculosis, are water soluble until they have bound ferric iron, when they can then be extracted by organic solvents such as chloroform. The iron molecule is thought to be exchanged

from the exochelin to mycobactin for transfer through the cell membrane into the cell. The process appears to be energy independent. Once inside the cell, the release of iron from mycobactin is carried out by a reductase that requires NAD(P)H (Brown and Ratledge, 1975).

MS-type exochelins are insoluble in organic solvents whether they are bound to ferric iron or not; these exochelins are synthesized by M. smegmatis, M. vaccae, M. parafortuitum, and M. neoaurum. The entire exochelin-iron complex is taken up by an energy-dependent process that is sensitive to inhibition by electron transport inhibitors and uncouplers of oxidative phosphorylation; mycobactins are not involved (Stephenson and Ratledge, 1979, 1980).

While mycobactins have been extensively characterized (Snow, 1970; Ratledge and Marshall, 1972; Barclay and Ratledge, 1988), little is known about the structure of the exochelins. Horowitz and coworkers have used mass spectrometry to analyze the chloroform-extractable exochelins of M. tuberculosis H37Ra and have found a mixture of low-molecular-weight peptides (Horowitz, personal communication). Those workers found a high yield of exochelins from M. tuberculosis cultures grown for 6 weeks in iron-limited medium. Indeed, Hall et al. (1987) have identified envelope proteins in M. smegmatis whose expression is induced by growth in such medium; antibodies raised against these proteins were used to evaluate their role in iron metabolism, and such experiments may lead to the cloning of the genes encoding the exochelins and mycobactins.

Calcium uptake in M. phlei was studied by Brodie and colleagues (Kumar et al., 1979). Active transport of calcium ions was first demonstrated in inside-out membrane vesicles (since these transport systems usually secrete Ca^{2+} to regulate internal levels); oxidation of respiratory-linked substrates or the hydrolysis of ATP generates a proton gradient sufficient to support the uptake of calcium ions in a Ca^{2+}-proton antiport system. Using techniques derived from studies of the Ca^{2+}-ATPase of sarcoplasmic reticulum, these workers were able to resolve and reconstitute Ca^{2+} transport protein in detergent-extracted membrane vesicles and proteoliposomes (Lee et al., 1979).

CONCLUSIONS

The need for new drug targets and drug designs has sparked renewed interest in the basic physiology, genetics, and metabolism of the mycobacteria. Permeability studies have provided increased understanding of the low permeability of the mycobacteria. In addition, structural studies of membrane transporters and their organization in the membrane are urgently needed, along with the cloning and sequencing of genes encoding these proteins.

Questions also remain concerning the intracellular metabolism of the mycobacteria. What nutrients are utilized within the macrophage? Are novel metabolic pathways induced during growth within the host cell, and are transport properties altered? Recent developments in mycobacterial genetics and molecular biology have offered new and exciting approaches to these kinds of questions, which are reviewed in other chapters of this volume.

REFERENCES

Asano, A., N. S. Cohen, R. F. Baker, and A. F. Brodie. 1973. Orientation of the cell membrane in ghosts and electron transport particles of *Mycobacterium phlei*. *J. Biol. Chem.* **248:**3386–3397.

Barclay, R., and C. Ratledge. 1988. Mycobactins and exochelins of *Mycobacterium tuberculosis*, *M. bovis*, *M. africanum*, and other related species. *J. Gen. Microbiol.* **134:**771–776.

Barrow, W. W., E. L. Wright, K. S. Goh, and N. Rastogi. 1993. Activities of fluoroquinolone, macrolide, and aminoglycoside drugs combined with inhibitors of glycosylation and fatty acid and peptide

biosynthesis against *Mycobacterium avium*. *Antimicrob. Agents Chemother.* **37:**652–661.

Bavoil, P., H. Nikaido, and K. von Meyenburg. 1977. Pleiotropic transport mutants of *Escherichia coli* lack porin, a major outer membrane protein. *Mol. Gen. Genet.* **158:**23–33.

Berger, E. D., and L. A. Heppel. 1975. Different mechanisms of energy coupling for the shock-sensitive and shock-resistant amino acid permeases of *Escherichia coli*. *J. Biol. Chem.* **249:**7747–7755.

Bisson, L. F., and D. G. Fraenkel. 1983. Transport of 6-deoxyglucose in *Saccharomyces cerevisiae*. *J. Bacteriol.* **155:**995–1000.

Blackwood, R. K., and A. R. English. 1970. Structure-activity relationships in the tetracycline series. *Adv. Appl. Microbiol.* **13:**237–266.

Brown, K. A., and C. Ratledge. 1975. Iron transport in *Mycobacterium smegmatis*: ferimycobactin reductase [NAD(P)H: ferimycobactin oxidoreductase], the enzyme releasing iron from its carrier. *FEBS Lett.* **53:**262–266.

Casal, M. J., F. C. Rodriguez, M. D. Luna, and M. C. Benavente. 1987. In vitro susceptibility of *Mycobacterium tuberculosis*, *Mycobacterium africanum*, *Mycobacterium bovis*, *Mycobacterium avium*, *Mycobacterium fortuitum*, and *Mycobacterium chelonae* to ticarcillin in combination with clavulanic acid. *J. Antimicrob. Chemother.* **31:**132–133.

Collins, C. H., and H. C. Hutley. 1988. In-vitro activity of seventeen antimicrobial compounds against seven species of mycobacteria. *J. Antimicrob. Chemother.* **22:**857–861.

Cowan, S. W., T. Schirmer, G. Rummel, M. Steiert, R. Ghosh, R. A. Pauptit, J. N. Jansonius, and J. P. Rosenbusch. 1992. Crystal structure explains functional properties of two *E. coli* porins. *Nature* (London) **358:**727–733.

Daffe, M., P. J. Brennan, and M. McNeil. 1990. Predominant structural features of the cell wall arabinogalactan of *Mycobacterium tuberculosis* as revealed through characterization of oligoglycosyl alditol fragments by gas chromatography/mass spectrometry and by ^{1}H and ^{13}C NMR analysis. *J. Biol. Chem.* **265:**6734–6743.

David, H. L., and N. Rastogi. 1985. Antibacterial action of colistin (polymyxin E) against *Mycobacterium aurum*. *Antimicrob. Agents Chemother.* **27:**701–707.

De Reuse, H., A. Kolb, and A. Danchin. 1992. Positive regulation of the expression of the *Escherichia coli pts* operon. *J. Mol. Biol.* **226:**623–635.

Dhariwal, K. R., A. Chander, and T. A. Venkitasubramanian. 1976. Alterations in lipid constituents during growth of *Mycobacterium smegmatis* CDC 46 and *Mycobacterium phlei* ATCC 354. *Microbios* **16:**169–182.

Edson, N. L. 1951. The intermediary metabolism of the

mycobacterium. *Bacteriol. Rev.* **15**:147–182.

Ellard, G. A., and P. H. Clarke. 1959. Acetate and fumarate permeases of *Mycobacterium smegmatis*. *J. Gen. Microbiol.* **21**:338–343.

Fernandes, P. B., D. J. Hardy, D. McDaniel, C. W. Hanson, and R. N. Swanson. 1989. In vitro and in vivo activities of clarithromycin against *Mycobacterium avium*. *Antimicrob. Agents Chemother.* **33**:1531–1534.

Franzblau, S. G. 1989. Drug susceptibility testing of *Mycobacterium leprae* in the BACTEC 460 system. *Antimicrob. Agents Chemother.* **33**:2115–2117.

Franzblau, S. G., and R. C. Hastings. 1988. In vitro and in vivo activities of macrolides against *Mycobacterium leprae*. *Antimicrob. Agents Chemother.* **32**:1758–1762.

Franzblau, S., and K. E. White. 1990. Comparative in vitro activities of 20 fluoroquinolones against *Mycobacterium leprae*. *Antimicrob. Agents Chemother.* **34**:229–231.

Furet, Y. X., J. Deshuisses, and J.-C. Péchère. 1992. Transport of pefloxacin across the bacterial cytoplasmic membrane in quinolone-susceptible *Staphylococcus aureus*. *Antimicrob. Agents Chemother.* **36**:2506–2511.

Gelber, R. H. 1987. Activity of minocycline in *Mycobacterium leprae*-infected mice. *J. Infect. Dis.* **156**:236–239.

Gelber, R. H., A. Iranmanesh, L. Murray, P. Siu, and M. Tsang. 1992. Activities of various quinolone antibiotics against *Mycobacterium leprae* in infected mice. *Antimicrob. Agents Chemother.* **36**:2544–2547.

Gilson, E., G. Alloing, T. Schmidt, J.-P. Claverys, R. Dudler, and M. Hofnung. 1988. Evidence for high-affinity binding protein-dependent transport systems in Gram-positive bacteria and in mycoplasma. *EMBO J.* **7**:3971–3974.

Gorzynski, E. A., S. I. Gutman, and W. Allen. 1989. Comparative antimycobacterial activities of difloxacin, temafloxacin, enoxacin, pefloxacin, reference fluoroquinolones, and a new macrolide, clarithromycin. *Antimicrob. Agents Chemother.* **33**:591–592.

Haemers, A., D. C. Leysen, W. Bollaert, M. Zhang, and S. R. Pattyn. 1990. Influence of N substitution on antimycobacterial activity of ciprofloxacin. *Antimicrob. Agents Chemother.* **34**:496–497.

Hall, R. M., M. Sritharan, A. J. M. Messenger, and C. Ratledge. 1987. Iron transport in *Mycobacterium smegmatis*: occurrence of iron-regulated envelope proteins as potential receptors for iron uptake. *J. Gen. Microbiol.* **133**:2107–2114.

Hancock, R. E. W. 1984. Alterations in outer membrane permeability. *Annu. Rev. Microbiol.* **38**:237–264.

Heifets, L. B., P. J. Lindholm-Levy, and M. A. Flory. 1990. Bactericidal activity in vitro of various rifamycins against *Mycobacterium avium* and *Mycobacterium tuberculosis*. *Am. Rev. Respir. Dis.* **141**:626–630.

Higgins, C. F. 1992. ABC transporters: from microorganisms to man. *Annu. Rev. Cell Biol.* **8**:67–113.

Higgins, C. F., S. C. Hyde, M. M. Mimmack, U. Gileadi, D. R. Gill, and M. P. Gallagher. 1990. Binding protein-dependent transport systems. *J. Bioenerg. Biomembr.* **22**:571–592.

Hirata, H., and A. F. Brodie. 1972. Membrane orientation and active transport of proline. *Biochem. Biophys. Res. Commun.* **47**:633–638.

Hirata, H., F. C. Kosmakos, and A. F. Brodie. 1974. Active transport of proline in membrane preparations from *Mycobacterium phlei*. *J. Biol. Chem.* **249**:6965–6970.

Horowitz, M. Personal communication.

Israeli, E., V. K. Kalra, and A. F. Brodie. 1977. Different binding sites for entry and exit of amino acids in whole cells of *Mycobacterium phlei*. *J. Bacteriol.* **130**:729–735.

Jarlier, V., L. Gutmann, and H. Nikaido. 1991. Interplay of cell wall barrier and β-lactamase activity determines high resistance to β-lactam antibiotics in *Mycobacterium chelonae*. *Antimicrob. Agents Chemother.* **35**:1937–1939.

Jarlier, V., and H. Nikaido. 1990. Permeability barrier to hydrophilic solutes in *Mycobacterium chelonae*. *J. Bacteriol.* **172**:1418–1423.

Jayanthi Bai, N., M. Ramachandra Pai, P. Suriyanarayana Murthy, and T. A. Venkitasubramanian. 1978. Uptake and transport of hexoses in *Mycobacterium smegmatis*. *Indian J. Biochem. Biophys.* **15**:369–372.

Kumar, G., R. Deves, and A. F. Brodie. 1979. Active transport of calcium in membrane vesicles from *Mycobacterium phlei*. *Eur. J. Biochem.* **100**:365–375.

Lee, S.-H., and A. F. Brodie. 1978. A model proteoliposomal system for proline transport using a purified proline carrier protein from *Mycobacterium phlei*. *Biochem. Biophys. Res. Commun.* **85**:788–794.

Lee, S.-H., N. S. Cohen, A. J. Jacobs, and A. F. Brodie. 1979. Isolation, purification, and reconstitution of a proline carrier protein from *Mycobacterium phlei*. *Biochemistry* **18**:2232–2238.

Lee, S.-H., V. K. Kalra, and A. F. Brodie. 1979. Resolution and reconstitution of active transport of calcium by a protein(s) from *Mycobacterium phlei*. *J. Biol. Chem.* **254**:6861–6864.

Lin, E. C. C. 1976. Glycerol dissimilation and its regulation in bacteria. *Annu. Rev. Microbiol.* **30**:535–578.

Lyon, R. H., W. H. Hall, and C. Costas-Martinez. 1970. Utilization of amino acids during growth of *Mycobacterium tuberculosis* in rotary cultures. *In-*

fect. Immun. **1**:513–520.

Macham, L. P., C. Ratledge, and J. C. Norton. 1975. Extracellular iron acquisition by mycobacteria: role of the exochelins and evidence against the participation of mycobactin. *Infect. Immun.* **12**:1242–1251.

McNeil, M., M. Daffe, and P. J. Brennan. 1991. Location of the mycolyl ester substituents in the cell walls of mycobacteria. *J. Biol. Chem.* **266**:13217–13223.

Meadow, N. D., D. K. Fox, and S. Roseman. 1990. The bacterial phosphoenolpyruvate:glucose phosphotransferase system. *Annu. Rev. Biochem.* **59**:497–542.

Minnikin, D. E. 1982. Lipids: complex lipids, their chemistry, biosynthesis, and roles, p. 95–184. *In* C. Ratledge and J. Stanford (ed.), *The Biology of the Mycobacteria*, vol. 1. Academic Press, London.

Mizuguchi, Y., M. Ogawa, and T. Udou. 1985. Morphological changes induced by β-lactam antibiotics in *Mycobacterium avium-intracellulare* complex. *Antimicrob. Agents Chemother.* **27**:541–547.

Naik, S., and R. Ruck. 1989. In vitro activities of several new macrolide antibiotics against *Mycobacterium avium* complex. *Antimicrob. Agents Chemother.* **33**:1614–1616.

Nikaido, H. 1990. Permeability of the lipid domains of bacterial membranes, p. 165–190. *In* R. C. Aloia, C. C. Curtain, and L. M. Gordon (ed.), *Advances in Membrane Fluidity*, vol. 4. *Membrane Transport and Information Storage*. Alan R. Liss, Inc., New York.

Nikaido, H. 1992. Porins and specific channels of bacterial outer membranes. *Mol. Microbiol.* **6**:435–442.

Nikaido, H., and V. Jarlier. 1991. Permeability of the mycobacterial cell wall. *Res. Microbiol.* **142**:437–443.

Nikaido, H., S.-H. Kim, and E. Y. Rosenberg. 1993. Physical organization of lipids in the cell wall of *Mycobacterium chelonae. Mol. Microbiol.* **8**:1025–1030.

Nikaido, H., and S. Normark. 1987. Sensitivity of Escherichia coli to various β-lactams is determined by the interplay of outer membrane permeability and degradation by periplasmic β-lactamases: a quantitative predictive treatment. *Mol. Microbiol.* **1**:29–36.

Nikaido, H., and E. Y. Rosenberg. 1983. Porin channels in *Escherichia coli*: studies with liposomes reconstituted from purified proteins. *J. Bacteriol.* **153**:241–252.

Nikaido, H., and D. G. Thanassi. 1993. Penetration of lipophilic agents of multiple protonation sites into bacterial cells: tetracyclines and fluoroquinolones as examples. *Antimicrob. Agents Chemother.* **37**:1393–1399.

Nikaido, H., and M. Vaara. 1985. Molecular basis of bacterial outer membrane permeability. *Microbiol. Rev.* **49**:1–32.

Pao, G. M., L.-F. Wu, K. D. Johnson, H. Hofte, M. J. Chrispeels, G. Sweet, N. N. Sandal, and M. H. Saier, Jr. 1991. Evolution of the MIP family of integral membrane transport proteins. *Mol. Microbiol.* **5**:33–37.

Perego, M., C. F. Higgins, S. R. Pearce, M. P. Gallagher, and J. A. Hoch. 1991. The oligopeptide transport system of *Bacillus subtilis* plays a role in the initiation of sporulation. *Mol. Microbiol.* **5**:173–185.

Plesiat, P., and H. Nikaido. 1992. Outer membranes of Gram-negative bacteria are permeable to steroid probes. *Mol. Microbiol.* **6**:1323–1333.

Prasad, R., V. K. Kalra, and A. F. Brodie. 1976. Different mechanisms of energy coupling for transport of various amino acids in cells of *Mycobacterium phlei. J. Biol. Chem.* **251**:2493–2498.

Ramasesh, N., J. L. Krahenbuhl, and R. C. Hastings. 1989. In vitro effects of antimicrobial agents on *Mycobacterium leprae* in mouse peritoneal macrophages. *Antimicrob. Agents Chemother.* **33**:657–662.

Rastogi, N., K. S. Goh, and H. L. David. 1990. Enhancement of drug susceptibility of *Mycobacterium avium* by inhibitors of cell envelope synthesis. *Antimicrob. Agents Chemother.* **34**:759–764.

Rastogi, N., K. S. Goh, and V. Labrousse. 1992. Activity of clarithromycin compared with those of other drugs against *Mycobacterium paratuberculosis* and further enhancement of its extracellular and intracellular activities by ethambutol. *Antimicrob. Agents Chemother.* **36**:2843–2846.

Rastogi, N., B. Moreau, M.-L. Capmau, K.-S. Goh, and H. L. David. 1988. Antibacterial action of amphipathic derivatives of isoniazid against the *Mycobacterium avium* complex. *Zentralbl. Bakteriol. Mikrobiol. Hyg. A* **268**:456–462.

Ratledge, C. 1982. Nutrition, growth and metabolism, p. 186–212. *In* C. Ratledge and J. Stanford (ed.), *The Biology of the Mycobacteria*, vol. 1. Academic Press, London.

Ratledge, C., and B. J. Marshall. 1972. Iron transport in *Mycobacterium smegmatis*: the role of mycobactin. *Biochim. Biophys. Acta* **279**:58–74.

Richey, D. P., and E. C. C. Lin. 1972. Importance of facilitated diffusion for effective utilization of glycerol by *Escherichia coli. J. Bacteriol.* **112**:784–790.

Romano, A. H. 1986. Microbial sugar transport systems and their importance in biotechnology. *Trends Biotechnol.* **4**:207–213.

Romano, A. H., S. J. Eberhard, S. L. Dingle, and T. D. McDowell. 1970. The distribution of the phosphoenolpyruvate:glucose phosphotransferase in bacteria. *J. Bacteriol.* **104**:808–813.

Rosenberg, E. Y., and H. Nikaido. Unpublished data.

Saier, M. H., Jr. 1985. *Mechanisms and Regulation of Carbohydrate Transport in Bacteria.* Academic Press, Inc., New York.

Snow, G. A. 1970. Mycobactins: iron-chelating growth factors from mycobacteria. *Bacteriol. Rev.* **34:**99–125.

Stahl, D. A., and J. W. Urbance. 1990. The division between fast- and slow-growing species corresponds to natural relationships among the mycobacteria. *J. Bacteriol.* **172:**116–124.

Stein, W. D. 1967. *The Movement of Molecules across Cell Membranes.* Academic Press, Inc., New York.

Stephenson, M. C., and C. Ratledge. 1979. Iron transport in *Mycobacterium smegmatis:* uptake of iron from ferriexochelin. *J. Gen. Microbiol.* **110:**193–202.

Stephenson, M. C., and C. Ratledge. 1980. Specificity of exochelins for iron transport in three species of mycobacteria. *J. Gen. Microbiol.* **116:**521–523.

Stock, J. B., A. J. Ninfa, and A. M. Stock. 1989. Protein phosphorylation and regulation of adaptive responses in bacteria. *Microbiol. Rev.* **53:**450–490.

Sweet, G., C. Gandor, R. Voegele, N. Wittekindt, J. Beuerle, V. Truniger, E. C. C. Lin, and W. Boos. 1990. Glycerol facilitator of *Escherichia coli:* cloning of *glpF* and identification of the *glpF* product. *J. Bacteriol.* **172:**424–430.

Tam, R., and M. H. Saier, Jr. 1993. Structural, functional and evolutionary relationship among extracellular solute-binding receptors in bacteria. *Microbiol. Rev.* **57:**320–246.

Tomioka, H., H. Saito, K. Fujii, K. Sato, and T. Hidaka. 1993. In vitro antimicrobial activity of benzoxazinorifamycin, KRM-1648, against *Mycobacterium avium* complex, determined by the radiometric method. *Antimicrob. Agents Chemother.* **37:**67–70.

Trias, J., and R. Benz. 1993. Characterization of the channel formed by the mycobacterial porin in lipid bilayer membranes. Demonstration of voltage gating and of negative point charges at the channel mouth. *J. Biol. Chem.* **268:**6234–6240.

Trias, J., and R. Benz. Permeability of the cell wall of *Mycobacterium smegmatis. Mol. Microbiol.,* in press.

Trias, J., V. Jarlier, and R. Benz. 1992. Porins in the cell wall of mycobacteria. *Science* **258:**1479–1481.

Truniger, V., W. Boos, and G. Sweet. 1992. Molecular analysis of the *glpFKX* regions of *Escherichia coli* and *Shigella flexneri. J. Bacteriol.* **174:**6981–6991.

Tuckman, D., and N. Connell. Unpublished data.

Voegele, R. T., G. D. Sweet, and W. Boos. 1993. Glycerol kinase of *Escherichia coli* is activated by interaction with the glycerol facilitator. *J. Bacteriol.* **175:**1087–1094.

Wallace, R. J., Jr., J. R. Dalovisio, and G. A. Pankey. 1979. Disk diffusion testing of susceptibility of *Mycobacterium fortuitum* and *Mycobacterium chelonei* to antibacterial agents. *Antimicrob. Agents Chemother.* **16:**611–614.

Weston, L. A., and R. J. Kadner. 1988. Role of *uhp* genes in expression of the *Escherichia coli* sugar-phosphate transport system. *J. Bacteriol.* **170:**3375–3383.

Yabu, K. 1967. The uptake of D-glutamic acid by *Mycobacterium avium. Biochim. Biophys. Acta* **135:**181–183.

Yabu, K. 1970. Amino acid transport in *Mycobacterium smegmatis. J. Bacteriol.* **102:**6–13.

Yabu, K. 1971. Aspartic acid transport in *Mycobacterium smegmatis. Jpn. J. Microbiol.* **15:**449–455.

Yang, Y. L., D. Goldrick, and J. S. Hong. 1988. Identification of the products and nucleotide sequences of two regulatory genes involved in the exogenous induction of phosphoglycerate transport in *Salmonella typhimurium. J. Bacteriol.* **170:**4299–4303.

Young, D. B., S. H. E. Kaufman, P. W. M. Hermans, and J. E. R. Thole. 1992. Mycobacterial protein antigens: a compilation. *Mol. Microbiol.* **6:**133–145.

Zimmermann, W., and A. Rosselet. 1977. The function of the outer membrane of *Escherichia coli* as a permeability barrier to B-lactam antibiotics. *Antimicrob. Agents Chemother.* **12:**368–372.

Tuberculosis: Pathogenesis, Protection, and Control
Edited by Barry R. Bloom
© 1994 American Society for Microbiology, Washington, DC 20005

Chapter 23

Metabolism of *Mycobacterium tuberculosis*

Paul R. Wheeler and Colin Ratledge

To understand its biochemistry is to understand *Mycobacterium tuberculosis*. Biochemistry seeks to describe in chemical terms all the reactions that are carried out by the cell. From such knowledge, it should be possible eventually to ascribe all the properties of the organism to its specific reactions: the organism can be no more than the integration of its own metabolism. Ultimately, the process of pathogenicity itself will be describable in terms of the chemistry of the mycobacterial cell. At the moment, though, it is very difficult to assert with confidence what reactions a virulent tubercle bacillus may carry out that are not found in the avirulent strains, or even in the nonpathogenic species of mycobacteria, and that may thus be uniquely associated with the causes of tuberculosis. However, it is not necessary to search for just the perhaps very few biochemical reactions that will be unique to *M. tuberculosis* if the purpose of gaining such knowledge is to use it for the rational design of antitubercular drugs. Many reactions of the mycobacterial cell are potential targets for interference by antimetabolite drugs, though as a conse-

quence, drugs that are effective against *M. tuberculosis* will also perforce inhibit a range of other mycobacteria. However, there is no disadvantage in this broad range of activity, provided, of course, that the antimycobacterial agents do not themselves inhibit key reactions in the host and thereby simultaneously harm the patient.

Basic biochemical knowledge of the organism gives vital information as to how the bacillus acquires its nutrients, converts these into the low-molecular-weight metabolites of the cell, and then assembles these metabolites into the macromolecules needed for cell multiplication. The aim of the microbial biochemist is to understand these processes and describe the growth of the cell in terms of its individual reactions. Even with well-studied bacteria, however, we are still some way from this goal. With mycobacterial biochemistry, our knowledge has been gained somewhat fragmentarily, principally because of the inherent difficulties of working with mycobacteria. All mycobacteria grow slowly: even the fastest-growing mycobacteria take 3 or 4 days to grow in the laboratory, whereas organisms such as *Escherichia coli* are easily cultivated in 16 to 18 h. Also, most mycobacteria do not grow as dispersed cultures, which produce cells in a uniform state. Instead, mycobacteria readily aggregate into clumps of cells that are clearly not

Paul R. Wheeler • Department of Clinical Sciences, London School of Hygiene and Tropical Medicine, Keppel Street, London WC1E 7HT, United Kingdom. ***Colin Ratledge*** • Department of Applied Biology, University of Hull, Hull HU6 7RX, United Kingdom.

all the same; these clumps are often so hydrophobic that attempts to cultivate them in simple, stirred, aerated vessels, as is common practice with other microorganisms, can lead to the bacteria gradually being thrown out of the culture medium itself and then colonizing the glass walls of the vessel above the medium. Thus, even the simple process of growing mycobacteria in the laboratory is fraught with difficulties. For these reasons, researchers interested in microbial biochemistry per se do not choose mycobacteria, even saprophytic ones, as their model organisms.

Researchers in mycobacterial biochemistry have almost exclusively concentrated their efforts on those aspects of metabolism that appear to be unique to members of the genus *Mycobacterium* and have, in the absence of information to the contrary, assumed that other aspects of metabolism will be more or less the same as those of other, more amenable bacteria.

In this short review, we have chosen to follow the same elective pathway, concentrating on those aspects of metabolism that appear to be at least in some way unique to the mycobacteria and are, moreover, of relevance to the growth of *M. tuberculosis* as a pathogen within the tissues and fluids of its host.

GENERAL METABOLISM

In broad terms, the metabolism of mycobacteria in general and of *M. tuberculosis* in particular is not exceptional. With respect to carbohydrate metabolism, energy production, and the biosynthesis of both low-molecular-weight metabolites and the macromolecules of the cell, this organism behaves like most other bacteria. Mycobacteria can utilize a wide range of carbon compounds for growth in the laboratory, which implies that when they are acting as pathogens within host tissues, they will be able to assimilate a range of host tissue

metabolites for their own purposes. In this way, mycobacteria are able to assimilate not only a range of carbohydrates but also a number of lipids, proteins, etc., by the production of lipases, proteases, etc., that may be associated with the cell surface or may even, in a laboratory culture, be found as extracellular enzymes. Aspects of mycobacterial metabolism have been reviewed in general by Ratledge (1982a, b) and, with respect to in vivo nutrition, by Barclay and Wheeler (1989).

It is worth repeating here the data assembled by Barclay and Wheeler (1989) that demonstrated the wide range of nutrients that would be available to *M. tuberculosis* and other pathogens in host tissues (Table 1). It is clear that a range of substrates is available to the pathogen in vivo. It may therefore be expected that all these materials will be used by the bacteria, since none of them present any problems of assimilation. How the bacteria may then organize their own metabolism with an array of substrates available to them is shown diagrammatically in Fig. 1.

As a consequence of this array of substrates, *M. tuberculosis* will probably rely principally on carbohydrates (primarily glucose) as a source of metabolic energy: glycolysis and the pentose phosphate pathway will not only generate a range of intermediates for macromolecular biosynthesis but will also culminate in the formation of acetyl coenzyme A (CoA) and oxaloacetate, from which citric acid is derived and with which the reactions of the tricarboxylic acid cycle (Krebs cycle) take place. This in turn will generate $NADH/FADH_2$, from which, by the process of oxidative phosphorylation, ATP will be produced. However, the role of exogenous lipids in the metabolism of mycobacteria can clearly be a major determinant in the economy of the cells. The amount of lipid that is potentially available for assimilation by *M. tuberculosis* is in excess of the quantity of carbohydrate (Table 1). Thus, cells will not be

Table 1. Substrates that may be available to mycobacteria growing in the host[a]

Substrate and location	Concn
Blood plasma	
Carbohydrates	
Glucose	3.6–5 mM
Glycogen (as glucose)	0.3–0.4 mM
Fructose	0.17–0.24 mM
Polysaccharides (as hexose)	3.8–5.4 mM
Glucosamine (in polysaccharides)	3–5.2 mM
Hexuronates (as glucuronic acid), including hyaluronic acid	0.02–0.07 mM
Pentose (total)	0.13–0.26 mM
Organic acids	
Lactate	890–1,900 μM
Acetoacetate	72–250 μM
Pyruvate	45–228 μM
Citrate	66–140 μM
2-Oxoglutarate	14–68 μM
Succinate	7.4–44 μM
Malate	7.5–67 μM
Lipids	
Total (nearly all present as lipoprotein)	3,850–6,750 mg/liter
Neutral (includes triacylglycerol)	800–2,400 mg/liter
Cholesterol, total	1,300–2,600 mg/liter[b]
Total fatty acids in lipids[c]	1,500–5,000 mg/liter
"Free" fatty acids[d]	80–300 mg/liter
Phospholipids, total[e]	1,500–2,500 mg/liter
Amino acids	
Glutamine	340–820 μM
Glutamate	28–81 μM
Alanine	330–420 μM
Valine	210–320 μM
Leucine	110–180 μm
Isoleucine	53–99 μM
Proline	160–290 μM
Glycine	170–230 μM
Lysine	170–210 μM
Threonine	100–140 μM
Serine	100–110 μm
Cysteine and cystine (as cysteine)	90–110 μM
Arginine	66–110 μM
Ornithine	45–61 μM
Histidine	52–96 μM
Tyrosine	44–83 μM
Phenylalanine	42–61 μM
Tryptophan	49–59 μM
Asparagine	40–55 μM
Aspartate	0.7–5 μM
Methionine	20–27 μM
α-Aminobutyrate	16–36 μM

Table 1—*Continued*

Substrate and location	Concn
Nucleic acid precursors, purines	
Hypoxanthine	1.6–19 μM
Inosine	0–11 μM
Xanthine	0.5–4.7 μM
Guanosine	0–2 μM
Guanine, adenine, adenosine	<0.1 μM (all)
Nucleic acid precursors, pyrimidines	
Uridine	1.0–5.4 μM
Thymidine	0.5–1.0 μM
In cells (but not in plasma)	
Nucleotides[f]	
GMP	160 μM
GDP	160 μM
GTP	1,100 μM
AMP	180 μM
ADP	450 μM
ATP	5,600 μM
UMP + dUMP	90 μM
UTP	850 μM

[a] Data are from Barclay and Wheeler (1989).
[b] Of which 900 to 1,900 mg/liter is esterified with fatty acids.
[c] $C_{18:1}$ (oleic) > $C_{16:0}$ (palmitic) > $C_{18:0}$ (stearic) > $C_{16:1}$ (palmitoleic) > $C_{10:0}$ (capric) > $C_{14:0}$ (myristic) > $C_{20:0}$ (arachidic) > $C_{24:0}$ (lignoceric).
[d] Fatty acids are nearly all complexed to serum albumin.
[e] Major acyl groups: $C_{16:0}$, $C_{18:0}$, $C_{18:1}$, $C_{18:2}$ (linoleic), $C_{20:4}$ (arachidonic).
[f] Purine deoxynucleotides are present at approximately 100 to 1,000 times lower concentrations.

lipogenic (that is, carrying out de novo lipid synthesis) but will be lipolytic. Assimilation of both carbohydrates and lipids can occur simultaneously in microbial cells; indeed, microorganisms in their own particular natural environments are probably all using a range of mixed substrates. For an organism using both lipids and carbohydrates, the presence of exogenous lipids will repress the enzymes of lipid syntheses so that the cell is able to take full advantage of its gratuitous carbon sources. Lipids of the mycobacterial cell will therefore be derived by elongation and transformation of the host's fatty acids once these acids have been acquired and transported into the cell. β-Oxidation of some of the fatty acids may simultaneously take place, thus providing

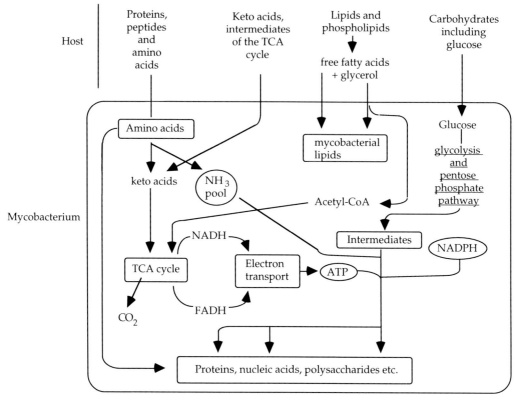

Figure 1. Metabolism of host carbon sources by intracellular mycobacteria (adapted from Barclay and Wheeler [1989]). In addition, mycobacteria may also assimilate purines and pyrimidines and use these for nucleic acid biosynthesis. TCA, tricarboxylic acid.

additional ATP as well as valuable acetyl-CoA units that can be used to augment the reactions of the tricarboxylic acid cycle. In some of the few observations to have been made with mycobacteria recovered from host tissues, Wheeler et al. (1990) were able to show that *M. leprae* recovered from armadillo liver could simultaneously elongate fatty acids and degrade them. A similar situation was found in both *M. avium* and *M. microti* (Wheeler et al., 1991) and consequently could be expected to apply to *M. tuberculosis* growing in a host animal.

In addition to using host lipids with which to synthesize its own cell components, *M. tuberculosis* could presumably derive most of its own amino acids not by de novo synthesis but by acquisition from the host (Table 1). Enough of all the principal amino acids are available that the mycobacteria need not express enzymes for amino acid synthesis. Indeed, it is more than likely that these amino acids will be the principal source of NH_3 within the bacterial cell that enables the cell to synthesize all other nitrogenous compounds it may require. However, even here, not every nitrogenous compound may need to be synthesized de novo: there may be sufficient purines and pyrimidines (as such or as their nucleotides) in host cells or fluids to satisfy the requirements of the mycobacteria in vivo (Wheeler, 1987a, 1990).

The picture therefore emerges of the in vivo mycobacterium being surrounded by a relative abundance of preformed metabolites, most of which can be readily assimilated and used for its own requirements.

Enzymes for the biosynthesis of amino acids, fatty acids, purines, and pyrimidines may all be repressed and will be detected only when the bacilli are regrown in laboratory medium that is devoid of these compounds. Not being obligate intracellular parasites (apart from *M. leprae* and *M. lepraemurium*), mycobacteria have clearly not lost the ability to synthesize all metabolites for themselves from a single, simple carbon substrate together with a supply of nitrogen and other essential elements such as are available when they are grown in laboratory media. Indeed, it is one of the features of mycobacteria that with few exceptions, none requires any preformed particular metabolite in order to grow in laboratory medium. We do not deny that growth can be enhanced by the addition of preformed metabolites to the medium, but such addition is only an enhancement and not a requirement. The mycobacteria to be excepted from this generalization are *M. paratuberculosis* and some strains of *M. avium* that require mycobactin or exochelin (see below) as a preformed growth factor; *M. haemophilum*, which requires hemin (Ratledge, 1982b); *M. lepraemurium*, which can be grown only at a very narrow pH range (Pattyn and Portaels, 1980); and *M. leprae*, which cannot yet be cultivated in laboratory medium free of host tissue cells. In the last two cases, the reason for their failure to grow is unknown. This failure may not be due just to an inability to synthesize some macromolecular precursors within their cells, since it could be argued that such precursors should have been found by now.

The only nutrient whose acquisition by in vivo mycobacteria remains uncertain is O_2. Mycobacteria are obligate aerobes and therefore require O_2 to grow. Oxygen itself is needed for the process of oxidative phosphorylation in order for the cell to produce ATP. Oxygen in host tissues is actively held by various heme-containing compounds (hemoglobin, myoglobin, cyto-

chromes, etc.), and mycobacteria must therefore rely on the low partial pressure of dissolved O_2 for their own supply. Mycobacteria in vivo therefore are probably oxygen limited in their metabolism, which may explain both their low rates of growth within tissues and their predilection for growing in lung tissues, where the partial pressure of O_2 is at its highest. Wayne and Lin (1982) have shown that intracellular mycobacteria are able to repress their respiratory metabolism, presumably in response to the low amounts of O_2 that are available. In the extreme case, where tissue necrosis has occurred, *M. tuberculosis* may be completely deprived of O_2 but can survive as an obligate aerobe by repressing all oxidative activities: the organism becomes completely dormant and may remain so for many years. It is possible, but by no means proven, that the rate of supply of O_2 to *M. tuberculosis* in vivo is the rate-limiting step for its multiplication: respiratory activities of tubercle bacilli grown in vitro are always considerably higher than those of cells grown in vivo, and furthermore, virulent strains have a lower respiration rate than avirulent strains (Wayne, 1976; Wayne and Lin, 1982), perhaps indicating successful adaptation to low partial pressures of O_2 in vivo (Barclay and Wheeler, 1989).

GROWTH RATES

Why Tubercle Bacilli Grow So Slowly

In the most favorable conditions yet devised, *M. tuberculosis* divides every 18 h on average (Wayne, 1976). *E. coli* requires only 20 min, and *M. smegmatis* requires 3 h.

Why mycobacteria grow slowly, like many basic facts about their bacteriology, is not really known. Originally, the envelope was implicated. It seemed that, being both thick and waxy, the envelope must be relatively impermeable to the uptake of nutrients. Then, starting in the late 1970s, a

Table 2. Growth and rates of synthesis of nucleic acids

Parameter	M. tuberculosis	M. smegmatis	E. coli	Reference(s)
Mean generation time (h)[a]	24	3	1.3	Harshey and Ramakrishnan, 1976; Hiriyanna and Ramakrishnan, 1986
Time to replicate genome DNA (h)	10–11	1.8–1.9	0.9–1.0	Hiriyanna and Ramakrishnan, 1986
Time to transcribe set of RNA genes (h)	0.12	ND[b]	0.013	Harshey and Ramakrishnan, 1976
No. of rRNA operons	1	2	7	Bercovier et al., 1986; Stahl and Urbance, 1990

[a] Times are for media used for study of DNA and RNA biosynthesis. Fastest mean generation times are given in the text.
[b] ND, not determined.

group at the Indian Institute for Sciences made a wide-ranging study of metabolism in *M. tuberculosis* and showed nucleic acid biosynthesis to be a strong candidate for limiting the growth rate. A biotechnologist's approach would be to ask whether slow growth is a result of limitation more by catabolism than by anabolism (Kell, 1987). This may (with caution) be determined by titrating inhibitors into a growing culture. The absence of a threshold with any one inhibitor suggests that there is no excess of the activity inhibited (Harvey and Koch, 1980), so this activity is limiting to growth. Such an approach has never been followed for any mycobacterium. However, the finding that the MIC of rifampin for *M. tuberculosis* is 200 nmol/liter (Woodley et al., 1972), thus in effect without a threshold, points to the importance of anabolism and of nucleic acid biosynthesis in particular.

RNA and DNA Biosynthesis

Both RNA and DNA polymerases from *M. tuberculosis* have been partially characterized, with the RNA polymerase being purified to homogeneity (Harshey and Ramakrishnan, 1976). This RNA polymerase is 1,000 times more sensitive to rifampin than the similar enzyme from *E. coli*, being inhibited 67% by 1 nmol of rifampin per liter. From the rate of activity of nucleic acid chain elongation, it can be shown that both the time to replicate the genome (Hiriyanna and Ramakrishnan, 1986) and the

time to transcribe RNA genes (Harshey and Ramakrishnan, 1976) are related to generation time (Table 2). Moreover, a further limitation is placed on such organisms as *M. tuberculosis* (Bercovier et al., 1986) and *M. lepraemurium* (Suzuki et al., 1987), which have only one set of rRNA genes (Table 2). Indeed, the division between fast- and slow-growing mycobacteria is a natural division reflected by the number of rRNA operons (Stahl and Urbance, 1990).

The Envelope

It is the lipid part of the cell wall that gives mycobacteria their unusually thick and waxy envelope. Structurally, the cell wall appears similar in all mycobacteria: mycolic acids attached to the outside of the arabinomannan-peptidoglycan cell wall presumably interact with variable amounts of more polar lipids, mainly mycosides, to form a permeability barrier (Minnikin, 1991; McNeil and Brennan, 1991; Rastogi, 1991). For *M. tuberculosis*, the outer layer containing the mycosides tends to be rather thin both in vivo (Frehel et al., 1988) and in vitro (Frehel et al., 1986), though a very small proportion of *M. tuberculosis* cells (compared with *M. avium*) have a very wide, 60-nm-thick, electron-transparent zone (Frehel et al., 1986) around individual cells.

Only recently has a convincing mechanism been suggested that could explain the observed differences in permeability between mycobacteria and other bacteria (see chapter 22 in this volume). Studies of *M. chelonae* reveal that it is considerably less permeable to hydrophilic substrates and agents than gram-negative bacteria (Jarlier and Nikaido, 1990; Jarlier et al., 1991). The only water-filled channels in its wall are formed by a single 59-kDa porin (Trias et al., 1992) that shows voltage gating such as is seen with the porins from gram-negative bacteria that exhibit ion selectivity (Trias and Benz, 1993). It will be interesting to see whether there are differences in permeability measurements between mycobacteria and what porins (if any) exist in *M. avium*. The special interest in *M. avium* is that it is impermeable to hydrophilic drugs (Rastogi et al., 1991) and is more selective in its ability to take up hydrophilic substrates than *M. microti* (one of the tubercle group) (Wheeler, 1987a, 1990; Wheeler and Ratledge, 1988). Only by modifying the substrates by fatty acylation to make them more hydrophobic (Rastogi and Goh, 1990) or by interfering with the biosynthesis of glycopeptidolipid in the outer layer (Rastogi et al., 1990) can hydrophilic agents readily enter *M. avium*.

The mycobacterial envelope therefore affects the rate at which agents, some harmful to the mycobacterium but also including growth substrates, enter the bacteria. That the low permeability to hydrophilic agents restrains the growth of at least some mycobacteria is conceivable but remains to be demonstrated. The question is, then, are the slow-growing mycobacteria, like *M. avium* and *M. tuberculosis*, able to evade this restriction when in vivo? As discussed above under General Metabolism, they could utilize lipophilic substrates such as phospholipids for their carbon requirements (Wheeler and Ratledge, 1992) and would need only more hydrophilic substrates to supply their nitrogen requirements. Purines (Wheeler, 1987a) and pyrimidines (Wheeler, 1990) may be acquired directly and used for nucleic acid biosynthesis, which is indeed related to generation time (Table 2).

A final comment on the envelope is that its biosynthesis might be rate limiting for growth. This would be awkward to prove, as production of envelope material and cell division must be coupled. Again, experiments with sublethal amounts of inhibitors may be useful here (Harvey and Koch, 1980), while quantifying the activities of enzymes involved in envelope biosynthesis must be preceded by characterizing the enzymes, in most cases for the first time. Alternatively, it may be possible to determine the number of operons for cell wall biosynthesis in fast- and slow-growing mycobacteria. Undoubtedly, with cell wall lipids making up about 10% of the dry weight of the mycobacterium (Dhariwal et al., 1976) and with each extra —$CH_2 \cdot CH_2$— added costing 1 ATP + 2 NADPH (Ratledge, 1982a), wall biosynthesis represents a massive effort on the part of *M. tuberculosis*.

The Stress Response

The stress response and the stringent response that occur in related environmental conditions but are differentially regulated both tend generally to downregulate growth. The stringent response depresses protein and ribosome synthesis (Lindquist, 1986), but it has barely been studied in mycobacteria except for a single observation of the presence of guanine nucleotides, which are characteristic of the response in *M. leprae* (Nam-Lee and Colston, 1985).

Mycobacteria are clearly capable of mounting a stress response. Several characteristic heat shock proteins have been cloned and identified for *M. tuberculosis* and other mycobacteria (Young et al., 1991). Their functions are mainly interactions with proteins such as those for translocation and protection (Table 3). Heat shock proteins are synthesized in tubercle bacilli (BCG) when the temperature is

Table 3. Heat shock proteins in *M. tuberculosis* and *M. bovis*

M_r (10^3)	Characteristic deduced from sequence similarity		Appearance	
	Homolog	Function(s)	On heat shock[a]	In vivo?[b]
90	Not known	Not known	↑	−
70–71	DnaK	Protein translocation/transport, ATPase activity	↑ ↑ (also ↑ on oxidative stress)	+
65	GroEL	Protein folding	↑	+
40	DnaJ	Interacts with DnaK	↑	−
23[c]	SodA	Superoxide dismutase	=	+
12	GroES	Interacts with GroEL	=	+

[a] ↑, new synthesis of protein or encoding mRNA (Monahan et al., 1993; Patel et al., 1991); =, no new synthesis.
[b] +, apparent as Coomassie blue-stained band on PAGE; −, did not stand out as Coomassie blue-stained band on PAGE.
[c] Not shown in *M. bovis*; all others are in both strains.

switched from 30 to 45°C (Patel et al., 1991), and a 65-kDa extracellular protein is produced in large amounts when growth in zinc-depleted conditions occurs (De Bruyn et al., 1989). We include in Table 3 a note on apparent heat shock proteins prevalent in host-grown *M. microti*, one of the tubercle group of bacteria. They were judged only by their intensities in gels stained for protein (Wheeler and Bulmer, unpublished work), so their identification needs to be confirmed using monoclonal antibodies. However, induction of the stress response may not be a key event in survival of *M. tuberculosis* on exposure to bactericidal efforts by the host.

In contrast to many microbes in which oxidative stress induces heat shock proteins, including superoxide dismutase (though differential responses to exposure in vitro to superoxide or peroxide have often been reported; Watson, 1980), only weak synthesis of a single stress protein of 71 kDa was observed when *M. bovis* was exposed to hydroxyl radicals (Monahan et al., 1993). Little or no protein synthesis was seen on exposure to peroxide or hypochlorite (Monahan et al., 1993). Moreover, new protein synthesis by BCG within 2 h of engulfment by macrophages could be observed, but this did not include any of the stress proteins in Table 3 (Monahan and Butcher, unpublished observations).

From the foregoing it can be seen that the stress response is clearly inducible in certain conditions. Furthermore, the heat shock proteins do not appear unusually prevalent in mycobacteria (Watson, 1990). Thus, the stress response in *M. tuberculosis* may be able to control growth rate, but it is not per se the reason the organism grows slowly.

IRON METABOLISM

General Observations

Of all the nutrients required by or available to *M. tuberculosis* (Table 1), only iron poses serious acquisition problems. Outside the animal body in aerobic environments, iron occurs in its oxidized ferric [Fe(III)] state and, as such, at neutral pH value has a solubility of about 10^{-18} mol/liter. The predominant forms of iron are the polymeric or colloidal ferric hydroxide, e.g., rust, or such complexes as insoluble ferric phosphate. Thus, since all forms of life require iron (the only exception being lactobacilli), there is a problem of abstracting ferric iron from its sources and then holding the iron in a soluble form for uptake and assimilation into a living organism.

Iron is used in conjunction with a variety of proteins for a wide range of functions: in animals, these functions include both oxygen transport (hemoglobin) and O_2 storage (myoglobin) and involve transport of iron around the body in the bloodstream while the iron is attached to transferrin (a glycoprotein of about 90 kDa) and storage within all cell types, but especially the liver, in the form of ferritin. Ferritin is a protein consisting of 24 equivalent subunits that surround a core of insoluble ferric hydroxide/phosphate such that the number of Fe atoms per molecule is about 4,500 (Harrison et al., 1987). The binding capacity of transferrin is only two atoms of Fe(III) per protein molecule, and even here, full saturation never occurs (the average content of Fe per molecule is only 0.7), because the body uses transferrin to ensure that there is no free circulating iron, as this iron would be directly and easily available to any invading pathogen (Kochan, 1976).

Bacteria, like animals, require iron for incorporation into cytochromes and all other heme-containing proteins as well as into enzymes such as aconitase, ribonucleoside reductase, various oxidases, and hydroxylases, which all use the iron as part of the catalytic site but without the involvement of a heme prosthetic group.

To be successful, therefore, a pathogen must acquire iron from one of the major iron-containing molecules of the host: from hemoglobin, which occurs in hemolytic diseases; from transferrin, which occurs in extracellular infections, or molecules related to it such as lactoferrin (as in saliva, tears, milk, and other secretions) or ovatransferrin (in oviparous animals); or from ferritin if the pathogen causes an intracellular infection.

The process of iron acquisition by bacteria has been elucidated mainly by using nonpathogenic organisms, but there is good evidence that in some infections, notably those caused by *Pseudomonas* spp. associated with infections in cystic fibrosis patients and those caused by pathogenic strains of *E. coli* and *Klebsiella* spp., the mechanisms described below will also be in operation (Griffiths, 1987). With mycobacteria, although the process of iron acquisition is known in some detail from laboratory studies, it can only be surmised that the in vitro process also represents the likely route of iron assimilation in pathogenic strains growing in vivo.

The process of iron acquisition by a microbial cell is shown in outline in Fig. 2. The key compound involved in the processes of iron solubilization and of subsequent transfer of iron into the cell is termed a siderophore. Siderophores are low-molecular-weight extracellular compounds

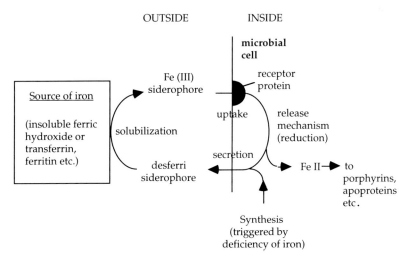

Figure 2. Iron assimilation in microorganisms.

produced in increased concentrations when the amount of available iron is limiting to growth: in other words, when a microorganism becomes deficient in iron, it derepresses the synthesis of its siderophore, which then sequesters any available iron for the microbe's use. The chemical nature of siderophores is very variable. They do not occur in animals, and the existence of counterparts in plants is uncertain. The most studied example of a siderophore is enterochelin, also known as enterobactin, which is produced by *E. coli* and other enterobacteria (*Salmonella* and *Klebsiella* spp., etc.). It is a cyclic triester of 2,3-dihydroxybenzoyl-*N*-serine and can remove iron from all iron-binding proteins, as it has a stability constant for Fe(III) of about 10^{50}. (EDTA has a stability constant of about 10^{24} for iron.) The entire area of microbial iron transport has been subject to many recent reviews, of which those by Neilands et al. (1987), Bagg and Neilands (1987), Winkelmann (1991), Braun (1990), and Nikaido (1993) can be recommended. Well over 100 different siderophores have now been reported.

Iron Metabolism in Mycobacteria

Iron assimilation in mycobacteria differs from the basic model (Fig. 2) in that the first siderophore identified, mycobactin, proved to be wholly intracellular (Snow, 1970). A family of mycobactins produced by mycobacteria have minor structural variations in the parent nucleus depending on the producing species (Fig. 3). It is possible to use these differences as a precise chemotaxonomic character for identifying mycobacteria at the species level (Hall, 1986; Hall and Ratledge, 1984). The presence of a long alkyl chain in the molecule ensures that the mycobactin remains within the cell envelope, probably at the boundary of the cytoplasmic membrane (Ratledge et al., 1982). Although mycobactin fulfills the criterion of a siderophore by having a high affinity for

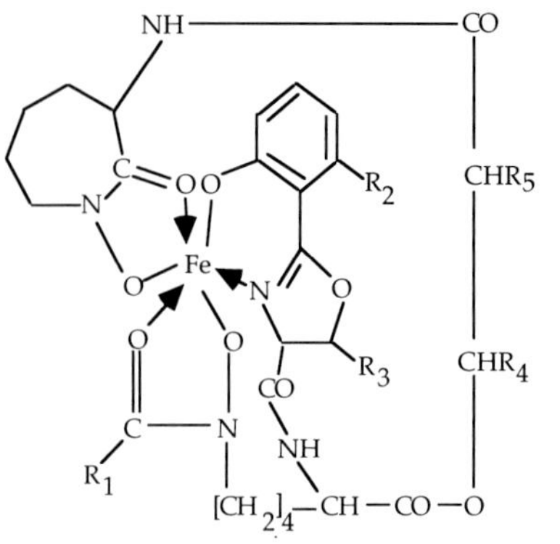

Figure 3. Structure of mycobactin, the intracellular siderophore of mycobacteria. For structures of other mycobactins, see Snow (1970) and Barclay et al. (1985). Substituents: R_1, alkyl chain up to C_{19}, often with double bond at *cis* $\Delta 2$ position, though occasionally, as with *M. marinum*, this can be CH_3; R_2, —H or —CH_3; R_3, —H or —CH_3; R_4, usually —CH_3 or —C_2H_5, though occasionally, as with *M. marinum*, a long alkyl chain up to C_{17}; R_5, —H or —CH_3. For *M. tuberculosis*, R_1 is —$C_{19}H_{37}$, $R_2 = R_3 = R_5 =$ —H, and R_4 is —CH_3.

iron (K_s of ca. 10^{36}) and is produced in greatly increased amounts (up to 10% of the cell dry weight) during iron-deficient growth, it nevertheless cannot be the agent for iron sequestration as it is not a secreted product (Macham et al., 1975), despite claims to the contrary (Kochan et al., 1971). This raises two questions: what is the role of mycobactin, and what is the extracellular siderophore that mycobacteria produce?

Extracellular iron solubilization: the exochelins

The initial candidate for the role of siderophore was salicylic acid (2-hydroxybenzoic acid), which is produced in increased quantities in the culture filtrates of a number of mycobacteria, including *M. tuberculosis* and BCG (Ratledge and Winder, 1962). However, later experiments showed that iron uptake as mediated by salicylate was ineffective in the presence of phosphate ions owing to the formation of the insoluble ferric phosphate (Ratledge et al., 1974). Further experiments (Macham and Ratledge, 1975) showed the presence of iron-solubilizing factors in the culture filtrates of *M. smegmatis* and BCG that, even in the presence of phosphate ions, still kept iron in a soluble form. These factors were termed "exochelins" (Macham and Ratledge, 1975) and were quickly shown to be the extracellular siderophores of mycobacteria (Macham et al., 1975).

The exochelins are small molecules (<1,000 Da) that can readily remove iron from ferritin and can reverse the bacteriostatic effects of serum due to the presence of transferrin. The ferric complexes of exochelin are freely diffusible and can rapidly transfer the chelated iron into the mycobacterial cell that had produced the exochelin with some specificity (Hall and Ratledge, 1987; Macham et al., 1977; Stephenson and Ratledge, 1980). Exochelins have been isolated from all laboratory-cultivated mycobacteria so far examined, including pathogenic strains. Their structures have been elusive to establish, though purified exochelins have been obtained from the saprophytes *M. smegmatis* and *M. neoaurum*, with both appearing to be pentapeptides containing ε-*N*-hydroxyornithine derivatives. The exochelin from the former species appears to contain ε-*N*-hydroxyornithine, β-alanine, and threonine in a 3:1:1 molar ratio.

Exochelins have been isolated (Barclay and Ratledge, 1983, 1988) from the following pathogenic mycobacteria: *M. tuberculosis* H37Rv and H37Ra and also fresh clinical isolates of *M. tuberculosis* (9 of 9 isolates), *M. africanum* (6 of 7 isolates), BCG (1 of 1 isolate), *M. intracellulare* (2 of 2 isolates), *M. scrofulaceum* (1 of 1 isolate), *M. avium* (13 of 13 isolates, including 8 strains that were dependent on mycobactin for growth), and *M. paratuberculosis* (4 of 4 mycobactin-requiring strains). These exochelins were chemically distinct from the ones from the saprophytes in that these ferriexochelins could be extracted into chloroform. No structural work was carried out at that time on these materials, though a number of exochelins were indicated to be present in each case (Barclay and Ratledge, 1983, 1988). The fact that exochelins were readily recovered from freshly isolated strains as well as from laboratory subcultured ones suggested that exochelins were the preferred means of acquiring iron from a host, thus confirming the initial properties found with the other exochelins (see above). This view was supported by the finding that mycobactin-dependent strains of *M. avium* and *M. paratuberculosis* could be grown in the absence of mycobactin but with an exochelin (from *M. avium*) now added to the medium (Barclay and Ratledge, 1983). Although when placed in laboratory medium these strains cannot initiate synthesis of exochelin or mycobactin, they obviously must be able to do so when a small amount of priming siderophore is included. In vivo, growth may be initiated by iron acquisition from another source, such as ferric citrate, which can be used by many mycobacteria (Messenger and Ratledge, 1982), and once growth is initiated, exochelin synthesis would quickly follow.

Exochelin is presumably essential for in vivo growth. The only alternative to its participation is (Lambrecht and Collins, 1992, 1993) an in vivo environment, i.e., the phagocytic vacuoles of the macrophage, in which the pH is between 4.5 and 6.0 and the dissociation of iron from ferritin or transferrin is consequently increased, perhaps sufficiently to sustain growth without the need for exochelin. Our view would be that while such conditions may pertain and could be responsible for initiation of growth, once growth has started, the pH seems likely to rise in accordance with the observations of Chicurel et al. (1988), and under such conditions, exochelin synthesis is likely to be essential for iron acquisition and further cell proliferation. The only certain way to establish the role of exochelin (and of mycobactin) in pathogens growing in vivo will be to produce exochelin (or mycobactin)-requiring auxotrophic mutants and then see if these mutants have lost their abilities to cause tuberculosis and other diseases.

Mycobactin

Although most mycobacteria produce a mycobactin (Snow, 1970), some species and strains are apparently deprived of this intracellular siderophore. For example, *M. paratuberculosis* and some strains of *M. avium*, as mentioned above, require mycobactin for laboratory culture, but since this requirement can also be satisfied by exochelin (Barclay and Ratledge, 1983), the absolute requirement for mycobactin is uncertain. In addition, a few strains of individual species of mycobacteria do not produce any discernible amount of mycobactin (Hall and Ratledge, 1984), but unlike *M. paratuberculosis*, these strains grow readily in laboratory media and under iron-deficient conditions produce exochelins (Messenger et al., 1986) without any priming of growth being needed.

Thus, mycobactin may not be absolutely necessary for growth of a mycobacterium

in laboratory medium, but the cells that produce it are probably at a considerable advantage in vivo, as they are able to use the mycobactin as a storage place for iron in the manner suggested in Fig. 4. Here mycobactin can store iron directly received from any low-molecular-weight forms of iron that can partially penetrate the cell envelope if these are suddenly available to the cell. Alternatively, mycobactin can hold any excess iron arriving in the cell via the exochelin route of uptake should the cell not be able to use all this iron. It is frequently envisaged that bacteria in their environments undergo a series of "feasts and famines" (Koch, 1971) as nutrients suddenly become available or are withheld for long periods. If iron were to be suddenly available to a pathogen such as *M. tuberculosis*, the organism would need to acquire and hold the iron until it could initiate synthesis of the necessary porphyrins and apoproteins to make the required heme groups and iron-containing proteins.

In reality, it has proved very difficult to isolate mycobactin from mycobacteria grown in vivo in order to demonstrate a positive role for it in vivo. Early studies

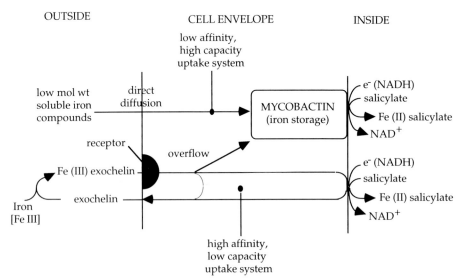

Figure 4. Mechanism of iron uptake in mycobacteria as mediated by the exochelins and mycobactins.

(McCready and Ratledge, 1977) failed to find mycobactin in *M. avium* recovered after growth in a rabbit, even though the strain produced copious amounts of mycobactin when grown iron deficiently in the laboratory. This failure was originally thought to be due to isolation of the bacilli at a very late stage of infection, when they may have become iron replete and thus repressed mycobactin biosynthesis and, indeed, degraded any mycobactin that remained. Later work with *M. leprae* (Kato, 1985) failed to locate any mycobactin in cells recovered from armadillo liver, and more recently, Lambrecht and Collins (1993) have failed to detect mycobactin in *M. tuberculosis*, *M. avium*, or *M. paratuberculosis* recovered from mouse spleen, flamingo liver and spleen, and bovine ileum, respectively. Clearly, in vivo-grown mycobacteria must produce very little if any mycobactin, implying that the bacilli may not always be restricted in their supply of iron. This, indeed, seems more than likely.

It can be argued that laboratory culture conditions have very little correlation with conditions that pertain in vivo. With regard to iron metabolism, the exaggerated response to iron deprivation is shown by growing cells in laboratory medium from which iron is permanently withheld. Consequently, cells derepress synthesis of all the components required for iron transport, but, as iron is never found within the culture flask, the cells never receive any metabolic signal to stop synthesis of some components of the uptake process. Consequently, the content of mycobactin within the cells continues to increase throughout growth and will, if left unchecked, reach up to 10% of the cell biomass. This is obviously a considerable waste of metabolic energy, but the cell has no means of stopping this useless synthesis since the situation is entirely contrived. When the same events occur in vivo at the commencement of an infection, the invading bacilli may

well express all the components for iron acquisition, but because the system is effective (it must be effective; otherwise the cells could not multiply), iron is gained by the invading bacilli. Then, as iron is effectively mobilized into the bacteria, supposedly by the exochelin and/or mycobactin system (Fig. 4), the bacteria repress synthesis of the uptake system in response to the apparent iron-sufficient conditions that they are now experiencing. Hence, it is to be expected that in vivo bacilli will be on the cusp of iron deficiency/sufficiency: their status will be synthesis of just enough exochelin, mycobactin, etc., to keep the cells supplied with a sufficient concentration of iron to enable growth to occur more or less unchecked.

This hypothesis is borne out when the putative iron uptake protein receptors (see below) are examined in in vivo bacilli. Certainly at the end of an infection with mycobacteria, it is to be expected that most of the bacilli will have obtained sufficient iron for them to be regarded as iron sufficient. It is perhaps therefore not too surprising that mycobactin has not been detected in such cells (Kato, 1985; Lambrecht and Collins, 1993). However, to suppose that mycobactin is never synthesized at all by mycobacteria in vivo is to beg the question of why mycobactin should be synthesized at all. Mycobactin biosynthesis did not evolve to allow mycobacteria to be grown in laboratory culture medium.

The alternative model to the exochelin/mycobactin process of iron uptake and storage is a model in which mycobacteria in vivo obtain their iron by direct acquisition from transferrin or lactoferrin (Lambrecht and Collins, 1993). That this can occur with other bacteria has been suggested for *Neisseria gonorrhoeae* (McKenna et al., 1988; Mickelsen et al., 1982), *Neisseria meningitidis* (Schryvers and Morris, 1988a, b), and, more recently, *Pasturella haemolytica* (Ogunnariwo and Schryvers, 1990) and *Helicobacter pylori* (Husson et al., 1993).

In all these cases, however, no extracellular production of any siderophore has ever been detected, whereas, as stated above, exochelin has been found in almost every single mycobacterium so far examined. Exochelin, though, cannot be detected in vivo, not just because of its low concentration, but because it will be lost during the recovery of tubercle bacilli from infected tissues. Interestingly, uptake of iron from transferrin and lactoferrin into *Neisseria*, *Pasturella*, and *Helicobacter* spp. (Husson et al., 1993; Mickelsen et al., 1982; Ogunnariwo and Schryvers, 1990; Schryvers and Morris, 1988a, b) involves the expression of specific uptake receptors. Transferrin or lactoferrin must anchor to these receptors, but how the iron is then removed remains unclear. With *Bordetella bronchiseptica*, it was initially suggested that iron could be taken up from transferrin and lactoferrin (Menozzi et al., 1991), and a direct route of acquisition was envisaged. More recent work, though, has shown that this process is mediated by a specific siderophore and that there is thus no direct interaction of the host iron-binding proteins and the receptors of the bacterial cell (Agiato Foster and Dyer, 1993).

Thus, direct transfer of iron from a host protein to a bacterium seems to occur only in those bacteria that apparently do not synthesize a siderophore. Mycobacteria clearly do synthesize siderophores, and this fact implies (but does not prove) that direct transfer of iron between host proteins and the bacterial cell does not take place. For the uptake of siderophores, including exochelins (Macham et al., 1977), other receptor proteins (Fig. 4) that can transfer the entire iron-siderophore complex across the cell envelope exist (see below).

Release of iron from exochelin and mycobactin

Although like most other siderophores both exochelin and mycobactin have rela-tively high stability constants with ferric iron (ca. 10^{25} and 10^{35}, respectively), the iron can easily be removed from them upon its reduction to ferrous [Fe(II)] iron. An NADH-dependent reductase that will reduce ferrimycobactin and ferriexochelin as well as other complexes such as ferriferrioxamine B and ferric ammonium citrate has been found in extracts of *M. smegmatis* (Brown and Ratledge, 1975a; McCready and Ratledge, 1979). The reaction assay requires anaerobic conditions [to prevent reoxidation of Fe(II) back to Fe(III)], an electron donor (NADH or NADPH), and an acceptor for the Fe(II), also to prevent reoxidation. Initially, EDTA was used as the Fe(II) acceptor, but it was subsequently found (McCready and Ratledge, 1979) that EDTA could be substituted for by salicy-late (Fig. 4), which of course occurs in mycobacteria (see above). Thus, the coupled reaction Fe(III)-mycobactin (or -exochelin) + NADH + salicylate → Fe(II)-salicylate + NAD^+ + mycobactin (or exochelin) was considered capable of effectively removing iron from the complex. It was hypothesized, but never established experimentally, that Fe(II)-salicylate could be the correct form for iron to be inserted into porphyrins or apoproteins, as it is known that such reactions require Fe(II) rather than Fe(III).

Work to characterize the reductase (McCready and Ratledge, 1979) indicated that it may not be a specific protein, in that reduction of ferrimycobactin could also be achieved by cell extracts from other microorganisms (*E. coli* and *Candida utilis*) besides mycobacteria. Even purified baker's yeast alcohol dehydrogenase, which contains 36 thiol groups per molecule, could reduce ferrimycobactin, suggesting that the reduction of iron may well be catalyzable by a number of enzymes. With this unpromising indication, further work on the reductase was abandoned.

Of possible relevance to the suggested role for salicylic acid in the transfer of iron from mycobactin or exochelin to heme or an apoprotein is the proposal that this could be the site of action of *p*-aminosalicylic acid (PAS). Brown and Ratledge (1975b) showed that PAS was always most effective against mycobacteria BCG and *M. smegmatis* when the intracellular concentration of salicylic acid was low. Furthermore, the metabolic consequences of PAS inhibition were very like those created by iron deficiency. It was concluded that the primary site of action of PAS could be at the transfer of Fe(II) from salicylate to some acceptor molecule (Fig. 4). Such a suggestion would then explain the specificity of PAS toward mycobacteria, as most other bacterial genera do not produce salicylate. Thus, by happenstance, there is already one antimycobacterial agent that acts by inhibiting iron metabolism.

Exochelin receptors: the iron-regulated envelope proteins

The uptake of ferri-siderophore complexes is known to be mediated by specific proteins that occur on the outer surfaces of microbial cells. These serve as physical receptors for the entire complex in order for it to be transported across the cell wall and membrane (Nikaido, 1993; Nikaido and Saier, 1992; Postle, 1990; Wooldridge et al., 1992; Zhou and van der Helm, 1993). These proteins, like all other components of the iron uptake systems, are found in increased amounts of cells that have been grown iron deficiently. They have now been recognized in a number of mycobacteria and have been characterized by using sodium dodecyl sulfate-polyacrylamide gel electrophoresis (SDS-PAGE) (Table 4). They are referred to here as iron-regulated envelope proteins (IREPs), as they can be recovered from both the wall (outer envelope) and the membrane (inner envelope) fractions (Hall et al., 1987; Sritharan and Ratledge, 1989, 1990). Prominent in all species examined is a 29-kDa protein. When antibodies to this protein isolated from *M. smegmatis* were raised (Hall et al., 1987), they subsequently prevented iron uptake into whole cells when ferriexochelin was presented. Antibodies raised to other IREPs (180, 84, and 25 kDa) were ineffective in stopping iron transport. Thus, the simple hypothesis is that the docking of ferriexochelin with its receptor (the 29-kDa IREP) was prevented by the antibody adhering to the IREP. A high specificity of siderophore for its receptor is therefore indicated.

The occurrence of the IREPs in mycobacteria is directly linked to the deprivation of iron from the cells (Kannan et al., unpublished data): their synthesis is not triggered by other deficiencies, such as, for example, zinc deficiency, where proteins of 32 and 65 kDa have been found in culture

Table 4. Occurrence of IREPs and HIPs as analyzed by SDS-PAGE in mycobacteria grown in vitro and in vivo[a]

Organism	HIPs of:		IREPs of:							
	250 kDa	240 kDa	180 kDa	120 kDa	84 kDa	29 kDa	25 kDa	21 kDa	14 kDa	11 kDa
M. smegmatis	*	*	+	−	+	+	+	−	+	−
M. neoaurum	*	*	+	*	−	+	−	+	+	−
ADM 8563	?	?	−	−	−	+	−	−	+	+
M. avium (in vitro)	*	*	+	−	−	+	−	+	+	−
M. avium (in vivo)	√	√	√	−	−	√	−	√	√	−
M. leprae (in vivo)	√	√	−	−	−	√	−	√	√	−

[a] Table is derived from work by Sritharan and Ratledge (1990). + and − denote the presence or absence of the IREP in iron deficiency-grown cells; *, presence of protein only in iron-sufficient cells; ?, very faint band, uncertain presence; √, present in vivo where iron status is uncertain; ADM, armadillo-derived mycobacterium.

filtrates (i.e., as extracellular proteins) of *M. tuberculosis* (De Bruyn et al., 1989). Nor are the IREPs heat shock proteins (Kannan et al., unpublished data), which are proteins associated with the cell's response to a sudden jump in temperature (Table 3) that might pertain in the initial stage of infection.

Since it is clearly impossible to recover exochelins from tissues infected with mycobacteria and since mycobactin has not been recovered from the cells recovered from various infected animals (Kato, 1985; Lambrecht and Collins, 1993), it is difficult to assert that the observations of iron transport in mycobacteria grown in vitro will necessarily apply to the in vivo situation. However, the IREPs have proved to be useful marker proteins for gauging what may be happening during mycobacterial infections.

By studying the same strain of *M. avium* grown both in the laboratory and in C57 mice, Sritharan and Ratledge (1990) were able to show the presence of IREPs of 180, 29, 21, and 14 kDa in the in vitro-grown bacteria and the appearance of proteins of the same sizes in the walls and membranes of the bacteria grown in vivo (Table 4). The 14- and 29-kDa proteins were particularly prominent in the wall fraction of in vivo mycobacteria. There is therefore a strong inference that the in vivo-grown mycobacteria have experienced an iron-deprived environment, which would account for the production of these IREP-like proteins. (The equivalence of the proteins from in vivo- and in vitro-grown *M. avium* is only presumptive at this stage.) Most curiously, however, two proteins (of 240 and 250 kDa) found only in cells grown under iron-sufficient conditions in laboratory media were also seen in *M. avium* recovered from the mouse liver (Sritharan and Ratledge, 1990). The presence of these two proteins indicates that the mycobacteria were not only iron deficient but also iron sufficient as well, a seeming contradiction. Similar proteins, both the high-molecular-weight high-iron proteins (HIPs) and the IREPs (29, 21, and 14 kDa), were also recognized in *M. leprae* recovered from infected armadillo livers (Sritharan and Ratledge, 1990) (Table 4).

An explanation for the simultaneous appearance of HIPs and "low-iron" proteins in the in vivo-grown mycobacteria can be proposed. This explanation may, if true, explain the iron status experienced by mycobacteria during infection. It has been suggested (Sritharan and Ratledge, 1990) that during the initial phase of infection, mycobacteria are probably deprived of iron principally in response to the nutritional immunity thought to be exercised by the host to ensure that all available iron is withheld from the invading bacteria (Kochan, 1973, 1976). Consequently, synthesis of all the components of iron uptake (exochelin, mycobactin, and the IREPs) may be coordinately expressed (Sritharan and Ratledge, 1989) under these conditions. However, because the exochelins are effective in gaining iron from transferrin, ferritin, etc. (Macham et al., 1975), the mycobacteria will quickly become iron replete and thus repress biosynthesis of the very molecules responsible for the assimilation of iron. Thus, the bacteria in vivo will be at the pivotal point of iron deprivation/iron sufficiency: the synthesis of the iron uptake components need never be extensive once the bacteria have established their niche. The uptake of iron will be at a rate sufficient to allow steady growth of the mycobacteria, but of course this is not a rampant infection as with other bacteria. Slow, steady growth of the bacilli will require participation of exochelins only in low quantities along with the attendant IREPs, but the cells will nevertheless "appear" to be almost iron sufficient. The absence of mycobactin in such cells (Lambrecht and Collins, 1993) may indicate merely that at the end of an infection, mycobacteria have acquired all the iron they could possibly need. What may have happened in the earlier stage of the infection remains an open question.

It also needs to be borne in mind that bacteria taken from an infected animal need not be all in the same nutritional state. If some are iron deprived and some are iron replete, as may occur in a tubercle, the simultaneous appearance of the HIPs along with the IREPs would be accounted for. HIPs may be produced in one set of cells and the IREPs may be produced by another set according to how the iron is available throughout the affected tissue.

Observations to date strongly suggest that mycobacteria, like other pathogens, are able to acquire iron from host sources of iron by the participation of specific siderophores, simultaneously requiring the presence of specific iron-regulated receptor proteins for the uptake of the iron-siderophore complex. Without exochelins, mycobacteria would not be able to overcome (Barclay and Ratledge, 1986a) the natural bacteriostatic effects of serum (Kochan, 1973, 1976; Kochan et al., 1971), which are attributed principally to the iron-withholding properties of transferrin. Interestingly, we (Barclay and Ratledge, 1986a) were able to show not only that the relief of the bacteriostatic effect of serum on *M. avium* and *M. paratuberculosis* required exochelin (or even mycobactin) but also that the mycobacteria for the inoculum had to be pregrown on low-iron medium. Under such conditions, the IREPs would be synthesized in increased amounts and would thus be able to function instantly with the added siderophore. Whether one of the IREPs (Table 4) could act as receptor for ferrimycobactin rather than ferriexochelin has not been examined, though mycobactin is clearly usable by mycobacteria if gratuiously supplied to them.

Conclusions: Prospects for Chemotherapy

Mycobacteria, like other pathogens, have developed highly coordinated systems for the acquisition of iron from the host. Although the host attempts to withhold iron from the pathogen by the process known as nutritional immunity (Kochan, 1973, 1976), successful pathogens such as *M. tuberculosis* are able to counter these defenses. It must be assumed that there are multiple mechanisms for uptake of iron in mycobacteria. It is highly unlikely that any organism relies on just one iron uptake system. *E. coli*, for example, possesses at least six different uptake systems (Nikaido, 1993; Nikaido and Saier, 1992; Wooldridge et al., 1992; Zhou and van der Helm, 1993), and though mycobacteria may not contain that many, the presence of several IREPs as putative siderophore receptors (Table 4) suggests a similar multiplicity of routes. Besides the uptake system described here for the major exochelins (Fig. 4), there exist separate transport processes for the uptake of ferric citrate (Messenger and Ratledge, 1982; Messenger et al., 1986) and even of ferric siderophores, such as ferrirhodotorulic acid, isolated from other organisms (Messenger and Ratledge, unpublished work).

Whether it is therefore possible to design an antitubercular agent that would prevent iron acquisition is an interesting proposition. As already mentioned above (Release of iron from exochelin and mycobactin), it is possible that PAS, the well-known and much-used antitubercular agent, exerts its inhibitory effect at some stage in iron metabolism (Brown and Ratledge, 1975b). PAS may be effective by acting at a point through which all iron, irrespective of its route of acquisition, must pass. Such a point could be the reductive assimilation into heme or apoproteins (Fig. 4). An alternative strategy would be to design an antimetabolite that would simultaneously inhibit all direct routes of iron uptake prior to the release and insertion of iron into cell components.

Attempts to use metal analogs (Sc, Y, W, Ga, Zr, etc.) of mycobactins and exochelins to inhibit growth of *M. tuberculosis* have been made (Barclay and Ratledge, 1986b) but without any significant success. Indeed, when metal complexes of an exochelin (from *M. intracellulare*) were used, these promoted rather than inhibited growth of *M. tuberculosis*. Presumably, the metal analog was displaced by iron during the incubation, and this change converted the potential inhibitor into a growth-promoting substance. Similar conclusions have been reached with other bacterial siderophores (Rogers et al., 1980, 1982), though here, because of the much shorter times of incubation (2 to 3 days compared to 42 days for *M. tuberculosis*), a greater initial success appeared to have occurred, as there was insufficient time for the metal analog to be displaced by iron. In long-term infections, however, metal analogs would probably prove ineffective agents because of the displacement of the analog by iron, which will always be the most tenaciously bound of all metal ions, as the siderophore has evolved to bind iron and not any other metal.

Bacterial iron metabolism remains an area of active research in many laboratories. Hopefully, this may provide the Achilles heel by which to attack the tubercle bacillus, but for the present, how this may be accomplished is not clear, though some opportunities are evidently being pursued with other bacteria (Miller, 1989; Miller and Malouin, 1993).

THE CELL ENVELOPE

The components of the mycobacterial envelope are well characterized, and their distribution in *M. tuberculosis* is elucidated elsewhere in this volume. Their arrangement has been partially elucidated, and physical restraints suggest limited possibilities for the structure of the entire envelope (Minnikin, 1991). A working model can be based on that of Minnikin (1991), whose proposal for an intercalating arrangement

of mycolic acids and other lipids in an outer barrier is now supported by recent X-ray diffraction studies of the wall of *M. chelonae* (Nikaido et al., 1993) (see chapter 19). However, hardly anything is known about cell envelope metabolism in any mycobacterium, let alone *M. tuberculosis*. Thus, we point to useful sources mainly with a view to stimulating research in this area.

The Plasma Membrane

The plasma membrane encloses the cytoplasmic contents and is the location of the extremely hydrophobic isoprenoid menaquinones (Minnikin, 1982; Ratledge, 1982a) and the rest of the respiratory system (Ratledge, 1982a). The lipid components are amphipathic lipids such as phospholipids and phosphatidylinositolmannosides that include fatty acyl chains usually 16 to 18 carbons long (Minnikin, 1982). It is important to note that the unusual long-chain acids, such as the multimethylated mycocerosates, cannot pack into the plasma membrane bilayer, though tuberculostearic acid (10-methyl stearate) is present in the plasma membrane. Indeed, the enzymatic methylation by *S*-methyladenosine of oleate (18:1*c*9) that yields tuberculostearate depends on the oleate being esterified to a phospholipid molecule (Akamatsu and Law, 1970).

Metabolic turnover of phospholipids can be demonstrated using spheroplasts from *M. smegmatis* (Dhariwal et al., 1978; Murty and Venkitasubramanian, 1984). In *M. microti* as well as in *M. leprae* and *M. avium*, phospholipase activity that hydrolyzed phosphatidylcholine had optimal activity when phosphatidylcholine was presented in mixed micelles, while phospholipase activity that hydrolyzed phosphatidylethanolamine had optimal activity only when high levels (5 mmol/liter) of Ca^{2+} were present (Wheeler and Ratledge, 1991, 1992). These differences could reflect the utilization of the predominantly host phosphatidylcho-

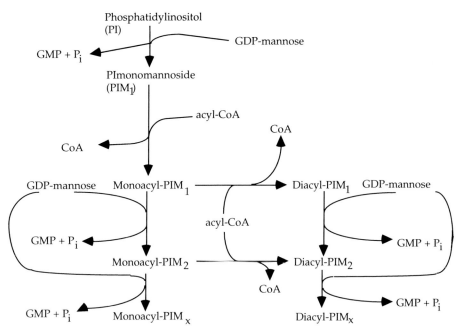

Figure 5. Possible biosynthetic pathways for phosphatidylinositolmannosides (PIM$_x$). PIM$_1$ is strictly an intermediate and does not accumulate.

line as a growth substrate and turnover of phosphatidylethanolamine, which occurs in mycobacterial plasma membranes.

Restricted to actinomycetes are the phosphatidylinositolmannosides (Minnikin and Goodfellow, 1980). It is characteristic that most of the research that led to the elucidation of the biochemical pathway for the biosynthesis of these molecules (Fig. 5) was done around 1970, using extracts from both *M. phlei* (Ballou, 1972) and *M. tuberculosis* (Takayama and Goldman, 1969, 1970). More recent findings show that phospholipid biosynthesis in general is affected by antibodies against phosphatidylinositolmannosides (Penumarti and Khuller, 1982), but such antibodies might have rather drastic, and probably pleiotropic, effects on the mycobacterial cell.

Finally, *M. tuberculosis* appears to lack the ability to regulate the fluidity of its plasma membrane. The classic mechanism operates in *M. phlei*: grown at low temperatures, it tends to have more saturated and therefore more fluid fatty acids in the 16- to 18-carbon range (Suntari and Laakso, 1993). Paradoxically, 18-carbon acids predominate at 10°C, while palmitate (16:0) predominates at 35°C, but the slight decrease in fluidity as a result of the additional two carbons would be outweighed by the prevalence of mono- and diunsaturated acids at 10°C. In contrast, there is no increase in unsaturated fatty acids in *M. tuberculosis*, and fatty acids of 24 to 26 carbons accumulate as mycolic acid biosynthesis breaks down and the tubercle bacilli die (Takayama et al., 1978a).

Peptidoglycan-Arabinogalactan

Peptidoglycan forms the basal layer of the cell wall to which arabinogalactan and, in turn, mycolate are covalently attached. The peptidoglycan in mycobacteria is of a type common in many bacteria (Draper, 1982) but with two slight differences. First, there are interpeptide linkages between two diaminopimelate residues as well as the usual D-alanyl-diaminopimelate linkages (Wietzerbin et al., 1975). Second, the usual N-acetylmuramic acid is replaced with N-glycolyl-muramic acid in *M. bovis* and in other mycobacteria (Azuma et al., 1970). Thus, peptidoglycan biosynthesis will probably prove to be similar to that in other bacteria, and those metabolic studies that have been carried out have concentrated on the unusual features of mycobacteria.

D D-Carboxypeptidase activity has been demonstrated in a membrane fraction of *M. smegmatis* (Eun et al., 1978). This enzyme breaks interpeptide bonds to enable new material to be inserted (mediated by enzymes not studied in mycobacteria) into growing cell walls. The enzyme is relatively insensitive to β-lactam antibiotics (Eun et al., 1978). However, it is a penicillin-binding protein and is most strongly inhibited by cefoxitin, a 7-α-methoxycephalosporin derivative (Basu et al., 1992). This property may be of general importance in mycobacteria; certainly, tubercle bacilli are resistant to penicillin, and the effectiveness only of 7-α-methoxycephalosporins was also clear in a detailed study of the susceptibility of *M. fortuitum* to β-lactams. Resistance of *M. tuberculosis* to β-lactams is partly due to the presence of a β-lactamase (Cynamon and Palmer, 1983), which can be induced (Zhang et al., 1992). However, more important may be the permeability of mycobacteria to β-lactams, which is very low (Jarlier et al., 1991). This low permeability is critical, because penicillin-binding proteins are located in the plasma membrane, so β-lactams must get through the cell wall permeability barrier to their site of action.

The enzymology underlying the insertion of N-glycolyl-muramic acid into peptidoglycan has not been studied. An approach that might be appropriate would be to make probes for *M. tuberculosis* DNA based on appropriate genes identified in muramic acid metabolism from other microbes, as these genes would be expected to have some sequence similarity in all bacteria. This approach should lead to cloning and characterizing the genes and then, it is hoped, elucidating the distinctive characteristics of the mycobacterial enzymes.

Almost nothing is known about the biosynthesis of the arabinogalactan, but the molecule has many distinctive motifs and an unusual region linking it to the peptidoglycan (McNeil and Brennan, 1991). A possible biosynthetic pathway features initial formation of N-acetylglucosamine-phosphoryl-polyprenol for the attachment of galactose and arabinose units (McNeil and Brennan, 1991). This seems feasible in light of the isolation of mannosylated phosphoryl-polyprenol in mycobacteria, including *M. tuberculosis* (Takayama and Goldman, 1969), and of the detection of a mannosyltransferase that transfers mannose residues to oligomannosides in an α 1→6-linked fashion (Yokoyama and Ballou, 1989). Interestingly, α 1→2 linkages in oligomannosides appear to be formed only when a mannosyltransferase acts on GDP-mannose as the mannosyl donor (Yokoyama and Ballou, 1989).

It seems probable that with complex and varied structures, including the saccharides, there will be several glycosyltransferases for each sugar to ensure correct linkage and placement of the sugars (Table 5). In this context, a further mannosyltransferase will be discussed below (see Methylated Mannose Oligosaccharides). A more general finding pertaining to arabinogalactan biosynthesis is the inhibition of incorporation of [^{14}C]glucose into arabinogalactan by ethambutol at 3 μg/ml, a pharmacological concentration (Takayama and Kilburn, 1989). Previously, this agent was thought to act on transfer of mycolate into the cell wall (Takayama and Armstrong, 1976), but inhibition of the transfer reaction is rationalized by there being less substrate, i.e., arabinan, for esterification by mycolate (Takayama and Kilburn, 1989). So far, the apparent primary effect of

Table 5. Mannosyltransferases detected in mycobacteria

Enzyme	Notes	Function	Reference(s)
GDP-mannose: polyprenol-1-P mannosyltransferase	Decaprenol-1-P is polyprenol principally used	Biosynthesis of mannosyl-phosphoryl-polyprenol	Takayama and Goldman, 1970
GDP-mannose: phosphatidylinositol mannosyltransferase	Not resolved; may be single enzyme	Biosynthesis of phosphatidylinositol mannosides with $\alpha\ 1\rightarrow2$ and $\alpha\ 1\rightarrow6$ linkages	Ballou, 1972; Takayama and Goldman, 1969
GDP-mannose:phosphatidylinositolmannoside mannosyltransferase	No involvement of polyprenol compounds	Biosynthesis of phosphatidylinositol mannosides with $\alpha\ 1\rightarrow2$ and $\alpha\ 1\rightarrow6$ linkages	
GDP-mannose: 3-O-methylmannoside mannosyltransferase	No polyprenol involvement; substrates are (Me-Man-OCH$_3$)$_{3-12}$; forms $\alpha\ 1\rightarrow4$ linkages	Biosynthesis of methylmannoside polysaccharide	Weisman and Ballou, 1984a
Mannosyl-phosphoryl-polyprenol:oligomannoside mannosyltransferase	Forms $\alpha\ 1\rightarrow6$ linkages	In mannan and arabinomannan biosynthesis, likely to be involved in synthesis of lipoarabinomannan and/or cell wall	Yokoyama and Ballou, 1989
GDP-mannose:oligomannoside mannosyltransferase	Forms $\alpha\ 1\rightarrow2$ linkages	In mannan and arabinomannan biosynthesis, likely to be involved in synthesis of lipoarabinomannan and/or cell wall	

ethambutol has been shown only in *M. smegmatis* (Takayama and Kilburn, 1989).

Biosynthesis and Attachment of Mycolic Acids

Mycolic acids are the outermost co-valently linked elements of the cell wall and thus the envelope. Each one is a β-hydroxy acid with an α side chain. The α side chain is a 24- or 26-carbon saturated fatty acyl chain, but the β-hydroxy acid is complex and long (up to 56 carbons) and may contain oxygen functions. This β-hydroxy acyl, or meromycolyl, unit gives different mycobacteria taxonomically distinct characteristics and characterizes the mycobacteria as a whole (Minnikin, 1982). Its attachment is specifically to terminal penta-arabinan motifs of the arabinogalactan, of which two-thirds are esterified (McNeil et al., 1991).

The first question related to metabolism in this section is, how do the mycolic acids get where they are? A possible mechanism for mycolate transfer with an enzyme, trehalose mycolyltransferase, purified from *M. smegmatis* (Sathyamoorthy and Takayama, 1987), has been shown in *M. tuberculosis* (Takayama and Armstrong, 1976) and *M. smegmatis* (Sathyamoorthy and Takayama, 1987). Though there has been no direct demonstration of this enzyme participating in the transfer of mycolate into cell wall, it is anticipated that it would have this activity, as it does not have mycolylhydrolase activity (Sathyamoorthy and Takayama, 1987). It is therefore not a catabolic enzyme and is thus presumably involved in anabolism. Another candidate for involvement in organizing the transfer of mycolate into the cell wall must be a recently discovered lectin (Kundu et al., 1991). Isolated and characterized from *M. smegmatis* but widely distributed, it binds strongly and specifically to mycobacterial arabinogalactan (Kundu et al., 1991). If it could also bind to mycolyltransferase, it might somehow have a role in directing mycolate placement in the cell wall.

Biosynthesis of mycolic acids themselves is an area of considerable research interest. However, establishing the essential starting point—a cell-free system—for sustained enzymology has been something of a holy grail for lipid biochemists. In one remarkable series of experiments, fatty acid-synthesizing and -elongating activities in soluble material from extracts of *M. tuberculosis* made fatty acids of up to 56 carbons but no mycolic acids (Qureshi et al., 1984). The breakthrough came by using a cell-free, principally cell wall extract (Lacave et al., 1990a). The material that catalyzed incorporation of [^{14}C]acetate into mycolates was shown by electron microscopy to contain discernible wall fragments (Lacave et al., 1990a) that could conceivably retain some of the structural organization of the intact organism. In our hands, similar material purified further on a Percoll gradient (Wheeler et al., 1993b) contained wall and at least some membrane material, as phosphatidylinositolmannoside and phosphatidylmannoside were present (Chatterjee, personal communication).

Deducing the biosynthetic pathways for mycolic acids remains an enormous challenge. However, there is now very strong evidence that the point of divergence from fatty acid biosynthesis in general is at the 24-carbon level, with principally a ω-19 acid, 24:1 *cis*-5, being elongated (Fig. 6). ω-19 acids have been detected at low concentrations in lipid extracts of mycobacteria including *M. tuberculosis* (Couderc et al., 1988; Takayama et al., 1972) and these acids correspond structurally to the methyl terminus of the meromycolate chain of native mycolic acids. The first clue that they were the building blocks for mycolates was the demonstration that when mycobacterial walls were incubated with labeled acetate and the resulting mycolate was extracted and oxidized to fragment the meromycolate chain at its double bonds, the methyl terminus and the next 18 C atoms were virtually unlabeled (Lacave et al., 1990b), indicating an endogenous ω-19 precursor. This reaction has now been demonstrated in an adaptation of the classical fatty-acyl elongase assay (Wheeler et al., 1993b). When wall material was extracted with hexane to remove endogenous fatty acids (an essential step), synthetic 24:1 *cis*-5 (Besra et al., 1993) significantly stimulated the incorporation of labeled acetate into mycolic acids, while a range of other acids, even some 24-carbon acids, had no effect (Wheeler et al., 1993b). Interestingly, a cyclopropenyl analog of the *cis*-5 acid appeared to be a specific inhibitor (Wheeler et al., 1993a), and although a high concentration of the analog (1 mg/ml in the hexane phase of a two-phase mycolate-synthesizing assay) was required, it may be that suitably de-

signed analogs will eventually lead to the effective inhibition of mycobacterial cell wall biosynthesis.

There remain to be solved problems in elucidating the early steps in the biosynthesis of mycolic acids. For example, it would be useful to show direct incorporation of appropriate labeled fatty acids such as 24:1 *cis*-5 into mycolic acids. The carrier molecule must be identified, since free fatty acids cannot function in these enzyme systems. CoA is the usual carrier, but it does not function in these cell-free assays (Lacave et al., 1990b; Wheeler et al., 1993b). Further, it is not known how mycobacteria synthesize 24:1 *cis*-5; frustratingly, a 24:0 desaturase has been characterized, but its product is the ubiquitous 24:1 *cis*-15 acid nervonic acid (Kikuchi and Kusaka, 1986). Finally, an assay for mycolate biosynthesis

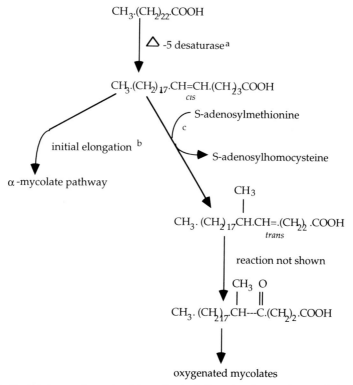

Figure 6. Early dedicated stages of mycolate biosynthesis. [a], Speculated—reaction sought but not shown; [b], see Wheeler et al., 1993b; [c], methylation reaction shown but not for 24:1 *cis*-5.

in *M. tuberculosis* itself remains to be devised.

α-Mycolate, which contains double bonds or cyclopropane rings as its only functional groups, is not a precursor of the more complex oxygenated mycolates. The dissociation of their biosynthesis was shown in synchronized cultures of *M. aurum*, in which label could appear in ketomycolate before α-mycolate (Lacave et al., 1989). Thus, any common intermediate must be at an early stage in biosynthesis (Fig. 6). For this, 24:1 *cis*-5 is a good candidate; judging from the structure of oxygenated mycolates, it would be expected to be oxidized and methylated to a 5-keto, 6-methyl, 24-carbon precursor (Besra et al., 1993). An assay for biosynthesis of oxygenated mycolates needs to be developed to test this hypothesis.

So far, we have concentrated on the early steps in mycolate biosynthesis. Deducing further stages in the pathways will depend on identifying intermediates, which do not substantially accumulate in cell-free assays done with *M. smegmatis* (Wheeler et al., 1993b). Mutants that are impaired in their abilities to synthesize mycolates will be useful. Prospects look good: there can be bacterial life without mycolates, as shown by the existence of mycolateless strains of actinomycetes (Embley et al., 1988). Also, one mutant of *M. smegmatis* that fails to make mycolate and synthesizes only the unbranched meromycolates has been isolated (Kundu et al., 1989). This mutant strain is, however, undoubtedly weakened, as it is particularly sensitive to penicillin (Kundu et al., 1989).

The starting 24- and 26-carbon fatty acids are synthesized by fatty acid synthases and elongases. In *M. tuberculosis*, these functions are linked in a multifunctional enzyme system that appears to be a de novo synthase (making principally 16-carbon acids from the 2-carbon acetyl-CoA) joined to an elongase that takes the 16-carbon acid and elongates it to 24 or 26 carbons (Kikuchi et al., 1992). It is speculated that this 500-kDa complex is a gene fusion product also found in *M. smegmatis*. These recent findings contrast with earlier isolation of separable activities for de novo fatty acid synthase (a 290-kDa multifunctional enzyme in *M. smegmatis*) and fatty acyl elongase in *M. smegmatis* (Rastogi, 1991) and *M. tuberculosis* (Medhi et al., 1979). A further complication is that the 500-kDa complex has no role for acyl carrier protein. Previous studies (Rastogi, 1991), including those of *M. tuberculosis* (Medhi et al., 1979), had suggested at least a partial role for separable functional enzymes linked to acyl carrier protein in fatty acyl elongation. Perhaps different strains, BCG (Kikuchi et al., 1992) and H37Rv (Medhi et al., 1979), which were used in these studies, express different enzymes for fatty acid metabolism; there is much to be learned from a genetic approach.

Predominantly 24-carbon acids accumulate in the presence of isoniazid (Takayama et al., 1978b). It has been suggested that at the pharmacological level of 0.5 μg/ml against *M. tuberculosis*, the agent exerts its effect on a Δ5 desaturase (discussed above). In *M. aurum*, a Schiffs base forms between isoniazid (incubated at 10 μg/ml) and the target enzyme, so that its effect becomes irreversible (Quemard et al., 1991). In all mycobacteria studied, isoniazid prevents mycolic acid biosynthesis. In *M. tuberculosis*, incubation at 15°C has an effect similar to that of isoniazid (Takayama et al., 1978a). Thus, while *M. smegmatis* regulates both the fluidity of its plasma membrane (see The Plasma Membrane) and its outer, mycolic acid-based permeability barrier by the classic method of increasing desaturation and, with the mycolates, decreasing the chain length at low temperatures (Toriyama et al., 1978), *M. tuberculosis* fails to regulate either and also fails to synthesize mycolic acids at all at low tem-

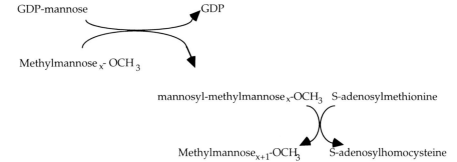

Figure 7. Biosynthesis of methylmannose polysaccharide. x = 3 to 12.

perature, with lethal consequences (Taka-yama et al., 1978a).

Methylated Mannose Oligosaccharides: Biosynthesis and Role in Fatty Acid Metabolism

Two classes of polysaccharide, based on 6-*O*-methylglucose and 3-*O*-methylman-nose, are found in all mycobacteria so far studied (Weisman and Ballou, 1984a). Their presence in *M. tuberculosis* is suggested by the isolation of a fatty acid synthase-stimu-lating factor that is polysaccharidic in na-ture (Medhi et al., 1979). Their role has been reviewed in detail by Ratledge (1982a). Briefly, they can relieve feedback inhibition of fatty acid synthase caused by fatty acyl-CoA by forming complexes with fatty acyl-CoA. By forming complexes and influencing the reaction rate of transacy-lases that release fatty acyl-CoAs from syn-thases, they have a powerful influence on the distribution of fatty acid chain length. To have these clear regulatory roles, the polysaccharides must be located in the cytoplasm, as this is where fatty acid syn-thases are found (Sathyamoorthy and Takayama, 1987; Kikuchi et al., 1992), and indeed, that is where the enzymes for their biosynthesis are located. The en-zymes for biosynthesis of the 3-*O*-methyl-mannose-based polysaccharide have been characterized (Fig. 7). First, an α 1→4 mannosyltransferase transfers mannose

from GDP-mannose to the growing saccha-ride chain (Weisman and Ballou, 1984a). Then the added mannose residue is methy-lated by a 3-*O*-methyltransferase that uses *S*-adenosylmethionine as methyl donor (Weisman and Ballou, 1984b). The consis-tent biosynthesis of 10- to 13-mer polysac-charides is attained by inhibition of the methyltransferase by palmitoyl-CoA when the potential polysaccharide substrate is 12 or more residues long (Weisman and Bal-lou, 1984b) and when it becomes func-tional, readily forming complexes with fatty acids and fatty acyl-CoA. The specificity of the mannosyltransferase for methylman-nose polysaccharide ensures that promiscu-ous formation of α 1→4 links does not occur (Weisman and Ballou, 1984a). How chain initiation occurs is still unresolved, since oligosaccharides with three or fewer residues are not substrates for this man-nosyltransferase (Weisman and Ballou, 1984a). Less is known about the biosynthe-sis of the 6-*O*-methylglucose-based poly-saccharides and lipopolysaccharides, but a similar mechanism appears to be involved, with the sequential addition of methyl groups derived from *S*-adenosylmethionine to preformed D-glucan (Walton and Jordan, 1988). The unusual α 1→4 linkages formed in both polysaccharides result in a helical polysaccharide that is the correct shape for complexing fatty acids and their CoA es-ters.

Biosynthesis of Envelope Components on the Mycobacterial Surface

The main components exposed on the surface of *M. tuberculosis* are lipoarabinomannan, sulfolipid, possibly cord factor, and phthiocerol dimycocerosate and, in most strains, its phenolic glycosylated form, phenolic glycolipid (see chapter 15). Lipoarabinomannan is a phosphatidylinositolpolysaccharide, and the structure of its phosphatidylinositol moiety indicates that it is anchored in the plasma membrane, while its terminal sugars, recognized by antibody and concanavalin A, are at the microbial surface (Hunter and Brennan, 1990).

Little is known about the metabolism of these surface components. Evidently, metabolism of these exotic lipids and glycolipids by the host is difficult if not impossible, as they can accumulate in mice following mycobacterial infections (Kondo and Kanai, 1972). Nothing is known about the biosynthesis of the first two components mentioned above. However, an intriguing property of lipoarabinomannan is that it contains a penta-arabinan motif identical to that found at the terminus of the cell wall arabinogalactan. This opens up two interesting areas of metabolism to investigate. First, similar enzymes must be involved in synthesizing this motif in two different locations in the envelope. Second, the enzyme for transferring mycolate to the cell wall must be able to distinguish penta-arabinan in arabinogalactan, the destination of mycolate, from penta-arabinan in lipoarabinomannan, which is not acylated.

Cord factor, trehalose dimycolate, is synthesized by the mycolyltransferase mentioned above (Sathyamoorthy and Takayama, 1987). The absence of trehalose dimycolate but the presence of trehalose monomycolate in *M. leprae* led to the suggestion that the former product accumulated only during periods of metabolic imbalance; otherwise, trehalose mycolates

were seen as being solely intermediates in cell wall assembly (Dhariwal et al., 1987) and turnover (Winder et al., 1972).

Parts of the biosynthetic pathway of phthiocerol dimycocerosate and the further phenolic glycolipid product have been elucidated. The enzyme for biosynthesis of the mycocerosate moieties has been purified (Rainwater and Kollatukudy, 1985), cloned, and sequenced (Mathur and Kollatukudy, 1992). Like the fatty acid synthase (Kikuchi et al., 1992), mycocerosate synthase is a multifunctional enzyme with domains that are recognized as being involved in fatty acid elongation (Mathur and Kollatukudy, 1992). Its unusual features are its substrate specificity for methyl-malonyl-CoA; an acyl carrier protein-like domain that is usually associated with aggregated enzyme systems such as those used for fatty acid biosynthesis in *E. coli*; and the product, 2,4,6,8-tetramethyloctacosanoate (mycocerosate), which remains bound to the pure enzyme. The role of the acyl carrier protein-like domain may be in binding the product, and there is no thioesterase domain to release the product. It seems likely that this arrangement prevents promiscuous acylation of lipids with mycocerosate. A specific thioesterase probably catalyzes the following reactions:

synthase-mycocerosate +

phthiocerol → phthiocerolmycocerosate +

synthase

synthase-mycocerosate +

phthiocerolmycocerosate →

phthioceroldimycocerosate + synthase

Methyl-malonyl-CoA is generated by the same acyl-CoA carboxylase that generates malonyl-CoA for straight-chain fatty acid elongation in *M. tuberculosis* (Rainwater and Kollatukudy, 1982). Mycobacteria that do not synthesize mycocerosates have acyl-CoA carboxylases with similar specificities (Wheeler et al., 1992), so the control in production of methyl-malonyl-CoA and malonyl-CoA must be in the availability of the respective substrates, propionyl-CoA and acetyl-CoA. Acyl-CoA carboxylase is also under metabolic control, its activity being depressed when mycobacteria are grown in media with a supply of lipids, when biotin is limited, or in the host (Wheeler et al., 1992). Depression of this activity is a way of avoiding wastefully synthesizing fatty acids when they can be scavenged, but the enzyme activity must presumably be sufficient to generate methyl-malonyl-CoA, as phthiocerol dimycocerosate-based lipids are readily found in host-grown tubercle (Kanai et al., 1970; Kondo and Kanai, 1972) as well as in leprosy bacilli (Cho et al., 1986).

IN CONCLUSION: METABOLIC STUDIES AND RATIONAL DESIGNS FOR VIABILITY ESTIMATION

We hope that in this chapter we have been able to show that the study of general metabolism provides an integrated view of mycobacteria and what the immune system sees of them. There are many interesting and important implications for the new field of mycobacterial genetics: the complex organization of these microbes demands multiple genes for fatty acid biosynthesis and seemingly innumerable glycosyltransferase genes. The data given in Table 5 must only be a start.

As enzymes that are drug targets are identified, they will no doubt be used as drug screens. However, more general metabolic activities can give an estimate of viability and thus can be used as rather general drug screens. Many proposed methods applicable to *M. leprae* have been reviewed before (Barclay and Wheeler, 1989). Metabolic activities can also be used in this way with *M. tuberculosis*. The BACTEC system, which allows growth of *M.*

tuberculosis to be demonstrated within a week, relies on one of its most readily detectable metabolic activities, the oxidation of palmitate to release CO_2. Palmitate oxidation can also be exploited in *M. leprae*, even though it is not growing; the BACTEC radiorespirometric assay can be used for drug screening, and a Buddemeyer-type system is even more efficient, giving rapid results (7 days) with 10^6 to 10^7 leprosy bacilli (Franzblau et al., 1992). The product of coupled oxidative metabolism is ATP. ATP can be measured directly (Barclay and Wheeler, 1989) or indirectly and ingeniously in *M. tuberculosis* by incubating drug, bacteria, and, after just 48 h of growth, a luciferase reporter phage. About 4 h later, resistant or untreated bacteria light up, as they have produced ATP; susceptible bacteria do not give a light signal (Jacobs et al., 1993).

A final illustration of the use of studies of metabolism in devising viability estimations and drug screens comes from the incorporation of labeled purines and pyrimidines into nucleic acids. Since thymidine is incorporated into DNA and not RNA, its incorporation might be an excellent viability correlate. This activity can be used, but for good biochemical reasons, it is slow and insensitive. Thymidine kinase is difficult to detect in mycobacteria (Wheeler, 1990), and thymidine is even more slowly incorporated than thymine in *M. avium*, *M. leprae*, *M. microti* (Wheeler, 1990), *M. tuberculosis* (Hiriyanna and Ramakrishnan, 1986), and *M. phlei* (Somogyi and Foldes, 1983). Uracil is more rapidly incorporated (Somogyi and Foldes, 1983; Wheeler, 1990), but purines appear to be the ideal substrate for nucleic acids. Adenosine is most rapidly incorporated of all the precursors, both by suspensions of mycobacteria (at 20 times the rate of thymidine in the case of *M. leprae* [Wheeler, 1987b]) and by leprosy bacilli resident in macrophages (Harshan et al., 1990). Rapid adenosine incorporation is not surprising: adenosine kinase is one of the easiest enzymes to detect in mycobacteria, even in extracts from *M. leprae* treated with sodium hydroxide to abolish any activities that might be adsorbed from the host (Wheeler, 1987b).

Our final comment must therefore be to emphasize the importance of metabolic studies not only in understanding the biology of mycobacteria but also in the application of applied scientific methods.

Acknowledgment. P.R.W. thanks K. Takayama for invaluable help on the literature concerning mannosyltransferases and its implications.

REFERENCES

Agiato Foster, L. A., and D. W. Dyer. 1993. A siderophore production mutant of *Bordetella bronchiseptica* cannot use lactoferrin as an iron source. *Infect. Immun.* **61:**2698–2702.

Akamatsu, Y., and J. H. Law. 1970. Enzymic alkylenation of phospholipid fatty acid chain by extracts of *Mycobacterium phlei. J. Biol. Chem.* **245:**701–708.

Azuma, I., D. W. Thomas, A. Adam, J. M. Ghuysen, R. Bonaly, J. F. Petit, and G. Lederer. 1970. Occurrence of N-glycolylmuramic acid in bacterial cell walls. *Biochim. Biophys. Acta* **208:**444–451.

Bagg, A., and J. B. Neilands. 1987. Molecular mechanism of siderophore-mediated iron assimilation. *Microbiol. Rev.* **51:**509–530.

Ballou, C. E. 1972. Biosynthesis of mannophosphoinositides in *Mycobacterium phlei. Methods Enzymol.* **28:**493–500.

Barclay, R., D. E. Ewing, and C. Ratledge. 1985. Isolation, identification and structural analysis of the mycobactins of *Mycobacterium avium, M. intracellulare, M. scrofulaceum,* and *M. paratuberculosis. J. Bacteriol.* **164:**896–905.

Barclay, R., and C. Ratledge. 1983. Iron-binding compounds of *Mycobacterium avium, M. intracellulare, M. scrofulaceum,* and mycobactin-dependent *M. paratuberculosis* and *M. avium. J. Bacteriol.* **153:**1138–1146.

Barclay, R., and C. Ratledge. 1986a. Participation of iron in the growth inhibition of pathogenic strain of *Mycobacterium avium* and *M. paratuberculosis* in serum. *Zentralbl. Bakteriol. Hyg. A* **262:**189–194.

Barclay, R., and C. Ratledge. 1986b. Metal analogues of mycobactin and exochelin fail to act as effective antimycobacterial agents. *Zentralbl. Bakteriol. Hyg. A* **264:**203–207.

Barclay, R., and C. Ratledge. 1988. Mycobactins and exochelins of *Mycobacterium tuberculosis, M. bo-*

vis, M. africanum and other related strains. *J. Gen. Microbiol.* **134:**771–776.

Barclay, R., and P. R. Wheeler. 1989. Metabolism of mycobacteria in tissues, p. 37–196. *In* C. Ratledge, J. Stanford, and J. M. Grange (ed.), *The Biology of the Mycobacteria,* vol. 3. Academic Press, London.

Basu, J., R. Chattopadhyay, M. Kundu, and P. Chakrabarti. 1992. Purification and partial characterization of a penicillin-binding protein from *Mycobacterium smegmatis. J. Bacteriol.* **174:**4829–4832.

Bercovier, H., O. Kafri, and S. Sela. 1986. Mycobacteria possess a surprisingly small number of RNA genes in relation to the size of their genome. *Biochem. Biophys. Res. Commun.* **136:**1136–1141.

Besra, G. S., D. E. Minnikin, P. R. Wheeler, and C. Ratledge. 1993. Synthesis of methyl (Z)-tetracos-5-enoate and both enantiomers of ethyl (E)-6-methyltetracos-4-enoate; possible intermediates in the biosynthesis of mycolic acids in mycobacteria. *Chem. Phys. Lipids* **66:**23–34.

Braun, V. 1990. Genetics of siderophore biosynthesis and transport, p. 103–129. *In* H. Kleinkauf and H. von Döhren (ed.), *Biochemistry of Peptide Antibiotics.* de Gruyter, Berlin.

Brown, K. A., and C. Ratledge. 1975a. Iron transport in *Mycobacterium smegmatis:* ferrimycobactin reductase (NAD(P)H:ferrimycobactin oxidoreductase), the enzyme releasing iron from its carrier. *FEBS Lett.* **53:**262–266.

Brown, K. A., and C. Ratledge. 1975b. The effect of *p*-aminosalicylic acid on iron transport and assimilation in mycobacteria. *Biochim. Biophys. Acta* **385:**207–220.

Chatterjee, D. Personal communication.

Chicurel, M., E. Garcia, and F. Goodsaid. 1988. Modulation of macrophage lysosomal pH by *Mycobacterium tuberculosis*-derived proteins. *Infect. Immun.* **56:**479–483.

Cho, S. N., S. W. Hunter, R. H. Gelber, T. H. Rea, and P. J. Brennan. 1986. Quantification of the phenolic glycolipid and relevance to glycolipid antigenemia in leprosy. *J. Infect. Dis.* **153:**560–569.

Couderc, F., H. Aurelle, D. Prome, A. Savagnac, and J. C. Prome. 1988. Analysis of fatty acids by negative ion gas chromatography/tandem mass spectrometry: structural correlations between α-mycolic acid chains and Δ-5-monounsaturated acids in *Mycobacterium phlei. Biomed. Environ. Mass Spectrom.* **16:**317–321.

Cynamon, M. H., and G. S. Palmer. 1983. In vitro activity of amoxicillin in combination with clavulanic acid against *Mycobacterium tuberculosis. Antimicrob. Agents Chemother.* **24:**429–431.

De Bruyn, J., R. Bosmano, J. Nyabenda, and J. P. van Vooren. 1989. Effect of zinc deficiency on the appearance of two immunodominant protein antigens

(32 kDa and 65 kDa) in culture filtrates of mycobacteria. *J. Gen. Microbiol.* **135**:79–84.

Dhariwal, K. R., A. Chander, and T. A. Venkitasubramanian. 1976. Alterations in lipid constituents during growth of *Mycobacterium smegmatis* CDC46 and *Mycobacterium phlei. Microbios* **16**:169–182.

Dhariwal, K. R., A. Chander, and T. A. Venkitasubramanian. 1978. Turnover of lipids in *Mycobacterium smegmatis* CDC 46 and *Mycobacterium phlei* ATCC 354. *Arch. Microbiol.* **116**:69–75.

Dhariwal, K. R., Y. M. Yang, H. M. Fildes, and M. B. Goren. 1987. Detection of trehalose monomycolate in *Mycobacterium leprae* grown in armadillo liver. *J. Gen. Microbiol.* **133**:201–209.

Draper, P. 1982. The anatomy of mycobacteria, p. 9–52. *In* C. Ratledge and J. L. Stanford (ed.), *Biology of the Mycobacteria*, vol. 1. Academic Press, Inc. (London) Ltd., London.

Embley, T. M., A. G. O'Donnell, J. Rostron, and M. Goodfellow. 1988. Chemotaxonomy of wall type IV actinomycetes which lack mycolic acids. *J. Gen. Microbiol.* **134**:953–960.

Eun, H. M., A. Yapo, and J.-F. Petit. 1978. D D-carboxypeptidase activity of membrane fragments of *Mycobacterium smegmatis*. Enzymic properties and sensitivity to β-lactam antibiotics. *Eur. J. Biochem.* **86**:97–103.

Franzblau, S. G., A. N. Biswas, P. Jenner, and M. J. Colston. 1992. Double-blind evaluation of BACTEC and Buddemeyer-type radiorespirometric assays for in vitro screening of antileprosy agents. *Lepr. Rev.* **63**:125–133.

Frehel, C., N. Rastogi, J. C. Benichou, and A. Ryter. 1988. Do test-tube grown pathogenic mycobacteria possess a protective capsule? *FEMS Microbiol. Lett.* **56**:225–230.

Frehel, C., A. Ryter, N. Rastogi, and H. L. David. 1986. The electron-transparent zone in phagocytosed *Mycobacterium avium* and other mycobacteria: formation, persistence and role in bacterial survival. *Ann. Inst. Pasteur (Microbiol.)* **137B**:239–257.

Griffiths, E. 1987. The iron-uptake systems of pathogenic bacteria, p. 69–138. *In* J. J. Bullen and E. Griffiths (ed.), *Iron and Infection: Molecular, Physiological and Clinical Aspects*. John Wiley & Sons, Chichester, United Kingdom.

Hall, R. M. 1986. Mycobactins: how to obtain them and how to employ them as chemotaxonomic characters for the mycobacteria and related organisms. *Actinomycetes* **19**:92–106.

Hall, R. M., and C. Ratledge. 1984. Mycobactins as chemotaxonomic characters for some rapidly growing mycobacteria. *J. Gen. Microbiol.* **130**:1883–1892.

Hall, R. M., and C. Ratledge. 1987. Exochelin-mediated iron acquisition by the leprosy bacillus, *Myco*-
bacterium leprae. J. Gen. Microbiol. **133**:193–199.

Hall, R. M., M. Sritharan, A. J. M. Messenger, and C. Ratledge. 1987. Iron transport in *Mycobacterium smegmatis*: occurrence of iron-regulated envelope proteins as potential receptors for iron uptake. *J. Gen. Microbiol.* **133**:2107–2114.

Harrison, P. M., S. C. Andrews, G. C. Ford, J. M. A. Smith, A. Treffry, and J. L. White. 1987. Ferritin and bacterioferritin: iron sequestering molecules from man to microbe, p. 445–475. *In* G. Winkelmann, D. van der Helm, and J. B. Neilands (ed.), *Iron Transport in Microbes, Plants and Animals.* VCH mbH, Weinheim, Germany.

Harshan, K. V., A. Mittal, H. K. Prasad, R. S. Misra, N. K. Chopra, and I. Nath. 1990. Uptake of purine and pyrimidine nucleosides by macrophage-resident *Mycobacterium leprae*: ^{3}H-adenosine as an indication of viability and antimicrobial activity. *Int. J. Lepr.* **58**:526–533.

Harshey, R. M., and T. Ramakrishnan. 1976. Purification and properties of DNA-dependent RNA polymerase from *Mycobacterium tuberculosis* H37Rv. *Biochim. Biophys. Acta* **432**:49–59.

Harvey, R. J., and A. L. Koch. 1980. How partially inhibitory concentrations of chloramphenicol affect the growth of *Escherichia coli. Antimicrob. Agents Chemother.* **18**:323–327.

Hiriyanna, K. T., and T. Ramakrishnan. 1986. DNA replication time in *Mycobacterium tuberculosis* H37Rv. *Arch. Microbiol.* **144**:105–109.

Hunter, S. W., and P. J. Brennan. 1990. Evidence for the presence of a phosphatidylinositol anchor on the lipoarabinomannan and lipomannan of *Mycobacterium tuberculosis. J. Biol. Chem.* **265**:9272–9279.

Husson, M. D., D. Legrand, G. Spik, and H. Leclerc. 1993. Iron acquisition by *Helicobacter pylori*: importance of human lactoferrin. *Infect. Immun.* **61**:2694–2697.

Jacobs, W. R., R. G. Barletta, R. Udani, G. Kalkut, G. Souse, T. Kieser, G. F. Hatfull, and B. R. Bloom. 1993. Rapid assessment of drug susceptibilities of *Mycobacterium tuberculosis* by means of luciferase reporter phages. *Science* **260**:819–822.

Jarlier, V., L. Gutmann, and H. Nikaido. 1991. Interplay of cell wall barrier and β-lactamase activity determines high resistance to β-lactam antibiotics in *Mycobacterium chelonae. Antimicrob. Agents Chemother.* **35**:1937–1939.

Jarlier, V., and H. Nikaido. 1990. Permeability barrier to hydrophilic solutes in *Mycobacterium chelonei. J. Bacteriol.* **172**:1418–1423.

Kanai, K., E. Wiegeshaus, and D. W. Smith. 1970. Demonstration of mycolic acid and phthiocerol dimycocerosate in "in vivo grown tubercle bacilli." *Jpn. J. Med. Sci. Biol.* **23**:327–333.

Kannan, K. B., L. G. Dover, and C. Ratledge. Unpublished data.

Kato, L. 1985. Absence of mycobactin in *Mycobacterium leprae*; probably a microbe dependent microorganism implications. *Int. J. Lepr.* **57**:58–70.

Kell, D. B. 1987. Forces, fluxes and the control of microbial growth and metabolism. *J. Gen. Microbiol.* **133**:1651–1665.

Kikuchi, K., D. L. Rainwater, and P. E. Kolattukudy. 1992. Purification and characterization of an unusually large fatty acid synthase from *Mycobacterium tuberculosis* var. bovis BCG. *Arch. Biochem. Biophys.* **295**:318–326.

Kikuchi, S., and T. Kusaka. 1986. Isolation and partial characterization of a fatty acid desaturation system from the cytosol of *Mycobacterium smegmatis*. *J. Biochem.* **99**:723–731.

Koch, A. L. 1971. The adaptive responses of *Escherichia coli* to a feast and famine existence. *Adv. Microb. Physiol.* **6**:147–217.

Kochan, I. 1973. The role of iron in bacterial infections with special consideration of host-tubercle bacillus interaction. *Curr. Top. Microbiol. Immunol.* **60**:1–30.

Kochan, I. 1976. Role of iron in the regulation of nutritional immunity. *Bioorg. Chem.* **2**:55–57.

Kochan, I., N. R. Pellis, and C. A. Golden. 1971. Mechanism of tuberculostasis in mammalian serum. III. Neutralization of serum tuberculostasis by mycobactin. *Infect. Immun.* **3**:553–558.

Kondo, E., and K. Kanai. 1972. Further demonstration of bacterial lipids in *Mycobacterium bovis* harvested from infected mouse lungs. *Jpn. J. Med. Sci. Biol.* **25**:249–257.

Kundu, M., J. Basu, and P. Chakrabarti. 1989. Purification and characterization of an extracellular lectin from *Mycobacterium smegmatis*. *FEBS Lett.* **256**:207–210.

Kundu, M., J. Basu, and P. Chakrabarti. 1991. Defective mycolic acid metabolism in mutant of *Mycobacterium smegmatis*. *J. Gen. Microbiol.* **137**:2197–2200.

Lacave, C., M.-A. Laneelle, M. Daffe, H. Montrozier, and G. Laneelle. 1989. Mycolic acid filiation and location in *Mycobacterium aurum* and *Mycobacterium phlei*. *Eur. J. Biochem.* **181**:459–466.

Lacave, C., M. A. Laneelle, and G. Laneelle. 1990a. Mycolic acid synthesis by *Mycobacterium aurum* cell-free extracts. *Biochim. Biophys. Acta* **1042**:315–323.

Lacave, C., A. Quemard, and G. Laneelle. 1990b. Cell-free synthesis of mycolic acids in *Mycobacterium aurum*: radioactivity distribution in newly synthesized acids and presence of cell wall in the system. *Biochim. Biophys. Acta* **1045**:58–65.

Lambrecht, R. S., and M. T. Collins. 1992. *Mycobacterium tuberculosis* factors that influence mycobactin dependence. *Diagn. Microbiol. Infect. Dis.* **15**:239–246.

Lambrecht, R. S., and M. T. Collins. 1993. Inability to detect mycobactin in Mycobacteria-infected tissues

suggests an alternative iron acquisition mechanism by Mycobacteria *in vivo*. *Microb. Pathog.* **14**:229–238.

Lindquist, S. 1986. The heat shock response. *Annu. Rev. Biochem.* **55**:1151–1192.

Macham, L. P., and C. Ratledge. 1975. A new group of water-soluble iron-binding compounds from mycobacteria: the exochelins. *J. Gen. Microbiol.* **89**:379–382.

Macham, L. P., C. Ratledge, and J. C. Nocton. 1975. Extracellular iron acquisition by mycobacteria: role of the exochelins and evidence against the participation of mycobactin. *Infect. Immun.* **12**:1242–1251.

Macham, L. P., M. C. Stephenson, and C. Ratledge. 1977. Iron transport in *Mycobacterium smegmatis*: the isolation, purification and function of exochelin MS. *J. Gen. Microbiol.* **101**:41–49.

Mathur, M., and P. E. Kolattukudy. 1992. Molecular cloning and sequencing of the gene for mycocerosic acid synthase, a novel fatty acid-elongating multifunctional enzyme, from *Mycobacterium tuberculosis* BCG. *J. Bacteriol.* **267**:19388–19395.

McCready, K. A., and C. Ratledge. 1977. Unpublished data.

McCready, K. A., and C. Ratledge. 1979. Ferrimycobactin reductase activity from *Mycobacterium smegmatis*. *J. Gen. Microbiol.* **113**:67–72.

McKenna, W. R., P. A. Mickelsen, P. F. Sparling, and D. W. Dyer. 1988. Iron uptake from lactoferrin and transferrin by *Neisseria gonorrhoeae*. *Infect. Immun.* **56**:785–790.

McNeil, M. R., and P. J. Brennan. 1991. Structure, function and biogenesis of the cell envelope of mycobacteria in relation to bacterial physiology, pathogenesis and drug resistance; some thoughts and possibilities arising from recent structural information. *Res. Microbiol.* **142**:451–463.

McNeil, M. R., M. Daffe, and P. J. Brennan. 1991. Location of the mycolyl ester subunits in the walls of mycobacteria. *J. Biol. Chem.* **266**:13217–13223.

Medhi, I., P. S. Murthy, and T. A. Venkitasubramanian. 1979. Demonstration and purification of three fatty acid synthases from *Mycobacterium tuberculosis* H37Rv. *Indian J. Biochem. Biophys.* **16**:216–222.

Menozzi, F. D., C. Gantiez, and C. Locht. 1991. Identification and purification of transferrin- and lactoferrin-binding proteins of *Bordetella pertussis* and *Bordetella bronchiseptica*. *Infect. Immun.* **59**:3982–3988.

Messenger, A. J. M., R. M. Hall, and C. Ratledge. 1986. Iron uptake processes in *Mycobacterium vaccae* R877R, a mycobacterium lacking mycobactin. *J. Gen. Microbiol.* **132**:845–852.

Messenger, A. J. M., and C. Ratledge. 1982. Iron transport in *Mycobacterium smegmatis*: uptake of iron from ferric citrate. *J. Bacteriol.* **149**:131–135.

Messenger, A. J. M., and C. Ratledge. Unpublished work.

Mickelsen, P. A., E. Blackman, and P. F. Sparling. 1982. Ability of *Neisseria gonorrhoeae, N. meningitidis*, and commensal *Neisseria* to obtain iron from lactoferrin. *Infect. Immun.* 35:915–920.

Miller, M. J. 1989. Syntheses and therapeutic potential of hydroxamic acid based siderophores and analogues. *Chem. Rev.* 89:1563–1579.

Miller, M. J., and F. Malouin. 1993. Microbial iron chelators as drug delivery agents: the rational design and synthesis of siderophore-drug conjugates. *Acc. Chem. Res.* 26:241–249.

Minnikin, D. E. 1982. Lipids: complex lipids, their chemistry, biosynthesis and roles, p. 95–185. *In* C. Ratledge and J. L. Stanford (ed.), *Biology of the Mycobacteria*, vol. 1. Academic Press, Inc. (London) Ltd., London.

Minnikin, D. E. 1991. Chemical principles in the organization of lipid components in the mycobacterial cell envelope. *Res. Microbiol.* 142:423–427.

Minnikin, D. E., and M. Goodfellow. 1980. Lipid composition in the classification and identification of acid-fast bacteria, p. 189–256. *In* M. Goodfellow and R. G. Board (ed.), *Microbiological Classification and Identification*. Academic Press, Inc. (London) Ltd., London.

Monahan, I. M., D. K. Banerjee, and P. D. Butcher. 1993. Gene expression of *Mycobacterium bovis* BCG induced *in-vitro* by stress stimuli associated with infection. *Biochem. Soc. Trans.* 22:89S.

Monahan, I. M., and P. D. Butcher. Unpublished observations.

Murty, M. V. V. S., and T. A. Venkitasubramanian. 1984. Turnover of phospholipids and glycerides in spheroplasts of *Mycobacterium smegmatis*. *Ann. Microbiol.* 135B:147–154.

Nam-Lee, Y., and M. J. Colston. 1985. Measurement of ATP generation and decay in *Mycobacterium leprae in vitro*. *J. Gen. Microbiol.* 131:3331–3338.

Neilands, J. B., K. Konopka, B. Schwyn, M. Coy, R. T. Francis, B. H. Paw, and A. Bagg. 1987. Comparative biochemistry of microbial iron assimilation, p. 3–33. *In* G. Winkelmann, D. van der Helm, and J. B. Neilands (ed.), *Iron Transport in Microbes, Plants and Animals*. VCH mbH, Weinheim, Germany.

Nikaido, H. 1993. Uptake of iron-siderophore complexes across the bacterial outer membrane. *Trends Microbiol.* 51:5–7.

Nikaido, H., S. H. Kim, and E. Y. Rosenberg. 1993. Physical organization of lipids in the cell wall of *Mycobacterium chelonae*. *Mol. Microbiol.* 8:1025–1030.

Nikaido, H., and M. H. Saier. 1992. Transport proteins in bacteria: common themes in their design. *Science* 258:936–942.

Ogunnariwo, J. A., and A. P. Schryvers. 1990. Iron acquisition in *Pasteurella haemolytica*: expression and identification of a bovine-specific transferrin receptor. *Infect. Immun.* 58:2091–2097.

Patel, B. K. R., D. K. Banerjee, and P. D. Butcher. 1991. Characterization of the heat shock response in *Mycobacterium bovis* BCG. *J. Bacteriol.* 173:7982–7987.

Pattyn, S. R., and F. Portaels. 1980. *In vitro* cultivation and characterization of *Mycobacterium lepraemurium*. *Int. J. Lepr.* 48:7–14.

Penumarti, N., and G. K. Khuller. 1982. Influence of antibodies to mannophosphoinositides on phospholipid synthesis in *Mycobacterium smegmatis* ATCC 607. *Infect. Immun.* 37:884–890.

Postle, K. 1990. Ton B and the Gram-negative dilemma. *Mol. Microbiol.* 4:2019–2025.

Quemard, A., C. Lacave, and G. Laneelle. 1991. Isoniazid inhibition of mycolic acid synthesis by extracts of sensitive and resistant strains of *Mycobacterium aurum*. *Antimicrob. Agents Chemother.* 35:1035–1039.

Qureshi, N., N. Sathyamoorthy, and K. Takayama. 1984. Biosynthesis of C_{30} to C_{56} fatty acids by an extract of *Mycobacterium tuberculosis* H37Ra. *J. Bacteriol.* 157:46–52.

Rainwater, D. L., and P. E. Kolattukudy. 1982. Isolation and characterization of acyl-CoA carboxylases from *Mycobacterium tuberculosis* and *M. bovis*, which produce multiple methyl branched mycocerosic acids. *J. Bacteriol.* 151:905–911.

Rainwater, D. L., and P. E. Kolattukudy. 1985. Fatty acid biosynthesis in *Mycobacterium tuberculosis var bovis* BCG: purification and characterization of a novel fatty acid synthase, mycocerosate synthase, which elongates n-fatty acyl-CoA with methylmalonyl-CoA. *J. Biol. Chem.* 260:616–623.

Rastogi, N. 1991. Recent observations concerning structure and function relationships in the mycobacterial cell envelope: elaboration of a model in terms of mycobacterial pathogenicity, virulence and drug-resistance. *Res. Microbiol.* 142:464–476.

Rastogi, N., C. Frehel, A. Ryter, H. Ohayou, M. Lesourd, and H. L. David. 1981. Multiple drug resistance in *Mycobacterium avium*: is the wall architecture responsible for the exclusion of antimicrobial agents? *Antimicrob. Agents Chemother.* 20:666–677.

Rastogi, N., and K. S. Goh. 1990. Antibacterial action of 1-isonicotinyl-2-palmitoyl hydrazine against the *Mycobacterium avium* complex and the enhancement of its activity by *m*-flurophenylalanine. *Antimicrob. Agents Chemother.* 34:2061–2064.

Rastogi, N., K. S. Goh, and H. L. David. 1990. Enhancement of drug susceptibility of *Mycobacterium avium* by inhibitors of cell envelope synthesis. *Antimicrob. Agents Chemother.* 34:759–764.

Ratledge, C. 1982a. Lipids: composition, fatty acid

biosynthesis, p. 53–94. *In* C. Ratledge and J. L. Stanford (ed.), *Biology of the Mycobacteria*, vol. 1. Academic Press, Inc. (London) Ltd., London.

Ratledge, C. 1982b. Nutrition, growth and metabolism, p. 186–212. *In* C. Ratledge and J. L. Stanford (ed.), *Biology of the Mycobacteria*, vol. 1. Academic Press, Inc. (London) Ltd., London.

Ratledge, C., L. P. Macham, K. A. Brown, and B. J. Marshall. 1974. Iron transport in *Mycobacterium smegmatis*: a restricted role for salicylic acid in the extracellular environment. *Biochim. Biophys. Acta* 372:39–51.

Ratledge, C., P. V. Patel, and J. Mundy. 1982. Iron transport in *Mycobacterium smegmatis*: the location of mycobactin by electron microscopy. *J. Gen. Microbiol.* 128:1559–1565.

Ratledge, C., and F. G. Winder. 1962. The accumulation of salicylic acid by mycobacteria during growth on an iron-deficient medium. *Biochem. J.* 84:501–506.

Rogers, H. J., C. Synge, and V. E. Woods. 1980. Antibacterial effect of scandium and indium complexes of enterochelin on *Klebsiella pneumoniae*. *Antimicrob. Agents Chemother.* 18:63–68.

Rogers, H. J., V. E. Woods, and C. Synge. 1982. Antibacterial effect of scandium and indium complexes of enterochelin on *Escherichia coli*. *J. Gen. Microbiol.* 128:2389–2394.

Sathyamoorthy, N., and K. Takayama. 1987. Purification and characterization of a novel mycolic acid exchange enzyme from *Mycobacterium smegmatis*. *J. Biol. Chem.* 262:13417–13423.

Schryvers, A. B., and L. J. Morris. 1988a. Identification and characterization of the transferrin receptor from *Neisseria meningitidis*. *Mol. Microbiol.* 2:281–288.

Schryvers, A. B., and L. J. Morris. 1988b. Identification and characterization of the human lactoferrin-binding protein from *Neisseria meningitidis*. *Infect. Immun.* 56:1144–1149.

Snow, G. A. 1970. Mycobactins: iron-chelating growth factors from mycobacteria. *Bacteriol. Rev.* 34:99–125.

Somogyi, P. A., and I. Foldes. 1983. Incorporation of thymine, thymidine, adenine and uracil into the nucleic acids of *Mycobacterium phlei* and its phage. *Ann. Microbiol.* 134a:19–28.

Sritharan, M., and C. Ratledge. 1989. Co-ordinated expression of the components of iron transport (mycobactin, exochelin and envelope proteins) in *Mycobacterium neoaurum*. *FEMS Microbiol. Lett.* 60:183–186.

Sritharan, M., and C. Ratledge. 1990. Iron-regulated envelope proteins of mycobacteria grown *in vitro* and their occurrence in *Mycobacterium leprae* grown *in vivo*. *Biol. Metals* 2:203–208.

Stahl, D. A., and J. W. Urbance. 1990. The division between fast- and slow-growing mycobacteria corresponds to natural relationships among the mycobacteria. *J. Bacteriol.* 172:116–124.

Stephenson, M. C., and C. Ratledge. 1980. Specificity of exochelins for iron transport in three species of mycobacteria. *J. Gen. Microbiol.* 116:521–523.

Suntari, M., and S. Laakso. 1993. Effect of growth temperature on the fatty acid composition of *Mycobacterium phlei*. *Arch. Microbiol.* 159:119–123.

Suzuki, Y., T. Mori, Y. Miyata, and T. Yamada. 1987. The number of ribosomal RNA genes in *Mycobacterium lepraemurium*. *FEMS Microbiol. Lett.* 44:73–76.

Takayama, K., and E. L. Armstrong. 1976. Isolation, characterization and function of 6-mycolyl-6′acetyl-trehalose in the H37Rv strain of *Mycobacterium tuberculosis*. *Biochemistry* 15:441–447.

Takayama, K., E. L. Armstrong, E. L. Davidson, K. A. Kunugi, and J. O. Kilburn. 1978a. Effect of low temperature on growth, viability, and synthesis of mycolic acids of *Mycobacterium tuberculosis* strain H37Ra. *Am. Rev. Respir. Dis.* 118:113–117.

Takayama, K., and D. S. Goldman. 1969. Pathway for the synthesis of mannophospholipids in *Mycobacterium tuberculosis*. *Biochim. Biophys. Acta* 176:196–198.

Takayama, K., and D. S. Goldman. 1970. Enzymatic synthesis of mannosyl-1-phosphoryl decaprenol by a cell-free system of *Mycobacterium tuberculosis*. *J. Bacteriol.* 245:6251–6257.

Takayama, K., and J. O. Kilburn. 1989. Inhibition of synthesis of arabinogalactan by ethambutol in *Mycobacterium smegmatis*. *Antimicrob. Agents Chemother.* 33:1493–1499.

Takayama, K., N. Qureshi, and H. K. Schnoes. 1978b. Isolation and characterization of the monounsaturated long chain fatty acids of *Mycobacterium tuberculosis*. *Lipids* 13:575–579.

Takayama, K., L. Wang, and H. L. David. 1972. Effect of isoniazid on the in vivo mycolic acid synthesis, cell growth and viability of *Mycobacterium tuberculosis*. *Antimicrob. Agents Chemother.* 2:29–35.

Toriyama, S., I. Yano, M. Matsui, M. Kusunose, and E. Kusunose. 1978. Separation of C50-60 and C70-80 mycolic acid molecular species and their changes by growth temperature in *Mycobacterium phlei*. *FEBS Lett.* 95:111–115.

Trias, J., and R. Benz. 1993. Characterization of the channel formed by the mycobacterial porin in lipid bilayer membranes. Demonstration of voltage gating and of negative point charges at the channel mouth. *J. Bacteriol.* 268:6234–6240.

Trias, J., V. Jarlier, and R. Benz. 1992. Porins in the cell wall of mycobacteria. *Science* 258:1479–1481.

Walton, D. J., and D. D. Jordan. 1988. Order of enzymic incorporation of *O*-methyl groups into the *O*-methyl-D-glucose containing polysaccharide of

Mycobacterium smegmatis: a tritium labelling study. *Carbohydr. Res.* **172**:267–274.

Watson, K. 1990. Microbial stress proteins. *Adv. Microb. Physiol.* **31**:183–223.

Wayne, L. G. 1976. Dynamics of submerged growth of *Mycobacterium tuberculosis* under aerobic and microaerophilic conditions. *Am. Rev. Respir. Dis.* **114**:807–811.

Wayne, L. G., and K.-Y. Lin. 1982. Glyoxylate metabolism and adaptation of *Mycobacterium tuberculosis* to survival under anaerobic conditions. *Infect. Immun.* **37**:1042–1049.

Weisman, L. S., and C. E. Ballou. 1984a. Biosynthesis of the mycobacterial methylmannose polysaccharide. Identification of an α 1-4 mannosyltransferase. *J. Biol. Chem.* **259**:3457–3463.

Weisman, L. S., and C. E. Ballou. 1984b. Biosynthesis of the mycobacterial methylmannose polysaccharide: identification of a 3-*O*-methyltransferase. *J. Biol. Chem.* **259**:3464–3469.

Wheeler, P. R. 1987a. Biosynthesis and scavenging of purines by pathogenic mycobacteria including *Mycobacterium leprae*. *J. Gen. Microbiol.* **133**:2999–3011.

Wheeler, P. R. 1987b. Enzymes for purine synthesis and scavenging in pathogenic mycobacteria and their distribution in *Mycobacterium leprae*. *J. Gen. Microbiol.* **133**:3013–3018.

Wheeler, P. R. 1990. Biosynthesis and scavenging of pyrimidines by pathogenic mycobacteria. *J. Gen. Microbiol.* **136**:189–201.

Wheeler, P. R., G. S. Besra, D. E. Minnikin, and C. Ratledge. 1993a. Inhibition of mycolic acid biosynthesis in a cell-wall preparation from *Mycobacterium smegmatis* by methyl 4-(2-octadecylcyclopropen-1-yl)butanoate, a structural analogue of a key precursor. *Lett. Appl. Microbiol.* **17**:33–36.

Wheeler, P. R., G. S. Besra, D. E. Minnikin, and C. Ratledge. 1993b. Stimulation of mycolic acid biosynthesis by incorporation of *cis*-tetracos-5-enoic acid in a cell-wall preparation from *Mycobacterium smegmatis*. *Biochim. Biophys. Acta* **1167**:182–188.

Wheeler, P. R., and K. Bulmer. Unpublished work.

Wheeler, P. R., K. Bulmer, and C. Ratledge. 1990. Enzymes for biosynthesis *de novo* and elongation of fatty acids in mycobacteria: is *Mycobacterium leprae* competent in fatty acid biosynthesis? *J. Gen. Microbiol.* **136**:211–217.

Wheeler, P. R., K. Bulmer, and C. Ratledge. 1991. Fatty acid oxidation and the β-oxidation complex in *Mycobacterium leprae* and two axenically cultivable mycobacteria that are pathogens. *J. Gen. Microbiol.* **137**:885–893.

Wheeler, P. R., K. Bulmer, C. Ratledge, J. W. Dale, and E. Norman. 1992. Control and location of acyl-CoA carboxylase activity in mycobacteria. *FEMS Microbiol. Lett.* **90**:169–172.

Wheeler, P. R., and C. Ratledge. 1988. Use of carbon sources for lipid biosynthesis in *Mycobacterium leprae*: a comparison with other pathogenic mycobacteria. *J. Gen. Microbiol.* **134**:2111–2121.

Wheeler, P. R., and C. Ratledge. 1991. Phospholipase activity of *Mycobacterium leprae* harvested from experimentally infected armadillo tissue. *Infect. Immun.* **59**:2781–2789.

Wheeler, P. R., and C. Ratledge. 1992. Control and location of acyl-hydrolysing phospholipase activity in mycobacteria. *J. Gen. Microbiol.* **138**:825–830.

Wietzerbin, J., B. C. Das, J. F. Petit, E. Lederer, L. M. Bouille, and J. M. Ghyusen. 1975. Occurrence of D-alanyl-(D)-meso-diaminopimelate and meso-diaminopimelyl-meso-diaminopimilate interpeptide linkages in the peptidoglycan of mycobacteria. *Biochemistry* **13**:3471–3476.

Winder, F. G., J. J. Tighe, and P. J. Brennan. 1972. Turnover of acylglucose, acyltrehalose and free trehalose during growth of *Mycobacterium smegmatis* on glucose. *J. Gen. Microbiol.* **73**:539–546.

Winkelmann, G. (ed.). 1991. *CRC Handbook of Microbial Iron Chelates*. CRC Press, Inc., Boca Raton, Fla.

Woodley, C. L., J. O. Kilburn, H. L. David, and V. A. Silcox. 1972. Susceptibility of mycobacteria to rifampin. *Antimicrob. Agents Chemother.* **2**:245–249.

Wooldridge, K. G., J. A. Morrissey, and P. H. Williams. 1992. Transport of ferric-aerobactin into the periplasm and cytoplasm of *Escherichia coli* K12: role of envelope-associated proteins and the effect of endogenous siderophores. *J. Gen. Microbiol.* **138**:597–603.

Yokoyama, K., and C. E. Ballou. 1989. Synthesis of a 1-6 mannooligosaccharides in *Mycobacterium smegmatis*: function of β-mannosylphosphoryldecaprenol as mannosyl donor. *J. Biol. Chem.* **264**:21621–21628.

Young, D. B., S. H. Kaufmann, P. W. Hermans, and J. F. Thole. 1991. Mycobacterial protein antigens: a compilation. *Mol. Microbiol.* **6**:133–145.

Zhang, Y., V. A. Steingrube, and R. J. Wallace. 1992. β-Lactamase inhibitors and the inducibility of β-lactamase of *Mycobacterium tuberculosis*. *Am. Rev. Respir. Dis.* **145**:657–660.

Zhou, X. H., and D. van der Helm. 1993. A novel purification of ferric citrate receptor (FecA) from *Escherichia coli* UT 5600 and further characterization of its binding capacity. *Biol. Metab.* **6**:37–44.

V. IMMUNOLOGY AND PATHOGENESIS OF TUBERCULOSIS

Tuberculosis: Pathogenesis, Protection, and Control
Edited by Barry R. Bloom
© 1994 American Society for Microbiology, Washington, DC 20005

Chapter 24

Immune Mechanisms of Protection

John Chan and Stefan H. E. Kaufmann

Acquired resistance against tuberculosis paradigmatically rests on cell-mediated immunity, with the major factors being mononuclear phagocytes (MP) and T lymphocytes. While the former cells act as the principal effectors, the latter ones serve as the predominant inducers of protection. At the same time, however, MP provide the preferred biotype for the etiologic agent of tuberculosis, *Mycobacterium tuberculosis*, and hence play a dual role in tuberculosis, promoting not only protection against the disease but also survival of the pathogen. Similarly, T cells not only are indispensable for protective immunity but also contribute to pathogenesis. A coordinated cross-talk between MP and T cells, therefore, is essential for optimum protection. Such coordination is best achieved in the granulomatous lesion, which provides the tissue site for defense against tuberculosis. Even in the face of coordinated T-cell–MP interactions, full eradication of the pathogen is frequently not achieved, so that the individual remains infected without developing active disease. Any later imbalance of the immune system will promote microbial reemergence and ultimately result in clinical disease. This chapter focuses on the immune mechanisms involved in protective immunity against tuberculosis, with the awareness that in most cases the immune response activated during infection with *M. tuberculosis* may be remarkably powerful yet insufficient.

A HISTORICAL NOTE

In his epoch-making description of the etiologic agent of tuberculosis in 1882, R. Koch noted the intracellular location of *M. tuberculosis* within giant cells (end-stage-differentiated MP) in granulomatous lesions (Koch, 1882). In his endeavor to develop an active vaccination protocol for treating tuberculosis, Koch found that after administration of glycerin extracts of *M. tuberculosis* culture supernatants, the lesions of tuberculous guinea pigs became heavily necrotized (Koch, 1890). In these necrotic reactions, many microorganisms died because of nutrient and oxygen deficiencies. Although Koch had already noted that *M. tuberculosis* organisms can be disseminated from such necrotizing lesions to other tissue sites, he underrated

John Chan • Department of Medicine, Montefiore Medical Center, Albert Einstein College of Medicine, Bronx, New York 10467. *Stefan H. E. Kaufmann* • Department of Immunology, University of Ulm, Albert-Einstein-Allee 11, D-89070 Ulm, Germany.

the detrimental consequences of this effect, which soon brought therapeutic vaccination with tuberculin to an end. E. Metchnikoff, a contemporary but not a close friend of Koch, was the first to fully realize the importance of MP in antibacterial immunity in general and in defense against tuberculosis in particular (Metchnikoff, 1905). The great success around the turn of the century in transferring protection against toxin-producing bacteria by using antisera from immune animals prompted numerous scientists to attempt passive vaccination against tuberculosis with antisera. Soon, however, it was realized that such antisera failed to transfer protection against tuberculosis. The first success in this direction was obtained in 1909 to 1910 by H. Helmholtz and O. Bail, who independently succeeded in adoptively transferring delayed-type hypersensitivity to tuberculosis with whole blood (containing leukocytes) or spleen homogenate, respectively (Helmholtz, 1909; Bail, 1910). Formal proof for the cellular dependence of delayed-type hypersensitivity to tuberculin was provided by M. Chase in 1945 (Chase, 1945). M. Lurie and E. Suter independently found that macrophages from immune animals expressed tuberculostatic activities, whereas those from normal animals permitted unrestricted bacillary multiplication (Suter, 1953; Lurie, 1964). Although these studies suggested involvement of specific immune mechanisms, the investigators did not contest alternative strategies when they realized that immune serum did not influence tuberculostasis by MP. It was the achievement of G. B. Mackaness to show that activation of antimycobacterial macrophage functions is controlled by lymphocytes (Mackaness and Blanden, 1967). That this activation is afforded by soluble mediators, now termed cytokines, was noted by B. R. Bloom and J. R. David (Bloom and Bennett, 1966; David, 1966).

IN VITRO ACTIVATION OF MACROPHAGE ANTIMYCOBACTERIAL FUNCTIONS

Evidence has long existed that murine macrophages have an antimycobacterial function in tissue culture systems (Lurie, 1942; Suter, 1952; Mackaness, 1969). Earlier work by various laboratories demonstrated that these cells, when activated in vitro by supernatants of immunologically stimulated lymphocytes, had various degrees of antimycobacterial activity (Patterson and Youmans, 1970; Klun and Youmans, 1973a, b; Cahall and Youmans, 1975a, b; Muroaka et al., 1976a, b; Turcotte et al., 1976). Soon, hydrogen peroxide (H_2O_2), one of the reactive oxygen intermediates (ROI) generated by macrophages during the oxidative burst (Sbarra and Karnovsky, 1959; Iyer et al., 1961; Klebanoff, 1980), was identified as the molecule that mediated mycobacteriocidal effects of MP (Walker and Lowrie, 1981). This finding marked the beginning of much debate concerning the significance of ROI in host defense against *M. tuberculosis*. Later, gamma interferon (IFN-γ) was found to be the key endogenous activating agent that triggers the antimycobacterial effects of murine macrophages (Rook et al., 1986; Flesch and Kaufmann, 1987), furnishing a better-defined system (compared to one using crude supernatants obtained from stimulated lymphocytes) in which to examine the antimycobacterial effects of macrophages. Recent remarkable advances made in the cloning, characterization, and production of numerous cytokines by recombinant DNA technology have facilitated similar in vitro experimentation designed to explore the potential of these interesting molecules in host defense against *M. tuberculosis*. Thus, tumor necrosis factor alpha (TNF-α), although ineffective when used alone, synergizes with IFN-γ to induce antimycobacterial effects of murine macrophages in vitro (Flesch and Kaufmann,

1990a). TNF-α also appears to play a critical role in the control of BCG infection in vivo, although its direct effect on the antimycobacterial capacity of macrophages has not been addressed in this model. Nevertheless, when TNF-α-specific monoclonal antibodies were used to probe the significance of this cytokine in defense against mycobacteria, deficient TNF-α resulted in poor granuloma formation and disseminated BCG infection in mice (Kindler et al., 1989). The significance of TNF-α in granuloma formation has been demonstrated in other infectious disease models (Chensue et al., 1989; Amiri et al., 1992). More importantly, preliminary studies suggest that anti-TNF-α antibodies markedly exacerbate disease progression in murine experimental tuberculosis (Flynn et al., personal communication).

Other cytokines have been implicated in macrophage defense against *M. tuberculosis*, although their roles are not as well established as those of IFN-γ and TNF-α. In vitro, interleukin-4 (IL-4) and IL-6 have the ability to induce macrophage antimycobacterial activity (Kaufmann et al., 1989; Flesch and Kaufmann, 1990a, b) by mechanisms presently undefined. Infection of the human myelomonocytic cell line THP-1 with *M. tuberculosis* enhances production of IL-6 (Friedland et al., 1993) compared to that in cells infected with *Toxoplasma gondii*, an intracellular protozoan known to elicit little inflammatory response even in immunocompetent patients. In the murine system, BCG or its subcellular components are capable of inducing production of IL-6 by splenocytes (Huygen et al., 1991). The antimycobacterial effects of IL-4 and IL-6 (Flesch and Kaufmann, 1990a, b) in the in vitro macrophage system are seen only when these cytokines are added to macrophage cultures after, but not before, the establishment of BCG infection. This phenomenon sharply contrasts with the ability of IFN-γ to induce antimycobacterial activity in macrophages, which is markedly blunted if it is given after initiation of infection (Flesch and Kaufmann, 1990a). The mechanism and the significance of this observation are currently obscure, but it illustrates well the complexity of the interaction between macrophages, cytokines, and the organisms as well as the limitations of existing in vitro systems in dissecting the likely complex cytokine network involved during tuberculous infection. Thus, it is known that THP-1 cells produce IL-8 in response to *M. tuberculosis* infection in vitro, but the role of this cytokine in host defense in tuberculosis is completely unknown (Friedland et al., 1992, 1993). Nevertheless, it has been postulated that IL-8 plays a role in granuloma formation by virtue of its ability to act as a chemotactic agent for T cells (Larsen et al., 1989; Friedland et al., 1992). IL-1 (Kobayashi et al., 1985; Dunn et al., 1988; Kasahara et al., 1988), IL-2 (Mathew et al., 1990; Cheever et al., 1992), IL-4 (McInnes and Rennick, 1988; Chensue et al., 1992), and IFN-γ (Squires et al., 1989; Chensue et al., 1992) may similarly contribute to resistance against *M. tuberculosis*, since these cytokines have been implicated in granulomatous reactions in various in vitro systems, including a murine schistosomiasis model. Recently, IL-10 (Bermudez and Champsi, 1993) and transforming growth factor beta1 (TGF-β1) (Denis and Ghadirian, 1991; Bermudez, 1993) have been shown to be associated with diminution of macrophage antimycobacterial effect in vitro and with disease exacerbation in mice infected with *M. avium*. In contrast, preliminary studies (Flynn and Bloom, personal communication) indicate that administration of recombinant IL-12, a recently characterized heterodimeric glycoprotein produced by various immune cells including macrophages (D'Andrea et al., 1992; Schoenhaut et al., 1992; Gazzinelli et al., 1993), may confer resistance to tuberculosis in mice. IL-12 has recently been shown to play an important role in resistance to *Leishmania major*, *T. gondii*, and *Listeria monocytogenes* (Gazzinelli et al., 1993; Heinzel et al., 1993; Locksley, 1993; Tripp et al., 1993). The events triggered by IL-12 help identify natural killer (NK) cells as a critical cellular component in defense against *M. tuberculosis*. By virtue of their ability to produce IFN-γ in response to IL-12 (Kobayashi et al., 1989; Wolf et al., 1991), NK cells can rapidly activate macrophages to express microbicidal functions during the early "nonimmune" phase of tuberculous infection, before the expansion and differentiation of specific T lymphocytes. As cytokines are being examined in experimental mycobacterial infection, it is becoming clear that these molecules interact dynamically to form a highly coordinated network that is configured by both host- and pathogen-specific factors, which together influence disease outcome and progression.

Compared to the murine system, much less is known about the activation of antimycobacterial activity in human macrophages. While it is clear that IFN-γ has the capability to induce significant antimycobacterial activity in murine macrophages, its role in the human system is unsettled. Thus, reports of the effect of IFN-γ-treated human macrophages on the replication of *M. tuberculosis* ranges from being inhibitory (Rook et al., 1986) to enhancing (Douvas et al., 1985). This inconsistency had cast considerable doubts on the antimycobacterial capability of human mononuclear phagocytes until the demonstration that 1,25-dihydroxy vitamin D_3 [1,25-$(OH)_2D_3$], alone or in combination with IFN-γ and TNF-α, was able to activate macrophages to inhibit and/or kill *M. tuberculosis* in the human system (Crowle et al., 1987; Rook, 1988; Denis, 1991b). Interestingly, IFN-γ stimulates human (Adams and Gacad, 1985; Koeffler et al., 1985; Reichel et al., 1987) but not murine (Rook, 1990) macrophages to produce 1,25-$(OH)_2D_3$, probably via induction of 25$(OH)D_3$-1α-hydroxylase, the enzyme that converts 25$(OH)D_3$ to the biologically more potent dihydroxylated form, which may explain the inability of 1,25$(OH)_2D_3$ to affect antimycobacterial activity in the murine system. This difference in 1,25$(OH)_2D_3$ metabolism between murine and human macrophages should serve as a reminder that species variations exist and a caution against the occasional readiness with which cross-species extrapolations of experimental results are made. The value of existing in vitro and in vivo murine models in understanding tuberculosis must, however, not be understated.

ANTIMYCOBACTERIAL EFFECTOR FUNCTIONS OF MACROPHAGES: HOW DOES *M. TUBERCULOSIS* SURVIVE?

The mononuclear phagocyte constitutes a potent antimicrobial component of cell-mediated immunity. The precise mechanisms by which these cells mediate killing or inhibition of bacterial pathogens are, however, not clearly understood. Nonetheless, in this section, some of the best-characterized antimicrobial effector functions of macrophages—phagosome-lysosome fusion, generation of ROI by the oxidative burst, and production of reactive nitrogen intermediates (RNI) via the L-arginine-dependent cytotoxic pathway—will be discussed in the context of tuberculous infection together with the possible evasion mechanisms employed by the tubercle bacillus to escape killing by activated macrophages (Fig. 1).

Phagosome-Lysosome Fusion

The lysosome is a highly complex organelle containing numerous enzymes within its own limiting membrane that are capable of degrading a whole range of macromolecules (reviewed in de Duve and Wattiaux [1966], Bainton [1981], and Kornfeld [1987]). To provide optimal conditions for the functioning of these degradative enzymes, the intralysosomal milieu is main-

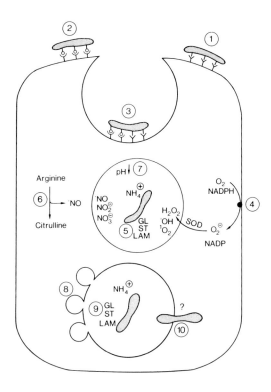

Figure 1. Antituberculous macrophage activities and evasion mechanisms. Accumulating evidence suggests that *M. tuberculosis* enters macrophages via specific binding to cell surface molecules of phagocytes. It has been reported that the tubercle bacillus can bind directly to the mannoase receptor via the cell wall-associated, mannosylated glycolipid LAM (1) or indirectly via complement receptors of the integrin family (CR1, CR3) or Fc receptors (2). Phagocytosis (3), triggered by engaging certain cell surface molecules such as the Fc receptor, stimulates the production of ROI via activation of the oxidative burst (4). Experimental data indicate that *M. tuberculosis* can interfere with the toxic effect of ROI by various mechanisms. First, various mycobacterial compounds including glycolipids (GL), sulfatides (ST), and LAM can downregulate the oxidative cytotoxic mechanism (5; see text for details). Second, uptake via CR1 bypasses activation of the respiratory burst. Cytokine-activated macrophages produce RNI that, at least in the mouse system, mediate potent antimycobacterial activity (6). The acidic condition of the phagolysosomal vacuole can be conducive to the toxic effect of RNI (7). However, NH_4^+ production by *M. tuberculosis* may attenuate the potency of the L-arginine-dependent antimycobacterial mechanism and that of lysosomal enzymes (8), which operate best at an acidic pH. In addition, mycobacterial products such as sulfatides and NH_4^+ may interfere with phagolysosomal fusion (9). Finally, the tubercle bacillus may evade the highly toxic environment by escaping into the cytoplasm via the production of hemolysin (10).

tained at a relatively acidic state (pH ~5) by an ATP-dependent proton pump (Ohkuma and Poole, 1978; Ohkuma et al., 1982). It is generally accepted that certain microorganisms, sequestered within the phagosome upon ingestion by phagocytic cells including macrophages, are subject to degradation by the various lysosomal digestive enzymes transferred into this subcellular compartment as a result of phagolysosomal fusion (Cohn, 1963). This fusion process, a highly regulated event, most likely constitutes a significant antimicrobial mechanism of phagocytes. Examination of the interaction between isotopically labeled bacteria and macrophages, using the generation of acid-soluble radioactive materials as an indicator of degradation, suggests that certain organisms are degraded extensively within

2 h after having been phagocytized (Cohn, 1963). Also, electron microscopic studies indicate that the cell wall of *Bacillus subtilis* is degraded extensively within 30 min after phagocytosis by polymorphonuclear leukocytes (Cohn, 1963). How, then, does *M. tuberculosis* survive the hostile environment of phagolysosomes?

M. tuberculosis has the ability to produce ammonia in abundance (Gordon et al., 1980). This volatile weak base accumulates in *M. tuberculosis* culture filtrates in concentrations of up to 20 mM and is thought to be responsible for the inhibitory effect of culture supernatants of virulent mycobacteria on phagolysosome fusion (Gordon et al., 1980). In addition, ammonium chloride (NH_4Cl) has been shown to affect the saltatory movement of lysosomes (D'Arcy

Hart et al., 1983) and to alkalinize the intralysosomal compartment (D'Arcy Hart et al., 1983). Thus, by virtue of its ability to produce a significant amount of ammonia, the tubercle bacillus can potentially evade the toxic environment within the lysosomal vacuole by (i) inhibiting phagosome-lysosome fusion and (ii) diminishing the potency of the intralysosomal enzymes via alkalinization. This latter attribute of raising intralysosomal pH might also be protective against the RNI cytotoxic mechanism of macrophages (see below).

Another mycobacterial product thought to have the ability to inhibit phagolysosomal fusion is the sulfatides (Goren et al., 1976b), derivatives of multiacylated trehalose 2-sulfate, a lysosomotropic polyanionic glycolipid produced by *M. tuberculosis* (Middlebrook et al., 1959; Goren et al., 1976a). Because of the ability of certain polyanionic compounds to entrap commonly used lysosomal markers employed to study phagolysosome fusion, artifactual "inhibition" of this process can occur and has spawned much controversy (Goren et al., 1987a, b). These entrapment phenomena could be secondary to the formation of gelatinous, sluggishly moving hydrocolloids that physically retain lysosomal markers or to ionic interaction with cationic markers such as acridine orange. Although sulfatides do not form hydrocolloids, the polyanionic nature of these glycolipids poses questions concerning their ability to inhibit phagolysosomal fusion (Goren et al., 1987a, b). Careful reanalysis of the effect of these glycolipids on phagolysosome fusion appears to be warranted. Regardless of the chemical components of the tubercle bacillus that contribute to the inhibition of phagolysosomal fusion, this phenomenon (controversy notwithstanding) has been extensively studied (Armstrong and D'Arcy Hart, 1971, 1975; Goren et al., 1976b; Myrvik et al., 1984; D'Arcy Hart et al., 1987) and is certainly a mechanism by which *M. tuberculosis* could evade cytotoxic ef-

fects of macrophages. This issue could perhaps be addressed more rigorously and definitively by direct immunohistochemical labeling of vacuolar membranes enclosing intracellular *M. tuberculosis* with antibodies specific to lysosomal glycoproteins (Joiner et al., 1990) or by using the "trap-resistant" ionic impermeant fluors (lucifer yellow, lissamine rhodamine, and sulforhodamine) as alternative lysosomal markers (Goren et al., 1987a, b). Finally, it is likely that virulent tubercle bacilli, like certain intracellular pathogens, including rickettsiae (Winkler, 1990), listeriae (Bielecki et al., 1990), and shigellae (Sansonetti et al., 1986), evade killing by escaping from phagocytic vacuoles into the cytoplasm (for a review, see Falkow et al. [1992]). Hemolytic activities capable of lysing vacuolar membranes are thought to be the common virulent determinant that enables successful parasitization of the cytoplasm (Falkow et al., 1992). Indeed, the translocation of *M. tuberculosis* from within phagocytic vacuoles into the cytoplasmic compartment has been reported (Myrvik et al., 1984; McDonough et al., 1993). These observations are reinforced by the presence of a hemolytic activity in the tubercle bacillus (King et al., 1993). Also, the cytoplasmic location made possible by this potential evasion mechanism could, in theory, facilitate the routing of mycobacterial components into the major histocompatibility class I (MHC I) pathway of antigen presentation, thus explaining at least in part the importance of MHC I molecules and CD8[+] T cells in defense against *M. tuberculosis* (Kaufmann, 1988; Flynn et al., 1992).

The Respiratory Burst

That ROI play a significant role in host defense against microbes is best exemplified by the frequent infectious complication experienced by chronic granulomatous disease patients (reviewed in Forrest et al. [1988]), whose phagocytes cannot mount an oxidative burst (Sbarra and Karnovsky, 1959; Iyer et al., 1961; Klebanoff, 1980). The significance of these toxic oxygen species in defense against *M. tuberculosis*, however, remains controversial. Since the report that H_2O_2 produced by lymphokine-activated murine macrophages kills *M. microti* (Walker and Lowrie, 1981), much effort has been focused on testing the role of the oxygen radical-dependent killing mechanism in defense against *M. tuberculosis*. Such effort, however, provided evidence indicating that oxygen radicals may not be sufficient to inhibit and/or kill *M. tuberculosis* (Flesch and Kaufmann, 1987, 1988; Chan et al., 1992). The validity of these findings has been reinforced by the demonstration of evasion mechanisms employed by the tubercle bacillus to elude the toxic effect of ROI. Of these mechanisms, those that are mediated by mycobacterial components lipoarabinomannan (LAM) and phenolicglycolipid I (PGL-I) are among the best studied and characterized (for reviews, see Brennan [1989] and Brennan et al. [1990]).

LAM, a major cell wall-associated, phosphatidylinositol-anchored complex lipopolysaccharide, is produced by *M. tuberculosis* in large amounts (15 mg/g of bacteria) (Hunter et al., 1986; Hunter and Brennan, 1991). Immunogold staining has demonstrated that LAM exists in a capsular sheath encasing *M. tuberculosis* (Hunter and Brennan, 1991). This strategic location places LAM at the frontline of attacks directed by the various antimicrobial mechanisms of macrophages. It has now been shown that LAM can incapacitate the oxygen radical-dependent antimicrobial mechanism at at least two levels: (i) studies using electron spin resonance spectroscopy and spin-trapping have shown that LAM is an effective ROI scavenger (Chan et al., 1991); and (ii) LAM can downregulate the oxidative burst by inhibiting protein kinase C (Chan et al., 1991), an enzyme that plays an important role in activation of the oxidative

burst in phagocytic cells (Gennaro et al., 1985; Pontyremoli et al., 1986; Wilson et al., 1986; Gavioli et al., 1987). In addition, since IFN-γ is a major factor for macrophage activation (Hamilton et al., 1984; Hamilton and Adams, 1987; Fan et al., 1988) and has the ability to enhance ROI production by phagocytic cells, it is possible that LAM, by virtue of its ability to inhibit transcriptional activation of IFN-γ-inducible genes (Chan et al., 1991), is able to block the expression of an as yet unidentified factor(s) inducible by this cytokine that is required for the oxidative burst. These results are in keeping with the findings that mouse peritoneal macrophages treated with LAM or infected with *M. leprae* (a LAM-producing pathogenic mycobacterium) are not responsive to IFN-γ activation as assessed by microbicidal and tumoricidal activities, O_2^- production, and surface Ia antigen expression (Sibley et al., 1988; Sibley and Krahenbuhl, 1988) and may partially explain the inability of IFN-γ-stimulated macrophages from both humans and mice to effectively kill *M. tuberculosis* in vitro (Rook et al., 1986; Flesch and Kaufmann, 1987).

Other mycobacterial components that interfere with the oxygen radical-dependent antimicrobial mechanism of macrophages are PGL-I and the sulfatides. PGL-I is an oligoglycosylphenolic phthiocerol diester with its species-specific trisaccharide moiety glycosidically linked to a phenyl group that in turn is attached to the branched glycolic chain, phthiocerol; two hydroxyl functions of the phthiocerol are esterified by methyl-branched fatty acids (mycocerosates) (Hunter and Brennan, 1981; Hunter et al., 1982). Although universally distributed among *M. leprae*, the expression of PGL-I in the various strains of *M. tuberculosis* is much restricted (Daffe et al., 1987; Brennan, 1989; Brennan et al., 1990). In contrast, the sulfatides, derivatives of multiacylated trehalose 2-sulfate (Middlebrook et al., 1959; Goren et al., 1976a), are widely expressed among different strains of *M. tuberculosis* (Middlebrook et al., 1959; Goren et al., 1974, 1976a). Because of its restricted distribution among tuberculous isolates, the significance of PGL-1 in the pathogenesis of tuberculosis remains to be determined. Nonetheless, both PGL-I and the sulfatides have the capacity to down-regulate ROI production in in vitro macrophage culture systems (Neill and Klebanoff, 1988; Pabst et al., 1988; Vachula et al., 1989; Brozna et al., 1991), and PGL-I directly scavenges oxygen radicals in a cell-free system (Chan et al., 1989). Another mechanism by which *M. tuberculosis* could evade the toxicity of ROI is to avoid binding to macrophage cell surface components, such as Fc receptors, that would provoke an oxidative burst. Instead, the tubercle bacillus parasitizes MP via complement receptors CR1 and CR3, molecules of the integrin family whose interaction with a ligand does not trigger ROI production (Wright and Silverstein, 1983), in resting macrophages (Schlesinger et al., 1990). Thus, as in other parasites (for reviews, see Isberg [1991] and Falkow et al. [1992]), including *Bordetella pertussis* (Relman et al., 1990), *Histoplasma capsulatum* (Bullock and Wright, 1987), *Legionella pneumophila* (Payne and Horwitz, 1987), and *Leishmania* spp. (Mosser and Edelson, 1987; Russell and Wright, 1988; Talamas-Rohana et al., 1990), exploitation of integrin receptors may be a common scheme of invasion among pathogenic mycobacteria.

Although these in vitro data provide substantive evidence to suggest pathogenetic roles of the various mycobacterial glycolipids, their in vivo significance is presently undefined and awaits rigorous genetic analyses. Nonetheless, it is undeniable that *Mycobacterium* spp. are extremely well adapted to the hostile environment of phagocytic cells, their deftness reflected by the alarming morbidity and mortality caused by tuberculosis worldwide (Murray et al., 1990). However, since infection with the tubercle bacillus does not equal disease, the host must be equally sophisticated in evolving effective defensive strategies against this formidable invader. It follows, then, that there must exist antimicrobial mechanisms to which the bacillus succumbs.

Reactive Nitrogen Oxides

The L-arginine-dependent cytotoxic pathway of activated macrophages constitutes an important antimicrobial mechanism against intracellular parasites (for reviews, see Nathan and Hibbs [1991], Liew and Cox [1991], and Nathan [1992]). The cytotoxic effect of this pathway is mediated through nitric oxide (NO) and related RNI generated from the substrate L-arginine via the action of the inducible form of the enzyme nitric oxide synthase (iNOS) (Nathan and Hibbs, 1991; Nathan, 1992). Recent studies have demonstrated an association between the antimycobacterial effect of cytokine-activated murine macrophages and the activation of the L-arginine-dependent cytotoxic pathway (Denis, 1991b; Flesch and Kaufmann, 1991; Chan et al., 1992). Thus, the capability of macrophages activated by IFN-γ and *Escherichia coli* lipopolysaccharide or TNF-α to kill and/or inhibit the virulent Erdman strain of *M. tuberculosis* correlates well with RNI production, and nitrogen oxides generated by acidification of nitrite are also mycobactericidal (Chan et al., 1992). Deletion analyses of the 5' flanking promoter sequence of murine iNOS indicate that IFN-γ alone is insufficient for transcriptional activation of this gene (Xie et al., 1993). The synergistic effect of IFN-γ and TNF-α in inducing macrophage antimycobacterial function via RNI production underscores the importance of these cytokines in defense against *M. tuberculosis*. Indeed, IFN-γ and IFN-γ receptor ''knockout'' mice that are deficient in mounting an RNI response to infection with the tubercle bacillus experience a fulminant course of tuberculosis (Dalton et al., 1993; Flynn et al., 1993; Cooper et al., 1993; Kamijo et al., 1993). In addition, in vitro studies using the ROI-deficient murine macrophage cell line D9 and its ROI-generating parental line J774.16 indicate that their antimycobacterial capacities are comparable, are independent of the amount of toxic oxygen species generated, and correlate well with RNI production. These data strongly suggest that L-arginine-dependent production of RNI is the principal effector mechanism in activated murine macrophages responsible for killing and inhibiting the growth of virulent *M. tuberculosis*. A role of ROI in defense against the tubercle bacillus cannot, however, be entirely excluded. For example, ROI may react with other compounds to generate effective toxic molecules that possess potent antimycobacterial activity. Although not yet tested for its effect on *M. tuberculosis*, peroxynitrite anion ($ONOO^-$), a product of NO and superoxide anion (O_2^-), has been shown to effectively kill *E. coli* (Beckman et al., 1990; Zhu et al., 1992; Stamler et al., 1992). Finally, the use of oxygen radical scavengers to probe the significance of ROI in the antimycobacterial function of macrophages can potentially generate misleading information because of nonspecific effects of these chemicals. Indeed, catalase has been shown to markedly inhibit RNI production by activated macrophages (Li et al., 1992; Chan and Bloom, unpublished observation). Although this inhibitory phenomenon could be reversed by tetrahydrobiopterin (Li et al., 1992), a cofactor for the macrophage nitric oxide synthase (Kwon et al., 1989; Tayeh and Marletta, 1989), the underlying mechanisms remain obscure. The original observation by Walker and Lowrie (1981) that catalase inhibited the antimycobacterial effect of activated macrophages is probably related to the ability of this H_2O_2 scavenger to suppress production of toxic nitrogen oxides.

The rapid unraveling of the nitric oxide puzzle has contributed substantially to the solution of many biological mysteries. However, much remains to be learned. More importantly, the role that RNIs play in defense against pathogens has not been established in humans. A not unreasonable skepticism about the role of RNI stems from the difficulty in activating human MP in vitro to generate nitrogen oxides. It is curious that while human macrophages had been reported to produce RNI in quantities sufficient to effect killing of *M. avium* in vitro (Denis, 1991c), efforts to demonstrate the activation of the L-arginine-dependent cytotoxic mechanism in these human cells have, in general, generated inconsistent results. Could this be due to the known insufficiency of tetrahydrobiopterin in human macrophages (Schoendon et al., 1987; Werner et al., 1989)? There is, however, evidence to suggest that human MP have the potential to generate RNI. Individuals experiencing sepsis (Ochoa et al., 1991) or undergoing cytokine therapy for tumors (Hibbs et al., 1992; Ochoa et al., 1992) generate large amounts of nitrate, suggesting the presence of iNOS in humans, although the cell types responsible for the production of RNI in these clinical settings have not been identified. Interestingly, while IFN-γ and TNF-α are sufficient to activate the L-arginine-dependent pathway in murine macrophages, optimal RNI production by human hepatocytes requires IL-1 and lipopolysaccharide in addition (Nussler et al., 1992). This variation in inducing agents required for RNI production by cells of different origins highlights the possibility that human macrophage iNOS may require as yet undefined inducing agents. Equally possible is the presence of an inhibitory molecule in the in vitro human system that prevent the activation of the L-arginine–NO pathway. In the murine system, RNI production by murine macrophages can be downregulated by various cytokines, including IL-4, IL-10, and TGF-β1 (Liew et al., 1991; Nelson et al.,

1991; Cunha et al., 1992; Gazzinelli et al., 1992; Oswald et al., 1992). More importantly, IL-10 and TGF-β have been shown to inhibit antimicrobial functions of activated macrophages in vitro as well as to exacerbate disease progression in certain infectious disease models whose pathogens are known to be susceptible to the toxic effects of RNI (Liew et al., 1991; Nelson et al., 1991; Cunha et al., 1992; Gazzinelli et al., 1992; Oswald et al., 1992). The widespread distribution of iNOS activity in tissues predicts tight regulation of the expression of this enzyme. Appraisal of iNOS gene expression, particularly in in vivo models, is likely to yield important information that may shed light on the intriguing mycobacterium-macrophage interaction.

From the mycobacterium's point of view, the development of strategies to evade the toxic effect of RNI seems prudent, if not absolutely required, for survival. Given the ability of microbes to mutate and the rapidity with which resistance to chemicals such as antibiotics can develop (Neu, 1992), it is not unreasonable to assume the existence of such RNI mutants. Recent chemical characterization of the mycobacterial glycolipid LAM indicates that the virulent H37Rv strain of *M. tuberculosis* produces a form (Man-LAM) that is mannosylated at the nonreducing end of the molecule. This is in contrast to the LAM of the relatively avirulent H37Ra strain, whose terminal arabinoses lack the mannose shield (Chatterjee et al., 1992a). More importantly, these two form of LAM differ in their biological function: LAM is a much more potent inducer of macrophage production of TNF-α than is Man-LAM (Chatterjee et al., 1992b; Chan and Bloom, unpublished observations). Since TNF-α is one of the key cytokines in the induction of macrophage RNI production, it appears that Man-LAM could have evolved under the selective pressure of RNI so as to evade the toxic effect of nitrogen oxides by intercepting the L-arginine-dependent cytotoxic pathway at the induction

level. Finally, the recent report that the susceptibility of *M. avium* to RNI varies among strains (Doi et al., 1993) further signals the existence of RNI-resistant mycobacteria. Characterization of such mutants will be a demanding task because of the incomplete understanding of the mammalian biochemical pathway of RNI production, the lack of information both on the precise nitrogen oxide species that mediate antimycobacterial activity and the targets that these molecules seek out, and the complexity of NO reactions (Stamler et al., 1992). Nevertheless, this is an important area of research that will most likely add significantly to the understanding of both NO chemistry in vivo and pathogenetic mechanisms of virulent mycobacteria and will possibly lead to new therapeutic interventions.

Before leaving the discussion of virulence factors and pathogenetic mechanisms as they relate to the intracellular survival of *M. tuberculosis*, a specific pathway of iron metabolism of the tubercle bacillus deserves mention. Although the relationship between iron and infection has been known for decades (Schade and Caroline, 1944; Weinberg, 1974, 1978, 1992; Griffiths et al., 1980), the mechanisms by which iron metabolism affect the outcome of infection are not clearly understood. Isolation and characterization of a class of iron-binding molecules termed siderophores in a wide variety of prokaryotes and eukaryotes (Nielands, 1981) have, however, shed considerable light on this subject. It has been reported that growth of certain bacteria, both in vitro and in vivo, is greatly enhanced in the presence of the iron-containing protein hemoglobin (Eaton et al. [1982] and references therein). The 50% lethal dose of *E. coli* in a rat model drops 3 logs when the organisms are given intraperitoneally with hemoglobin. The virulence-enhancing effect of this heme compound can be reversed by heptaglobin, a protein that binds specifically to hemoglobin (Eaton et al., 1982). Since inorganic iron salts can achieve the same effect as hemoglobin, a direct connection of iron and infection is made (Eaton et al., 1982). In human diseases, the mortality rate of *Vibrio vulnificus* is markedly increased in patients suffering from iron overload as a result of conditions such as hemochromatosis and alcoholism (Brennt et al., 1991; Bullen et al., 1991). These experimental data thus suggest a possible role of siderophores in bacterial virulence.

Mycobactins, a group of iron-chelating growth factors of mycobacteria, have been considered a possible virulence factor of *M. tuberculosis* (Snow, 1970). These hydroxamate derivatives chelate ferric ions with a stability constant exceeding 10^{30} (Snow, 1970). Thus, mycobactins compete favorably for chelating Fe^{3+} with human ferritin and transferrin, the major iron storage and iron-transporting proteins, respectively. The significance of these mycobacterial iron-binding agents in the pathogenesis of tuberculosis, however, remains to be established. Recently, the L-arginine–NO pathway has been reported to participate in posttranscriptional regulation of the expression of ferritin, transferrin receptor, and 5-aminolevulinate synthase (a rate-limiting enzyme in erythroid heme synthesis) in macrophages (Drapier et al., 1993; Weiss et al., 1993). It is fascinating that the very same pathway that produces potent antimycobacterial activities in macrophages participates also in the regulation of the metabolism of iron, whose availability is essential to the optimum growth of *M. tuberculosis*. Dissecting this likely complex tangle may uncover additional roles for the NO pathway in tuberculous infection and shed light on the significance of iron in the pathogenicity of *M. tuberculosis*.

DOES *M. TUBERCULOSIS* INVADE CELLS OTHER THAN PROFESSIONAL PHAGOCYTES?

There is little doubt that *M. tuberculosis* has the ability to establish infection in and replicate inside of a wide variety of mammalian cells in vitro (Sheppard, 1958). Yet in infected tissues, the tubercle bacillus is to be found only in polymorphonuclear leukocytes and MP (Filley and Rook, 1991). The findings by Filley and Rook that endothelial cells and fibroblasts infected by *M. tuberculosis* exhibit increased sensitivity to the cytolytic effect of TNF have led to the hypothesis that this cytokine contributes significantly to the immunopathology of tuberculosis (Filley and Rook, 1991). The enhanced susceptibility of nonphagocytic cells to TNF upon mycobacterial infection may also partially explain the difficulties encountered in identifying such target cells in vivo. It is also possible that these nonphagocytic cells serve as a reservoir for bacterial multiplication and thus aid in disease dissemination upon lysis by TNF. Research in these areas is just beginning to draw attention and is likely to help provide insight into the pathogenic strategies of *M. tuberculosis*. Finally, unlike the processes of other pathogenic bacteria such as the enteric shigellae and salmonellae and the gram-positive listeriae (for reviews see Isberg [1991] and Falkow et al. [1992]), the processes of adhesion and invasion by which *M. tuberculosis* enters host cells are just beginning to be understood. *M. tuberculosis* gains entry into MP via cell surface molecules, including the integrin family CR1 and CR3 complement receptors (Schlesinger et al., 1990) and the mannose receptor (Schlesinger, 1993). Recently, *M. avium* has been shown to enter macrophages via $\alpha_v\beta_3$, another molecule of the integrin family (Rao et al., 1993). Parasitization of phagocytes via the CR1 and CR3 receptors by various pathogens avoids triggering the oxidative burst (Wright and Silverstein, 1983). Whether the same advantage is gained by engaging the mannose receptor or the $\alpha_v\beta_3$ integrin is presently unclear. Since the cytoplasmic domain of β subunit of integrin is coupled to the cytoskeleton (Albelda and Buck, 1990), it is possible that binding to such cell surface receptors serves to initiate the process of internalization by the host cell (Isberg, 1991). Does the recently described mycobacterial invasin (Arruda et al., 1993) bind also to integrin receptors? Comprehension of these adhesion and invasion events is very important in advancing our understanding of the pathogenicity of *M. tuberculosis*.

CONTRIBUTION OF T CELLS TO ACQUIRED RESISTANCE

T lymphocytes are obligatory mediators of protection. They do not act alone but must interact with other cells of the immune system to achieve optimum resistance. All T-cell populations (CD4 α/β T cells, CD8 α/β T cells, and γ/δ T cells) contribute to protection. The central role of T lymphocytes has been exemplified by experiments showing that *nu/nu* and *scids* mice suffer more severely from experimental *M. tuberculosis* and BCG infections than their control counterparts (Sher et al., 1975; Izzo and North, 1992).

T-Cell Populations

T cells expressing an α/β-T-cell receptor constitute more than 95% of postthymic T cells in peripheral organs and blood. In contrast, γ/δ T cells are a minority at these sites, but they are more prominent in mucosal tissues such as the lung. Formal proof that α/β T cells are crucial for acquired resistance against tuberculosis was provided recently with mutant mice lacking all α/β T cells. In these mice, the gene encoding the T-cell receptor β chain had been deleted by homologous recombination (Mombaerts et al., 1992). Although these α/β-T-cell-deficient mice are relatively resistant to sublethal BCG infection during the first 4 weeks of infection, growth of BCG markedly increases afterwards, and ultimately the α/β-T-cell-deficient mice succumb to BCG infection (Ladel and Kauf-

mann, unpublished data). α/β T cells can be further divided into CD4 T cells, which recognize antigenic peptides in the context of MHC class II molecules, and CD8 T cells, which respond to peptides presented by the MHC class I gene products. Mycobacterium-specific CD4 T lymphocytes have been identified consistently in experimental and human tuberculosis (Kaufmann and Flesch, 1986; Ottenhoff et al., 1988; Barnes et al., 1989). Furthermore, CD4 T-cell depletion by specific monoclonal antibodies exacerbates experimental infection of mice with *M. tuberculosis* and BCG (Müller et al., 1987; Pedrazzini et al., 1987). Conversely, adoptive protection against *M. tuberculosis* and BCG largely depends on transfer of selected CD4 T cells (Orme and Collins, 1984; Orme, 1987). Consistent with these findings, mutant mice with a deficiency in the MHC class II gene that are devoid of functionally active CD4 T cells die of BCG (Ladel and Kaufmann, unpublished data) and *M. tuberculosis* (Flynn et al., unpublished observation) infections. In conclusion, these experiments strongly point to an essential role of CD4 T cells in protection against tuberculosis. Consistent with these data, CD4 depletion as a result of human immunodeficiency virus infection frequently results in clinical tuberculosis in AIDS patients.

A substantial role for CD8 T cells in protection against tuberculosis is indicated by several lines of experimental studies. Depletion of CD8 T cells with specific monoclonal antibodies exacerbates *M. tuberculosis* infection in mice, and selected CD8 T cells transfer adoptive protection against tuberculosis (Orme and Collins, 1984; Müller et al., 1987; Orme, 1987; Pedrazzini et al., 1987). These findings have been further substantiated recently by application of mutant mice in which the $\beta2$-microglobulin ($\beta2m$) gene had been deleted (Flynn et al., 1992). Because $\beta2m$ is required for MHC class I surface expression, $\beta2m$-deficient mutant mice are devoid of functionally active CD8 T cells. These mice die rapidly from *M. tuberculosis* but not from BCG infection. Impressive as these studies are, it should be kept in mind that β2m not only serves to stabilize MHC class I surface expression but may also perform other functions that could influence survival of *M. tuberculosis* in β2m-deficient mice. Furthermore, mycobacterium-specific CD8 T cells have been isolated from *M. tuberculosis*- and BCG-immune mice (DeLibero et al., 1988). In contrast, such mycobacterium-specific CD8 T cells were rarely identified in patients suffering from human tuberculosis (Rees et al., 1988). CD8 T-cell lines derived from *M. tuberculosis*- and BCG-immune mice are MHC class I restricted, thus raising the question of how *M. tuberculosis* and BCG proteins gain access to the MHC class I processing pathway (DeLibero et al., 1988). Although it is generally assumed that *M. tuberculosis* remains in the endosomal compartment, clear evidence for escape of *M. tuberculosis* from phagolysosomes into the cytoplasm has been presented (Leake et al., 1984; McDonough et al., 1993). Microbes residing in the cytoplasm could then produce proteins that contact MHC class I molecules, as has been clearly shown for *Listeria monocytogenes*. Alternatively, it can be assumed that during persistent replication within the phagosome, mycobacterial proteins or peptides are translocated into the cytoplasm, where they contact the MHC class I processing machinery. Recent evidence indicates that MHC class I processing can occur independently of microbial egression into the cytoplasm (Pfeifer et al., 1993).

Besides conventional MHC class I-restricted CD8 T cells, T cells that are apparently MHC class I nonrestricted have been described (DeLibero et al., 1988). Similar T cells have been identified in the listeriosis system, where these T lymphocytes are focused on peptides containing the *N*-formylmethionine (*N*-fMet) sequence pre-sented by nonconventional MHC class Ib molecules (Kaufmann et al., 1988; Kurlander et al., 1992; Pamer et al., 1992). The *N*-fMet sequence probably serves as a secretion signal in prokaryotic cells. In mammals, the *N*-fMet sequence is present only in proteins encoded by the mitochondrial genome (probably of prokaryotic origin). Furthermore, nonconventional MHC class Ib gene products are highly conserved and vary in only few mouse strains. Thus, it appears that a subset of bacterium-specific CD8 T cells is focused on (i) conserved bacterial peptides and (ii) nonpolymorphic presentation elements. If these observations can be generalized to human tuberculosis, important consequences for peptide vaccination against bacteria with few peptides and independent of human lymphocyte antigen polymorphism can be envisaged.

A contribution of γ/δ T cells to protection is suggested by indirect evidence. They have been identified in reversal reactions of leprosy patients and in tuberculous lymphadenitis lesions (Falini et al., 1989; Modlin et al., 1989). No evidence for increased γ/δ T cell numbers, however, has been observed in lymph node granulomas of tuberculosis patients (Tazi et al., 1991). In mice, γ/δ T cells accumulate early at the site of BCG replication, in draining lymph nodes after immunization with complete Freund's adjuvant, and in the lung after aerosol immunization with mycobacterial components (Augustin et al., 1989; Janis et al., 1989; Inoue et al., 1991). Furthermore, the progressive BCG infection in *scid* mice compared to *nu/nu* mice and mice depleted of CD4 and CD8 T cells has been taken as evidence for a role of γ/δ T cells (Izzo and North, 1992). Direct proof, however, has to await experiments with mutant mice devoid of γ/δ T cells. The γ/δ T cells from healthy individuals proliferate vigorously in response to mycobacterial components (Kabelitz et al., 1990; Munk et al., 1990). Although preferential γ/δ-T-cell expansion by mycobacteria is caused to a large degree by low-molecular-weight nonproteinaceous components that act in a superantigen-like fashion, γ/δ T cells also appear to be stimulated by *M. tuberculosis* antigens (Munk et al., 1990; Pfeffer et al., 1990). Thus far, the kind of antigens and presentation molecules required for γ/δ-T-cell stimulation remain virtually unknown. Evidence from other systems indicates that the relevant peptides are presented by nonconventional MHC molecules (Pamer et al., 1993). Perhaps the MHC class Ib molecules involved in CD8 T-cell stimulation also participate in γ/δ-T-cell stimulation.

T-Cell Functions

Various in vitro studies of the human and murine systems show that mycobacterium-reactive CD4 T cells are potent IFN-γ producers (Emmrich et al., 1986; Kaufmann and Flesch, 1986). IFN-γ is also produced by murine CD8 T cells with mycobacterial specificity (DeLibero et al., 1988). As described above, this cytokine is the principal mediator of antituberculous resistance. Mycobacterium-reactive CD4 T cells and CD8 T cells also express specific cytolytic activities; i.e., they lyse macrophages primed with mycobacterial antigens or infected with BCG or *M. tuberculosis* (De-Libero et al., 1988; Ottenhoff et al., 1988). It appears that these two functions not only are demonstrable in vitro but also contribute to protection in vivo. Besides the well-characterized α/β T cells, other cells also produce IFN-γ and express cytolytic activities, suggesting their participation in acquisition of resistance. In particular, both NK cells and γ/δ T cells produce IFN-γ and lyse mycobacterium-pulsed target cells (Munk et al., 1990; Bancroft et al., 1991; Follows et al., 1992; Molloy et al., 1993). In addition, polymorphonuclear granulocytes (PNG) produce highly proteolytic enzymes causing tissue liquefaction (Weiss, 1989). At the site of *M. tuberculosis* growth, these cells appear sequentially in the following order: PNG, NK cells, γ/δ T cells, α/β T cells.

Evidence has been presented elsewhere that T-cell lysis of BCG-infected macrophages causes bacterial growth inhibition in vitro (DeLibero et al., 1988). Perhaps target cell lysis promotes discharge of toxic macrophage products that inhibit mycobacterial growth. This in vitro observation may be taken as evidence for a direct protective effect afforded by cytolytic T cells. More importantly, a coordinated interplay between macrophage activation by IFN-γ (probably in conjunction with additional mediators) and target cell lysis appears to be required for optimum protection (Kaufmann, 1988). *M. tuberculosis* is extremely resistant to macrophage killing. The persistence of *M. tuberculosis* in healthy individuals for years without causing disease indicates that the immune system generally fails to sterilely eradicate this pathogen and must rely on mycobacterial containment and growth inhibition. Not only prior to but also after IFN-γ stimulation, macrophages are largely abused as habitat. Lysis of such macrophages promotes bacillary release from a shelter. Provided that the microorganisms are taken up by more efficient phagocytes soon after their liberation, this mechanism should improve host defense against tuberculosis. Such an interplay between lysis and activation of MP would best be controlled in productive granulomas (see below). At the same time, target cell lysis causes tissue damage, affects organ functions, and, in the absence of phagocytosis, promotes microbial dissemination. Lysis of infected MP, therefore, is a double-edged sword that, depending on the general situation, has a beneficial or a detrimental outcome.

T-Cell Antigens

At least two characteristics of *M. tuberculosis* and BCG influence the type of antigens that are recognized by protective T cells. First, the intracellular location (phagosome versus cytosol) dictates processing via the MHC class I or class II pathway. Second, the intracellular viability of the pathogen determines availability of polypeptides for processing (Fig. 2). MHC class I versus MHC class II processing has been discussed above. Because soluble protein antigens are not introduced into the MHC class I pathway, the design of subunit vaccines requires use of appropriate adjuvants or viable carriers capable of targeting both the MHC class I and the MHC class II pathway. As long as MP fail to kill significant numbers of intracellular *M. tuberculosis*, secreted proteins and metabolically produced peptides are the main, if not the sole, source of antigens. Later, when *M. tuberculosis* and *M. bovis* die in the activated macrophage, somatic proteins become a major source of T-cell antigens. The less metabolically active bacteria are, the lower the relative proportion of secreted protein antigens will be. Dormant tubercle bacilli without significant metabolic activity but resisting macrophage killing will be an ineffectual source of any antigen. Both features may be relevant to the low effectiveness of the only vaccine against tuberculosis available, BCG. First, BCG seems to primarily activate CD4 T cells (Pedrazzini et al., 1987). While this seems to be sufficient for protection against BCG, it appears to be insufficient for effective vaccination against tuberculosis. Perhaps the shorter intracellular survival of BCG together with a deficiency in cytolysins restricts access of BCG-derived proteins to the MHC class I pathway. Second, owing to the shorter survival time of BCG, somatic antigens will predominate early after infection. Early recognition of *M. tuberculosis*-infected macrophages, however, primarily depends on T cells that recognize secreted proteins. Thus, the preponderance of CD4 T cells and somatic antigens may explain, at least in part, the insufficient protection against *M. tuberculosis* afforded by BCG vaccination.

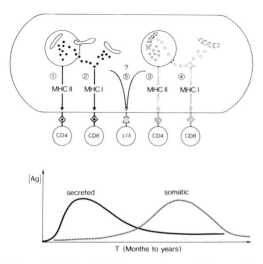

Figure 2. Relationship between intracellular persistence of *M. tuberculosis*, antigen type, and T-cell subset activation. (1) *M. tuberculosis* replicating in the phagosome secretes proteins that are degraded into peptides and then translocated to the cell surface by MHC class II molecules. (2) MHC class I molecules capture *M. tuberculosis* peptides derived from secreted proteins in the cytoplasm. Either the proteins or peptides had been translocated from the endosomal into the cytoplasmic compartment, or they were secreted into the cytoplasm by *M. tuberculosis* after its evasion of the phagosome. Later, *M. tuberculosis* is killed and degraded, thus giving rise to somatic proteins. (3) Peptides derived from *M. tuberculosis* killed in the phagosome contact MHC class II molecules. (4) Peptides from somatic proteins present in the cytoplasm are charged to MHC class I molecules. (5) Neither the source of peptides nor the presentation molecules involved in γ/δ T-cell stimulation are fully understood. This sequence of events leads to a first wave of T cells with specificity for secreted proteins followed by a second wave of T cells with specificity for somatic proteins. Ag, antigen.

THE IN VIVO SITUATION

In tuberculosis, the port of entry as well as the major organ of disease is the lung. After being inhaled, the pathogen is engulfed by alveolar macrophages that appear to be insufficiently equipped for microbial killing. Probably these alveolar macrophages transport the pathogen into the lung parenchyma and into draining lymph nodes, where the microbe replicates. Infected macrophages produce chemokines that cause the extravasation of additional phagocytes (Oppenheim et al., 1991; Friedland et al., 1992). These inflammatory phagocytes (PNG and blood monocytes) secrete significant amounts of proteolytic enzymes, generating an exudative lesion. Activated MP also secrete TNF, which initiates granuloma formation (Kindler et al., 1989). Eventually, T cells activated in draining lymph nodes as well as NK cells are attracted to the site of inflammation. Although NK cells and γ/δ T lymphocytes seem to precede α/β T cells, the former two are soon outnumbered by the last. The α/β T cells and γ/δ T cells interact with MP that present mycobacterial peptides in the context of adequate MHC molecules. They produce IFN-γ, as do NK cells, which in turn activates tuberculostatic macrophage functions. A productive granuloma with a high cellular turnover develops; bacteria are confined in it, and their growth is restrained. Although these granulomas effectively inhibit bacterial replication, they are generally unable to sterilely eradicate the pathogens. In particular, the multinucleated giant cells harbor *M. tuberculosis* and seem to be unable to eradicate their intracellular predators. Lysis of such cells, therefore, may contribute to protection by allowing uptake by more efficient phagocytes. Later, the productive granuloma may become encapsulated by a fibrotic wall, and the center of the granuloma may necrotize. TNF seems to play a notable role in fibrotic encapsulation and central necrosis (Vassalli, 1992). Encapsulation further contributes to microbial containment, and the low partial O_2 pressure (pO_2) in the necrotic center provides unfavorable growth conditions for *M. tuberculosis*. Uncontrolled cell destruction by cytolytic T cells, NK cells, activated MP, and/or PNG

may promote granuloma liquefaction and rupture into the bronchoalveolar and vascular systems. The cellular detritus and the elevated pO_2 thus arising provide an excellent medium for *M. tuberculosis* that favors its uncontrolled multiplication. Rupture of the granuloma promotes microbial dissemination through the bronchoalveolar system into the environment and through the vascular system to other tissue sites.

WHY DO WE NEED MORE THAN ONE T-CELL POPULATION FOR PROTECTION?

Given that in vitro CD4 T cells, CD8 T cells, and γ/δ T cells are so highly similar with respect to their functional competence, why do we need several T-cell subsets for optimum protection to occur? At the moment, this question cannot be fully answered. A first advantage of CD8 T cells and γ/δ T cells over CD4 T cells is their restriction by MHC class I molecules, which are expressed on virtually all host cells, while MHC class II expression is restricted to certain host cells such as MP. Although *M. tuberculosis* preferentially resides in MP, a few parenchyma cells, typically in the lung, may become infected. These cells remain unnoticed by CD4 T cells and are identified only by CD8 T cells (and perhaps γ/δ T cells). Second, the three T-cell populations may differ in their activation kinetics, with γ/δ T cells probably arriving first at the site of mycobacterial growth. Thus, γ/δ T cells may perform essential effector functions before α/β T cells do. Although γ/δ T cells may be less effective, their faster kinetics of mobilization and activation may give them some advantage. Third, these T-cell populations may differ in effector functions thus far unclear, e.g., in their capacity to leave the vascular bed or in their responsiveness to inflammatory signals. Fourth, α/β T cells and γ/δ T cells vary remarkably in their tissue distributions. In mucosal tissues, including the lung, as preferred port of entry and site of disease manifestation in tuberculosis, the percentage of γ/δ T cells is markedly higher than in peripheral blood and central lymphoid organs. Finally, regulatory interactions between these T-cell subsets may be required. In support of this last possibility, evidence has been presented that γ/δ T cells control activation of α/β T cells not only in vitro but also in vivo (Kaufmann et al., 1993). Most impressively, in the model of experimental listeriosis of γ/δ T-cell-deficient mutant mice, huge, abscess-like lesions develop that are strikingly different from the granulomatous lesions at the site of listerial implantation in healthy controls (Mombaerts et al., 1993).

GENETIC DETERMINANTS FOR SUSCEPTIBILITY AND RESISTANCE IN TUBERCULOSIS

While there is little formal genetic evidence in humans, data obtained from epidemiological investigations suggest that susceptibility to many infectious diseases, including tuberculosis, is under some genetic control (Motulsky, 1979; Skamene, 1986). The annual death rate from tuberculosis reached 10% when the disease first became prevalent in the Qu'appelle Valley Indian Reservation in Canada, eliminating half the Indian families in the first three generations; yet 40 years later, the annual death rate had dwindled to 0.2%, suggesting selection for host resistance (Goodman and Motulsky, 1979). Clearly, it is conceivable that different genetic strains of the same pathogen cause diseases in different geographical regions, so that with continued passage, as could be in the case of tuberculosis in the Qu'appelle Valley, attenuated virulence and thus in a drastic drop in death rate over time result. While this confounding factor is difficult to rule out, nonetheless, the higher degree of concordance of tuberculosis among monozygotic than dizygotic twins (Comstock, 1978) and the tragic incident of Lubeck in 1927 (Anonymous, 1935), in which infants inadvertently immunized with a single viable virulent *M. tuberculosis* strain displayed marked differences in susceptibility ranging from death to recovery, argue for a genetic basis for resistance to mycobacterial diseases.

In contrast to work with the human system, experimental studies on the genetics of resistance to an enormous variety of infectious agents (salmonellae, leishmaniae, mycobacteria, murine leukemia viruses, rickettsiae, etc.) in inbred strains of mice are abundant (Skamene, 1985). In the case of resistance to *Salmonella typhimurium*, *Leishmania donovani*, and BCG, compelling experimental evidence obtained from backcross linkage analyses (Skamene et al., 1982) suggests that resistance against these three pathogens is under monogenic control. This allele has been designated *Ity*, *Lsh*, and *Bcg* in the resistance models of *S. typhimurium*, *Leishmania donovani*, and BCG, respectively. Through typing for resistance and susceptibility to BCG among recombinant inbred mouse strains together with linkage analyses and detailed dissection of a 30-centimorgan segment on murine chromosome 1, the cloning of the cDNA for the *Bcg* gene, designated *Nramp* (natural-resistance-associated macrophage protein), has recently been achieved (Vidal et al., 1993). Sequence analysis of the *Nramp* cDNA reveals a 1,452-nucleotide open reading frame that encodes a 484-amino-acid protein with structural homology to a eukaryotic nitrate transporter. Analysis of *Nramp* cDNAs from seven Bcg^r and six Bcg^s mouse strains indicates that BCG susceptibility is the result of a G-to-A transition at position 783 associated with a nonconservative substitution of Asp-105 for Gly-105 within a predicted transmembrane domain of *Nramp*. Comparison of amino acid sequences of the murine *Nramp* and a human homolog deduced from a partial cDNA clone reveals 89% homology between the two species. Nucleic acid sequence analysis indicates that Gly-105 of murine *Nramp* is conserved in the human sequence.

While it is known that the *Bcg*[r] gene confers resistance against mycobacteria by acting early during the nonimmune phase of infection in mice (in contrast to the MHC genes, which appear to be associated with recovery after infection), the precise biochemical and molecular mechanisms of how *Nramp* regulates resistance and susceptibility to infection remain to be defined (reviewed in Skamene [1986]). Experimental evidence strongly suggests that the *Nramp* phenotype is mediated via macrophages. It has been demonstrated that the cell type expressing the *Nramp* phenotype is derived from the bone marrow and is relatively radioresistant. In addition, the phenotypic expression of *Nramp* can be inactivated by chronic exposure of mice to silica, a macrophage poison (Gros et al., 1983). Finally, *Nramp* mRNAs are preferentially expressed in the reticuloendothelial system, particularly in macrophages. The recent finding that RNI generated via the macrophage L-arginine-dependent cytotoxic mechanism is effectively antimycobacterial (Denis, 1991a; Flesch and Kaufmann, 1991; Chan et al., 1992) and the demonstration of marked structural resemblance of *Nramp* protein to a eukaryotic nitrate transporter (Vidal et al., 1993) lend support to the hypothesis that regulation of RNI trafficking in macrophages might be one way by which the resistance phenotype of this gene is expressed. It is thus possible that *Nramp* participates in the L-arginine-dependent antimycobacterial pathway by transporting NO_2^-, a relatively stable and nontoxic nitrogen oxide formed via the oxidation of nitric oxide in the aqueous phase, into the phagolysosomal compartment, whose acidic environment is requisite to and allows the formation of nitrous acid,

which dismutates to generate NO (Shank et al., 1962) and other more reactive and perhaps more toxic reactive nitrogen species such as the nitrogen dioxide radical. A corollary of this possibility is that ammonia production by *M. tuberculosis* (Gordon et al., 1980) is a means by which generation of toxic RNI could be intercepted via alkalinization of the phagolysosomal content. The existence of a human homolog of *Nramp*, at least by cDNA analyses (Vidal et al., 1993), together with the presence on human chromosome 2q of a region syntenic to the 30-centimorgan segment on murine chromosome 1 that contains the *Bcg* allele (Schurr et al., 1990) should presage optimism in unraveling the genetic basis for resistance and susceptibility to mycobacterial diseases, at least at the early phase of infection. It is hoped that the elucidation of one aspect of this difficult question will form a firm springboard for understanding other as yet unknown genetic factors, e.g., the MHC molecules (Skamene, 1986), that aid in determining the outcome of mycobacterial infection.

CONCLUDING REMARKS

Around the world, as many as 60 million people suffer from tuberculosis. This high figure may lead to the false conclusion that protective immunity is totally insufficient for control of this disease. The figure, however, is clearly qualified by the even higher number of more than 1.7 billion infected individuals, i.e., one-third of the world population, illustrating that in the vast majority of infected individuals, disease does not develop in the face of an ongoing infection. Hence, protective immunity is extraordinarily inefficient in terminating infection and, at the same time, highly efficacious in preventing disease. Because the relationship between *M. tuberculosis* and host immunity underlying infection is a labile one, any diminution of protective immunity will cause progression into clinical disease.

Acknowledgments. S. H. E. Kaufmann acknowledges financial support from SFB 322, Landesschwerpunkt "Chronic Infectious Diseases," and from the German Ministry of Science and Technology (BMFT).

REFERENCES

Adams, J. S., and M. A. Gacad. 1985. Characterization of 1-alpha hydroxylation of vitamin D₃ sterols by cultured alveolar macrophages from patients with sarcoidosis. *J. Exp. Med.* **161**:755–765.

Albelda, S. M., and C. A. Buck. 1990. Integrins and other cell adhesion molecules. *FASEB J.* **4**:2868–2880.

Amiri, P., R. M. Locksley, T. G. Parslow, M. Sadick, E. Rector, D. Ritter, and J. H. McKerrow. 1992. Tumor necrosis factor α restores granulomas and induces parasite egg-laying in schistosome-infected SCID mice. *Nature* (London) **356**:604–607.

Anonymous. 1935. *Die Sauglingstuberkulose in Lubeck.* Julius Springer, Berlin.

Armstrong, J. A., and P. D'Arcy Hart. 1971. Response of cultured macrophages to *Mycobacterium tuberculosis*, with observations on fusion of lysosomes with phagosomes. *J. Exp. Med.* **134**:713–740.

Armstrong, J. A., and P. D'Arcy Hart. 1975. Phagosome-lysosome interactions in cultured macrophages infected with virulent tubercle bacilli. Reversal of the usual fusion pattern and observations on bacterial survival. *J. Exp. Med.* **142**:1–16.

Arruda, S., G. Bomfim, R. Knights, T. Huima-Byron, and L. W. Riley. 1993. Cloning of an *M. tuberculosis* DNA fragment associated with entry and survival inside cells. *Science* **261**:1454–1457.

Augustin, A., R. T. Kubo, and G.-K. Sim. 1989. Resident pulmonary lymphocytes expressing the c/d T-cell receptor. *Nature* (London) **340**:239–241.

Bail, O. 1910. Übertragung der Tuberkulinempfindlichkeit. *Z. Immunitaetsforsch.* **4**:470–485.

Bainton, D. F. 1981. The discovery of lysosomes. *J. Cell Biol.* **91**:66S–76S.

Bancroft, G. J., R. D. Schreiber, and E. R. Unanue. 1991. Natural immunity: a T-cell-independent pathway of macrophage activation defined in the scid mouse. *Immunol. Rev.* **124**:5–24.

Barnes, P. F., S. D. Mistry, C. L. Cooper, C. Pirmez, T. H. Rea, and R. L. Modlin. 1989. Compartmentalization of a CD4+ T lymphocyte subpopulation in tuberculous pleuritis. *J. Immunol.* **142**:1114–1119.

Beckman, J. S., T. W. Beckman, J. Chen, P. A. Marshall, and B. A. Freeman. 1990. Apparent hydroxyl radical production by peroxynitrite: implications for endothelial injury from nitric oxide and superoxide. *Proc. Natl. Acad. Sci. USA* **87**:1620–1624.

Bermudez, L. E. 1993. Production of transforming growth factor-β by *Mycobacterium avium*-infected human macrophages is associated with unresponsiveness to IFN-γ. *J. Immunol.* **150**:1838–1845.

Bermudez, L. E., and J. Champsi. 1993. Infection with *Mycobacterium avium* induces production of interleukin-10 (IL-10), and administration of anti-IL-10 antibody is associated with enhanced resistance to infection in mice. *Infect. Immun.* **61**:3093–3097.

Bielecki, J., P. Youngman, P. Connelly, and D. A. Portnoy. 1990. *Bacillus subtilis* expressing a haemolysin gene from *Listeria monocytogenes* can grow in mammalian cells. *Nature* (London) **345**:175–176.

Bloom, B. R., and B. Bennett. 1966. Mechanism of a reaction in vitro associated with delayed-type hypersensitivity. *Science* **153**:80–82.

Brennan, P. J. 1989. Structure of mycobacteria: recent developments in defining cell wall carbohydrates and proteins. *J. Infect. Dis.* **11**:S420–S430.

Brennan, P. J., S. W. Hunter, M. McNeil, D. Chatterjee, and M. Daffe. 1990. Reappraisal of the chemistry of mycobacterial cell walls, with a view to understanding the roles of individual entities in disease processes, p. 55–75. *In* E. M. Ayoub, G. H. Cassell, W. C. Branche, Jr., and T. J. Henry (ed.), *Microbial Determinants of Virulence and Host Response.* American Society for Microbiology, Washington, D.C.

Brennt, C. E., A. C. Wright, S. K. Dutta, and J. G. Morris, Jr. 1991. Growth of *Vibrio vulnificus* in serum from alcoholics: association with high transferrin iron saturation. *J. Infect. Dis.* **164**:1030–1032.

Brozna, J. P., M. Horan, J. M. Rademacher, K. A. Pabst, and M. J. Pabst. 1991. Monocyte responses to sulfatide from *Mycobacterium tuberculosis*: inhibition of priming for enhanced release of superoxide, associated with increased secretion of interleukin-1 and tumor necrosis factor alpha, and altered protein phosphorylation. *Infect. Immun.* **59**:2542–2548.

Bullen, J. J., P. B. Spalding, C. G. Ward, and J. M. C. Gutteridge. 1991. Hemochromatosis, iron, and septicemia caused by *Vibrio vulnificus*. *Arch. Intern. Med.* **151**:1606–1609.

Bullock, W. E., and S. D. Wright. 1987. Role of the adherence-promoting receptors, CR3, LFA-1, and p150,95 in binding of *Histoplasma capsulatum* by human macrophages. *J. Exp. Med.* **165**:195–210.

Cahall, D. L., and C. P. Youmans. 1975a. Conditions for production, and some characteristics, of mycobacterial growth inhibitory factor produced by spleen cells from mice immunized with viable cells of the attenuated H37Ra strain of *Mycobacterium tuberculosis*. *Infect. Immun.* **12**:833–840.

Cahall, D. L., and C. P. Youmans. 1975b. Molecular weight and other characteristics of mycobacterial growth inhibitory factor produced by spleen cells obtained from mice immunized with viable cells of the attenuated mycobacterial cells. *Infect. Immun.* **12**:841–850.

Chan, J., and B. R. Bloom. Unpublished observations.

Chan, J., X.-D. Fan, S. W. Hunter, P. J. Brennan, and B. R. Bloom. 1991. Lipoarabinomannan, a possible virulence factor involved in persistence of *Mycobacterium tuberculosis* within macrophages. *Infect. Immun.* **59**:1755–1761.

Chan, J., T. Fujiwara, P. Brennan, M. McNeil, S. J. Turco, J.-C. Sibille, M. Snapper, P. Aisen, and B. R. Bloom. 1989. Microbial glycolipids: possible virulence factors that scavenge oxygen radicals. *Proc. Natl. Acad. Sci. USA* **86**:2453–2457.

Chan, J., Y. Xing, R. S. Magliozzo, and B. R. Bloom. 1992. Killing of virulent *Mycobacterium tuberculosis* by reactive nitrogen intermediates produced by activated murine macrophages. *J. Exp. Med.* **175**: 1111–1122.

Chase, M. W. 1945. The cellular transfer of cutaneous hypersensitivity to tuberculin. *Proc. Soc. Exp. Biol. Med.* **59**:134–135.

Chatterjee, D., K. Lowell, B. Rivoire, M. R. McNeil, and P. J. Brennan. 1992a. Lipoarabinomannan of *Mycobacterium tuberculosis*. Capping with mannosyl residues in some strains. *J. Biol. Chem.* **267**: 6234–6239.

Chatterjee, D., A. D. Roberts, K. Lowell, P. J. Brennan, and I. M. Orme. 1992b. Structural basis of capacity of lipoarabinomannan to induce secretion of tumor necrosis factor. *Infect. Immun.* **60**:1249–1253.

Cheever, A. W., F. D. Finkelman, P. Caspar, S. Heiny, J. G. Macedonia, and A. Sher. 1992. Treatment with anti-IL-2 antibodies reduces hepatic pathology and eosinophilia in *Schistosoma mansoni*-infected mice while selectively inhibiting T cell IL-5 production. *J. Immunol.* **148**:3244–3248.

Chensue, S. W., I. G. Otterness, G. I. Higashi, C. S. Forsch, and S. L. Kunkel. 1989. Monokine production by hypersensitivity (*Schistosoma mansoni* egg) and foreign body (Sephadex bead)-type granuloma macrophages. Evidence for sequential production of IL-1 and tumor necrosis factor. *J. Immunol.* **142**: 1281–1286.

Chensue, S. W., P. D. Terebuh, K. S. Warmington, S. D. Hershey, H. L. Evanoff, S. L. Kunkel, and G. I. Higashi. 1992. Role of IL-4 and IFN-γ in *Schistosoma mansoni* egg-induced hypersensitivity granuloma formation. Orchestration, relative contribution, and relationship to macrophage function. *J. Immunol.* **148**:900–906.

Cohn, Z. A. 1963. The fate of bacteria within phagocytic cells. I. The degradation of isotopically labeled bacteria by polymorphonuclear leucocytes and macrophages. *J. Exp. Med.* **117**:27–42.

Comstock, G. W. 1978. Tuberculosis in twins: a reanalysis of the Prophit survey. *Am. Rev. Respir. Dis.* **117**:621–624.

Cooper, A. M., D. K. Dalton, T. A. Stewart, J. P. Griffin, D. G. Russell, and I. M. Orme. 1993. Disseminated tuberculosis in interferon-γ gene-disrupted mice. *J. Exp. Med.* **178**:2243–2247.

Crowle, A. J., E. J. Ross, and M. H. May. 1987. Inhibition by 1,25(OH)$_2$-vitamin D$_3$ of the multiplication of virulent tubercle bacilli in cultured human macrophages. *Infect. Immun.* **55**:2945–2950.

Cunha, F. Q., S. Moncada, and F. Y. Liew. 1992. Interleukin-10 (IL-10) inhibits the induction of nitric oxide synthase by interferon-gamma in murine macrophages. *Biochem. Biophys. Res. Commun.* **182**: 1155–1159.

Daffe, M., C. Lacave, M.-A. Laneelle, and G. Laneelle. 1987. Structure of the major triglycosyl phenol-phthiocerol of *Mycobacterium tuberculosis* (strain Canetti). *Eur. J. Biochem.* **167**:144–160.

Dalton, D., S. Pitts-Meek, S. Keshav, I. S. Figari, A. Bradley, and T. A. Stewart. 1993. Multiple defects of immune cell function in mice with disrupted interferon-γ genes. *Science* **259**:1739–1742.

D'Andrea, A., M. Rengaraju, N. M. Valiente, J. Chehimi, M. Kubin, M. Aste, S. H. Chan, M. Kobayashi, D. Young, E. Nickbarg, R. Chizzonite, S. F. Wolf, and G. Trinchieri. 1992. Production of natural killer cell stimulatory factor (interleukin 12) by peripheral blood mononuclear cells. *J. Exp. Med.* **176**:1387–1398.

D'Arcy Hart, P., M. R. Young, A. H. Gordon, and K. H. Sullivan. 1987. Inhibition of phagosome-lysosome fusion in macrophages by certain mycobacteria can be explained by inhibition of lysosomal movements observed after phagocytosis. *J. Exp. Med.* **166**:933–946.

D'Arcy Hart, P., M. R. Young, M. M. Jordan, W. J. Perkins, and M. J. Geisow. 1983. Chemical inhibitors of phagosome-lysosome fusion in cultured macrophages also inhibit saltatory lysosomal movements. A combined microscopic and computer study. *J. Exp. Med.* **158**:477–492.

David, J. R. 1966. Delayed hypersensitivity in vitro: its mediation by cell-free substances formed by lymphoid cell-antigen interaction. *Proc. Natl. Acad. Sci. USA* **56**:72–77.

de Duve, C., and R. Wattiaux. 1966. Functions of lysosomes. *Annu. Rev. Physiol.* **28**:435–492.

DeLibero, G., I. Flesch, and S. H. E. Kaufmann. 1988. Mycobacteria reactive Lyt2+ T cell lines. *Eur. J. Immunol.* **18**:59–66.

Denis, M. 1991a. Killing of *Mycobacterium tuberculosis* within human monocytes: activation by cytokines and calcitriol. *Clin. Exp. Immunol.* **84**:200–206.

Denis, M. 1991b. Interferon-gamma-treated murine macrophages inhibit growth of tubercle bacilli via the generation of reactive nitrogen intermediates. *Cell. Immunol.* **132**:150–157.

Denis, M. 1991c. Tumor necrosis factor and granulo-cyte macrophage colony-stimulating factor stimulate human macrophages to restrict growth of virulent *Mycobacterium avium* and to kill avirulent *M. avium*: killing effector mechanism depends on the generation of reactive nitrogen intermediates. *J. Leukocyte Biol.* **49:**380–387.

Denis, M., and E. Ghadirian. 1991. Transforming growth factor (TGF-β1) plays a detrimental role in the progression of experimental *Mycobacterium avium* infection; in vivo and in vitro evidence. *Microb. Pathog.* **11:**367–372.

Doi, T., M. Ando, T. Akaike, M. Suga, K. Sato, and H. Maeda. 1993. Resistance to nitric oxide in *Mycobacterium avium* complex and its implication in pathogenesis. *Infect. Immun.* **61:**1980–1989.

Douvas, G. S., D. L. Looker, A. E. Vatter, and A. J. Crowle. 1985. Gamma interferon activates human macrophages to become tumoricidal and leishmanicidal but enhances replication of macrophage-associated mycobacteria. *Infect. Immun.* **50:**1–8.

Drapier, J.-C., H. Hirling, J. Wietzerbin, P. Kaldy, and L. C. Kuhn. 1993. Biosynthesis of nitric oxide activates iron regulatory factor in macrophages. *EMBO J.* **12:**3643–3649.

Dunn, C. J., M. M. Hardee, A. J. Gibbons, N. D. Staite, and K. A. Richard. 1988. Interleukin-1 induces chronic granulomatous inflammation, p. 329–334. *In* M. C. Powanda, J. J. Oppenheim, M. J. Kluger, and C. A. Dinarello (ed.), *Monokines and Other Non-lymphocytic Cytokines*. Alan R. Liss, Inc., New York.

Eaton, J. W., P. Brandt, and J. R. Mahoney. 1982. Haptoglobin: a natural bacteriostat. *Science* **215:**691–693.

Emmrich, F., J. Thole, J. D. A. Van Embden, and S. H. E. Kaufmann. 1986. A recombinant 64 kilodalton protein of Mycobacterium bovis BCG specifically stimulates human T4 clones reactive to mycobacterial antigens. *J. Exp. Med.* **163:**1024–1029.

Falini, B., L. Flenghi, S. Pileri, P. Pelicci, M. Fagioli, M. F. Martelli, L. Moretta, and E. Ciccone. 1989. Distribution of T cells bearing different forms of the T cell receptor c/d in normal and pathological human tissues. *J. Immunol.* **143:**2480–2488.

Falkow, S., R. R. Isberg, and D. A. Portnoy. 1992. The interaction of bacteria with mammalian cells. *Annu. Rev. Cell Biol.* **8:**333–363.

Fan, X.-D., M. Goldberg, and B. R. Bloom. 1988. Interferon-gamma-induced transcriptional activation is mediated by protein kinase C. *Proc. Natl. Acad. Sci. USA* **85:**5122–5125.

Filley, E. A., and G. A. W. Rook. 1991. Effect of mycobacteria on sensitivity to the cytotoxic effects of tumor necrosis factor. *Infect. Immun.* **59:**2567–2572.

Flesch, I. E. A., and S. H. E. Kaufmann. 1987. Myco-bacterial growth inhibition by interferon-γ-activated bone marrow macrophages and differential susceptibility among strains of *Mycobacterium tuberculosis*. *J. Immunol.* **138:**4408–4413.

Flesch, I. E. A., and S. H. E. Kaufmann. 1988. Attempts to characterize the mechanisms involved in mycobacterial growth inhibition by gamma-interferon-activated bone marrow macrophages. *Infect. Immun.* **56:**1464.

Flesch, I. E. A., and S. H. E. Kaufmann. 1990a. Activation of tuberculostatic macrophage functions by gamma interferon, interleukin-4, and tumor necrosis factor. *Infect. Immun.* **58:**2675–2677.

Flesch, I. E. A., and S. H. E. Kaufmann. 1990b. Stimulation of antibacterial macrophage activities by B-cell stimulatory factor 2 (interleukin-6). *Infect. Immun.* **58:**269–271.

Flesch, I. E. A., and S. H. E. Kaufmann. 1991. Mechanisms involved in mycobacterial growth inhibition by gamma interferon-activated bone marrow macrophages: role of reactive nitrogen intermediates. *Infect. Immun.* **59:**3213–3218.

Flynn, J. L., and B. R. Bloom. Personal communication.

Flynn, J. L., J. Chan, K. J. Triebold, D. K. Dalton, T. A. Stewart, and B. R. Bloom. 1993. An essential role for IFN-γ in resistance to *Mycobacterium tuberculosis* infection. *J. Exp. Med.* **178:**2249–2254.

Flynn, J. L., M. A. Goldstein, K. J. Treibold, B. Koller, and B. R. Bloom. 1992. Major histocompatibility complex class I-restricted T cells are required for resistance to *Mycobacterium tuberculosis* infection. *Proc. Natl. Acad. Sci. USA* **89:**12013–12017.

Flynn, J. L., D. Mathis, and B. R. Bloom. Unpublished observations.

Flynn, J. L., R. Schreiber, and B. R. Bloom. Personal communication.

Follows, G. A., M. E. Munk, A. J. Gatrill, P. Conradt, and S. H. E. Kaufmann. 1992. Interferon-γ and interleukin 2 but no detectable interleukin 4 in γ/δ T-cell cultures after activation with bacteria. *Infect. Immun.* **60:**1229–1231.

Forrest, C. B., J. R. Forehand, R. A. Axtell, R. L. Roberts, and R. B. Johnston, Jr. 1988. Clinical features and current management of chronic granulomatous disease. *Hematol. Oncol. Clin. N. Am.* **2:**253–265.

Friedland, J. S., D. G. Remick, R. Shattock, and G. E. Griffin. 1992. Secretion of interleukin-8 following phagocytosis of *Mycobacterium tuberculosis* by human monocyte cell lines. *Eur. J. Immunol.* **22:**1373–1378.

Friedland, J. S., R. J. Shattock, J. D. Johnson, D. G. Remick, R. E. Holliman, and G. E. Griffin. 1993. Differential cytokine gene expression and secretion after phagocytosis by a human monocytic cell line of *Toxoplasma gondii* compared with *Mycobacterium tuberculosis. Clin. Exp. Immunol.* **91**:282–286.

Gavioli, R., S. Spisani, A. Giuliani, and S. Traniello. 1987. Protein kinase C mediates human neutrophil cytotoxicity. *Biochem. Biophys. Res. Commun.* **148**:1290–1294.

Gazzinelli, R. T., S. Hieny, T. A. Wynn, S. Wolf, and A. Sher. 1993. Interleukin 12 is required for the T-lymphocyte-independent induction of interferon γ by an intracellular parasite and induces resistance in T-cell-deficient hosts. *Proc. Natl. Acad. Sci. USA* **90**:6115–6119.

Gazzinelli, R. T., I. P. Oswald, S. L. James, and A. Sher. 1992. IL-10 inhibits parasite killing and nitrogen oxide production by IFN-gamma-activated macrophages. *J. Immunol.* **148**:1792–1796.

Gennaro, R., C. Florio, and D. Romeo. 1985. Activation of protein kinase C in neutrophil cytoplasts. *FEBS Lett.* **180**:185–190.

Goodman, R. M., and A. G. Motulsky. 1979. *Genetic Diseases among Askenazi Jews*, p. 301. Raven Press, Inc., New York.

Gordon, A. H., P. D'Arcy Hart, and M. R. Young. 1980. Ammonia inhibits phagosome-lysosome fusion in macrophages. *Nature* (London) **286**:79–81.

Goren, M. B., O. Brokl, P. Roller, H. M. Fales, and B. C. Das. 1976a. Sulfatides of *Mycobacterium tuberculosis*: the structure of the principal sulfatide (SL-1). *Biochemistry* **15**:2728.

Goren, M. B., O. Brokl, and W. B. Schaeffer. 1974. Lipids of putative relevance to virulence in *Mycobacterium tuberculosis*: correlation of virulence with elaboration of sulfatides and strongly acidic lipids. *Infect. Immun.* **9**:142–149.

Goren, M. B., P. D'Arcy Hart, M. R. Young, and J. A. Armstrong. 1976b. Prevention of phagosome-lysosome fusion in cultured macrophages by sulfatides of *Mycobacterium tuberculosis*. *Proc. Natl. Acad. Sci. USA* **73**:2510–2514.

Goren, M. B., A. E. Vatter, and J. Fiscus. 1987a. Polyanionic agents as inhibitors of phagosome-lysosome fusion in cultured macrophages: evolution of an alternative interpretation. *J. Leukocyte Biol.* **41**:111–121.

Goren, M. B., A. E. Vatter, and J. Fiscus. 1987b. Polyanionic agents do not inhibit phagosome-lysosome fusion in cultured macrophages. *J. Leukocyte Biol.* **41**:122–129.

Griffiths, E., H. J. Rogers, and J. J. Bullen. 1980. Iron, plasmids and infection. *Nature* (London) **284**:508–509.

Gros, P., E. Skamene, and A. Forget. 1983. Cellular mechanisms of genetically controlled host resistance to *Mycobacterium bovis* (BCG). *J. Immunol.* **131**:1966–1973.

Hamilton, T. A., and D. O. Adams. 1987. Molecular mechanisms of signal transduction in macrophages. *Immunol. Today* **8**:151–158.

Hamilton, T. A., D. L. Becton, S. D. Somers, P. W. Gray, and D. O. Adams. 1984. Interferon-γ modulates protein kinase C activity in murine peritoneal macrophages. *J. Biol. Chem.* **260**:1378–1381.

Heinzel, F. P., D. S. Schoenhaut, R. M. Rerko, L. E. Rosser, and M. K. Gately. 1993. Recombinant interleukin 12 cures mice infected with *Leishmania major. J. Exp. Med.* **177**:1505–1509.

Helmholz, H. F. 1909. Über passive Übertragung der Tuberkulin-Überempfindlichkeit bei Meerschweinchen. *Z. Immunitaetsforsch.* **3**:371–375.

Hibbs, J. B., C. Westenfelder, R. Taintor, Z. Vavrin, C. Kablitz, R. L. Baranowski, J. H. Ward, R. L. Menlove, M. P. McMurry, J. P. Kushner, and W. E. Samlowski. 1992. Evidence for cytokine-inducible nitric oxide synthesis from L-arginine in patients receiving interleukin-2 therapy. *J. Clin. Invest.* **89**:867–877.

Hunter, S. W., and P. J. Brennan. 1981. A novel phenolic glycolipid from *Mycobacterium leprae* possibly involved in immunogenicity and pathogenicity. *J. Bacteriol.* **147**:728–735.

Hunter, S. W., and P. J. Brennan. 1991. Evidence for the presence of a phosphatidylinositol anchor on the lipoarabinomannan and lipomannan of *Mycobacterium tuberculosis. J. Biol. Chem.* **265**:9272–9279.

Hunter, S. W., T. Fujiwara, and P. J. Brennan. 1982. Structure and antigenicity of the major specific glycolipid antigen of *Mycobacterium leprae. J. Biol. Chem.* **257**:15072–15078.

Hunter, S. W., H. Gaylord, and P. J. Brennan. 1986. Structure and antigenicity of the phosphorylated lipopolysaccharide antigens from the leprosy and tubercle bacilli. *J. Biol. Chem.* **261**:12345–12351.

Huygen, K., P. Vandenbussche, and H. Heremans. 1991. Interleukin-6 production in *Mycobacterium bovis* BCG-infected mice. *Cell. Immunol.* **137**:224–231.

Inoue, T., Y. Yoshikai, G. Matsuzaki, and K. Nomoto. 1991. Early appearing γ/δ-bearing T cells during infection with Calmette Guérin bacillus. *J. Immunol.* **146**:2754–2762.

Isberg, R. R. 1991. Discrimination between intracellular uptake and surface adhesion of bacterial pathogens. *Science* **252**:934–938.

Iyer, G. Y. N., M. F. Islam, and J. H. Quastel. 1961. Biochemical aspects of phagocytosis. *Nature* (London) **192**:535–541.

Izzo, A. A., and R. J. North. 1992. Evidence for an α/β T cell-independent mechanism of resistance to mycobacteria. Bacillus-Calmette-Guérin causes progressive infection in severe combined immunodeficient mice, but not in nude mice or in mice depleted of CD4+ and CD8+ T cells. *J. Exp. Med.* **176**:581–586.

Janis, E. M., S. H. E. Kaufmann, R. H. Schwartz, and A. M. Pardoll. 1989. Activation of γ/δ T cells in the primary immune response to Mycobacterium tuberculosis. *Science* **244**:713–717.

Joiner, K. A., S. A. Fuhrman, H. M. Miettinen, L. H. Kasper, and I. Mellman. 1990. *Toxoplasma gondii*: fusion competence of parasitophorous vacuoles in Fc receptor-transfected fibroblasts. *Science* **249**: 641–646.

Kabelitz, D., A. Bender, S. Schondelmaier, B. Schoel, and S. H. E. Kaufmann. 1990. A large fraction of human peripheral blood γ/δ+ T cells is activated by Mycobacterium tuberculosis but not by its 65-kD heat shock protein. *J. Exp. Med.* **171**:667–679.

Kamijo, R., J. Le, D. Shapiro, E. A. Havell, S. Huang, M. Aguet, M. Bosland, and J. Vilcek. 1993. Mice that lack the interferon-γ receptor have profoundly altered responses to infection with Bacillus Calmette-Guerin and subsequent challenge with lipopolysaccharide. *J. Exp. Med.* **178**:1435–1440.

Kasahara, K., K. Kobayashi, Y. Shikama, I. Yoneya, K. Soezima, H. Ide, and T. Takahashi. 1988. Direct evidence for granuloma-inducing activity of interleukin-1. Induction of experimental pulmonary granuloma formation in mice by interleukin-1-coupled beads. *Am. J. Pathol.* **130**:629–638.

Kaufmann, S. H. E. 1988. CD8+ T lymphocytes in intracellular microbial infections. *Immunol. Today* **9**:168–174.

Kaufmann, S. H. E., C. Blum, and S. Yamamoto. 1993. Crosstalk between α/β T cells and γ/δ T cells in vivo: activation of α/β T cell responses after γ/δ T cell modulation with the monoclonal antibody GL3. *Proc. Natl. Acad. Sci. USA* **90**:9620–9624.

Kaufmann, S. H. E., and I. Flesch. 1986. Function and antigen recognition pattern of L3T4+ T cell clones from Mycobacterium tuberculosis-immune mice. *Infect. Immun.* **54**:291–296.

Kaufmann, S. H. E., M. E. Munk, T. Koga, et al. 1989. Effector T cells in bacterial infections, p. 963–970. *In* F. Melchers (ed.), *Progress in Immunology*. Spring Verlag, Stuttgart, Germany.

Kaufmann, S. H. E., H. R. Rodewald, E. Hug, and G. DeLibero. 1988. Cloned Listeria monocytogenes specific non-MHC-restricted Lyt2+ T cells with cytolytic and protective activity. *J. Immunol.* **140**: 3173–3179.

Kindler, V., A.-P. Sappino, G. E. Gran, P.-F. Piquet, and P. Vassalli. 1989. The inducing role of tumor necrosis factor in the development of bactericidal granulomas during BCG infection. *Cell* **56**:731–740.

King, C., M. Sathish, J. T. Crawford, and T. M. Shinnick. 1993. Expression of contact-dependent cytolytic activity of *Mycobacterium tuberculosis* and isolation of the locus encoding the activity. *Infect. Immun.* **61**:2708–2712.

Klebanoff, S. J. 1980. *In* R. Van Furth (ed.), *Mononuclear Phagocytes, Functional Aspects*, part 2, p. 1105–1141. Nijhoff, Boston.

Klun, C. L., and G. P. Youmans. 1973a. The effect of lymphocyte supernatant fluids on the intracellular growth of virulent tubercle bacilli. *J. Reticuloendothel. Soc.* **13**:263–274.

Klun, C. L., and G. P. Youmans. 1973b. The induction by *Listeria monocytogenes* and plant mitogens of lymphocyte supernatant fluids which inhibit the growth of *Mycobacterium tuberculosis* within macrophages in vitro. *J. Reticuloendothel. Soc.* **13**:275–285.

Kobayashi, K., C. Allred, S. Cohen, and T. Yoshida. 1985. Role of interleukin 1 in experimental granuloma in mice. *J. Immunol.* **134**:358–364.

Kobayashi, M., L. Fitz, M. Ryan, R. M. Hewick, S. C. Clark, S. Chan, R. Loudon, F. Sherman, B. Perussia, and G. Trinchieri. 1989. Identification and purification of natural killer cell stimulatory factor (NKSF), a cytokine with multiple biologic effects on human lymphocytes. *J. Exp. Med.* **170**:827.

Koch, R. 1882. Die Ätiologie der Tuberkulose. *Berliner Klin. Wochenschr.* **19**:221–230.

Koch, R. 1890. Weitere Mitteilungen über ein Heilmittel gegen Tuberkulose. *Dtsch. Med. Wochenschr.* **16**:1029–1032.

Koeffler, H. P., H. Reichel, J. E. Bishop, and A. W. Norman. 1985. Gamma interferon stimulates production of 1,25-dihydroxyvitamin D_3 by normal human macrophages. *Biochem. Biophys. Res. Commun.* **127**:596–603.

Kornfeld, S. 1987. Trafficking of lysosomal enzymes. *FASEB J.* **1**:462–468.

Kurlander, R. J., S. M. Shawar, M. L. Brown, and R. R. Rich. 1992. Specialized role for a murine class I-b MHC molecule in prokaryotic host defenses. *Science* **257**:678–679.

Kwon, N. S., C. F. Nathan, and D. J. Stuehr. 1989. Reduced biopterin as a cofactor in the generation of nitrogen oxides by murine macrophages. *J. Biol. Chem.* **264**:20496–20501.

Ladel, C., and S. H. E. Kaufmann. Unpublished data.

Larsen, C. A., A. O. Anderson, E. Apella, J. J. Oppenheim, and K. Matsushima. 1989. The neutrophil-activating protein (NAP-1) is also chemotactic for T lymphocytes. *Science* **243**:1464.

Leake, E. S., Q. N. Myrvik, and M. J. Wright. 1984. Phagosomal membranes of *Mycobacterium bovis* BCG-immune alveolar macrophages are resistant to disruption by *Mycobacterium tuberculosis*. *Infect. Immun.* **45**:443–446.

Li, Y., A. Severn, M. V. Rogers, R. M. J. Palmer, S. Moncada, and F. Y. Liew. 1992. Catalase inhibits nitric oxide synthesis and the killing of intracellular *Leishmania major* in murine macrophages. *Eur. J. Immunol.* **22**:441–446.

Liew, F. Y., and F. E. G. Cox. 1991. Nonspecific defence mechanism: the role of nitric oxide. *Immunol. Today* **12A**:17–21.

Liew, F. Y., Y. Li, A. Severn, S. Millott, J. Schmidt, M. Salter, and S. Moncada. 1991. A possible novel pathway of regulation by murine T helper type-2 (Th2) cells of a Th1 cell activity via the modulation of the induction of nitric oxide synthase on macrophages. *J. Immunol.* **21:**2489–2494.

Locksley, R. M. 1993. Interleukin 12 in host defense against microbial pathogens. *Proc. Natl. Acad. Sci. USA* **90:**5879–5880.

Lurie, M. B. 1942. Studies on the mechanism of immunity in tuberculosis. The fate of tubercle bacilli ingested by mononuclear phagocytes derived from normal and immunized animals. *J. Exp. Med.* **75:** 247.

Lurie, M. B. 1964. *Resistance to Tuberculosis.* Harvard University Press, Cambridge, Mass.

Mackaness, G. B. 1969. The influence of immunologically committed lynphoid cells on macrophage activation in vivo. *J. Exp. Med.* **129:**973.

Mackaness, G. B., and R. V. Blanden. 1967. Cellular immunity. *Prog. Allergy* **11:**89–140.

Mathew, R. C., S. Ragheb, and D. L. Boros. 1990. Recombinant IL-2 therapy reverses diminished granulomatous responsiveness in anti-L3T4-treated, *Schistosoma mansoni*-infected mice. *J. Immunol.* **144:**4356–4361.

McDonough, K. A., Y. Kress, and B. R. Bloom. 1993. Pathogenesis of tuberculosis: interaction of *Mycobacterium tuberculosis* with macrophages. *Infect. Immun.* **61:**2763–2773.

McInnes, A., and D. M. Rennick. 1988. Interleukin 4 induces cultured monocytes/macrophages to form giant multinucleated cells. *J. Exp. Med.* **167:**598–611.

Metchnikoff, E. 1905. *Immunity to Infectious Diseases.* Cambridge University Press, London.

Middlebrook, G., C. M. Coleman, and W. B. Schaeffer. 1959. Sulfolipid from virulent tubercle bacilli. *Proc. Natl. Acad. Sci. USA* **45:**1801–1804.

Modlin, R. L., C. Pirmez, F. M. Hofmann, V. Torigian, K. Uyemura, T. H. Rea, B. R. Bloom, and M. B. Brenner. 1989. Lymphocytes bearing antigen-specific c/d T-cell receptors accumulate in human infectious disease lesions. *Nature* (London) **339:**544–548.

Molloy, A., P. A. Meyn, K. D. Smith, and G. Kaplan. 1993. Recognition and destruction of bacillus Calmette-Guérin-infected human monocytes. *J. Exp. Med.* **177:**1691–1698.

Mombaerts, P., J. Arnoldi, F. Russ, S. Tonegawa, and S. H. E. Kaufmann. 1993. Differential roles of α/β and γ/δ T cells in immunity against an intracellular bacterial pathogen. *Nature* (London) **365:**53–56.

Mombaerts, P., A. R. Clarke, M. A. Rudnicki, J. Iacomini, S. Itohara, J. J. Lafaille, L. Wang, Y. Ichikawa, R. Jaenisch, M. L. Hooper, and S. Tonegawa. 1992. Mutations in T-cell antigen receptor genes a and b block thymocyte development at different stages. *Nature* (London) **360:**225–231.

Mosser, D. M., and P. J. Edelson. 1987. The third component of complement (C3) is responsible for the intracellular survival of *Leishmania major*. *Nature* (London) **327:**329–331.

Motulsky, A. G. 1979. *Human Genetics*. Raven Press, Inc., New York.

Müller, I., S. P. Cobbold, H. Waldmann, and S. H. E. Kaufmann. 1987. Impaired resistance against *Mycobacterium tuberculosis* infection after selective in-vivo depletion of L3T4$^+$ and Lyt2$^+$ T cells. *Infect. Immun.* **55:**2037–2041.

Munk, M. E., A. Gatrill, and S. H. E. Kaufmann. 1990. Antigen-specific target cell lysis and interleukin-2 secretion by *Mycobacterium tuberculosis*-activated γ/δ T cells. *J. Immunol.* **145:**2434–2439.

Muroaka, S., K. Takeya, and K. Nomoto. 1976a. In vitro studies on the mechanism of acquired resistance to tuberculous infection. I. The relationship between lymphocytes and macrophages in cellular immunity to tuberculous infection. *Jpn. J. Microbiol.* **20:**115–122.

Muroaka, S., K. Takeya, and K. Nomoto. 1976b. In vitro studies on the mechanism of acquired resistance to tuberculous infection. II. The effects of the culture supernatants of specifically-sensitized lymphocytes on the growth of tubercle bacilli within macrophages. *Jpn. J. Microbiol.* **20:**365–373.

Murray, C. J. L., K. Styblo, and A. Rouillon. 1990. Tuberculosis in developing countries: burden, intervention, and cost. *Bull. Int. Union Tuberc.* **65:**2.

Myrvik, Q. N., E. S. Leake, and M. J. Wright. 1984. Disruption of phagosomal membranes of normal alveolar macrophages by the H37Rv strain of *Mycobacterium tuberculosis*. *Am. Rev. Respir. Dis.* **129:**322–328.

Nathan, C. 1992. Nitric oxide as a secretory product of mammalian cells. *FASEB J.* **6:**3051–3064.

Nathan, C. F., and J. B. Hibbs, Jr. 1991. Role of nitric oxide synthesis in macrophage antimicrobial activity. *Curr. Opin. Immunol.* **3:**65.

Neilands, J. B. 1981. Microbial iron compounds. *Annu. Rev. Biochem.* **50:**715–731.

Neill, M. A., and S. J. Klebanoff. 1988. The effect of phenolic glycolipid-I from *Mycobacterium leprae* on the antimicrobial activity of human macrophages. *J. Exp. Med.* **167:**30–42.

Nelson, B. J., P. Ralph, S. J. Green, and C. A. Nacy. 1991. Differential susceptibility of activated macrophage cytotoxic effector reactions to the suppressive effects of transforming growth factor-β1. *J. Immunol.* **146:**1849–1857.

Neu, H. C. 1992. The crisis in antibiotic resistance. *Science* **257:**1064–1073.

Nussler, A., M. Di Silvio, T. R. Billiar, R. A. Hoffman, D. A. Geller, R. Selby, J. Madariaga, and R. L. Simmons. 1992. Stimulation of nitric oxide synthase pathway in human hepatocytes by cytokines and endotoxin. *J. Exp. Med.* **176:**261–266.

Ochoa, J. B., B. Curti, A. B. Peitzman, R. L. Simmons, T. R. Billiar, R. Hoffman, R. Rault, D. L. Longo, W. J. Urba, and A. C. Ochoa. 1992. Increased circulating nitrogen oxides after human tumor immunotherapy: correlation with toxic hemodynamic changes. *J. Natl. Cancer Inst.* **84:**864–867.

Ochoa, J. B., A. O. Udekwu, T. R. Billiar, R. D. Curran, F. B. Cerra, R. L. Simmons, and A. B. Peitzman. 1991. Nitrogen oxide levels in patients after trauma and during sepsis. *Ann. Surg.* **214:**621–626.

Ohkuma, S., Y. Moriyama, and T. Takano. 1982. Identification and characterization of a proton pump on lysosomes by fluorescein isothiocyanate-dextran fluorescence. *Proc. Natl. Acad. Sci. USA* **79:**2758–2762.

Ohkuma, S., and B. Poole. 1978. Fluorescence probe measurement of the intralysosomal pH in living cells and the perturbation of pH by various agents. *Proc. Natl. Acad. Sci. USA* **75:**3327–3331.

Oppenheim, J. J., C. O. C. Zachariae, N. Mukaida, and K. Matsushima. 1991. Properties of the novel proinflammatory supergene "intercrine" cytokine family. *Annu. Rev. Immunol.* **9:**617–648.

Orme, I. M. 1987. The kinetics of emergence and loss of mediator T lymphocytes acquired in response to infection with *Mycobacterium tuberculosis*. *J. Immunol.* **138:**293–298.

Orme, I. M., and F. M. Collins. 1984. Adoptive protection of the Mycobacterium tuberculosis-infected lung. Dissociation between cells that passively transfer protective immunity and those that transfer delayed type hypersensitivity to tuberculin. *Cell. Immunol.* **84:**113–120.

Oswald, I. P., R. T. Gazzinelli, A. Sher, and S. L. James. 1992. IL-10 synergizes with IL-4 and transforming growth factor-beta to inhibit macrophage cytotoxic activity. *J. Immunol.* **148:**3578–3582.

Ottenhoff, T. H. M., A. B. Kale, J. D. A. Van Embden, J. E. R. Thole, and R. Kiessling. 1988. The recombinant 65 kD heat shock protein of Mycobacterium bovis BCG/M. tuberculosis is a target molecule for CD4+ cytotoxic T lymphocytes that lyse human monocytes. *J. Exp. Med.* **168:**1947–1952.

Pabst, M. J., J. M. Gross, J. P. Prozna, and M. B. Goren. 1988. Inhibition of macrophage priming by sulfatide from *Mycobacterium tuberculosis*. *J. Immunol.* **140:**634–640.

Pamer, E. G., M. J. Bevan, and K. Fischer Lindahl. 1993. Do nonclassical, class Ib MHC molecules present bacterial antigens to T cells? *Trends Microbiol.* **1:**35–38.

Pamer, E. G., C.-R. Wang, L. Flaherty, K. Fischer Lindahl, and M. J. Bevan. 1992. H-2M3 presents a Listeria monocytogenes peptide to cytotoxic T lymphocytes. *Cell* **70:**215–223.

Patterson, R. J., and G. P. Youmans. 1970. Demonstration in tissue culture of lymphocyte-mediated immunity to tuberculosis. *Infect. Immun.* **1:**600–603.

Payne, N. R., and M. A. Horwitz. 1987. Phagocytosis of *Legionella pneumophila* is mediated by human monocyte complement receptors. *J. Exp. Med.* **166:**1377–1389.

Pedrazzini, T., K. Hug, and J. A. Louis. 1987. Importance of L3T4+ and Lyt-2+ cells in the immunologic control of infection with Mycobacterium bovis strain bacillus Calmette-Guérin in mice. Assessment by elimination of T cell subsets in vivo. *J. Immunol.* **139:**2032–2037.

Pfeffer, K., B. Schoel, H. Gulle, S. H. E. Kaufmann, and H. Wagner. 1990. Primary responses of human T cells to mycobacteria: a frequent set of γ/δ T cells are stimulated by protease-resistant ligands. *Eur. J. Immunol.* **20:**1175–1179.

Pfeifer, J. D., M. J. Wick, R. L. Robert, K. Findlay, S. J. Normark, and C. V. Harding. 1993. Phagocytic processing of bacterial antigens for class I MHC presentation to T cells. *Nature* (London) **361:**359–362.

Pontyremoli, S., E. Melloni, F. Salamino, B. Sparatore, M. Michetti, O. Sacco, and B. L. Horecker. 1986. Activation of NADPH oxidase and phosphorylation of membrane proteins in human neutrophils: coordinate inhibition by a surface antigen-directed monoclonal. *Biochem. Biophys. Res. Commun.* **140:**1121–1126.

Rao, S. P., K. Ogata, and A. Catanzaro. 1993. *Mycobacterium avium-M. intracellulare* binds to the integrin receptor $\alpha_v\beta_3$ on human monocytes and monocyte-derived macrophages. *Infect. Immun.* **61:**663–670.

Rees, A. D. M., A. Scoging, A. Mehlert, D. B. Young, and J. Ivanyi. 1988. Specificity of proliferative response of human CD8 clones to mycobacterial antigens. *Eur. J. Immunol.* **18:**1881–1887.

Reichel, H., H. P. Koeffler, and A. W. Norman. 1987. Synthesis in vitro of 1,25-dihydroxyvitamin D_3 and 24,25-dihydroxyvitamin D_3 by interferon-γ-stimulated normal human bone marrow and alveolar macrophages. *J. Biol. Chem.* **262:**10931–10987.

Relman, D., E. Yuomanen, S. Falkow, D. T. Golenbock, K. Saukkonen, and S. D. Wright. 1990. Recognition of a bacterial adhesin by an integrin: macrophage CR3 ($\alpha_M\beta_2$, CD11b/CD18) binds filamentous hemagglutinin of Bordetella pertussis. *Cell* **61:**1375–1382.

Rook, G. A. W. 1988. The role of vitamin D in tuberculosis. *Am. Rev. Respir. Dis.* **138:**768–770.

Rook, G. A. W. 1990. The role of activated macrophages in protection and immunopathology in tuberculosis. *Res. Microbiol.* **141:**253–256.

Rook, G. A. W., J. Steele, M. Ainsworth, and B. R.

Champion. 1986. Activation of macrophages to inhibit proliferation of *Mycobacterium tuberculosis*: comparison of the effects of recombinant gamma interferon on human monocytes and murine peritoneal macrophages. *Immunology* **59**:333–338.

Russell, D. G., and S. D. Wright. 1988. Complement receptor type 3 (CR3) binds to an Arg-Gly-Sap-containing region of the major surface glycoprotein, gp63, of *Leishmania* promastigotes. *J. Exp. Med.* **168**:279–292.

Sansonetti, P. J., A. Ryer, P. Clerc, A. T. Maurelli, and J. Mounier. 1986. Multiplication of *Shigella flexneri* within HeLa cells: lysis of the phagocytic vacuole and plasmid-mediated contact hemolysis. *Infect. Immun.* **51**:461–469.

Sbarra, A. J., and M. L. Karnovsky. 1959. The biochemical basis of phagocytosis. I. Metabolic changes during the ingestion of particles by polymorphonuclear leukocytes. *J. Biol. Chem.* **234:** 1355–1362.

Schade, A. L., and L. Caroline. 1944. Raw hen egg white and the role of iron in growth inhibition of *Shigella dysenteriae, Staphylococcus aureus, Escherichia coli,* and *Saccharomyces cerevisiae. Science* **100**:14–15.

Schlesinger, L. S. 1993. Macrophage phagocytosis of virulent but not attenuated strains of *Mycobacterium tuberculosis* is mediated by mannose receptors in addition to complement receptors. *J. Immunol.* **150**:2920–2930.

Schlesinger, L. S., C. G. Bellinger-Kawahara, N. R. Payne, and M. A. Horwitz. 1990. Phagocytosis of *Mycobacterium tuberculosis* is mediated by human monocyte complement receptors and complement component C3. *J. Immunol.* **144**:2771–2780.

Schoendon, G., J. Troppmair, A. Fontana, C. Huber, H.-C. Curtis, and A. Neiderwieser. 1987. Biosynthesis and metabolism of pterins in peripheral blood mononuclear cells and leukemia lines of man and mouse. *Eur. J. Biochem.* **166**:303–310.

Schoenhaut, D. S., A. O. Chua, A. G. Wolitzky, P. M. Quinn, C. M. Dwyer, W. McMomas, P. C. Familletti, M. K. Gately, and U. Gubler. 1992. Cloning and expression of murine IL-12. *J. Immunol.* **148**:3433–3440.

Schurr, E., E. Skemene, K. Morgan, M.-L. Chu, and P. Gros. 1990. Mapping of *Col3a1* and *Col6a3* to proximal murine chromosome 1 identifies conserved linkage of structural protein genes between murine chromosome 1 and human chromosome 2q. *Genomics* **8**:477–486.

Shank, J. L., J. H. Silliker, and R. H. Harper. 1962. The effect of nitric oxide on bacteria. *Appl. Microbiol.* **10**:185.

Sheppard, C. C. 1958. A comparison of the growth of selected mycobacteria in HeLa, monkey kidney, and human amnion cells in tissue culture. *J. Exp.*

Med. **107**:237–245.

Sher, N. A., S. D. Chaparas, L. F. Greenberg, E. M. Merchant, and J. H. Vickers. 1975. Response of congenitally athymic (nude) mice to infection with *Mycobacterium bovis* (strain BCG). *J. Natl. Cancer Inst.* **54**:1419–1426.

Sibley, L. D., S. W. Hunter, P. J. Brennan, and J. L. Krehenbuhl. 1988. Mycobacterial lipoarabinomannan inhibits gamma interferon-mediated activation of macrophages. *Infect. Immun.* **56**:1232–1236.

Sibley, L. D., and J. L. Krahenbuhl. 1988. Induction of unresponsiveness to gamma interferon in macrophages infected with *Mycobacterium leprae. Infect. Immun.* **56**:1912–1919.

Skamene, E. 1985. Genetic control of host resistance to infection and malignancy. *Prog. Leukocyte Biol.* **3**:111–159.

Skamene, E. 1986. Genetic control of resistance to mycobacterial infection. *Curr. Top. Microbiol. Immunol.* **124**:49–66.

Skamene, E., P. Gros, A. Forget, P. A. L. Kongshavn, C. St. Charles, and B. A. Taylor. 1982. Genetic regulation of resistance to intracellular pathogens. *Nature* (London) **297**:506–509.

Snow, G. A. 1970. Mycobactins: iron-chelating growth factors from mycobacteria. *Bacteriol. Rev.* **34**:99–125.

Squires, K. E., R. D. Schreiber, M. J. McElrath, B. Y. Rubin, S. L. Anderson, and H. W. Murray. 1989. Experimental visceral leishmaniasis: role of endogenous IFN-γ in host defense and tissue granulomatous response. *J. Immunol.* **143**:4244–4249.

Stamler, J. S., D. J. Singel, and J. Loscalzo. 1992. Biochemistry of nitric oxide and its redox-activated forms. *Science* **258**:1898–1902.

Suter, E. 1952. The multiplication of tubercle bacilli within normal phagocytes in tissue cultures. *J. Exp. Med.* **96**:137.

Suter, E. 1953. Multiplication of tubercle bacilli within mononuclear phagocytes in tissue cultures derived from normal animals and animals vaccinated with BCG. *J. Exp. Med.* **97**:235.

Talamas-Rohana, P., S. D. Wright, M. R. Lennartz, and D. G. Russell. 1990. Lipophosphoglycan (LPG) from *Leishmania mexicana* promastigotes binds to members of the CR3, p150,95 and LFA-1 family of leukocyte integrins. *J. Immunol.* **144**:4817–4824.

Tayeh, M. A., and M. A. Marletta. 1989. Macrophage oxidation of L-arginine to nitric oxide, nitrite and nitrate. Tetrahydrobiopterin is required as a cofactor. *J. Biol. Chem.* **264**:19654–19658.

Tazi, A., I. Fajac, P. Soler, D. Valeyre, J. P. Battesti, and A. J. Hance. 1991. Gamma/delta T lymphocytes are not increased in number in granulomatous lesions of patients with tuberculosis or sarcoidosis. *Am. Rev. Respir. Dis.* **144**:1373–1375.

Tripp, C. S., S. F. Wolf, and E. R. Unanue. 1993.

Interleukin 12 and tumor necrosis factor α are costimulators of interferon γ production by natural killer cells in severe combined immunodeficiency mice with listeriosis, and IL-10 is a physiologic antagonist. *Proc. Natl. Acad. Sci. USA* **90**:3725–3729.

Turcotte, R., Y. Des Ormeaus, and A. F. Borduas. 1976. Partial characterization of a factor extracted from sensitized lymphocytes that inhibits the growth of *Mycobacterium tuberculosis* within macrophages in vitro. *Infect. Immun.* **14**:337–344.

Vachula, M., T. J. Holzer, and B. R. Anderson. 1989. Suppression of monocyte oxidative response by phenolic glycolipid I of *Mycobacterium leprae. J. Immunol.* **142**:1696–1701.

Vassalli, P. 1992. The pathophysiology of tumor necrosis factors. *Annu. Rev. Immunol.* **10**:411–452.

Vidal, S. M., D. Malo, K. Vogan, E. Skamene, and P. Gros. 1993. Natural resistance to infection with intracellular parasites: isolation of a candidate for *Bcg. Cell* **73**:469–485.

Walker, L., and D. B. Lowrie. 1981. Killing of *Mycobacterium microti* by immunologically activated macrophages. *Nature* (London) **293**:69–70.

Weinberg, E. D. 1974. Iron and susceptibility to infectious disease. *Science* **184**:952–956.

Weinberg, E. D. 1978. Iron and infection. *Microbiol. Rev.* **42**:45–66.

Weinberg, E. D. 1992. Iron depletion: a defense against intracellular infection and neoplasia. *Life Sci.* **50**:1289–1297.

Weiss, G., B. Goossen, W. Doppler, D. Fuchs, K. Pantopoulos, G. Werner-Felmayer, H. Wachter, and M. W. Hentze. 1993. Translational regulation via iron-responsive elements by the nitric oxide/NO-synthase pathway. *EMBO J.* **12**:3651–3657.

Weiss, S. J. 1989. Tissue destruction by neutrophils. *N. Engl. J. Med.* **320**:365–376.

Werner, E. R., G. Verner-Felmayer, D. Fuchs, A. Hausen, G. Reibnegger, and H. Wachter. 1989. Parallel induction of tetrahydrobiopterin biosynthesis and indoleamine 2,3-dioxygenase activity in human cells and cell lines by interferon-γ. *Biochem. J.* **262**:861–866.

Wilson, E., M. C. Olcott, R. M. Bell, A. H. Merrill, Jr., and J. D. Lambeth. 1986. Inhibition of the oxidative burst in human neutrophils by sphingoid long-chain bases. *J. Biol. Chem.* **261**:12616–12623.

Winkler, H. H. 1990. *Rickettsia* species (as organisms). *Annu. Rev. Microbiol.* **44**:131–153.

Wolf, S. F., P. A. Temple, M. Kobayashi, D. Young, M. Dicig, L. Lowe, R. Dzialo, L. Fitz, C. Ferenz, R. M. Hewick, K. Kelleher, S. H. Herrmann, S. C. Clark, L. Azzoni, S. H. Chan, G. Trinchieri, and B. Perussia. 1991. Cloning of cDNA for natural killer cell stimulatory factor, a heterodimeric cytokine with multiple biologic effects on T and natural killer cells. *J. Immunol.* **146**:3074–3081.

Wright, S. D., and S. C. Silverstein. 1983. Receptors for C3b and C3bi promote phagocytosis but not the release of toxic oxygen from human phagocytes. *J. Exp. Med.* **158**:2016–2023.

Xie, Q. W., R. Whisnant, and C. Nathan. 1993. Promoter of the mouse gene encoding calcium-independent nitric oxide synthase confers inducibility by interferon gamma and bacterial lipopolysaccharide. *J. Exp. Med.* **177**:1779–1784.

Zhu, L., C. Gunn, and J. S. Beckman. 1992. Bactericidal activity of peroxynitrite. *Arch. Biochem. Biophys.* **298**:452–457.

Tuberculosis: Pathogenesis, Protection, and Control
Edited by Barry R. Bloom
© 1994 American Society for Microbiology, Washington, DC 20005

Chapter 25

T-Cell Responses and Cytokines

Peter F. Barnes, Robert L. Modlin, and Jerrold J. Ellner

The immune response to tuberculosis is a double-edged sword that may contribute to both clearance of infection and tissue damage. In addition, recent evidence suggests that tuberculosis promotes progression of disease due to human immunodeficiency virus (HIV) (Toossi et al., 1993). Development of antituberculosis vaccines, of modalities to enhance the immune response, and of approaches to mitigate immunopathology requires a comprehensive understanding of the human immune response to *Mycobacterium tuberculosis*. In view of the increasing frequency of multidrug-resistant tuberculosis unresponsive to treatment (Centers for Disease Control, 1991; Fischl et al., 1992), immunomodulatory approaches may serve as important adjuncts or alternatives to chemotherapy.

SPECTRUM OF CLINICAL MANIFESTATIONS OF TUBERCULOSIS INFECTION

Most persons who become infected with *M. tuberculosis* mount a protective immune response and remain clinically well, the only evidence of infection being development of a positive tuberculin skin test. Five to 10% develop tuberculosis disease within the first 2 years after infection (primary tuberculosis) or thereafter (reactivation tuberculosis). Miliary tuberculosis is the most serious form of the disease; it is characterized by hematogenous dissemination of large numbers of organisms throughout the body and severe disease that is almost invariably fatal if untreated. Disseminated tuberculosis reflects an ineffective immune response, manifested by a high frequency of negative tuberculin skin tests and failure of T lymphocytes to proliferate in vitro in response to *M. tuberculosis* antigens. Between the extremes of healthy tuberculin reactors and patients with miliary tuberculosis, two other common manifestations of tuberculosis can also be considered to reflect the efficacy of the immune response. Tuberculous pleuritis results when a small focus of organisms ruptures into the pleural space, triggering an exudative pleural effusion through a vigorous in situ delayed-type hypersensitivity response. Patients with pleuritis mount a resistant immune re-

Peter F. Barnes • HMR 904, University of Southern California School of Medicine, 2025 Zonal Avenue, Los Angeles, California 90033. *Robert L. Modlin* • Division of Dermatology, 52-121 CHS, University of California Los Angeles School of Medicine, 10833 Le Conte Avenue, Los Angeles, California 90024. *Jerrold J. Ellner* • Division of Infectious Diseases, University Hospitals of Cleveland, Case Western Reserve University School of Medicine, 10900 Euclid Avenue, Cleveland, Ohio 44106-4984.

sponse to infection, reflected by resolution of pleuritis without therapy in most cases (Roper and Waring, 1955). In contrast, patients with advanced pulmonary tuberculosis have an ineffective immune response and develop severe disease manifestations that are often life-threatening.

IMMUNE DEFENSES AGAINST TUBERCULOSIS

The clinical outcomes of infection with *M. tuberculosis* depend on the efficacy of cell-mediated immunity rather than humoral immunity. Persons with defective cell-mediated immunity, such as those with HIV infection and chronic renal failure, are at markedly increased risk for tuberculosis (American Thoracic Society, 1986). In contrast, persons with defective humoral immunity, such as those with sickle cell disease and multiple myeloma, show no increased predisposition to tuberculosis.

Experimental evidence indicates that antimycobacterial immune defenses are mediated primarily by T lymphocytes and macrophages, and adoptive transfer of resistance against tuberculosis in animal models is mediated by T cells (Orme and Collins, 1983). Although neutrophils and natural killer cells can exhibit mycobacteriostatic effects in vitro (May and Spagnuolo, 1987; Bermudez and Young, 1991) and eosinophils can ingest mycobacteria (Castro et al., 1991), their role in immune defenses in vivo is uncertain. Therefore, the interplay of T lymphocytes and macrophages in the immune response against tuberculosis will be discussed in detail.

THE ROLE OF MONONUCLEAR PHAGOCYTES

When *M. tuberculosis* organisms are inhaled into the lung, they are engulfed by alveolar macrophages, which perform three important functions. First, the macro-

Table 1. Cytokines produced by macrophages and by Th1 and Th2 cells

Cytokine	Production by:		
	Macrophage	Th1	Th2
IL-2	−	+	−
IFN-γ[a]	−	+	−
Lymphotoxin	−	+	−
IL-4	−	−	+
IL-5	−	−	+
IL-6	+	−	+
IL-10	+	−[b]	+
IL-3	−	+	+
GM-CSF	+	+	+
TNF	+	+	+
IL-1	+	−	−
IL-8	+	−	−
TGF-β	+	−	−

[a] IFN-γ, gamma interferon.
[b] IL-10 is produced by human but not murine Th1 cells.

phages produce proteolytic enzymes and other metabolites that exhibit mycobactericidal effects, described in detail elsewhere in this volume (chapter 19). Second, macrophages produce a characteristic pattern of soluble mediators (cytokines) in response to *M. tuberculosis* (Table 1), including interleukin-1 (IL-1), IL-6, IL-10, tumor necrosis factor alpha (TNF-α), and transforming growth factor beta (TGF-β) (Valone et al., 1988; Toossi et al., 1991; Barnes et al., 1992a). These cytokines have the potential to exert potent immunoregulatory effects and to mediate many of the clinical manifestations of tuberculosis. IL-1 is an endogenous pyrogen that may contribute to the fever that is characteristic of tuberculosis (Dinarello, 1984). IL-6, which enhances immunoglobulin production by activated B cells (Hirano et al., 1990), may mediate the hyperglobulinemia that is common in tuberculosis patients. TNF synergizes with gamma interferon to increase production of nitric oxide metabolites (Ding et al., 1988) and mycobacterial killing (Bermudez and Young, 1988) and is essential for granuloma formation to contain mycobacterial infection (Kindler et al., 1989). On the other hand, TNF may cause the immunopathologic effects such as fever, weight loss, and tissue necrosis that are typical of tuberculosis (Beutler and Cerami, 1987). IL-10 inhibits cytokine production by monocytes and lymphocytes (Mosmann and Moore, 1991; de Waal Malefyt et al., 1991), and TGF-β suppresses T-cell proliferation and inhibits macrophage effector function (Tsunawaki et al., 1988; Ding et al., 1990; Palladino et al., 1990). These two cytokines may prevent excessive inflammation and tissue damage from an uncontrolled inflammatory response. The third critical function of macrophages is to process and present mycobacterial antigens to T lymphocytes. Macrophages phagocytose mycobacteria or ingest secreted mycobacterial proteins by pinocytosis and then degrade these proteins into peptides that are expressed on the cell surface in association with self molecules of the major histocompatibility complex (MHC). Expression of antigens through this pathway induces expansion of specific CD4$^+$ lymphocytes, the cell population that is central to acquired resistance to *M. tuberculosis*.

Immunoregulatory Effects Mediated by Mononuclear Phagocytes

A significant minority of tuberculosis patients have negative tuberculin skin tests and generalized anergy associated with failure of T cells to proliferate in response to *M. tuberculosis* antigens (Ellner, 1978). This defect in purified protein derivative (PPD)-stimulated lymphocyte proliferation and in IL-2 production is reversed at least in part by depletion of monocytes (Ellner, 1978; Toossi et al., 1986). These effects were observed specifically with PPD but not with nonmycobacterial antigens. The "antigen-specific" suppressive activity exerted by monocytes from tuberculosis patients appears to result from overexpression of suppressive factors that are produced when monocytes primed during the course of tuberculosis are stimulated in

vitro with PPD. Patients in whom lymphocyte proliferation in response to *M. tuberculosis* is depressed have elevated percentages of circulating monocytes that are abnormally activated in terms of expression of class II MHC determinants (Tweardy et al., 1984), producing large amounts of IL-1 when stimulated with *M. tuberculosis* PPD (Fujiwara et al., 1986) and constitutively expressing IL-2 receptors (Toossi et al., 1990). Monocyte production of TNF and IL-6 is also increased in tuberculosis patients (Takashima et al., 1990; Ogawa et al., 1991). Monocytes from tuberculosis patients may exert their effects partially through consumption of IL-2, which is a critical T-cell growth factor. In addition, suppressor monocytes may inhibit lymphocyte proliferation through secretion of immunosuppressive cytokines such as IL-10 and TGF-β. IL-10 mRNA is selectively increased at the site of disease in tuberculosis and is expressed predominantly by macrophages rather than T cells (Barnes et al., 1993b). TGF-β is produced constitutively by monocytes from patients with tuberculosis, and production is increased in response to PPD. Langhans giant cells and epithelioid cells in tuberculous granulomas also express mRNA for TGF-β (Toossi et al., 1991), suggesting that local production of TGF-β may result in deactivation of macrophages and immunopathology.

Carbohydrate and glycolipid components of the mycobacterial cell wall as well as secreted proteins may trigger the immunosuppressive effects of macrophages in tuberculosis patients. Lipoarabinomannan, a complex heteropolysaccharide, is embedded in the mycobacterial cell membrane and suppresses proliferative responses to *M. tuberculosis* (Moreno et al., 1988), perhaps through inducing macrophages to release immunosuppressive cytokines such as IL-10 (Barnes et al., 1992a). Lipoarabinomannan inhibits gamma interferon-mediated activation of macrophages and scavenges oxygen-free radicals, inhibiting a major pathway for destruction of intracellular pathogens (Chan et al., 1991). Lipoarabinomannan from virulent *M. tuberculosis* Erdman has arabinan side chains masked by mannan residues, whereas that from a nonpathogenic mycobacterial strain lacks mannan moieties. Lipoarabinomannan from virulent *M. tuberculosis* does not induce macrophage early activation genes and does not elicit production of large amounts of the antimycobacterial cytokine TNF (Chatterjee et al., 1992; Roach et al., 1993). By avoiding macrophage activation, lipoarabinomannan from virulent *M. tuberculosis* may act as a virulence factor that allows the organism to evade cytokine-mediated mechanisms of elimination.

Secretory proteins of *M. tuberculosis* can also induce cytokine production by macrophages and may therefore contribute to systemic immunosuppression and local immunopathology. Both the 30-kDa α antigen and a 58-kDa constituent of *M. tuberculosis* culture filtrates induce production of TNF by monocytes (Aung et al., 1993; Wallis et al., 1993a). It is likely that carbohydrates, glycolipids, and proteins of *M. tuberculosis* act in concert to modulate expression of the host immune response.

ANTIGEN RECOGNITION BY T CELLS

T cells recognize antigen through an antigen receptor composed of α and β or γ and δ polypeptide chains. Changes in the amino acid sequences of the variable (V) regions of these polypeptides alter the shape of the antigen-binding groove that confers antigen specificity to individual T cells (Davis and Bjorkman, 1988). Once antigen is bound, signal transduction into the cytoplasm triggers functions such as cytokine production and cytolytic activity. Most $\alpha\beta$ T cells bear the CD4 or CD8 determinants. CD4$^+$ cells recognize antigens associated with self MHC class II glycoproteins, whereas CD8$^+$ $\alpha\beta$ T cells recognize antigen in the context

of MHC class I products. $\gamma\delta$ T cells make up less than 5% of resting human T cells, and most are CD4$^-$ CD8$^-$, although a minority are CD8$^+$. The restriction molecules for $\gamma\delta$ T cells remain undefined but are thought to include MHC-like molecules (Strominger, 1989).

CD4$^+$ T CELLS

Dominance of CD4$^+$ Cells in Immune Defenses against Tuberculosis

The bulk of experimental and clinical data favor a dominant but not exclusive role for CD4$^+$ cells in immune defenses against tuberculosis. Mice depleted of CD4$^+$ cells prior to infection with *M. bovis* are unable to control mycobacterial growth, whereas depletion of CD8$^+$ cells shows variable effects (Pedrazzini et al., 1987; Muller et al., 1987). In addition, adoptive transfer of CD4$^+$ cells from sensitized animals confers protection against tuberculosis (Orme, 1988a, 1987). In humans, CD4$^+$ T cells are selectively expanded at the site of disease in patients with a resistant immune response, such as those with tuberculous pleuritis (Barnes et al., 1989a). Depletion of CD4$^+$ cells by HIV infection markedly increases susceptibility to primary and reactivation tuberculosis (Barnes et al., 1991). Furthermore, in HIV-infected patients, clinical indicators of severe tuberculosis, such as extrapulmonary involvement, mycobacteremia, and positive acid-fast smears, become progressively more common as the CD4 cell count declines (Jones et al., 1993). For example, the frequency of mycobacteremia rises from 4% in patients with more than 200 CD4 cells/μl to 49% in those with 100 or fewer CD4 cells/μl (Jones et al., 1993).

CD4$^+$ Memory Cells

CD4$^+$ cells can be divided into "memory" and "naive" cells according to their expression of CD45. CD4$^+$ cells that express the CD45RO isoform are memory T cells with prior exposure to antigen, whereas cells that express the CD45RA isoform are naive T cells that have not previously encountered antigen (Akbar et al., 1991). CD4$^+$ memory T cells are selectively concentrated in the pleural spaces of patients with tuberculous pleuritis, whereas naive T cells are not (Barnes et al., 1989a). Furthermore, memory but not naive T cells proliferate in response to *M. tuberculosis* antigens and produce gamma interferon (Barnes et al., 1989a), a macrophage-activating cytokine that enhances antimycobacterial activity in experimental systems. These findings suggest that memory T cells predominate in local immune defenses against tuberculosis, probably through recognition of specific mycobacterial antigens and production of cytokines.

Cytokines Produced by CD4$^+$ Cells

Th1 and Th2 cells in murine models of infectious disease

Murine CD4$^+$ T cells comprise two functionally distinct subpopulations that differ in patterns of cytokine production and in requirements for costimulatory factors and antigen-presenting cells (Street and Mosmann, 1991). Th1 cells produce gamma interferon, IL-2, and lymphotoxin; enhance microbicidal activity of macrophages; and augment delayed-type hypersensitivity responses (Table 1). Th2 cells produce IL-4, IL-5, IL-6, and IL-10; support B-cell growth and differentiation; and augment humoral immune responses. Both Th1 and Th2 cells produce IL-3, granulocyte macrophage–colony-stimulating factor (GM-CSF), and TNF. IL-1 is an important growth factor for Th2 but not Th1 cells (Greenbaum et al., 1988), and macrophages are optimal antigen-presenting cells for Th1 cells, whereas B cells are optimal for Th2 cells (Gajewski et al., 1991). In the course of an immune response to a specific pathogen, Th1 and Th2 cells exert cross-regula-

tory influences that favor predominance of one subpopulation. Gamma interferon produced by Th1 cells inhibits proliferation by Th2 cells, IL-10 produced by Th2 cells inhibits cytokine synthesis by Th1 cells, and IL-4 inhibits generation of Th1 cells (Maggi et al., 1992).

Predominance of Th1 or Th2 cells has striking effects on the manifestations of infection by intracellular pathogens. In murine leishmaniasis, Th1 cells mediate immunologic resistance to infection through production of gamma interferon, whereas Th2 cells exacerbate disease through production of IL-4 (Heinzel et al., 1989; Scott et al., 1988). Immunologic resistance to mycobacterial infection in mice is probably also mediated by Th1 cells. Lymphocytes from mice with immune resistance to BCG produce high concentrations of gamma interferon and IL-2 but low levels of IL-4, whereas susceptible mice produce high levels of IL-4 and low levels of gamma interferon and IL-2 (Huygen et al., 1992). In addition, production of gamma interferon is a functional marker of murine T cells that confer adoptive immunity against *M. tuberculosis* (Orme et al., 1992).

Th1 and Th2 responses in humans

Human T cells can exhibit dichotomous patterns of cytokine production similar to those of murine Th1 and Th2 cells (Table 1). IL-10 is produced by human Th1 and Th2 cells both and inhibits proliferation and cytokine production by both subpopulations (Yssel et al., 1992; Del Prete et al., 1993). In humans, IL-4 may be the main Th2 cytokine that specifically inhibits growth of Th1 cells through selective effects on antigen-presenting cells or through direct effects on T cells (Salgame et al., 1991). Patterns of cytokine production in humans correlate with clinical manifestations of infectious disease. For example, CD4$^+$ T cells derived from patients with helminthic infections preferentially pro-

422   Barnes et al.

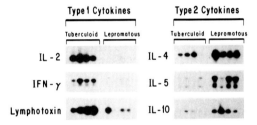

Figure 1. Cytokine patterns in mycobacterial disease. Reverse transcriptase polymerase chain reaction was used to quantify cytokine mRNA in skin lesions of patients with tuberculoid and lepromatous leprosy. Type 1 cytokines predominate in tuberculoid lepromatous patients, whereas type 2 cytokines are dominant in patients with lepromatous leprosy. IFN-γ, gamma interferon.

duce the Th2 cytokines IL-4 and IL-5 (Del Prete et al., 1991), which is consistent with the capacities of IL-4 to stimulate production of immunoglobulin E and of IL-5 to promote eosinophil growth and differentiation. In patients with leprosy, the Th1 cytokines gamma interferon and IL-2 predominate in the skin lesions of tuberculoid leprosy patients who mount a resistant immune response to *M. leprae*, whereas the Th2 cytokines IL-4 and IL-10 are prominent in lepromatous leprosy patients with ineffective immunity and enormous bacillary burdens (Fig. 1) (Yamamura et al., 1991). Because IL-4 and IL-10 suppress T-cell responses and lepromatous leprosy patients showed immunologic unresponsiveness to *M. leprae*, it is intriguing to speculate that parallel mechanisms may explain the anergy that is common in patients with advanced tuberculosis.

Published data on cytokine production by human T cells in response to *M. tuberculosis* are conflicting. Some studies have indicated that most CD4$^+$ *M. tuberculosis*-reactive T-cell clones propagated in vitro are Th1-like, producing high concentrations of gamma interferon but low concentrations of IL-4 and IL-5 (Del Prete et al., 1991; Haanen et al., 1991). In contrast, one study demonstrated that most *M. tuberculosis*-

reactive T-cell clones secrete gamma interferon and IL-4 (Boom et al., 1991), and another report indicated that most *M. tuberculosis*-reactive T-cell clones produce both Th1 and Th2 cytokines, including gamma interferon, IL-2, IL-5, and IL-10 (Barnes et al., 1993a). In the latter study, some clones expressed mRNA for IL-4, although IL-4 was not detectable in cell culture supernatants. Because these disparate results may reflect selection of T-cell subpopulations by culture conditions in vitro and may not reflect events in vivo, it is critical to evaluate the cytokine response at the site of mycobacterial disease. In patients with tuberculous pleuritis, expression of mRNA for the Th1 cytokines gamma interferon and IL-2 is greater in pleural fluid mononuclear cells than in blood mononuclear cells, and concentrations of gamma interferon are 15-fold higher than those in serum (Barnes et al., 1993b). In contrast, expression of mRNA for the Th2 cytokine IL-4 is lower in pleural fluid than in blood. Pleural fluid lymphocytes stimulated with *M. tuberculosis* produce 6-fold more gamma interferon and 40-fold more IL-2 than do peripheral blood lymphocytes. These results provide strong evidence for selective concentration of Th1-like cells at the site of disease in persons with a resistant immune response and suggest that Th1 cells play an important role in human antimycobacterial defenses.

Gamma interferon in combination with TNF-α enhances the antimycobacterial activity of murine macrophages, probably through increased production of reactive nitric oxide metabolites (Flesch and Kaufmann, 1991; Chan et al., 1992). Although the capacity of gamma interferon to augment mycobacterial killing in human macrophages remains controversial, gamma interferon stimulates human macrophages to produce TNF and 1,25-dihydroxyvitamin D, both of which facilitate mycobacterial elimination (Rook et al., 1986; Bermudez and Young, 1988). IL-2 causes T-cell division, further increasing the local concentration of macrophage-activating factors secreted by T cells. In contrast to the effects of Th1 cytokines, IL-4 deactivates macrophages (Lehn et al., 1989; Ho et al., 1992), blocks T-cell proliferation by downregulation of IL-2 receptor expression (Martinez et al., 1990), and may therefore inhibit the immune response to *M. tuberculosis*.

Dominance of Th1 or Th2 cells in the course of an immune response

A growing body of evidence indicates that Th1 and Th2 cells are derived from common precursors (Rocken et al., 1992; Seder et al., 1992). Distinct microbial antigens may favor dominance of Th1 or Th2 cells (Scott et al., 1988). Alternatively, the interplay of cytokines may control skewing toward a Th1 or Th2 response. IL-12 may be pivotal in favoring a Th1 response, as it induces differentiation of Th1 cells in vitro and in murine leishmaniasis in vivo (Manetti et al., 1993; Hsieh et al., Scott, 1993; Heinzel et al., 1993). IL-12 mRNA and protein were present at the site of disease in pleural tuberculosis, and bioactive IL-12 was produced by pleural fluid mononuclear cells in response to *M. tuberculosis* (Zhang et al., in press). It is therefore intriguing to speculate that alveolar macrophages ingest mycobacteria and produce IL-12, favoring development of Th1 cells.

Cytolytic Activity of CD4+ Cells

Although most research has focused on the capacity of CD4+ T cells to mediate antimycobacterial effects through cytokine production and activation of macrophages, an alternative mechanism by which T cells contribute to immune defense is through direct cytolysis of macrophages and nonphagocytic cells infected with *M. tuberculosis*. Human *M. tuberculosis*-specific cytolytic T cells cultured in vitro are CD4+ (Ottenhoff and Mutis, 1990; Lorgat et al., 1992), and *M. tuberculosis*-specific cyto-

lytic activity of CD4+ cells at the site of disease is greatly enhanced compared to that of peripheral blood cells (Lorgat et al., 1992). Kaufmann (1988) has suggested that many macrophages infected with *M. tuberculosis* have low antimycobacterial potential, allowing the bacilli to evade host defenses. Cytolytic T cells that specifically recognize mycobacterial antigens can lyse these macrophages, releasing bacilli to be engulfed and killed by macrophages with greater antimycobacterial activity. Alternatively, cytolytic T cells may play a scavenger role by lysing dead macrophages containing large numbers of dead bacilli so that they can be catabolized by surrounding mononuclear cells (Orme et al., 1992). Another hypothesis is that cytolytic T cells cause immunopathology by destroying infected macrophages, which in turn release toxic products that result in caseous necrosis (Dannenberg, 1991).

CD8+ T LYMPHOCYTES

CD8+ T cells constitute the major cytolytic T-cell population in defenses against many intracellular pathogens in animal models of infection, including listeriae and shigellae. Unlike CD4+ cells, CD8+ cells do not produce high levels of IL-2 but depend on an exogenous source of this critical T-cell growth factor. Murine CD8+ T cells can directly lyse *M. tuberculosis*-infected cells in an antigen-specific manner in vitro, depletion of CD8+ cells increases the severity of murine tuberculosis (Kaufmann, 1988), and mice that lack functional CD8+ T cells because of a disrupted β_2-microglobulin gene exhibit severe manifestations of tuberculosis (Flynn et al., 1992). These data suggest that murine CD4+ and CD8+ T cells play complementary roles in the immune response to *M. tuberculosis*. CD4+ T cells may produce cytokines that activate macrophages to kill most mycobacteria and produce sufficient IL-2 to activate CD8+ T cells, which in turn lyse additional myco-bacterium-infected cells.

Despite the importance of CD8$^+$ cells in murine models of tuberculosis, their role in human antimycobacterial defenses remains uncertain. On the one hand, human *M. tuberculosis*-specific cytolytic T cells evaluated to date are not CD8$^+$ (Ottenhoff and Mutis, 1990; Lorgat et al., 1992), CD8$^+$ T cells are not selectively concentrated at the site of disease in tuberculosis patients (Barnes et al., 1989a), and the severity of tuberculosis in HIV-infected patients is unaffected by the CD8 cell count (Jones et al., 1993). On the other hand, the lack of correlation between positive tuberculin skin tests and protection against tuberculosis could be explained by the failure of tuberculin skin tests to evaluate CD8$^+$ cytotoxic activity. More comprehensive studies are needed to assess the role of CD8$^+$ cells in human antituberculosis defenses.

γδ T CELLS

Several lines of evidence suggest that γδ T cells play a role in the initial immune response to *M. tuberculosis* infection. The percentage of γδ T cells is markedly elevated in draining lymph nodes and lungs of mice after primary infection with *M. tuberculosis* (Janis et al., 1989; Augustin et al., 1989), and culture of human peripheral blood lymphocytes with live *M. tuberculosis* results in selective expansion of γδ T cells (Havlir et al., 1991a; Boom et al., 1992). γδ T cells from tuberculin-negative persons and from newborns proliferate in response to *M. tuberculosis*, and limiting dilution analysis has demonstrated that the frequency of *M. tuberculosis*-reactive γδ T cells ranges from 5 to 40%, indicating that human γδ T cells have an innate capacity to recognize mycobacterial antigens (O'Brien et al., 1989; Kabelitz et al., 1990; Tsuyuguchi et al., 1991). Rechallenge with *M. tuberculosis* does not expand γδ T cells, suggest-ing that they do not contribute to the anamnestic response (Janis et al., 1989; Griffin et al., 1991). The percentage of γδ T cells is not increased in the blood of healthy tuberculin reactors or of tuberculosis patients (Tazi et al., 1992; Barnes et al., 1992b) or pleural fluid or lymph nodes at the site of disease in tuberculosis patients (Tazi et al., 1991; Ohmen et al., 1991). However, this does not exclude a role for γδ T cells during the early phases of the immune response, such as in the lungs and lymph nodes of persons recently infected with *M. tuberculosis*. Expansion of *M. tuberculosis*-reactive γδ T cells is greater in healthy tuberculin reactors and in patients with tuberculous pleuritis than in those with advanced pulmonary and miliary tuberculosis, suggesting that γδ T cells contribute to immune resistance (Barnes et al., 1992b).

Although the functional role of γδ T cells in human immunity remains uncertain, it is generally believed that they contribute to control of primary infection before the αβ T-cell response has become established. *M. tuberculosis*-reactive γδ T-cell clones produce gamma interferon, TNF, IL-2, IL-4, IL-5, and IL-10, a group similar to the cytokines produced by αβ T cells (Barnes et al., 1993a), and lyse target cells infected with *M. tuberculosis* (Munk et al., 1990). γδ T cells recognize mycobacterial protease-resistant antigens distinct from the proteins recognized by αβ T cells (Pfeffer et al., 1990; Tsuyuguchi et al., 1991; Boom et al., 1992). In addition, supernatants from *M. tuberculosis*-stimulated γδ T cells enhance macrophage aggregation and may therefore contribute to granuloma formation (Modlin et al., 1989).

MYCOBACTERIAL ANTIGENS RECOGNIZED BY T CELLS

M. tuberculosis is a complex organism with a wide variety of protein antigens that can be broadly divided into structural antigens that are present in the cytoplasm or cell wall and secreted antigens (chapter 20). Immunization of animals with live mycobacteria confers protective immunity against tuberculosis, whereas immunization with killed organisms does not (Orme, 1988b). Because similar structural antigens are present in both live and killed bacilli, secreted antigens produced only by live organisms are likely to be the most important targets of T cells that confer protective immunity. Further support for this hypothesis comes from the recent demonstration that immunization of guinea pigs with secreted proteins of *M. tuberculosis* confers substantial protection against respiratory challenge with *M. tuberculosis* (Pal and Horwitz, 1992).

Of the wide variety of proteins secreted by *M. tuberculosis*, three are of the greatest interest from the standpoint of potentially eliciting protective immunity in humans. Two of these proteins are the 30- and 32-kDa members of the BCG 85 complex that are secreted in large quantities by rapidly growing mycobacteria. Because these proteins can bind fibronectin, a major component of human extracellular matrix, they may mediate adhesion of bacilli to mucosal surfaces and subsequent intracellular invasion through macrophage fibronectin receptors (Abou-Zeid et al., 1988a). These proteins may therefore be critical virulence factors that are important targets of the immune response. The 30-kDa antigen (also referred to as BCG 85B, α antigen, and antigen 6) elicits proliferation by lymphocytes from healthy tuberculin reactors but not by those from tuberculosis patients, raising the intriguing possibility that failure to recognize this antigen, perhaps a genetically determined characteristic, predisposes patients to development of tuberculosis (Havlir et al., 1991c). Alternatively, the 30-kDa antigen may activate suppressive circuits that inhibit the proliferative response in tuberculosis patients. The 32-kDa antigen (also known as BCG 85A or P32) elicits greater proliferation and gamma interferon production in lymphocytes from healthy tuberculin reactors than in those from tuberculosis patients (Huygen et al., 1988).

The 10-kDa antigen, also referred to as BCG-a, is a secreted antigen that is associated with the cell wall of *M. tuberculosis* (Abou-Zeid et al., 1988b; Barnes et al., 1992c). This antigen elicits the greatest level of proliferation and gamma interferon production by lymphocytes from healthy tuberculin reactors compared with other culture filtrate antigens (Barnes et al., 1992c). In addition, proliferative responses to the 10-kDa antigen of pleural fluid lymphocytes from tuberculous pleuritis patients are significantly greater than those of peripheral blood lymphocytes, indicating that this antigen is an important target for T cells at the site of disease.

The mycobacterial antigen that has been studied most intensively is the 65-kDa heat shock protein, a highly conserved molecule that has both bacterial and human homologs. Heat shock proteins are generated in large quantities by cells under stressful conditions and are thought to be produced by mycobacteria in the harsh intracellular environment of the macrophage. The 65-kDa protein is essential for many cellular processes, playing a major role in folding, unfolding, and translocation of polypeptides. It is a potent immunogen for generation of antibody by murine B cells and is recognized by a high proportion of *M. tuberculosis*-reactive murine T cells (Kaufmann, 1990). Despite initial hopes that the 65-kDa protein would elicit protective immunity in humans, this is now believed to be unlikely. First, the 65-kDa antigen is not a secreted antigen and is present at a high concentration in killed mycobacterial preparations that do not elicit protective immunity. Second, murine T cells that confer protective immunity against tuberculosis do not recognize the 65-kDa antigen (Orme et al., 1992). Third, the 65-kDa antigen does not elicit proliferation by lymphocytes from most healthy tuberculin reactors (Havlir et al., 1991c; Barnes et al., 1992c).

Expansion of Specific T-Cell Subpopulations by *M. tuberculosis* Antigens

Some microbial antigens, termed superantigens, do not bind to the groove formed by the two chains of the T-cell receptor but instead bind to the outer surface of a specific V region(s). These superantigens are recognized by all T cells that express these V regions and therefore stimulate a much larger fraction of T cells than do peptide antigens that bind in the groove (Zumla, 1992). Although a mycobacterial superantigen has not been isolated, some data suggest that a superantigen is involved in the pathogenesis of tuberculosis. T cells from healthy tuberculin-negative persons that bear the Vβ8 T-cell receptor proliferate in vitro in response to *M. tuberculosis* (Ohmen et al., submitted). This response does not require antigen processing but requires MHC class II molecules in a manner consistent with superantigen responses. *M. tuberculosis* induces Vβ8$^+$ cells to produce both Th1 and Th2 cytokines, and Vβ8$^+$ T cells are expanded in the pleural fluid of patients with tuberculous pleuritis. The capacity of *M. tuberculosis* to act as a superantigen and stimulate a large fraction of T cells to secrete cytokines may result in the tissue injury characteristic of the disease.

Delayed-Type Hypersensitivity and Protective Immunity

The delayed-type hypersensitivity response to *M. tuberculosis* is evaluated by the tuberculin skin test, which involves intradermal injection of tuberculin PPD. T cells that have been previously sensitized to mycobacterial antigens are attracted to the skin test site. These cells are predominantly activated CD4$^+$ cells (Platt et al., 1983) that are probably memory cells, although this has not been formally demonstrated. T cells proliferate in response to mycobacterial antigens at the skin test site and produce predominantly Th1 cytokines (Tsicopoulos et al., 1992). Because tuberculin contains many antigens that are shared with nontuberculous environmental mycobacteria, sensitization with these organisms can yield a positive skin test in the absence of tuberculous infection.

A negative tuberculin skin test in a healthy person usually indicates the absence of prior infection with *M. tuberculosis* and lack of an expanded population of *M. tuberculosis*-reactive memory T cells. In patients with tuberculous infection or disease, negative tuberculin skin tests can result from processes that interfere with the Th1 delayed-type hypersensitivity response, such as HIV infection, malnutrition, glucocorticoid therapy, and tuberculosis itself. In some persons with prior positive tuberculin skin tests, particularly those with small positive skin tests (<15 mm), there is spontaneous reversion to negative tests in the absence of known immunosuppressive factors (Havlir et al., 1991b).

Delayed-type hypersensitivity is associated with but is not identical to protective immunity (chapters 24 and 31). This association is supported by the clinical observation that persons with positive tuberculin skin tests display substantial resistance to tuberculosis from exogenous reinfection (Stead et al., submitted). On the other hand, separate cell populations transfer delayed-type hypersensitivity and protective immunity to *M. tuberculosis* in some experimental systems (Orme and Collins, 1984), and many patients with severe tuberculosis have positive tuberculin skin tests.

CYTOKINES: PROTECTION AND IMMUNOPATHOLOGY

The human immune response eliminates microbial pathogens through an inflammatory response that may be harmful to host tissue. In tuberculosis, tissue necrosis and fibrosis are characteristic manifestations that are thought to result in part from cytokines produced during the inflammatory response. Inhaled *M. tuberculosis* organisms are initially engulfed by alveolar macrophages that can produce a plethora of cytokines, including IL-1, IL-8, IL-10, TNF, and GM-CSF. IL-1, IL-8, TNF, and GM-CSF are proinflammatory molecules that facilitate recruitment of lymphocytes and monocytes. TNF and GM-CSF also activate macrophages and may augment mycobactericidal activity. In animal models, TNF-α and gamma interferon regulate production of nitric oxide, which is bactericidal for *M. tuberculosis* (Chan et al., 1992). T lymphocytes recruited to the site of infection can produce cytokines that include gamma interferon and IL-2 (Barnes et al., 1993b), and recruited macrophages can produce TNF and 1,25-dihydroxyvitamin D (Barnes et al., 1989b; Cadranel et al., 1988). Gamma interferon and 1,25-dihydroxyvitamin D further enhance macrophage activation and monokine production. The protective immune response may also cause significant tissue necrosis as well as systemic effects such as fever and wasting from release of cytokines such as TNF into the circulation.

To reduce excessive inflammation and tissue damage, immunosuppressive cytokines such as IL-10 and TGF-β, both of which are produced by macrophages at the site of disease in tuberculosis (Barnes et al., 1993b; Toossi et al., 1991; Maeda et al., 1993), may downregulate the immune response and limit the extent of tissue injury. On the other hand, excessive production of immunosuppressive cytokines may result in failure to control infection.

SPECTRUM OF TUBERCULOUS INFECTION AND RELATIONSHIP TO THE IMMUNE RESPONSE

It is intriguing to speculate that the consequences of exposure to *M. tuberculosis*, from establishment of infection to primary and reactivation tuberculosis, reflect the interplay between macrophages, T cells, and *M. tuberculosis*. The likelihood of establishment of tuberculous infection upon inhalation of tubercle bacilli is influenced by genetic host factors. For example, blacks are more susceptible to tuberculous infection than are whites, despite equivalent exposure (Stead et al., 1990), perhaps because macrophages from blacks are more permissive for growth of *M. tuberculosis* (Crowle and Elkins, 1990). If alveolar macrophages eliminate all tubercle bacilli, T cells do not encounter mycobacterial antigens, *M. tuberculosis*-reactive memory T cells are not expanded, and the tuberculin skin test remains negative. Therefore, innate resistance may control infection without development of acquired resistance or expansion of memory T cells.

Primary Tuberculosis

Persons in whom tuberculous infection is established have primary tuberculosis and develop a positive tuberculin skin test. Most remain well, but a minority develop hilar adenopathy, which usually resolves without therapy. In these individuals, macrophages do not eliminate the mycobacteria but present mycobacterial antigens to *M. tuberculosis*-reactive T cells. γδ T cells may predominate in the initial immune response and produce proinflammatory cytokines, attracting and activating a second wave of αβ T cells. One might speculate that the mild clinical manifestations of primary tuberculosis reflect rapid expansion of protective Th1 cells, which recognize secreted mycobacterial antigens. Some become memory cells that mediate delayed-type hypersensitivity. Persistence of memory cells may explain the relative resistance of tuberculin-positive persons to exogenous reinfection with *M. tuberculosis* (Stead et al., submitted).

Rarely, patients develop progressive primary tuberculosis with extensive pulmonary disease and cavitation. These findings may reflect a marked inflammatory response that fails to eliminate bacilli, perhaps because T cells that recognize secreted mycobacterial antigens are not expanded. Both Th1 and Th2 cells may be activated, and immunosuppressive factors such as IL-4, IL-10, and TGF-β produced by Th2 cells and/or macrophages may inhibit bacillary clearance. IL-4, IL-5, and IL-6 may induce polyclonal B-cell immunoglobulin production and the hyperglobulinemia characteristic of patients with extensive tuberculosis. Alternatively, there may be minimal activation of Th1 or Th2 cells, and the immune response may be dominated by macrophages that produce inflammatory mediators but are unable to clear the infection in the absence of a Th1 response.

Miliary tuberculosis, characterized by disseminated disease, anergy, and lack of a T-cell proliferative response to *M. tuberculosis*, reflects a poor inflammatory and delayed-type hypersensitivity response, suggesting a defective Th1 response and predominance of immunosuppressive cytokines such as IL-4, IL-10, and TGF-β produced by Th2 cells and/or macrophages, although this important issue has not been studied.

Reactivation Tuberculosis

After resolution of primary tuberculosis, most persons remain well, but 5 to 10% develop reactivation tuberculosis. One may speculate that rapid development of a Th1 memory cell response may result in self-healing lesions such as in minimal pulmonary tuberculosis or tuberculous pleuritis. Activation of both Th1 and Th2 cells or predominance of macrophage inflammatory mediators may result in advanced pulmonary tuberculosis, which is clinically similar to progressive primary tuberculosis. Absence of a Th1 response and predominance of immunosuppressive cytokines may be associated with miliary tuberculosis.

INTERACTION BETWEEN *M. TUBERCULOSIS* AND HIV

Infection with HIV markedly increases the risk of primary and reactivation tuberculosis, reflecting the dominant role of the $CD4^+$ lymphocyte in protective immunity and in preventing recrudescence of latent infection. It will be of interest to determine whether antimycobacterial immunity and CD4 cell function deteriorate before CD4 cell numbers decline, as such studies may provide insight into protective immune mechanisms.

Clinical, epidemiologic, and experimental evidence suggest that tuberculosis may accelerate the course of HIV infection by activating cells that harbor latent virus. Patients coinfected with tuberculosis and HIV have shortened survival times compared to controls matched for CD4 cell counts (Whalen et al., 1993) and die from complications of progressive HIV infection rather than from tuberculosis (Vjecha et al., 1992). Peripheral blood mononuclear cells from dually infected patients produce more TNF in response to PPD than do those from patients with tuberculosis or HIV infection alone (Wallis et al., 1993b). TNF produced in response to *M. tuberculosis* may promote HIV replication through activation of NFkB (Matsuyama et al., 1991). Mycobacteria and their soluble products activate HIV replication in the latently infected cell line U1 (Lederman et al., submitted), and monocytes from tuberculosis patients show enhanced susceptibility to productive infection with HIV in vitro (Toossi et al., 1993). In addition, HIV-infected tuberculosis patients have higher serum levels of β_2-microglobulin, a surrogate marker of HIV activity (Wallis et al., 1993b). If tuberculosis facilitates progression of HIV disease, then preventive therapy of tuberculosis assumes critical importance, and inhibitors of TNF production such as pentoxifylline and thalidomide may be important adjuncts to chemotherapy.

POTENTIAL APPROACHES TO IMMUNOTHERAPY

Although chemotherapy will remain the mainstay of antituberculosis treatment, the use of adjunctive immunotherapeutic modalities is attractive, particularly in persons with drug-resistant tuberculosis. One approach to immunotherapy is to administer vaccine preparations that stimulate immune defenses and predominance of Th1 cytokines. Such vaccines could include purified or recombinant mycobacterial antigens or live vaccine vector organisms that secrete specific mycobacterial proteins. An alternative approach is to use whole mycobacteria as vaccines. *M. vaccae*, a rapidly growing nonpathogenic organism, is thought by some investigators to be a potential immunotherapeutic agent. *M. vaccae* may possess cross-reactive antigens that elicit protective immunity against *M. tuberculosis* but may lack *M. tuberculosis* antigens that induce delayed-type hypersensitivity and possibly tissue necrosis (Stanford et al., 1990), although biochemical evidence supporting this interpretation is currently lacking.

An alternative immunotherapeutic strategy is to administer cytokines that enhance bacillary elimination, such as gamma interferon or IL-2. Administration of these cytokines to lepromatous leprosy patients decreases the bacillary burden, but gamma interferon increases the frequency of erythema nodosum leprosum (Nathan et al., 1986; Sampaio et al., 1992; Kaplan et al.,

1991). Therapeutic use of cytokines may be limited by high cost and by toxicity of the large parenteral doses required to attain effective tissue levels.

A third approach is to administer antagonists or neutralizing antibodies to immunosuppressive cytokines such as IL-4, IL-10, and TGF-β or to cytokines that may cause immunopathology, such as TNF. An example of this approach is the use of thalidomide to treat erythema nodosum leprosum by reducing *M. leprae*-induced TNF release (Sampaio et al., 1992).

DEVELOPMENT OF ANTITUBERCULOSIS VACCINES

Widespread use of BCG has not controlled tuberculosis, and more effective vaccines are clearly needed. Strategies to construct recombinant vaccines against intracellular pathogens (Stover et al., 1991; Aldovini and Young, 1991) have been devised, but ultimate development of antituberculosis vaccines hinges on an improved understanding of the human immune response to *M. tuberculosis*. One can imagine at least two types of vaccines: one to prevent primary infection in tuberculin-negative persons and another to prevent reactivation tuberculosis in tuberculin reactors.

One strategy for developing antituberculosis vaccines is to characterize the T cells and cytokines that mediate clearance of bacilli during the primary immune response as well as the memory T-cell subpopulations and cytokines that protect against tuberculosis from exogenous reinfection and endogenous reactivation. Mycobacterial antigens that are recognized by these T cells and that elicit production of protective cytokines are potentially important vaccine antigens. Because antigen recognition is often linked to expression of specific MHC molecules, which are highly polymorphic in the population, an effective vaccine would include different antigens that elicit protective immunity in the context of a broad variety of MHC molecules.

Because secreted antigens are most likely to elicit protective immunity, a live vaccine vector that secretes immunogenic antigens is appealing. Mycobacterial genes coding for protective mycobacterial antigens can be incorporated into a vector organism such as BCG, which will have the potential to secrete multiple immunogenic proteins. Development and widespread administration of such a vaccine may play a major role in the eventual control and elimination of tuberculosis throughout the world.

Acknowledgments. This work was supported in part by grants from the National Institutes of Health (AI27285, AI31066, AI22553, AR40312, AI18471, and AI24298) and the World Health Organization (IMM TUB).

REFERENCES

Abou-Zeid, C., T. L. Ratliff, H. G. Wiker, M. Harboe, J. Bennedsen, and G. A. W. Rook. 1988a. Characterization of fibronectin-binding antigens released by *Mycobacterium tuberculosis* and *Mycobacterium bovis* BCG. *Infect. Immun.* **56**:3046–3051.

Abou-Zeid, C., I. Smith, J. M. Grange, T. L. Ratliff, J. Steele, and G. A. W. Rook. 1988b. The secreted antigens of *Mycobacterium tuberculosis* and their relationship to those recognized by the available antibodies. *J. Gen. Microbiol.* **134**:531–538.

Akbar, A. N., M. Salmon, and G. Janossy. 1991. The synergy between naive and memory T cells during activation. *Immunol. Today* **12**:184–188.

Aldovini, A., and R. A. Young. 1991. Humoral and cell-mediated immune responses to live recombinant BCG-HIV vaccines. *Nature* (London) **351**:479–482.

American Thoracic Society. 1986. Treatment of tuberculosis and tuberculosis infection in adults and children. *Am. Rev. Respir. Dis.* **134**:355–363.

Augustin, A., R. T. Kubo, and G. K. Sim. 1989. Resident pulmonary lymphocytes expressing the gamma/delta T-cell receptor. *Nature* (London) **340**:239–241.

Aung, H., L. E. Averill, Z. Toossi, and J. J. Ellner. 1993. Induction of TNF-α from human monocytes stimulated with native 30 kDa antigen of *Mycobacterium tuberculosis*. *Clin. Res.* **41**:323A.

Barnes, P. F., J. S. Abrams, S. Lu, P. A. Sieling, T. H. Rea, and R. L. Modlin. 1993a. Patterns of cytokine production by mycobacterium-reactive human T cell clones. *Infect. Immun.* **61**:197–203.

Barnes, P. F., A. B. Bloch, P. T. Davidson, and D. E. Snider, Jr. 1991. Tuberculosis in patients with human immunodeficiency virus infection. *N. Engl. J. Med.* **324**:1644–1650.

Barnes, P. F., D. Chatterjee, J. S. Abrams, S. Lu, E. Wang, M. Yamamura, P. J. Brennan, and R. L. Modlin. 1992a. Cytokine production induced by *Mycobacterium tuberculosis* lipoarabinomannan: relationship to chemical structure. *J. Immunol.* **307**:1593–1597.

Barnes, P. F., C. L. Grisso, J. S. Abrams, H. Band, T. H. Rea, and R. L. Modlin. 1992b. γδ T lymphocytes in human tuberculosis. *J. Infect. Dis.* **165**:506–512.

Barnes, P. F., S. Lu, J. S. Abrams, E. Wang, M. Yamamura, and R. L. Modlin. 1993b. Cytokine production at the site of disease in human tuberculosis. *Infect. Immun.* **61**:3482–3489.

Barnes, P. F., V. Mehra, B. Rivoire, S.-J. Fong, P. J. Brennan, M. S. Voegtline, P. Minden, R. A. Houghten, B. R. Bloom, and R. L. Modlin. 1992c. Immunoreactivity of a 10 kD antigen of *Mycobacterium tuberculosis*. *J. Immunol.* **148**:1835–1840.

Barnes, P. F., S. D. Mistry, C. L. Cooper, C. Pirmez, T. H. Rea, and R. L. Modlin. 1989a. Compartmentalization of a CD4+ T lymphocyte subpopulation in tuberculous pleuritis. *J. Immunol.* **142**:1114–1119.

Barnes, P. F., R. L. Modlin, D. D. Bikle, and J. S. Adams. 1989b. Transpleural gradient of 1,25-dihydroxyvitamin D in tuberculous pleuritis. *J. Clin. Invest.* **83**:1527–1532.

Bermudez, L. E. M., and L. S. Young. 1988. Tumor necrosis factor, alone or in combination with IL-2, but not IFN-γ, is associated with macrophage killing of *Mycobacterium avium* complex. *J. Immunol.* **140**:3006–3013.

Bermudez, L. E. M., and L. S. Young. 1991. Natural killer cell-dependent mycobacteriostatic and mycobactericidal activity in human macrophages. *J. Immunol.* **146**:265–270.

Beutler, B., and A. Cerami. 1987. Cachectin: more than a tumor necrosis factor. *N. Engl. J. Med.* **316**:379–385.

Boom, W. H., K. A. Chervenak, M. A. Mincek, and J. J. Ellner. 1992. Role of the mononuclear phagocyte as an antigen-presenting cell for human γδ T cells activated by live *Mycobacterium tuberculosis*. *Infect. Immun.* **60**:3480–3488.

Boom, W. H., R. S. Wallis, and K. A. Chervenak. 1991. Human *Mycobacterium tuberculosis*-reactive CD4+ T-cell clones: heterogeneity in antigen recognition, cytokine production, and cytotoxicity for mononuclear phagocytes. *Infect. Immun.* **59**:2737–2743.

Cadranel, J., A. J. Hance, B. Milleron, F. Paillard, G. M. Akoun, and M. Garabedian. 1988. Production of 1,25(OH)$_2$D$_3$ by cells recovered by bronchoalveolar lavage and the role of this metabolite in calcium homeostasis. *Am. Rev. Respir. Dis.* **138**:984–989.

Castro, A. G., N. Esaguy, P. M. Macedo, A. P. Aguas, and M. T. Silva. 1991. Live but not heat-killed mycobacteria cause rapid chemotaxis of large numbers of eosinophils in vivo and are ingested by the attracted granulocytes. *Infect. Immun.* **59**:3009–3014.

Centers for Disease Control. 1991. Nosocomial transmission of multidrug-resistant tuberculosis among HIV-infected persons—Florida and New York, 1988–1991. *Morbid. Mortal. Weekly Rep.* **40**:585–591.

Chan, J., X. Fan, S. W. Hunter, P. J. Brennan, and B. R. Bloom. 1991. Lipoarabinomannan, a possible virulence factor involved in persistence of *Mycobacterium tuberculosis* within macrophages. *Infect. Immun.* **59**:1755–1761.

Chan, J., Y. Xing, R. S. Magliozzo, and B. R. Bloom. 1992. Killing of virulent *Mycobacterium tuberculosis* by reactive nitrogen intermediates produced by activated murine macrophages. *J. Exp. Med.* **175**:1111–1122.

Chatterjee, D., A. D. Roberts, K. Lowell, P. J. Brennan, and I. M. Orme. 1992. Structural basis of capacity of lipoarabinomannan to induce secretion of tumor necrosis factor. *Infect. Immun.* **60**:1249–1253.

Crowle, A. J., and N. Elkins. 1990. Relative permissiveness of macrophages from black and white people for virulent tubercle bacilli. *Infect. Immun.* **58**:632–638.

Dannenberg, A. M. 1991. Delayed-type hypersensitivity and cell-mediated immunity in the pathogenesis of tuberculosis. *Immunol. Today* **12**:228–233.

Davis, M. M., and P. J. Bjorkman. 1988. T-cell antigen receptor genes and T-cell recognition. *Nature* (London) **334**:395–402.

de Waal Malefyt, R., J. Abrams, B. Bennett, C. Figdor, and J. E. De Vries. 1991. IL-10 inhibits cytokine synthesis by human monocytes: an autocrine role of IL-10 produced by monocytes. *J. Exp. Med.* **250**:1302–1305.

Del Prete, G., M. De Carli, F. Almerigogna, M. G. Giudizi, R. Biagotti, and S. Romagnani. 1993. Human IL-10 is produced by both type 1 helper (Th1) and type 2 helper (Th2) T cell clones and inhibits their antigen-specific proliferation and cytokine production. *J. Immunol.* **150**:353–360.

Del Prete, G. F., M. De Carli, C. Mastromauro, R. Biagotti, D. Macchia, P. Falagiani, M. Ricci, and S. Romagnani. 1991. Purified protein derivative of *Mycobacterium tuberculosis* and excretory-secretory antigen(s) of *Toxocara canis* expand *in vitro* human T cells with stable and opposite (type 1 T helper or type 2 T helper) profile of cytokine production. *J. Clin. Invest.* **88**:346–350.

Dinarello, C. 1984. Interleukin-1 and the pathogenesis of the acute-phase response. *N. Engl. J. Med.* **311**:1413–1418.

Ding, A. H., C. Nathan, J. Graycar, R. Dernyck, D. J. Stuehr, and S. Srimal. 1990. Macrophage deactivating factor and transforming growth factors- B$_1$, B$_2$, and B$_3$, inhibit macrophage nitrogen oxide synthesis by interferon-γ. *J. Immunol.* **145**:940–944.

Ding, A. H., C. F. Nathan, and D. J. Stuehr. 1988. Release of reactive nitrogen intermediates and reactive oxygen intermediates from mouse peritoneal macrophages: comparison of activating cytokines and evidence for independent production. *J. Immunol.* **141**:2407–2412.

Ellner, J. J. 1978. Suppressor adherent cells in human tuberculosis. *J. Immunol.* **121**:2573–2578.

Fischl, M. A., G. L. Daikos, R. B. Uttamchandani, R. B. Poblete, J. N. Moreno, R. R. Reyes, A. M. Boota, L. M. Thompson, T. J. Cleary, S. A. Oldham, M. J. Saldana, and S. Lai. 1992. Clinical presentation and outcome of patients with HIV infection and tuberculosis caused by multiple-drug-resistant bacilli. *Ann. Intern. Med.* **117**:184–190.

Flesch, I. E., and S. H. E. Kaufmann. 1991. Mechanisms involved in mycobacterial growth inhibition by gamma interferon-activated bone marrow macrophages: role of reactive nitrogen intermediates. *Infect. Immun.* **59**:3213–3218.

Flynn, J. L., M. M. Goldstein, K. J. Triebold, B. Koller, and B. R. Bloom. 1992. Major histocompatibility complex class I-restricted T cells are required for resistance to *Mycobacterium tuberculosis* infection. *Proc. Natl. Acad. Sci. USA* **89**:12013–12017.

Fujiwara, H., M. E. Kleinhenz, R. S. Wallis, and J. J. Ellner. 1986. Increased interleukin-1 production and monocyte suppressor cell activity associated with human tuberculosis. *Am. Rev. Respir. Dis.* **133**:73–77.

Gajewski, T. F., M. Pinnas, T. Wong, and F. W. Fitch. 1991. Murine Th1 and Th2 clones proliferate optimally in response to distinct antigen-presenting cell populations. *J. Immunol.* **146**:1750–1758.

Greenbaum, L. A., J. B. Horowitz, A. Woods, T. Pasqualini, E.-P. Reich, and K. Bottomly. 1988. Autocrine growth of CD4$^+$ T cells: differential effects of IL-1 on helper and inflammatory T cells. *J. Immunol.* **140**:1555–1560.

Griffin, J. P., K. V. Harshan, W. K. Born, and I. M. Orme. 1991. Kinetics of accumulation of gamma/delta receptor-bearing T lymphocytes in mice infected with live mycobacteria. *Infect. Immun.* **59**:4263–4265.

Haanen, J. B. A. G., R. de Waal Malefijt, P. C. M. Res, E. M. Kraakman, T. H. M. Ottenhoff, R. R. P. de Vries, and H. Spits. 1991. Selection of a human T helper type 1-like T cell subset by mycobacteria. *J. Exp. Med.* **174:**583–592.

Havlir, D. V., J. J. Ellner, K. Chervenak, and W. H. Boom. 1991a. Selective expansion of human γδ T cells by monocytes infected with live *Mycobacterium tuberculosis*. *J. Clin. Invest.* **87:**729–733.

Havlir, D. V., F. van der Kuyp, E. Duffy, R. Marshall, D. Hom, and J. J. Ellner. 1991b. A 19-year follow-up of tuberculin reactors: assessment of skin test reactivity and *in vitro* lymphocyte responses. *Chest* **99:**1172–1176.

Havlir, D. V., R. S. Wallis, W. H. Boom, T. M. Daniel, K. Chervenak, and J. J. Ellner. 1991c. Human immune response to *Mycobacterium tuberculosis* antigens. *Infect. Immun.* **59:**665–670.

Heinzel, F. P., M. D. Sadick, B. J. Holaday, R. L. Coffman, and R. M. Locksley. 1989. Reciprocal expression of interferon gamma or interleukin 4 during the resolution or progression of murine leishmaniasis: evidence for expansion of distinct helper T cell subsets. *J. Exp. Med.* **169:**59–72.

Heinzel, F. P., D. S. Schoenhaut, M. Rerko, L. E. Rosser, and M. K. Gately. 1993. Recombinant interleukin 12 cures mice infected with *Leishmania major*. *J. Exp. Med.* **177:**1505–1509.

Hirano, T., S. Akira, T. Taga, and T. Kishimoto. 1990. Biological and clinical aspects of interleukin 6. *Immunol. Today* **11:**443–449.

Ho, L. H., S. H. He, M. J. C. Rios, and E. A. Wick. 1992. Interleukin-4 inhibits human macrophage activation by tumor necrosis factor, granulocyte-monocyte colony-stimulating factor, and interleukin-3 for antileishmanial activity and oxidative burst capacity. *J. Infect. Dis.* **165:**344–351.

Hsieh, C. S., S. E. Macatonia, C. S. Tripp, S. F. Wolf, A. O'Garra, and K. M. Murphy. 1993. Development of T_H1 CD4⁺ T cells through IL-12 produced by Listeria-induced macrophages. *Science* **260:**547–549.

Huygen, K., D. Abramowicz, P. Vandenbussche, F. Jacobs, J. DeBruyn, A. Kentos, A. Drowart, J. P. VanVooren, and M. Goldman. 1992. Spleen cell cytokine secretion in *Mycobacterium bovis* BCG-infected mice. *Infect. Immun.* **60:**2880–2886.

Huygen, K., J. P. Van Vooren, M. Turneer, R. Bosmans, P. Dierckx, and J. De Bruyn. 1988. Specific lymphoproliferation, gamma interferon production, and serum immunoglobulin G directed against a purified 32 kDa mycobacterial protein antigen (P32) in patients with active tuberculosis. *Scand. J. Immunol.* **27:**187–194.

Janis, E. M., S. H. Kaufmann, R. H. Schwartz, and D. M. Pardoll. 1989. Activation of γδ T cells in the primary immune response to *Mycobacterium tuberculosis*. *Science* **244:**713–716.

Jones, B. E., S. M. M. Young, D. Antoniskis, P. T. Davidson, F. Kramer, and P. F. Barnes. 1993. Rela-
tionship of the manifestations of tuberculosis to CD4 cell counts in patients with human immunodeficiency virus infection. *Am. Rev. Respir. Dis.* **148:**1292–1297.

Kabelitz, D., A. Bender, S. Schondelmaier, B. Schoel, and S. H. E. Kaufmann. 1990. A large fraction of human peripheral blood γδ⁺ T cells is activated by *Mycobacterium tuberculosis* but not by its 65-kD heat shock protein. *J. Exp. Med.* **171:**667–679.

Kaplan, G., W. J. Britton, G. E. Hancock, W. J. Theuvenet, K. A. Smith, C. K. Job, P. W. Roche, A. Molloy, R. Burkhardt, J. Barker, H. M. Pradhan, and Z. A. Cohn. 1991. The systemic influence of recombinant interleukin 2 on the manifestations of lepromatous leprosy. *J. Exp. Med.* **173:**993–1006.

Kaufmann, S. H. E. 1988. CD8+ T lymphocytes in intracellular microbial infections. *Immunol. Today* **9:**168–174.

Kaufmann, S. H. E. 1990. Heat shock proteins and the immune response. *Immunol. Today* **11(4):**129–136.

Kindler, V., A.-P. Sappino, G. E. Grau, P.-F. Piguet, and P. Vassalli. 1989. The inducing role of tumor necrosis factor in the development of bactericidal granulomas during BCG infection. *Cell* **56:**731–740.

Lederman, M. M., D. Georges, D. Kusher, C. Z. Giam, and Z. Toossi. *Mycobacterium tuberculosis* and its purified protein derivative activate expression of the human immunodeficiency virus. Submitted for publication.

Lehn, M., W. Y. Weisner, S. Engelhorn, S. Gillis, and H. G. Remold. 1989. IL-4 inhibits H₂O₂ production and antileishmanial capacity of human cultured monocytes mediated by IFN-gamma. *J. Immunol.* **143:**3020–3024.

Lorgat, F., M. M. Keraan, P. T. Lukey, and S. R. Ress. 1992. Evidence for in vivo generation of cytotoxic T cells: PPD-stimulated lymphocytes from tuberculous pleural effusions demonstrate enhanced cytotoxicity with accelerated kinetics of induction. *Am. Rev. Respir. Dis.* **145:**418–423.

Maeda, J., N. Ueki, T. Ohkawa, N. Iwahashi, T. Nakano, T. Hada, and K. Higashino. 1993. Local production and localization of transforming growth factor-β in tuberculous pleurisy. *Clin. Exp. Immunol.* **92:**32–38.

Maggi, E., P. Parronchi, R. Manetti, C. Simonelli, M.-P. Piccinni, F. S. Rugiu, M. De Carli, M. Ricci, and S. Romagnani. 1992. Reciprocal regulatory effects of IFN-γ and IL-4 on the *in vitro* development of human Th1 and Th2 clones. *J. Immunol.* **148:**2142–2147.

Manetti, R., P. Parronchi, M. G. Giudizi, M. P. Piccinni, E. Maggi, G. Trinchieri, and S. Romagnani. 1993. Natural killer cell stimulatory factor (interleukin 12 [IL-12]) induces T helper type 1 (Th1)-specific immune responses and inhibits the development of

IL-4-producing Th cells. *J. Exp. Med.* **177:**1199–1204.

Martinez, O. M., R. S. Gibbons, M. R. Garovoy, and F. R. Aronson. 1990. IL-4 inhibits IL-2 receptor expression and IL-2-dependent proliferation of human T cells. *J. Immunol.* **144:**2211–2215.

Matsuyama, T., N. Kobayashi, and N. Yamamoto. 1991. Cytokines and HIV infection: is AIDS a tumor necrosis factor disease? *AIDS* **5:**1405–1417.

May, M. E., and P. J. Spagnuolo. 1987. Evidence for activation of a respiratory burst in the interaction of human neutrophils with *Mycobacterium tuberculosis. Infect. Immun.* **55:**2304–2307.

Modlin, R. L., C. Pirmez, F. M. Hofman, V. Torigian, K. Uyemura, T. H. Rea, B. R. Bloom, and M. B. Brenner. 1989. Lymphocytes bearing antigen-specific γδ T-cell receptors accumulate in human infectious disease lesions. *Nature* (London) **339:**544–548.

Moreno, C., A. Mehlert, and J. Lamb. 1988. The inhibitory effects of mycobacterial lipoarabinomannan and polysaccharides upon polyclonal and monoclonal human T cell proliferation. *Clin. Exp. Immunol.* **74:**206–210.

Mosmann, T. R., and K. W. Moore. 1991. The role of IL-10 in crossregulation of Th1 and Th2 responses. *Immunol. Today* **12:**A49–A53.

Muller, I., S. P. Cobbold, H. Waldmann, and S. H. E. Kaufmann. 1987. Impaired resistance to *Mycobacterium tuberculosis* infection after selective *in vivo* depletion of L3T4$^+$ and Lyt-2$^+$ T cells. *Infect. Immun.* **55:**2037–2041.

Munk, M. E., A. J. Gatrill, and S. H. E. Kaufmann. 1990. Target cell lysis and IL-2 secretion by gamma/delta T lymphocytes after activation with bacteria. *J. Immunol.* **145:**2434–2439.

Nathan, C. F., G. Kaplan, W. R. Levis, A. Nusrat, M. D. Witmer, S. A. Sherwin, C. K. Job, C. R. Horowitz, R. M. Steinman, and Z. A. Cohn. 1986. Local and systemic effects of intradermal recombinant interferon-γ in patients with lepromatous leprosy. *N. Engl. J. Med.* **315:**6–15.

O'Brien, R. L., M. P. Happ, A. Dallas, E. Palmer, R. Kubo, and W. K. Born. 1989. Stimulation of a major subset of lymphocytes expressing T cell receptor gamma delta by an antigen derived from *Mycobacterium tuberculosis. Cell* **57:**667–674.

Ogawa, T., H. Uclieda, Y. Kusumoto, Y. Mori, Y. Yamamura, and S. Hamada. 1991. Increase in tumor necrosis factor alpha and interleukin-6 secreting cells in peripheral blood mononuclear cells from subjects infected with *Mycobacterium tuberculosis. Infect. Immun.* **59:**3021–3025.

Ohmen, J. D., P. F. Barnes, C. L. Grisso, B. R. Bloom, and R. L. Modlin. Expansion of T cells bearing the Vβ8 T cell receptor by *Mycobacterium tuberculosis.* Submitted for publication.

Ohmen, J. D., P. F. Barnes, K. Uyemura, S. Lu, C. L. Grisso, and R. L. Modlin. 1991. The T-cell receptor of human γδ T-cells reactive to *Mycobacterium tuberculosis* are encoded by specific V genes but diverse V-J junctions. *J. Immunol.* **50:**361–362.

Orme, I. M. 1987. The kinetics of emergence and loss of mediator T lymphocytes acquired in response to infection with *Mycobacterium tuberculosis. J. Immunol.* **138:**293–298.

Orme, I. M. 1988a. Characteristics and specificity of acquired immunologic memory to *Mycobacterium tuberculosis* infection. *J. Immunol.* **140:**3589–3593.

Orme, I. M. 1988b. Induction of nonspecific acquired resistance and delayed-type hypersensitivity, but not specific acquired resistance, in mice inoculated with killed mycobacterial vaccines. *Infect. Immun.* **56:**3310–3312.

Orme, I. M., and F. M. Collins. 1983. Protection against *Mycobacterium tuberculosis* infection by adoptive immunotherapy. *J. Exp. Med.* **158:**74–83.

Orme, I. M., and F. M. Collins. 1984. Adoptive protection of the *Mycobacterium tuberculosis*-infected lung: dissociation between cells that passively transfer protective immunity and those that transfer delayed-type hypersensitivity. *Cell. Immunol.* **84:**113–120.

Orme, I. M., E. S. Miller, A. D. Roberts, S. K. Furney, J. P. Griffin, K. M. Dobos, D. Chi, B. Rivoire, and P. J. Brennan. 1992. T lymphocytes mediating protection and cellular cytolysis during the course of *Mycobacterium tuberculosis* infection. *J. Immunol.* **148:**189–196.

Ottenhoff, T. H. M., and T. Mutis. 1990. Specific killing of cytotoxic T cells and antigen-presenting cells by CD4$^+$ cytotoxic T cell clones. *J. Exp. Med.* **171:**2011–2024.

Pal, P. G., and M. A. Horwitz. 1992. Immunization with extracellular proteins of *Mycobacterium tuberculosis* induces cell-mediated immune responses and substantial protective immunity in a guinea pig model of pulmonary tuberculosis. *Infect. Immun.* **60:**4781–4792.

Palladino, M. A., R. E. Morris, and A. D. Levinson. 1990. TGFβs: a new family of immunoregulatory molecules. *Ann. N.Y. Acad. Sci.* **593:**181–187.

Pedrazzini, T., K. Hug, and J. A. Louis. 1987. Importance of L3T4+ and Lyt-2+ cells in the immunologic control of infection with *Mycobacterium bovis* strain bacillus Calmette-Guerin in mice. *J. Immunol.* **139:**2032–2037.

Pfeffer, K., B. Schoel, H. Gulle, S. H. E. Kaufmann, and H. Wagner. 1990. Primary responses of human T cells to mycobacteria: a frequent set of γδ T cells are stimulated by protease-resistant ligands. *Eur. J. Immunol.* **20:**1175–1179.

Platt, J., B. W. Grant, A. A. Eddy, and A. F. Michael. 1983. Immune cell populations in cutaneous de-

434   Barnes et al.

layed-type hypersensitivity. *J. Exp. Med.* **158**:1227–1242.

Roach, T. I., C. H. Barton, D. Chatterjee, and J. M. Blackwell. 1993. Macrophage activation: lipoarabinomannan from avirulent and virulent strains of *Mycobacterium tuberculosis* differentially induces the early genes c-fos, KC, JE, and tumor necrosis factor-α. *J. Immunol.* **150**:1886–1896.

Rocken, M., J.-H. Saurat, and C. Hauser. 1992. A common precursor for CD4+ T cells producing IL-2 or IL-4. *J. Immunol.* **148**:1031–1036.

Rook, G. A. W., J. Steele, L. Fraher, S. Barker, R. Karmali, and J. O'Riordan. 1986. Vitamin D_3, gamma interferon, and control of proliferation of *Mycobacterium tuberculosis* by human monocytes. *Immunology* **57**:159–163.

Roper, W. H., and J. J. Waring. 1955. Primary serofibrinous pleural effusion in military personnel. *Am. Rev. Tuberc.* **71**:616–634.

Salgame, P., J. Abrams, C. Clayberger, H. Goldstein, J. Convit, R. L. Modlin, and B. R. Bloom. 1991. Differing lymphokine profiles of functional subsets of human CD4 and CD8 T cell clones. *Science* **254**:279–281.

Sampaio, E. P., A. L. Moreira, E. N. Sarno, A. M. Malta, and G. Kaplan. 1992. Prolonged treatment with recombinant interferon gamma induces erythema nodosum leprosum in lepromatous leprosy patients. *J. Exp. Med.* **175**:1729–1737.

Scott, P. 1993. IL-12: initiation cytokine for cell-mediated immunity. *Science* **260**:496–497.

Scott, P., P. Natovitz, R. L. Coffman, E. Pearce, and A. Sher. 1988. Immunoregulation of cutaneous leishmaniasis. *J. Exp. Med.* **168**:1675–1684.

Seder, R. A., W. E. Paul, M. M. Davis, and B. Fazekas de St. Groth. 1992. The presence of interleukin 4 during in vitro priming determines the lymphokine-producing potential of CD4+ T cell receptor transgenic mice. *J. Exp. Med.* **176**:1091–1098.

Stanford, J. L., G. M. Bahr, G. A. W. Rook, M. A. Shaaban, T. D. Chugh, M. Gabriel, B. Al-Shimali, Z. Siddiqui, F. Ghardani, A. Shahin, and K. Behbehani. 1990. Immunotherapy with *Mycobacterium vaccae* as an adjunct to chemotherapy in the treatment of pulmonary tuberculosis. *Tubercle* **71**:87–93.

Stead, W. W., J. P. Lofgren, H. L. Masters, G. L. Templeton, M. D. Cave, and L. A. Illing. An attempt to quantify protection against exogenous reinfection tuberculosis in healthy persons. Submitted for publication.

Stead, W. W., J. W. Senner, W. T. Reddick, and J. P. Lofgren. 1990. Racial differences in susceptibility to infection by *Mycobacterium tuberculosis*. *N. Engl. J. Med.* **322**:422–427.

Stover, C. K., V. F. de la Cruz, T. R. Fuerst, J. E. Burlein, L. A. Benson, L. T. Bennett, G. P. Bansai, J. F. Young, M. H. Lee, G. F. Hatfull, S. B. Snapper, **R. G. Barletta, W. R. Jacobs, Jr., and B. R. Bloom.** 1991. New use of BCG for recombinant vaccines. *Nature* (London) **351**:456–460.

Street, N. E., and T. R. Mosmann. 1991. Functional diversity of T lymphocytes due to secretion of different cytokine patterns. *FASEB J.* **5**:171–175.

Strominger, J. L. 1989. The gamma delta T cell receptor and class Ib MHC-related proteins: enigmatic molecules of immune recognition. *Cell* **57**:895–898.

Takashima, S., C. Ueta, I. Tsuyuguchi, and S. Kishimuto. 1990. Production of tumor necrosis factor by monocytes from patients with pulmonary tuberculosis. *Infect. Immun.* **58**:3286–3292.

Tazi, A., F. Bouchonnet, D. Valeyre, J. Cadranel, J. P. Battesti, and A. J. Hance. 1992. Characterization of γδ T-lymphocytes in the peripheral blood of patients with active tuberculosis: a comparison with normal subjects and patients with sarcoidosis. *Am. Rev. Respir. Dis.* **146**:1216–1221.

Tazi, A., I. Fajac, P. Soler, D. Valeyre, J. P. Battesti, and A. J. Hance. 1991. Gamma/delta T-lymphocytes are not increased in number in granulomatous lesions of patients with tuberculosis or sarcoidosis. *Am. Rev. Respir. Dis.* **144**:1373–1375.

Toossi, Z., M. E. Kleinhenz, and J. J. Ellner. 1986. Defective interleukin-2 production and responsiveness in human pulmonary tuberculosis. *J. Exp. Med.* **163**:1162–1172.

Toossi, Z., J. R. Sedor, J. P. Lapurge, R. J. Ondash, and J. J. Ellner. 1990. Expression of functional interleukin 2 receptors by peripheral blood monocytes from patients with active pulmonary tuberculosis. *J. Clin. Invest.* **85**:1777–1784.

Toossi, Z., J. G. Sierra-Madero, R. A. Blinkhorn, M. A. Mettler, and E. A. Rich. 1993. Enhanced susceptibility of blood monocytes from patients with pulmonary tuberculosis to productive infection with human immunodeficiency virus type 1. *J. Exp. Med.* **177**:1511–1516.

Toossi, Z., T. Young, P. Gogate, and J. J. Ellner. 1991. Expression of transforming growth factor-β in lung granulomas and peripheral blood monocytes of patients with tuberculosis, abstr., p. 57–62. Twenty-Sixth Joint Conf. Tuberc. Lepr.

Tsicopoulos, A., Q. Hamid, V. Varney, S. Ying, R. Moqbel, S. R. Durham, and A. B. Kay. 1992. Preferential messenger RNA expression of Th1-type cells (IFN-gamma+, IL-2+) in classical delayed-type (tuberculin) hypersensitivity reactions in human skin. *J. Immunol.* **148**:2058–2061.

Tsunawaki, S., M. Sporn, A. Ding, and C. Nathan. 1988. Deactivation of macrophages by transforming growth factor β. *Nature* (London) **334**:260–262.

Tsuyuguchi, I., H. Kawasumi, C. Ueta, I. Yano, and S. Kishimoto. 1991. Increase of T-cell receptor gamma/delta-bearing T cells in cord blood of newborn babies obtained by in vitro stimulation with mycobacterial cord factor. *Infect. Immun.* **59**:3053–3059.

Tweardy, D. J., B. Z. Schacter, and J. J. Ellner. 1984. Association of altered dynamics of monocyte expression of human leukocyte antigen-DR with immunosuppression in tuberculosis. *J. Infect. Dis.* **149**:31–37.

Valone, S. E., E. A. Rich, R. S. Wallis, and J. J. Ellner. 1988. Expression of tumor necrosis factor in vitro by human mononuclear phagocytes stimulated with whole *Mycobacterium bovis* BCG and mycobacterial antigens. *Infect. Immun.* **56**:3313–3315.

Vjecha, M., A. Okwera, F. Byekwaso, J. Kakibali, S. Nyole, M. Okot-Nwang, T. Avu, P. Eriki, R. Mujeuwa, T. Daniel, R. Huebner, and J. J. Ellner. 1992. Predictors of mortality and drug toxicity in HIV-infected patients from Uganda treated for pulmonary tuberculosis, abstr. B180. Abstr. VIII Int. Conf. AIDS/III STD World Congr.

Wallis, R. S., R. Paranjape, and M. Phillips. 1993a. Identification by two-dimensional gel electrophoresis of a 58-kilodalton tumor necrosis factor-inducing protein of *Mycobacterium tuberculosis*. *Infect. Immun.* **61**:627–632.

Wallis, R. S., M. Vjecha, M. Amir-Tahmasseb, A. Okwera, F. Byekwaso, S. Nyole, S. Kabengera, R. D. Mugerwa, and J. J. Ellner. 1993b. Influence of tuberculosis on human immunodeficiency virus (HIV-1): enhanced cytokine expression and elevated β_2-microglobulin in HIV-1-associated tuberculosis. *J. Infect. Dis.* **167**:43–48.

Whalen, C., C. R. Horsburgh, Jr., D. Hom, C. Labart, S. Simberkoff, and J. J. Ellner. 1993. Accelerated clinical course of human immunodeficiency virus infection following active tuberculosis. *Clin. Res.* **41**:290A.

Yamamura, M., K. Uyemura, R. J. Deans, K. Weinberg, T. H. Rea, B. R. Bloom, and R. L. Modlin. 1991. Defining protective responses to pathogens: cytokine profiles in leprosy lesions. *Science* **254**:277–279.

Yssel, H., R. de Waal Malefyt, M. G. Roncarolo, J. S. Abrams, R. Lahesmaa, H. Spits, and J. E. deVries. 1992. IL-10 is produced by subsets of human CD4 T cell clones and peripheral blood T cells. *J. Immunol.* **149**:2378–2384.

Zhang, M., M. K. Gately, E. Wang, S. F. Wolf, S. Lu, R. L. Modlin, and P. F. Barnes. Interleukin-12 at the site of disease in tuberculosis. *J. Clin. Invest.*, in press.

Zumla, A. 1992. Superantigens, T cells, and microbes. *Clin. Infect. Dis.* **15**:313–320.

Tuberculosis: Pathogenesis, Protection, and Control
Edited by Barry R. Bloom
© 1994 American Society for Microbiology, Washington, DC 20005

Chapter 26

Specificity and Function of T- and B-Cell Recognition in Tuberculosis

Juraj Ivanyi and Jelle Thole

Infection with *Mycobacterium tuberculosis* triggers a broad spectrum of immune responses, but little is known about the specificities involved in the elimination of the pathogen or in the mechanisms of disease-associated pathology. The thick bacterial cell wall of tubercle bacilli is probably conducive to survival within host macrophages, but it is the nature of T-cell-mediated immune reactions that determines the outcome of infection. Although the key role is played by CD4 T cells, the exact role of cytokines derived from T cells in the host-parasite relationship is poorly understood. Gamma interferon (IFN-γ), which is characteristic for Th1 cells, may be involved in protection as well as pathogenesis, although the pathological features of infections with intracellular microbial pathogens have generally been attributed to the effects of cytokines derived from Th2 cells. The individual epitopes of protein antigens from tubercle bacilli are recognized by major histocompatibility (MHC) class II-restricted CD4 T cells as well as by MHC class I-restricted CD8 T cells. Moreover,

γδ T cells have been implicated in the early response to mycobacterial infection. Protective immunity involves activation and perhaps lysis of infected macrophages as well as containment of the infection in granulomas. While the protective coordinated reactions of multiple functionally different T cells secreting a complex array of cytokines represent a labile balance between the host and the infecting bacteria, disturbance of this balance may lead to immunopathology manifested by overt disease.

Patients with tuberculosis have abundant T-cell immunity and antibodies to several antigens of the infecting organism. Since it is not known whether the protective and pathogenic host immune responses are of distinct specificity, the study of the molecular nature of mycobacterial antigens and of their immunogenicity in the infected or diseased host is of major interest. The experimental analysis is difficult, however, because protection can be imparted only by a live attenuated vaccine such as the bacillus Calmette-Guérin (BCG). The complexity of immune responses to multiple antigens also imposes a formidable obstacle to the design of novel immunodiagnostic reagents. In this chapter we discuss progress in the study of immune reactions mainly to

Juraj Ivanyi • MRC Tuberculosis and Related Infections Unit, Clinical Sciences Centre, London W12 ONN, United Kingdom. *Jelle Thole* • Department of Immunohaematology and Blood Bank, University Hospital, 2300 RC Leiden, The Netherlands.

antigens of *M. tuberculosis* that have been firmly identified and of the largely characterized protein structure.

PROTEIN ANTIGENS OF
M. TUBERCULOSIS

Previous efforts to isolate the constituents of the purified protein derivative (PPD), representing a crude extract from the culture filtrate of *M. tuberculosis* that is still in routine use for human skin testing, have focused attention on the analysis of individual structural constituents (Daniel and Janicki, 1978). Several antigenic components of mycobacteria were classified in a reference system on the basis of reactivity with hyperimmune rabbit antisera. Using crossed immunoelectrophoresis, initially only 11 but later more than 50 complex or single antigens had been defined (Wiker et al., 1988). A number of identified antigens have been isolated from mycobacterial culture filtrates, and the complete amino acid sequence or N-terminal sequences from several other proteins have been determined (Daniel and Janicki, 1978; Wiker and Harboe, 1992). However, protein and subsequent DNA sequencing produced different results, at least in the case of the MPB70 protein from *M. bovis* (Patarroyo et al., 1986; Terasaka et al., 1989).

An important breakthrough in the characterization of antigens was achieved initially by the production of monoclonal antibodies to mycobacterial antigens (Coates et al., 1981; Ivanyi et al., 1985; Engers et al., 1986) and particularly by the development of recombinant DNA systems for efficient expression of mycobacterial genes in *Escherichia coli* (Young et al., 1985; Thole and Van der Zee, 1990). The screening of genomic expression libraries of mycobacteria by using monoclonal antibodies allowed the isolation of antigen-expressing DNA clones and subsequent analysis of the amino acid sequences. Other probes, such

as polyclonal antibodies, T cells, and oligonucleotides deduced from partial amino acid sequences, have been used to isolate and characterize mycobacterial antigens. Purification from overexpressing *E. coli* bacteria has been initiated through immunological evaluation of T-cell as well as B-cell responses induced by these antigens. The combined use of subgene libraries and synthetic peptides allowed the exact characterization of B-cell and T-cell determinants involved. Structural and immunological analyses of many of these antigens is in progress (Young et al., 1992) but has been focused in particular on the following three groups of proteins that reside in different locations of the tubercle bacilli.

Cytoplasmic Stress Proteins

Heat shock proteins (hsp) have highly conserved amino acid sequences. Their functions as molecular chaperones in the assembly and disassembly of proteins into oligomers during transport through the cell or as proteases that degrade misfolded or foreign proteins are vital for each cell. Protein families classified on the basis of their molecular weight, such as hsp65 (GroEL), hsp10 (GroES), hsp70 (DnaK), and hsp90, have been identified in both prokaryotes and eukaryotes. Other families, such as 16-kDa α-crystallins, seem to have somewhat less conserved sequences. The cellular expression of stress proteins is enhanced by a variety of stimuli, such as heat, nutrient deprivation, and oxygen radicals, and this response probably protects the cell during adverse conditions by maintaining a functional conformation of essential proteins or by assisting in the removal of denatured proteins.

In *M. tuberculosis*, the antigenic structure and biochemical function have been characterized for hsp70, hsp65, and hsp 10 (Shinnick et al., 1988; Baird et al., 1989; Garsia et al., 1989; Young and Garbe, 1991b; McKenzie et al., 1991). However, the 16-kDa constituents were classified as stress proteins merely on the basis of sequence homology (Verbon et al., 1992b), while a mycobacterial homolog of the hsp90 family has not as yet been identified. Interestingly, two genes that code for related hsp65 molecules were identified; one of them is localized in an operon with hsp10 (Rinke de Wit et al., 1992; Kong et al., 1993). The first *M. tuberculosis* hsp65 is approximately 60% homologous to the second hsp65 of this species, whereas the counterparts of these proteins in other mycobacteria show significantly higher homologies. Both hsp65 proteins display approximately 40 to 60% homology to other bacterial and eukaryotic species, while the 16-kDa protein displays only 20 to 30% homology with other α-crystallins, including the *M. leprae* 18-kDa antigen (Verbon et al., 1992b). hsp65 has been found to be immunogenic in various experimental models and in humans (Thole and Van der Zee, 1990; Kiessling et al., 1991). A large number of T-cell clones generated against mycobacteria were found to react with hsp65 (Boom et al., 1991). This outcome may have been influenced by enhanced cellular expression of bacterial hsp65 in infected cells or by cross-stimulation by the homologous proteins from commensal organisms. The special immunogenicity of hsp70 even in the absence of adjuvants and without prior mycobacterial sensitization has recently been documented (Barrios et al., 1992).

Since the regions of homology and of species-specific residues are randomly distributed throughout the hsp65 sequence, the positions of species and cross-reactive epitopes are spread out. The majority of monoclonal antibodies (MAbs) are directed against common mycobacterial epitopes. However, certain epitopes react even more broadly with other bacterial genera (Ivanyi et al., 1988; Thole and Van der Zee, 1990), and one antibody (ML30; peptide specificity, 286–299) reacts with the human ho-

molog (Kiessling et al., 1991). Recently, antigenic mimicry between hsp65 and functionally and evolutionary nonhomologous proteins was observed (Aguas et al., 1990; Rambukkana et al., 1992), but the implications of these findings for the role of hsp65 in disease is currently unclear. In contrast, restricted binding to hsp65 from organisms of the *M. tuberculosis* complex and from merely a few other mycobacterial species applies only to MAb TB78, which binds to a conformational epitope, and antibody DC16, which reacts to a linear epitope mapping to sequence 154–164. One T-cell epitope with specificity for the *M. tuberculosis* complex has been localized to the peptide sequence 231–245 with a DR2-restricted human T-cell clone (Oftung et al., 1988). This clone fails to react with the homologous sequence from *M. leprae*, which differs in two residues (G-Q and P-S), both of which have potentials for changing the peptide's conformation. Competition studies indicated that both residues were involved in binding to DR2 rather than to the T-cell receptor.

Membrane Lipoproteins

The significance of lipoproteins for the immune response to mycobacteria has been in focus in view of reports that acylation of proteins enhances their ability to induce delayed-type hypersensitivity (DTH) (Coon and Hunter, 1975) and that synthetic lipopeptides have the ability to prime cytotoxic T cells (Deres et al., 1989). The latter finding is of particular interest for class I-restricted responses. Moreover, vaccination with recombinant BCG expressing OspA as a lipoprotein protected against *Borrelia burgdorferi* infection, in marked contrast to the lack of protective potency of the same antigen when expressed as an intracellular protein (Stover et al., 1993).

By detergent phase separation and metabolic labeling, four lipoproteins with molecular masses of 19, 26, 27, and 38 kDa have been identified in *M. tuberculosis* (Young and Garbe, 1991a). The 19- and 38-kDa proteins are identical to previously identified strong immunogens (Ivanyi et al., 1988; Harboe and Wiker, 1992). They contain a signal peptide and a cysteine motif, characteristic of bacterial lipoproteins (Ashbridge et al., 1990; Anderson and Hansen, 1989). The 38-kDa lipoprotein has 30% sequence identity with the PstS or PhoS periplasmic binding protein with a role in phosphate transport in *E. coli*. Accordingly, increased expression of the 38-kDa protein in the cell wall of mycobacteria has been observed upon growth at limiting phosphate concentration (Espitia et al., 1992a). Antigens corresponding to the 19-kDa protein have been identified in *M. avium* and other mycobacterial species (Nair et al., 1992; Booth et al., 1993).

Lipoylation of peptides can also affect the in vitro T-cell proliferative responses (Rees et al., 1993). Modification of peptide side chains by a lipid tail was investigated in respect to the N-terminal epitopes located close to the natural consensus motif for lipidation of the 19-kDa antigen. Lipoylation of epitopic peptides had variable effects on the responses of several of the human clones tested and therefore could not constitute the mechanism for the genetically permissive recognition of several apparently distinct epitopes within that region of the molecule. In addition, several linear and conformational B-cell epitopes have been mapped on the 19-kDa molecule that involves the lipidated region, indicating its recognition by T cells as well as antibodies (Ashbridge et al., 1992). Furthermore, it is of interest that peptides corresponding to the leader sequences of the 19- and 38-kDa lipoproteins have been found to be immunogenic in humans (Faith et al., 1991; Vordermeier et al., 1992a).

Glycosylation during biosynthesis in mycobacteria was suggested for the 38-kDa protein on the basis of concanavalin A-binding studies (Espitia and Mancilla, 1989) and for the 19-kDa protein on the basis of genetic and biochemical experiments (Garbe et al., 1993). These findings are of interest, since glycosylation of particular residues involved in the interactions with MHC molecules can inhibit presentation of peptide determinants for T-cell recognition (Ishioka et al., 1992). The involvement of sugar moieties in antibody recognition was suggested by the inhibition of MAb TB72 binding following the chemical removal of sugar molecules from the 38-kDa antigen (Espitia and Mancilla, 1989). The effects of lipid and sugar moieties on the immunogenicity of protein antigens of mycobacteria deserve further study.

Secreted Antigens

Proteins secreted from viable bacteria could be available for immune recognition at an early stage of infection and may therefore play a special role in protective immune mechanisms. Although it is generally thought that only infection with live attenuated bacilli (e.g., BCG) induces effective protective immunity, it has been claimed that secreted antigens give at least a limited amount of protection in an animal model for tuberculosis (Pal and Horwitz, 1992). Although antigens containing the signal peptide are classically defined as secreted proteins, several constituents translated without a signal peptide also accumulate in early culture filtrates under some conditions. Hence, superoxide dismutase and hsp65 may be secreted by other not-yet-identified mechanisms. Moreover, a proportion of lipoproteins is found in culture filtrate.

Of the antigens isolated from mycobacterial culture filtrates, molecular and immunological analyses have been focused on two prominent components, represented by the 22-kDa MPB70 protein of *M. bovis* (Billman-Jacobe et al., 1990) and the antigen 85 complex of fibronectin-binding proteins (Abou-Zeid et al., 1988; Wiker and Harboe, 1992). Both molecules contain a signal sequence compatible with their secreted nature (Content et al., 1991). An apparently new secreted protein of 27 kDa that carries at least one epitope with specificity for the *M. tuberculosis* complex has been reported recently (Rambukkana et al., 1993).

The antigen 85 complex comprises three different but closely related proteins of approximately 30-kDa molecular mass that have been designated 85A, 85B, and 85C (Wiker and Harboe, 1992; Thole et al., 1992). The A, B, and C molecules have approximately 70 to 80% identical sequences and are encoded by three genes separately localized on the chromosome. These proteins are present in several species of mycobacteria, although a related protein has also been identified in corynebacteria (Joliff et al., 1992). All three components have been localized in the cell membrane, but differences exist in the relative amount of each molecule that is secreted. A related, fourth member of this family, designated MPT51 and showing approximately 40% sequence identity with the 85A, B, and C molecules, was recently shown to be localized very close to the gene for the A component, and it was suggested that MPT51 and the 85A gene are localized within the same operon (Rinke de Wit et al., 1993). The antigen 85 complex molecules bind fibronectin, and this characteristic could be involved in the colonization and uptake of mycobacteria by host cells. The antigen 85 complex molecules are known to be immunogenic: they elicit DTH reactions in sensitized guinea pigs (Worsaae et al., 1987) and stimulate IFN-γ production by peripheral blood mononuclear cells of tuberculosis patients (Huygen et al., 1988) and spleen cells from infected mice (Huygen et al., 1990).

GENETIC CONTROL OF ANTIBODY RESPONSES

Studies in Mice

Antibody levels following immunization with soluble extracts of tubercle bacilli in adjuvant demonstrated the codominant control by the *H-2* IA locus of the response to individual epitopes (Ivanyi et al., 1988; Huygen et al., 1990; Ljungqvist et al., 1988). In one instance, however, F_1 hybrids of high- and low-responder strains showed low antibody titers to the TB68 epitope of the 16-kDa antigen; the mechanisms of this uncommon dominant low responsiveness remain unresolved. The idiotypic markers of several MAbs have also been described elsewhere (Ivanyi, 1990).

In contrast to the MHC-controlled response to individual epitopes, non-MHC genes influence the overall heterogeneity of the antibody repertoire. Multi- or oligo-banded Western blots (immunoblots) were found in mice of BALB and B10 genetic backgrounds, respectively, following systemic tuberculous infection (Brett and Ivanyi, 1990; Huygen et al., 1990). The non-*H-2* genetic phenotypes have been best reflected by differences in antibody levels to the hsp65 and hsp71 antigens. These phenotypes segregate in backcross animals, indicating a role for possibly one yet-unidentified gene (Ivanyi, unpublished results). The mechanisms that lead to the serological differences observed between mouse strains have tentatively been attributed to differences in the extent of granuloma formation (Orrell et al., 1992), which could influence the release and recognition of native mycobacterial proteins by B cells. The overall representation of the antibody repertoire in these studies probably results from a combined effect of non-*H-2* and *H-2* genes.

Studies in Humans

Significant HLA-DR15 (DR2) association was reported for the incidence of pulmonary tuberculosis and for the antibody levels to the 38-kDa protein antigen of *M. tuberculosis* (Bothamley et al., 1989). Furthermore, DR2 has been linked most prominently with the severe multibacillary form of tuberculosis (Brahmajothi et al., 1991), which also manifests the highest antibody levels. The joint association of DR15 with both higher antibody levels and higher incidence of pulmonary disease raises the possibility of a pathogenic role for the 38-kDa antigen. This could be based on mechanisms whereby Th2-type cytokines (e.g., interleukin-4 [IL-4] and IL-10), while helping the stimulation of antibody-forming B cells, would also cause the decline in the macrophage-activating, i.e., protective, immune function of Th1 cells (Bloom et al., 1992). Furthermore, antigen presentation by B cells (instead of macrophages) was recently reported to favor the induction of Th2 responsiveness to *Leishmania* antigens as evidence for the regulatory potential of B cells to divert T-cell maturation toward the pathogenic pathway (Rossi-Bergmann et al., 1993). On the assumption of a reciprocal relationship between humoral and protective immunity, the target of antibody specificity may represent an important clue about the critical antigens that serve both as protective antigens and as targets of pathogenic immunoregulation.

The high-affinity expression of the 2B3 epitope on DQ molecules has been associated with antibody levels and implicated as a restricting element for the serological response to the 19-kDa antigen (Bothamley et al., 1993). Since anti-38-kDa antibodies are associated with severe tuberculosis and anti-19-kDa antibodies are associated with limited disease, it has been proposed that the relatively common linkage of DR15 and DQ5 haplotypes in Java, which is associated with high anti-38-kDa and low anti-19-kDa antibody levels, could represent a genetic basis for the fulminant form of disease in that population. Further study of genetic associations with the immune repertoire

and clinical forms of tuberculosis may bring to light epidemiological data relevant for control programs in certain geographical regions.

THE T-CELL REPERTOIRE

Studies in Mice

Both cytoplasmic and log-phase culture filtrate proteins were stimulatory in several functional assays, such as assays of IFN-γ secretion, cellular cytotoxicity, and DTH reactions (Orme et al., 1992). These activities seemed to be somewhat restricted in Western blot fractions, although T-cell proliferation assays showed a very broad distribution of stimulatory activity to fractions throughout the whole range of molecular weights (Brett and Ivanyi, 1990). Lambda gt11 clone lysates could initially be used only for the in vitro analysis of cloned T cells due to the *E. coli* contaminants. Subsequent purification of recombinant proteins produced in various high-expression systems resulted in antigenic materials that were suitable for immunization but were not always devoid of contaminant-derived nonspecific mitogenicity for uncloned lymph node or spleen lymphocytes. The systematic study of the T-cell repertoire at the level of individual epitopes has been helped by the introduction of synthetic peptides for the in vitro stimulation of primed mouse T cells.

The first study of primed lymph node T-cell responses involved seven peptides selected from the sequence of hsp65 on the basis of the Rothbard-Taylor epitope prediction motif (Brett et al., 1989). The results of in vitro proliferative responses revealed the existence of immunodominant as well as cryptic epitopes and demonstrated the effect of genetic restriction factors. Interestingly, two immunodominant peptides (153–171 and 180–196) have been found to be permissively stimulatory in hsp65-primed mouse strains of multiple *H-2* haplotypes, while the magnitude of proliferation following immunization with peptides was *H-2* restricted. Analysis using L-cell transfectants suggested that peptide 65–85 could be presented by both I-A^d and IE^d molecules.

A corresponding experimental approach allowed the identification of T-cell stimulatory epitopes of the 38-kDa antigen (Vordermeier et al., 1991). Of the seven peptides selected for analysis on the basis of their high score in forming amphipathic helices, only one peptide located at the C-terminal end of the molecule (350–369) was found to be immunodominant and genetically permissive in *H-2*^{b}, *H-2*^{k}, and *H-2*^{d} haplotypes. Another peptide (285–304) was strongly immunogenic but behaved merely as a cryptic epitope. In contrast, responsiveness to peptide 201–220 could be induced only with the whole antigen but not by the peptide alone, thus indicating the role of flanking regions in immunogenicity. Subsequent study has shown that responsiveness to p350–369 can be induced in mice that have been primed by tubercle but not nontuberculous mycobacteria and that this peptide can effectively elicit footpad enlargement as an expression of DTH reaction in presensitized mice (Vordermeier et al., 1992b). Specificity toward the *M. tuberculosis* complex and genetic permissiveness of T-cell recognition qualify this peptide as a candidate reagent for early detection of tuberculous infection.

The most comprehensive mapping analysis of murine T-cell stimulatory epitopes with overlapping peptides stretching across the whole sequence of the 19-kDa antigen was carried out in two separate laboratories in London and Auckland (Harris et al., 1991; Ashbridge et al., 1992). Both groups consistently localized the most prominent genetically permissive epitope to a peptide of the sequence 61–80. However, there are several significant discrepancies in the identification of T-cell proliferation stimulatory immunodominant peptides within sequences 1–20, 46–64, 76–95, and 121–159. Surprisingly, several peptides had different potencies when T-cell proliferation and DTH responses were compared (Ashbridge et al., 1992). It appears, however, from the immunization protocol that mice were sensitized with whole protein for the proliferation but with peptides for the DTH reactions; the latter could have engaged additional cryptic T-cell epitopes in the DTH readout. In reference to the genetically permissive recognition, two epitopes (46–64 and 61–80) were scanned by using closely overlapping peptides, demonstrating that the same position was recognized by T cells of different *H-2* haplotypes (Harris et al., 1993).

The proliferative T-cell repertoire of responses to epitopes of the 16-kDa antigen was compared in mice that had been immunized with individual peptides, with the whole antigen, or with live *M. tuberculosis* (Vordermeier et al., 1993). Lymph node and splenic T cells from infected mice reacted only with two epitopes (31–40 and 71–91), although immunization with antigen and peptides revealed four immunodominant and as many as six cryptic epitopes, respectively. Focusing of T-cell recognition in infected animals could take place at the level of antigen-presenting cells, perhaps owing to elevated activities of proteolytic enzymes in the activated macrophages.

Studies in Humans

T-cell responses are abundant in infected healthy subjects as well as in tuberculosis patients. Consequently, it has been of interest to identify differences in the T-cell repertoire as a possible basis for explaining defective resistance in patients. Proliferative T-cell responses to PPD are known to be diminished in tuberculosis patients with advanced disease, and this anergy has been at least partly attributed to the failure of T cells to produce IL-2 and to express the IL-2 receptor (Shiratsuchi et al., 1987). As an alternative mechanism, inhibition of DTH reactions was attributed to the neutralization of T-cell fibronectin, which is involved in the initiation of DTH reactions, by the fibronectin-binding antigen 85 protein complex of *M. tuberculosis* (Godfrey et al., 1992).

It has been of interest whether the diminished responsiveness of tuberculosis patients involves any element of antigenic specificity. The proliferative T-cell stimulatory assay of fractions that had been separated by single- or two-dimensional Western blots failed to identify any significant differences in specificity between tuberculosis patients and healthy sensitized subjects (Havlir et al., 1991; Schoel et al., 1992). Analysis of proliferation and IFN-γ production in response to purified whole antigens such as the 30- to 32-kDa fibronectin-binding protein were correlated with responsiveness to PPD in both tuberculosis patients and sensitized healthy controls (Huygen et al., 1988). These results indicate that the search for possible differences in specificity needs to be done at the level of individual T-cell stimulatory epitopes. Such an analysis has so far been performed only with synthetic peptides derived from the sequences of the 19- and 38-kDa antigens.

Responsiveness to peptides of the 19-kDa antigen when a complete set of 15 peptides was used was highest for healthy controls with two peptides at the N terminus (1–20 and 11–30) and with peptides 51–70 and 61–80 (Faith et al., 1991). Patients showed a somewhat diminished response to peptide 11–30. Further evaluation showed more then 90% responsiveness to peptide 46–64 in healthy subjects as well as in tuberculosis patients (Harris et al., 1993). Interestingly, enhanced responsiveness to peptide 61–80 was observed in patients with lymphatic tuberculosis. Three genetically permissive epitopes of the 38-kDa antigen have been identified on the basis of more than 80% frequency of responsiveness in a group of 30 genetically random healthy tu-berculin responders (Vordermeier et al., 1992a). It is of special interest that proliferative responsiveness to peptide G (350–369) was severely impaired in patients with active pulmonary and extrapulmonary (nonlymphatic) tuberculosis but not in those with lymphatic tuberculosis. T-cell anergy to this epitope was selective, as it was demonstrable in individuals with undiminished responsiveness to peptide A (1–20) and to PPD. However, responsiveness to four other peptides that stimulated only 10 to 20% of healthy sensitized individuals did not significantly vary between controls and any group of patients.

In order to find out whether antigenic specificity influences the phenotype of CD4 T cells, IFN-γ- and IL-4-secreting cells responding to the 19- or 38-kDa antigen and corresponding peptide epitopes have been examined by the "elispot" assay (Surcel et al., 1994). The results demonstrated that compared to sensitized healthy subjects, tuberculosis patients had raised IL-4 responses and decreased proliferation but no significant change in IFN-γ-producing cells. However, none of the antigens or peptides showed preferential stimulation of any of the T-cell phenotypes, and proliferation was not correlated with either IL-4 or IFN-γ production. Since antibody levels to both 19- and 38-kDa antigens are known to be elevated in tuberculosis patients, demonstration of IL-4-secreting Th2 cells of corresponding specificity corroborates their like role as helpers for antibody formation.

The systematic analysis of large panels of T-cell clones reacting with the hsp65 protein was addressed, particularly regarding the role of genetic restriction by HLA-DR molecules. The most striking finding has been that all DR3 individuals exclusively recognized one epitopic peptide, 2–12, while individuals with other haplotypes, such as DR1 and DR5, recognized several distinct epitopic regions (Van Schooten et al., 1989). Thus, five T-cell epitopes were presented only in the context of DR1, three epitopes were present only in the context of DR5, and two epitopes were present only in the context of DR2. Cytolysis of PPD-pulsed targets was attributed exclusively to HLA class II-restricted but not to class I-restricted T cells from healthy sensitized subjects and was decreased in patients with disseminated tuberculosis (Kumararatne et al., 1990). However, cytotoxicity is a common property of several cloned CD4 T cells, irrespective of their cytokine profiles and specificities (Boom et al., 1991). Cloned human CD8 cells have been characterized by the proliferation assay (Rees et al., 1988).

By using clones of a patient with reactive arthritis, it was found that the DR3/p4-13 complex is recognized by a Vβ5 overrepresented TcR repertoire (Henwood et al., 1993). The TcR chain usage, identical for blood- and synovial fluid-derived clones, was stable over a period of 3 years. However, the third complementarity-determining region of the β chain was not conserved and was associated with two different Vα chain families. In contrast, DP4-restricted clones to peptide 456–466 showed conserved usage of the Vα1 chain in association with multiple Vβ families. Another study of TcR gene usage in anti-BCG clones from synovial fluid indicated a generally heterogeneous repertoire, although with an overrepresentation of the Vβ8 gene family (Wilson et al., 1993).

STIMULATION OF γδ T CELLS BY MYCOBACTERIA

Studies in Mice

Intraperitoneal BCG infection elevated the numbers of γδ T cells in the peritoneal exudate and lymph nodes after 7 days. This elevation was followed by a gradual decline, which coincides with the rise of αβ T cells (Inoue et al., 1991). These γδ T cells were of the Vγ1,2/Vδ6 TcR family and

responded in vitro oligoclonally to PPD, polyclonally to BCG lysate, but not at all to the hsp65 protein. In contrast, only modest effects were found following footpad inoculation, and furthermore, doubts were raised about the specificity of this response, since incomplete Freund's adjuvant was also effective (Griffin et al., 1991).

Extensive analysis of γδ T-cell hybridomas showed cells reacting with hsp65 originally in the newborn murine thymus and representing a major population comprising 10 to 20% of all γδ T cells in mouse spleen and lymph nodes (O'Brien et al., 1992). These hybridoma cells of the Vγ1/Vδ6 TcR family recognize a single peptide, 180–196, in the absence of presenting cells. It is of particular interest that much stronger stimulation is obtained with the mycobacterial than with the mammalian 180–196 sequence. Despite some similarity to superantigenic stimulation, such classification has not been favored in view of the small size of the stimulatory ligand, lack of presentation by class II molecules, and need for more than one V gene for reactivity.

Studies in Humans

About 10% of all γδ T cells from healthy human peripheral blood is represented by the Vγ9/Vδ2 TcR family, which can be expanded by incubation with heat-killed cells of *M. tuberculosis* (Kabelitz et al., 1991; De Libero et al., 1991). These cells are targeted to a protease-resistant ligand of low molecular weight, and their stimulation depends on HLA class II-presenting cells, although they are not restricted by genetically polymorphic regions (Pfeffer et al., 1992). Nevertheless, hsp60 has been implicated in other studies on the basis of the stimulation-inhibitory effect of a polyclonal anti-hsp65 antiserum (Fisch et al., 1990). The ligand apparently lacks specificity for *M. tuberculosis* in view of cross-stimulation with other bacteria or with human lymphoid cell lines. Interestingly, γδ T cells from cord blood but not from the blood of adult tuberculin-positive individuals proliferate in vitro following incubation with trehalose dimycolate (cord factor) (Tsuyuguchi et al., 1991). This glycolipid constituent of *Mycobacterium* spp. and related genera has granulomapoietic and other immunomodulatory activities, and its toxicity has been implicated in the wasting associated with tuberculosis. It seems reasonable for the time being to speculate that the low-molecular-weight mycobacterial constituents stimulate enhanced expression of host hsp60 as the specific ligand recognized by $\gamma\delta$ T cells. This explanation could reconcile most of the presently available experimental data for both mice and humans.

IMMUNODIAGNOSIS OF TUBERCULOSIS

Skin Testing

The DTH reaction following intracutaneous injection of tuberculin (PPD) is a well-established and widely used test for determining infection with tubercle bacilli. It has practical value for contact tracing in previously nonsensitized individuals, but test specificity is ablated in subjects previously sensitized by BCG vaccination or by intensive exposure to environmental mycobacteria. Hence, the test is of little value in the countries of Asia and Africa where tuberculosis is endemic, where most of the adult population is normally tuberculin positive. Tuberculin skin testing in the United States is of unsatisfactory specificity for distinguishing pulmonary disease caused by tubercle bacilli from that caused by nontuberculous opportunistic mycobacterial pathogens (Huebner et al., 1992), and its conversion rate in Spain has been considered to overestimate the true risk of tuberculous infection (De March-Ayuela, 1990). However, the purified "antigen 5," which is known to contain the 38-kDa antigen as its main constitu-

ent, was no more specific than PPD in geographic areas where nonspecific tuberculin reactivity is frequently encountered (Daniel et al., 1982).

Synthetic peptides derived from the sequences of various mycobacterial antigens are effective in eliciting DTH skin reactions in sensitized guinea pigs, mice, and human volunteers (Minden et al., 1986; Vordermeier et al., 1992b; Ashbridge et al., 1992). Of the immunogenic peptides, the C-terminal 350–369 "G" epitope of the 38-kDa antigen has the attribute of genetic permissiveness as well as of specificity, demonstrated by the lack of DTH in mice that had been sensitized by nontuberculous mycobacteria. Furthermore, the anergy to this peptide, observed in patients with active tuberculosis (Vordermeier et al., 1992a), could discriminate between patients and sensitized healthy individuals. Hence, there is a need for further study of optimal formulation of peptide "tuberculins" followed by diagnostic and epidemiological evaluation.

Serology

Interest in developing a specific and sensitive serodiagnostic test encouraged the initial searches for tubercle-specific MAbs. Their application in a competition assay against sera from patients with tuberculosis firstly identified the 38-, 19-, and 16-kDa proteins as prominent immunogens (Ivanyi et al., 1985). Titration of antibody levels using the MAb competition and enzyme-linked immunosorbent assay (ELISA) techniques revealed significant differences in the specificity of the antibody repertoire between various clinical forms of tuberculosis. Thus, antibody levels to the 38-kDa antigen are elevated in multibacillary pulmonary tuberculosis patients, while antibodies to hsp71 have been found equally increased in sputum smear-negative pulmonary disease patients (Elsaghier et al., 1991). Antibodies to the 16-kDa antigen were selectively increased in chronically exposed household contacts of patients and hospital workers (Jackett et al., 1988; Bothamley et al., 1992a), while only antibodies to lipoarabinomannan and the 16-kDa antigen were elevated in the cerebrospinal fluid of patients with tuberculous meningitis (Chandramuki et al., 1989). The potential clinical value of the combined measurement of several epitope-specific antibody levels for patient management rather than for diagnosis was proposed on the basis of the following observations (Bothamley et al., 1992b). Recurrent and extensive radiographic pulmonary tuberculosis with poor prognosis was associated with high anti-38-kDa and low anti-16-kDa antibody levels. Patients with less pulmonary cavitation had high anti-19-kDa titers, while bacteriological relapse during treatment was indicated by a rise in 16-kDa–TB68 epitope antibodies. On the basis of higher antibody levels to lipoarabinomannan and other antigens in children with localized tuberculosis compared with levels in children with disseminated tuberculosis, the possible role of antibodies in preventing the disseminated forms of disease was proposed (Costello et al., 1992).

The antigen of first choice for diagnostic serology is undoubtedly the 38-kDa protein, although a specificity caveat is represented by the presence of *M. tuberculosis*-specific anti-38-kDa "original antigenic sin" antibodies in patients with lepromatous leprosy (Bothamley et al., 1991). Of the other antigens, the 19-kDa protein is compromised by its cross-reactivity with *M. avium* (Nair et al., 1992), while antibodies to the 16-kDa protein can be detected also in a significant fraction of infected healthy subjects. Antibodies to the 30- to 32-kDa fibronectin-binding protein, which is cross-reactive with other species of mycobacteria, have been demonstrated in two-thirds of tuberculosis patients but in an even larger proportion of lepromatous lep-

rosy patients (Turneer et al., 1988; Espitia et al., 1992b; Van Vooren et al., 1992).

The pronounced immunogenicity of hsp71 during paucibacillary infection (Elsaghier et al., 1991) could be attributed to enhanced secretion during intracellular replication, to surface expression enabling recognition by B cells, and/or to the adjuvant independence of this antigen (Barrios et al., 1992). Antibodies to hsp71 are directed to both linear and conformational epitopes localized at the polymorphic and largely species-specific carboxy-terminal part of the molecule (Elsaghier et al., 1992; Peake et al., 1993). The proportion between antibodies to the respective epitopes is yet to be determined, but the bulk of antibodies to most antigens in the sera of tuberculosis patients is thought to be directed to conformational epitopes (Ivanyi, 1991; Verbon et al., 1992a).

The main diagnostic benefit from serology rests in the rapid detection of approximately 50% of cases with smear-negative pulmonary and extrapulmonary tuberculosis (Wilkins and Ivanyi, 1991). This was achieved with the modified MAb TB72 (anti-38-kDa antigen) competition test, which enables testing of human sera at a much lower dilution (one-half to one-third) than a standard ELISA does (1/100), making possible the detection of low levels of specific antibodies. However, in view of about 30% seronegativity of smear-positive pulmonary tuberculosis cases, serology cannot replace sputum microscopy. A combination of tests using several antigens may be needed in view of the large individual variations demonstrable by Western blot analysis (Verbon et al., 1990). There is priority for improving the diagnosis of tuberculosis meningitis in view of the life-saving impact of early therapy (Chandramuki et al., 1989; Radhakrishnan and Mathai, 1991). However, in children with tuberculosis and in immunocompromised patients, such as AIDS patients, serology has a predictably diminished sensitivity.

The potential practical usefulness of serology needs to be considered also in relation to distinct operational factors of tuberculosis diagnosis in advanced and developing countries. These need to be evaluated prospectively in clinical suspects, since all serological studies reported so far merely represent retrospective surveys.

Bovine Tuberculosis

Tuberculosis in cattle is controlled in several countries by the statutory policy of eliminating not only diseased but all infected animals. However, tuberculin skin testing in cattle is thought to produce about 30% false-positive reactions, resulting in considerable economic losses that could be avoided if there was a test with improved specificity but undiminished sensitivity. IFN-γ responses to PPD in whole-blood cultures were reported to be of 97% specificity and 77 to 94% sensitivity (Wood et al., 1991). The basis for the better specificity of IFN-γ compared with the skin DTH test, however, is not known, and stimulation of IFN-γ with the 22-kDa MPB70 protein that is considered to be the major *M. bovis*-specific immunogen resulted in a serious loss of diagnostic sensitivity (Wood et al., 1992).

Serological tests have generally received less attention than skin testing, but a comprehensive study showed that the best specificity and the highest sensitivity (60%) were obtained with the MPB70 antigen (Fifis et al., 1992). The glycosylated 25-kDa form appeared to give stronger but also more cross-reactive ELISA binding than the 22-kDa nonglycosylated form of this antigen. Moreover, a high proportion of sera from both tuberculous and nontuberculous infected cattle reacted with a 70-kDa fraction. Nevertheless, field evaluation of the MPB70 antigen showed only 18% diagnostic sensitivity (Wood et al., 1992). Therefore, it is of interest that a pronounced rise in MPB70 antibody levels could be achieved in *M. bovis*-presensitized animals by prior skin testing with PPD (Harboe et al., 1990). MPB70 has been evaluated also for the immunodiagnosis of farmed deer (Griffin, 1991).

PROTECTIVE AND AUTOIMMUNE INTERACTIONS

Protective Immunity to Tuberculous Infection

Firm evidence that protection is mediated by T cells rather than antibodies has been provided by adoptive transfer experiments, and the role of protection has been allocated mainly to the $\alpha\beta$ TCR CD4 subset (reviewed by Orme et al. [1993]). Although the protective cells are clearly distinct from cells that mediate DTH (Lovik and Closs, 1982), the discriminating cytokines have not yet been defined. The protective role of CD8 T cells has been a subject of debate, but such a role has been supported recently by a demonstration that mice with genetically disrupted class I *H-2* expression had higher mortality and a higher bacterial load in the lungs following infection with *M. tuberculosis* (Flynn et al., 1992).

An analysis of the antigenic specificity of protective immunity has been difficult because of the lack of a suitable in vitro assay. Furthermore, consistent protection can be induced only by an attenuated infection, e.g., with BCG, while the potency of various antigenic fractions (Pal and Horwitz, 1992) of tubercle bacilli is yet uncorroborated. It has been argued that the protective epitopes could be identified with those T-cell clones that can respond to antigen-presenting cells previously infected with live bacilli (Rook et al., 1986). However, analysis of several CD4 clones by cytotoxicity failed to distinguish between the lysis of infected and PPD-pulsed target monocytes (Boom et al., 1991). Another attempt in this direction has been using a complex antigenic extract to stimulate T cells to block the intracellular replication of phago-cytosed mycobacteria (Beschin et al., 1991).

The selective nature of antibody specific-ities in guinea pigs was investigated follow-ing either live infection or immunization with dead tubercle bacilli (Romain et al., 1993b). Interestingly, an antigenic complex of 45 to 47 kDa reacting with antibodies exclusively in infected animals was identi-fied in the culture medium of logarithmi-cally growing BCG but only in trace amounts from bacilli. Its N-terminal se-quence is of high alanine-and-proline con-tent, and studies from another laboratory indicated that the molecule is probably gly-cosylated (Espitia and Mancilla, 1989). An-other protein of similar molecular weight and of unusual (40% proline, 12% threo-nine) composition was found to be eliciting DTH reactions 100 times more efficiently in guinea pigs that had been infected with *M. tuberculosis* than in those immunized with dead bacilli (Romain et al., 1993a).

Comparison of the infected or immunized mice showed that the most prominent infec-tion-dependent proliferative response of splenic T cells was directed to the 32-kDa fibronectin-binding protein (Andersen et al., 1991). In contrast, IFN-γ production by splenic T cell from mice that had been challenged following prior infection and chemotherapy was most prominently stim-ulated by a secreted protein of 3- to 9-kDa molecular mass (Anderson and Heron, 1993). Taking a different experimental ap-proach, the specificity of protective T cells that had been stimulated by BCG vaccina-tion was directly analyzed by adoptive pro-tection following an antigen-dependent T-cell culture stage in vitro (D'Souza and Ivanyi, 1993). Since killed tubercle bacilli or a crude soluble extract maintained the protective capacity of BCG-primed T cells, one may conclude that the protective epitopes are at least adequately expressed by tubercle bacilli grown in bacteriological

culture and do not require selective expres-sion during growth in the infected host.

γδ T cells have been assigned to the first line of defense, acting before the expansion of αβ T cells (Inoue et al., 1991). Thus, γδ T cells recognizing a ligand that is common for several bacterial genera expand with age in response to environmental organisms and may protect against the invading patho-gens by elimination of infected cells with overexpressed stress proteins (Tsuyuguchi et al., 1991). This mechanism has been postulated as an important host defense against murine salmonellosis on the basis of the finding that the ability of *Salmonella* spp. to induce hsp60 synthesis in infected macrophages and expansion of Vγ1/Vδ6 T cells correlated inversely with virulence (Emoto et al., 1992). The lack of γδ T-cell response to virulent salmonellae has been tentatively attributed to an inhibition of hsp60 synthesis by the cell respiratory burst or to inhibition of its processing/presentation by phagosome-lysosome fu-sion. However, it has also been proposed that efficient IL-2 secretion by stimulated γδ T cells may also activate self-reactive αβ CD4⁻ CD8⁻ T cells and thus lead to auto-immunity (Yuuki et al., 1990).

The Role of hsp65 in Autoimmunity

Analysis of the specificity of T-cell re-sponses to the mycobacterial 65-kDa heat shock protein has so far attracted more attention in relation to its potential role in autoimmunity than in respect to tuberculo-sis. The role of T cells reacting with the 180–188 peptide have been associated with both protection and pathogenicity in the rat model of adjuvant arthritis (Hogervorst et al., 1991). However, anti-p180–188 T cells do not react with the corresponding peptide of the human hsp60 homolog but rather with the link protein part of the synovial cartilage proteoglycan. The pathogenic function of T-cell recognition of this single epitope has been based on (i) association of responsiveness to p180–188 with the genetic susceptibility to arthritis in the Lewis strain of rats and (ii) inhibition of anti-p180–188 responsiveness following immunization with the whole hsp65 protein, which protects against subsequent induction of adjuvant and other forms of experimental arthritis. In contrast, the protective function of T cells of the same specificity was suggested on the grounds that immunization of Lewis rats with p180–188 itself is immunogenic but (i) does not lead to arthritis and (ii) protects against subsequent induction of adjuvant arthritis (Yang et al., 1990). Furthermore, it should be borne in mind that T cells cross-reacting between mycobacterial and other bacterial genera but unrelated to hsp65 have also been implicated in the immunopathogenesis of experimental rat arthritis (De Joy et al., 1989).

T-cell responses to mycobacterial hsp65 in human autoimmunity have been reviewed comprehensively elsewhere (Res et al., 1991b). Contrary to earlier studies, synovial fluid T cells in rheumatoid arthritis patients were shown to react to multiple mycobacterial antigens, predominantly to those other than hsp65 and to contaminants from *E. coli* (Res et al., 1991a; Life et al., 1991), thus failing to support the original contention of preferential homing on the basis of hsp65 specificity. Indeed, no hsp65-reactive T cells were detected in the synovial fluid by limiting dilution analysis (Crick and Gatenby, 1992). Nevertheless, a number of anti-hsp65 T clones derived from either blood or synovial fluid were shown to be directed to epitopes shared between bacterial and mammalian hsp65 (Lamb et al., 1989; Munk et al., 1989; Hermann et al., 1991) or to be species specific to bacteria (Gaston et al., 1990; Shanafelt et al., 1991). These clones can be found in healthy individuals but have also been associated with juvenile chronic arthritis (De Graeff-Meeder et al., 1991).

CONCLUSIONS AND FUTURE PROSPECTS

Advancements in the molecular definition of immunogenic subunits of tubercle bacilli have been instrumental in better understanding of several areas of the host-parasite relationship that are of interest and potentially for shifting the balance in favor of the host.

(i) Biochemical functions in bacteria and immunogenicity. The roles of three distinct categories of constituents represented by stress proteins, lipoproteins, and secreted proteins have been highlighted. Stress proteins attracted interest particularly in relation to autoimmunity. However, evidence that tuberculous infection could upregulate their synthesis has yet to be provided. Lipoproteins are potent immunogens, but it is not clear whether the lipid chains are instrumental merely in the distribution of the protein within the bacterial compartments or whether they are directly involved in interactions with the cells of the immune system. It will be desirable to expand the knowledge of protein secretion in organisms that are either replicating or persisting within host macrophages. Moreover, the function of other posttranslational modifications, such as glycosylation, needs to be examined.

(ii) Species specificity for the *M. tuberculosis* complex. This specificity exists only at the level of individual epitopes, but no protein antigens with exclusive representation in tubercle bacilli have been identified. The specificity should be qualified as relative, because testing has invariably been carried out with only a limited set of other mycobacterial species, and cross-reactivity with a few nontuberculous mycobacteria (as in the case of some MAbs) cannot be ruled out. T-cell epitope specificity is determined by both the positions and the nature of substituted residues and cannot be estimated from sequence homology alone.

(iii) Which are the "major" antigens? The initial selection of the "prominent" immunogens was based on serological studies with MAbs. This selection was due to technical feasibility, although it may seem paradoxical in the light of knowledge of the mandatory role of T cells. Attempts for a broadening of the collection of immune "targets" and searches for constituents that would stimulate only T cells did not yield any substantial data. Instead, all serologically active antigens also turned out to be powerful T-cell stimulants, thus vindicating the guiding role of antibodies. Whether B cells play even a regulatory function in respect of the T-cell phenotype remains to be explored.

(iv) Specificity of the T-cell repertoire. Work in the field of specificity progressed with the realization that T-cell clones are poorly representative and that bulk lymphocyte cultures give satisfactory responses to synthetic peptides. Unexpectedly, the majority of immunodominant epitopes (i.e., active after priming with whole antigen) have been found to be permissively stimulatory between individuals with diverse MHC gene composition. It is not known whether this outcome is of any evolutionary significance. Further study is needed on the structural determinants of the genetically permissive recognition in terms of key residues within the epitope as well as within the MHC class II molecules.

(v) Protective subunits. The general trend in favor of subunit vaccine development is problematic for tuberculous infections. The question is still whether many or few antigens are protective rather than which antigen is protective. Proteins secreted by live bacilli during infection had justifiably come to be the focus of attention. Experimental analysis is difficult, however, because protection has consistently been imparted only by a live attenuated organism such as BCG. Individual antigenic constituents delivered within a live recombinant vector have so far not been protective.

However, the requirement of live vaccination may not be due to a critical antigenic specificity but rather to an association with suitable immunomodulatory stimuli from the mycobacterial cell wall. The finding of overlapping repertoire when patients and healthy subjects are compared indicates that the key discriminatory function between the pathogenic and protective host response may rest in the phenotype rather than the epitope specificity of T cells. Experimental evidence suggests that neither DTH nor any of the existing in vitro lymphocyte responses represent a satisfactory protection test. This aspect may be the main reason for our inconclusive knowledge about the efficacy of BCG vaccination in humans.

(vi) Antibody formation. Many MAbs were derived from fusions with B cells from mice that had been invariably immunized with various antigenic preparations or killed organisms rather than with B cells from infected mice. Nevertheless, some of these specificities overlap those of antibodies of tuberculosis patients, indicating the immunogenicity of corresponding antigens during infection. It is puzzling why as many as 30% of sputum-positive cases of pulmonary tuberculosis have low antibody levels. It would be of interest to know whether genetic factors are involved and whether "seronegative tuberculosis" has any characteristic clinical features. Perhaps the phenotype of T cells in these patients will reveal distinct immunoregulatory mechanisms. Diagnostic application of serology, represented by present knowledge of the immunogenic and specific constituents, seems most beneficial for smear-negative tuberculosis and tuberculosis meningitis. However, its practical value needs to be evaluated in the context of relevant operational aspects of clinical diagnosis.

REFERENCES

Abou-Zeid, C., I. Smith, J. M. Grange, T. L. Ratliff, J. Steele, and G. A. W. Rook. 1988. The secreted antigens of *M. tuberculosis* and their relationship to those recognised by the available antibodies. *J. Gen. Microbiol.* **134**:531–538.

Aguas, A. P., N. Esaguy, C. E. Sunkel, and M. T. Silva. 1990. Cross-reactivity and sequence homology between the 65-kilodalton mycobacterial heat shock protein and human lactoferrin, transferrin, and DR$_\beta$ subsets of major histocompatibility complex class II molecules. *Infect. Immun.* **58**:1461–1470.

Andersen, Å. B., and E. B. Hansen. 1989. Structure and mapping of antigenic domains of protein antigen b, a 38,000-molecular-weight protein of *Mycobacterium tuberculosis. Infect. Immun.* **57**:2481–2488.

Andersen, P., and I. Heron. 1993. Specificity of protective memory immune response against *Mycobacterium tuberculosis. Infect. Immun.* **61**:844–851.

Andersen, P., L. Ljungqvist, K. Haslov, M. W. Bentzon, and I. Heron. 1991. Proliferative response to seven affinity purified mycobacterial antigens in eight strains of inbred mice. *Int. J. Lepr.* **59**:58–67.

Ashbridge, K. R., B. T. Backstrom, H.-X. Liu, T. Vikerfors, D. R. Englebretsen, D. R. K. Harding, and J. D. Watson. 1992. Mapping of T helper cell epitopes by using peptides spanning the 19-kDa protein of *Mycobacterium tuberculosis. J. Immunol.* **148**:2248–2255.

Ashbridge, K. R., R. L. Prestidge, R. J. Booth, and J. D. Watson. 1990. The mapping of an antibody-binding region on the *Mycobacterium tuberculosis* 19 kilodalton antigen. *J. Immunol.* **144**:3137–3142.

Baird, P. N., L. M. C. Hall, and A. R. M. Coates. 1989. Cloning and sequence analysis of the 10 kDa antigen gene of *Mycobacterium tuberculosis. J. Gen. Microbiol.* **135**:931–940.

Barrios, C., A. R. Lussow, J. Van Embden, R. Van der Zee, R. Rappuoli, P. Costantino, J. A. Louis, P.-H. Lambert, and G. Del Giudice. 1992. Mycobacterial heat-shock proteins as carrier molecules. II. The use of the 70-kDa mycobacterial heat-shock protein as carrier for conjugated vaccines can circumvent the need for adjuvants and Bacillus Calmette Guerin priming. *Eur. J. Immunol.* **22**:1365–1372.

Beschin, A., L. Brijs, P. De Baetselier, and C. Cocito. 1991. Mycobacterial proliferation in macrophages is prevented by incubation with lymphocytes activated *in vitro* with a mycobacterial antigen complex. *Eur. J. Immunol.* **21**:793–797.

Billman-Jacobe, H., A. J. Radford, J. S. Rothel, and P. R. Wood. 1990. Mapping of the T and B cell epitopes of the *Mycobacterium bovis* protein, MPB70. *Immunol. Cell Biol.* **68**:359–365.

Bloom, B. R., P. Salgame, and B. Diamond. 1992. Revisiting and revising suppressor T cells. *Immunol. Today* **31**:131–136.

Boom, W. H., R. S. Wallis, and K. A. Chervenak. 1991. Human *Mycobacterium tuberculosis*-reactive CD4$^+$ T-cell clones: heterogeneity in antigen recognition,

cytokine production, and cytotoxicity for mononuclear phagocytes. *Infect. Immun.* **59**:2737–2743.

Booth, R. J., D. L. Williams, K. D. Moudgil, L. C. Noonan, P. M. Grandison, J. J. McKee, R. L. Prestidge, and J. D. Watson. 1993. Homologs of *Mycobacterium leprae* 18-kilodalton and *Mycobacterium tuberculosis* 19-kilodalton antigens in other mycobacteria. *Infect. Immun.* **61**:1509–1515.

Bothamley, G., J. Swanson Beck, W. Britton, and J. Ivanyi. 1991. Antibodies to M. tuberculosis specific epitopes in lepromatous leprosy. *Clin. Exp. Immunol.* **86**:426–432.

Bothamley, G., J. Swanson Beck, R. C. Potts, J. M. Grange, T. Kardjito, and J. Ivanyi. 1992a. Specificity of antibody and tuberculin response after occupational exposure to tuberculosis. *J. Infect. Dis.* **166**:182–186.

Bothamley, G. H., G. M. T. Schreuder, R. R. P. de Vries, and J. Ivanyi. 1993. Association of antibody responses to the 19-kDa antigen of *Mycobacterium tuberculosis* and the HLA-DQ locus. *J. Infect. Dis.* **167**:992–993.

Bothamley, G. H., J. S. Beck, G. M. T. Schreuder, J. D'Amaro, R. R. P. de Vries, T. Kardjito, and J. Ivanyi. 1989. Association of tuberculosis and M. tuberculosis-specific antibody levels with HLA. *J. Infect. Dis.* **159**:549–555.

Bothamley, G. H., R. Rudd, F. Festenstein, and J. Ivanyi. 1992b. Clinical value of the measurement of M. tuberculosis-specific antibody in pulmonary tuberculosis. *Thorax* **47**:270–275.

Brahmajothi, S., R. M. Pitchappan, V. N. Kakkanaiah, M. Sashidhar, K. Rajaram, S. Ramu, K. Palanimurugan, C. N. Paramasivan, and R. Prabhakar. 1991. Association of pulmonary tuberculosis and HLA in South India. *Tubercle* **72**:123–132.

Brett, S. J., and J. Ivanyi. 1990. Genetic influences on the immune repertoire following tuberculous infection in mice. *Immunology* **71**:113–119.

Brett, S. J., J. R. Lamb, J. H. Cox, J. B. Rothbard, A. Mehlert, and J. Ivanyi. 1989. Differential pattern of T cell recognition of the 65-kDa mycobacterial antigen following immunization with the whole protein or peptides. *Eur. J. Immunol.* **19**:1303–1310.

Chandramuki, A., G. H. Bothamley, P. J. Brennan, and J. Ivanyi. 1989. Levels of antibody to defined antigens of *Mycobacterium tuberculosis* in tuberculous meningitis. *J. Clin. Microbiol.* **27**:821–825.

Coates, A. R. M., J. Hewitt, B. W. Allen, J. Ivanyi, and D. A. Mitchison. 1981. Antigenic diversity of *Mycobacterium tuberculosis* and *Mycobacterium bovis* detected by means of monoclonal antibodies. *Lancet* **ii**:167–169.

Content, J., A. De La Cuvellerie, L. De Wit, V. Vincent-Levy-Frebault, J. Ooms, and J. De Bruyn. 1991. The genes coding for the antigen 85 complexes of *Mycobacterium tuberculosis* and *Mycobacterium bovis* BCG are members of a gene family: cloning, sequence determination, and genomic organization of the gene coding for antigen 85-C of *M. tuberculosis*. *Infect. Immun.* **59**:3205–3212.

Coon, J., and R. Hunter. 1975. Properties of conjugated protein immunogens which selectively stimulate delayed-type hypersensitivity. *J. Immunol.* **114**:1518–1522.

Costello, A. M. L., A. Kumar, V. Narayan, M. S. Akbar, S. Ahmed, C. Abou-Zeid, G. A. W. Rook, J. Stanford, and C. Moreno. 1992. Does antibody to mycobacterial antigens, including lipoarabinomannan, limit dissemination in childhood tuberculosis? *Proc. R. Soc. Trop. Med. Hyg.* **86**:686–692.

Crick, F. D., and P. A. Gatenby. 1992. Limiting-dilution analysis of T cell reactivity to mycobacterial antigens in peripheral blood and synovium from rheumatoid arthritis patients. *Clin. Exp. Immunol.* **88**:424–429.

Daniel, T. M., E. A. Balestrino, O. C. Balestrino, P. T. Davidson, S. M. Debanne, S. Kataria, Y. P. Kataria, and J. B. Scocozza. 1982. The tuberculin specificity in humans of *Mycobacterium tuberculosis* antigen 5. *Am. Rev. Respir. Dis.* **126**:600–606.

Daniel, T. M., and B. W. Janicki. 1978. Mycobacterial antigens: a review of their isolation, chemistry, and immunological properties. *Microbiol. Rev.* **42**:84–113.

De Graeff-Meeder, D. E., V. D. R. Zee, G. T. Rijkers, H. J. Schuurman, J. W. J. Bijlsma, B. J. M. Wegers, and W. Van Eden. 1991. Recognition of human 60 kDa heat shock protein by mononuclear cells from patients with juvenile chronic arthritis. *Lancet* **337**:1369–1373.

De Joy, S. Q., K. M. Ferguson, T. M. Sapp, J. B. Zabriskie, A. L. Oronsky, and S. S. Kerwar. 1989. Passive transfer of disease with a T cell line and crossreactivity of streptococcal cell wall antigens with *Mycobacterium tuberculosis*. *J. Exp. Med.* **170**:369–382.

De Libero, G., G. Casorati, C. Giachino, C. Carbonara, N. Migone, P. Matzinger, and A. Lanzavecchia. 1991. Selection by two powerful antigens may account for the presence of the major population of human peripheral γ/δ T cells. *J. Exp. Med.* **173**:1311–1322.

De March-Ayuela, P. 1990. Choosing an appropriate criterion for true or false conversion in serial tuberculin testing. *Am. Rev. Respir. Dis.* **141**:815–820.

Deres, K., H. Schild, K.-H. Wiesmuller, G. Jung, and H. G. Rammensee. 1989. *In vivo* priming of virus-specific cytotoxic T lymphocytes with synthetic lipopeptide vaccine. *Nature* (London) **342**:561–564.

D'Souza, S., and J. Ivanyi. 1993. Antigen-dependent *in vitro* culture of protective T cells from BCG-primed mice. *Clin. Exp. Immunol.* **91**:68–72.

Elsaghier, A., R. Lathigra, and J. Ivanyi. 1992.

Epitope-scan of *Mycobacterium tuberculosis*-specific carboxy-terminal residues of the hsp71 stress protein. *Mol. Immunol.* **29**:1153–1156.

Elsaghier, A. A. F., E. G. L. Wilkins, P. K. Mehrotra, S. Jindal, and J. Ivanyi. 1991. Elevated antibody levels to stress protein HSP70 in smear-negative tuberculosis. *Immunol. Infect. Dis.* **1**:323–328.

Emoto, M., H. Danbara, and Y. Yoshikai. 1992. Induction of γ/δ T cells in murine salmonellosis by an avirulent but not by a virulent strain of *Salmonella cholerasuis*. *J. Exp. Med.* **176**:363–372.

Engers, H. D., V. Houba, J. Bennedsen, T. M. Buchanan, S. D. Chapars, G. Kadival, O. Closs, J. R. David, J. D. A. van Embden, T. Godal, S. A. Mustafa, J. Ivanyi, D. B. Young, S. H. E. Kaufmann, A. G. Komenko, A. H. J. Kolk, M. Kubin, J. A. Louis, P. Minden, T. M. Shinnick, L. Trnka, and R. A. Young. 1986. Results of a World Health Organisation-sponsored workshop to characterize antigens recognized by mycobacterium-specific monoclonal antibodies. *Infect. Immun.* **51**:718–720.

Espitia, C., M. Elinos, R. Hernandez-Pando, and R. Mancilla. 1992a. Phosphate starvation enhances expression of the immunodominant 38-kilodalton protein antigen of *Mycobacterium tuberculosis*: demonstration by immunogold electron microscopy. *Infect. Immun.* **60**:2998–3001.

Espitia, C., and R. Mancilla. 1989. Identification, isolation and partial characterization of *Mycobacterium tuberculosis* glycoprotein antigens. *Clin. Exp. Immunol.* **77**:378–383.

Espitia, C., E. Sciutto, O. Bottasso, R. Gonzalez-Amaro, R. Hernandez-Pando, and R. Mancilla. 1992b. High antibody levels to the mycobacterial fibronectin-binding antigen of 30–31 kDa in tuberculosis and lepromatous leprosy. *Clin. Exp. Immunol.* **87**:362–367.

Faith, A., C. Moreno, R. Lathigra, E. Roman, D. Mitchell, J. Ivanyi, and A. D. M. Rees. 1991. Analysis of human T cell epitopes in the 19,000 MW antigen of *Mycobacterium tuberculosis*: influence of HLA-DR. *Immunology* **74**:1–7.

Fifis, T., I. C. Costopoulos, L. A. Corner, and P. R. Wood. 1992. Serological reactivity to *Mycobacterium bovis* protein antigens in cattle. *Vet. Microbiol.* **30**:343–354.

Fisch, P., M. Malkovsky, S. Kovats, E. Sturm, E. Braakman, B. S. Klein, S. D. Voss, L. W. Morrissey, R. DeMars, W. J. Welch, R. L. H. Bolhuis, and P. M. Sondel. 1990. Recognition by human Vγ9/Vδ2 T cells of a GroEL homolog on Daudi Burkitt's lymphoma cells. *Science* **250**:1269–1273.

Flynn, J. L., M. M. Goldstein, K. J. Triebold, B. Koller, and B. R. Bloom. 1992. Major histocompatibility complex class I-restricted T cells are required for resistance to *Mycobacterium tuberculosis* infection. *Proc. Natl. Acad. Sci. USA* **89**:12013–12017.

454   Ivanyi and Thole

Garbe, T., D. Harris, M. Vordermeier, R. Lathigra, J. Ivanyi, and D. Young. 1993. Expression of the *Mycobacterium tuberculosis* 19-kilodalton antigen in *Mycobacterium smegmatis*: immunological analysis and evidence of glycosylation. *Infect. Immun.* **61**:260–267.

Garsia, R. J., L. Hellqvist, R. J. Booth, A. J. Radford, W. J. Britton, L. Astbury, R. J. Trent, and A. Basten. 1989. Homology of the 70-kilodalton antigens from *Mycobacterium leprae* and *Mycobacterium tuberculosis* 71-kilodalton antigen and with the conserved heat shock protein 70 of eucaryotes. *Infect. Immun.* **57**:204–212.

Gaston, J. S. H., P. J. Life, P. J. Jenner, M. J. Colston, and P. A. Bacon. 1990. Recognition of a mycobacterial-specific epitope in the 65 kilodalton heat shock protein by synovial fluid derived T cell clones. *J. Exp. Med.* **171**:831–834.

Godfrey, H. P., Z. Feng, S. Mandy, K. Mandy, K. Huygen, J. de Bruyn, C. Abou-Zeid, H. G. Wiker, S. Nagal, and H. Tasaka. 1992. Modulation of expression of delayed hypersensitivity by mycobacterial antigen 85 fibronectin-binding proteins. *Infect. Immun.* **60**:2522–2528.

Griffin, J. F. T. 1991. Tuberculosis in domesticated red deer: comparison of purified protein derivative and the specific protein MPB70 for *in vitro* diagnosis. *Res. Vet. Sci.* **50**:279–285.

Griffin, J. P., K. V. Harshan, W. K. Born, and I. M. Orme. 1991. Kinetics of accumulation of γδ receptor-bearing T lymphocytes in mice infected with live mycobacteria. *Infect. Immun.* **59**:4263–4265.

Harboe, M., and H. G. Wiker. 1992. The 38-kDa protein of *Mycobacterium tuberculosis*: a review. *J. Infect. Dis.* **166**:874–884.

Harboe, M., H. G. Wiker, J. R. Duncan, M. M. Garcia, T. W. Dukes, B. W. Brooks, C. Turcotte, and S. Nagai. 1990. Protein G-based enzyme-linked immunosorbent assay for anti-MPB70 antibodies in bovine tuberculosis. *J. Clin. Microbiol.* **28**:913–921.

Harris, D. P., H. M. Vordermeier, G. Friscia, E. Roman, H.-M. Surcel, G. Pasvol, C. Moreno, and J. Ivanyi. 1993. Genetically permissive recognition of adjacent epitopes from the 19-kDa antigen of *Mycobacterium tuberculosis* by human and murine T cells. *J. Immunol.* **150**:5041–5050.

Harris, D. P., H. M. Vordermeier, E. Roman, R. Lathigra, S. J. Brett, C. Moreno, and J. Ivanyi. 1991. Murine T cell-stimulatory peptides from the 19-kDa antigen of *Mycobacterium tuberculosis*: epitope-restricted homology with the 28-kDa protein of *Mycobacterium leprae*. *J. Immunol.* **147**:2706–2712.

Havlir, D. V., R. S. Wallis, W. H. Boom, T. M. Daniel, K. Chervenak, and J. J. Ellner. 1991. Human immune response to *Mycobacterium tuberculosis* antigens. *Infect. Immun.* **59**:665–670.

Henwood, J., J. Loveridge, J. I. Bell, and J. S. H. Gaston. 1993. Restricted T cell receptor expression by human T cell clones specific for mycobacterial 65-kDa heat-shock protein: selective *in vivo* expansion of T cells bearing defined receptors. *Eur. J. Immunol.* **23**:1256–1265.

Hermann, E., A. W. Lohse, W. Van der Zee, W. Van Eden, W.-J. Mayet, P. Probst, T. Poralla, K.-H. M. zum Buschenfelde, and B. Fleischer. 1991. Synovial fluid-derived Yersinia-reactive T cells responding to human 65-kDa heat-shock protein and heat-stressed antigen-presenting cells. *J. Immunol.* **21**:2139–2143.

Hogervorst, E. J. M., C. J. P. Boog, J. P. A. Wagenaar, M. H. M. Wauben, R. Van der Zee, and W. Van Eden. 1991. T cell reactivity to an epitope of the mycobacterial 65-kDa heat-shock protein (hsp 65) corresponds with arthritis susceptibility in rats and is regulated by hsp 65-specific cellular responses. *J. Immunol.* **21**:1289–1296.

Huebner, R. E., M. F. Schein, G. M. Cauthen, L. J. Geiter, M. J. Selin, R. C. Good, and R. J. O'Brien. 1992. Evaluation of the clinical usefulness of mycobacterial skin test antigens in adults with pulmonary mycobacterioses. *Am. Rev. Respir. Dis.* **145**:1160–1166.

Huygen, K., L. Ljungqvist, R. Berg, and J. V. Vooren. 1990. Repertoires of antibodies to culture filtrate antigens in different mouse strains infected with *Mycobacterium bovis* BCG. *Infect. Immun.* **58**:2192–2197.

Huygen, K., J. P. van Vooren, M. Turneer, R. Bosmans, P. Dierckx, and J. De Bruyn. 1988. Specific lymphoproliferation, gamma-interferon production and serum immunoglobulin G directed against a purified 32-kDa mycobacterial antigen (P32) in patients with active tuberculosis. *Scand. J. Immunol.* **27**:187–194.

Inoue, T., Y. Yoshikai, G. Matsuzaki, and K. Nomoto. 1991. Early appearing γ/δ-bearing T cells during infection with Calmette Guerin bacillus. *J. Immunol.* **146**:2754–2762.

Ishioka, G. Y., A. G. Lamont, D. Thomson, A. Bulbow, F. C. A. Gaeta, A. Sette, and H. M. Grey. 1992. MHC interaction and T cell recognition of carbohydrate and glycopeptides. *J. Immunol.* **148**:2446–2451.

Ivanyi, J. 1990. Idiotypic markers of the immune response to mycobacterial antigens, p. 121–132. *In* J. Cerny and J. Hiermaux (ed.), *Idiotypic Network and Diseases*. American Society for Microbiology, Washington, D.C.

Ivanyi, J. 1991. Serological tests for the diagnosis of tuberculosis and leprosy, p. 267–277. *In* A. Vaheri, R. C. Tilton, and A. Balows (ed.), *Rapid Methods and Automation in Microbiology and Immunology*, Springer-Verlag, Heidelberg.

Ivanyi, J. Unpublished results.

Ivanyi, J., J. A. Morris, and M. Keen. 1985. Studies

with monoclonal antibodies to mycobacteria, p. 59–90. *In* A. J. L. Macario and E. C. Macario (ed.), *Monoclonal Antibodies against Bacteria.* Academic Press, Orlando, Fla.

Ivanyi, J., K. Sharp, P. Jackett, and G. Bothamley. 1988. Immunological study of the defined constituents of mycobacteria. *Springer Semin. Immunopathol.* **10:**279–300.

Jackett, P. S., G. H. Bothamley, H. V. Batra, A. Mistry, D. B. Young, and J. Ivanyi. 1988. Specificity of antibodies to immunodominant mycobacterial antigens in pulmonary tuberculosis. *J. Clin. Microbiol.* **26:**2313–2318.

Joliff, G., L. Mathieu, V. Hahn, N. Bayan, F. Duchiron, M. Renaud, E. Schechter, and G. Leblon. 1992. Cloning and nucleotide sequence of the csp1 gene encoding PS1, one of the two major secreted proteins of *Corynebacterium glutamicum*: the deduced N-terminal region of PS1 is similar to the *Mycobacterium* antigen 85 complex. *Mol. Microbiol.* **6:**2349–2362.

Kabelitz, D., A. Bender, T. Prospero, S. Wesselborg, O. Janssen, and K. Pechhold. 1991. The primary response of human γ/δ^+ T cells to *Mycobacterium tuberculosis* is restricted to Vg9-bearing cells. *J. Exp. Med.* **173:**1331–1338.

Kiessling, R., A. Grönberg, J. Ivanyi, K. Söderström, M. Ferm, S. Kleinau, F. Nilsson, and L. Klareskog. 1991. Role of hsp60 during autoimmune and bacterial inflammation. *Immunol. Rev.* **121:**91–111.

Kong, T. H., A. R. M. Coates, P. D. Butcher, C. J. Hickman, and T. M. Shinnick. 1993. *Mycobacterium tuberculosis* expresses two chaperonin-60 homologs. *Proc. Natl. Acad. Sci. USA* **90:**2608–2612.

Kumararatne, D. S., A. S. Pithie, P. Drysdale, J. S. H. Gaston, R. Kiessling, P. B. Iles, C. J. Ellis, J. Innes, and R. Wise. 1990. Specific lysis of mycobacterial antigen-bearing macrophages by class II MHC-restricted polyclonal T cell lines in healthy donors or patients with tuberculosis. *Clin. Exp. Immunol.* **80:**314–323.

Lamb, J. R., V. Bal, P. Mendez-Sampario, A. Mehlert, A. So, J. B. Rothbard, S. Jindal, R. A. Young, and D. B. Young. 1989. Stress proteins may provide a link between the immune response to infection and autoimmunity. *Int. Immunol.* **1:**191–196.

Life, P. F., E. O. E. Bassey, and J. S. H. Gaston. 1991. T cell recognition of bacterial heat shock proteins in inflammatory arthritis. *Immunol. Rev.* **121:**113–135.

Ljungqvist, L., A. Worsaae, and I. Heron. 1988. Antibody responses against *Mycobacterium tuberculosis* in 11 strains of inbred mice: novel monoclonal antibody specificities generated by fusions, using spleens from BALB.B10 and CBA/J mice. *Infect. Immun.* **56:**1994–1998.

Lovik, M., and O. Closs. 1982. Repeated delayed-type hypersensitivity reactions against *Mycobacterium lepramurium* antigens at the infection site do not affect bacillary multiplication in C3H mice. *Infect. Immun.* **36:**768–774.

McKenzie, K. R., E. Adams, W. J. Britton, R. J. Garsia, and A. Basten. 1991. Sequence and immunogenicity of the 70-kDa heat shock protein of *Mycobacterium leprae*. *J. Immunol.* **147:**312–319.

Minden, P., R. A. Houghten, J. R. Spear, and T. M. Shinnick. 1986. A chemically synthesized peptide which elicits humoral and cellular immune response to mycobacterial antigens. *Infect. Immun.* **53:**560–564.

Munk, M. E., B. Schoel, S. Modrow, R. W. Karr, R. A. Young, and S. H. E. Kaufmann. 1989. T lymphocytes from healthy individuals with specificity to self epitopes shared by the mycobacterial and human 65KDa heat-shock protein. *J. Immunol.* **143:**2844–2849.

Nair, J., D. A. Rouse, and S. L. Morris. 1992. Nucleotide sequence analysis and serologic characterization of the *Mycobacterium intracellulare* homologue of the *Mycobacterium tuberculosis* 19 kDa antigen. *Mol. Microbiol.* **6:**1431–1439.

O'Brien, R. L., Y.-X. Fu, R. Cranfill, A. Dallas, C. Ellis, C. Reardon, J. Lang, S. R. Carding, R. Kubo, and W. Born. 1992. Heat shock protein Hsp60-reactive γδ cells: a large, diversified T-lymphocyte subset with highly focused specificity. *Proc. Natl. Acad. Sci. USA* **89:**4348–4352.

Oftung, F., A. S. Mustafa, T. M. Shinnick, R. A. Houghten, G. Kvalheim, M. Degre, K. E. A. Lundin, and T. Godal. 1988. Epitopes of the *Mycobacterium tuberculosis* 65-kilodalton protein antigen as recognized by human T cells. *J. Immunol.* **141:**2749–2754.

Orme, I. M., P. Andersen, and W. H. Boom. 1993. T cell responses to *Mycobacterium tuberculosis*. *J. Infect. Dis.* **167:**1481–1497.

Orme, I. M., E. S. Miller, A. D. Roberts, S. K. Furney, J. P. Griffin, K. M. Dobos, D. Chi, B. Rivoire, and P. J. Brennan. 1992. T lymphocytes mediating protection and cellular cytolysis during the course of *Mycobacterium tuberculosis* infection. *J. Immunol.* **148:**189–196.

Orrell, J. M., S. J. Brett, J. Ivanyi, G. Coghill, A. Grant, and J. S. Beck. 1992. Measurement of the immunoperoxidase staining of macrophages within liver granulomata of mice infected with *Mycobacterium tuberculosis*. *Anal. Quant. Cytol. Histol.* **14:**451–458.

Pal, P. G., and H. A. Horwitz. 1992. Immunization with extracellular proteins of *Mycobacterium tuberculosis* induces cell-mediated immune responses and substantial protective immunity in a guinea pig model of pulmonary tuberculosis. *Infect. Immun.* **60:**4781–4792.

Patarroyo, M. E., C. A. Parra, C. Pinilla, P. D. Portillo, M. L. Torres, P. Clavijo, L. M. Salazar, and

C. Jimenez. 1986. Immunogenic synthetic peptides against mycobacteria of potential immunodiagnostic and immunoprophylactic value. *Lepr. Rev.* **57**:163–168.

Peake, P. W., W. J. Britton, M. P. Davenport, P. W. Roche, and K. R. McKenzie. 1993. Analysis of B-cell epitopes in the variable C-terminal region of the *Mycobacterium leprae* 70-kilodalton heat shock protein. *Infect. Immun.* **61**:135–141.

Pfeffer, K., B. Schoel, N. Plesnila, G. B. Lipford, S. Kromer, and H. Wagner. 1992. A lectin binding, protease resistant mycobacterial ligand specifically activates Vγ9 + human γδ T cells. *J. Immunol.* **148**:575–583.

Radhakrishnan, V. V., and A. Mathai. 1991. Detection of *Mycobacterium tuberculosis* antigen 5 in cerebrospinal fluid by inhibition ELISA and its diagnostic potential in tuberculous meningitis. *J. Infect. Dis.* **163**:650–652.

Rambukkana, A., P. K. Das, J. D. Burggraaf, W. R. Faber, P. Teeling, S. Krieg, J. E. R. Thole, and M. Harboe. 1992. Identification and characterization of epitopes shared between the mycobacterial 65-kilodalton heat shock protein and the actively secreted antigen 85 complex: their in situ expression on the cell wall surface of *Mycobacterium leprae*. *Infect. Immun.* **60**:4517–4527.

Rambukkana, A., P. K. Das, A. H. J. Kolk, J. D. Burggraaf, S. Kuijper, and M. Harboe. 1993. Identification of a novel 27-kDa protein from *Mycobacterium tuberculosis* culture fluid by a monoclonal antibody specific for the *Mycobacterium tuberculosis* complex. *Scand. J. Immunol.* **37**:471–478.

Rees, A., A. Scoging, A. Mehlert, D. B. Young, and J. Ivanyi. 1988. Specificity of proliferative response of human CD8 clones to mycobacterial antigens. *Eur. J. Immunol.* **18**:1881–1887.

Rees, A. D. M., A. Faith, E. Roman, M. Fernandez, J. Ivanyi, K.-H. Wiesmuller, and C. Moreno. 1993. The effect of lipoylation on human epitope-specific CD4 T-cell recognition of the 19kDa mycobacterial antigen. *Immunology* **80**:407–414.

Res, P. C. M., D. L. M. Orsini, J. M. Van Laar, A. A. M. Janson, C. Abou-Zeid, and R. R. P. De Vries. 1991a. Diversity in antigen recognition by *Mycobacterium tuberculosis*-reactive T cell clones from the synovial fluid of rheumatoid arthritis patients. *Eur. J. Immunol.* **21**:1297–1302.

Res, P. C. M., J. Thole, and R. de Vries. 1991b. Heat-shock proteins and autoimmunity in humans. *Curr. Opin. Immunol.* **13**:81–98.

Rinke de Wit, T. F., S. Bekelie, A. Osland, T. L. Miko, P. W. M. Hermans, D. van Sooligen, J.-W. Drijfhout, R. Schoningh, A. A. M. Janson, and J. E. R. Thole. 1992. Mycobacteria contain two GroEL genes: the second *Mycobacterium leprae* GroEL gene is arranged in an operon with GroES. *Mol.*

Microbiol. **6**:1995–2007.

Rinke de Wit, T. F., S. Bekelie, A. Osland, B. Wieles, A. A. M. Janson, and J. E. R. Thole. 1993. The *Mycobacterium leprae* antigen 85 complex gene family: identification of the genes for the 85a, 85c, and related MPT51 proteins. *Infect. Immun.* **61**:3642–3647.

Romain, F., J. Augier, P. Pescher, and G. Marchal. 1993a. Isolation of a proline-rich mycobacterial protein eliciting delayed-type hypersensitivity reactions only in guinea pigs immunized with living mycobacteria. *Proc. Natl. Acad. Sci. USA* **90**:5322–5326.

Romain, F., A. Laqueyrerie, P. Militzer, P. Pescher, P. Chavarot, M. Lagranderie, G. Auregan, M. Gheorghiu, and G. Marchal. 1993b. Identification of a *Mycobacterium bovis* BCG 45/47-kilodalton antigen complex, an immunodominant target for antibody response after immunization with living bacteria. *Infect. Immun.* **61**:742–750.

Rook, G. A. W., J. Steele, S. Barnass, J. Mace, and J. L. Stanford. 1986. Responsiveness to live *M. tuberculosis*, and common antigens, of sonicate-stimulated T cell lines from normal donors. *Clin. Exp. Immunol.* **63**:105–110.

Rossi-Bergmann, B., I. Muller, and E. B. Godinho. 1993. TH1 and TH2 T-cell subsets are differentially activated by macrophages and B cells in murine leishmaniasis. *Infect. Immun.* **61**:2266–2269.

Schoel, B., H. Gulle, and S. H. E. Kaufmann. 1992. Heterogeneity of the repertoire of T cells of tuberculosis patients and healthy contacts to *Mycobacterium tuberculosis* antigens separated by high-resolution techniques. *Infect. Immun.* **60**:1717–1720.

Shanafelt, M.-C., P. Hindersson, C. Soderberg, N. Mensi, C. W. Turck, D. Webb, H. Yssel, and G. Peltz. 1991. T cell and antibody reactivity with the *Borrelia burgdorferi* 60-kDa heat shock protein in lyme arthritis. *J. Immunol.* **146**:3985–3992.

Shinnick, T. M., M. H. Vodkin, and J. C. Williams. 1988. The *Mycobacterium tuberculosis* 65-kilodalton antigen is a heat shock protein which corresponds to common antigen and to the *Escherichia coli* GroEL protein. *Infect. Immun.* **56**:446–451.

Shiratsuchi, H., Y. Okuda, and I. Tsuyuguchi. 1987. Recombinant human interleukin-2 reverses *in vitro*-deficient cell-mediated immune responses to tuberculin purified protein derivative by lymphocytes of tuberculous patients. *Infect. Immun.* **55**:2126–2131.

Stover, C. K., G. P. Bansal, M. S. Hanson, J. E. Burlein, S. R. Palaszynski, J. F. Young, S. Koenig, D. B. Young, A. Sadziene, and A. G. Barbour. 1993. Strategy to express chimeric lipoproteins on the surface of recombinant BCG: a candidate lyme disease vaccine. *J. Exp. Med.* **178**:197–209.

Surcel, H. M., M. Troye-Blomberg, S. Paulie, G. Andersson, C. Moreno, G. Pasvol, and J. Ivanyi.

1994. T_h1/T_h2 profiles in tuberculosis, based on proliferation and cytokine response of blood lymphocytes to mycobacterial antigens and peptides. *Immunology* **81:**171–176.

Terasaka, K., R. Yamaguchi, K. Matsuo, A. Yamazaki, S. Nagai, and T. Yamada. 1989. Complete nucleotide sequence of immunogenic protein MPB70 from *Mycobacterium bovis* BCG. *FEMS Microbiol. Lett.* **58:**273–276.

Thole, J. E. R., and R. Van der Zee. 1990. The 65 kD antigen: molecular studies on a ubiquitous antigen, p. 37–67. *In* J. McFadden (ed.), *Molecular Biology of the Mycobacteria.* Surrey University Press, London.

Thole, J. E. R., W. C. A. van Schooten, A. A. M. Janson, T. Garbe, Y. E. Cornelisse, J. E. Clarke-Curtiss, A. H. J. Kolk, T. II. M. Ottenhoff, R. R. P. De Vries, and C. Abou-Seid. 1992. Molecular and immunological analysis of a fibronectin-binding protein antigen secreted by *Mycobacterium leprae.* *Mol. Microbiol.* **6:**153–163.

Tsuyuguchi, I., H. Kawasumi, C. Ueta, I. Yano, and S. Kishimoto. 1991. Increase of T-cell receptor γ/δ-bearing T cells in cord blood of newborn babies obtained by in vitro stimulation with mycobacterial cord factor. *Infect. Immun.* **59:**3053–3059.

Turneer, M., J.-P. Van Vooren, J. De Bruyn, E. Serruys, P. Dierckx, and J.-C. Yernault. 1988. Humoral immune response in human tuberculosis: immunoglobulins G, A, and M directed against the purified P32 protein antigen of *Mycobacterium bovis* bacillus Calmette-Guérin. *J. Clin. Microbiol.* **26:**1714–1719.

Van Schooten, W. C. A., D. G. Elferink, J. Van Embden, D. C. Anderson, and R. R. P. De Vries. 1989. DR3-restricted T cells from different HLA-DR3-positive individuals recognize the same peptide (amino acids 2–12) of the mycobacterial 65-kDa heat-shock protein. *Eur. J. Immunol.* **19:**2075–2079.

Van Vooren, J.-P., A. Drowart, J. De Bruyn, P. Launois, J. Millan, E. Delaporte, M. Develoux, J.-C. Yernault, and K. Huygen. 1992. Humoral responses against the 85A and 85B antigens of *Mycobacterium bovis* BCG in patients with leprosy and tuberculosis. *J. Clin. Microbiol.* **30:**1608–1610.

Verbon, A., R. A. Hartskeerl, C. Moreno, and A. H. J. Kolk. 1992a. Characterization of B cell epitopes on the 16K antigen of *Mycobacterium tuberculosis.* *Clin. Exp. Immunol.* **89:**395–401.

Verbon, A., R. A. Hartskeerl, A. Schuitema, A. H. J. Kolk, D. B. Young, and R. Lathigra. 1992b. The 14,000-molecular-weight antigen of *Mycobacterium tuberculosis* is related to the alpha-crystallin family of low-molecular-weight heat shock proteins. *J. Bacteriol.* **174:**1352–1359.

Verbon, A., S. Kuijper, H. M. Jansen, P. Speelman, and A. H. J. Kolk. 1990. Antigens in culture supernatant of *Mycobacterium tuberculosis*: epitopes defined by monoclonal and human antibodies. *J. Gen. Microbiol.* **136:**955–964.

Vordermeier, H. M., D. P. Harris, G. Friscia, E. Roman, H.-M. Surcel, C. Moreno, G. Pasvol, and J. Ivanyi. 1992a. T cell repertoire in tuberculosis: selective anergy to an immunodominant epitope of the 38kDa antigen in patients with active disease. *Eur. J. Immunol.* **22:**2631–2637.

Vordermeier, H. M., D. P. Harris, R. Lathigra, E. Roman, C. Moreno, and J. Ivanyi. 1993. Recognition of peptide epitopes of the 16,000 MW antigen of *Mycobacterium tuberculosis* by murine T cells. *Immunology* **80:**6–12.

Vordermeier, H. M., D. P. Harris, P. K. Mehrotra, E. Roman, A. Elsaghier, C. Moreno, and J. Ivanyi. 1992b. *M. tuberculosis*-complex specific T cell stimulation and DTH reactions induced with a peptide from the 38 kDa protein. *Scand. J. Immunol.* **35:**711–718.

Vordermeier, H. M., D. P. Harris, E. Roman, R. Lathigra, C. Moreno, and J. Ivanyi. 1991. Identification of T-cell stimulatory peptides from the 38 kilodalton protein of *Mycobacterium tuberculosis.* *J. Immunol.* **147:**1023–1029.

Wiker, H. G., and M. Harboe. 1992. The antigen 85 complex: a major secretion product of *Mycobacterium tuberculosis.* *Microbiol. Rev.* **56:**648–661.

Wiker, H. G., M. Harboe, J. Bennedsen, and O. Closs. 1988. The antigens of *Mycobacterium tuberculosis*, H37Rv, studied by crossed immunoelectrophoresis: comparison with a reference system for *Mycobacterium bovis* BCG. *Scand. J. Immunol.* **27:**223–239.

Wilkins, E. G. L., and J. Ivanyi. 1991. Potential value of serology for diagnosis of extrapulmonary tuberculosis. *Lancet* **336:**641–643.

Wilson, K. B., A. J. Quayle, S. Suleyman, J. Kjeldsen-Kragh, O. Forre, J. B. Natvig, and J. D. Capra. 1993. Heterogeneity of the TCR repertoire in synovial fluid T lymphocytes responding to BCG in a patient with early rheumatoid arthritis. *Scand. J. Immunol.* **38:**102–112.

Wood, P. R., L. A. Corner, J. S. Rothel, C. Baldock, S. L. Jones, D. B. Cousins, B. S. McCormick, B. R. Francis, J. Creeper, and N. A. Tweedle. 1991. Field comparison of the interferon-gamma assay and the intradermal tuberculin test for the diagnosis of bovine tuberculosis. *Aust. J. Med.* **68:**286–290.

Wood, P. R., L. A. Corner, J. S. Rothel, J. L. Ripper, T. Fifis, B. S. McCormic, B. Francis, L. Melville, K. Small, K. De Witte, J. Tolson, T. J. Ryan, G. W. de Lisle, J. C. Cox, and S. L. Jones. 1992. A field evaluation of serological and cellular diagnostic tests for bovine tuberculosis. *Vet. Microbiol.* **31:**71–79.

Worsaae, A., L. Ljungqvist, K. Haslov, I. Heron, and J. Bennedsen. 1987. Allergenic and blastogenic reactivity of three antigens from *Mycobacterium tuberculosis* in sensitized guinea pigs. *Infect. Immun.* **55**:2922–2927.

Yang, X.-D., J. Gasser, and U. Feige. 1990. Prevention of adjuvant arthritis in rats by a nonapeptide from the 65-kD mycobacterial heat-shock protein. *Clin. Exp. Immunol.* **81**:189–194.

Young, D. B., and T. R. Garbe. 1991a. Lipoprotein antigens of *Mycobacterium tuberculosis*. *Res. Microbiol.* **142**:55–65.

Young, D. B., and T. R. Garbe. 1991b. Heat shock proteins and antigens of *Mycobacterium tuberculosis*. *Infect. Immun.* **59**:3086–3093.

Young, D. B., S. H. E. Kaufmann, P. W. M. Hermans, and J. E. R. Thole. 1992. Mycobacterial protein antigens: a compilation. *Mol. Microbiol.* **6**:133–145.

Young, R. A., B. R. Bloom, C. M. Grosskinsky, J. Ivanyi, and R. W. Davis. 1985. Dissecting *Mycobacterium tuberculosis* antigens using recombinant DNA. *Proc. Natl. Acad. Sci. USA* **82**:2583–2587.

Yuuki, H., Y. Yoshikai, K. Kishihara, A. Iwasaki, G. Matsuzaki, H. Takimoto, and K. Nomoto. 1990. Clonal anergy in self-reactive α/β T cells is abrogated by heat-shock protein-reactive γ/δ T cells in aged athymic nude mice. *Eur. J. Immunol.* **20**:1475–1482.

Tuberculosis: Pathogenesis, Protection, and Control
Edited by Barry R. Bloom
© 1994 American Society for Microbiology, Washington, DC 20005

Chapter 27

Pathogenesis of Pulmonary Tuberculosis: an Interplay of Tissue-Damaging and Macrophage-Activating Immune Responses—Dual Mechanisms That Control Bacillary Multiplication

Arthur M. Dannenberg, Jr., and Graham A. W. Rook

The development of pulmonary tuberculosis from its onset to its various clinical manifestations may be pictured as a series of battles between host and invader. (i) The inhaled bacillus may multiply, or it may be eliminated by alveolar macrophages before any lesion is produced. (ii) Small caseous lesions (a few millimeters in diameter) may progress or may heal or stabilize before they are detectable by radiograph. (iii) Larger caseous lesions may grow locally and shed bacilli into the blood and lymph, or they may heal or stabilize. (iv) Alternatively, caseous lesions may liquefy and introduce bacilli and their products into the bronchial tree, making arrest of the disease more difficult. In general, each successive battle is won by the host with increasing difficulty. Furthermore, in a given lung, each tuberculous lesion is independent;

i.e., each lesion (or even parts of large lesions) may be engaged in any battle in this series, regardless of which battle the other lesions (or parts) are engaged in.

Once the first small caseous tuberculous lesion is established, all subsequent battles occur in a host capable of both tissue-damaging and macrophage-activating immune responses. The former causes caseous necrosis if high local concentrations of the tuberculin-like bacillary products are present. The latter, often called cell-mediated immunity (CMI) or acquired cellular resistance, causes an accumulation of activated microbicidal macrophages around the caseous center of the lesion. The interplay between multiplication of bacilli and these responses of the host to various bacillary components determines whether the disease will progress or regress and, if it does progress, what form it will take.

Detailed information on the pathogenesis of tuberculosis may be obtained from the classic texts in the field written by those who worked with the disease before the antimicrobial era: Lurie (1964), Canetti (1955), Rich (1951), Dubos and Dubos (1952), Poole and Florey (1970), and Long

Arthur M. Dannenberg, Jr. • Department of Environmental Health Sciences, The Johns Hopkins University School of Hygiene and Public Health, 615 North Wolfe Street, Room 4001, Baltimore, Maryland 21205. *Graham A. W. Rook* • Department of Medical Microbiology, School of Pathology, University College London Medical School, 67-73 Riding House Street, London W1P 7LD, United Kingdom.

(1958). This pathogenesis was recently reviewed by Dannenberg and Tomashefski (1988).

DEFINITIONS OF TISSUE-DAMAGING AND MACROPHAGE-ACTIVATING IMMUNE RESPONSES AND THEIR ROLES IN THE PATHOGENESIS OF TUBERCULOSIS

The tissue-damaging response is often produced during delayed-type hypersensitivity (DTH) reactions to the tuberculin-like products of the bacillus. It is used during the course of the disease to destroy nonactivated macrophages within which the bacillus is multiplying (Dannenberg, 1991, 1993, 1994). The macrophage-activating response is a cell-mediated response that activates macrophages, so that they can kill and digest the bacilli they ingest (Dannenberg, 1968, 1989; Ando et al., 1977; Mackaness, 1968). Both tissue-damaging and macrophage-activating immune responses can stop the growth (i.e., multiplication) of tubercle bacilli, because these bacilli do not multiply appreciably in nonliquefied caseous necrotic tissue. In both responses, specific antigens locally stimulate T lymphocytes to produce lymphokines that attract and activate macrophages and lymphocytes (Dannenberg, 1968; Dannenberg et al., 1968).

Both the tissue-damaging and macrophage-activating immune processes are complex, each with many interactions and checks and balances. Various inflammatory mediators, e.g., clotting factors, eicosanoids, cytokines, hydrolytic enzymes, and reactive oxygen and nitrogen intermediates, are frequently involved in one or both processes. However, the principles described in this article are most easily understood if the reader accepts our simplified definitions, namely, that the tissue-damaging hypersensitivity process kills nonactivated macrophages that have allowed tubercle bacilli to multiply within them and

that the CMI process makes the microbicidal power of macrophages strong enough to kill or inhibit mycobacteria.

In tuberculosis, the tissue-damaging response causes both caseous necrosis and cavity formation. In other words, the pulmonary damage that is present in clinical tuberculosis appears to be almost entirely due to the tissue-damaging response (Lurie, 1964; Rich, 1951). Why, then, did such a detrimental process develop during the evolution of mammalian species? Bacillary growth curves provide the answer (Fig. 1) (Lurie, 1964; Lurie et al., 1955; Allison et al., 1962). Tubercle bacilli grow logarithmically within the cytoplasm of immature nonactivated macrophages. The killing of such bacilli-laden macrophages by the tissue-damaging immune response immediately stops this logarithmic multiplication of the bacillus, enabling the host to survive at the expense of some of its own tissues.

This tissue-damaging immune response is therefore a quick and powerful mechanism for keeping the number of tubercle bacilli at low levels. It does not eradicate the bacilli, but it does stop their multiplication and provide an unfavorable environment in which many of the bacilli die.

The balance between the macrophage-activating and tissue-damaging immune responses throughout the course of this disease determines what form the disease takes. The tissue-damaging response produces caseous necrosis within which the bacilli are inhibited extracellularly; the macrophage-activating response produces activated macrophages within which the bacilli are killed intracellularly. They are two distinct effective immune responses for inhibiting the progression of the disease. For the successful management of tuberculosis, there is a real need to study the interplay between these two immune responses and alter the ratio between them, so that the host can control bacillary growth with minimal tissue destruction (Dannenberg, 1990). In other words, the

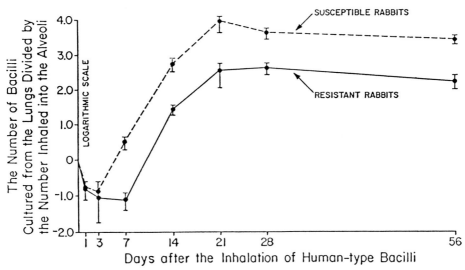

Figure 1. Changes in the number of human-type tubercle bacilli in the lungs of natively resistant rabbits and natively susceptible rabbits at different intervals after infection by quantitative airborne inhalation. By 7 days after infection, the resistant animals had inhibited the growth of the bacilli 20 to 30 times more effectively than did the susceptible animals, but from then on, the two curves ran parallel. At 4 to 5 weeks, susceptible animals had about 13 times more primary pulmonary tubercles than were present in resistant animals. Means and standard errors are shown. The number of bacilli in the lungs of the resistant group failed to decrease during the period illustrated, because liquefaction, with extracellular multiplication of the bacillus, readily occurs in these rabbits (Lurie, 1964; Lurie et al., 1955). Liquefaction rarely occurs in the susceptible group (Lurie, 1964; Lurie et al., 1955) because their macrophages apparently develop only low levels of hydrolytic enzymes. (Reprinted with permission from Lurie et al. [1955].)

tissue-damaging immune reaction is probably excessive in many cases of this disease, and the control of this excess would reduce much of the pulmonary destruction that occurs.

Note that in previous publications (Dannenberg, 1991, 1993, 1994), the senior author of this chapter used the term DTH for the tissue-damaging immune response and used the term CMI for the macrophage-activating immune response. This terminology (derived from the pathology) has caused some confusion. Therefore, in this chapter we have usually used DTH with modifiers, e.g., necrotizing or tissue-damaging DTH.

STAGES IN THE PATHOGENESIS OF TUBERCULOSIS

The different stages of human tuberculosis were reproduced by Max B. Lurie over 30 years ago in his susceptible and resistant strains of inbred rabbits (Lurie, 1964; Lurie and Dannenberg, 1965). Tuberculosis in rabbits resembles the disease in humans more closely than does tuberculosis in any other common laboratory animal species (Lurie, 1964; Dannenberg, 1984). Newborn infants and immunosuppressed individuals (including those with AIDS) develop a form of tuberculosis similar to that found in Lurie's susceptible rabbits (Lurie, 1964; Dannenberg and Tomashefski, 1988). Immunocompetent adult human beings develop a form of tuberculosis similar to that found in Lurie's resistant rabbits (Lurie, 1964; Dannenberg and Tomashefski, 1988). Early primary lesions of tuberculosis can be studied histologically only in experimental animals, because specimens of such early human lesions are almost never available. Nonetheless, the following sequence of pathogenesis should also occur in human beings.

Stage I: Onset

The first stage (Lurie, 1964; Dannenberg and Tomashefski, 1988; Dannenberg, 1991) begins following the inhalation of the tubercle bacillus into an alveolus. There, an alveolar macrophage ingests the bacillus and often destroys it. This destruction depends on the inherent microbicidal power of the alveolar macrophage and the genetic and phenotypic virulence of the ingested bacillus. A virulent bacillus in a relatively weak alveolar macrophage seems to be able to multiply and initiate the disease, but a weak bacillus in a strong alveolar macrophage seems to be readily destroyed or inhibited before bacillary multiplication can occur.

Alveolar macrophages are cells that have been nonspecifically activated by a variety of inhaled particles, by ingestion of occasional extravasated erythrocytes, and possibly by any general stimulation of the mononuclear phagocyte system. Therefore, the microbicidal ability of the alveolar macrophage exists before tubercle bacilli are inhaled.

CMI (in which antigens stimulate specific T cells to activate macrophages) is not involved in the immediate destruction of inhaled tubercle bacilli. The only particles small enough to reach the alveolar spaces contain no more than three bacilli (Lurie, 1964; Riley et al., 1962). So few bacilli do not possess enough antigen to elicit either a primary or a secondary immune response. The number of units containing one to three bacilli that must be inhaled by the average human being to establish the infection is not known. It depends on the virulence of the bacilli (Riley et al., 1962) and the resistance of the recipient, but it is probably between 10 and 50 units.

Persons with AIDS have an increased susceptibility to tuberculosis (see chapter 29). Infection of alveolar macrophages with the AIDS virus (Salahuddin et al., 1986) may have decreased the ability of these cells to prevent disease. However, most cases of tuberculosis in AIDS patients are caused by the reduced ability of the host to produce CMI. This immunodeficiency allows a new pulmonary lesion to reach clinical proportions or a dormant endogenous infection to reactivate. The latter is the most common source of active disease in these patients (Selwyn et al., 1989).

Resistance to the establishment of tuberculosis is partly under genetic control; i.e., some individuals probably have a more effective alveolar macrophage population than others. Because blacks convert to tuberculin positive more frequently than whites following the same exposure to tubercle bacilli (Stead et al., 1990), the alveolar macrophages of blacks may be less effective in destroying inhaled tubercle bacilli than those of whites. Among the converters, however, the incidence of clinical disease is the same.

Seven days after the inhalation of human tubercle bacilli, the lungs of Lurie's resistant rabbits contained significantly fewer viable bacilli than did the lungs of his susceptible rabbits (Lurie, 1964; Lurie et al., 1955; Allison et al., 1962); there was a 20- to 30-fold difference, which was subsequently maintained for many weeks (Fig. 1). The alveolar macrophages of the resistant rabbits evidently destroyed some bacilli and inhibited the growth of others to a much greater degree than did those of the susceptible host.

Stage II: Symbiosis

If the original alveolar macrophage fails to destroy or inhibit the inhaled unit of one to three bacilli, the bacilli multiply until that macrophage (or its progeny) bursts. Its bacillary load is then ingested by other alveolar macrophages and by nonactivated macrophages, i.e., monocytes emigrating

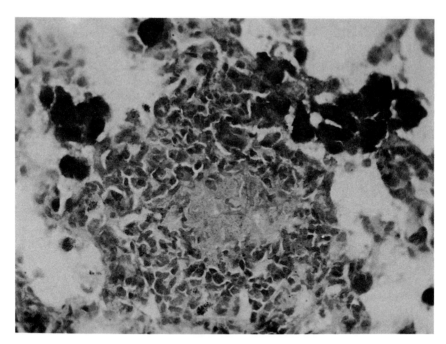

Figure 2. A 10-day rabbit pulmonary BCG lesion. In the small caseous center are disintegrated β-galactosidase-negative epithelioid cells containing more than 10 faintly stained tubercle bacilli. Around the small caseous center are viable, young, β-galactosidase-negative macrophages from the bloodstream, which control the fate of the tuberculous lesion. Alveolar macrophages, staining 3+ and 4+ for β-galactosidase (a marker for macrophage activation), have accumulated in the surrounding alveolar area (rather far from the bacilli in the center). Although this lesion was produced by the intravenous injection of tubercle bacilli, tubercles produced by the inhalation of bacilli should show the same pattern. Specifically, bacilli would be released from the initial alveolar macrophages, which in this case had failed to control bacillary multiplication. These bacilli would chemotactically attract from the bloodstream new macrophages, which cannot control the multiplication of tubercle bacilli in their cytoplasm until they become activated by T cells. Magnification, ×400. (Photograph reprinted with permission from Shima et al. [1972].)

from the bloodstream. Both types of macrophage are attracted to the site by released bacilli, cellular debris, and a variety of chemotactic factors of host origin, e.g., the complement component C5a and the cytokine monocyte chemoattractant protein (MCP-1). In time, macrophages from the circulation become completely responsible for the fate of the early lesion. In such a lesion, the alveolar macrophages rarely participate, because they remain peripheral, rather far from the bacilli, which are almost always located more centrally (Fig. 2).

The new immature macrophages from the bloodstream readily ingest the released

bacilli. Then, a symbiotic relationship develops (Lurie, 1964; Lurie et al., 1955; Allison et al., 1962), in which neither the macrophages of the host nor the bacilli injure each other: the new macrophages have not yet been activated, so they cannot inhibit or destroy the bacilli (Fig. 3), and the bacilli cannot injure the macrophages because the host has not yet developed tuberculin-type hypersensitivity. With time, more and more macrophages and more and more bacilli accumulate in the lesion.

In this symbiotic stage (Fig. 3), between 7 and 21 days after infection, the bacilli multiply logarithmically at the same rate in both resistant and susceptible rabbits (Fig.

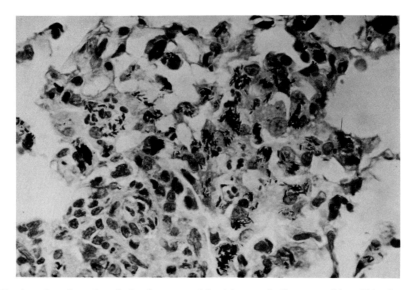

Figure 3. Portion of a tuberculous lesion from one of Lurie's genetically susceptible rabbits 2 weeks after the inhalation of human-type tubercle bacilli. The blood-borne nonactivated macrophages depicted contain numerous (rod-shaped) acid-fast bacilli. Two weeks is near the end of stage II, the stage of symbiosis: the bacilli have grown logarithmically within macrophages with no apparent damage to these cells. Magnification, ×850. (Photograph reprinted with permission from Lurie et al. [1955].)

1). Evidently, the intracellular bacilli do not stimulate the microbicidal mechanisms of immature macrophages in either type of host. Smith and Harding (1977) observed the same parallelism in BCG-vaccinated and control guinea pigs.

Only activated macrophages of resistant and susceptible rabbits show differences in their abilities to inhibit the growth of tubercle bacilli; alveolar macrophages are activated nonspecifically prior to inhalation of tubercle bacilli, while blood-borne monocytes/macrophages are activated by specific T cells and their lymphokines (see below).

Histologically, macrophages in the lesions of the susceptible host contain more visible bacilli (Fig. 3) and tend to be located intra-alveolarly (Lurie, 1964; Lurie et al., 1955). Macrophages in the lesions of the resistant host contain fewer bacilli and usually are located interstitially, i.e., within the alveolar walls (Lurie, 1964; Lurie et al., 1955). However, during this symbiotic stage, these histological differences have no

apparent effect on the rate of bacillary multiplication (Fig. 1). In both resistant and susceptible rabbits, the newly arrived macrophages from the bloodstream support such bacillary growth equally well in their cytoplasm. The interstitial inflammatory areas in the resistant rabbits probably contain greater numbers of T lymphocytes, attracted there by chemotactants, such as the cytokine neutrophil (and lymphocyte) attractant/activating protein (NAP-1, also called interleukin 8). Such T cells play a major role in the immune response, which terminates the second (symbiotic) stage of this disease.

Stage III: Initial Caseous Necrosis

The third stage of the disease begins when the logarithmic bacillary multiplication stops (Fig. 1). At that time (2 to 3 weeks after the inhalation of the bacilli), the host becomes tuberculin positive and the lesions undergo caseous necrosis in their centers (Fig. 2). The first three stages of this disease are depicted diagrammatically in Fig. 4.

When the second (symbiotic) stage ends, the lungs of Lurie's susceptible rabbits contain 20 to 30 times more bacilli than do the lungs of his resistant rabbits (Fig. 1). Most of these bacilli are probably in developing lesions. At 5 weeks, the susceptible rabbits have 13 times more grossly visible lesions than resistant rabbits have. At this time, each "susceptible" lesion therefore contains about two times more bacilli (assuming that all the tubercle bacilli in the lungs are in these lesions). Yet in spite of this numerical difference, the susceptible hosts inhibit further bacillary growth just as efficiently as do the resistant hosts (Fig. 1). The macrophage-activating immune response (CMI) could not be responsible, because the susceptible host develops only weak CMI, and at this stage of the disease,

the CMI of the resistant host is not yet fully developed. The marked inhibition of bacillary growth in both strains of rabbits must therefore be due to another mechanism.

This mechanism is quite apparent when one studies tissue sections of the lesions. The logarithmic phase of bacillary multiplication stops abruptly as soon as caseous necrosis develops (Fig. 2 and 4). The caseous centers are larger in the susceptible host (Lurie et al., 1955), apparently because each "susceptible" lesion probably contains roughly twice as many bacilli. Thus, by killing the nonactivated macrophages in which the bacilli are growing, the host eliminates the intracellular environment that is so favorable to such growth. This phenomenon had been predicted many years ago (Koch, 1891; Canetti, 1955) and has recently been advocated by several

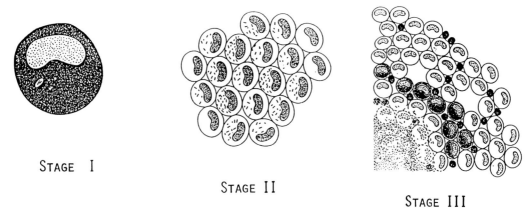

STAGE I

STAGE II

STAGE III

Figure 4. The sketch of stage I depicts an alveolar macrophage that has ingested and destroyed the two tubercle bacilli in the phagocytic vacuole. The cytoplasm of this macrophage is darkly shaded to depict a high degree of activation, i.e., high levels of lysosomal and oxidative enzymes (Dannenberg, 1968). The sketch of stage II depicts an early primary tubercle in which tubercle bacilli multiply logarithmically within the macrophages that had emigrated from the bloodstream into the developing lesion. These newly arriving phagocytes are nonactivated and incompetent. The cytoplasm of these macrophages is unshaded to depict the lack of activation. In fact, the phagocytic vacuoles in the cytoplasm of these nonactivated macrophages seem to provide an ideal environment for mycobacterial growth. Stage II is called the stage of symbiosis (Lurie, 1964; Dannenberg, 1991), since the bacilli are multiplying, the macrophages are accumulating, and neither is destroyed by the other. The sketch of stage III depicts a tubercle 3 weeks of age with a caseous necrotic center and a peripheral accumulation of partly activated macrophages (lightly shaded) and lymphocytes (small dark cells). The first stages of caseation occur when the tissue-damaging immune response (to the tuberculin-like products of the bacilli) kills the nonactivated macrophages that have allowed the bacilli to grow logarithmically within them (Fig. 1 and 3). The dead and dying macrophages are depicted by fragmented cell membranes. Intact and fragmented bacilli are present, both within macrophages and within the caseum.

research groups (Kaufmann, 1988; Lowrie, 1990; Boom et al., 1991).

The tubercle bacillus can survive in this solid caseous material, but it apparently cannot multiply because of anoxic conditions, reduced pH, and the presence of inhibitory fatty acids (Poole and Florey, 1970; Hemsworth and Kochan, 1978). (In fact, tubercle bacilli may survive for years in solid caseous foci.) Thus, the host locally destroys its own tissues to control the uninhibited intracellular multiplication of bacilli that would otherwise be fatal (Canetti, 1955; Poole and Florey, 1970; Dannenberg, 1991). Only after such control is established can the activated macrophages (produced by CMI) that accumulate around the caseous focus prevent the extension of the disease (see below).

At 2 to 3 weeks, when the second (symbiotic) stage of pulmonary tuberculosis is ended by the development of the tissue-damaging immune response, a small caseous center is present (Fig. 4, stage III). If the bacilli are few, the lesions will probably regress. However, if the bacilli are numerous, the lesions will probably enlarge to become the grossly visible tubercles with caseous centers that Lurie counted at 4 to 5 weeks. The microscopic lesions present at 2 to 3 weeks have never been counted, so no information is available on the progression and regression of tuberculous lesions at this stage of the primary infection.

Secondary lesions of hematogenous origin always originate from very few bacilli. The same is true of lesions of reinfection from exogenous inhaled bacilli. In both situations, the rapid accumulation and activation of macrophages often arrest the lesions before they become grossly visible (Lurie, 1964). This is especially true in organs in which the multiplication of tubercle bacilli is inhibited more efficiently than in the lung (see below).

Mononuclear phagocytes (MN) have a continual turnover in the caseous tuberculous lesion (Tsuda et al., 1976). Numerous MN enter the lesion, and numerous MN die in it (or leave via the lymphatics). In spite of this turnover, numerous MN accumulate there and become activated. Both the macrophage turnover rate and the accumulation of activated macrophages peak when the T-cell-mediated responses first develop. At that time, a large amount of bacillary antigen is present, and it stimulates local lymphokine production.

Stage IVa or IVb: Interplay of Tissue-Damaging and Macrophage-Activating Immune Responses

From 3 weeks on, the multiplication of the bacillus (in caseous tubercles) is controlled equally well in both resistant and susceptible rabbits; hence, the bacillary growth curve is flat (Fig. 1). However, the two rabbit strains apparently achieve this plateau by somewhat different mechanisms, which are depicted diagrammatically in Fig. 5.

Stage IVa is illustrated by the susceptible rabbits, which develop only weak CMI (Lurie, 1964; Dannenberg, 1991; Lurie and Dannenberg, 1965). Tubercle bacilli released from the edge of the caseous center are ingested by incompetent (nonactivated and poorly activated) macrophages (Fig. 5 and 6). Therefore, the susceptible rabbits must continue to use the tissue-damaging immune response (necrotizing DTH) to stop the intracellular bacillary multiplication. The caseous center enlarges, and local lung tissue is destroyed.

Similar to the susceptible rabbits, human infants and immunosuppressed adults (including nonterminal AIDS patients) also have many poorly activated macrophages around the caseous centers of the tuberculous lesions. These incompetent macrophages allow the bacillus to continue to multiply intracellularly (Lurie, 1964; Lurie and Dannenberg, 1965; Dannenberg, 1991). These macrophages die (because of the tissue-damaging immune reaction), and the

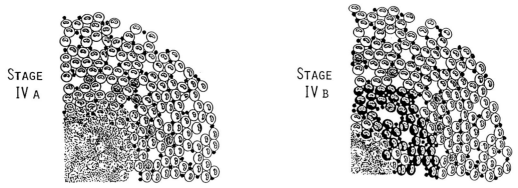

Figure 5. The sketch of stage IVa depicts an established tubercle 4 to 5 weeks of age representing that found in one of Lurie's susceptible rabbits. It has an enlarging caseous center. The bacilli escaping from the edge of this center are ingested by nonactivated incompetent macrophages. In such macrophages, they again find a favorable intracellular environment in which to multiply. They do so until again the tissue-damaging immune response kills these new bacilli-laden macrophages and the area of caseous necrosis enlarges. This sequence may be repeated many times. The lung is destroyed, and the bacilli spread by the lymphatic and hematogenous routes to other sites, where the tissue destruction continues. Several partly activated macrophages (lightly shaded) are included to show that these susceptible rabbits develop only weak CMI. (This pattern of tuberculosis is seen in immunosuppressed individuals, including nonterminal AIDS patients.) The sketch of stage IVb depicts an established tubercle 4 to 5 weeks of age representing that found in one of Lurie's resistant rabbits. The caseous center remains small because the bacilli escaping from its edge are ingested by highly activated (competent) macrophages (darkly shaded), which surrounded the caseum. In such activated macrophages, the bacilli cannot multiply and are eventually destroyed. Such effective (activated) macrophages are produced by T cells and their lymphokines (Fig. 9). If the caseous center remains solid and does not liquefy, the disease will be arrested by this CMI process, because further tissue destruction does not occur. (This scenario occurs in healthy immunocompetent human beings who show positive tuberculin reactions and yet no clinical and often even no X-ray evidence of the disease.)

caseous center enlarges. With virulent bovine-type bacilli in susceptible rabbits (and both human and bovine bacilli in infants and immunosuppressed adults), bacilli lodging in the draining tracheobronchial lymph nodes and elsewhere in the body are not destroyed. Multiple uncontrolled tubercles (of hematogenous origin) with extensive caseation develop in many organs, especially in the lungs (Fig. 7), and the host eventually dies of the disease (Lurie, 1964; Lurie and Dannenberg, 1965; Dannenberg and Tomashefski, 1988).

In human beings, this type of hematogenous spread of tubercle bacilli may cause miliary tuberculosis. Many small tubercles of uniform size and hematogenous origin occur simultaneously in the lungs (Fig. 7B) and/or in the liver, spleen, and kidneys. A miliary tubercle is 2 to 4 mm in diameter,

the size of a millet seed, from which the term miliary is derived. Bacilli are distributed to both lungs after entering the right side of the heart from caseous hilar nodes. These lymph nodes discharge infective particles into efferent lymphatic trunks, which drain into the systemic veins. These veins carry them into the right side of the heart, from which they are pumped into the lungs. Therefore, most of the lesions of hematogenous origin in the lungs are caused by bacilli once present in the hilar lymph nodes. Bacilli are distributed to the extrapulmonary organs of the body by blood from the left side of the heart. Therefore, most of the lesions of hematogenous origin in the extrapulmonary organs are caused by bacilli once present in lung lesions.

These secondary lesions of hematogenous origin, i.e., miliary tubercles, may be

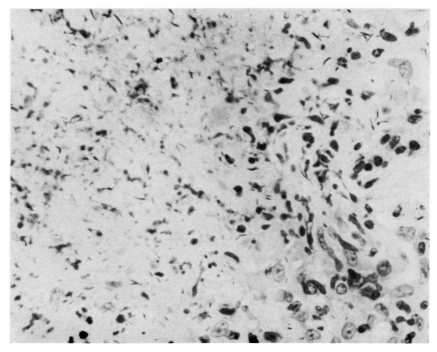

Figure 6. Photograph of stage IVa: a caseous tubercle in the lungs of one of Lurie's susceptible rabbits 5 weeks after the inhalation of human-type tubercle bacilli. Bacilli escaping from the caseous center (left) are ingested by the surrounding nonactivated macrophages, i.e., incompetent immature epithelioid cells (right), where they again find a favorable intracellular environment in which to grow (Fig. 5). Magnification, ×660. (Photograph reprinted with permission from Lurie et al. [1952].)

of two types, depending on the resistance of the host: (i) a compact "hard" tubercle, i.e., a proliferative type with epithelioid cells and occasional giant cells with (or without) a caseous center (Fig. 8A), and (ii) a "soft" tubercle, i.e., a loosely formed, exudative type (Fig. 8B). The exudative type often enlarges rapidly, usually contains more bacilli than the hard tubercle, and often undergoes early and complete caseation. Tubercles with mixed hard and soft characteristics are common in human beings.

Stage IVb is illustrated by Lurie's resistant rabbits, which develop strong CMI, i.e., many macrophages capable of inhibiting the multiplication of the bacilli within them (Lurie, 1964; Dannenberg, 1991). The bacillary antigens apparently expand specific T-cell populations. These T cells (when stimulated by the same antigens)

release gamma interferon and probably other lymphokines that activate local macrophages (Fig. 9). Therefore, a mantle of highly activated macrophages accumulates around the caseous center (Fig. 5 and 10). Such macrophages ingest and destroy the bacilli that escape from the edge of the caseum (Fig. 11), so that little or no further tissue destruction occurs. Thirty years ago, Lurie (1964) had no histochemical test for activated macrophages capable of destroying tubercle bacilli, but he identified them histologically as mature epithelioid cells. They were subsequently found to contain high levels of β-galactosidase and other histochemically demonstrable marker enzymes (Fig. 12) (Dannenberg, 1968; Dannenberg et al., 1968; Ando et al., 1977).

In a resistant host, the primary tubercle eventually becomes walled off, the caseous center inspissates, and the disease is ar-

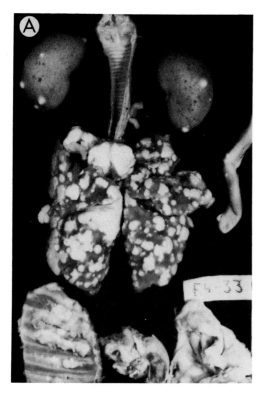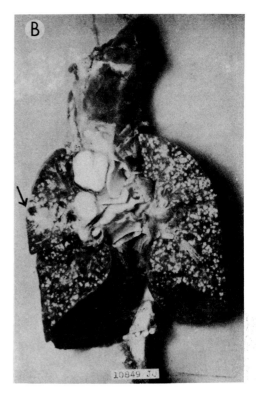

Figure 7. (A) Multiple caseous foci of hematogenous origin in the lungs of one of Lurie's susceptible rabbits. A large, completely caseous (nonliquefied) primary lesion is present in the middle of the left lung. It was caused by the inhalation of a single unit of one to three virulent bovine-type tubercle bacilli. The hilar nodes were infected by the lymph draining from this primary lesion. Bacilli in the efferent lymph of these infected (caseous) lymph nodes entered the venous circulation to the right side of the heart and then seeded the lungs via branches of the pulmonary artery. Tuberculous lesions were also present in the pleura, in the kidneys, and in the knee joint. (Reprinted with permission from Lurie [1941].) (B) Rapidly progressing miliary tuberculosis in an 11-month-old infant. This specimen is the human counterpart of panel A. Most of the multiple caseous areas are of hematogenous origin. The primary lesion is marked by an arrow.

rested, frequently for a lifetime. The few bacilli that disseminate via the lymphatic system or the bloodstream are rapidly destroyed at their site of lodgment by accelerated tubercle formation, i.e., a rapid CMI response producing many locally activated macrophages (Fig. 9 and 10) (Dannenberg, 1968, 1989; Mackaness, 1968) and relatively little caseation. Thus, in resistant hosts, the disease is usually well controlled and is even arrested. (In Fig. 1, however, the number of bacilli did not decrease, because in this experiment, liquefaction and extracellular multiplication of bacilli occurred in the resistant rabbits [see Stage V below].)

Similar to susceptible rabbits, resistant rabbits continue to use the tissue-damaging immune response to kill macrophages (along with normal lung tissue) whenever intracellular bacillary multiplication is not controlled; but the ratio of "activated macrophages" to "caseous necrosis" is much higher in resistant rabbits than in susceptible ones. In other words, both resistant and susceptible rabbits develop strong tuberculin reactions, and both show caseous necrosis (due to the tissue-damaging immune response), but only resistant rabbits develop large numbers of highly activated macrophages (mature epithelioid cells)

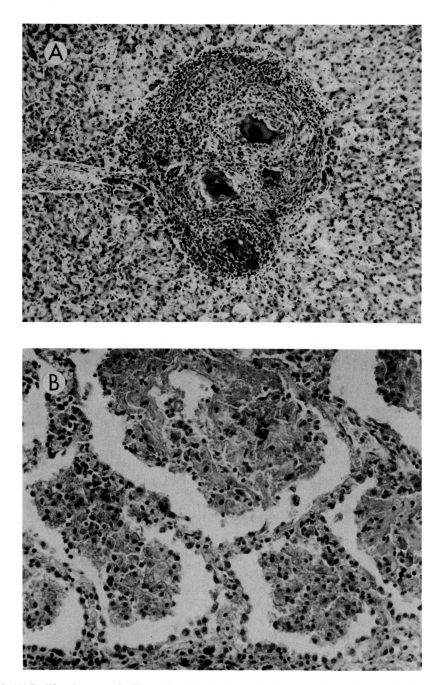

Figure 8. (A) Proliferative type of miliary tubercle in the liver of an 8-month-old male infant. The lesion consists predominantly of a cellular infiltrate composed of macrophages, lymphocytes, plasma cells, and fibroblasts, none of which are distinguishable at this magnification. Part of four Langhans giant cells are seen. They are thought to be formed by several macrophages surrounding a bit of caseous tissue too large for one macrophage to ingest. Hematoxylin and eosin stain. Magnification, ×116. (B) Exudative type of tuberculous lesion in the lung of a 47-year-old black male. Depicted is an area of tuberculous pneumonia. A large proportion of the cellular exudate in the alveolar spaces has undergone caseous necrosis, and the intervening alveolar septa are thickened by infiltrating cells. Hematoxylin and eosin stain. Magnification, ×200.

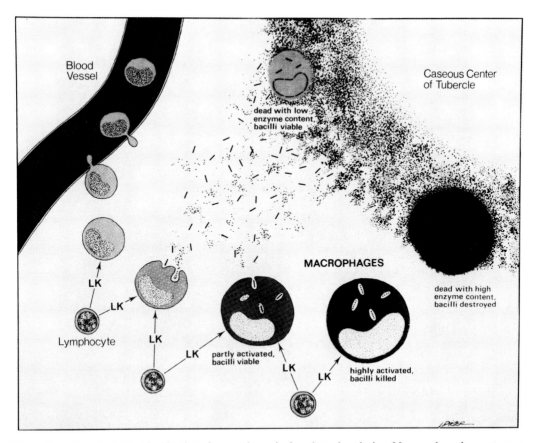

Figure 9. CMI producing local activation of macrophages in the tuberculous lesion. Mononuclear phagocytes are attracted from the bloodstream and are activated locally by lymphocytes and their lymphokines (LK) (probably the most efficient mechanism), by endotoxin-like bacillary products, and also by the ingestion of dead cells and tissue debris. Lymphokines are produced when lymphocytes (mainly T cells) with antigen-specific receptors are stimulated by the bacillus and its products. Only activated macrophages seem capable of destroying the tubercle bacillus. (Reprinted with permission from Dannenberg [1978].)

around the caseous areas. These mature phagocytes readily destroy the tubercle bacilli that they ingest.

With human-type bacilli, the disease in both resistant and susceptible strains of rabbits healed after many months. However, before such healing could take place, the susceptible rabbits often developed metastatic hematogenous lesions, and the resistant rabbits often developed cavities (Lurie, 1964). (See chapter 10 for a description of tuberculosis produced by human-type and bovine-type tubercle bacilli in rabbits.)

Stage V: Liquefaction and Cavity Formation

Unfortunately, even if the CMI is strong, progression of the disease may still occur in Lurie's resistant rabbits as well as in immunocompetent adult human beings. Such progression is caused by liquefaction and cavity formation (Fig. 13) (Lurie, 1941, 1964; Lurie and Dannenberg, 1965; Rich, 1951; Canetti, 1955; Dannenberg and Tomashefski, 1988). (Liquefied caseous foci and cavities do not occur in Lurie's susceptible rabbits [Lurie, 1964; Lurie and Dan-

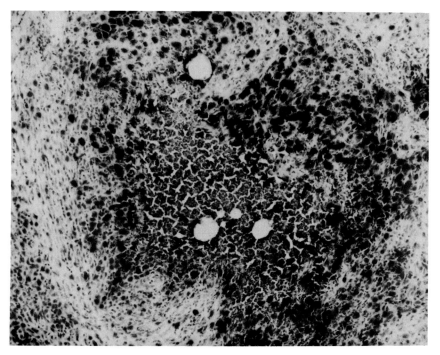

Figure 10. Highly activated (strongly β-galactosidase-positive) macrophages surrounding the caseous center of a 12-day rabbit dermal BCG lesion. This figure illustrates a major aspect of effective CMI, namely, that large numbers of highly activated macrophages accumulate around a caseous focus, so that bacilli released from dead and dying cells will be ingested by competent rather than incompetent cells. Magnification, ×115. (Photograph reprinted with permission from Shima et al. [1972].)

nenberg, 1965] and are not common in infants and immunosuppressed individuals [Dannenberg and Tomashefski, 1988].)

The liquefied material is an excellent growth medium for the tubercle bacillus, and (for the first time during the course of the disease) the bacillus multiplies extracellularly, often reaching tremendous numbers (Fig. 14). Because the host is now highly sensitive to the tuberculin-like products of the bacillus, this large antigenic load is quite toxic to the tissues. The walls of nearby bronchi often become necrotic and rupture, forming a cavity (Fig. 13 and 15). Then, the bacilli and the liquefied caseous material are discharged into the airways and reach other parts of the lung and the outside environment (Fig. 15 and 16).

The walls of most cavities consist of an external zone of collagen, the cavity's capsule (which in humans is occasionally hyalinized), and a caseous (often liquefying) internal zone where the high oxygen content from the ambient air nurtures the growth of bacilli (Canetti, 1955; Dannenberg and Tomashefski, 1988). By coughing, the patient aerosolizes this infectious material, disseminating bacilli to other parts of the lung and to the outside world. Rabbits do not cough, but bronchogenic spread of bacilli from the cavities occurs during normal respiration.

In humans, between the external and internal zones of the cavity wall, there is a zone of granulation tissue rich in capillaries, granulocytes, macrophages, lymphocytes, and fibroblasts (Canetti, 1955; Dannenberg and Tomashefski, 1988). At times, typical tubercles are present. The three zones are of various thicknesses and are

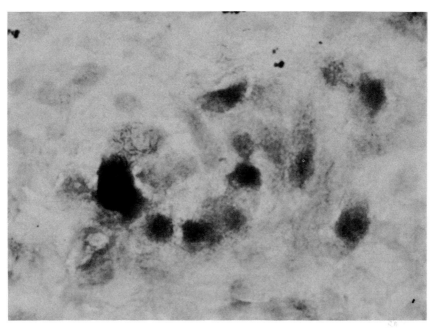

Figure 11. Macrophages stained for β-galactosidase activity and acid-fast bacilli in a BCG lesion of a rabbit injected intradermally 21 days previously. On the left, one of these macrophages shows negligible β-galactosidase activity. It contains numerous bacilli and has ruptured. Another macrophage (just adjacent) shows high β-galactosidase activity. It contains no bacilli but is apparently ingesting the bacilli released from the ruptured cell. This figure illustrates an effective CMI response, namely, highly activated macrophages ingesting (and destroying) bacilli released from ineffectual macrophages. The section was stained with 5-bromo-4-chloroindol-3-yl-β-D-galactopyranoside for β-galactosidases and with carbol fuchsin for acid-fast bacilli and then lightly counterstained with hematoxylin. Magnification, ×1,000. (Photograph reprinted with permission from Dannenberg [1968].)

not clearly demarcated from each other. With newly formed cavities, the internal caseous zone is thickest. With older, still-active cavities, the external capsule is thickest. Around the capsule, usually between the pleura and the cavity, an area of atelectasis is often present. This atelectatic area may prevent perforation into the pleural spaces. Erosion of incompletely thrombosed vessels in the intermediate zone leads to hemorrhage into the wall of the cavity. There, blood may pool and thereby give rise to some hemoptysis. Massive hemoptysis, however, is usually due to the leakage or rupture of a fully patent blood vessel located in the wall of the cavity or traversing its lumen.

A liquefied caseous lesion in the lung (or in a hilar lymph node) may discharge its contents into the air passages and cause small to large pneumonic foci or bronchopneumonia (Fig. 8B and 16) or even lobar pneumonia. The extent of the disease is determined by the number of bacilli and their viability, the quantity of tuberculin-like products in the liquefied caseous material, and the amount of aspiration of this material throughout the bronchial tree. Local deposits, containing bacilli and their components in low concentrations, commonly cause scattered, compact proliferative-type tubercles (Fig. 8A) or (rarely) confluent proliferative tubercles with small foci of encapsulated caseous pneumonia. However, local deposits containing bacilli and their components in high concentra-

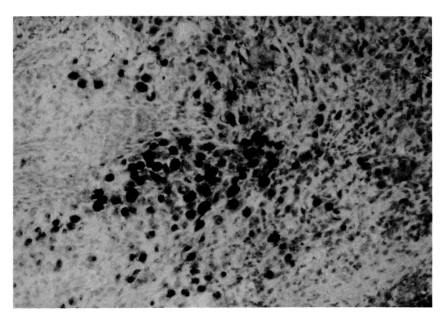

Figure 12. Group of activated macrophages (epithelioid cells) in a 21-day dermal BCG lesion from a rabbit, stained darkly for the lysosomal enzyme β-galactosidase (Dannenberg, 1968; Dannenberg et al., 1968). Although the perifocal tuberculous granulation tissue contains thousands of macrophages, only those macrophages in locations where tubercle bacilli (and their products) are present seem to become activated and develop the power to destroy the bacillus. In other words, CMI is mainly a localized phenomenon. The darker the macrophage is stained for β-galactosidase, the more it resembles Lurie's mature epithelioid cell, which has destroyed tubercle bacilli. The relationship between β-galactosidase activity and destruction of tubercle bacilli was confirmed with ^{14}C-labeled bacilli and autoradiography (Ando et al., 1977). The section was lightly counterstained with hematoxylin. Magnification, ×200. (Photograph reprinted with permission from Dannenberg [1968].)

tions cause exudative-type lesions, which soon caseate, so that small or large areas of tuberculous pneumonia result (Fig. 8B and 16). Whether the disease heals or progresses depends on the extent of the disease, the number of bacilli, and their rate of multiplication. Small scattered foci readily heal or encapsulate, but areas of tuberculous pneumonia may progress into adjacent alveoli and bronchi.

Cavitary tuberculous lesions may never heal during the life of the patient. They may enlarge or shrink or may remain in a more or less stable condition. Spontaneous healing may be caused by a gradual collapse of the cavity, a progressive fibrosis from without, and/or an obstruction of the bronchocavitary junction followed by absorption of the air within the cavity and fibrotic organization. Fibrosis is often incomplete, and variable amounts of caseous and fibrocaseous material may remain within the fibrotic lesion. Calcium deposition is frequent, and occasionally ossification occurs. A "healed" cavity, like a "healed" caseous focus, is seldom completely free of tubercle bacilli, which may persist for years, often in a dormant state.

Since the advent of effective antimicrobial agents, "open healing" of cavities occurs. Successful treatment with antimicrobial agents eliminates most of the bacilli from the cavity. Inflammation then decreases, and much or all of the necrotic contents drains through the still patent bronchocavitary junction. Such drainage is facilitated if the cavity is located in an upper lobe (the usual place). Metaplastic bronchial epithe-

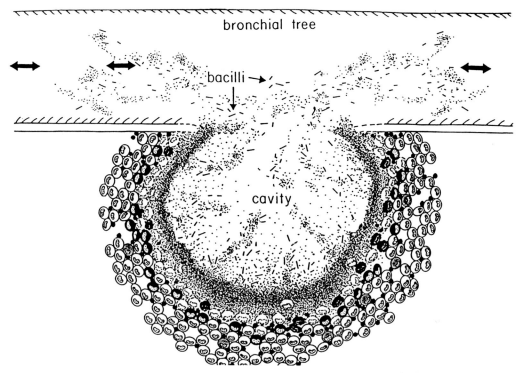

Figure 13. Stage V: a recently formed small cavity discharging liquefied caseous material into a bronchus. In this liquefied material, the bacilli have multiplied profusely and extracellularly. With such large numbers of bacilli, there is an increased likelihood of a mutation resulting in antimicrobial resistance. Also, the large quantities of bacilli and their antigens in the liquefied caseum overwhelm a formerly effective CMI, causing progression of the disease and the destruction of local tissues, including the wall of an adjacent bronchus (illustrated here). The liquefied caseous material is then discharged into the airways, so that the bacilli disseminate to other parts of the lung and to the environment.

lium (squamous with no cilia) may eventually line the cavity. The "open healed" cavity may persist as one with a thick or thin fibrotic wall or as an emphysematous bleb or bulla.

Ultimately, it is liquefaction that perpetuates the disease in mankind. Among the large number of bacilli, mutants resistant to antimicrobial agents may arise. For this reason, tuberculosis is often treated with four or even five antimicrobial agents simultaneously.

Macrophages do not survive in liquefied (or even solid) caseous material. Possibly, they have been passively sensitized to tuberculin and other antigens that are present there in high (lethal) concentrations. Possibly, the macrophages entering the liquefied caseum are killed by toxic fatty acids originating from host cells and/or the bacilli (Poole and Florey, 1970; Hemsworth and Kochan, 1978). Thus, activated macrophages (produced by well-developed CMI) are completely ineffective in controlling the extracellular multiplication of bacilli within a cavity.

The factors that cause liquefaction are largely unknown, but in experimental animals, liquefaction is associated with high levels of tuberculin reactivity (Yamamura et al., 1974) and elevated hydrolytic enzymes (probably proteinases, nucleases, and lipases) (Dannenberg and Sugimoto, 1976). A subtle change in the nature of the

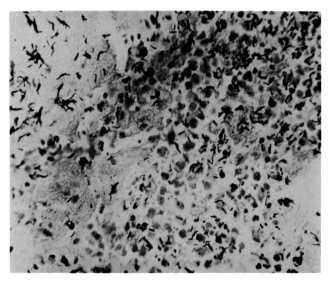

Figure 14. Wall of a cavity from one of Lurie's genetically resistant rabbits 8 weeks after the inhalation of human-type tubercle bacilli. The liquefied caseous tissue (right) and liquefying caseous tissue (left) are both swarming with (rod-shaped) acid-fast bacilli. Such bacilli were formerly inhibited in solid caseous tissue, but they now grow profusely in the liquefied menstruum present in the wall of the cavity. Magnification, ×600. (Photograph reprinted with permission from Lurie et al. [1955].)

tissue-damaging pathways may be involved (Yamamura, 1958; Yamamura et al., 1974). The breakdown products of caseous material are osmotically active, so that water is absorbed from the surrounding tissue, and an excellent culture medium for tubercle bacilli is created. At present, no therapeutic agent exists to prevent liquefaction, but appropriate antimicrobial therapy can markedly reduce the number of viable bacilli and in time arrest the disease.

BASIC TYPES OF TUBERCULOUS LESIONS AND DISEASE

The majority of pulmonary tuberculous infections of human beings are arrested before they cause clinical disease. In such cases, the inhalation of tubercle bacilli causes an inapparent lesion that is sufficient to produce a positive tuberculin reaction but is usually not large enough to be detected in a chest radiograph.

The various types of lesions and disease found in human pulmonary tuberculosis are listed in Table 1 (Rich, 1951; Dannenberg and Tomashefski, 1988). The lesions sometimes change from one type to another or are a composite of several. Also, one type of lesion may coexist in the lung with other types. Tuberculosis is a local disease in that each lesion is handled by the host almost as if the other lesions did not exist. Thus, lesions in one area of the lung may progress while lesions in another area stabilize or even regress. Even parts of a single lesion may progress while other parts remain stable. Finally, the disease as a whole may fluctuate between periods of exacerbation and remission.

APPLICATIONS OF TISSUE-DAMAGING AND MACROPHAGE-ACTIVATING IMMUNE RESPONSES TO CLINICAL TUBERCULOSIS

CMI, Cellular Immunity, and Acquired Cellular Resistance

The terms CMI, cellular immunity, and acquired cellular resistance are often used

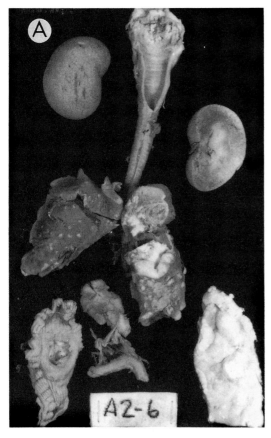
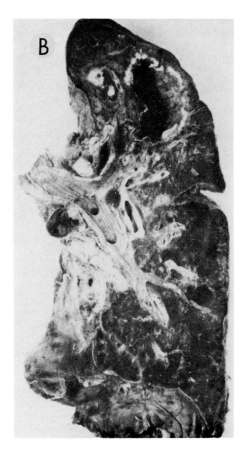

Figure 15. (A) Cavity in one of Lurie's natively resistant inbred rabbits that had inhaled a single unit of one to three virulent bovine-type tubercle bacilli 9 months previously. The primary lesion eventually formed the cavity, from which large numbers of bacilli infected the larynx and the gut. The tracheobronchial lymph nodes and the kidneys show no overt tuberculous lesions. (Photograph reprinted with permission from Lurie [1941].) (B) Single large cavity in the upper lobe of an adult human being. The hilar lymph nodes are only slightly involved, and the rest of the lung has only a few tuberculous lesions.

interchangeably. However, Mackaness (1968) used the term acquired cellular resistance and Dannenberg (1968) used the term cellular immunity to designate the existence of many activated macrophages in the host, usually at the site where the bacilli are located. In contrast, the term CMI is a more inclusive term. It designates a clonally expanded T-lymphocyte population (specific for the antigens of the tubercle bacillus) whether or not increased numbers of activated macrophages are also present. In other words, the term CMI is used to represent the potential for a rapid development

of acquired cellular resistance because of the expanded specific T-cell population. In addition, CMI often (but not always) includes the actual presence of such acquired resistance, i.e., large numbers of locally activated macrophages produced by the expanded specific T-cell population and their lymphokines.

Duration and Specificity of CMI and Its Recall upon Reinfection

The following principles were established by Mackaness and his associates by infect-

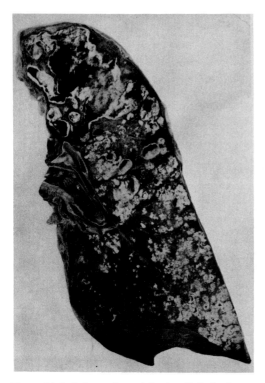

Figure 16. Left lung of an adult who died of tuberculosis. A large cavity is present in the upper lobe. Bacilli and their tuberculin-like antigens from this cavity caused the caseous bronchopneumonia found in the rest of the lung.

Table 1. Basic types of pulmonary tuberculosis[a]

Types of lesions
  Encapsulated caseous, liquefied, or calcified nodules
  Proliferative type lesions
  Exudative type lesions
  Cavities

Types of disease
  Small discrete tubercles of hematogenous origin; focally localized or scattered diffusely throughout both lungs (miliary tuberculosis)
  Liquefied caseous lesions with cavity formation and bronchogenic spread
  Progressive, locally destructive lesions

[a] Table is adapted from Rich (1951).

ing mice with several kinds of facultative intracellular bacteria (Mackaness, 1968; briefly reviewed by Dannenberg [1968]).

After immunization with BCG, acquired cellular resistance (i.e., the number of activated macrophages) decreases with time. Such resistance, however, can be rapidly recalled to full strength by reexposure to the BCG immunizing antigens. From the first exposure, the host retains increased numbers of (clonally expanded) T cells with specific receptors for these antigens. Upon reexposure to BCG antigens, these T cells rapidly produce lymphokines, which cause local macrophage (and lymphocyte) accumulation and activation.

The injection of other types of facultative intracellular bacteria does not recall the host's immunity to the tubercle bacillus.

However, once macrophages have been activated in local sites (by BCG, the specific antigen), these macrophages can nonspecifically destroy a variety of facultative intracellular microorganisms (in the same local sites). The specificity of CMI resides entirely in the T lymphocyte, not the macrophage. Macrophages kill facultative intracellular microorganisms only nonspecifically.

Mackaness (1968) gave the immunizing (and recalling) BCG intravenously. In this case, most of the bacilli were deposited in the liver and spleen, where many local sites containing activated macrophages developed. Such macrophages could readily destroy other types of facultative intracellular bacilli that would be deposited mainly in the liver and spleen by a subsequent intravenous injection.

The number of specific T cells in the blood and tissues decreases with time, and the tuberculin reaction may even disappear. These events may occur if the tubercle bacilli and their antigens are eliminated. Nonetheless, an expanded specific T-cell population remains, and upon antigenic stimulation, this population further expands to a point at which CMI and tuberculin reaction are again apparent.

Effect of Vaccines on Establishment of Pulmonary Tuberculous Lesions

Vaccination cannot prevent the establishment of an infection with the tubercle bacillus; it can prevent only the disease (Dannenberg, 1990). Inhaled virulent tubercle bacilli are ingested by alveolar macrophages. These highly activated cells usually destroy the inhaled tubercle bacillus before it has a chance to multiply (in both vaccinated and nonvaccinated individuals). Vaccination with BCG may initially increase the microbicidal power of the alveolar macrophages, because BCG produces a systemic infection. However, 1 or 2 years after vaccination with BCG, almost all but a small residuum of the BCG has been eliminated. At that time, one would expect vaccinated and nonvaccinated individuals to show no difference in the number of alveolar macrophages or in the microbicidal abilities of these macrophages. Thus, both the vaccinated and the nonvaccinated host would initially destroy the same number of inhaled virulent bacilli or allow the same number to multiply.

When first inhaled, a unit of one to three bacilli (which is the only size that can stay suspended in the airstream long enough to reach the alveolar spaces) contains insufficient antigen to stimulate the immune system. However, once this bacillary unit begins to multiply, sufficient antigen is produced to be recognized by lymphocytes. From this point on, vaccinated and nonvaccinated individuals show different responses. Vaccinated hosts show accelerated tubercle formation, i.e., a rapid local accumulation of activated lymphocytes and activated macrophages. These cells usually arrest the early microscopic focus of infection, thereby preventing clinical disease. In nonvaccinated hosts, the activation of lymphocytes and macrophages develops at a much slower pace, so that clinical disease occurs more frequently.

Because of the high incidence of tuberculosis in urban teaching hospitals, vaccination of the house staff with currently available BCG vaccines is again being considered in the United States (Greenberg et al., 1991).

Helpful and Harmful Effects of the Immune Processes

High sensitivity to tuberculin and the CMI response that accompanies it are always beneficial to the host in controlling the progression of beginning lesions arising from exogenous or hematogenously spread endogenous bacilli. (Such lesions always contain relatively few bacilli.) The strongly tuberculin-positive host responds with an accelerated accumulation of macrophages and specific T lymphocytes before the number of bacilli and their antigens reach high local concentrations. These immune responses can therefore stop the progression of such beginning lesions before much tissue damage and caseous necrosis can occur.

The presence of high sensitivity to tuberculin is harmful, however, when tubercle bacilli and their tuberculin-like antigens are present in high concentrations. Then, much caseation and tissue destruction result. Such high concentrations occur in areas of the lung that are seeded by liquefied caseous material discharging from a cavity into the bronchial tree. They also occur when bacilli grow logarithmically intracellularly within macrophages in genetically susceptible hosts and in hosts with immunodeficiencies.

The composition of the antigen, or antigen-adjuvant complex, may favor macrophage activation (CMI) over tissue damage (necrotizing DTH), or vice versa. (Tubercle bacilli contain built-in adjuvants.) In other words, some bacillary components (probably certain proteins complexed with certain carbohydrates and lipids) may stimulate CMI with minimal tissue damage, whereas other proteins, e.g., the tuberculopeptides that produce the tuberculin reaction, may produce more tissue damage with less CMI. Such relationships need further study.

One of the challenges to researchers developing new tuberculosis vaccines will be to purify components of the bacilli that produce more activated (microbicidal) macrophages and less tissue destruction. Animal models, such as tuberculous rabbits and guinea pigs, which develop high levels of tuberculin sensitivity, would be a prerequisite for efficient screening of such components.

Local Immunity

Acquired cellular resistance, i.e., activated microbicidal macrophages, produced by the CMI process is a local phenomenon (Dannenberg, 1968; Dannenberg et al., 1968). Macrophages enter the tuberculous lesion in a nonimmune, nonactivated state. They become activated and develop acquired resistance only locally, wherever T cells are stimulated to produce cytokines by the bacilli and their antigens (Fig. 12). The greater the local accumulation of macrophages and the greater their activation, the greater will be their ability to destroy the tubercle bacillus.

In a regressing tuberculous lesion, macrophages and bacilli usually interact in the following manner. A poorly activated macrophage that contains numerous bacilli dies and releases its bacillary load (Fig. 11). Then, the highly activated (microbicidal) macrophages (that have accumulated nearby due to the immune response) ingest and kill the released bacilli, thereby stopping the progression of the lesion and furthering its resolution.

Systemic Immunity

Greater numbers of T lymphocytes with specific receptors for the bacillary antigens are present in the blood and lymphoid tissues of individuals with DTH and CMI than in the blood and tissues of nonimmune individuals (Dannenberg, 1968, 1989; Mackaness, 1968). These T cells had clonally expanded during the immunizing exposure. Therefore, at sites where the bacilli are deposited, greater numbers of specific (and nonspecific) T cells accumulate and produce lymphokines. The resulting high local concentration of lymphokines accelerates macrophage accumulation and activation. The activated macrophages destroy the bacilli before they multiply appreciably, so that the lesions remain small and heal rapidly. As mentioned above, such accelerated tubercle formation (Mackaness, 1968) is the reason small secondary tubercles of either exogenous or endogenous (Balasubramanian et al., 1992) origin usually do not progress in immunocompetent adult human beings.

In immune infection-free individuals, the only systemic immunity may be an expanded specific T-cell population. This T-cell population causes an accelerated tubercle formation at sites where tubercle bacilli are deposited. Thus, systemic immunity is in reality the ability to rapidly produce local immunity.

CONCLUSIONS

(i) Activated macrophages can kill the tubercle bacilli they ingest. Under normal conditions, i.e., before infection begins, most of the alveolar macrophages are nonspecifically activated.

(ii) During infection, tubercle bacilli multiply logarithmically in nonactivated macrophages. Their cytoplasm provides a very fertile "soil" for such bacillary growth.

(iii) The tissue-damaging immune response is the main mechanism by which the host stops bacillary growth in nonactivated macrophages. It kills the bacilli-laden macrophages (and nearby tissues), forming a caseous necrotic focus. Tubercle bacilli do not multiply appreciably in such solid caseous material.

(iv) This favorable result occurs at the expense of host tissues. In susceptible hosts, when the bacilli escape from the edge of the caseous focus, they are ingested by immature nonactivated macrophages (from the bloodstream). In the cytoplasm of these nonactivated cells, the bacilli again find fertile soil in which to grow. And again, the host's tissue-damaging immune response will kill the bacilli-laden macrophages (and nearby tissues). If continued, so much viable lung tissue is sacrificed that the host will die.

(v) Only the macrophage-activating immune response, also called CMI or acquired cellular resistance, can stop this continued destruction of host tissues caused by the tissue-damaging reaction to bacillary antigens. In hosts that develop good CMI, immunologically specific T cells and their lymphokines (especially gamma interferon) produce a perifocal mantle of highly activated macrophages around the caseous center. These macrophages ingest and destroy the bacilli that escape from the edge of the caseous center. Continued destruction of host tissue is no longer required to stop the multiplication of the bacillus, because the bacillus now resides in highly activated macrophages.

(vi) When solid caseous tissue liquefies, the tubercle bacillus again finds fertile soil in which to multiply logarithmically. For the first time during the course of the disease, the bacillus multiplies extracellularly, frequently reaching tremendous numbers. Such numbers may not be controlled even in a highly immune host. Due to the tissue-damaging immune response, the bacilli and/or their tuberculin-like products often cause extensive necrosis. One (or more) bronchi is eroded, a cavity forms, and the bacilli can spread throughout the airways to other parts of the lung and to the outside environment. Also, mutants resistant to antimicrobial agents may arise because of the large numbers of bacilli present.

(vii) Therapeutic agents to prevent lique- faction or to prevent its continuation are greatly needed to treat tuberculosis and limit the spread of this disease to other people.

Acknowledgments. We are grateful to the late Max B. Lurie, of the University of Pennsylvania, for the fundamental understanding of tuberculosis that he personally gave to one of us (A.M.D., Jr.). We are also indebted to Ilse M. Harrop for superb editorial assistance; to Joseph M. Dieter, Jr., who drew Fig. 9; and to Roberta R. Proctor and Lester J. Dyer, who drew Fig. 1, 4, and 5 (all from The Johns Hopkins Medical Institutions). Figures 7B, 8A, 8B, 15B, and 16 are from the collection of the late A. R. Rich and W. G. MacCallum, Department of Pathology, School of Medicine, The Johns Hopkins University.

Financial support for the studies in the laboratory of A.M.D., Jr. came from the following grants: AI-27165 from the National Institute of Allergy and Infectious Diseases; ES-03819 for The Johns Hopkins Environmental Health Sciences Center from the National Institute of Environmental Health Sciences, Research Triangle Park, N.C.; and HL-10342 from the National Heart, Lung, and Blood Institute, Bethesda, Md. G.A.W.R. acknowledges support from the World Health Organization, the British Medical Research Council, and the Wellcome Trust.

REFERENCES

Allison, M. J., P. Zappasodi, and M. B. Lurie. 1962. Host-parasite relationships in natively resistant and susceptible rabbits on quantitative inhalation of tubercle bacilli. *Am. Rev. Respir. Dis.* **85:**553–569.

Ando, M., A. M. Dannenberg, Jr., M. Sugimoto, and B. S. Tepper. 1977. Histochemical studies relating the activation of macrophages to the intracellular destruction of tubercle bacilli. *Am. J. Pathol.* **86:**623–634.

Balasubramanian, V., E. H. Wiegeshaus, and D. W. Smith. 1992. Growth characteristics of recent sputum isolates of *Mycobacterium tuberculosis* in guinea pigs infected by the respiratory route. *Infect. Immun.* **60:**4762–4767.

Boom, W. H., R. S. Wallis, and K. A. Chervenak. 1991. Human *Mycobacterium tuberculosis*-reactive CD4+ T-cell clones: heterogeneity in antigen recognition, cytokine production, and cytotoxicity for mononuclear phagocytes. *Infect. Immun.* **59:**2737–2743.

Canetti, G. 1955. *The Tubercle Bacillus in the Pulmonary Lesion of Man*, p. 130. Springer Publishing Co., Inc., New York.

Dannenberg, A. M., Jr. 1968. Cellular hypersensitivity and cellular immunity in the pathogenesis of tuberculosis: specificity, systemic and local nature, and associated macrophage enzymes. *Bacteriol. Rev.* **32:**85–102.

Dannenberg, A. M., Jr. 1978. Pathogenesis of pulmonary tuberculosis in man and animals: protection of personnel against tuberculosis, p. 65–75. *In* R. J. Montali (ed.), *Mycobacterial Infection of Zoo Animals*. Smithsonian Institution Press, Washington, D.C.

Dannenberg, A. M., Jr. 1984. Pathogenesis of tuberculosis: native and acquired resistance in animals and humans, p. 344–354. *In* L. Leive and D. Schlessinger (ed.), *Microbiology—1984*. American Society for Microbiology, Washington, D.C.

Dannenberg, A. M., Jr. 1989. Immune mechanisms in the pathogenesis of pulmonary tuberculosis. *Rev. Infect. Dis.* **11**(Suppl. 2):S369–S378.

Dannenberg, A. M., Jr. 1990. Controlling tuberculosis: the pathologist's point of view. *Res. Microbiol.* **141:**192–196, 262–263.

Dannenberg, A. M., Jr. 1991. Delayed-type hypersensitivity and cell-mediated immunity in the pathogenesis of tuberculosis. *Immunol. Today* **12:**228–233.

Dannenberg, A. M., Jr. 1993. Immunopathogenesis of pulmonary tuberculosis. *Hosp. Pract.* **28:**33–40 or 51–58.

Dannenberg, A. M., Jr. 1994. Pathogenesis of pulmonary tuberculosis: host-parasite interactions, cell-mediated immunity, and delayed-type hypersensitivity: basic principles, p. 17–39. *In* D. Schlossberg (ed.), *Tuberculosis*, 3rd ed. Springer Verlag, New York.

Dannenberg, A. M., Jr., O. T. Meyer, J. R. Esterly, and T. Kambara. 1968. The local nature of immunity in tuberculosis, illustrated histochemically in dermal BCG lesions. *J. Immunol.* **100:**931–941.

Dannenberg, A. M., Jr., and M. Sugimoto. 1976. Liquefaction of caseous foci in tuberculosis. *Am. Rev. Respir. Dis.* **113:**257–259. (Editorial.)

Dannenberg, A. M., Jr., and J. F. Tomashefski, Jr. 1988. Pathogenesis of pulmonary tuberculosis, p. 1821–1842. *In* A. P. Fishman (ed.), *Pulmonary Diseases and Disorders*, 2nd ed., vol. 3. McGraw-Hill Book Co., New York.

Dubos, R., and J. Dubos. 1952. *The White Plague: Tuberculosis, Man and Society*. Little, Brown & Co., Boston.

Greenberg, P. D., K. G. Lax, and C. B. Schechter. 1991. Tuberculosis in house staff: a decision analysis comparing the tuberculin screening strategy with the BCG vaccination. *Am. Rev. Respir. Dis.* **143:**490–495.

Hemsworth, G. R., and I. Kochan. 1978. Secretion of antimycobacterial fatty acids by normal and activated macrophages. *Infect. Immun.* **19:**170–177.

Kaufmann, S. H. E. 1988. CD8$^+$ T lymphocytes in intracellular microbial infections. *Immunol. Today* **9:**168–174.

Koch, R. 1891. Fortsetzung der Mittheilungen über ein Heilmittel gegen Tuberculose. (Continuation of the communication concerning a treatment for tuberculosis.) *Dtsch. Med. Wochenschr.* **1891**(Jan. 15):101–102.

Long, E. R. 1958. *The Chemistry and Chemotherapy of Tuberculosis*, 3rd ed., p. 106–108, 122–124. The Williams & Wilkins Co., Baltimore.

Lowrie, D. B. 1990. Is macrophage death on the field of battle essential to victory, or a tactical weakness in immunity against tuberculosis? *Clin. Exp. Immunol.* **80:**301–303.

Lurie, M. B. 1941. Heredity, constitution and tuberculosis: an experimental study. *Am. Rev. Tuberc.* **44**(3)(Suppl.):1–125.

Lurie, M. B. 1964. *Resistance to Tuberculosis: Experimental Studies in Native and Acquired Defensive Mechanisms*. Harvard University Press, Cambridge, Mass.

Lurie, M. B., S. Abramson, and A. G. Heppleston. 1952. On the response of genetically resistant and susceptible rabbits to the quantitative inhalation of human-type tubercle bacilli and the nature of resistance to tuberculosis. *J. Exp. Med.* **95:**119–134.

Lurie, M. B., and A. M. Dannenberg, Jr. 1965. Macrophage function in infectious disease with inbred rabbits. *Bacteriol. Rev.* **29:**466–476.

Lurie, M. B., P. Zappasodi, and C. Tickner. 1955. On the nature of genetic resistance to tuberculosis in the light of the host-parasite relationships in natively resistant and susceptible rabbits. *Am. Rev. Tuberc. Pulm. Dis.* **72:**297–323.

Mackaness, G. B. 1968. The immunology of antituberculous immunity. *Am. Rev. Respir. Dis.* **97:**337–344. (Editorial.)

Poole, J. C. F., and H. W. Florey. 1970. Chronic inflammation and tuberculosis, p. 1183–1224. *In* H. W. Florey (ed.), *General Pathology*, 4th ed. The W. B. Saunders Co., Philadelphia.

Rich, A. R. 1951. *The Pathogenesis of Tuberculosis*, 2nd ed. Charles C Thomas, Publisher, Springfield, Ill.

Riley, R. L., C. C. Mills, F. O'Grady, L. U. Sultan, F. Wittstadt, and D. N. Shivpuri. 1962. Infectiousness of air from a tuberculosis ward. Ultraviolet irradiation of infected air: comparative infectiousness of different patients. *Am. Rev. Respir. Dis.* **85:**511–525.

Salahuddin, S. Z., R. M. Rose, J. E. Groopman, P. D. Markham, and R. C. Gallo. 1986. Human T lymphotropic virus type III infection of human alveolar macrophages. *Blood* **68:**281–284.

Selwyn, P. A., D. Hartel, V. A. Lewis, E. E. Schoenbaum, S. H. Vermund, R. S. Klein, A. T. Walker, and G. H. Friedland. 1989. A prospective study of the risk of tuberculosis among intravenous drug users with human immunodeficiency virus infection. *N. Engl. J. Med.* **320**:545–550.

Shima, K., A. M. Dannenberg, Jr., M. Ando, S. Chandrasekhar, J. A. Seluzicki, and J. I. Fabrikant. 1972. Macrophage accumulation, division, maturation, and digestive and microbicidal capacities in tuberculous lesions. I. Studies involving their incorporation of tritiated thymidine and their content of lysosomal enzymes and bacilli. *Am. J. Pathol.* **67**:159–180.

Smith, D. W., and G. E. Harding. 1977. Animal model of human disease: experimental airborne tuberculosis in the guinea pig. *Am. J. Pathol.* **89**:273–277.

Stead, W. W., J. W. Senner, W. T. Reddick, and J. P. Lofgren. 1990. Racial differences in susceptibility to infection by *Mycobacterium tuberculosis*. *N. Engl. J. Med.* **322**:422–427.

Tsuda, T., A. M. Dannenberg, Jr., M. Ando, H. Abbey, and A. R. Corrin. 1976. Mononuclear cell turnover in chronic inflammation: studies on tritiated thymidine-labeled cells in blood, tuberculin traps, and dermal BCG lesions of rabbits. *Am. J. Pathol.* **83**:255–268.

Yamamura, Y. 1958. The pathogenesis of tuberculous cavities. *Adv. Tuberc. Res.* **9**:13–37.

Yamamura, Y., Y. Ogawa, H. Maeda, and Y. Yamamura. 1974. Prevention of tuberculous cavity formation by desensitization with tuberculin-active peptide. *Am. Rev. Respir. Dis.* **109**:594–601.

Tuberculosis: Pathogenesis, Protection, and Control
Edited by Barry R. Bloom
© 1994 American Society for Microbiology, Washington, DC 20005

Chapter 28

Mechanisms of Pathogenesis in Tuberculosis

Graham A. W. Rook and Barry R. Bloom

KOCH PHENOMENON, TISSUE DAMAGE, AND PROTECTIVE IMMUNITY IN THE PATHOGENESIS OF TUBERCULOSIS

In the 1890s, Robert Koch observed that a primary infection of guinea pigs with *Mycobacterium tuberculosis* in the skin produced a nonhealing lesion and that reinoculation of the animals after several weeks produced only a firm, red nodule that necrosed and finally healed. These observations first suggested the existence of immunity to tuberculosis infection. When tuberculous guinea pigs were challenged intradermally with a culture supernatant of *M. tuberculosis* (old tuberculin) or with live organisms, there was necrosis both locally in the challenge site and at a distance in the preexisting tuberculous lesion (Koch, 1891). This reaction, now known as "the Koch phenomenon," protected against virulent organisms, perhaps among other reasons because the local necrosis caused sloughing of the tissue containing the organisms, since similar necrosis in deep sites

or in the lungs failed to eliminate the bacteria. Thus, if guinea pigs were preimmunized by protocols that gave rise to necrotizing skin test reactivity equivalent to the local necrosis elicited by Koch, they were rendered more rather than less susceptible to infection by intramuscular injection of a small number of virulent organisms. In contrast, immunization protocols priming small tuberculin reactions were protective (Wilson et al., 1940). These observations led to endless confusion. For instance, is the Koch phenomenon an exaggerated version of the tissue-damaging process seen routinely in tuberculosis lesions? If so, what is the relationship between this tissue-damaging response and protection? The problem is that we do not know the mechanisms involved at the cellular or molecular level. Therefore, we do not know whether the tissue damage, the Koch phenomenon, and the protection are "excessive" and "regulated" manifestations of similar pathways or whether they are the results of qualitatively different immunological mechanisms (Dannenberg, 1968). The balance between cell-mediated immunity and tissue damage throughout the course of this disease determines what form the disease takes and may not be dissimilar to the spectrum in leprosy that has been correlated to the balance of Th1 and Th2 lymphocyte subsets (Salgame et al., 1992; Bloom et al., 1992). In the ideal

Graham A. W. Rook • Department of Medical Microbiology, University College London Medical School, 67-73 Riding House Street, London W1P 7PP, United Kingdom. *Barry R. Bloom* • Howard Hughes Medical Institute, Albert Einstein College of Medicine, 1300 Morris Park Avenue, Bronx, New York 10461.

case, which is the situation for the large proportion of tuberculin-positive individuals who have been infected but show no evidence of disease, an early and appropriate cell-mediated immune response develops and controls the infection. While the tissue-damaging component is excessive in only a small number of individuals infected with *M. tuberculosis*, it is largely responsible for the clinical manifestations of the disease, and the control of this excess would reduce much of the pulmonary destruction that occurs. The little that we do know about these mechanisms is discussed in this chapter and in chapter 27.

Activated Macrophages: Discrepancy between Mouse and Human

The topic of activated macrophages is discussed in detail in chapter 27, but in brief, the microbicidal mechanism is uncertain, particularly in relation to humans. Since the work of Mackaness (1968), mostly with *Listeria monocytogenes*, demonstrated the enhanced nonspecific bactericidal activity of macrophages activated by mediators released from lymphocytes primed and stimulated to specific antigens, activated macrophages have usually been assumed to be important effectors in mycobacterial diseases as well. This view is compatible with histological evidence, as outlined above. However, most of the published work involves mouse macrophages. Murine macrophages can be activated to inhibit or destroy virulent *M. tuberculosis* in vitro. This can be achieved with class II major histocompatibility complex (MHC)-restricted T-cell lines (Rook et al., 1985) or with lymphokines (Rook et al., 1986a; Flesch and Kaufmann, 1990). More recently, it has become apparent that by activation with gamma interferon (IFN-γ) and either lipopolysaccharide or tumor necrosis factor alpha (TNF-α), murine macrophages can be triggered to release nitric oxide (NO), which is required for the my-

cobactericidal activity of macrophages (Denis, 1991a; Chan et al., 1992).

The situation is still less clear when we consider human macrophages. To our knowledge, only two authors have claimed to be able to induce killing of virulent *M. tuberculosis* by human monocytes or monocyte-derived macrophages in vitro (Denis, 1991b; Crowle, 1990). The authors of this chapter have been unable to demonstrate such killing. At best, a slowing of the rate of intracellular replication by about one generation in four was achieved following addition of recombinant IFN-γ and calcitriol (Rook et al., 1986b). IFN-γ alone frequently causes increased growth of *M. tuberculosis* in human cells (Rook et al., 1986a, b). Moreover, it seems that human monocytes are unable to generate tetrahydrobiopterin, which is an essential cofactor for arginine-dependent NO synthesis (Stuehr et al., 1991). We are careful to note that these studies have been carried out with blood monocytes, not tissue macrophages. Since other human cell types, e.g., endothelial cells and liver cells, can produce this NO in large quantities, it is not clear whether human macrophages are unable to do so or whether the correct combination of cytokines and culture conditions or tissue sources has simply not yet been found.

Cytotoxic T Cells

While T-cell-derived lymphokines and the activated macrophage represent a necessary condition for protection, it is certainly not the whole story even in the mouse. In vitro evidence exists that cytotoxic T cells recognizing mycobacterial antigens do develop in both humans and mice (Kaufmann, 1988; Ottenhoff et al., 1988; Orme et al., 1992). Transgenic animals whose gene for β2-microglobulin is disrupted and who are unable to express class I MHC on the cell membrane have greatly increased susceptibility to tuberculosis

(Flynn et al., 1992). This implies a role for CD8$^+$ T cells, possibly cytotoxic cells. Interestingly, β2-microglobulin "knockout" mice were unaffected by infection with BCG or avirulent *M. tuberculosis* H37Ra. One way that an antigen known initially to be taken up into an endosomal compartment could be presented to MHC class I-restricted cytotoxic lymphocytes (CTL) would be by its ability to escape from phagolysosomes into the cytoplasm, as has been found for *Listeria* and *Shigella* spp. In mycobacterial infeciton, the issue remains controversial. There is electron microscopic evidence that virulent *M. tuberculosis* can escape from the phagosome (Myrvik et al., 1984; McDonough et al., 1993). In the latter work, it is noteworthy that in the 7-day macrophage cultures studied, only the virulent H37Rv and not the avirulent *M. tuberculosis* H37Ra or BCG strain was observed in the cytoplasmic compartment. On the other hand, when rapid freezing techniques are used to preserve membranes, there is evidence that *M. tuberculosis* retains host lysosomal membrane antigens and may still be within a vesicle (Xu et al., in press). It is possible that processing of antigen via the class I pathway is important, allowing the host to kill parasitized cells that are failing to exert bactericidal effects. This failure could result from an unusual intracellular location of the organisms or, according to a recent report, from a failure to present the antigens of such organisms (Pancholi et al., 1993) (further discussed below).

γδ T Cells

A large proportion of human peripheral blood γδ T cells, even from PPD-negative donors, will proliferate in response to mycobacteria (Kabelitz et al., 1990; Uyemura et al., 1991). In vitro, these cells secrete a pattern of cytokines similar to those of Th1 cells (see below) and are cytotoxic. It is reasonable to speculate that they may be involved early in immunity to tuberculosis, but there is only circumstantial evidence for this (Barnes et al., 1992). Knockout mice unable to generate these T cells may reveal their relevance to the control of mycobacterial infection.

Lymphokines and Cytokines

Recent experiments involving *M. tuberculosis* infection of transgenic mice are providing new and interesting information on the role of some lymphokines and cytokines. As would be expected, knockout mice with a disruption in the gene for IFN-γ succumb rapidly (within 3 weeks) to *M. tuberculosis* infection. In contrast, mice will eventually die, although after many weeks, from BCG (Dalton et al., 1993; Cooper et al., 1993; Flynn et al., 1993). While knockout mice for TNF-α are not yet available, it has been possible to treat mice with neutralizing anti-TNF antibodies. This has led to dissemination of BCG infection (Kindler et al., 1989) and rapid death of *M. tuberculosis* (Flynn et al., submitted). Thus, TNF is a necessary condition for protection, again suggesting the importance of NO and reactive nitrogen intermediates in protection. Together, these data suggest to us that multiple immune mechanisms are required for protection. On the basis of available data, we believe that both MHC class II-restricted T-cell-derived cytokines, at least IFN-γ, macrophage-derived TNF-α, and MHC class I-restricted T-cell responses, probably CTL, are necessary conditions for protection; none is sufficient, and the roles of γδ T cells and other cytokines remain to be elucidated.

TISSUE-DAMAGING MECHANISMS IN TUBERCULOSIS

Direct Toxicity and Enhanced Susceptibility of Individual Cells to TNF-α

M. tuberculosis has some toxicity for cells in vitro. This is particularly noticeable with monocytes, which often die if they take up more than five bacilli. Conversely, monocytes or macrophages can take up very large numbers of *M. avium* without obvious toxic effects. It had previously been suggested that *M. tuberculosis* has the ability to inhibit lysosomal fusion, which could contribute to the survival of the pathogen in macrophages (Armstrong and Hart, 1975). In those studies, fusion could be blocked by agents that prevented lysosomal acidification, and *M. tuberculosis* produced ammonia in abundance (Gordon et al., 1980). In this context, recent studies by Sturgill-Koszycki et al. (in press) indicate that vacuoles formed around *M. avium* fail to acidify below pH 6.3 to 6.5. Immunoelectron microscopy indicated that the vacuoles containing the mycobacteria contain lysosomal proteins but not the proton-ATPase responsible for acidification. Because other lysosomal membrane markers were present, this result indicates remarkably selective fusion of vesicular membrane proteins. Because of the difficulty in securing *M. tuberculosis* cultures that are 100% viable, it is always difficult to ascertain with certainty whether fused vesicles contain primarily nonviable organisms and whether the bacilli found in nonfused vesicles are responsible for most of the damage. Recent studies by McDonough et al. (1993) indicate that lysosomal fusion occurred very rapidly in murine or human macrophages infected in vitro with live or dead *M. tuberculosis* or BCG. However, the intracellular fates differed. BCG essentially remained in fused phagolysomes for the entire 7-day observation period. Both H37Rv and H37Ra *M. tuberculosis* strains rapidly appeared to bud or extrude from the fused phagolysosome to form a unique vesicle, with the organisms enclosed by a very tightly apposed membrane. Over time, fusion of secondary lysosomes failed to occur in these tightly membrane-apposed containing vesicles, and much of the multiplication of *M. tuberculosis* occurred in these vesicles. Between

4 and 7 days, only the virulent strain of *M. tuberculosis*, H37Rv, escaped from these tightly apposed membrane vesicles and entered the cytoplasm. These results, with electron-dense markers used for lysosomes, thus confirmed and extended the earlier observations by Myrvik et al. (1984) indicating that *M. tuberculosis* could escape from phagolysosomes into the cytoplasm. However, using immunoelectron micrographic techniques designed to preserve membranes, Xu et al. (in press) found that all bacilli appear to be surrounded with host cell membrane and membrane antigen and may not be free within the cytoplasm. Escape from phagolysosomes would represent one of the few biological differences between avirulent and virulent strains of *M. tuberculosis* that could be directly related to virulence, and so the issue is an important one to resolve. Not only is it relevant for antigen presentation to MHC class I-restricted CTL, but *M. tuberculosis* that enters the cytoplasm of macrophages could exert direct toxic effects on the cells or may increase the susceptibility of infected cells to TNF-α that is discussed below.

M. tuberculosis is readily taken up by a wide variety of nonmacrophage cell types in vitro (Shepard, 1958; Filley and Rook, 1991; Filley et al., 1992), and such cells are much less susceptible to the toxicity of the organism. This has been shown for several cell lines and also for human endothelial cells and fibroblasts. This is paradoxical, because unlike *M. leprae*, *M. tuberculosis* is not seen inside such cells in vivo. One possibility is that in vivo these cells are killed quickly, so that parenchymal cells infected with bacilli are rarely seen in histological sections of tissues. An alternative answer may lie in the observation that cells containing *M. tuberculosis* are rendered exquisitely sensitive to killing by TNF-α (Filley and Rook, 1991; Filley et al., 1992). Therefore, macrophages infected in vitro may be killed by their own production of TNF-α, while nonmacrophage cells survive in vitro in the absence of TNF-α but are rapidly killed in vivo, since TNF-α is probably abundant in lesions, as discussed below. The ability to increase sensitivity to TNF-α was prominent in virulent strains of *M. tuberculosis* but weak in H37Ra and virtually absent from *M. avium* and BCG strains (Filley and Rook, 1991). Finally, if CTL are engaged, they would have the capability of lysing parenchymal cells expressing mycobacterial antigens in association with MHC class I.

The Koch Phenomenon

As outlined above, Koch noted that 4 to 6 weeks after establishment of infection in guinea pigs, intradermal challenge with whole organisms or culture filtrate resulted in necrosis locally and in the original tuberculous lesion (Koch, 1891). Similar phenomena occur in humans. The tuberculin test is frequently necrotic in subjects who are or have been tuberculous. This is not an inevitable consequence of the delayed hypersensitivity response to tuberculin, because necrosis does not occur when the same test is performed in healthy BCG recipients or in tuberculoid leprosy patients. Moreover, Koch sought to exploit this phenomenon for the treatment of tuberculosis and found that injection of larger quantities of culture filtrate (old tuberculin) subcutaneously into tuberculosis patients would evoke necrosis in established tuberculous lesions at distant sites (Anderson, 1891). This resulted in necrosis and sloughing of the lesions of skin tuberculosis (lupus vulgaris, usually caused by bovine strains), but when similar necrosis was evoked in deep lesions in the spine or lungs, the results were disastrous and merely provided further necrotic tissue in which the bacteria could proliferate. This treatment was therefore abandoned.

This phenomenon shows parallels with the Shwartzman reaction. Shwartzman observed that a site primed by an injection of gram-negative bacteria (though endotoxin will substitute) undergoes necrosis if a second dose of gram-negative organisms (or endotoxin) is injected intravenously 24 h later (Shwartzman, 1937). Several early workers demonstrated that mycobacterial lesions will undergo necrosis if the animal is subsequently challenged intravenously or subcutaneously with endotoxin-rich bacteria (Bordet, 1931), endotoxin (Shands and Senterfitt, 1972), or muramyl dipeptide (Nagao and Tanaka, 1985), and this necrosis is accompanied by massive systemic release of TNF-α (Carswell et al., 1975). It is thought that the "prepared" inflammatory site is abnormally susceptible to circulating cytokines and activated cells resulting from the second challenge injection. Direct injection of cytokines, particularly TNF-α, into such sites will cause similar necrosis (Rothstein and Schreiber, 1988). Recent studies suggest, however, that the susceptibility of mycobacterial lesions to such necrosis differs in one fundamental way from that studied by Shwartzman. The injection of mycobacterial components (if genuinely endotoxin free) will not prepare a site for TNF-α-mediated necrosis unless CD4[+] T-cell reactivity has previously been primed (Al Attiyah et al., 1992). Moreover, recent studies have revealed that such sites undergo necrosis only if the CD4[+] T-cell-mediated response involved is mixed Th1-Th2 or Th0, while in contrast, mycobacterial immunization schedules leading exclusively to Th1 cytokine release yield T-cell-mediated inflammatory sites that are not sensitive to TNF-α-mediated damage (Hernandez-Pando and Rook, unpublished data). Perhaps, therefore, the role of TNF-α depends on what the T cells are doing. Is the Koch phenomenon a "T-cell-dependent" Shwartzman reaction in a susceptible, mixed Th1-Th2 inflammatory site?

A second set of mediators that must be considered is reactive oxygen intermediates and reactive nitrogen intermediates. Much evidence has shown that macrophages can be activated by IFN-γ to release reactive oxygen intermediates, O_2, H_2O_2, and hydroxyl radicals. Chan et al. (1992) showed that these compounds were not microbicidal for *M. tuberculosis*. They further showed that IFN-γ and TNF-α activated mouse macrophages to release reactive nitrogen intermediates that were mycobactericidal. One mechanism by which NO is cytotoxic for mammalian cells is by binding to the Fe-S centers present in some critical enzymes, including ribonucleotide reductase (Nathan and Hibbs, 1991). The triggering of oxygen radicals and nitric oxide release by infected macrophages could in fact damage those and adjacent cells and contribute to tissue pathology.

Even if these speculations are correct, they do not provide a complete account of the mechanism of tissue damage in tuberculosis. More important, they leave us uncertain as to the link between the acute necrotic phenomenon evoked by Koch and the slowly evolving necrosis leading to caseation, liquefaction, calcification, and cavity formation described above.

We cannot rule out several other possible mechanisms. CTL were considered above as possible components of the protective pathway, but increased activity of such cells could also contribute to the increased killing of infected macrophages. Indeed, we know too little to rule out any effector cell type.

Excessive Cytokine Release

In view of the ability of *M. tuberculosis* to increase the sensitivity to TNF-α of individual cells, the ability of the CD4$^+$ T-cell-mediated response to render a whole tissue sensitive to the same cytokine, and the Shwartzman-like nature of Koch's "cure" for tuberculosis, we must consider the possibility that TNF-α in synergy with other cytokines is a component of tissue destruction in humans. The bacteria produce potent triggers of cytokine release

(Rook et al., 1987; Valone et al., 1988; Moreno et al., 1989; Silva and Faccioli, 1988). Blood monocytes (Takashima et al., 1990) and alveolar macrophages (Rook and Al Attiyah, 1991) from tuberculosis patients release TNF-α "spontaneously" in large quantities, and the cytokine is present in the lung (Barnes et al., 1990). In view of the weight loss seen in humans, it is interesting that cytokine-induced wasting can be evoked by injecting very small quantities of trehalose dimycolate (cord factor) dissolved in oil into the peritoneal cavities of mice (Silva and Faccioli, 1988). Circulating levels of TNF-α inhibitors are also high in the serum of tuberculosis patients (Foley et al., 1990). These are extracellular domains of receptors shed in response to TNF-α release. Thus, TNF-α is certainly released in the human disease. Its role is uncertain, but recent studies show that administration of thalidomide, which reduces mRNA levels for TNF-α, to tuberculosis patients causes rapid symptomatic improvement and weight gain (Kaplan, 1993), as it did for reducing erythema nodosum in leprosy (Sampaio et al., 1991). In the mouse, on the other hand, TNF-α is clearly necessary for protection, though as discussed in the previous section, this is probably not the whole story, and protection may depend on the type of T-cell reactivity at the site into which TNF is released. Studies by Kindler et al. (1989) showed that treatment of mice with polyclonal anti-TNF-α antibodies inhibited granuloma formation, leading to disseminated infection with BCG. However, in *M. tuberculosis*-infected mice treated with neutralizing monoclonal antibodies to TNF-α, Flynn et al. (submitted) have evidence that granuloma-like structures formed, but the mice were unable to control the infection. Interestingly, the granulomas in the anti-TNF-α-treated mice were necrotizing, while the control mice, which were able to restrict the growth of *M. tuberculosis*, had nonnecrotizing granulomas. Thus, although TNF-α probably plays a role, these data indicate that high levels of TNF-α are not necessary for induction of tissue necrosis in mice. It will be crucial to resolve the discrepancies between the results using the polyclonal and monoclonal anti-TNF antibodies through transgenic knockout mice unable either to express the appropriate TNF receptors or to produce TNF-α itself.

Tuberculin Shock

As will be discussed below, tuberculosis patients have defective adrenal function, and some have reduced ability to increase cortisol levels in response to adrenocorticotropin, so they have little "adrenal reserve." This adrenal deficit may explain a tendency to go into "tuberculin shock" (systemic Koch phenomenon?) if chemotherapy causes rapid release of bacterial antigens and cytokine triggers (Scott et al., 1990). This complication is most often seen in patients with severe disseminated disease and in patients with protein malnutrition and liver damage. It may be relevant that in experimental models, liver damage greatly enhances susceptibility to the toxicity of TNF-α released in response to bacterial components (Freudenberg and Galanos, 1991).

REGULATION OF PROTECTIVE AND TISSUE-DAMAGING RESPONSES IN TUBERCULOSIS

In the absence of certainty about the effector mechanisms involved, any discussion of the regulation of the protective and tissue-damaging responses must be somewhat speculative.

Th1 and Th2 Cells: Selection of Functional T-Cell Subsets and Disease Progression

Functional T-cell subsets in mice (Mosmann and Moore, 1991) and humans (Romagnani, 1991; Salgame et al., 1991) have been defined by the patterns of lympho-

kines they produce (see chapter 25 for more detailed discussion). Type 1 CD4$^+$ and CD8$^+$ CTL produce IFN-γ, interleukin-2 (IL-2), and lymphotoxin. Type 2 CD4$^+$ (Th2) cells and CD8$^+$ T cells produce predominantly IL-4. Each subset exerts negative regulation upon the other (Romagnani, 1991; Maggi et al., 1992), and together with the major regulatory cytokines IL-12 and IL-10 produced primarily by macrophages, they largely determine the type of T-cell response that ensues. Thus, the cytokine profile observed in mycobacterium-responsive human cells from healthy donors may be influenced by the conditions used (Haanen et al., 1991; Barnes et al., 1993) and can be altered by the addition of cytokines or cytokine-neutralizing antibodies (Maggi et al., 1992). In many experimental intracellular infections, e.g., with *Leishmania* spp., the type 1 response is protective and the type 2 response leads to disease progression. In helminth infections, the reverse may be true. In human leprosy, the type 1 response is associated with resistance and the type 2 response is associated with the lepromatous or unresponsive form (Bloom et al., 1992). One wonders whether the anergy seen in a quarter of tuberculosis patients may be related to Th2 function, and evidence for effects of type 2 cytokines in tuberculosis has been discussed by Rook (1991; Rook et al., 1993b).

In many chronic infections or inflammatory diseases, there is a permanent or transient switch from a Th1 pattern of response to Th2. Such a switch appears to occur, for example, in schistosomiasis (Grzych et al., 1991) and syphilis (Fitzgerald, 1992) patients. Does the evidence for a Th2 component in the response of tuberculosis patients mentioned above suggest a similar trend in this disease? It is certainly interesting that the necrosis that occurs around the ova in murine schistosomiasis occurs at precisely the time when a Th2 response becomes superimposed on a preexisting Th1 pattern (Grzych et al., 1991). It is not impossible that a similar mixed pattern of response lies behind the necrosis seen in tuberculosis (Barnes et al., 1993), and as pointed out above, it is these "mixed" responses that are TNF-α sensitive in one murine model.

Current dogma states that the cytokines released by Th1 cells enhance Th1 activity and inhibit Th2. Why, then, does the Th1 → Th2 shift occur? We should remember that the Th1/Th2 ratio is not determined only by cytokines. The release of prostaglandins from activated macrophages downregulates Th1 cells (Phipps et al., 1991), and there are two striking endocrine changes in tuberculosis patients that would indeed be expected to have this effect.

(i) Formation of calcitriol in mycobacterial lesions. The macrophages of tuberculosis patients, following activation by IFN-γ, express an active 1a-hydroxylase and rapidly convert 25(OH)-vitamin D3 to calcitriol (Rook et al., 1986b; Rook, 1988). Their T cells may also produce this enzyme (Cadranel et al., 1990). This is a potent phenomenon, leading occasionally to leakage of calcitriol into the periphery and to hypercalcemia, though it has in the past been difficult to understand its role in the disease (Rook, 1988). It now seems possible that this is a feedback mechanism that tends to downregulate Th1 and enhance Th2 responses, because the active vitamin D3 metabolite, $1,25(OH)_2$ cholecalciferol (calcitriol), inhibits production of IFN-γ and IL-2 and increases production of IL-4 and IL-5 (Daynes et al., 1991).

(ii) Adrenal dysfunction in tuberculosis. The pituitary-adrenal axis is disturbed in patients with tuberculosis (Sarma et al., 1990; Ellis and Tayoub, 1986; Barnes et al., 1989a). There is a striking reduction in adrenal function, reflected by low levels of essentially all steroid metabolites in 24-h urine collections (Rook et al., unpublished data). Most significantly, patients have very low or absent levels of dehydroepiandrosterone sulfate (DHEA-S) (Ellis and Tayoub, 1986; Rook et al., unpublished data). This may have serious consequences, because the desulfated form, DHEA, is a genuine antiglucocorticoid, the specific receptors for which are found in T cells (Meikle et al., 1992). DHEA enhances Th1 activity (Suzuki et al., 1991; Daynes et al., 1990) and inhibits the effects of glucocorticoids, including their tendency to suppress Th1 lymphocytes and enhance Th2 (Blauer et al., 1991; Daynes et al., 1990; Fischer and Konig, 1991). For instance, a single dose of DHEA given before dexamethasone can block the ability of the latter to cause depletion of thymocytes and temporary unresponsiveness of peripheral T cells to mitogens (Blauer et al., 1991). Therefore, the T cells of tuberculosis patients may be chronically exposed to glucocorticoid effects unopposed by the antiglucocorticoid influence of DHEA. This may not only encourage a Th1-to-Th2 switch but even contribute to the fall in $CD4^+$ T-cell count and in CD4/CD8 ratio that is well documented in tuberculosis patients (Singhal et al., 1989; Ainslie et al., 1992) and of course in human immunodeficiency virus-infected patients, in whom DHEA is also low and correlates directly with CD4 counts (Wisniewski et al., 1993). This has been developed further as a hypothesis elsewhere (Rook et al., 1993b).

At present, no information exists on the patterns of lymphokines and T-cell subsets in healing and progressing lesions in tuberculosis. It is clear that there is anergy associated with a significant proportion of tuberculosis patients and that the prognosis for these patients prior to chemotherapy was generally poorer than for those with tuberculin hypersensitivity. That picture is suggestive of the type 2 (Th2) predominance in many patients with lepromatous leprosy. We suggest the hypothesis that in the proportion of individuals infected with *M. tuberculosis* who progress to primary progressive or recrudescent forms of disease, the relative ratios of type 1 (Th1) to type 2 (Th2) are altered. We propose further, on the basis of the requirement for MHC class I-restricted T-cell function for resistance to tuberculosis in mice and the finding that protection can be engendered by the 65-kDa antigen presented in transfected mammalian cells (Silva and Lowrie, in press), that the number of $CD8^+$ CTL may similarly be critical.

Roles of Different Antigenic Components of *M. tuberculosis*

Is there any evidence that protective cell-mediated immunity and the Koch phenomenon or tissue-damaging pathways represent responses to different components of the organism? It has long been the dream of many workers to create a novel vaccine, perhaps a modified BCG, that primes bactericidal cell-mediated immunity but not necrosis. The practical advantages would be even greater if nonnecrotizing skin test responsiveness could also be dissociated from induction of protective immunity. Such a vaccine, if achievable, would have many potential benefits (adapted from Dannenberg [1990]). (i) Vaccinated individuals would not be appreciably tuberculin positive, so that tuberculin testing of such persons would still be a useful procedure for diagnosing infection with virulent tubercle bacilli. (ii) A vaccine that evoked little or no delayed hypersensitivity could be given more than once to create high levels of immunity (especially in high-risk groups). (iii) If available, such a vaccine might replace isoniazid in preventive therapy for persons who recently became tuberculin positive, obviating hepatotoxicity and possibly bacillary resistance to the drug. (iv) Such a vaccine could be given to patients with active disease in order to boost the bactericidal pathways (immunotherapy). Tuberculin and BCG cannot be used for immunotherapy, because they evoke the Koch phenomenon, as Robert Koch discovered to his cost (Anderson, 1891).

How realistic a proposal is this? First, as discussed in detail in chapter 28, there is unambiguous evidence that tuberculin skin test reactivity can be dissociated from protection in humans. For example, while greater than 85% skin test conversion was observed in most of the controlled trials of BCG against tuberculosis, protection varied from 0 to 77%. Similarly, in the British Medical Research Council trials, one lot of vole bacillus vaccine produced very few skin test conversions yet protected well against tuberculosis. This and other studies with different strains of BCG (Fine, 1989) suggest that tuberculin positivity may not correlate with protective immunity in humans. At present, there is no evidence that different antigens are involved. If, as suggested by Kaufmann (1988) and Flynn et al. (1992, 1993), both type 1 CD4 T-cell function and lymphokines and $CD8^+$ MHC class I-restricted T cells are required for protection, it might be expected that different antigens and certainly different T-cell epitopes would be involved. On the other hand, there is good evidence that the necrosis-inducing components can be separated from at least some potentially protective antigens, as explained below.

The tissue-damaging responses are evoked by tuberculin, which is a very crude culture supernatant from old autolysing bacterial cultures precipitated by trichloroacetic acid or ammonium sulfate. Such supernatants contain fragments of essentially all the antigens of *M. tuberculosis*. Therefore, it is not meaningful to speak of removing the "tuberculin" antigens from BCG. However, the Koch phenomenon (manifested as a necrotic skin test reaction) appears to be targeted preferentially toward the species-specific epitopes of *M. tuberculosis*. When tuberculosis patients are skin tested with antigens derived from other mycobacteria, they do not exhibit necrotic responses. In fact, their responses to the common, cross-reactive mycobacterial antigens or epitopes (which must include the heat shock proteins [HSPs]) are diminished (Kardjito et al., 1986). Moreover, there is strong evidence that cell-mediated immunity to mycobacteria can be initiated, perhaps mediated, by responses to the common, cross-reactive epitopes. The more obvious reasons for this assertion are as follows. (i) BCG protects against leprosy as well as or better than it does against tuberculosis (Fine et al., 1986). (ii) Small positive tuberculin reactions in non-BCG recipients correlate with protection (Palmer and Long, 1966; Fine, 1994). These reactions are caused by contact with environmental mycobacteria. (iii) A common cross-reactive protein (the 65-kDa HSP) from *M. leprae* that is expressed in murine macrophages can engender protection against tuberculosis in a murine model (Silva and Lowrie, in press). (iv) Tuberculosis patients may lose their skin test responses to common cross-reactive antigens (Kardjito et al., 1986).

At present, the simplest way to achieve a preparation with suitable adjuvant properties that contains a broad spectrum of common but not species-specific antigens of *M. tuberculosis* appears to be use of related mycobacterial species. Preliminary results of immunotherapy with an autoclaved member of the fast-growing subgenus *M. vaccae* are encouraging (Onyebujoh and Rook, 1991; Rook et al., 1994). For immunotherapy as an adjunct to chemotherapy, such preparations are at present the only possibility. It is dangerous to administer species-specific components of *M. tuberculosis* to patients, since they may trigger the Koch phenomenon and tuberculin shock (Anderson, 1891).

Tuberculin Skin Test: Significance in Apparently Healthy People

One must consider at the outset, from the presently available evidence, that the tuberculin test, like the lepromin skin test, represents the consequences primarily of type 1 (Th1) CD4 T cells in response to mycobacterial antigens. If CD8 CTL are necessary for protection, their presence is unlikely to be readily detected by skin testing with tuberculoproteins that do not have access to the cytoplasmic compartment of antigen-presenting cells and are not presented in the context of MHC class I antigens.

In countries with a high standard of living, a positive test can be a diagnostic clue, but in developing countries, much tuberculin skin test positivity is due to frequent contact with ubiquitous environmental species. In such populations, a positive test has little validity as a diagnostic tool. On the other hand, a negative test (unless the patient has evidence of advanced disease or AIDS and is anergic) renders tuberculosis unlikely. Nevertheless, epidemiologically, even in developing countries, the test has some predictive power in healthy people. As already mentioned, small nonnecrotizing responses in people who have not received BCG correlate with a significantly decreased risk of developing tuberculosis, while large reactions (Koch phenomena?) correlate with an increased risk of disease, perhaps because many such individuals are in fact already infected (Palmer and Long, 1966; Fine, 1994).

A large or necrotic tuberculin reaction, remaining years after the primary disease has healed, probably signifies that a few dormant bacilli are still present in inapparent caseous foci. Such bacilli may be released from time to time and then rapidly destroyed, which gives a booster effect to the whole immune system, including to the level of tuberculin sensitivity.

Individuals who have been infected with the tubercle bacillus can in time become tuberculin negative with or without antimicrobial treatment. In some of these individuals, the tubercle bacillus may have been eradicated. In many, a recall of tuberculin sensitivity is produced by the antigens in tuberculin (purified protein derivative) injected for skin testing. When retested with intermediate-strength purified protein derivative, a person who was negative 3 weeks earlier may now be tuberculin positive as a result of the booster effect of tuberculin itself (Thompson et al., 1979).

Significance in Patients with Active Tuberculosis

The size of the dermal tuberculin reaction in patients is of limited prognostic significance (Lurie, 1964), though individuals who are very ill with tuberculosis may show a negative tuberculin skin test. However, when they are recovering, they again show a positive skin test. Several mechanisms could be involved, including compartmentalization of T cells, Th2 cell dominance, or suppressive cytokines from infected macrophages. Regarding compartmentalization, tuberculous lesions may collect most of the relevant circulating T cells, so that few are available to participate in the tuberculin reaction. This concept receives support from the fact that lymphocytes in bronchoalveolar lavage and pleural fluids (and presumably in other diseased tissues) contain a greater proportion of antigen-specific T cells, secrete greater quantities of lymphokines, and show a greater tendency to proliferate (in the presence of specific antigen) than T lymphocytes in the peripheral blood (Barnes et al., 1989b, 1990). Tuberculin-negative patients with active tuberculosis also have a greater number of monocytes and lymphocytes in their peripheral blood that exert apparently suppressive effects in vitro (Ellner and Wallis, 1989). Production of prostaglandin E_2 (Ellner and Wallis, 1989), or possibly IL-10 or transforming growth factor β, by these monocytes may contribute to their suppressive effects. Finally, as mentioned above, the balance of type 1 (Th1) to type 2 (Th2) T-cell subsets may be critical, and a switch from type 1 to type 2 responses (or to mixed responses) could result in anergy or sup-pressive effects on type 1 T-cell function and macrophage activation.

Persisting Viable Tubercle Bacilli

In human beings, after even an inapparent tuberculous infection heals, the lungs may contain one or more small encapsulated caseous foci. In such foci, tubercle bacilli may persist in a dormant and nonmetabolizing state, insusceptible to sterilization by antimicrobial agents. The bacilli may remain viable in the host for life and cause active disease when resistance is lowered by old age, corticosteroids, immunosuppressants, AIDS, or other factors. It is the presence of these bacilli that necessitates prolonged (6-month) courses of chemotherapy, with the resulting problems of cost, compliance, and drug resistance. It is not certain that drugs able to kill dormant or stationary-phase mycobacteria can be devised, since most microbicidal agents depend on actively metabolizing or dividing cells. Persistence of viable tubercle bacilli may also be the reason the positive tuberculin reaction is usually maintained for life. Each time the bacillus multiplies, the immune system may be stimulated.

In addition, tubercle bacilli may possibly persist within macrophages as forms with unusual cell walls (Stanford, 1987), and there are reports of mycobacterial genomic material in the tissues of some patients with sarcoidosis (Bocart et al., 1992; Fidler et al., 1993), in spite of the absence of bacteria detectable by conventional means. It is conceivable that similar forms exist in tuberculosis patients, and new studies with in situ polymerase chain reactions should help us explore this point.

Mycobacteria and Idiopathic or "Autoimmune" Diseases

Tuberculosis patients have a spectrum of autoantibodies that is remarkably similar to that seen in rheumatoid arthritis patients (Shoenfeld and Isenberg, 1988). They also have a striking change in the glycosylation of the immunoglobulin G heavy chain, and this is also characteristic of patients with rheumatoid arthritis or Crohn's disease and a subset of patients with sarcoidosis (Rook et al., 1993a). The immunotherapy discussed above leads to a rapid fall in percent agalactosyl immunoglobulin G in tuberculosis patients (Rook et al., 1994), though the significance of this remains to be elucidated.

The known capacity of mycobacterium-containing adjuvants (Freund's complete adjuvant) to facilitate experimental induction of autoimmunity and evidence that mycobacterial disease can be accompanied by a sterile arthropathy (reviewed by Rook et al. [1993a]) have reawakened speculation that some autoimmune syndromes may be cryptic infections or may be triggered by past encounters with mycobacterium-like organisms (Rook et al., 1993a). Interest was further increased by the discovery that T cells that will passively transfer the arthritis evoked in susceptible rat strains by Freund's complete adjuvant are able to recognize the mycobacterial 65-kDa HSP (van Eden et al., 1988).

HSPs are involved in assembly, folding, and transport of other cellular proteins and are expressed under various conditions of stress. These functions are fundamental to the survival of all life-forms, particularly under stressful conditions, when synthesis of HSPs may increase while synthesis of other proteins is reduced. HSPs are highly conserved throughout evolution, and there is striking sequence homology between the HSPs of microorganisms and those of higher animals. These facts, together with the demonstration that T cells mediating an experimental autoimmune disorder recognize the mycobacterial HSP65, have led to the following hypotheses, for each of which there is some evidence (compare reviews by Young and Elliott [1989], Polla [1991], and Cohen and Young [1991]). (i) The immune response to bacterial HSPs may

cross-react with host HSPs, leading to autoimmune disease. (ii) The immune response may focus its attention on HSPs because they are so conserved and may be induced by the stress of infection or inflammation. This may enable rapid recognition of any pathogen. (Inadvertent autoimmunity is a consequent risk.) (iii) Self-HSP-derived peptides presented by MHC molecules may be targets for cytotoxic cells. This would enable the immune response to detect and eliminate stressed autologous cells, which might facilitate recognition of transformed or infected cells.

At present, the evidence for recognition of HSPs by T cells from synovia of joints of patients with inflammatory arthritides or from thyroid tissue of patients with thyroiditis (reviewed by Young [1992]), despite the best efforts of several laboratories, have mostly been unsupportive of the HSP cross-reactivity hypothesis as the basis for autoimmunity, and sporadic reports of reactivity to the human homolog in juvenile chronic arthritis (De Graeff-Meeder et al., 1991) or in *Yersinia*-associated reactive arthritis (Hermann et al., 1991) are unconvincing, rely on few cell lines, and fail to exclude the possibility of contamination of the recombinant protein with the *Escherichia coli* products.

In tuberculosis, such autoimmune reactions could contribute to both caseous necrosis and liquefaction, but there is at present no direct evidence for this. In fact, desensitization to mycobacterial antigens prevented cavity formation in animals (Yamamura et al., 1974), indicating that if there is any autoimmune component, it is dependent on initiation by a mycobacterium-specific cellular immune response. We suggest that although the evidence for recognition of HSPs by CD4 Th cells is negligible, possibility must be considered that common cross-reactive HSP antigens could be recognized by MHC class I-restricted CTL. The logic is that HSPs are expressed as cytoplasmic antigens and would be expected to be presented in association with MHC class I antigens. Since any pathogen—viral, bacterial, or protozoal—that invaded the cytoplasm of infected cells would induce the same conserved antigens, there would be existing memory for CTL activity that could provide an early response. Cytotoxic CD4 T cells in humans have been reported to kill macrophages pulsed with the mycobacterial 65-kDa HSP (Ottenhoff et al., 1988) and stressed autologous cells in the absence of mycobacterial antigen, presumably through cross-reactive recognition of the autologous HSP (Koga et al., 1989), although this has not yet been confirmed. Finally, the results of Silva and Lowrie (in press) indicate that expression of the 65-kDa heat shock cognate protein of BCG in mouse macrophages provided effective immunization against challenge with *M. tuberculosis* and suggest that there must be some immune responses against HSP65 that can provide protection. While definitive evidence for a role of HSPs in either protection or autoimmunity is lacking, the available data are consistent with the hypothesis that if HSPs are involved, rather than being important at the level of MHC class II-restricted CD4 cells, they would preferentially engage $CD8^+$ MHC class I-restricted CTL. They could then exert cytotoxic activity on infected macrophages containing more bacilli than they are able to kill and presumably could liberate the bacilli to enable them to be phagocytosed by infiltrating macrophages that may be activated by the IFN-γ released locally by the $CD8^+$ CTL or $CD4^+$ Th1 cells in granulomas and be more effective in killing at lower multiplicities of infection. CTL might also kill somatic cells in the vicinity either infected with *M. tuberculosis* or stressed to express endogenous HSPs in association with MHC class I. Events that can be interpreted in this manner are seen in histopathological studies (Dannenberg, 1991). Clearly, it will be important to undertake experiments to establish the existence of human CTL, the nature of the antigens they recognize, and their relation to protection, tissue damage, and autoimmunity.

Acknowledgments. G.A.W.R. acknowledges support from the World Health Organization, the British Medical Research Council, and the Wellcome Trust.

REFERENCES

Ainslie, G. M., J. A. Solomon, and E. D. Bateman. 1992. Lymphocyte and lymphocyte subset numbers in blood and in bronchoalveolar lavage and pleural fluid in various forms of human pulmonary tuberculosis at presentation and during recovery. *Thorax* **47:**513–518.

Al Attiyah, R., C. Moreno, and G. A. W. Rook. 1992. TNF-alpha-mediated tissue damage in mouse footpads primed with mycobacterial preparations. *Res. Immunol.* **143:**601–610.

Anderson, M. C. 1891. On Koch's treatment. *Lancet* **i:**651–652.

Armstrong, J. A., and P. D. Hart. 1975. Phagosome-lysosome interactions in cultured macrophages infected with virulent tubercle bacilli: reversal of the usual nonfusion pattern and observations on bacterial survival. *J. Exp. Med.* **142:**1–16.

Barnes, D. J., S. Naraqi, P. Temu, and J. R. Turtle. 1989a. Adrenal function in patients with active tuberculosis. *Thorax* **44:**422–424.

Barnes, P. F., J. S. Abrams, S. Lu, P. A. Sieling, T. H. Rea, and R. L. Modlin. 1993. Patterns of cytokine production by mycobacterium-reactive human T cell clones. *Infect. Immun.* **61:**197–203.

Barnes, P. F., S.-J. Fong, P. J. Brennan, P. E. Twomey, A. Mazumder, and R. L. Modlin. 1990. Local production of tumor necrosis factor and IFN-gamma in tuberculous pleuritis. *J. Immunol.* **145:** 149–154.

Barnes, P. F., C. L. Grisso, J. S. Abrams, H. Band, T. H. Rea, and R. L. Modlin. 1992. Gamma delta T lymphocytes in human tuberculosis. *J. Infect. Dis.* **165:**506–512.

Barnes, P. F., S. D. Mistry, C. L. Cooper, C. Pirmez, T. H. Rea, and R. L. Modlin. 1989b. Compartmentalization of a CD4+ T lymphocyte subpopulation in tuberculous pleuritis. *J. Immunol.* **142:**1114–1119.

Blauer, K. L., M. Poth, W. M. Rogers, and E. W. Bernton. 1991. Dehydroepiandrosterone antagonises the suppressive effects of dexamethasone on lymphocyte proliferation. *Endocrinology* **129:**3174–3179.

Bloom, B. R., R. L. Modlin, and P. Salgame. 1992. Stigma variations: observations on suppressor T cells and leprosy. *Annu. Rev. Immunol.* **10:**453–488.

Bocart, D., D. Lecossier, A. de Lassence, D. Valeyre,

J.-P. Battesti, and A. Hance. 1992. A search for mycobacterial DNA in granulomatous tissues from patients with sarcoidosis using the polymerase chain reaction. *Am. Rev. Respir. Dis.* **145**:1142–1148.

Bordet, P. 1931. Contribution à l'étude de l'allergie. *C.R. Soc. Biol.* **107**:622–623.

Cadranel, J., M. Garabedian, B. Milleron, H. Guillozo, G. Akoun, and A. J. Hance. 1990. 1,25(OH)2 D3 production by T lymphocytes and alveolar macrophages recovered by lavage from normocalcaemic patients with tuberculosis. *J. Clin. Invest.* **85**:1588–1593.

Carswell, E. A., L. J. Old, R. L. Kassel, S. Green, W. Fiore, and B. Williamson. 1975. An endotoxin-induced serum factor that causes necrosis of tumours. *Proc. Natl. Acad. Sci. USA* **72**:3666–3670.

Chan, J., Y. Xing, R. S. Magliozzo, and B. R. Bloom. 1992. Killing of virulent Mycobacterium tuberculosis by reactive nitrogen intermediates produced by activated murine macrophages. *J. Exp. Med.* **175**:1111–1122.

Cohen, I. R., and D. B. Young. 1991. Autoimmunity, microbial immunity and the immunological homunculus. *Immunol. Today* **12**:105–110.

Cooper, A. M., D. K. Dalton, T. A. Stewart, J. P. Griffin, D. G. Russell, and I. M. Orme. 1993. Disseminated tuberculosis in interferon-γ gene-disrupted mice. *J. Exp. Med.* **178**:2242–2248.

Crowle, A. J. 1990. Intracellular killing of mycobacteria. *Res. Microbiol.* **141**:231–236.

Dalton, D. K., A. Pitts-Meek, S. Keshaw, I. S. Figari, A. Bradley, and T. A. Stewart. 1993. Multiple defects of immune cell function in mice with disrupted interferon-gamma genes. *Science* **259**:1739–1742.

Dannenberg, A. M., Jr. 1968. Cellular hypersensitivity and cellular immunity in the pathogenesis of tuberculosis: specificity, systemic and local nature, and associated macrophage enzymes. *Bacteriol. Rev.* **32**:85–102.

Dannenberg, A. M. 1990. Killing intracellular bacteria: dogmas and realities. *Res. Microbiol.* **141**:193–196.

Dannenberg, A. M. 1991. Delayed-type hypersensitivity and cell-mediated immunity in the pathogenesis of tuberculosis. *Immunol. Today* **12**:228–233.

Daynes, R. A., B. A. Araneo, T. A. Dowell, K. Huang, and D. Dudley. 1990. Regulation of murine lymphokine production in vivo. III. The lymphoid tissue microenvironment exerts regulatory influences over T helper cell function. *J. Exp. Med.* **171**:979–996.

Daynes, R. A., A. W. Meikle, and B. A. Araneo. 1991. Locally active steroid hormones may facilitate compartmentalization of immunity by regulating the types of lymphokines produced by helper T cells. *Res. Immunol.* **142**:40–45.

De Graeff-Meeder, E. R., R. van der Zee, G. T. Rijkers, H. J. Schuurman, W. Kuis, J. W. Bijlsma, B. J. Zegers, and W. van Eden. 1991. Recognition of human 60 kD heat shock protein by mononuclear cells from patients with juvenile chronic arthritis. *Lancet* **337**:1368–1372.

Denis, M. 1991a. Interferon-gamma-treated murine macrophages inhibit growth of tubercle bacilli via the generation of reactive nitrogen intermediates. *Cell. Immunol.* **132**:150–157.

Denis, M. 1991b. Killing of Mycobacterium tuberculosis within human monocytes: activation by cytokines and calcitriol. *Clin. Exp. Immunol.* **84**:200–206.

Ellis, M. E., and F. Tayoub. 1986. Adrenal function in tuberculosis. *Br. J. Dis. Chest* **80**:7–12.

Ellner, J. J., and R. S. Wallis. 1989. Immunologic aspects of mycobacterial infections. *Rev. Infect. Dis.* **11**(Suppl. 2):S455–S459.

Fidler, H. M., G. A. W. Rook, N. M. Johnson, and J. McFadden. 1993. Mycobacterium tuberculosis DNA in tissue affected by sarcoidosis. *Br. Med. J.* **306**:546–549.

Filley, E. A., H. A. Bull, P. M. Dowd, and G. A. W. Rook. 1992. The effect of Mycobacterium tuberculosis on the susceptibility of human cells to the stimulatory and toxic effects of tumour necrosis factor. *Immunology* **77**:505–509.

Filley, E. A., and G. A. W. Rook. 1991. Effect of mycobacteria on sensitivity to the cytotoxic effects of tumor necrosis factor. *Infect. Immun.* **59**:2567–2572.

Fine, P. E. M. 1989. The BCG story: lessons from the past and implications for the future. *Rev. Infect. Dis.* **11**(Suppl. 2):S353–S359.

Fine, P. E. M. 1994. Immunities in and to tuberculosis: implications for pathogenesis and vaccination, p. 53–74. *In* K. P. W. J. McAdam and J. D. H. Porter (ed.), *Tuberculosis: Back to the Future: Proceedings of the London School of Hygiene and Tropical Medicine 3rd Annual Public Health Forum.* John Wiley, Chichester.

Fine, P. E. M., J. M. Ponnighaus, N. Maine, J. A. Clarkson, and L. Bliss. 1986. The protective efficacy of BCG against leprosy in northern Malawi. *Lancet* **ii**:499–502.

Fischer, A., and W. Konig. 1991. Influence of cytokines and cellular interactions on the glucocorticoid-induced Ig (E, G, A, M) synthesis of peripheral blood mononuclear cells. *Immunology* **74**:228–233.

Fitzgerald, T. J. 1992. The TH1/TH2 switch in syphilitic infection: is it detrimental? *Infect. Immun.* **60**:3475–3479.

Flesch, I. E. A., and S. H. E. Kaufmann. 1990. Activation of tuberculostatic macrophage functions by gamma interferon, interleukin-4, and tumor necrosis factor. *Infect. Immun.* **58**:2675–2677.

Flynn, J. L., J. Chan, K. J. Triebold, D. K. Dalton, T. A. Steward, and B. R. Bloom. 1993. An essential role for IFN-γ in resistance to *Mycobacterium tu-*

berculosis infection. *J. Exp. Med.* **178**:2249–2254.

Flynn, J. L., M. M. Goldstein, K. J. Triebold, B. Koller, and B. R. Bloom. 1992. Major histocompatibility complex class I-restricted T cells are required for resistance to Mycobacterium tuberculosis infection. *Proc. Natl. Acad. Sci. USA* **89**:12013–12017.

Flynn, J. L., K. Pfeffer, R. Schreiber, K. J. Triebold, M. M. Goldstein, T. W. Mak, and B. R. Bloom. TNF-α is necessary for resistance to *Mycobacterium tuberculosis* in mice. Submitted for publication.

Foley, N., C. Lambert, M. McNicol, N. M. I. Johnson, and G. A. W. Rook. 1990. An inhibitor of the toxicity of tumour necrosis factor in the serum of patients with sarcoidosis, tuberculosis and Crohn's disease. *Clin. Exp. Immunol.* **80**:395–399.

Freudenberg, M. A., and C. Galanos. 1991. Tumor necrosis factor alpha mediates lethal activity of killed gram-negative and gram-positive bacteria in D-galactosamine-treated mice. *Infect. Immun.* **59**:2110–2115.

Gordon, A. H., P. D'Arcy Hart, and M. R. Young. 1980. Ammonia inhibits phagosome-lysosome fusion in macrophages. *Nature* (London) **286**:79–81.

Grzych, J. M., E. Pearce, A. Cheever, Z. A. Caulada, P. Caspar, S. Henry, F. Lewis, and A. Sher. 1991. Egg deposition is the stimulus for the production of TH2 cytokines in murine schistosomiasis mansoni. *J. Immunol.* **146**:1322–1340.

Haanen, J. B., R. de Waal-Malefijt, P. C. Res, E. M. Kraakman, T. H. Ottenhoff, R. R. de Vries, and H. Spits. 1991. Selection of a human T helper type 1-like T cell subset by mycobacteria. *J. Exp. Med.* **174**:583–592.

Hermann, E., A. W. Lohse, R. Van der Zee, W. Van Eden, W. J. Mayet, P. Probst, T. Poralla, K. H. Meyer zum Buschenfelde, and B. Fleischer. 1991. Synovial fluid-derived Yersinia-reactive T cells responding to human 65-kDa heat-shock protein and heat-stressed antigen-presenting cells. *Eur. J. Immunol.* **21**:2139–2143.

Kabelitz, D., A. Bender, S. Schondelmaier, B. Schoel, and S. H. E. Kaufmann. 1990. A large fraction of human peripheral blood gamma/delta positive T cells is activated by Mycobacterium tuberculosis but not by its 65-kD heat shock protein. *J. Exp. Med.* **171**:667–679.

Kaplan, G. 1993. Therapy trials in tuberculosis patients. *Robert-Koch-Symposium 1993 on Progress in Tuberculosis Research, Berlin.* (Abstract.)

Kardjito, T., J. S. Beck, J. M. Grange, and J. L. Stanford. 1986. A comparison of the responsiveness to four new tuberculins among Indonesian patients with pulmonary tuberculosis and healthy subjects. *Eur. J. Respir. Dis.* **69**:142–145.

Kaufmann, S. H. E. 1988. CD8+ T lymphocytes in

intracellular microbial infections. *Immunol. Today* **9**:168–174.

Kindler, V., A.-P. Sappino, G. E. Grau, P.-F. Piguet, and P. Vassalli. 1989. The inducing role of tumor necrosis factor in the development of bacterial granulomas during BCG infection. *Cell* **56**:731–740.

Koch, R. 1891. Fortsetzung über ein Heilmittel gegen Tuberculose. *Dtsch. Med. Wochenschr.* **17**:101–102.

Koga, T., A. Wand-Wurttenberger, J. DeBruyn, M. E. Munk, B. Schoel, and S. H. Kaufmann. 1989. T cells against a bacterial heat shock protein recognise stressed macrophages. *Science* **245**:1112–1115.

Lurie, M. B. 1964. *Resistance to Tuberculosis: Experimental Studies in Native and Acquired Defensive Mechanisms.* Harvard University Press, Cambridge, Mass.

Mackaness, G. B. 1968. The immunology of antituberculous immunity. *Am. Rev. Respir. Dis.* **97**:337–344.

Maggi, E., P. Parronchi, R. Manetti, C. Simonelli, M. P. Piccinni, F. S. Rugui, M. De Carli, M. Ricci, and S. Romagnani. 1992. Reciprocal regulatory effects of IFN-gamma and IL-4 on the in vitro development of human TH1 and TH2 clones. *J. Immunol.* **148**:2142–2147.

McDonough, K. A., Y. Kress, and B. R. Bloom. 1993. Pathogenesis of tuberculosis: interaction of *Mycobacterium tuberculosis* with macrophages. *Infect. Immun.* **61**:2763–2773.

Meikle, A. W., R. W. Dorchuck, B. A. Araneo, J. D. Stringham, T. G. Evans, S. L. Spruance, and R. A. Daynes. 1992. The presence of a dehydroepiandrosterone-specific receptor-binding complex in murine T cells. *J. Steroid Biochem. Mol. Biol.* **42**:293–304.

Moreno, C., J. Taverne, A. Mehlert, C. A. Bate, R. J. Brealey, A. Meager, G. A. W. Rook, and J. H. L. Playfair. 1989. Lipoarabinomannan from Mycobacterium tuberculosis induces the production of tumour necrosis factor from human and murine macrophages. *Clin. Exp. Immunol.* **76**:240–245.

Mosmann, T. R., and K. W. Moore. 1991. The role of IL-10 in crossregulation of TH1 and TH2 responses. *Immunol. Today* **12**(3):A49–A53.

Myrvik, Q. N., E. S. Leake, and M. J. Wright. 1984. Disruption of phagosomal membranes of normal alveolar macrophages by the H37Rv strain of Mycobacterium tuberculosis: a correlate of virulence. *Am. Rev. Respir. Dis.* **129**:322–328.

Nagao, S., and A. Tanaka. 1985. Necrotic inflammatory reaction induced by muramyl dipeptide in guinea-pigs sensitized by tubercle bacilli. *J. Exp. Med.* **162**:401–412.

Nathan, C. F., and J. B. Hibbs, Jr. 1991. Role of nitric oxide synthesis in macrophage antimicrobial activity. *Curr. Opin. Immunol.* **3**:65.

Onyebujoh, P., and G. A. W. Rook. 1991. Letter. *Lancet* **338**:1534.

Orme, I. M., E. S. Miller, A. D. Roberts, S. K. Furney,

J. P. Griffin, K. M. Dobos, D. Chi, B. Rivoire, and P. J. Brennan. 1992. T lymphocytes mediating protection and cellular cytolysis during the course of Mycobacterium tuberculosis infection: evidence for different kinetics and recognition of a wide spectrum of protein antigens. *J. Immunol.* **148**:189–196.

Ottenhoff, T. H., B. K. Ab, J. D. van Embden, J. E. Thole, and R. Kiessling. 1988. The recombinant 65kDa heat shock protein of Mycobacterium bovis Bacillus Calmette-Guerin/M. tuberculosis is a target molecule for CD4+ cytotoxic T lymphocytes that lyse human monocytes. *J. Exp. Med.* **168**:1947–1952.

Palmer, C. E., and M. W. Long. 1966. Effects of infection with atypical mycobacteria on BCG vacination and tuberculosis. *Am. Rev. Respir. Dis.* **94**:553–568.

Pancholi, P., A. Mirza, N. Bhardwaj, and R. M. Steinman. 1993. Sequestration from immune CD4+ T cells of mycobacteria growing in human macrophages. *Science* **260**:984–986.

Phipps, R. P., S. H. Stein, and R. L. Roper. 1991. A new view of prostaglandin E regulation of the immune response. *Immunol. Today* **12**:349–352.

Polla, B. S. 1991. Heat shock proteins in host-parasite interactions. *Immunol. Today* **12**(3):A38–A41.

Romagnani, S. 1991. Human TH1 and TH2 subsets: doubt no more. *Immunol. Today* **12**:256–257.

Rook, G. A. W. 1988. The role of vitamin D in tuberculosis. *Am. Rev. Respir. Dis.* **138**:768–770. (Editorial.)

Rook, G. A. W. 1991. Mobilising the appropriate T-cell subset: the immune response as taxonomist. *Tubercle* **72**:253–254.

Rook, G. A. W., et al. Unpublished data.

Rook, G. A. W., and R. Al Attiyah. 1991. Cytokines and the Koch phenomenon. *Tubercle* **72**:13–20.

Rook, G. A. W., B. R. Champion, J. Steele, A. M. Varey, and J. L. Stanford. 1985. I-A restricted activation by T cell lines of anti-tuberculosis activity in murine macrophages. *Clin. Exp. Immunol.* **59**: 414–420.

Rook, G. A. W., P. M. Lydyard, and J. L. Stanford. 1993a. A reappraisal of the evidence that rheumatoid arthritis, and several other idiopathic diseases, are slow bacterial infections. *Ann. Rheum. Dis.* **52**(Suppl. 1):S30–S38.

Rook, G. A. W., P. Onyebujoh, and J. L. Stanford. 1993b. TH1→TH2 switch and loss of CD4 cells in chronic infections; an immuno-endocrinological hypothesis not exclusive to HIV. *Immunol. Today* **14**:568–569.

Rook, G. A. W., P. Onyebujoh, E. Wilkins, H. M. Ly, R. Al Attiyah, G. M. Bahr, T. Corrah, H. Hernandez, and J. L. Stanford. 1994. A longitudinal study of % agalactosyl IgG in tuberculosis patients receiving chemotherapy, with or without immunotherapy. *Immunology* **81**:149–154.

Rook, G. A. W., J. Steele, M. Ainsworth, and B. R. Champion. 1986a. Activation of macrophages to inhibit proliferation of Mycobacterium tuberculosis: comparison of the effects of recombinant gamma-interferon on human monocytes and murine peritoneal macrophages. *Immunology* **59**:333–338.

Rook, G. A. W., J. Steele, L. Fraher, S. Barker, R. Karmali, J. O'Riordan, and J. Stanford. 1986b. Vitamin D3, gamma interferon, and control of proliferation of *Mycobacterium tuberculosis* by human monocytes. *Immunology* **57**:159–163.

Rook, G. A. W., J. Taverne, C. Leveton, and J. Steele. 1987. The role of gamma-interferon, vitamin D3 metabolines and tumor necrosis factor in the pathogenesis of tuberculosis. *Immunology* **62**:229–234.

Rothstein, J., and H. Schreiber. 1988. Synergy between tumor necrosis factor and bacterial products causes hemorrhagic necrosis and lethal shock in normal mice. *Proc. Natl. Acad. Sci. USA* **85**:607–611.

Salgame, P. R., J. S. Abrams, C. Clayberger, H. Goldstein, R. L. Modlin, J. Convit, and B. R. Bloom. 1991. Differing lymphokine profiles of functional subsets of human CD4 and CD8 T cell clones. *Science* **254**:279–282.

Sampaio, E. P., E. N. Sarno, R. Galilly, Z. A. Cohn, and G. Kaplan. 1991. Thalidomide selectively inhibits TNFα production by stimulated human monocytes. *J. Exp. Med.* **173**:699–703.

Sarma, G. R., I. Chandra, G. Ramachandran, P. V. Krishnamurthy, V. Kumaraswami, and R. Prabhakar. 1990. Adrenocortical function in patients with pulmonary tuberculosis. *Tubercle* **71**:277–282.

Scott, G. M., P. G. Murphy, and M. E. Gemidjioglu. 1990. Predicting deterioration of treated tuberculosis by corticosteroid reserve and C-reactive protein. *J. Infect.* **21**:61–69.

Shands, J. W., and V. C. Senterfitt. 1972. Endotoxin-induced hepatic damage in BCG-infected mice. *Am. J. Pathol.* **67**:23–40.

Shepard, C. C. 1958. A comparison of the growth of selected mycobacteria in HeLa, monkey kidney, and human amnion cells in tissue culture. *J. Exp. Med.* **107**:237–246.

Shoenfeld, Y., and D. A. Isenberg. 1988. Mycobacteria and autoimmunity. *Immunol. Today* **9**:178–182.

Shwartzman, G. 1937. *Phenomenon of Local Tissue Reactivity and Its Immunological, Pathological, and Clinical Significance*, p. 461. Paul B. Hoeber, New York.

Silva, C. L., and L. H. Faccioli. 1988. Tumor necrosis factor (cachectin) mediates induction of cachexia by cord factor from mycobacteria. *Infect. Immun.* **56**: 3067–3071.

Silva, C. L., and D. B. Lowrie. A single mycobacterial protein (hsp60) expressed by a transgenic antigen-presenting cell vaccinates mice against tuberculosis. *Immunology*, in press.

Singhal, M., J. N. Banavalikar, S. Sharma, and K. Saha. 1989. Peripheral blood T lymphocyte subpopulations in patients with tuberculosis and the effect of chemotherapy. *Tubercle* **70**:171–178.

Stanford, J. L. 1987. Much's granules revisited. *Tubercle* **68**:241–242.

Stuehr, D. J., H. J. Cho, N. S. Kwon, M. F. Weise, and C. F. Nathan. 1991. Purification and characterization of the cytokine-induced macrophage nitric oxide synthase: an FAD- and FMN-containing flavoprotein. *Proc. Natl. Acad. Sci. USA* **88**:7773–7777.

Sturgill-Koszycki, S., P. H. Schlesinger, P. Chakraborty, P. L. Haddix, H. L. Collins, A. K. Fok, R. D. Allen, S. L. Gluck, J. Heuser, and D. G. Russell. *Mycobacterium* phagosomes fail to acidify through exclusion of the vesicular proton-ATPase. *Science*, in press.

Suzuki, T., N. Suzuki, R. A. Daynes, and E. G. Engleman. 1991. Dehydroepiandrosterone enhances IL2 production and cytotoxic effector function of human T cells. *Clin. Immunol. Immunopathol.* **61**:202–211.

Takashima, T., C. Ueta, I. Tsuyuguchi, and S. Kishimoto. 1990. Production of tumor necrosis factor alpha by monocytes from patients with pulmonary tuberculosis. *Infect. Immun.* **58**:3286–3292.

Thompson, N. J., J. L. Glassroth, D. E. Snider, Jr., and L. S. Farer. 1979. The booster phenomenon in serial tuberculin testing. *Am. Rev. Respir. Dis.* **119**:587–597.

Uyemura, K., R. J. Deans, H. Band, J. Ohmen, G.

Panchamoorthy, C. T. Morita, T. H. Rea, and R. L. Modlin. 1991. Evidence for clonal selection of gamma/delta T cells in response to a human pathogen. *J. Exp. Med.* **174**:683–692.

Valone, S. E., E. A. Rich, R. S. Wallis, and J. J. Ellner. 1988. Expression of tumor necrosis factor in vitro by human mononuclear phagocytes stimulated with whole *Mycobacterium bovis* BCG and mycobacterial antigens. *Infect. Immun.* **56**:3313–3315.

van Eden, W., J. E. R. Thole, R. van der Zee, A. Noordzij, J. D. A. van Embden, E. J. Yamamura, E. J. Hensen, and I. R. Cohen. 1988. Cloning of the mycobacterial epitope recognised by T lymphocytes in adjuvant arthritis. *Nature* (London) **331**:171–173.

Wilson, G. S., H. Schwabacher, and I. Maier. 1940. The effect of the desensitisation of tuberculous guinea-pigs. *J. Pathol. Bacteriol.* **50**:89–109.

Wisniewski, T. L., C. W. Hilton, E. V. Morse, and F. Svec. 1993. The relationship of serum DHEA-S and cortisol levels to measures of immune function in human immunodeficiency virus-related illness. *Am. J. Med. Sci.* **305**:79–83.

Xu, S., S. Sturgill-Koszycki, T. van Heyningen, A. Cooper, D. Chatterjee, I. Orme, P. Allen, and D. G. Russell. Intracellular trafficking and the *Mycobacterium*-infected macrophage. *J. Immunol.*, in press.

Yamamura, Y., Y. Ogawa, H. Maeda, and Y. Yamamura. 1974. Prevention of tuberculous cavity formation by desensitization with tuberculin-active peptide. *Am. Rev. Respir. Dis.* **109**:594–601.

Young, D. B. 1992. Heat-shock proteins: immunity and autoimmunity. *Curr. Opin. Immunol.* **4**:396–400.

Young, R. A., and T. J. Elliott. 1989. Stress proteins, infection, and immune surveillance. *Cell* **59**:5–8.

Tuberculosis: Pathogenesis, Protection, and Control
Edited by Barry R. Bloom
© 1994 American Society for Microbiology, Washington, DC 20005

Chapter 29

Pathogenesis of Tuberculosis in Human Immunodeficiency Virus-Infected People

Sebastian Lucas and Ann Marie Nelson

BACKGROUND EPIDEMIOLOGY

Tuberculosis among human immunodeficiency virus (HIV)-infected people has become an epidemic within an epidemic. In industrialized countries, the overall proportion of patients with AIDS who have tuberculosis is <10% (De Cock et al., 1992; Louie et al., 1986). However, in developing countries, particularly in Africa, where more than two-thirds of all HIV-positive adults and 90% of all HIV-positive children reside (Mann et al., 1992), tuberculosis presents an overwhelming public health problem. In such countries, the 1.0 to 2.5% annual risk of tuberculous infection means that by the time of infection with HIV, half of the adults or more have already had a primary infection with tubercle bacilli.

HIV infection is the strongest known risk factor for the development of tuberculosis. In comparison with the 5 to 10% lifetime risk of developing a later tuberculosis lesion incurred by HIV-negative people with primary lesions, HIV-positive people who are Mantoux skin test positive have an 8%

annual risk of tuberculosis (Selwyn et al., 1989). In Rwanda, the rate ratio for the development of tuberculosis over a 2-year period among HIV-positive women was 22 compared with HIV-negative women (Allen et al., 1992). The proportion of tuberculosis patients in Africa who are HIV positive ranges from 25 to 67%. While HIV type 1 (HIV-1) is the predominant global HIV infection, the association with tuberculosis pertains for HIV-2-infected and dually infected people also (De Cock et al., 1992). Autopsy studies in Africa (Abidjan and Kinshasa) found that 38% of all HIV-positive cadavers and 43 to 54% of those dying with AIDS-defining pathology had active tuberculosis (Lucas et al., 1993; Nelson et al., 1993). Clearly, tuberculosis is the single most important opportunistic HIV-related disease in the developing world.

REACTIVATION VERSUS REINFECTION

Because of the known high incidence of infection by *Mycobacterium tuberculosis* in developing countries, it is usually assumed that the postprimary tuberculous disease follows from reactivation of latent infection. Autopsy of HIV-positive tuberculosis patients frequently reveals old fibrous or

Sebastian Lucas • Department of Histopathology, University College London Medical School, London WC1, United Kingdom. *Ann Marie Nelson* • Division of AIDS Pathology M003B, Armed Forces Institute of Pathology, Washington, D.C. 20306-6000.

calcified lesions of tuberculosis in the thorax that are adjacent to recent active lesions with bacilli. Studies in the pre-AIDS era found 26% of primary complex lesions (lung and hilar node) to contain cultivable bacilli (Opie and Aronson, 1927). However, this does not prove the reactivation hypothesis, since new lesions may also represent reinfection. Recent observations in Kenya suggest that at least some HIV-associated tuberculosis in adults is reinfection; relapse has been observed with a different genotype of *M. tuberculosis* (Hawken et al., 1993). Primary infection with *M. tuberculosis* in previously HIV-infected adult patients is observed in countries of low tuberculosis endemicity.

CD4 COUNTS AND TUBERCULOSIS

It is evident from several studies of the clinical presentation of HIV-positive patients that the HIV-associated opportunistic diseases develop at different levels of declining immunocompetence. Tuberculosis, being the most virulent, is often the earliest infection to present, while *M. avium* complex infection becomes prevalent only when the blood $CD4^+$ T-lymphocyte count is $<<100 \times 10^6$/liter (Nightingale et al., 1992). CD4 counts are used as a marker of the state of cellular immunocompetence of the host (normal range, 500 to $2,000 \times 10^6$/liter).

Table 1 and Fig. 1 indicate the relationships between CD4 count and presentation of tuberculosis in HIV-positive people. There are no correlated clinical, pathological, and immunological longitudinal studies of HIV-positive tuberculosis patients, all the data available being derived from cross-sectional studies. Figure 1 does not necessarily represent an individual but indicates at what point of immunodepression the various patterns of clinical and histological tuberculosis are encountered.

An autopsy study in Abidjan found that the median CD4 counts for patients who had disseminated tuberculosis with tuberculous meningitis were significantly higher

Table 1. Representative correlations of blood $CD4^+$ T-lymphocyte counts with clinicopathological presentation of tuberculosis

Clinical category	Location of study	Median CD4 count (10^6/liter)	Reference
HIV positive			
Pulmonary tuberculosis	Melbourne, Australia	250–500	Crowe et al., 1991
	San Francisco	367	Theuer et al., 1990
	New York City	299	Shafer et al., 1991
	Abidjan, Côte d'Ivoire	262	Ackah et al., 1993
	Kinshasa, Zaire	316	Mukadi et al., 1993
	Harare, Zimbabwe	251	Pozniak et al., 1992
Localized extrapulmonary tuberculosis	New York City	242	Shafer et al., 1991
	Abidjan, Côte d'Ivoire	197	Ackah et al., 1993
Lymph node tuberculosis	Kinshasa, Zaire	218	Lewin-Smith et al., 1993
Tuberculous meningitis	Abidjan, Côte d'Ivoire	137	Lucas et al., 1993
Disseminated miliary tuberculosis	New York City	79	Shafer et al., 1991
	Boston	70	Barber et al., 1990
	Abidjan, Côte d'Ivoire	40	Lucas et al., 1993
HIV negative			
Pulmonary tuberculosis	Abidjan, Côte d'Ivoire	824	Lucas et al., 1993
	Kinshasa, Zaire	830	Mukadi et al., 1993
	Harare, Zimbabwe	847	Pozniak et al., 1992

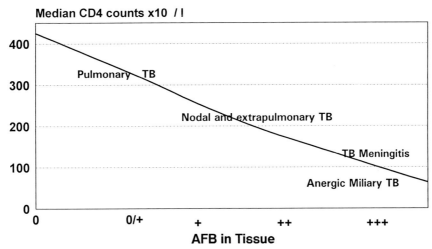

Figure 1. Clinical and immunopathological courses of HIV-associated tuberculosis. The figure does not represent one patient but is a composite of cross-sectional data (Table 1).

$(137 \times 10^6/\text{liter})$ than those for tuberculosis patients without meningitis $(40 \times 10^6/\text{liter})$ (De Cock et al., 1992; Lucas et al., 1993). This suggests that patients presenting with tuberculous meningitis are arriving at health centers earlier, because the meningitis causes a more notable symptomatology than the gradual debilitating effect of non-meningitic tuberculosis.

Some caution may be needed in interpreting the correlations of CD4 counts with tuberculosis clinical pathology. From the pre-AIDS era, there is evidence that pulmonary tuberculosis itself is immunosuppressive and causes a depression in blood CD4 counts that reverts on appropriate chemotherapy (Onsuaballi and Palmer, 1987; Beck et al., 1985). This is also seen in HIV-positive patients: one study in Zimbabwe found that in HIV-positive pulmonary tuberculosis patients, the presenting median CD4 count of $251 \times 10^6/\text{liter}$ had risen to $389 \times 10^6/\text{liter}$ after 1 year (Pozniak et al., 1992). Nonetheless, despite being derived from several continents, the CD4 data in Table 1 are remarkably consistent and comparable, indicating that the relative values do follow a systematic pattern.

CLINICAL PATTERNS OF TUBERCULOSIS IN HIV-POSITIVE PATIENTS

Many reviews compare the clinical presentation of tuberculosis in HIV-positive and HIV-negative people (Elliot et al., 1990). Tuberculosis precedes other AIDS-defining illnesses by up to 2 years in about half of the cases (Chaisson et al., 1987). Differences in HIV-positive patients include a higher proportion of cases with extrapulmonary or disseminated disease, a higher frequency of false-negative tuberculin skin tests, atypical features on chest radiographs, fewer cavitating lung lesions, a higher rate of adverse drug reactions, the presence of other AIDS-associated manifestations, and a higher death rate. The rate of sputum positivity for acid-fast bacilli (AFB) is not significantly affected by HIV status.

PATTERNS OF TUBERCULOSIS FOUND AT AUTOPSY IN HIV-POSITIVE PATIENTS

Table 2 shows the distribution of tuberculous lesions found at autopsy in two

Table 2. Distribution of tuberculosis lesions in HIV-positive patients at autopsy in Zaire and Côte d'Ivoire

Site of lesions	% of cadavers with active tuberculosis[a]	
	Kinshasa, Zaire (n = 27)	Abidjan, Côte d'Ivoire (n = 107)
Disseminated (>1 organ affected)	96	87
Lungs	93	93
Lungs only	4	5
Lymph nodes (any)	85	97
Hilar nodes	NA	96
Liver	78	84
Spleen	85	84
Kidney	56	55
Intestines	26	20
Meninges	NA	18
Adrenals	19	45
Thyroid	NA	10
Bone marrow	NA	80
Skin	NA	1
Pericardium	NA	8

[a] NA, data not available.

studies in Africa, from Kinshasa, Zaire, and Abidjan, Côte d'Ivoire. In the Abidjan study, tuberculosis was the prime cause of death (and single commonest cause) in 32% of HIV-positive cadavers. The overall prevalence of tuberculosis was 38% (Lucas et al., 1993). In 87% of cadavers, tuberculosis was disseminated to more than one organ, nearly always involving the lungs, liver, spleen, multiple internal lymph nodes, and bone marrow. The commonest gross pattern was miliary nodules in lung (Fig. 2), liver, and spleen and greatly enlarged, necrotic mesenteric and para-aortic nodes. One-half of the tuberculous lungs also showed consolidation, and half of these showed cavitation (insufficient HIV-negative tuberculous cadavers were encountered to compare rates of cavitation at autopsy). In these terminal cases, the peripheral cervical, axillary, and inguinal lymph nodes were infrequently enlarged and on section had only inconspicuous mil-iary lesions. The intestine, usually the small bowel but also the colorectum and esophagus, had focal tuberculous lesions in 20% of cadavers. The meninges had tuberculosis in 18% of tuberculosis cases. In only 5 of 107 cases was there solely pulmonary tuberculous disease without nodal or more distal spread. Obviously, it is easier to identify extrapulmonary tuberculosis at autopsy than clinically, but this cadaveric evidence highlights the artificiality of such distinctions and supports the recent decision to include pulmonary as well as extrapulmonary tuberculosis as an AIDS-defining disease (Buehler and Ward, 1993).

HISTOPATHOLOGY OF HIV-ASSOCIATED TUBERCULOSIS

The histologic patterns of tuberculosis reflect the integrity of the cellular immune response of the patient. Although changes occur on a continuum, we have identified three histologic stages of cellular immune response that correlate well with the stage of HIV infection (Fig. 3).

Early HIV Infection (Granulomatous)

Patients with relatively intact cellular immunity have a typical granulomatous response. Epithelioid macrophages and Langhans giant cells are abundant, and numbers of mycobacteria are low (Nambuya et al., 1988; Nelson et al., 1991). Immunostaining shows clustering of CD4$^+$ lymphocytes around epithelioid macrophages and Langhans giant cells. The majority of macrophages have abundant cytoplasm that, as one of us (A.M.N.) has shown, stains intensely with KP-1 (CD68) macrophage markers.

HIV with Moderate Immunosuppression (Hyporeactive)

As the CD4$^+$ lymphocyte count drops, cellular immunity decreases. The first obvi-

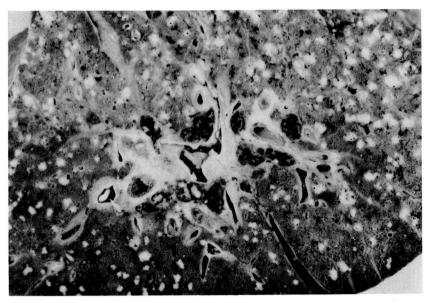

Figure 2. Miliary tuberculosis. Cut section of lung shows seeding of the parenchyma and peribronchial lymph nodes by small ("millet seed") nodules.

ous changes in tissue sections are loss of Langhans giant cells and a subsequent decrease in epithelioid macrophages (Table 3). Immunostaining shows a decrease in numbers of $CD4^+$ lymphocytes. The proportion of macrophages with abundant, intensely staining (CD68) cytoplasm is also decreased. The decreased number of activated macrophages results in poor intracellular killing of mycobacteria (Dannenberg, 1991). The caseous centers enlarge centrifugally, and lesions coalesce. Necrosis is

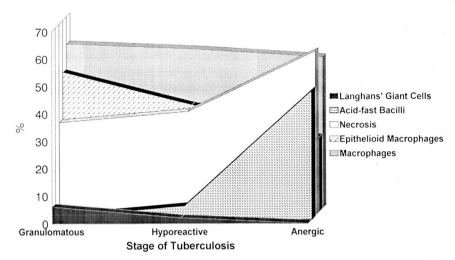

Figure 3. Spectrum of histological responses in HIV-associated tuberculosis patients. As HIV disease progresses, there is a loss of the normal cellular immune response (granulomatous reaction) and a concomitant increase in numbers of mycobacteria and in necrosis.

Table 3. Density of Langhans giant cells in tuberculosis lesions of HIV-positive cadavers in Abidjan correlated with premortem blood CD4$^+$ T-lymphocyte counts

Langhans giant cells	CD4$^+$ count (10^6/liter)		
	No. of patients	Median	Range
Absent	15	34	4–221
Scanty	12	72	14–359
>1/granuloma	11	167	26–537

mixed suppurative and caseous. AFB are numerous (Table 4).

Advanced HIV Disease with Severe Immunosuppression (Anergic Miliary)

In the final stages of AIDS, miliary or disseminated anergic disease is present at autopsy in almost all patients (Table 2). CD68 immunostaining reveals no decrease in the relative number of macrophages in the tuberculous lesion, but there is decreased staining. Epithelioid macrophages, Langhans giant cells, and granuloma formation are absent. There are few remaining CD4$^+$ lymphocytes in tissue sections. Suppuration and coagulative necrosis have replaced the typical caseating granulomatous response. AFB are myriad. The large number of AFB within macrophages is reminiscent of proliferation in the naive host.

Meningitis versus Visceral AFB Densities

Histological examination of the tissues in HIV-positive tuberculosis patients at au-

Table 4. Density of AFB in untreated tuberculosis lesions of HIV-positive cadavers in Abidjan correlated with premortem blood CD4$^+$ T-lymphocyte counts[a]

No. of AFB/hpf[b]	No. of patients	CD4$^+$ count (10^6/liter)	
		Median	Range
>100	16	28	4–130
≤100	22	151	26–537

[a] Histological scale is that of Nambuya et al. (1988).
[b] hpf, high-power field.

topsy shows that the qualitative patterns and the densities of AFB are broadly comparable throughout the active lesions in the viscera. However, a significant difference exists between the densities of AFB in the viscera and the meninges in those patients with disseminated and meningeal tuberculosis. The meninges contain 10- to 100-fold more AFB than the visceral lesions (Lucas, unpublished data).

CAUSES OF DEATH IN HIV-POSITIVE TUBERCULOSIS PATIENTS

It has been noted that in the United States, the great majority of treated tuberculosis patients with AIDS who died had another AIDS-defining cause of death (Chaisson et al., 1987). In a large series of HIV-positive tuberculosis patients in Africa, one of the most striking features is the high mortality among HIV-positive patients compared with that among HIV-negative patients after antituberculosis therapy is commenced. These data derive from chest clinics, not in-patient hospitals; thus, the patients differ from those terminal cases of HIV-associated tuberculosis that are studied at autopsy. In Nairobi, the relative risk of death within 1 year of diagnosis and starting treatment was 3.8 (Nunn et al., 1992); in Kinshasa, it was 7.0 (Perriëns et al., 1991), while in Abidjan, it was 14.9 for HIV-1-positive patients (Kassim et al., 1992). It is unclear what underlies this high mortality. A small proportion of deaths may follow a lethal drug reaction (if, for example, thiacetazone is used [Perriëns et al., 1991; Nunn et al., 1991]). Clinical observations suggest that other HIV-related opportunistic diseases such as gram-negative bacteremia, toxoplasmosis, diarrhea, and bacterial pneumonia are responsible (Nunn et al., 1992; Gilks et al., 1992). The Abidjan autopsy study, which was not designed to address this specific problem, suggested that in advanced active tuberculosis, the fibrotic sequelae of tuberculosis and nontuberculosis AIDS-defining conditions are all important (Lucas, unpublished data). Unpublished observations from Abidjan indicate that this increased mortality occurs in patients with low CD4 counts (Ackah et al., 1993). A formal autopsy study is required to investigate the underlying reasons for this serious problem.

IMMUNOPATHOGENESIS OF TUBERCULOSIS

A large body of in vivo and in vitro data on the patterns of T-cell subsets, antigen responses, cytokine production and effects, and macrophage activation following infection with *M. leprae* has been gathered (Modlin et al., 1988; Yamamura et al., 1991). These data have greatly aided our understanding of leprosy, but comparable information for tuberculosis is lacking.

T lymphocytes may have a helper/inducer function ($CD4^+$, Th), which enhances immune response, or a cytotoxic function ($CD8^+$). Two subsets of T helper cells (Th1 and Th2) have been described (chapter 25). Th1 cells secrete interleukin-2 and gamma interferon and are thought to be responsible for macrophage activation in response to various antigens in the tubercle bacillus. Th2 cells secrete interleukins-4, -5, and -10, which stimulate B cells. These two T-cell subsets seem to regulate each other negatively (Mosmann and Coffman, 1989).

Recent studies of HIV-infected individuals show that Th1 cells are progressively lost, shifting the ratio to a Th2-dominant population (Clerici and Shearer, 1993). Understanding the timing of Th1 function loss is key to understanding the altered host response in tuberculosis and to developing strategies for prophylaxis.

EFFECT OF TUBERCULOSIS ON HIV DISEASE

It has long been suspected that tuberculosis infection accelerates the progression of HIV disease from asymptomatic infection to AIDS to death. Supporting epidemiological data come from the Haiti isoniazid prophylaxis trial (see below), in which antituberculosis prophylaxis delayed both phases of this progression among people previously infected by tuberculosis (purified protein derivative positive) (Pape et al., 1993). A potent activator of HIV replication within T cells is tumor necrosis factor alpha (Matsuyama et al., 1991), and infection load with HIV increases in the later stages of HIV disease. This cytokine is produced by activated macrophages within granulomas as a response to tubercle infection. Levels of tumor necrosis factor alpha in the blood of patients coinfected with HIV and tuberculosis are 3- to 10-fold higher than levels in the blood of those infected with HIV only (Wallis et al., 1993). Thus, *M. tuberculosis* is probably a cofactor for progression of HIV disease.

TREATMENT OF TUBERCULOSIS IN HIV-INFECTED PATIENTS

Aside from the recent focal outbreaks of multidrug-resistant tuberculosis in the United States (Fischl et al., 1992), drug resistance is not a major problem in industrialized countries, and relapses are uncommon in compliant HIV-positive patients (Small et al., 1991). However, in Africa, relapse of pulmonary tuberculosis patients is frequent. In Kinshasa, using the standard streptomycin-based regimen, HIV-positive patients relapsed three times more often than HIV-negative patients; in Nairobi, the same rate ratio was 33, and from DNA fingerprinting, it appeared that both relapse and reinfection may have produced recurrence of tuberculosis (Hawken et al., 1993; Perriëns et al., 1991).

Autopsy studies emphasize advanced presentations of tuberculous disease in HIV-positive patients. In Abidjan, half of the adult patients admitted to general medical wards were HIV positive; 38% died, their modal survival was 1 day, and multibacillary tuberculosis was the commonest cause of death (Lucas, unpublished data). The response to therapy of patients with disseminated tuberculosis lesions containing vast numbers of AFB is unclear. In the pre-AIDS era, it was frequently observed that patients with advanced tuberculosis died rapidly despite therapy, with a form of Herxheimer reaction claimed as being responsible (Ellis and Webb, 1983; Barss, 1983). It is therefore possible that much of the tuberculosis being seen in such hospitals is untreatable even with better facilities.

PROPHYLAXIS OF TUBERCULOSIS IN HIV-INFECTED PEOPLE

Because of the high risk of developing tuberculosis by reactivation or reinfection, trials in Africa and elsewhere are under way to assess the value of antituberculosis prophylaxis in preventing or deferring the development of tuberculosis. In Haiti, asymptomatic HIV-positive adults were given isoniazid or placebo for 12 months and then monitored for 3 to 6 years. Isoniazid reduced the risk of tuberculosis by 71% overall and by 83% among the purified protein derivative skin test-positive subgroup (Pape et al., 1993). The possibility of increased drug resistance through use of isoniazid alone awaits evaluation.

PEDIATRIC TUBERCULOSIS AND HIV INFECTION

Even in areas where tuberculosis is highly endemic, the prevalence of childhood tuberculosis is low, since the infection rate is 1 to 2.5% per annum from birth. In the United States, there is some evidence that HIV is associated with an increased incidence of pediatric tuberculosis (Braun and Cauthen, 1992). Case reports have found that mainly black children are affected; they present at a median age of 42 months and with a median $CD4^+$ lymphocyte count of 120×10^6/liter. The proportion with extrapulmonary tuberculosis is greater than that expected in historical (HIV-negative) controls (Khouri et al., 1992). In Africa, the data are scanty. In Abidjan, children seen at tuberculosis centers were 6% of newly diagnosed cases; 12% were HIV positive, with the highest age-specific seroprevalence (20%) in those aged 1 to 4 years. The majority were diagnosed as having primary pulmonary or extrapulmonary tuberculosis (De Cock et al., 1992). However, in an autopsy series of consecutive children (age, <15 years) examined in the main mortuary of the same city, only 1 of 77 HIV-positive and 2 of 78 HIV-negative children were found to have tuberculosis (Lucas, unpublished data). Such data suggest that in Africa, pediatric HIV-associated tuberculosis is not a major problem. A possible cause for this discrepancy is overdiagnosis of tuberculosis in childhood. Most cases are negative for AFB in samples, and the diagnosis is made clinically and radiologically. More sensitive means of establishing the diagnosis are required.

DIFFERENTIAL DIAGNOSIS

The radiographic appearances of advanced pulmonary tuberculosis with or without cavitation are well recognized. An important differential diagnosis both radiographically and histopathologically is nocardiosis, a disease that is also more frequent in HIV-positive patients because of immunosuppression (Kim et al., 1991). In nocardiosis, a granulomatous reaction may be present, but in HIV-positive patients, the reaction is usually polymorphic. A silver impregnation technique (such as Grocott methenamine silver) will readily demonstrate the branching bacterial filaments that can then be identified by their partial acid-fast-staining characteristics (these are better seen with the Coates-Fite modification of the carbol fuchsin stain).

In our experience, HIV-associated miliary pulmonary tuberculosis is readily missed as a clinical diagnosis because the lesions are often too small to be visualized and sputum negativity is common. Similarly, extrapulmonary tuberculosis is always a diagnostic problem (the old epithet "cryptic miliary tuberculosis" is appropriate) (O'Brien, 1954). In Abidjan, tuberculous meningitis often (in 12 of 19 patients autopsied) had caused a neutrophil polymorphic response in the cerebrospinal fluid rather than the classical lymphocytosis (Lucas et al., 1993); this may lead to the overdiagnosis of purulent bacterial infection instead of tuberculosis.

Where sophisticated technology is available, ultrasound or computed tomography scan-guided needle aspiration can be used to obtain material for smears, culture, and light microscopy. In the developing world, wide-needle aspiration has been reported for diagnosis of lymphadenitis (Bem et al., 1993). Similar techniques could be used for liver biopsy to detect dissemination, since this organ was found to be involved in approximately 80% (Table 2) of patients dying with tuberculosis. Adequate clinical information on whether patients with tuberculous liver involvement have symptoms such as hepatomegaly, jaundice, or hepatic tenderness would be helpful.

CHALLENGES FOR FUTURE HIV/TUBERCULOSIS RESEARCH

The challenges for future research on tuberculosis in HIV-infected people include the following: (i) to determine the causes of the excess mortality in HIV-positive tuberculosis patients; (ii) to correlate $CD4^+$ T-lymphocyte counts with the premortem histopathology and bacteriology of tuberculosis lesions; (iii) to determine the immunopathogenesis of tuberculosis by in situ study of macrophages, T cells, cytokines, and bacilli in both HIV-positive and HIV-negative people; (iv) to evaluate the correct modes of managing very advanced tuberculosis infection (highly multibacillary) in HIV-positive patients; (v) to characterize the genotypes of *M. tuberculosis* infecting patients in order to pursue the reactivation versus reinfection hypotheses in tuberculosis pathogenesis; (vi) to devise more sensitive methods of diagnosing tuberculosis, particularly in children; and (vii) to evaluate the logistics and microbiological consequences of mass prophylaxis against tuberculosis in HIV-positive populations at risk.

REFERENCES

Ackah, A., K. Diallo, H. Digbeu, E. Boateng, D. Coulibaly, and K. M. De Cock. 1993. $CD4^+$ T-lymphocyte counts, clinical disease, and outcome in tuberculosis patients in Abidjan, Côte d'Ivoire, abstr. WS-B09-2. 9th Int. Conf. AIDS.

Allen, S., J. Batungwanayo, K. Kerlikowske, A. R. Lifson, W. Wolf, R. Granich, H. Taelman, P. van der Perre, A. Serufilira, and J. Bogaerts. 1992. Two-year incidence of tuberculosis in cohorts of HIV-infected and uninfected urban Rwandan women. *Am. Rev. Respir. Dis.* **146**:1439–1443.

Barber, T. W., D. E. Craven, and W. R. McCabe. 1990. Bacteremia due to *Mycobacterium tuberculosis* in patients with human immunodeficiency virus infection: a report of 9 cases and a review of the literature. *Medicine* **69**:375–383.

Barss, P. 1983. Unexpected deaths in pulmonary tuberculosis. *Lancet* **i**:1437.

Beck, J. S., R. C. Potts, T. Kardjito, and J. M. Grange. 1985. T4 lymphopenia in patients with active pulmonary tuberculosis. *Clin. Exp. Immunol.* **60**:49–54.

Bem, C., P. S. Patil, A. M. Elliot, K. M. Namaambo, H. Bharucha, and J. D. H. Porter. 1993. The value of wide-needle aspiration in the diagnosis of tuberculous lymphadenitis in Africa. *AIDS* **7**:1221–1225.

Braun, M. M., and G. Cauthen. 1992. Relationship of the human immunodeficiency virus epidemic to pediatric tuberculosis and Bacille Calmette-Guérin immunization. *Pediatr. Infect. Dis. J.* **11**:220–227.

Buehler, J. W., and J. W. Ward. 1993. A new case definition for AIDS surveillance. *Ann. Intern. Med.* **118**:390–392.

Chaisson, R. E., G. F. Schecter, C. P. Theuer, G. W. Rutherford, D. F. Echenberg, and P. C. Hopewell. 1987. Tuberculosis in patients with the acquired immunodeficiency syndrome: clinical features, response to therapy, and survival. *Am. Rev. Respir. Dis.* **136**:570–574.

Clerici, M., and G. M. Shearer. 1993. A TH1-TH2 switch is a critical step in the etiology of HIV infection. *Immunol. Today* **14**:107–111.

Crowe, S. M., J. B. Carlin, K. I. Stewart, C. R. Lucas, and J. F. Hoy. 1991. Predictive value of CD4 lymphocyte numbers for the development of opportunistic infections and malignancies in HIV-infected persons. *J. Acquired Immune Defic. Syndr.* **4**:770–776.

Dannenberg, A., Jr. 1991. Delayed-type hypersensitivity and cell-mediated immunity in the pathogenesis of tuberculosis. *Immunol. Today* **12**:228–233.

De Cock, K. M., B. Soro, I. M. Coulibaly, and S. B. Lucas. 1992. Tuberculosis and HIV infection in sub-Saharan Africa. *JAMA* **268**:1581–1587.

Elliott, A. M., N. L. Luo, G. Tembo, B. Halwiindi, G. Steenbergen, L. Machiels, J. Pobee, P. Nunn, R. J. Hayes, and K. P. W. J. McAdam. 1990. Impact of HIV on tuberculosis in Zambia: a cross sectional study. *Br. Med. J.* **301**:412–415.

Ellis, M. E., and A. K. Webb. 1983. Cause of death in patients admitted to hospital for pulmonary tuberculosis. *Lancet* **i**:665–667.

Fischl, M. A., R. B. Uttamchandari, G. L. Daikos, R. G. Poblete, J. N. Moreno, R. R. Reyes, A. M. Boota, L. M. Thompson, T. J. Cleary, and S. Lai. 1992. An outbreak of tuberculosis caused by multiple-drug resistant tubercle bacilli among patients with HIV infection. *Ann. Intern. Med.* **117**:177–183.

Gilks, C. F., L. S. Otieno, R. J. Brindle, R. S. Newnham, G. N. Lule, J. B. O. Were, P. M. Simani, S. M. Bhatt, G. B. A. Okelo, P. G. Waiyaki, and D. A. Warrell. 1992. The presentation and outcome of HIV-related disease in Nairobi. *Q. J. Med.* **82**:25–32.

Hawken, M., P. Nunn, S. Gathua, R. Brindle, P. Godfrey-Faussett, W. Githui, J. Odhiambo, B. Batchelor, C. Gilks, J. Morris, and K. McAdam. 1993. Increased recurrence of tuberculosis in HIV-1-infected patients in Kenya. *Lancet* **342**:332–337.

Kassim, S., M. Sassan-Moroko, and R. Doorly. 1992. Prospective study of pulmonary tuberculosis and HIV-1 and HIV-2 infections, Abidjan, Côte d'Ivoire, abstr. PoB 3086. 8th Int. Conf. AIDS.

Khouri, Y. F., M. T. Mastrucci, C. Hutto, C. D. Mitchell, and G. B. Scott. 1992. Mycobacterium tuberculosis in children with human immunodefi-

ciency virus type 1 infection. *Pediatr. Infect. Dis. J.* **11**:950–955.

Kim, J., G. Y. Minamoto, and M. H. Grieco. 1991. Nocardial infection as a complication of AIDS: report of six cases and review. *Rev. Infect. Dis.* **13**:624–629.

Lewin-Smith, M. R., A. M. Nelson, and W. M. Meyers. 1993. A semi-quantitative assessment of cellular immune response to tuberculosis in HIV-infected patients. *Int. J. Leprosy* **61**:123A.

Louie, E., L. B. Rice, and R. S. Holgman. 1986. Tuberculosis in non-Haitian patients with acquired immunodeficiency syndrome. *Chest* **90**:542–545.

Lucas, S. Unpublished data.

Lucas, S. B., A. Hounnou, C. S. Peacock, A. Beaumel, G. Djomand, J.-M. N'Gbichi, K. Yeboue, M. Hondé, M. Diomande, C. Giordano, R. Doorly, K. Brattegaard, L. Kestens, R. W. Smithwick, A. Kadio, N. Ezani, A. Yapi, and K. M. De Cock. 1993. The mortality and pathology of HIV disease in a West African city. *AIDS* **7**:1569–1579.

Mann, J. M., D. J. M. Tarantola, and T. W. Netter. 1992. *AIDS in the World.* Harvard University Press, Cambridge, Mass.

Matsuyama, T., N. Kobayashi, and N. Yamamoto. 1991. Cytokines and HIV infection: is AIDS a tumour necrosis factor disease? *AIDS* **5**:1405–1417.

Modlin, R. L., J. Melancon-Kaplan, S. M. M. Young, C. Permez, H. Kino, J. Convit, T. H. Rea, and B. R. Bloom. 1988. Learning from lesions: patterns of tissue inflammation in leprosy. *Proc. Natl. Acad. Sci. USA* **85**:1213–1217.

Mosmann, T. R., and R. L. Coffman. 1989. TH1 and TH2 cells: different kinds of lymphokine secretion lead to different functional properties. *Annu. Rev. Immunol.* **7**:145–173.

Mukadi, Y., J. H. Perriëns, M. E. St. Louis, C. Brown, J. Prignot, J.-C. Willame, F. Pouthier, K. Kabota, R. W. Ryder, F. Portaels, and P. Piot. 1993. Spectrum of immunodeficiency in HIV-1-infected patients with pulmonary tuberculosis in Zaire. *Lancet* **342**:143–146.

Nambuya, A., N. Sewankambo, J. Mugerwa, R. W. Goodgame, and S. B. Lucas. 1988. Tuberculous lymphadenitis associated with human immunodeficiency virus (HIV) in Uganda. *J. Clin. Pathol.* **41**:93–96.

Nelson, A. M., L. Okonda, Y. Mukadi, C. Moran, L. Mbuyamba, B. Kabongo, C. Brown, and F. G. Mullick. 1991. Histologic patterns of tuberculosis in HIV-1 infected Zairians, abstr. W.B. 2260. 7th Int. Conf. AIDS.

Nelson, A. M., J. H. Perriëns, B. Kapita, L. Okonda, N. Lusamuno, M. R. Kalengayi, P. Angritt, T. C. Quinn, and F. G. Mullick. 1993. A clinical and pathological comparison of the WHO and CDC case definitions for AIDS in Kinshasa, Zaire: is passive surveillance valid? *AIDS* **7:**1241–1245.

Nightingale, S. D., L. T. Byrd, P. M. Southern, J. D. Jockusch, S. X. Cal, and B. A. Wynne. 1992. Incidence of *Mycobacterium avium-intracellulare* complex bacteremia in human immunodeficiency virus-positive patients. *J. Infect. Dis.* **165:**1082–1085.

Nunn, P., R. Brindle, L. Carpenter, J. Odhiambo, K. Wasunna, R. Newnham, W. Githui, S. Gathua, M. Omwega, and K. McAdam. 1992. Cohort study of HIV infection in tuberculosis patients, Nairobi, Kenya: analysis of early (6 months) mortality. *Am. Rev. Respir. Dis.* **146:**849–854.

Nunn, P., D. Kibuga, S. Gathua, R. Brindle, A. Imalingat, K. Wasunna, S. Lucas, C. Gilks, M. Omwega, J. Were, and K. McAdam. 1991. Cutaneous hypersensitivity reactions due to thiacetazone in HIV-1 seropositive patients treated for tuberculosis. *Lancet* **337:**627–630.

O'Brien, J. R. 1954. Non-reactive tuberculosis. *J. Clin. Pathol.* **7:**216–225.

Onsuaballi, J. E., and L. Palmer. 1987. T4 lymphopenia in human tuberculosis. *Tubercle* **68:**195–200.

Opie, E. L., and J. D. Aronson. 1927. Tubercle bacilli in latent tuberculosis lesions and in lung tissue without tuberculous lesions. *Arch. Pathol.* **4:**1–21.

Pape, J. W., S. S. Jean, A. Hafner, and W. D. Johnson. 1993. Effect of isoniazid prophylaxis on incidence of active tuberculosis and progression of HIV infection. *Lancet* **342:**268–272.

Perriëns, J. H., R. L. Colebunders, C. Karahunga, J. C. Willame, J. Jeugmans, M. Kabota, Y. Mukadi, P. Pauwels, R. W. Ryder, J. Prignot, and P. Piot. 1991. Increased mortality and tuberculosis treatment failure rate among human immunodeficiency virus (HIV) seropositive compared with HIV seronegative patients with pulmonary tuberculosis

treated with "standard" chemotherapy in Kinshasa, Zaire. *Am. Rev. Respir. Dis.* **144:**750–755.

Pozniak, A., P. Neill, B. Ndmere, A. S. Malin, A. Phillips, L. Chidede, and A. Latif. 1992. Is tuberculosis a co-factor in HIV immunosuppression?, abstr. PoA 2121. 8th Int. Conf. AIDS.

Selwyn, P. A., D. Hartel, V. A. Lewis, E. E. Schoenbaum, S. H. Vermund, R. S. Klein, A. T. Walker, and G. H. Friedland. 1989. A prospective study of the risk of tuberculosis among intravenous drug users with HIV. *N. Engl. J. Med.* **320:**545–550.

Shafer, R. W., K. D. Chirgwin, A. E. Glatt, M. A. Dahsouh, S. H. Landesman, and B. Suster. 1991. HIV prevalence, immunosuppression, and drug resistance in patients with tuberculosis in an area endemic for AIDS. *AIDS* **5:**399–405.

Small, P. M., G. F. Schecter, P. C. Goodman, M. A. Sande, R. E. Chaisson, and P. C. Hopewell. 1991. Treatment of tuberculosis in patients with advanced human immunodeficiency virus infection. *N. Engl. J. Med.* **324:**289–294.

Theuer, C. P., P. C. Hopewell, D. Elias, G. F. Schecter, G. W. Rutherford, and R. F. Chaisson. 1990. Human immunodeficiency virus infection in tuberculosis patients. *J. Infect. Dis.* **162:**8–12.

Wallis, R. S., M. Vjecha, M. Amir-Tahmasseb, A. Okwera, F. Byekwaso, S. Nyole, S. Kabengera, R. D. Mugerwa, and J. J. Ellner. 1993. Influence of tuberculosis on human immunodeficiency virus (HIV-1): enhanced cytokine expression and elevated β2-microglobulin in HIV-1 associated tuberculosis. *J. Infect. Dis.* **167:**43–48.

Yamamura, M., K. Uyemura, R. J. Deans, K. Weinberg, T. H. Rea, B. R. Bloom, and R. L. Modlin. 1991. Defining protective response to pathogens: cytokine profiles in leprosy lesions. *Science* **254:**277–279.

VI. NEW APPROACHES TO PREVENTION AND TREATMENT OF TUBERCULOSIS

Tuberculosis: Pathogenesis, Protection, and Control
Edited by Barry R. Bloom
© 1994 American Society for Microbiology, Washington, DC 20005

Chapter 30

Molecular Approaches to the Diagnosis of Tuberculosis

Thomas M. Shinnick and Vivian Jonas

The timely identification of persons infected with *Mycobacterium tuberculosis* and the rapid laboratory confirmation of tuberculosis are two key ingredients of effective public health measures to combat the resurgence of tuberculosis and the outbreaks of nosocomially transmitted tuberculosis (National MDR-TB Task Force, 1992). Current procedures for identifying infected persons are limited by a lack of sensitivity or specificity, and the laboratory confirmation of an infection can require many weeks (reviewed in chapter 7). Indeed, a workshop of tuberculosis experts concluded that all "current techniques for the diagnosis of *M. tuberculosis* are beset by serious limitations" and that "the rapid and specific diagnosis of *M. tuberculosis* is one of the most pressing needs in efforts to eradicate the disease" (Bates et al., 1986). In this chapter, we review progress in developing new tools and procedures for the rapid and reliable diagnosis of tuberculosis.

Thomas M. Shinnick • Division of Bacterial and Mycotic Diseases, National Center for Infectious Diseases, Centers for Disease Control and Prevention, Atlanta, Georgia 30333. ***Vivian Jonas*** • Gen-Probe Incorporated, 9880 Campus Point Drive, San Diego, California 92121.

DETECTION OF INFECTED PERSONS

The timely identification of persons with active *M. tuberculosis* infection is important, because only about 10% of infected immunocompetent persons will develop active tuberculosis during their lifetimes, and overt disease symptoms appear fairly late in the infection (Stead et al., 1987; American Thoracic Society and Centers for Disease Control [hereinafter referred to as ATS-CDC], 1990). Appropriate preventive chemotherapy for persons whose infection is progressing toward overt disease can dramatically reduce the development of infectious tuberculosis (Stead et al., 1987; Centers for Disease Control [hereinafter referred to as CDC], 1990). Indeed, preventive therapy for these infected persons may be the most cost-effective way to reduce the general public health impact of tuberculosis in populations in which the incidence is low.

Historically, the detection of infected persons has relied upon procedures that use rather crude preparations of antigens to detect the cell-mediated immune response to the infecting mycobacterium: the tuberculin, or purified protein derivative, skin test (Koch, 1891; ATS-CDC, 1981, 1990). However, the usefulness of tuberculin is limited by its lack of specificity for tuberculosis and by its inability to distinguish between active disease, prior sensitization by contact with *M. tuberculosis*, BCG vaccination, and cross-sensitization by other *Mycobacterium* species (Palmer and Edwards, 1967; Huebner et al., 1993b). The tuberculin skin test also fails to detect a substantial proportion of persons coinfected with human immunodeficiency virus (HIV) and *M. tuberculosis* and of persons with advanced tuberculosis (ATS-CDC, 1981; CDC, 1991; Huebner et al., 1993b). Despite these limitations, the tuberculin skin test is still a very useful tool, especially when conversion to a positive skin test is used to identify recently infected persons for preventive therapy or to help confirm a physician's suspicion of tuberculosis.

In populations with high rates of tuberculosis, antibody detection tests are reasonably specific and have predictive values similar to that of the acid-fast smear (reviewed in chapter 26). However, the specificity of the assays is a concern in populations with a low incidence of tuberculosis, because of a large number of false-positive results due presumably to an immune response to cross-reactive antigens carried by environmental mycobacteria (Grange, 1984; Ivanyi, 1991). Also, the published assays do not clearly distinguish active infections or disease from inactive infections or prior exposure.

Antigen detection tests have received relatively little attention for tuberculosis (reviewed in chapter 26). In general, antigen detection assays can detect patients with multibacillary disease but have difficulty detecting those with paucibacillary disease. This apparent requirement for a large bacterial load reduces the potential utility of these assays in identifying recently infected persons or high-risk groups for preventive therapy but may be useful for monitoring the efficacy of chemotherapy.

The ELISPOT test, which measures antibody-secreting cells (Czerkinsky et al., 1983; Sedgewick and Holt, 1983), may be able to distinguish active infections from inactive infections, prior exposure, and BCG vaccination. The basic premise of this test is that a person with an active or recent infection will have many more antibody-secreting cells (especially immunoglobulin M [IgM]-secreting cells) than a person whose immune response is due to an inactive infection or prior exposure. ELISPOT assays have been quite useful for the diagnosis of active HIV infections and for monitoring the response to anti-HIV therapy (Lee et al., 1989; Nesheim et al., 1992). With respect to tuberculosis, Lu et al. (1990) found that 24 of 25 patients with tuberculous meningitis had elevated levels of lymphocytes secreting IgM or IgG antibodies against BCG in the cerebrospinal fluid and peripheral blood. Although this assay seems promising, it is a difficult and expensive assay that will need much work to convert it to a reliable assay for use in a clinical laboratory.

In summary, there still is a critical need for assays to detect infection with *M. tuberculosis* prior to the onset of clinical symptoms. An ideal test should be simple, inexpensive, and noninvasive. The test should also be applicable to immunocompetent and immunocompromised adults and children. Such a test also needs to distinguish persons with active *M. tuberculosis* infection from persons whose immune systems have controlled a prior infection.

LABORATORY CONFIRMATION OF INFECTIONS

A definitive diagnosis of tuberculosis requires the identification of *M. tuberculosis* bacilli in patient specimens. Conventional procedures for detecting *M. tuberculosis* in specimens usually start with microscopic examination of smears for the presence of acid-fast bacilli and continue with culture of the organisms and then biochemical tests on the cultured organisms to identify which

Mycobacterium species was present (Kent and Kubica, 1985; see also chapter 7). The entire process often requires 4 to 6 weeks from the time of specimen collection to provide species identification, primarily because of the slow growth rate of mycobacteria (Huebner et al., 1993a). Determination of drug susceptibility of an isolate by culturing can add 3 to 6 weeks to this already long process.

EXISTING RAPID DIAGNOSTIC PROCEDURES

Species Identification of Cultured Organisms

Several methods that allow for more rapid determination of the species of a cultured organism have been developed recently. One such method is based on the observations that each *Mycobacterium* species synthesizes a unique set of mycolic acids and that a species-specific pattern of mycolic acids can be produced by a variety of chromatographic procedures such as high-performance liquid chromatography (HPLC) (Minniken and Goodfellow, 1980; Butler and Kilburn, 1988; see also chapter 7). HPLC can provide definitive species identification for any of more than 50 *Mycobacterium* species in less than 4 h after the culture is available. The test not only is rapid but also can replace an entire battery of biochemical tests.

A second family of rapid species identification procedures involves nucleic acid hybridization (reviewed by Kohne [1989]). Nucleic acid probes that react specifically with *M. tuberculosis*, *M. avium*, or *M. intracellulare* or with any member of the genus *Mycobacterium* have been developed. In general, the commercially available assays display sensitivities and specificities approaching 100% for the detection and identification of these species and can usually be completed in a few hours. One drawback is that they require $>10^5$ organisms to give clear-cut results. This requirement is easily met with pure cultures but reduces the utility of the approach with clinical specimens, which often contain many fewer bacilli. Nonetheless, combining a nucleic acid identification system with a rapid culture system such as BACTEC can shorten the time required for detecting and identifying *M. tuberculosis* to as little as 4 to 7 days (Evans et al., 1992; see also chapter 7).

FUTURE RAPID DIAGNOSTIC PROCEDURES

The goal of research into rapid diagnostics is to develop reliable procedures that can detect and identify mycobacteria directly from clinical specimens and thereby avoid the many weeks required for culturing. This goal has been difficult to achieve, since clinical specimens usually contain only small numbers of bacilli. Thus, the direct detection of mycobacteria or mycobacterial components in specimens requires either an extremely sensitive and specific assay or a process by which a diagnostically useful mycobacterial component can be "amplified" to a detectable level.

Tuberculostearic Acid

One easily detected component of *M. tuberculosis* is tuberculostearic acid, which can be detected in femtomole quantities by gas-liquid chromatography (Brooks et al., 1987). The presence of tuberculostearic acid in cerebrospinal fluid is thought to be diagnostic for tuberculous meningitis (Mardh et al., 1983; French et al., 1987; Brooks et al., 1990) and has been suggested to be useful in diagnosing pulmonary tuberculosis (Larsson et al., 1981; Savic et al., 1992). However, an important concern with pulmonary specimens is that organisms other than *M. tuberculosis* may produce components that will generate a false-positive signal.

Improved Nucleic Acid Probes

The sensitivity of nucleic acid hybridization assays can be increased by using a signal amplification system such as branched DNA signal amplification (Urdea, 1991). In this procedure, one constructs a bifunctional oligonucleotide probe that contains a sequence specific for the target species and a sequence to which a second oligonucleotide can bind. The key feature of the second oligonucleotide is that it has many binding sites for a third oligonucleotide that carries an enzyme (e.g., alkaline phosphatase) that produces the detectable signal. Theoretically, such a procedure could amplify a hybridization signal 10- to 100-fold, which might improve the detection limit of the hybridization assays to as few as 100 to 1,000 organisms per specimen. These tests have yet to be evaluated on clinical specimens or in a clinical trial.

Gene Amplification

An alternative to a very sensitive detection system is a procedure that amplifies a target molecule to a detectable level. Several procedures have been described for use with *M. tuberculosis* and include strand displacement amplification (SDA) (Walker et al., 1992a), polymerase chain reaction (PCR) amplification (Mullis and Faloona, 1987), transcription-mediated amplification (TMA) (Jonas et al., 1993a), reporter phage systems (Jacobs et al., 1993), oligonucleotide ligation amplification (Iovannisci and Winn-Deen, 1993), and Q-beta replicase amplification (Kramer et al., 1991). The first four of these amplification systems are the best developed of the systems for mycobacteria and are described in detail below.

In the research laboratory, the *M. tuberculosis*-specific amplification assays display excellent specificity and sensitivity. In general, each amplification system can (i) produce a clear positive signal from specimens containing as few as 1 to 10 bacilli, (ii)

clearly distinguish *M. tuberculosis* from other *Mycobacterium* species and common respiratory specimen contaminants, (iii) detect *M. tuberculosis* in specimens containing a large excess of nucleic acids from human cells or from other *Mycobacterium* species, and (iv) be completed in less than 1 day. The assays have been used with a variety of clinical specimens, including sputum, gastric lavage fluid, cerebrospinal fluid, and tissue biopsy specimens. Because of the need to culture organisms for drug susceptibility testing or for identifying *Mycobacterium* species other than *M. tuberculosis*, the assays usually are designed to be used with specimens that have been processed for culture, such as by the N-acetyl-L-cysteine/NaOH procedure for sputum specimens (Kent and Kubica, 1985; see also chapter 7). The second step for most assays is lysis of the mycobacteria, which can be accomplished by a variety of methods, including sonication, boiling, sodium dodecyl sulfate (SDS) plus lysozyme plus heat, proteinase K, chaeotropic salts, etc. Because inhibitors of enzymatic amplification reactions are found in a small percentage (1 to 5%) of processed sputum specimens, the lysis step is often followed by a nucleic acid purification step. Also, most assays include internal controls to assess amplification efficiency and the presence of inhibitors.

SDA

SDA is an isothermal amplification process developed by Becton Dickinson (Research Triangle Park, N.C.) that takes advantage of the ability of the Klenow fragment of *Escherichia coli* DNA polymerase to start at the site of a single-stranded nick in double-stranded DNA, extend one strand from the 3' end, and displace the downstream strand of DNA (Walker et al., 1992a, b). The replicated DNA and the displaced strands are then substrates for additional rounds of oligonucleotide annealing, nicking, and strand displacement such that the amplification proceeds in a geometric manner and can produce a 10^7- to 10^8-fold amplification in about 2 h. The specificity of the SDA reaction is based on the choice of primers to direct the DNA synthesis. When coupled with a chemiluminescence-based hybridization detection system, the entire assay can be completed within 4 h of obtaining a processed specimen (Spargo et al., in press; Nycz et al., submitted).

Species-specific SDA assays have been developed for *M. tuberculosis*, *M. avium*, and *M. kansasii*. An assay that detects many members of the *Mycobacterium* genus (a genus-specific assay) has also been developed (Walker et al., submitted). These assays can be multiplexed (i.e., the amplifications can be done in a single tube, and the products can be distinguished by the detection system) without significant loss of sensitivity (Walker et al., submitted). Thus, one can have a single two-step assay to detect and differentiate the two most commonly encountered acid-fast bacteria in smear-positive specimens, *M. tuberculosis* and *M. avium* (Schram et al., submitted). One potential concern with genus-specific assays is that the signal produced by one species (e.g., *M. gordonae*, a common contaminant of sputum specimens) may mask the signal from a second species (e.g., *M. tuberculosis*). Thus, the ability to detect mixed infections is an important but untested feature of the assay.

Additional performance characteristics of the SDA assay are that (i) autoclaving can be used to sterilize a sample and lyse the bacteria, (ii) internal controls can be included to assess amplification efficiency and the presence of inhibitors, (iii) the assay is semiquantitative, and (iv) the detection system can be conveniently batched in 96-well microtiter plates. The assay has not yet been evaluated in a clinical setting.

PCR

PCR uses oligonucleotide primers to direct the amplification of target nucleic acid sequences via repeated rounds of denaturation, primer annealing, and primer extension (Mullis and Faloona, 1987). The specificity of the amplification process lies in the choice of primers. Descriptions of numerous PCR-based assays for the detection and identification of individual *Mycobacterium* species, such as *M. tuberculosis*, *M. leprae*, or *M. avium*, have been published recently (e.g., Brisson-Noel et al., 1989; Böddinghaus et al., 1990; Eisenach et al., 1990; DeWit et al., 1990; Fries et al., 1990; Hermans et al., 1990; Pao et al., 1990; Patel et al., 1990; Plikaytis et al., 1990; Sjobring et al., 1990; Del Portillo et al., 1991; Manjunath et al., 1991; Sritharan and Barker, 1991; Altamirano et al., 1992; Cousins et al., 1992; Kolk et al., 1992; Soini et al., 1992; Victor et al., 1992). Many target sequences have been used, but the most thoroughly evaluated assays target the *M. tuberculosis*-specific repeated DNA element IS*6110* (Eisenach et al., 1990, 1991). In addition, a variety of two-step PCR-based assays have been described in which the first step amplifies a target sequence common to all *Mycobacterium* species and the second step determines which species gave rise to the amplified product. The second step can involve species-specific hybridization probes (Hance et al., 1989), restriction fragment length polymorphism analysis (Plikaytis et al., 1992), or nucleic acid sequencing (Rogall et al., 1990). In general, the amplification process can be completed in 2 to 4 h of obtaining a processed specimen, and the detection assay can be completed in an additional 2 to 24 h. Additional performance characteristics are that (i) the assay requires a thermocycler and a thermostable DNA polymerase, (ii) internal controls can be included to assess amplification efficiency and the presence of inhibitors, and (iii) the assay is semiquantitative.

Most of the published PCR-based tests have been shown to work well only in the research laboratory. However, three recent publications address the transfer of these research-oriented tests to the clinical laboratory (Clarridge et al., 1993; Nolte et al., 1993; Shawar et al., 1993). For these studies, the clinical laboratories were provided with reagents and a PCR system that amplified a portion of IS6110. The laboratories analyzed all sputum specimens sent to them for testing for mycobacteria. The specimens were decontaminated using routine procedures, and 70 to 90% of the processed samples were used for culture. The remaining 10 to 30% were processed for the PCR-based assay by centrifuging to pellet any bacilli, suspending the pellet in a low-salt buffer containing 1% Triton X-100, and boiling it for 30 min (Sritharan and Barker, 1991). Portions of these lysates were used directly in the PCR reactions, and amplification products were analyzed by agarose gel electrophoresis.

The general conclusions from these studies were that (i) this PCR-based assay easily fit into the daily routine of the clinical laboratory with a turnaround time of 24 to 36 h from the time of specimen collection, (ii) existing clinical laboratory personnel were able to perform the assay, and (iii) false-positive results due to end product contamination were relatively rare with the use of appropriate precautions. Also, in the clinical laboratories, the specificity of the PCR-based assay was essentially 100%. However, its sensitivity was less than that in the research laboratory. That is, while about 95% of smear-positive, culture-positive samples were also PCR positive, only about 60% of the smear-negative, culture-positive samples were also PCR positive. (A smear-positive specimen contains $>5 \times 10^3$ bacilli [Smithwick, 1976].) Most of this apparent lack of sensitivity was probably due to so little of the sample actually making it into the PCR assay tube. Only 1 to 5% of the sputum specimen was analyzed by

PCR, while up to 90% was analyzed by culture. Some of the lack of sensitivity was due to the presence of PCR inhibitors in the processed sputum specimens, particularly in smear-positive specimens. Nonetheless, in these trials, the overall positive predictive value of the test was ~98%, and most important, the PCR-based assay correctly confirmed *M. tuberculosis* infection in all patients for whom three or more sputum specimens were tested (Clarridge et al., 1993).

TMA

TMA, an isothermal target-based amplification system developed by Gen-Probe Incorporated (San Diego, Calif.), has been combined with a homogeneous detection method to detect *M. tuberculosis* in clinical specimens (Jonas et al., 1993a). This test (the Gen-Probe Amplified Mycobacterium Tuberculosis Direct Test, or MTD test) uses the sediments prepared by the standard NALC/NaOH method (Kent and Kubica, 1985) and lyses the mycobacteria by sonication of the cells in a water bath sonicator. rRNA is amplified via TMA in which the rRNA target sequences are copied into a transcription complex by using reverse transcriptase and then RNA polymerase is used to make numerous RNA transcripts of the target sequence from the transcription complex. The process then repeats autocatalytically. Detection of the amplified sequences is achieved by using an acridinium ester-labeled DNA probe specific for *M. tuberculosis* in a homogeneous solution hybridization assay format similar to that used in the Gen-Probe Accuprobe species identification system. An important feature of the MTD assay is that it can be done entirely in one test tube, which minimizes sample manipulations and the possibility of laboratory-introduced contamination. Also, the entire assay can be completed within 3 to 4 h of obtaining a processed specimen.

In the research laboratory (Jonas et al., 1993a), the MTD assay is able to detect as few as ~1,000 copies of rRNA, which is about one-half the number of copies of rRNA in a single *M. tuberculosis* bacillus, and is capable of greater than 10^9-fold amplification. Even when ~290,000 cells of closely related organisms or respiratory pathogens were present, the detection of 10,000 copies (about five bacilli) of *M. tuberculosis* rRNA is still achievable. Furthermore, of the 65 species from 42 genera representing a cross-section of phylogeny and the 60 strains from 55 *Mycobacterium* species tested, only members of the *M. tuberculosis* complex give positive signals.

Six clinical laboratories in the United States have participated in an evaluation of the Gen-Probe MTD test (Jonas et al., 1993b; Miller et al., 1994). The six clinical laboratories analyzed 2,258 processed specimens by the MTD test, acid-fast bacillus smear, culture, and clinical history of the patient. The sensitivity and specificity of the MTD test for detecting *M. tuberculosis* when compared specimen by specimen with culture were 90 and 96%, respectively. When compared patient by patient with culture, the MTD test displayed 94% sensitivity and 93% specificity. However, culture may not be the best "gold standard" for comparison, because it is not 100% sensitive, since the decontamination process can kill >90% of the tubercle bacilli and thereby produce false-negative culture results. Such dead bacilli may contain sufficiently intact nucleic acids to allow detection by an amplification procedure. Indeed, some of the MTD-positive, culture-negative specimens were also smear positive, indicating that the nonviable staining bacilli in the specimen contained intact target nucleic acids. Therefore, additional analyses are necessary to determine the actual sensitivity and specificity of the MTD test for detecting a patient infected with *M. tuberculosis*. If one uses a physician's diagnosis of tuberculosis as the gold standard (deter-

mined by a chart review), then the MTD test displayed 95% sensitivity and 96% specificity for correctly identifying persons as having tuberculosis. In fact, the sensitivity of the MTD test and the sensitivity of culture with respect to detecting the presence of *M. tuberculosis* bacilli in a specimen were not statistically significantly different ($0.1 < P < 0.2$). However, the critical, highly significant difference here was that the MTD test allowed the detection of *M. tuberculosis* in patient specimens in 1 day compared to the 14 to 28 days required by the culturing procedure.

A seventh laboratory in Switzerland also evaluated the MTD test with NALC/NaOH-processed specimens ($n = 515$) as well as SDS-processed specimens ($n = 423$) (Pfyffer et al., 1994). The MTD test displayed 93% sensitivity and 96% specificity when the NALC/NaOH-processed specimens were compared specimen by specimen with culture and 97% sensitivity and 96% specificity when the SDS-processed specimens were compared specimen by specimen with culture. After discrepant-result analysis using patient history, the sensitivity and specificity of the MTD test with the NALC/NaOH series were 94 and 98%, respectively, and those with the SDS series were 98 and 98%, respectively. Overall, the MTD test performed equally well with specimens processed by the two methods.

A general question that arises from these clinical evaluations is why culture-positive specimens occasionally yield negative amplification results, given that the analytic sensitivities of the amplification tests are one cell or less (Eisenach et al., 1990; Jonas et al., 1993b). One possible answer is that specimens containing few bacilli may be subject to sampling variation. For example, Miller et al. (1994) found that simply repeating the MTD assay increased the sensitivity from 84 to 90%. Similarly, Jonas et al. (1993b) found that 18 of the 24 MTD test-negative, culture-positive specimens had fewer than 100 bacilli per ml of sediment and that 6 of the 18 were positive upon retesting. Another explanation for false-negative results is the presence of inhibitors of the amplification reaction, which was observed by Jonas et al. (1993b) in 6 of 199 culture-positive specimens. Clearly, additional clinical evaluations of amplification-based tests will be necessary to reveal the ultimate utility of such a test in making patient management decisions.

Reporter Mycobacteriophage

A reporter mycobacteriophage is a virus that infects the desired *Mycobacterium* species and produces an easily measured product. The specificity of this approach lies in the host range specificity of the reporter phage. There are phage that can infect only *M. tuberculosis* as well as ones that can grow in several species of *Mycobacterium* (Jones, 1988). The sensitivity of the system lies in the synthesis of large amounts of the reporter product during phage growth (i.e., amplification of the product) and in the sensitivity of the assay in detecting the reporter product. Jacobs et al. (1993) recently constructed a reporter phage for detecting *M. tuberculosis* that carries the gene for the firefly enzyme luciferase. In the presence of ATP, this enzyme oxidizes luciferin to generate light, which is the reaction that makes fireflies glow in the dark (de Wet et al., 1987). As expected, mycobacteria infected with this reporter phage produce light when luciferin is added, and samples containing as few as 500 to 5,000 mycobacteria generate a clear positive signal (Jacobs et al., 1993). Although much work needs to be done to complete the development and evaluation of this assay (e.g., construction of an *M. tuberculosis*-specific reporter phage), it does hold promise for being an inexpensive, easy, and specific assay for detecting *M. tuberculosis* directly from specimens.

This assay may also be useful in distinguishing live and dead bacilli.

RAPID DRUG SUSCEPTIBILITY TESTING

A key limitation of the nucleic acid amplification assays described above is that they cannot distinguish drug-resistant bacilli from drug-susceptible bacilli. Given the importance of drug-resistant tuberculosis, it would be advantageous to determine drug susceptibilities directly from clinical specimens and avoid the time required for culture. At the very least, it would help to be able to determine drug susceptibility from organisms cultured from the specimen without the necessity of subculture.

Genetic Approach

One approach to determining drug susceptibility is based on potential differences between the genetic materials of a resistant strain and a susceptible strain. For example, if kanamycin resistance is due to the acquisition of a gene that encodes an enzyme that destroys kanamycin, then one could use a PCR-based assay to detect the presence of that gene. The assumption would be that if the gene were present, the strain would be kanamycin resistant. If it were absent, the strain would be susceptible to kanamycin. So, theoretically at least, one could develop gene amplification assays for each of the drug resistance alleles. Unfortunately, we are just beginning to learn about the genes that encode drug resistance in *M. tuberculosis* and do not yet know precisely what is different about the genes in resistant strains and those in susceptible strains, although great progress is being made in identifying mechanisms of resistance to isoniazid, ethionamide, and rifampin (Zhang et al., 1992; Banerjee et al., 1994; Telenti et al., 1993).

In many bacteria, rifampin resistance is due to changes in the sequence of a small region of the beta subunit of RNA polymerase so that the enzyme no longer binds rifampin (Jun Jin and Gross, 1988). Recently, the sequences of the genes (*rpoB*) encoding the corresponding region of the *M. tuberculosis* RNA polymerase beta subunit have been determined for resistant and susceptible strains, and a number of mutations thought to cause rifampin resistance have been identified (Telenti et al., 1993). Using this information, Telenti et al. (1993) developed a rapid assay to detect changes in this region of the *rpoB* gene by combining a PCR amplification step with a detection system called single-strand conformation polymorphism electrophoresis (Ilayashi, 1991). They successfully identified changes in 64 of the 66 rifampin-resistant *M. tuberculosis* isolates tested. Thus, this assay holds promise for the rapid identification of most rifampin-resistant strains directly from specimens.

A critical limitation of the genetic approach is that a different assay will be required for each of the possible mechanisms of drug resistance. For example, if isoniazid resistance can result from the loss of the catalase gene or from failure of a key enzyme to bind isoniazid or from a process that blocks the entry of isoniazid into the cell, then at least three different genetic assays would be needed to assess isoniazid resistance.

Functional Approach

The key feature of a drug-resistant strain is that it can grow in the presence of the drug. One rapid way to distinguish growing and nongrowing cells is by measuring the amount of nucleic acids in a culture. For example, Kawa et al. (1989) used the Gen-Probe Rapid Diagnostic System for *M. tuberculosis* to monitor rRNA levels in cultures of *M. tuberculosis* treated with isoniazid, and they could distinguish isoniazid-resistant isolates from isoniazid-susceptible isolates in 3 to 5 days compared to

the 21 to 28 days required for conventional culture assays. The performance of this system with other antituberculosis drugs or with mixed populations of resistant and susceptible bacilli has not been reported. Theoretically, a more rapid differentiation of resistant and susceptible strains might be achieved by targeting a more labile RNA population, such as mRNA. Also, by adding a gene amplification step, this assay might be applicable to the small numbers of bacilli in a clinical specimen.

Reporter mycobacteriophage such as the one described above can also be used to assess drug susceptibility because (i) the production of luciferase activity is sensitive to the metabolic state of the bacterium in that luciferase activity is dependent on both the synthesis of the luciferase enzyme and the ATP levels in the cell, and (ii) antimicrobial agents decrease cellular metabolic activity and can thereby interfere with the synthesis of the luciferase enzyme or can reduce ATP levels in the cell. Consequently, the inhibition of luciferase activity or light production can be used as a surrogate marker for drug susceptibility.

In one possible assay for measuring drug susceptibility (Jacobs et al., 1993), media with or without drugs are inoculated with an isolate and the samples are incubated to allow the drug activity to be realized. The samples are then infected with the luciferase reporter phage and incubated for 1 to 3 h to allow the luciferase enzyme to be produced. Finally, luciferin is added, and luciferase activity is measured. In the absence of any drug, light production is detectable within 15 to 30 min of adding the luciferase reporter phage to the culture, and light production reaches a plateau level by 1 to 3 h (Jacobs et al., 1993). Pretreatment of cultures of a pansusceptible strain of *M. tuberculosis* with isoniazid, rifampin, or streptomycin for 48 h completely abolished light production. Pretreatment of an isoniazid-resistant *M. tuberculosis* strain with isoniazid did not significantly reduce luciferase activity, while pretreatment of this strain with rifampin or streptomycin abolished light production (Jacobs et al., 1993). Thus, this assay can distinguish drug-resistant strains from drug-susceptible strains and can do so in a matter of days compared to the weeks required for conventional drug susceptibility tests.

These preliminary studies used $\sim 10^6$ to 10^8 bacteria per sample. This number is achievable from pure cultures but rarely achievable directly from patient specimens, so the detection limit of this assay must be improved before the assay will be usable with specimens directly. Also, additional important studies will be needed to determine whether the assay can identify specimens that contain a mixture of resistant and susceptible organisms: a patient producing a specimen containing >1% resistant bacilli is considered to have drug-resistant tuberculosis. Despite these concerns, the reporter phage approach does hold great promise for producing a dramatic improvement in drug susceptibility testing for *M. tuberculosis*.

RAPID TESTS FOR DETERMINING DRUG ACTIVITIES

Research to develop new antituberculosis drugs has been greatly hampered by the difficulty and expense of screening compounds for antituberculosis activity. Conventional methods using solid media or radiometric procedures are satisfactory for testing small numbers of highly promising agents but are quite labor intensive, are not suitable for screening large numbers of compounds, and require large amounts of test compounds. The availability of a rapid assay should facilitate and accelerate the screening of the thousands of existing compounds and may even encourage the search for new classes of agents, which are urgently needed to control this reemerging disease.

The luciferase reporter technology described above has been used to develop simple and rapid screening procedures to identify new antituberculosis agents (Cooksey et al., 1993; Jacobs et al., 1993). Once again, the inhibition of luciferase activity is used as a surrogate marker for antimicrobial activity to shorten the time required for determining antituberculosis activity from weeks to hours. These assays require either a luciferase reporter phage to introduce the luciferase genes into an *M. tuberculosis* strain or a well-characterized strain of *M. tuberculosis* that expresses the firefly luciferase enzyme. For example, Cooksey et al. (1993) generated a luciferase-expressing *M. tuberculosis* strain by first constructing a plasmid, pLUC10, that stably replicates and expresses luciferase activity in mycobacteria and then electroporating it into *M. tuberculosis* H37Ra. Sonicates of 10^9 *M. tuberculosis* H37Ra(pLUC10) cells produce ~800 relative light units of activity, which is more than 5 orders of magnitude above background, and significant light production can be detected from samples containing as few as 10^4 bacilli.

One way to use a luciferase-expressing *M. tuberculosis* strain to determine drug activities is to place samples of the strain in the wells of a microtiter plate, add various dilutions of the compounds to be tested, incubate to allow the drug activity to be realized, add luciferin, and measure luciferase activity. An active drug prevents light production, while an inactive drug does not block light production. The microtiter plate format allows the screening of large numbers of compounds and minimizes the amount of candidate agent required for evaluation. Also, by assaying a range of drug concentrations, this procedure can provide an estimate of the MICs of the effective antimicrobial agents.

Cooksey et al. (1993) have shown that this procedure could clearly distinguish active from inactive drugs in as few as 48 h. For example, incubation of the luciferase-expressing *M. tuberculosis* strain with 0.06 μg of isoniazid, rifampin, rifabutin, or streptomycin per ml completely abolished light production. For each of the other five drugs they tested (ciprofloxacin, cycloserine, ethambutol, ethionamide, and kanamycin), bioluminescence readings in samples containing small amounts of the drugs were similar to those in the drug-free controls but then sharply decreased at higher drug concentrations. These decreases in luciferase activity occurred at drug concentrations that correlated well with the MICs determined by conventional susceptibility testing methods. However, the luciferase assay provided results in 2 days, whereas the conventional tests required 3 weeks to provide results, and the luciferase assay required only a single microtiter plate, whereas the conventional assays required dozens of tubes and plates.

SUMMARY

Before the recent nosocomial outbreaks and resurgence of tuberculosis, the standardly used culturing procedures required 4 to 6 weeks to identify *M. tuberculosis* and another 2 to 4 weeks to determine drug susceptibilities. Adoption of available rapid techniques (BACTEC, rapid species identification methods, and direct drug susceptibility testing) has allowed some laboratories to reduce the time required to report results to physicians from 2 months to as few as 10 days, a rather impressive improvement that has helped tremendously in reducing the impact of tuberculosis in some hospitals. The assays described in this chapter are designed to shorten this response time even further.

In general, the results to date clearly demonstrate that the new systems are feasible and that the next generation of rapid diagnostic tests is on the horizon. Perhaps the greatest promise is held by the gene amplification systems that are nearing the marketplace (at least one of these tests has

been submitted to the Food and Drug Administration). If the assays behave as well in routine use as they have in preliminary clinical evaluations, a clinical diagnostic laboratory may soon be able to report the confirmation of an *M. tuberculosis* infection to the physician within hours of receiving a specimen. At the very least, such rapid identification of *M. tuberculosis* in a specimen will allow the physician to promptly initiate proper infection control procedures and therapeutic regimens. These steps alone should help limit the nosocomial transmission of *M. tuberculosis* and may help bring the resurgence of tuberculosis under control.

Acknowledgments. We thank Robert Good, Robin Huebner, William Jacobs, Jr., Douglas Moore, Tim Cleary, G. Pfyffer, and Terry Walker for helpful comments and for providing information prior to publication.

REFERENCES

Altamirano, M., M. T. Kelly, A. Wong, E. T. Bessuille, W. A. Black, and J. A. Smith. 1992. Characterization of a DNA probe for detection of *Mycobacterium tuberculosis* complex in clinical samples by polymerase chain reaction. *J. Clin. Microbiol.* **30:** 2173–2176.

American Thoracic Society and Centers for Disease Control. 1981. The tuberculin skin test. *Am. Rev. Respir. Dis.* **124:**356–363.

American Thoracic Society and Centers for Disease Control. 1990. Diagnostic standards and classification of tuberculosis. *Am. Rev. Respir. Dis.* **142:**725–735.

Banerjee, A., E. Dubnau, A. Quemard, V. Balasubramanian, K. S. Um, T. Wilson, D. Collins, G. de Lisle, and W. R. Jacobs, Jr. 1994. *inhA*, a gene encoding a target for isoniazid and ethionamide in *Mycobacterium tuberculosis. Science* **263:**227–230.

Bates, J., P. J. Brennan, G. W. Douglas, J. C. Feeley, J. Glassroth, D. E. Kohne, W. J. Martin, L. G. Wayne, and C. R. Zeiss. 1986. Subcommittee report on improvements in the diagnosis of tuberculosis. *Am. Rev. Respir. Dis.* **134**(Suppl.):415–417.

Böddinghaus, B., T. Rogall, T. Flohr, H. Blöcker, and E. C. Böttger. 1990. Detection and identification of mycobacteria by amplification of rRNA. *J. Clin. Microbiol.* **28:**1751–1759.

Brisson-Noel, A., B. Gicquel, D. Lecossier, V. Levy-Frebault, X. Nassif, and A. J. Hance. 1989. Rapid diagnosis of tuberculosis by amplification of mycobacterial DNA in clinical samples. *Lancet* **ii**:1069–1071.

Brooks, J. B., M. I. Daneshvar, D. M. Fast, and R. C. Good. 1987. Selective procedures for detecting femtomole quantities of tuberculostearic acid in serum and cerebrospinal fluid by frequency-pulsed electron-capture gas-liquid chromatography. *J. Clin. Microbiol.* **25**:1201–1206.

Brooks, J. B., M. I. Daneshvar, R. L. Haberberger, and I. A. Mikhail. 1990. Rapid diagnosis of tuberculous meningitis by frequency-pulsed electron-capture gas-liquid chromatography detection of carboxylic acids in cerebrospinal fluid. *J. Clin. Microbiol.* **28**:989–997.

Butler, W. R., and J. O. Kilburn. 1988. Identification of major slow growing pathogenic mycobacteria and *Mycobacterium gordonae* by high-performance liquid chromatography of their mycolic acids. *J. Clin. Microbiol.* **26**:50–53.

Centers for Disease Control. 1990. The use of preventive therapy for tuberculosis infection in the United States. Recommendations of the Advisory Committee for the Elimination of Tuberculosis. *Morbid. Mortal. Weekly Rep.* **39**(RR-8):9–12.

Centers for Disease Control. 1991. Purified protein derivative (PPD)-tuberculin anergy and HIV infection: guidelines for anergy testing and management of anergic persons at risk of tuberculosis. *Morbid. Mortal. Weekly Rep.* **40**:27–33.

Clarridge, J. E., R. M. Shawar, T. M. Shinnick, and B. B. Plikaytis. 1993. Large-scale use of polymerase chain reaction for detection of *Mycobacterium tuberculosis* in a routine mycobacteriology laboratory. *J. Clin. Microbiol.* **31**:2049–2056.

Cooksey, R. C., J. T. Crawford, W. R. Jacobs, Jr., and T. M. Shinnick. 1993. A rapid method for screening antimicrobial agents for activity against a strain of *Mycobacterium tuberculosis* expressing firefly luciferase. *Antimicrob. Agents Chemother.* **37**:1348–1352.

Cousins, D. V., S. D. Wilton, B. R. Francis, and B. L. Gow. 1992. Use of polymerase chain reaction for rapid diagnosis of tuberculosis. *J. Clin. Microbiol.* **30**:255–258.

Czerkinsky, C. C., L. A. Nilsson, H. Nygren, O. Ouchterlony, and A. Tarkowski. 1983. A solid-phase enzyme-linked immunospot (ELISPOT) assay for enumeration of specific antibody-secreting cells. *J. Immunol. Methods* **65**:109–121.

Del Portillo, P., L. A. Murillo, and M. E. Patarroyo. 1991. Amplification of species-specific DNA fragment of *Mycobacterium tuberculosis* and its possible use in diagnosis. *J. Clin. Microbiol.* **29**:2163–2168.

de Wet, J. R., K. V. Wood, M. DeLuca, D. R. Helinski, and S. Subramani. 1987. Firefly luciferase gene: structure and expression in mammalian cells. *Mol. Cell. Biol.* **7**:725–737.

DeWit, D., L. Steyn, S. Shoemaker, and M. Sogin. 1990. Direct detection of *Mycobacterium tuberculosis* in clinical specimens by DNA amplification. *J. Clin. Microbiol.* **28**:2437–2441.

Eisenach, K. D., M. D. Cave, J. H. Bates, and J. T. Crawford. 1990. Polymerase chain reaction amplification of a repetitive DNA sequence specific for *Mycobacterium tuberculosis*. *J. Infect. Dis.* **161**:977–981.

Eisenach, K. D., M. D. Sifford, M. D. Cave, J. H. Bates, and J. T. Crawford. 1991. Detection of *Mycobacterium tuberculosis* in sputum samples using a polymerase chain reaction. *Am. Rev. Respir. Dis.* **144**:1160–1163.

Evans, K. D., A. S. Nakasome, P. A. Sutherland, L. M. DeLaMaza, and E. M. Peterson. 1992. Identification of *Mycobacterium tuberculosis* and *Mycobacterium avium-M. intracellulare* directly from primary BACTEC cultures by using acridinium ester labeled DNA probes. *J. Clin. Microbiol.* **30**:2427–2431.

French, G. A., R. Teoh, C. Y. Chan, M. J. Humphries, S. W. Cheung, and G. O'Mahoney. 1987. Diagnosis of tuberculous meningitis by detection of tuberculostearic acid in cerebrospinal fluid. *Lancet* **2**:117–119.

Fries, J. W. U., R. J. Patel, W. F. Piessens, and D. F. Wirth. 1990. Genus- and species-specific DNA probes to identify mycobacteria using the polymerase chain reaction. *Mol. Cell. Probes* **4**:87–105.

Grange, J. M. 1984. The humoral immune response in tuberculosis: its nature, biological role, and diagnostic usefulness. *Adv. Tuberc. Res.* **21**:1–78.

Hance, A. J., B. Grandchamp, V. Levy-Frebault, D. Lecossier, J. Rauzier, D. Bocart, and B. Gicquel. 1989. Detection and identification of mycobacteria by amplification of mycobacterial DNA. *Mol. Microbiol.* **3**:843–849.

Hermans, P. W. M., A. R. J. Schuitema, D. van Soolingen, C. P. H. J. Verstynen, E. M. Bik, J. E. R. Thole, A. H. J. Kolk, and J. D. A. van Embden. 1990. Specific detection of *Mycobacterium tuberculosis* complex strains by polymerase chain reaction. *J. Clin. Microbiol.* **28**:1204–1213.

Huebner, R. E., R. C. Good, and J. I. Tokars. 1993a. Current practices in mycobacteriology: results of a survey of state public health laboratories. *J. Clin. Microbiol.* **31**:771–775.

Huebner, R. E., M. F. Schein, and J. B. Bass, Jr. 1993b. The tuberculin skin test. *Clin. Infect. Dis.* **17**:968–975.

Ilayashi, K. 1991. PCR-SSCP: a simple and sensitive method for detection of mutations in genomic PCR. *PCR Methods Appl.* **1**:34–38.

Iovannisci, D. M., and E. S. Winn-Deen. 1993. Ligation amplification and fluorescence detection of *Myco-*

bacterium tuberculosis DNA. *Mol. Cell. Probes* 7:35–43.

Ivanyi, J. 1991. Serologic tests for the diagnosis of tuberculosis and leprosy, p. 267–279. *In* A. Vaheri, R. C. Tilton, and A. Balows (ed.), *Rapid Methods and Automation in Microbiology and Immunology.* Springer-Verlag, Berlin.

Jacobs, W. R., R. G. Barletta, R. Udani, J. Chan, G. Kalkut, G. Sosne, T. Kieser, G. J. Sarkis, G. F. Hatfull, and B. R. Bloom. 1993. Rapid assessment of drug susceptibilities of *Mycobacterium tuberculosis* by means of luciferase reporter phages. *Science* 260:819–822.

Jonas, V., M. Alden, T. Endozo, P. Hammond, K. Kamisango, C. Knott, R. Lankford, D. McAllister, L. Wood, Y. Yang, S. McDonough, and D. Kacian. 1993a. Rapid direct detection of *Mycobacterium tuberculosis* in respiratory specimens, abstr. U-44, p. 176. *Abstr. 93rd Gen. Meet. Am. Soc. Microbiol.*

Jonas, V., M. J. Alden, J. I. Curry, K. Kamisango, C. A. Knott, R. Lankford, J. M. Wolfe, and D. F. Moore. 1993b. Detection and identification of *Mycobacterium tuberculosis* directly from induced sputum specimens using amplification of rRNA. *J. Clin. Microbiol.* 31:2410–2416.

Jones, W. D., Jr. 1988. Bacteriophage typing of *Mycobacterium tuberculosis* cultures from incidents of suspected laboratory cross-contamination. *Tubercle* 69:43–46.

Jun Jin, D., and C. A. Gross. 1988. Mapping and sequencing of mutations in the *Escherichia coli rpoB* gene that lead to rifampin resistance. *J. Mol. Biol.* 202:45–58.

Kawa, D. E., D. R. Pennel, L. N. Kubista, and R. F. Schell. 1989. Development of a rapid method for determining the susceptibility of *Mycobacterium tuberculosis* to isoniazid using the Gen-Probe DNA hybridization system. *Antimicrob. Agents Chemother.* 33:1000–1005.

Kent, B. D., and G. P. Kubica. 1985. Public health mycobacteriology: a guide for the level III laboratory, 207 p. U.S. Department of Health and Human Services. Centers for Disease Control, Atlanta.

Koch, R. 1891. Weitere Mittheilung uber das Tuberkulin. *Dtsch. Med. Wochenschr.* 17:1189–1192.

Kohne, D. E. 1989. The use of DNA probes to detect and identify microorganisms, p. 11–35. *In* B. Kleger, D. Jungkind, E. Hinks, and L. A. Miller (ed.), *Rapid Methods in Clinical Microbiology.* Plenum Press, New York.

Kolk, A. H. J., A. R. J. Schuitema, S. Kuijper, J. van Leeuwen, P. W. M. Hermans, J. D. A. van Embden, and R. A. Hartskeerl. 1992. Detection of *Mycobacterium tuberculosis* in clinical samples by using polymerase chain reaction and the nonradioactive detection system. *J. Clin. Microbiol.* 30:2567–2575.

Kramer, F. R., S. Tyagi, C. E. Guerra, H. Lomeli, and

P. M. Lizardi. 1991. Q-beta amplification assays, p. 17–22. *In* A. Vaheri, R. C. Tilton, and A. Balows (ed.), *Rapid Methods and Automation in Microbiology and Immunology.* Springer-Verlag, Berlin.

Larsson, L., P. A. Mardh, G. Odham, and G. Westerdahl. 1981. Use of selected ion monitoring for detection of tuberculostearic and C_{32} mycocerosic acid in mycobacteria and in five-day-old cultures of sputum specimens from patients with pulmonary tuberculosis. *Acta Pathol. Microbiol. Scand. Sect. B* 89:245–251.

Lee, F. K., A. J. Nahmias, S. A. Lowery, S. E. Reef, S. E. Thompson, J. Oleske, A. Vahline, and C. Czerkinsky. 1989. ELISPOT—a new approach to the study of the dynamics of virus-immune system interaction for diagnosis and monitoring of HIV infection. *AIDS Res. Hum. Retroviruses* 5:517–523.

Lu, C. Z., J. Qiao, T. Shen, and H. Link. 1990. Early diagnosis of tuberculosis meningitis by detection of anti-BCG secreting cells in cerebrospinal fluid. *Lancet* 336:10–13.

Manjunath, N., P. Shankara, L. Rajan, A. Bhargava, S. Saluja, and Shriniwas. 1991. Evaluation of a polymerase chain reaction for the diagnosis of tuberculosis. *Tubercle* 72:21–27.

Mardh, P. A., L. Larson, N. Hoiby, H. C. Engbaek, and G. Oldham. 1983. Tuberculostearic acid as a diagnostic marker in tuberculous meningitis. *Lancet* i:367.

Miller, N., S. G. Hernandez, and T. Cleary. 1994. Evaluation of the Gen-Probe Amplified Mycobacterium Tuberculosis Direct Test and PCR for direct detection of *Mycobacterium tuberculosis* in clinical specimens. *J. Clin. Microbiol.* 32:393–397.

Minniken, D. E., and M. Goodfellow. 1980. Lipid composition in the classification and identification of acid-fast bacteria, p. 189–256. *In* M. Goodfellow and R. G. Board (ed.), *Microbiological Classification and Identification.* Academic Press, London.

Mullis, K. B., and F. A. Faloona. 1987. Specific synthesis of DNA in vitro via a polymerase-catalyzed chain reaction. *Methods Enzymol.* 155:335–350.

National MDR-TB Task Force. 1992. National action plan to combat multidrug-resistant tuberculosis. *Morbid. Mortal. Weekly Rep.* 41(RR-11):1–48.

Nesheim, S., F. Lee, M. Sawyer, D. Jones, B. Slade, N. Shaffer, R. Holmes, V. Grimes, M. Rogers, and A. Nahmias. 1992. Diagnosis of human immunodeficiency virus infection by enzyme-linked immunospot (ELISPOT) assays in a prospectively followed cohort of infants of HIV-seropositive women. *Pediatr. Infect. Dis. J.* 11:635–639.

Nolte, F. S., B. Metchock, J. E. McGowan, Jr., A. Edwards, O. Okwumabua, C. Thurmond, P. S. Mitchell, B. Plikaytis, and T. Shinnick. 1993. Direct detection of *Mycobacterium tuberculosis* in sputum by polymerase chain reaction and DNA hybridization. *J. Clin. Microbiol.* 31:1777–1782.

Nycz, C. M., G. P. Vonk, J. L. Schram, G. D. Shank, and G. T. Walker. Detection of *Mycobacterium avium/intracellulare* complex specific DNA using strand displacement amplification. Submitted for publication.

Palmer, C. E., and L. B. Edwards. 1967. Tuberculin test in retrospect and prospect. *Arch. Environ. Health* 15:792–808.

Pao, C. C., T. S. B. Yen, J.-B. You, J.-S. Maa, E. H. Fiss, and C.-H. Chang. 1990. Detection and identification of *Mycobacterium tuberculosis* by DNA amplification. *J. Clin. Microbiol.* 28:1877–1880.

Patel, R. J., J. W. U. Fries, W. F. Piessens, and D. F. Wirth. 1990. Sequence analysis and amplification by polymerase chain reaction of a cloned DNA fragment of *Mycobacterium tuberculosis*. *J. Clin. Microbiol.* 28:513–518.

Pfyffer, G. E., P. Kissling, R. Wirth, and R. Weber. 1994. Direct detection of *Mycobacterium tuberculosis* complex in respiratory specimens by a target-amplified test system. *J. Clin. Microbiol.* 32:918–923.

Plikaytis, B. B., R. H. Gelber, and T. M. Shinnick. 1990. Rapid and sensitive detection of *Mycobacterium leprae* using a nested primer gene amplification assay. *J. Clin. Microbiol.* 28:1913–1917.

Plikaytis, B. B., B. D. Plikaytis, M. A. Yakrus, W. R. Butler, C. L. Woodley, V. A. Silcox, and T. M. Shinnick. 1992. Differentiation of slow growing *Mycobacterium* species including *Mycobacterium tuberculosis* by gene amplification and restriction fragment length polymorphism. *J. Clin. Microbiol.* 30:1815–1822.

Rogall, T., T. Flohr, and E. C. Böttger. 1990. Differentiation of *Mycobacterium* species by direct sequencing of amplified DNA. *J. Gen. Microbiol.* 136:1915–1920.

Savic, B., U. Sobring, S. Alugupalli, L. Larsson, and H. Miörner. 1992. Evaluation of polymerase chain reaction, tuberculostearic acid analysis, and direct microscopy for the detection of *Mycobacterium tuberculosis* in sputum. *J. Infect. Dis.* 166:1177–1180.

Schram, J. L., D. D. Shank, and G. T. Walker. DNA probe detection of *Mycobacterium avium* and *Mycobacterium intracellulare* genomic DNA using strand displacement amplification (SDA). Submitted for publication.

Sedgewick, J. D., and P. G. Holt. 1983. A solid phase immunoenzymatic technique for the enumeration of specific antibody-secreting cells. *J. Immunol. Methods* 65:301–309.

Shawar, R. M., F. A. K. El Zaatari, A. Nataraj, and J. E. Clarridge. 1993. Detection of *Mycobacterium tuberculosis* in clinical samples by two-step polymerase chain reaction and nonisotopic hybridization methods. *J. Clin. Microbiol.* 31:61–65.

Sjobring, U., M. Mecklenburg, A. B. Andersen, and H. Miörner. 1990. Polymerase chain reaction for detection of *Mycobacterium tuberculosis*. *J. Clin. Microbiol.* 28:2200–2204.

Smithwick, R. W. 1976. *Laboratory Manual for Acid-Fast Microscopy*, 2nd ed. Center for Disease Control, Atlanta.

Soini, H., M. Skurnik, K. Liippo, E. Tala, and M. K. Viljanen. 1992. Detection and identification of mycobacteria by amplification of a segment of the gene coding for the 32-kDa protein. *J. Clin. Microbiol.* 30:2025–2028.

Spargo, C. A., P. D. Haaland, S. R. Jurgensen, D. D. Shank, and G. T. Walker. 1993. Chemiluminescent detection of strand displacement amplified DNA from species comprising the *Mycobacterium tuberculosis* complex. *Mol. Cell. Probes* 7:395–404.

Sritharan, V., and R. H. Barker. 1991. A simple method for diagnosing *Mycobacterium tuberculosis* infections in clinical samples using PCR. *Mol. Cell. Probes* 5:385–395.

Stead, W. W., T. To, R. W. Harrison, and J. H. Abraham. 1987. Benefit-risk consideration in preventive treatment for tuberculosis in elderly persons. *Ann. Intern. Med.* 107:834–845.

Telenti, A., P. Imboden, F. Marchesi, D. Lowrie, S. Cole, M. J. Colston, L. Matter, K. Schopfer, and T. Bodmer. 1993. Detection of rifampin-resistance mutations in *Mycobacterium tuberculosis*. *Lancet* 341:647–650.

Urdea, M. S. 1991. Controlled synthetic oligonucleotide networks for the detection of pathogenic organisms, p. 1–5. *In* A. Vaheri, R. C. Tilton, and A. Balows (ed.), *Rapid Methods and Automation in Microbiology and Immunology*. Springer-Verlag, Berlin.

Victor, T., R. DuToit, and P. D. VanHeiden. 1992. Purification of sputum samples through sucrose improves detection of *Mycobacterium tuberculosis* by polymerase chain reaction. *J. Clin. Microbiol.* 30:1514–1517.

Walker, G. T., M. S. Fraiser, J. L. Schram, M. C. Little, J. D. Nadeau, and D. P. Malinowski. 1992a. Strand displacement amplification—an isothermal in vitro DNA amplification technique. *Nucleic Acids Res.* 20:1691–1696.

Walker, G. T., M. C. Little, J. D. Nadeau, and D. D. Shank. 1992b. Isothermal in vitro amplification of DNA by a restriction enzyme/DNA polymerase system. *Proc. Natl. Acad. Sci. USA* 89:392–396.

Walker, G. T., J. D. Nadeau, P. A. Spears, J. L. Schram, C. M. Nycz, and D. D. Shank. A DNA probe test for *M. tuberculosis* and other mycobacterial pathogens. Submitted for publication.

Zhang, J., B. Heym, B. Allen, D. Young, and S. Cole. 1992. The catalase-peroxidase gene of *Mycobacterium tuberculosis*. *Nature* (London) 358:591–593.

Tuberculosis: Pathogenesis, Protection, and Control
Edited by Barry R. Bloom
© 1994 American Society for Microbiology, Washington, DC 20005

Chapter 31

The BCG Experience: Implications for Future Vaccines against Tuberculosis

Barry R. Bloom and Paul E. M. Fine

More people alive today have been vaccinated with BCG (bacille Calmette-Guérin) than have received any other vaccine. Approximately 100 million newborns and children received BCG in 1992 through the World Health Organization (WHO)/ United Nations Children's Emergency Fund (UNICEF) Expanded Program for Immunization (WHO, 1992). It has many advantages for a vaccine: it can be given at birth or any time thereafter; a single inoculation can produce long-lasting sensitization; it is safe; it is relatively stable; it produces a scar, which is useful for epidemiological surveillance; and it is inexpensive. In addition, though BCG is generally considered a vaccine against tuberculosis, it has also provided protection against leprosy in four major trials and in observational studies in Asia, Africa, and Latin America (Fine and Rodrigues, 1990). However, despite its wide usage and these many advantages, BCG remains the most controversial of all currently used vaccines, as its protective efficacy has varied widely in different parts of the world and its impact on tuberculosis

trends worldwide remains unclear. At a time when tuberculosis is increasing in both developing and industrialized countries, when the risk for tuberculosis has increased in many populations, particularly among individuals infected with human immunodeficiency virus (HIV), and when multidrug-resistant strains are emerging, there is renewed interest in and urgency about understanding the lessons of BCG.

ORIGINS

In 1906, Calmette observed that oral infection of guinea pigs with a weakly virulent equine strain of tubercle bacilli that persisted in the lymph nodes conferred resistance to reinfection by the intravenous route (Calmette, 1927; Guérin, 1957). Calmette and Guérin then turned their attention to a virulent strain of the bovine tubercle bacillus previously isolated by Nocard from a heifer with tuberculous mastitis. They fortuitously observed that they could prevent its aggregation in culture on a potato-glycerin medium by the addition of ox bile, and after 39 passages, they noted a change in colony morphology. Knowing that numerous investigators had tried to attenuate the tubercle bacillus (using methods devised by Pasteur for attenuation of

Barry R. Bloom • Howard Hughes Medical Institute, Albert Einstein College of Medicine, Bronx, New York 10461. *Paul E. M. Fine* • London School of Tropical Medicine and Hygiene, London WC1E 7HT, United Kingdom.

viruses as vaccines), they proceeded to test the virulence of this variant strain. Over the next 13 years, they reported that infection of bovines, guinea pigs, mice, rhesus monkeys, and chimpanzees with this strain produced no evidence of reversion to virulence but instead conferred resistance, after 30 days, to challenge with virulent bovine or human tubercle bacilli. In 1921, this bacillus was administered orally on the third, fifth, and seventh days of life to a newborn in the Hôpital de la Charité in Paris (Weill-Halle, 1980). The child was deemed at extremely high risk of tuberculosis, as his mother had died of the disease and the child was destined to live with a grandmother who was also suffering from tuberculosis. That child was to remain free of tuberculosis for his entire life. Calmette (1927) later reported that of 969 children who were born of tuberculous mothers or otherwise had close tuberculous contacts and were vaccinated with BCG between 1921 and 1927, only 3.9% died of tuberculosis or unspecified causes, while the comparable mortality rate for unvaccinated children was 32.6%. Despite some controversy about such evidence (Greenwood, 1928), BCG was recommended by the League of Nations in 1928 for widespread use in the prevention of tuberculosis.

BCG VACCINES TODAY

Formally, the WHO, in addition to national regulatory authorities, oversees the quality control of BCG vaccines by means of regular in vitro testing and clinical trials (WHO, 1966; Milstien and Gibson, 1989). Three parent strains (Glaxo-1077, Tokyo-172, and Pasteur-1173P2) account for over 90% of the BCG vaccines in use in the world today. Though these strains were all derived from the original uncloned culture of Calmette and Guérin, they have since been grown under very different conditions in different reference laboratories and pro-duction facilities and are known to differ in a variety of characteristics, including growth rate, morphology, antigen expression, and viability (Osborn, 1983; Milstien and Gibson, 1989). The vaccines have traditionally been grown as pellicles on the surface of liquid Sauton medium and harvested at 6 to 9 days (ten Dam et al., 1976). The semidry mass (obtained after filtering and pressing) is homogenized in a ball mill. The exact degree of homogenization is variable but critical, as it determines the degree of dispersion and viability of the organisms. Some producers, such as Glaxo (now Evans) and Pasteur, have grown the bacilli dispersed in liquid cultures. Homogenized vaccine suspensions are now typically freeze-dried and suspended in saline or distilled water before use. In order to prevent continued genetic changes in the strains, WHO in 1966 recommended that no batch of vaccine be prepared from any culture carried more than 12 passages beyond a defined frozen "seed lot" (WHO, 1966).

The viability of BCG vaccines is defined by convention as the number of colony-forming organisms (or units; thus, CFU) relative to the total mass or number of acid-fast organisms; this number ranges from 5 to 45%. Thus, a fresh vaccine suspension containing approximately 10^8 bacilli per mg of BCG (moist weight) may yield only 5×10^6 to 45×10^6 CFU. The viable proportion may decrease by half after freeze-drying. Vaccines produced as dispersed cultures tend to have higher viability than do those produced as surface pellicles (Gheorghiu et al., 1988). It is possible that increased viability is responsible for the higher reactigenicity associated with some dispersed culture vaccines and also that the presence of nonviable organisms may not be entirely detrimental, as they may elicit a local cell-mediated immune response that retards systemic dissemination of the bacilli (Gheorghiu et al., 1988; Mackaness et al., 1973).

SAFETY OF BCG

A major catastrophe that cast a cloud over the reputation of BCG vaccines occurred in 1929. In Lubeck, Germany, 251 children received a BCG vaccine prepared at a local institute, and 72 of these children died. Subsequent investigation revealed that the institute also maintained cultures of virulent tubercle bacilli and that the batch of BCG vaccine given to the children had accidently been contaminated with one of these strains of *Mycobacterium tuberculosis* (Lubeck, 1935). By virtue of its peculiar metabolic characteristic of turning Sauton's medium green, the contaminating strain was demonstrated unequivocally to be the Kiel strain of *M. tuberculosis*. BCG was thus vindicated, but public confidence in the vaccine was severely damaged, and Calmette died in 1933 a disheartened man.

Use of BCG vaccines increased in Europe after World War II and in developing countries starting in the 1950s to the extent that the vaccines have now been given to over 3 billion people. In a major evaluation of BCG's safety, Lotte attempted to catalog all adverse events reported as attributed to BCG vaccination (Lotte et al., 1984, 1988). Two of her conclusions are notable. First, the reports of severe neurologic or fatal sequelae, in particular from Europe, where the likelihood of ascertainment is greatest, indicate that the risk of such events is extremely rare, far less than that reported for the smallpox vaccine (Lotte et al., 1984, 1988; ten Dam et al., 1976). This estimate is considerably lower than that reported for smallpox vaccine (Fenner et al., 1988). Second, BCG vaccines are associated with a variety of more common minor adverse effects in addition to induration and ulceration of the vaccination site, which occur in almost all vaccinees. Prominent among these adverse effects are regional suppurative adenitis, reported at a frequency of 0.1 to 38/1,000, and osteitis (0.01 to 330/10^6). The risk of such adverse effects appears to vary with the strain of BCG, some strains apparently being more reactigenic. While such condition are not life-threatening, they constitute an important problem for vaccination programs. Given that BCG is the first vaccine a child receives in the Expanded Program for Immunization, the reactions may discourage families from completing the recommended vaccination schedule, thereby placing children at unnecessary risk for other vaccine-preventable diseases.

A new question has arisen regarding the safety of BCG in HIV-infected individuals. A small number of cases of disseminated BCG-osis have been reported among children who received BCG vaccine and were subsequently found to be HIV seropositive (von Reyn et al., 1987; Braun and Cauthen, 1992; Weltman and Rose, 1993). While *M. bovis*-type strains were identified in several cases, it was not always established that the organism was in fact a BCG vaccine strain rather than virulent *M. bovis* infection unrelated to vaccination. Given the very large number of children vaccinated each year, one might take some comfort in the fact that the reported rate of disseminated BCG-osis is not greater. This may be due in part to the attenuation of the BCG strains but may also reflect inefficient recognition and reporting of vaccine-related complications in developing countries, particularly in Africa, where many thousands of HIV-infected infants receive BCG each year. Several studies have revealed no increase in complications of BCG in HIV-seropositive compared to HIV-seronegative children (Lallemant-Le Coeur et al., 1991; Centers for Disease Control, 1991). There thus appears to be a window in time allowing safe vaccination of newborns before congenitally HIV-infected infants become so immunodeficient that BCG-osis becomes a substantial risk. WHO currently recommends that BCG immunization of newborns continue, excluding only children showing overt signs of immunodeficiency (WHO, 1987).

BCG AND PROTECTION AGAINST TUBERCULOSIS

The conventional measure of the utility of a vaccine is its protective efficacy, which is defined as the percent reduction in disease risk associated with a vaccine or, more formally,

examined, irrespective of whether or not that individual had actually received a scar-producing vaccine. The rarity of tuberculosis (an annual incidence of 1/1,000 is high) means that large trials are necessary in order to obtain sufficient cases to measure vaccine efficacy with reasonable precision.

$$\text{protective efficacy} = \frac{(\text{incidence rate in unvaccinated} - \text{incidence rate in vaccinees})}{\text{incidence rate in unvaccinated}} \times 100\%$$

A major concern in interpreting differences in disease incidence between vaccinated and unvaccinated individuals is the possibility that observed differences are due to factors not directly related to the vaccine but in fact attributable to underlying differences in susceptibility, exposure, follow-up, or diagnosis between the two groups (Smith, 1988). Factors such as socioeconomic status and gender can affect both susceptibility and access to medical services and can thus bias outcomes. In addition to variables that one may readily predict, there may be other confounding factors that are difficult to anticipate.

Recognition of the need to eliminate or at least minimize biases has led to emphasis on randomized controlled trials as the "gold standard" method for vaccine evaluation. Random allocation ensures that the groups who receive one or another vaccine or placebo are comparable. To avoid biases on the part of the staff conducting the trial, it is desirable that the test be double blind, so that neither the recipient nor the investigator knows which vaccine any particular individual received. Though randomization of trial participants is relatively straightforward, the fact that BCG produces a local ulcer followed by a scar makes blinding particularly difficult. Nevertheless, some trials have achieved this, for example, by ensuring that a bandage is placed over the site of vaccination before each individual is

Furthermore, in order to evaluate the duration of protection, such trials must continue for many years. Randomized controlled trials of antituberculosis vaccines are thus very major undertakings.

The results of the major randomized controlled trials are summarized in Table 1, and those of the major observational studies are summarized in Fig. 1. (The reader is referred to Hart [1967], ten Dam [1984], Fine [1988, 1989], and Smith [in press] for more discussion of these studies and to Rosenthal [1980] for reference to many other observational studies, e.g., large volunteer studies by Dahlstrom and Difs [1951].) A meta-analysis of BCG in the prevention of tuberculosis that considers 13 prospective studies and 10 case control studies has recently been completed (Colditz et al., in press). While it concluded that on average BCG was about 50% protective in preventing tuberculosis, the biological and operational significance of averaging, in essence, such widely divergent results is itself arguable. A complete review of the design, results, and analyses of all these trials is not feasible here, but a few summary comments are in order. In some of the trials (e.g., in Chicago), newborns or infants were vaccinated, and thus the trials assessed protection against disease in young children. Other trials (in Puerto Rico and Great Britain) targeted schoolchildren and thus evaluated protection in adoles-

Table 1. Summary of major randomized BCG trials

Trial or study	BCG vaccine	Age	No. studied		No. of tuberculosis cases		Protective efficacy (%)	Follow-up (yr)	Atypical exposure[a]	Reference
			Unvaccinated	Vaccinated	Control	BCG				
Haiti	Montreal and isoniazid	<20 yr	629	2,545	15	25	80	3	?	Vandiviere et al., 1973
Canada, Qu'appelle Cree Indians	Montreal	<3 mo	303	306	29	6	80	6.5	Low	Ferguson and Simes, 1949
British MRC	Danish and vole	14 yr	12,867	13,598	93	56	77	20	(Low)	Hart and Sutherland, 1977
North American Indians	Phipps	0–19 yr	1,451	1,541	372	108	75	20	(Low)	Aronson et al., 1958
Chicago, high risk	Tice	<3 mo	1,665	1,716	65	17	75?	23	Low	Rosenthal et al., 1961
South Africa, miners	Glaxo	30 yr	17,135	20,623	74	48	37	3	?	Coetzee and Berjak, 1968
Puerto Rico	Birkhaug	1–18 yr	27,338	50,634	141	186	31	6.3	(High)	Comstock et al., 1974
India, Madanapalle	Madras	All ages	5,808	5,069	46	28	31	14	High	Frimodt-Moller et al., 1973
Georgia	Tice	6–17 yr	2,341	2,398	3	5	None	20	High	Comstock and Webster, 1969
Georgia and Alabama	Tice	>5 yr	17,854	16,913	32	26	14	14	High	Comstock et al., 1976
India, Chingleput	Danish and Paris	>1 yr	79,398	272,455			None	12.5	High	Tuberculosis Prevention Trial, Madras, 1980
<7 mm			30,000	60,000	93	192	None			

[a] Parentheses indicate presumed, not reported, exposure.

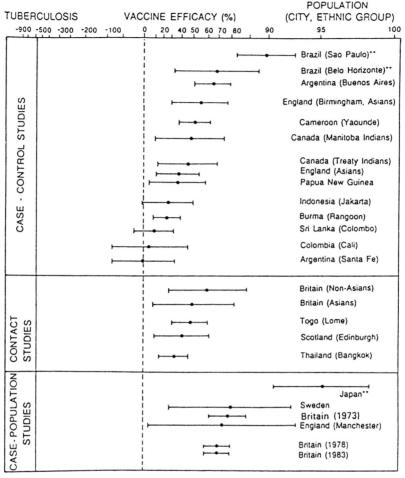

Figure 1. Estimation of protective efficacy of BCG vaccination against tuberculosis derived from case-control studies, contact studies, and comparisons between vaccination rate among patients and the general population. Vaccine efficacy is shown on a logarithmic scale, and the bars indicate 95% confidence intervals. (From Rodrigues and Smith, 1990.)

cents and young adults. Yet other trials (in Georgia and Alabama in the United States and in Chingleput and Bangalore in South India) included all ages. All of the vaccines in Table 1 were applied intradermally, but different methods were used, e.g., multiple puncture (Chicago, Georgia, Alabama) or injection (Puerto Rico, Great Britain, Madanapalle, Chingleput). Some of the trials compared different vaccines (the Great Britain trial included a Danish BCG and a vaccine prepared from *M. microti*, and the Chingleput trial in-

cluded two different dosages of both Paris and Danish BCGs). In all but the Chingleput trial, individuals assessed to be positive to one or another dose of tuberculin were excluded from the randomization, as it was felt that such individuals would not benefit from BCG (on the assumption that tuberculin positivity implied prior infection with the tubercle bacillus) and would suffer particularly large local reactions. In most trials, clinical as well as radiographic or laboratory diagnosis was included, although the

Chingleput trial in South India emphasized bacteriological confirmation as well.

The most striking aspect of these trial results is the enormous variability in protective efficacy, ranging from −57 to over 75%. A second obvious feature is that despite the large size of these trials and the effort devoted to them, the actual numbers of cases detected were small. This is most dramatic in the Georgia-Alabama and the Chingleput trials. In the latter, although it had been anticipated that at least 350 cases would be detected in the 97,000 individuals who were skin test "negative" (less than 7-mm response) at intake, only 52 cases were detected in the first 7.5 years of follow-up (Tuberculosis Prevention Trial, Madras, 1980).

The cost, time, and difficulty of conducting randomized controlled trials and the confusing results shown in Table 1 have encouraged the use of observational studies to evaluate the efficacy of BCG vaccines. They are known as "observational" because they are based on passive observation alone, without active intervention in the population as in trials. There are basically two sorts of such trials: cohort and case-control. In cohort-type studies, one compares incidence rates of disease in vaccinated and unvaccinated individuals, but the allocation of vaccines is determined not by the investigator but by the prevailing situation in the population concerned. Several variants of this design have been used depending on whether records that allow follow-up of large numbers of vaccinated and unvaccinated individuals and tracing of tuberculosis incidence are available (as in the United Kingdom [Sutherland and Springett, 1987] and in Malawi [Ponnighaus et al., 1992]) or whether the analysis concentrates on special high-risk groups such as household contacts of known cases (a design encouraged by the WHO [Tidjani et al., 1986; Padungchan et al., 1986]).

The case-control approach is different, being based upon a comparison of prior vaccination status of cases (preferably recently diagnosed) with that of a group of controls, generally selected so as to be similar to the cases in age, sex, and socioeconomic status (Smith, 1982). It is then possible to estimate the vaccine efficacy on the basis of the ratio of the odds of vaccination (i.e., number vaccinated divided by number not vaccinated) in the cases and the controls. It is ideal to have a vaccine registration system for later ascertainment of whether an individual did or did not receive vaccine. Because that is currently seldom available in developing countries, an approximation is made by examining the individuals for a BCG scar, even though one is fully aware that not all BCG vaccinations leave a scar that is detectable years later and that there are not infrequently scars that mimic those of a BCG vaccination. Nevertheless, with care, it is possible to obtain meaningful data from case-controlled methods, although the degree of confidence varies with the percentage of the population that is actually covered by vaccines. It is recognized that both of these observational study designs are open to a variety of biases owing to the fact that neither vaccination, disease risk, nor disease ascertainment is randomly or independently distributed in populations. For example, it is known that BCG was introduced into many countries in mass campaigns, which concentrated on schools. In many of these countries, only better-off families send their children to school, providing a confounding situation in which better-off children, who are probably less likely than average to contract tuberculosis on account of their socioeconomic advantages, are also preferential recipients of the vaccine. It would thus be unwise to attribute a low incidence of tuberculosis in such children solely to BCG vaccination. For such reasons, the design and analysis of all these types of studies are difficult, and particular care must be taken to assess the comparability of the various groups. Once again, we are struck by the wide range of estimates of vaccine efficacy.

If a principal aim of any global or national vaccine program is to prevent disease, either directly in the vaccinated individual or indirectly from a reduction in transmission, then analysis of trends in tuberculosis incidence after the adoption of a BCG program should provide a measure of impact. Using such an approach, Bjartveit and Waaler (1965) provided evidence for a direct protective effect of BCG but not for the indirect effect. Unfortunately, vaccination data and disease reporting have been too inconsistent in most countries to allow convincing interpretation of impact on recorded incidence over time. In most wealthy countries, the incidence of tuberculosis has been declining for at least a century, and thus it is unreasonable to attribute recent declines to BCG vaccination alone. This is illustrated in comparisons between The Netherlands (which never employed BCG vaccination on a large scale but relied on tuberculin screening, outbreak investigation, and chemoprophylaxis, as in the United States) and the United Kingdom and Scandinavia (which instituted national BCG vaccination in the 1950s and placed less emphasis on tuberculin screening and chemoprophylaxis). The declines in tuberculosis reported in these countries were similar, despite the very different approaches to tuberculosis control (Styblo, 1991; Sutherland, 1981). Of course, one reason for this similarity is the fact that most tuberculous disease and most sources of transmission in the communities in these countries are among older individuals, who were born too early to be eligible for the BCG vaccination programs that began in the 1950s.

It is these results, in particular those summarized in Table 1, that have led to uncertainty about the protective efficacy of BCG and to controversy about its appropriate use. The dilemma is that BCG, or at least some vaccine strains, appears to have imparted appreciable protection in some populations, even in some areas of the United States, but this is not true of all the vaccines or all the populations.

It should be emphasized that the results discussed above relate mainly to pulmonary tuberculosis. This form of the disease represents the majority of all tuberculous disease and is important also for its role in transmission of infection. However, despite the variability in BCG's protection against pulmonary disease in adults, studies of the effect of BCG vaccination on preventing the serious forms of tuberculosis in children (tuberculous meningitis and disseminated tuberculosis) have shown consistently high protection (Rodrigues et al., in press).

INTERPRETING THE VARIABLE EFFICACY OF BCG

The inconsistencies in BCG's observed protection have long been the subject of debate. We believe it is important to review the principal interpretations that have been offered, because careful consideration of them will be necessary if improved vaccines and trials against tuberculosis are to be undertaken.

Methodological Flaws

Clemens et al. (1983) argued that the variation in results reflected methodological differences between the major trials. They concentrated on four types of bias: (i) susceptibility bias, which occurs if subjects allocated to receive or not receive BCG are not distributed similarly with respect to their susceptibility to tuberculosis; (ii) surveillance bias, which occurs if the vaccinated and unvaccinated individuals do not receive equal attention in follow-up examinations; (iii) diagnostic-testing bias, which occurs if the criteria for soliciting of diagnostic tests are not equivalent in both groups; and (iv) diagnostic-interpretation bias, which occurs if diagnostic information is not evaluated independently of knowledge of the patients' vaccination status. The authors attempted to grade eight trials by each of these categories and concluded that the three trials (North American Indians, Great Britain, and Chicago) that showed the highest efficacies were in general better protected against bias and had greater statistical precision (narrower confidence intervals) than did the trials showing lower efficacies. Though this exercise was useful in pointing out some of the potential pitfalls of BCG evaluation, it did not explain away all of the observations of low efficacy in the trials (and did not consider the observational studies at all). Most experts believe that the major differences in protective efficacy as observed in the several studies cannot be explained on methodological grounds alone. The weight of evidence indicates that the differences also reflect biological factors.

Differences between Vaccines

The recognized heterogeneity between BCG vaccines provides one obvious potential explanation for observed differences in protective efficacy (Osborn, 1983; Comstock, 1988). Calmette's original culture was not preserved, and until the 1960s, there was no seed lot system to reduce the increasing variation of individual vaccine strains grown under different conditions in different laboratories.

There is some direct evidence consistent with the vaccine strain hypothesis. Comstock (1988) has pointed out that reanalysis of case-control studies in Cali, Colombia, and in Indonesia by date of vaccination suggests that efficacy fell in each of these populations when the programs shifted from Japanese or Glaxo to Danish or Paris vaccines. A study in Hong Kong revealed statistically significant differences between protection associated with Paris and Japanese vaccines (ten Dam, 1993).

The hypothesis that the trial differences were due primarily to differences in vaccines is challenged by the finding that apparently similar vaccines have given very different efficacies in different trials. For example, the Danish strain gave high protection in the Medical Research Council (MRC) trial in the United Kingdom but no protection in the Chingleput trial. In contrast, quite different vaccines, for example, the Danish BCG and *M. microti* (the vole bacillus), gave identical high levels of protection in the British MRC trial, and both Paris and Danish vaccines gave equally poor protection in the South India trial. Even though three of the four trials with Tice vaccine in the United States failed to show protection, the vaccine appeared to impart 75% protection in a trial of high-risk infants in Chicago (Rosenthal et al., 1961). There are close parallels in the leprosy literature. For example, the same Glaxo freeze-dried BCG gave very different results in Uganda and Burma (Fine, 1989).

Attempts to correlate efficacy with microbiological characteristics of the several vaccines or with animal protection studies have thus far been discouraging. Animal studies have proved particularly difficult to interpret (Chamberlayne, 1972). Smith (1988) and his colleagues (Wiegeshaus and Smith, 1989) have pointed out that there are a large number of experimental variables, including animal species, challenge organism, dose and route, vaccination schedule, and outcome measure. Comparative studies by Frappier et al. (1972) and by Smith et al. (1972) and his colleagues (Wiegeshaus and Smith, 1989) have shown poor correlations both between the parameters assessed in the laboratory and the results of studies and trials in humans. The absence of any confirmed and consistent measurable laboratory correlate of protection in humans remains a major challenge to research on mycobacterial vaccines.

Genetic Differences within and between Populations

That susceptibility to tuberculosis is determined in part by genetic factors is supported by observed differences in susceptibility between racial groups (Stead et al., 1990; Stead, 1992) as well as by twin (Comstock, 1978) and HLA (Fine, 1981) studies. It has thus been reasoned that there might be similar genetic differences in response to BCG vaccination.

There are some experimental data in support of this hypothesis. Experiments in mice have revealed a genetic locus on chromosome 1 that controls resistance to BCG and to *Salmonella* and *Leishmania* spp. (Schurr et al., 1991). Of particular interest is the finding that there is a high degree of synteny between this region of mouse chromosome 1 and a region of human chromosome 2, suggesting that there may be a human counterpart to this gene. The mouse gene has recently been cloned, sequenced, and found to be homologous to a lower eukaryotic nitrate transporter (Vidal et al., 1993). We might relate this to the studies by Chan et al. (1992) demonstrating that mouse macrophages activated by gamma interferon (IFN-γ) and tumor necrosis factor alpha (TNF-α) to produce nitric oxide were cytocidal for virulent tubercle bacilli (see chapter 24). The function of the nitrate transporter might include also the transport of nitrite, which in the acidified compartment of endosomes and phagolysosomes could generate nitric oxide. One must be cautious in extrapolating such interpretations to humans, however, because it has not yet been established that human monocytes, in contrast to macrophages of the mouse, can be activated to produce significant levels of nitric oxide.

There is little epidemiological support for the possibility that human genetic differences are responsible for the variable behavior of BCG. Comstock and Palmer (1966) noted a slightly higher efficacy among whites than among blacks in the Public Health Service trials in Georgia and Alabama, but the significance of the finding and whether it reflected genetic or other differences were unclear. More recently, two case-control studies in England have examined the effect of BCG in the immigrant Asian community to test the hypothesis that genetic differences determined the poor performance of BCG in the Chingleput trial. Both of these studies found far greater protection associated with BCG vaccination of Asians in England than had been observed in Chingleput (Packe and Innes, 1988; Rodrigues et al., 1991).

Differences in Virulence between *M. tuberculosis* Strains

There is little information on variability in the virulence characteristics of *M. tuberculosis* isolates in different parts of the world. From restriction fragment length polymorphism (RFLP) and DNA fingerprinting analyses, it is clear that there are different strains within and between different countries (see chapter 33). Whether and, if so, how these differences relate to the biological properties of the strains remain unknown. There is evidence that a higher proportion of *M. tuberculosis* isolates from South India than of strains from Europe and elsewhere are of low virulence in guinea pigs, and it has been suggested that this difference might be associated with the poor performance of BCG in the Chingleput trial (Mitchison, 1964). However, while the virulence of these strains may be low in guinea pigs, it is not clear that it would be low in other experimental animals; the fact that these strains were isolated from tuberculosis patients in South India indicates that they are not without virulence in humans. Hank et al. (1981) were unable to show any difference in the ability of BCG to protect guinea pigs challenged with either low-virulence South Indian or high-virulence European strains. At present, there is thus no direct evidence to support the view that BCG is more protective against some isolates of *M. tuberculosis* than against others. Given the rapid development of molecular genetic tools that will enable characterization of virulence determinants in molecular terms (see chapter 18), it will be important to search for such differences in *M. tuberculosis* isolates from vaccinated and unvaccinated individuals in different parts of the world.

BCG Protects against Endogenous but Not Exogenous Infection

Another explanation for the observed variation in BCG's performance is based on a hypothesis that BCG is effective against primary infection in children and endogenous reactivation of long-standing infections but not against exogenous reinfection (ten Dam, 1984; ten Dam and Pio, 1988). According to this view, the proportion of disease attributable to these several mechanisms varies between populations, and hence, so does the effectiveness of BCG.

Epidemiological data suggest that BCG vaccination imparts greater or more consistent protection against systemic disease, in particular miliary tuberculosis and tuberculous meningitis in children, than against pulmonary disease (Rodrigues et al., in press). There is evidence, primarily from studies of the guinea pig, that BCG acts at least in part by preventing the spread of infection from an initial site of implantation in the lung. Other experimental evidence, particularly in guinea pigs, indicates that one effect of BCG is to restrict either the transit or the seeding of hematogenously spread *M. tuberculosis* (Fok et al., 1976; Legranderie et al., 1993). This process has been considered analogous to that underlying endogenous reactivation or secondary breakdown (though there is still much confusion regarding the pathogenesis of tuberculosis in adults; see chapters 3 and 28). In addition, studies by Lurie (1964) of tuber-

culosis in rabbits and by Sutherland and Lindgren (1979) of human autopsy material provide evidence that BCG imparts greater protection against disease than against primary infection with the tubercle bacillus. Lurie's studies indicated that the number of CFU of *M. tuberculosis* isolated from lungs of BCG-immunized versus unimmunized rabbits showed no difference in the number of organisms reaching and capable of being cultured from lung and other tissues. Thus, BCG did not protect against infection but did protect against disease. One of the major limitations in experimental animal models, however, is the lack of a model for endogenous reactivation and study of reinfection.

The high incidence and prevalence of tuberculin sensitivity in the Chingleput population have suggested to some investigators that the apparent low protective efficacy of BCG may have been related to a very high risk of exogenous reinfection disease in the population (ten Dam, 1984). Recent RFLP studies on isolates from tuberculosis patients in Hong Kong indicate that an appreciable proportion of recurrent disease episodes in adults is due to new infections (Das et al., 1993). On the other hand, it is not clear what sort of immunological mechanism would protect against primary exogenous infection and endogenous reactivation but not against exogenous reinfection. In this context, it is relevant that analyses of data from England and Wales have shown that the protection imparted by BCG remained constant over a 20-year period during which the tuberculosis notification rate fell from 250 to 10.5/100,000 (British Thoracic Association, 1980; Sutherland and Springett, 1987). These findings indicate that the protective ability of BCG vaccination, at least in this context, was independent of the prevailing infection and disease incidence rates, which should have determined the risk of exogenous reinfection. Conversely, although the trial was small and is not included in Table 1, BCG was found to be 80% protective in a study among the Qu'appelle Cree Indians in Saskatchewan (Ferguson and Simes, 1949), a population in which the incidence of tuberculosis was among the highest reported (Grzybowski, 1980). For such reasons and despite the paucity of critical data, we find it unlikely that the disparities in BCG's protective ability can be explained primarily on the basis of its failure to protect against exogenous reinfection.

Interference with or Masking of Protection by Environmental Mycobacterial Infections

One of the most compelling explanations for the variability in protective efficacy of BCG in different geographic areas is based on the recognition that infection with environmental or atypical mycobacteria differs in frequency and intensity between different populations and that prior exposure to some of these mycobacteria can provide a degree of protection against tuberculosis. This led Palmer and colleagues to argue that if BCG cannot add to protection already imparted by environmental mycobacterial infections, then the observed protective effect of BCG should be low in populations with high prevalence of such exposure (Palmer and Long, 1966).

Many species of environmental mycobacteria have been described (Woods and Washington, 1987), though only a few have been associated with human disease. These organisms are known to vary widely in their ecological requirements and geographical distributions (Kirschner et al., 1992). Available data indicate that the prevalence of human exposure to these antigens is greatest in the warmer, tropical regions of the globe. Such a trend was shown in studies of sensitivity to tuberculins made from *M. avium-M. intracellulare* purified protein derivative B ([PPD-B], named for the Battey bacillus [Edwards and Palmer, 1958]) among U.S. naval recruits, which revealed much higher prevalence of sensitivity in the southeastern than in the northern United States (Edwards et al., 1969, 1973).

There are both human and animal data showing that infection with various environmental mycobacteria can impart some protection against tuberculosis. Follow-up of U.S. naval personnel revealed that the incidence rate of tuberculosis was lower in individuals whose initial sensitivity to PPD-B was greater than that to tuberculin (PPD-S) compared to individuals with no sensitivity to either antigen or with greater sensitivity to PPD-S than to PPD-B (Edwards et al., 1973). These data were interpreted as evidence that those individuals with prior sensitivity to PPD-B had thereby naturally acquired some heterologous protection against tuberculosis. In addition, studies of several populations (e.g., U.S. nurses, unvaccinated controls in the British BCG trial, a general population in Malawi) have shown that individuals with low levels of tuberculin sensitivity (e.g., approximately 5-mm response to 2 to 5 tuberculin units [TU]) are at lower risk of disease than are individuals with either no or very strong tuberculin sensitivity (Palmer, 1957; MRC, 1972; Fine et al., submitted). This has been interpreted as evidence that the low level of tuberculin sensitivity reflects prior exposure to environmental mycobacteria, which in turn provides some heterologous protection against tuberculosis.

Further support for the hypothesis comes from a monumental experimental study by Palmer and Long (1966) that involved 1,722 guinea pigs exposed to four different species of atypical mycobacteria: *M. fortuitum*, *M. avium*, *M. kansasii*, and a scotochromogen known as *M. gauss*. The results indicated (i) that infection with different atypical mycobacteria provided different degrees of protection against *M. tuberculosis* challenge, with *M. kansasii* being almost as effective as BCG itself; (ii) that the protective effect of BCG was not additive to that which the animals had already acquired from prior infection with atypical mycobacteria; and (iii) that the observed protective effect of BCG was its potential capacity in unexposed animals minus the protection acquired from other mycobacterial infections. Thus, the heterologous protection induced by the atypical mycobacterial infections reduced the observed (apparent) effectiveness of BCG.

If this evidence relating to the immunizing potential of environmental mycobacterial infections is relevant for trials of BCG against tuberculosis, one might expect that trials carried out in populations most exposed to such infections would find lower protection associated with BCG than would trials carried out in areas relatively free of such infections. This is in fact the case. Several authors have noted a correlation between observed protection and distance from the equator (Fine, 1984), a differential that is consistent with the greater prevalence of environmental mycobacterial infections in the warmer latitudes. This could explain the high protection observed among North American Indians, Chicago infants, and British schoolchildren in contrast to the lower protection observed in the southeastern United States, Puerto Rico, and South India. The high prevalence of environmental mycobacteria in Georgia, Alabama, and South India was demonstrated by extensive skin testing with PPD-B. For example, in the Chingleput trial, two-thirds of the individuals were positive to PPD-B by the age of 9, and 97% were positive by the ages of 15 to 19 years. Both the Georgia schoolchild trials and the British trials excluded individuals who were positive to a high dose (100 TU) of tuberculin, a precaution assumed to have removed most individuals previously infected with environmental mycobacteria. However, the Georgia and South Indian populations would have been constantly exposed to such infections after vaccination, thereby reducing any difference in immunity between the vaccinated and control populations. The exposure of the British trial population to such infections must have been far less than that in the southeastern United States. On the other hand, a steady decrease in apparent protection was observed in the British trial over 20 years (Smith, in press), a fact consistent with gradual exposure of the unvaccinated controls to natural immunization by environmental mycobacterial infections over time.

It should be admitted that not all data are consistent with the environmental mycobacteria hypothesis. Hart (1967) argued that the hypothesis could not explain all the differences between the trials. Comstock et al. (1974) have noted that the protection imparted by BCG in the Puerto Rico trial was similar (approximately 30%) regardless of prior sensitivity to strong tuberculin (in individuals either negative to 100 TU or positive to 100 or 10 TU). A simple interpretation of the environmental mycobacterial hypothesis might have predicted that individuals with prior sensitivity to the strong tuberculin should have benefitted less from the BCG and hence provided lower estimates of BCG's protection than those completely lacking in prior sensitivity. While the observation is inconsistent with the prediction, it is not a refutation.

We believe that the arguments against this hypothesis are based on two assumptions that may not be valid. The first is that it is possible to predict exposure to atypical mycobacteria by skin testing with tuberculin PPD prepared from *M. tuberculosis*. The second is that failure to react to high-dose PPD indicates a lack of exposure to atypical mycobacteria. There are experimental data that challenge both assumptions. In the British MRC trial, protection (75%) equal to that achieved with BCG was obtained by using a vaccine prepared from *M. microti* (the vole bacillus), which induced fewer than 30% positive skin test conversions in response to PPD derived from *M. tuberculosis*, establishing that immunological protection that could not be detected by tuberculin skin test was induced. In the animal studies of Palmer and Long (1966), a significant percentage of the guinea pigs immunized to various atypical mycobacteria failed to respond not only to PPDs prepared from *M. tuberculosis* but even to those prepared from homologous species, yet these guinea pigs showed degrees of protection comparable to those of the guinea pigs that did respond to homologous-species PPD. Additionally, the little-known studies by Edwards et al. (1973) with over a million U.S. naval recruits found that the incidence of tuberculosis in individuals whose skin test responses to PPDs prepared from atypical mycobacteria (Edwards and Palmer, 1958) were greater than the responses to PPD-S from *M. tuberculosis* was only 1/10 the incidence in those with stronger reactions to PPD-S. These data point out real limitations on interpretation of results of skin tests that use only PPD derived from *M. tuberculosis*. Finally, if other immunological mechanisms, for example, cytotoxic T lymphocytes (CTL), were necessary for protection, their existence would probably not be ascertained by PPD testing.

There is ample evidence that tuberculin sensitivity is not a simple correlate of protection against tuberculosis. Comstock (1988) has himself shown that protection observed in the several trials was not correlated with rates of tuberculin conversion associated with the vaccinations, and Hart et al. (1967) demonstrated that protection within the British trial was independent of postvaccination tuberculin status. Brown et al. (1985) have reported that prior exposure to *M. vaccae* can affect responses in a variety of ways depending on the route, dose, and timing of the challenge. It is quite possible that some atypical mycobacteria provide protection as effectively as does BCG while others do not, and there is no assurance that immunological priming, or even "sensitization" by such organisms,

can reliably be detected by standard tuberculin testing.

Though some experts have commented that the disparate results for BCG's protection against tuberculosis cannot be explained on the basis of any single hypothesis, we believe that interference by environmental mycobacteria provides the best available explanation for results of BCG immunization observed in experimental animals and for the pattern of protection observed in different areas of the world. This is not to claim that other factors play no role in determining the effect of BCG or that the evidence is complete. Our point is simply to state that we are not convinced that any of the existing data formally refute the environmental mycobacteria hypothesis, and we believe that of all those proposed thus far, this hypothesis is the most consistent with the available data.

LESSONS FOR THE FUTURE

Importance of Understanding Mechanisms of Pathogenesis and Protection

Vaccination with BCG generally induces hypersensitivity to soluble mycobacterial antigens that is demonstrable by conventional tuberculin skin testing. This fact and the ease with which tuberculin testing is performed have encouraged many investigators in the past to equate the induction of such sensitivity with the provision of protective immunity. Unfortunately, there is little evidence in favor of this association and much evidence against it. To summarize the arguments: (i) BCG-induced tuberculin sensitivity does not correlate with vaccine-induced protection on the basis of data from within the British trial (Hart et al., 1967), between all the trials (Comstock, 1988), and in a general population in Africa (Fine et al., submitted); (ii) in all of the trials (Table 1, Fig. 1) in which skin test conversion to PPD positivity was achieved in over 85% of the populations tested, the protective efficacies varied enormously; (iii) conversely, the ability of the *M. microti* vaccine in the MRC trial to engender protection under circumstances where it failed to generate significant delayed-type hypersensitivity (MRC, 1972) revealed that the tuberculin test is not a sufficient indicator or surrogate for protective immunological mechanisms; and (iv) studies in experimental animals have described a "dissociation" between the cells and mechanisms responsible for hypersensitivity and those responsible for protective immunity (Youmans, 1979; Orme and Collins, 1984). Clearly, one of the most important challenges in the immunology of tuberculosis is to find more convincing correlates of vaccine-induced protective immunity than that which is provided (or not provided) by tuberculin testing. This leads us to consider recent developments in cellular immunology of mycobacterial infections.

A pragmatic approach is illustrated by a recent report that BCG-induced antimycobacterial activity of monocytes may correlate to some degree with protective capability of the vaccine in different populations (Cheng et al., 1993). This study used a standardized protocol to compare children vaccinated in Great Britain with children vaccinated (with the same vaccine) in Madras, South India. This result fits nicely with evidence that immunological background, perhaps reflecting exposure to environmental mycobacteria, determines the effectiveness of the response to BCG vaccination.

On a more theoretical level, detailed analyses of T-cell subsets and lymphokine mRNAs within tuberculin reaction sites and within lesions of tuberculoid relative to lepromatous leprosy patients give some insight into possible mechanisms of protective immunity. It is now known that tuberculin hypersensitivity reflects the production, particularly by CD4 T cells, of various lymphokines, in particular IFN-γ, interleukin-2 (IL-2), granulocyte macrophage–colony-stimulating factor, and lymphotoxin (TNF-β) (see chapter 25). Macrophages within these sites also produce mRNAs for TNF-α, IL-1, and IL-12. Studies of murine macrophages indicate that IFN-γ and TNF are in turn necessary for activation of macrophages to produce sufficient reactive nitrogen intermediates to kill virulent *M. tuberculosis* (Chan et al., 1992). We know from studies of transgenic mice in which the gene for IFN-γ has been disrupted (Flynn et al., 1993; Cooper et al., 1993) that this lymphokine is necessary both for resistance to *M. tuberculosis* infection and for NO formation (Flynn et al., 1993). Despite these interesting findings, we again note that the production of NO by activated human monocytes has yet to be demonstrated, and one must thus be cautious about extrapolation of mechanisms from mouse to humans.

IFN-γ is produced by the type 1 (Th1) subset of human CD4 and CD8 T cells (Salgame et al., 1991; Parronchi et al., 1991) and by NK cells and leads to activation of macrophages. It is possible that some individuals infected with *M. tuberculosis* or with BCG develop a predominantly type 2 (Th2) response, characterized by production of the cytokines IL-4 and IL-10 that in turn suppress CD4 T-cell expansion and transcription of IFN-γ and IL-2 and block macrophage activation, all of which serve to inhibit clearance of intracellular pathogens. Production of IL-4 by CD8 T suppressor cells from blood and lesions of lepromatous leprosy suggests that the type 2 response may be largely responsible for the unresponsiveness associated with this form of the disease (Bloom et al., 1992). Such an inappropriate response to the tubercle bacillus could play a similar role in PPD-negative tuberculosis patients. The factors that determine whether the type 1 (Th1) subset of T cells, thought to be required for protection, will be generated in most infectious diseases, and certainly in tuberculosis, remain to be established. In this context, failure of BCG to protect some vaccinated individuals could be a function of the inappropriate induction of type 2 rather than type 1 T-cell responses.

Early studies by Orme and Collins (1984) indicated that mice depleted of either CD4 or CD8 cells by prior administration of specific antibodies were more susceptible to challenge with *M. tuberculosis*. Recently, Silva and Lowrie (in press) have shown that T cells generated by immunization of mice with antigen-presenting cells transfected with a mycobacterial hsp60 gene are protective and cytotoxic for mycobacterium-infected macrophages. More recent studies using transgenic mice, whose genes for β2-microglobulin (required for major histocompatibility complex [MHC] class 1 expression [Flynn et al., 1992]) or CD8 have been disrupted (Flynn et al., unpublished data), indicate that the presence of functioning MHC class I-restricted CD8$^+$ T cells is also necessary for mice to resist *M. tuberculosis* challenge. Since MHC class 1 molecules are required for presentation of antigens to CTL and since Kaufmann (1988, 1993) and colleagues have detected MHC class 1-restricted cytotoxic T lymphocytes that are capable of lysing murine macrophages infected with mycobacteria, it follows that development of CTL may also be a necessary condition for protection against infection with *M. tuberculosis*. However, since CD8 T cells are known to be dependent for their expansion on IL-2 production by CD4 cells and since CD4 transgenic "knockout" mice die rapidly from *M. tuberculosis* challenge (Flynn et al., unpublished data), the data suggest that neither CD4 nor CD8 T cells alone are sufficient—and both may be necessary—for protection against *M. tuberculosis* infection.

In this context, it is of interest to note findings for transgenic β2-microglobulin knockout mice (Flynn et al., 1992) that reveal a major difference in immunological requirements for resistance to challenge with BCG relative to *M. tuberculosis*. Although 75% of the β2-microglobulin or CD8 knockout animals died within 24 days of challenge with *M. tuberculosis* (Flynn et al., 1992), none of those challenged with BCG died even after 30 weeks postinfection, and there was no difference between the β2M$^-$ and control mice with respect to their abilities to restrict the growth of BCG. We interpret these data to indicate that MHC class II-restricted CD4 T cells, lymphokine production, and macrophage activation are sufficient for resistance to BCG but not to *M. tuberculosis* infection.

Another insight is provided by the intracellular location of the mycobacteria. Electron microscopic findings indicate that BCG remains essentially entirely within the phagolysosomes after in vitro infection of macrophages, whereas virulent *M. tuberculosis* (strain H37Rv) can escape from the phagolysosome and enter the cytoplasm (McDonough et al., 1993). This may be relevant insofar as it is the antigens in the endosomal compartment of antigen-presenting cells that are presented in conjunction with MHC class II determinants to CD4 T helper cells, whereas cytoplasmic antigens are presented in association with the MHC class 1 determinants to CD8 CTL. If these findings in vitro are general, they would explain why *M. tuberculosis* is more dependent for its elimination on MHC class I-restricted CTL than BCG and suggest that BCG may not be very effective in eliciting MHC class I-restricted CTL. It should be noted that recombinant BCG expressing β-galactosidase as a model antigen was able to induce MHC class I-restricted CTL to β-galactosidase, but only many weeks after vaccination (Stover et al., 1991). In this context, it is interesting to recall that several of the elder statesmen of the tuberculosis, including Rich (1951), Canetti (1955), and Lurie (1964), all commented that recovery from infection with *M. tuberculosis* provided stronger protection against future tuberculosis than could

BCG. It is our view that effective resistance to *M. tuberculosis* infection will require participation both of specific CD8 CTL to lyse macrophages or parenchymal cells unable to restrict their infection and of specific CD4 T cells able to produce IFN-γ, TNF-α, and other lymphokines involved in macrophage activation.

This has profound implications for vaccination against tuberculosis. While the tuberculin skin test has been the most useful epidemiological tool for detecting prior exposure to *M. tuberculosis* infection and may be a valid surrogate marker for the CD4 T-cell component producing lymphokines such as IFN-γ required for protection, this test is probably not effective in measuring an MHC class I-restricted cytotoxic T-cell response. At present, there exist very few data from experimental animals that demonstrate existence of cytotoxic T cells against mycobacterial antigens, and it is important to emphasize that there is no evidence for the existence of MHC class I-restricted CTL in humans. We thus believe some priority in research ought to be given to ascertaining whether CTL are present in tuberculosis patients and in "healthy" individuals exposed to infection, whether these cells are generated by BCG vaccination, and what antigens are recognized and presented to cytotoxic cells, be they CD8 cells, γδ cells, or double-negative T cells. We believe that such studies may identify useful surrogate markers for the evaluation of different preparations of BCG or new vaccines against tuberculosis.

DEVELOPING BETTER VACCINES AGAINST TUBERCULOSIS

Identification of the immunological mechanisms required for protection and of the antigens recognized by those protective responses would provide a variety of opportunities for the development of new and possibly more effective vaccines against tuberculosis.

Recombinant BCG Vaccines

One approach would be the development of recombinant BCG vaccines based on the stable introduction and expression of the appropriate protective antigens of *M. tuberculosis* in BCG. Although BCG is effective in developing type I CD4 T-cell responses, it is still unclear how effective it is in generating MHC class I-restricted CTL responses. It may ultimately be necessary to identify the molecules, either enzymes or lysins, that enable *M. tuberculosis* to escape from phagolysosomes into the cytoplasm in order to develop recombinant BCG vaccines that are effective in inducing both CD8- and CD4-type protective responses. However, it is conceivable that enabling BCG to enter the cytoplasm of infected cells will render it pathogenic. Evidence has recently been presented that a hemolysin activity similar to activities found in *Listeria* and *Shigella* spp., which are also able to escape from the phagolysosomes to invade the cytoplasm of infected macrophages, is found in *M. tuberculosis* but not BCG (King et al., 1993).

It might also be possible by recombinant DNA technology to express and deliver protective antigens of *M. tuberculosis* in other recombinant vaccine vectors, such as attenuated poxvirus or salmonella vaccine vectors.

Genetically Attenuated *M. tuberculosis* Vaccines

At least in theory, another rational strategy would be to identify the genes of *M. tuberculosis* required for virulence, perhaps by mutational analysis, and then delete them, thereby creating a new attenuated vaccine strain. The availability of molecular techniques for creating random mutations in the *M. tuberculosis* genome by means of transposons or illegitimate recombination (McAdam et al., in press; Ganjam et al., 1991; see also chapter 14) provides new opportunities for defining and marking genes necessary for virulence and protection. While this approach will be critical to understanding the molecular basis of mycobacterial pathogenesis, such an approach has several obvious drawbacks in ensuring the development of new vaccines superior to BCG. Some of these drawbacks are theoretical. For example, how is one to identify such genes in the absence of a convincing animal model of tuberculosis in humans? Since it has not yet been possible to demonstrate homologous recombination or allelic exchange in the slow-growing mycobacteria, how would it be possible to specifically delete or replace virulence genes? Furthermore, if any of the products of virulence genes were necessary for developing a protective immune response (and this is at present unknown), the deletion of such genes might create an attenuated strain but one that could not provide adequate protection. A more practical problem is that in the absence of a good animal model of human tuberculosis, the initial testing of any such live mutants in people would raise serious ethical questions and concerns.

An Atypical Mycobacterial Vaccine

The findings of Palmer and Long (1966) that certain environmental mycobacteria can provide protection against tuberculosis, the evidence that *M. microti* provided protection as good as that of BCG in the MRC trial (Hart and Sutherland, 1977), and recent anecdotal evidence that killed *M. vaccae* may reduce the severity of clinical tuberculosis without eliciting tissue damage (Onyebujoh and Rook, 1991; Etemadi et al., 1992) provide suggestive evidence that various species of nonpathogenic mycobacteria could serve as effective vaccines. Some protection in mice against challenge with tuberculosis has been found with another killed atypical mycobacterium, *Mycobacterium W* (Singh et al., 1991). If there were appropriate immunological markers

for the identification of protective responses, it would be possible to screen systematically for candidate killed or viable atypical mycobacterial vaccines.

Auxotrophic or Killed Vaccines

Given the increased prevalence of HIV disease, there are concerns over the use of live vaccines in potentially immunocompromised recipients. One approach to this problem would be to use molecular genetic techniques to create BCG or *M. tuberculosis* "auxotrophs," that is, mutants that lack one or more of the enzymes essential for continued growth. An ideal auxotrophic vaccine might be a double mutant in which the probability of reversion to a fully viable organism is statistically remote and that is capable of surviving for 1 to 3 months in the host before being lost. During that time, this ideal vaccine would be antigenically indistinguishable from wild-type virulent or attenuated *M. tuberculosis* and would target the appropriate antigen-presenting cells and lymphoid tissues and thus immunize the host before the auxotrophic mutation rendered it nonviable. Even after the organism was no longer capable of replication, it might continue for some time to serve as a source of antigens that continue the immunization process. While immunity induced by such vaccines might not be as long-lasting as that induced by fully viable recombinant or attenuated vaccines, auxotrophic vaccines should be safe even in immunocompromised populations.

Experience with killed mycobacterial vaccines in experimental animals indicates that viable organisms are generally more protective and better able to induce cell-mediated immune responses. However, it is worth recalling in this context that Anacker et al. (1969) found that cell wall vaccines coated in oil and administered intravenously were able to protect mice from aerosol challenge almost as effectively as living BCG. Remarkably, the experiments with *M. vaccae* mentioned above were all carried out with killed organisms.

Subunit or DNA Vaccines That Do Not Compromise Skin Tests

It is at least conceivable that a protective vaccine that does not compromise assessment of the risk of infection by skin tests could be developed. There is evidence that BCG and *M. microti* can, at least in some populations, impart protection without inducing hypersensitivity to tuberculin (Comstock, 1988; Hart et al., 1967, Fine et al., 1993). One hopes, therefore, that if antigens necessary for protection can be defined, they could be used selectively in assays of vaccine-induced protective immunity. Conversely, it might also be possible to develop skin or other tests based on antigens that are not necessary for protection and which could thus detect tuberculous infection per se but could be excluded from a protective vaccine.

Advances in recombinant DNA technology now make it possible to produce large amounts of individual recombinant protein antigens of *M. tuberculosis* and *M. leprae*, and some of these antigens have already been established in an antigen bank under the auspices of the IMMYC program at WHO. While purified protein antigens are generally ineffective in engendering high levels of cell-mediated immunity or cytotoxic T-cell responses, their ability to do so can be enhanced by the use of lipid adjuvants. Recently, Anderson and colleagues (in press) have shown that a combination of the recombinant 6- and 32-kDa protein antigens in a lipophilic adjuvant are almost as effective as live BCG in protecting mice against *M. tuberculosis* challenge. In other systems, it is possible to convert proteins and peptides into effective immunogens for stimulating both antibody and CTL by cou-

pling to them specific lipid moieties, particularly the tripalmitoyl group (Lex et al., 1986). Finally, one of the most extraordinary new approaches to immunization is the use of naked DNA as a vaccine. When antigen genes are placed under the control of strong promoters and injected on plasmids into muscle cells, in the limited number of instances reported, there has been production of specific antibodies and CTL for remarkably long periods, i.e., up to 2 years in mice (Tang et al., 1992; Wang et al., 1993). Since it is a great deal less expensive to prepare pure DNA than proteins, this technology is very appealing. However, there are many safety concerns relating to the possibility that the DNA will integrate into the host chromosome and perhaps mutate tumor suppressor genes that in some low but real frequency could result in tumor formation.

ROUTE AND DOSE OF IMMUNIZATION

Developing Better Vaccines

BCG was first given orally, and this route of administration was continued in some populations for more than 50 years. Calmette et al. (1933) observed that a bacillemia sometimes occurred within 4 h of ingestion of viable BCG and that this could generate a systemic immune response. This suggests that bacilli are able to attach to and be engulfed by M cells of the intestine, a situation that has now been confirmed by electron photomicrographic evidence of BCG bacilli residing in M cells of rabbits immunized orally with BCG (Fujimura, 1986; Momotani et al., 1988).

Oral administration of BCG was discontinued for two reasons. One was that the viability of BCG is reduced 1 to 2 logs by exposure to gastric secretions and low pH (Gaudier and Gernez-Rieux, 1962), and thus very high concentrations of bacilli were required. Second, oral administration was frequently associated with cervical lymphadenopathy.

Given the important role of the lung in the pathogenesis of tuberculosis, it may be helpful to consider direct engagement of the secretory immune system by antituberculosis vaccines. It was shown long ago that as few as 10 CFU of aerosolized BCG could protect guinea pigs as well as or better than much larger doses given either intradermally or subcutaneously (Cohn et al., 1958; Middlebrook, 1961). Recent studies indicate that intranasal exposure of mice to recombinant BCG expressing the OspA antigen of *Borrelia burgdorferi* is more immunogenic than is exposure by oral or other routes (Langermann et al., submitted). Several studies of protection of primates against aerosol *M. tuberculosis* challenge provided evidence that aerosol BCG immunization was superior to vaccination by other routes (Good, 1968; Barclay et al., 1973; Anacker et al., 1972). Although the number of monkeys studied was small, aerosolized BCG and BCG cell walls both appeared to protect rhesus monkeys without eliciting tuberculin reactivity (on the other hand, it must be noted that rhesus monkeys are notorious for giving poor skin test responses). Surprisingly, aerosol BCG was associated with fewer pathologic lesions in the lungs than were seen after intravenous BCG, which was also found to be protective (Good, 1968; Barclay et al., 1973). No adverse effects were found when BCG was given by aerosol to human volunteers in doses as high as 4×10^4 CFU (Rosenthal et al., 1968).

Given these results, it is important that future research on tuberculosis vaccines consider carefully the implications of the various compartments of the immune response for protection. Comparative studies of pulmonary, oral, rectal, and intranasal exposures to new and old vaccines could provide important insights into mechanisms of protection.

Finally, consideration of the doses of vaccines used may be important. Bretscher (1992a) has argued that the dose of antigen in mice can be a critical factor in determining the degree to which Th1 or Th2 responses are generated and that higher doses are inhibitory to development of cell-mediated immunity. In immunization studies with *Leishmania major* in BALB/c mice (Bretscher, 1992b), very low doses of parasites generated protective cell-mediated immunity, while higher doses led to Th2 responses, antibody formation, and diminished protection. In preliminary studies with BCG, similar findings were apparently seen.

WHO SHOULD BE VACCINATED, AND WHERE SHOULD TRIALS BE CONDUCTED?

Despite the large number of trials and observational studies of BCG that have been carried out, we still do not understand the behavior, efficacy, and impact of BCG vaccines. Though we have argued above that environmental mycobacteria are likely to be important determinants of apparent vaccine efficacy, we are still not able confidently to predict the utility of a given BCG vaccine in a population for which it has not been studied. Given the availability of effective drugs and the declining incidence of tuberculosis in many countries, it will not be easy to undertake long-term large-scale trials. However, assuming that there will be new vaccines that will have the ability to engender all the appropriate protective mechanisms in experimental models, how would we evaluate them?

The first prerequisite is a study population that is at high risk of tuberculosis yet can be followed up thoroughly. The fact that BCG vaccine is now employed in most populations in the world, at least outside the United States, will impose important ethical and practical constraints (Fine, 1989). It may be difficult to identify appropriate high-risk populations free of BCG vaccine, and there may be arguments to provide BCG to trial participants or at least to the control group. The possibility of studying high-risk groups in the United States may be considered but is likely to raise logistic difficulties.

The apparent geographic variation observed in studies of BCG will pose a difficulty in interpreting and extrapolating the results of any future tuberculosis vaccine trials. Given the evidence that environmental mycobacteria are an important determinant of BCG's apparent efficacy, it will be essential to assess the frequency and pattern of exposure/sensitivity to these organisms in future trial populations.

The possibility of new vaccines, particularly auxotrophic or killed vaccines, raises the possibility of therapeutic vaccination aimed at providing individuals already infected or clinically ill with tuberculosis with an appropriate protective immune response. Uncontrolled studies in Venezuela have suggested that multiple injections with BCG plus *M. leprae* can improve the immunological status of previously unresponsive lepromatous leprosy patients (Convit et al., 1982). It has been argued that in order to be beneficial in tuberculosis, a therapeutic vaccine must avoid responses associated with tissue-damaging sequelae (Onyebujoh and Rook, 1991). These responses posed a devastating problem for Koch in his attempts to cure tuberculosis with *M. tuberculosis* culture filtrates (Bloom and Murray, 1992).

Finally, there is the vexing question of immunizing individuals or groups at high risk for multiple-drug-resistant tuberculosis. In areas where tuberculosis infection rates are high, concerns about the compromise of the tuberculin test by BCG immunization have not been compelling. For example, in a survey of rural households in India in the absence of BCG immunization, the prevalence of infected individuals (PPD skin test positive) in households with a bacillary case was 77%, and the prevalence in households with no infected cases was 54% (Narain et al., 1966). There has been reluctance to use BCG in populations in low-incidence countries such as the United States, as this would compromise the tuberculin skin test, which is an important element of tuberculosis control strategy. This reluctance is being challenged by the increases in tuberculosis, in particular multidrug-resistant tuberculosis, with its associated risks to intimate contacts, HIV-infected individuals, hospital patients, and health care providers as well as to correctional facility inmates and personnel. Health care givers have traditionally been at high risk for acquiring tuberculosis (Geiseler et al., 1986), and if there were a more effective vaccine than BCG, its use in such defined risk populations might be encouraged. In a controversial decision analysis, Greenberg et al. (1991) argued that because compliance with isoniazid prophylaxis and annual tuberculin testing was so poor in the at-risk health care population, it might be advisable, even if the protective efficacy were as low as 17%, to recommend BCG vaccination of such groups.

EXPECTATIONS

It was once hoped that BCG immunization of children as a matter of public health policy would provide long-lasting protection against tuberculosis and would ultimately have an impact on the overall population patterns of disease. There is little evidence that BCG vaccination has had such an impact thus far. For example, the declines in annual risk of infection in the United Kingdom and Sweden, which had national BCG vaccine programs, were no greater than those in The Netherlands, which did not (Styblo and Meijer, 1976; Styblo, 1991). The fact that most transmission is attributable to older adults means that there will be a long delay before population effects are manifest. Even in Europe today, where BCG has been used for the longest time, the older age groups were born too early to have been eligible for BCG vaccination. In addition, the expectation of a long-term population impact presupposes that any protection imparted by BCG will last for many decades. In fact, we know very little about the long-term duration of immunity imparted by any vaccine, let alone by BCG. There was some evidence for a decline in protection associated with BCG in the MRC trial (MRC, 1972), but it is not clear whether this decline reflected a true waning of protection or just a progressive masking of the effect of BCG by the accumulation of heterologous protection attributable to exposure to environmental mycobacteria in the control group (Rodrigues and Smith, 1990). Although several countries (in particular, those in Eastern Europe) have recommended repeated BCG vaccination, there have to date been no evaluations whatever of the efficacy of repeated BCG vaccination against tuberculosis. A trial currently in progress in Malawi will provide the first controlled evaluation of one versus two BCG vaccinations (Fine and Ponnighaus, 1988).

Many of the vaccines in common use (e.g., tetanus, diphtheria, measles, and polio) provide very high levels of protection through neutralization of toxins or viruses. It is significant that the least effective of the common vaccines are those against pertussis and tuberculosis. Indeed, it may be unrealistic to expect that vaccines can deliver high levels of protection against chronic or intracellular bacterial, fungal, and protozoal infections, given the complexity of the agents, their relationships to host cells and tissues, and the multifaceted immune responses required to engender protection. For this reason, we should be cautious in our expectations of candidate vaccines against tuberculosis.

Both Sutherland (1981) and Murray et al. (1990) have pointed out that even in circumstances in which BCG provides high protection, as the incidence of disease declines, the cost-effectiveness of vaccination as a tuberculosis control strategy decreases relative to that of an alternative policy based on case finding and treatment. This is so in part because with declining incidence, more and more vaccinations are required to prevent each single case of disease and in part because childhood BCG vaccination does not directly affect the older segment of the population, which carries the most pulmonary disease and is hence most responsible for transmission of infection.

However, with the recent increases in single-drug- and multidrug-resistant tuberculosis and the high cost of adding second-line and newer drugs to existing regimens, the potential value of immunization, even if it is not highly effective on an individual basis, should not be minimized. New strategies for identifying individuals and populations at risk together with selective use of antituberculosis vaccines could yet represent a cost-effective strategy for preventing or ameliorating disease.

Modern scientific advances are providing important opportunities to understand the mechanisms involved in the pathogenesis of and protection against tuberculosis. Just as the BCG trials have provided our most detailed studies of the epidemiology of tuberculosis, so basic research directed at tuberculosis vaccines is leading the way in understanding pathogenesis of the disease. Research on vaccines continues to represent a key approach to understanding and ultimately controlling tuberculosis.

Acknowledgments. We express our appreciation to J. Flynn for her critical reading of the manuscript and helpful suggestions; to G. Comstock, T. Brewer, and G. A. Colditz for providing us with their unpublished data relating to trials; and to C. J. L. Murray for helpful discussions.

REFERENCES

Anacker, R. L., W. R. Barclay, W. Brehwer, G. Goude, R. H. List, E. Ribi, and D. F. Tarmina. 1969. Effectiveness of cell walls of *Mycobacterium bovis* strain BCG administered by various routes and in different adjuvants in protecting mice against airborne infection with *Mycobacterium tuberculosis* strain H37Rv. *Am. Rev. Respir. Dis.* **99:**242–248.

Anacker, R. L., W. Brehmer, W. R. Barclay, W. R. Leif, E. Ribi, J. H. Simmons, and A. W. Smith. 1972. Superiority of intravenous BCG and BCG cell walls in protecting rhesus monkeys (*Macaca mulatta*) against airborne tuberculosis. *Z. Immunitaetsforsch.* **143:**363.

Andersen, P. Vaccination of mice against *M. tuberculosis* infection: protective immunity obtained with a soluble mixture of secreted mycobacterial proteins. Submitted for publication.

Aronson, J. D., C. F. Aronson, and H. C. Taylon. 1958. A twenty-year appraisal of BCG vaccination in the control of tuberculosis. *Arch. Intern. Med.* **101:**881–893.

Barclay, W. R., W. M. Busey, D. W. Dalgard, R. C. Good, B. W. Janicki, J. E. Kasik, E. Ribi, C. E. Ulrich, and E. Wolinsky. 1973. Protection of monkeys against airborne tuberculosis by aerosol vaccination with Bacillus Calmette-Guerin. *Am. Rev. Respir. Dis.* **107:**351–358.

Bjartveit, K., and H. Waaler. 1965. Some evidence of the efficacy of mass BCG vaccination. *Bull. W.H.O.* **33:**289–319.

Bloom, B. R., R. L. Modlin, and P. Salgame. 1992. Stigma variations: observations on suppressor T cells and leprosy. *Annu. Rev. Immunol.* **10:**453–488.

Bloom, B. R., and C. J. L. Murray. 1992. Tuberculosis: commentary on a reemergent killer. *Science* **257:**1055–1064.

Braun, M. M., and G. Cauthen. 1992. Relationship of the human immunodeficiency virus epidemic to pediatric tuberculosis and Bacillus Calmette-Guerin immunization. *Pediatr. Infect. Dis. J.* **11:**220–227.

Bretcher, P. A. 1992a. A strategy to improve the efficacy of vaccination against tuberculosis and leprosy. *Immunol. Today* **13:**342–345.

Bretcher, P. A. 1992b. Establishment of stable, cell-mediated immunity that makes ''susceptible'' mice resistant to *Leishmania major*. *Science* **260:**539–542.

British Thoracic Association. 1980. Effectiveness of BCG vaccination in Great Britain in 1978. *Br. J. Chest Dis.* **74:**215–227.

Brown, C. A., I. N. Brown, and S. Swinburne. 1985. The effect of oral *Mycobacterium vaccae* on subsequent responses to BCG sensitization. *Tubercle* **66:**251–260.

Calmette, A. 1927. *La Vaccination Preventive contra la Tuberculosis*, 250 p. Masson et Cie, Paris.

Calmette, A., B. Weill-Halle, A. Saenz, and L. Costil. 1933. Demonstration experimentale du passage des bacilles vaccines BCG a travers la muquese intestinale chez l'infant et chez le singe. *Bull. Acad. Med.* **110:**203–206.

Canetti, G. 1955. *The Tubercle Bacillus in the Pulmonary Lesion of Man*, 226 p. Springer, New York.

Centers for Disease Control. 1991. BCG vaccination and pediatric HIV infection—Rwanda, 1988–90. *Morbid. Mortal. Weekly Rep.* **40:**833–835.

Chamberlayne, E. C. (ed.). 1972. *Status of Immunization in Tuberculosis in 1971*, 249 p. Department of Health, Education and Welfare, Washington, D.C.

Chan, J., Y. Xing, R. S. Magliozzo, and B. R. Bloom. 1992. Killing of virulent *M. tuberculosis* by reactive nitrogen intermediates produced by activated murine macrophages. *J. Exp. Med.* **175:**1111–1122.

Cheng, S. H., K. B. Walker, D. B. Lowrie, D. A. Mitchison, R. Swamy, M. Datta, and R. Prabhaka. 1993. Monocyte antimycobacterial activity before and after *Mycobacterium bovis* BCG vaccination in Chingleput, India, and London, United Kingdom. *Infect. Immun.* **61:**4501–4503.

Clemens, J. D., J. H. Jackie, J. H. Chuong, and A. R. Feinstein. 1983. The BCG controversy: a methodological and statistical reappraisal. *JAMA* **249:**2362–2369.

Coetzee, A. M., and J. Berjak. 1968. BCG in the prevention of tuberculosis in an adult population. *Proc. Mine Med. Officers Assoc.* **48:**41–53.

Cohn, M. L., C. L. Davis, and G. Middlebrook. 1958. Airborne immunization against tuberculosis. *Science* **128:**1282–1283.

Colditz, G. A., T. Brewer, C. Berkey, M. Wilson, E. Burdick, H. V. Fineberg, and F. Mosteller. The efficacy of BCG in the prevention of tuberculosis: meta-analyses of the published literature. *JAMA*, in press.

Comstock, G. W. 1978. Tuberculosis in twins: a reanalysis of the Prophit survey. *Am. Rev. Respir. Dis.* **117:**621–624.

Comstock, G. W. 1988. Identification of an effective vaccine against tuberculosis. *Am. Rev. Respir. Dis.* **138:**479–480.

Comstock, G. W., V. T. Livesay, and S. F. Woolpert. 1974. Evaluation of BCG vaccination among Puerto Rican Children. *Am. J. Public Health* **64:**283–291.

Comstock, G. W., and C. E. Palmer. 1966. Long-term results of BCG vaccination in the southern United States. *Am. Rev. Respir. Dis.* **93:**171–183.

Comstock, G. W., and R. G. Webster. 1969. Tuberculosis studies in Muscogee County, Georgia. VII. A twenty-year evaluation of BCG vaccination in a school population. *Am. Rev. Respir. Dis.* **100:**839–845.

Comstock, G. W., S. F. Woolpert, and V. T. Livesay. 1976. Tuberculosis studies in Muscogee County,

Georgia. Twenty-year evaluation of a community trial of BCG vaccination. *Public Health Rep.* **91:** 276–280.

Convit, J., N. Aranzazu, M. Ulrich, M. E. Pinardi, O. Reyes, and J. Alvarado. 1982. Immunotherapy with a mixture of Mycobacterium leprae and BCG in different forms of leprosy and Mitsuda negative contacts. *Int. J. Lepr.* **50:**415.

Cooper, A. M., D. K. Dalton, T. A. Stewart, D. G. Griffin, D. G. Ressell, and I. M. Orme. 1993. Disseminated tuberculosis in IFN-γ gene-disrupted mice. *J. Exp. Med.* **178:**2242–2248.

Dahlstrom, G., and H. Difs. 1951. The efficacy of BCG vaccination: a study on vaccinated and tuberculin-negative conscripts. *Acta Tuberc. Scand. Suppl.* **27:**1.

Das, S., S. L. Chan, B. W. Allan, D. A. Mitchison, and D. B. Lowrie. 1993. Application of DNA fingerprinting with IS986 to sequential mycobacterial isolates from pulmonary tuberculosis patients in Hong Kong before, during and after short-course chemotherapy. *Tuberc. Lung Dis.* **74:**47–51.

Edwards, L. B., F. A. Acquaviva, and V. T. Livesay. 1973. Identification of tuberculous infected. Dual tests and density of reaction. *Am. Rev. Respir. Dis.* **108:**1334–1339.

Edwards, L. B., F. A. Acquaviva, V. T. Livesay, F. W. Cross, and C. E. Palmer. 1969. An atlas of sensitivity to tuberculin, PPD-B, and histoplasmin in the United States. *Am. Rev. Respir. Dis.* **99:**1–132.

Edwards, L. B., and C. E. Palmer. 1958. Epidemiologic studies of tuberculin sensitivity. I. Preliminary results from purified protein derivatives prepared from atypical acid-fast organisms. *Am. J. Hyg.* **68:**213–231.

Etemadi, A., R. Farid, and J. L. Stanford. 1992. Immunotherapy for drug resistant tuberculosis. *Lancet* **340:**1360–1361. (Letter.)

Fenner, F., D. A. Henderson, I. Arita, Z. Jezek, and I. D. Ladnyi. 1988. *Smallpox and Its Eradication*, 1,460 p. World Health Organization, Geneva.

Ferguson, R. G., and A. B. Simes. 1949. BCG vaccination of Indian infants in Saskatchewan. *Tubercle* **30:**5–11.

Fine, P. E. M. 1981. Immunogenetics of susceptibility to leprosy, tuberculosis and leishmnaniasis: an epidemiological perspective. *Int. J. Lepr.* **49:**337–454.

Fine, P. E. M. 1984. Leprosy and tuberculosis—an epidemiological comparison. *Tubercle* **65:**137–153.

Fine, P. E. M. 1988. BCG vaccination against tuberculosis and leprosy. *Br. Med. Bull.* **44:**691–703.

Fine, P. E. M. 1989. The BCG story: lessons from the past and implications for the future. *Rev. Infect. Dis.* **11**(Suppl. 2):S353–S359.

Fine, P. E. M., and J. M. Ponnighaus. 1988. Background, design and prospects of the Karonga Prevention Trial, a leprosy vaccine trial in Northern Malawi. *Trans. R. Soc. Trop. Med. Hyg.* **82:**810–817.

Fine, P. E. M., and L. C. Rodrigues. 1990. Modern vaccines: mycobacterial diseases. *Lancet* **335:**1016–1020.

Fine, P. E. M., J. A. C. Sterne, J. M. Ponnighaus, and R. J. W. Rees. Delayed-type hypersensitivity, mycobacterial vaccines and protective immunity. Submitted for publication.

Flynn, J. L., D. Mathis, C. Benoist, T. Mak, and B. R. Bloom. Unpublished data.

Flynn, J. L., J. Chan, K. J. Triebold, D. K. Dalton, T. A. Stewart, and B. R. Bloom. 1993. An essential role for interferon-γ in resistance to *M. tuberculosis*. *J. Exp. Med.* **178:**2249–2254.

Flynn, J. L., M. Goldstein, K. J. Triebold, B. Koller, and B. R. Bloom. 1992. MHC class I restricted T cells are required for resistance to *M. tuberculosis* infection. *Proc. Natl. Acad. Sci. USA* **89:**12013–12017.

Fok, J. S., R. S. Ho, P. K. Arora, G. E. Harding, and D. W. Smith. 1976. Host-parasite relationships in experimental airborne tuberculosis. V. Lack of hematogenous dissemination of *Mycobacterium tuberculosis* to the lungs in animals vaccinated with Bacille Calmette-Guerin. *J. Infect. Dis.* **133:**137–144.

Frappier, A., V. Portelance, J. St.-Pierre, and M. Panisset. 1972. BCG strains: characteristics and relative efficacy, p. 157–178. *In* E. C. Chamberlayne (ed.), *Status of Immunization in Tuberculosis in 1971*. Department of Health, Education and Welfare publication no. (NIH) 72-68. Government Printing Office, Washington, D.C.

Frimodt-Moller, J., G. S. Acharyulu, and K. Kesava Pillai. 1973. Observations on the protective effect of BCG vaccination in a South Indian rural population: fourth report. *Bull. Int. Union Tuberc.* **48:**40–52.

Fujimura, Y. 1986. Functional morphology of microfold cells (M cells) in Peyer's patches—phagocytosis and transport of BCG by M cells into rabbit Peyer's patches. *Gastroenterol. Jpn.* **21:**325–335.

Ganjam, K., B. R. Bloom, and W. R. Jacobs, Jr. 1991. Insertional mutagenesis and illegitimate recombination in mycobacteria. *Proc. Natl. Acad. Sci. USA* **88:**5433–5437.

Gaudier, B., and C. Gernez-Rieux. 1962. Étude experimentale de la vitalité du B.C.G. au cours de la traversée gastro-intestinale chez des enfants non allergiques vaccinés par voie digestive. *Ann. Inst. Pasteur* (Lille) **13:**77–87.

Geiseler, R. J., K. E. Nelsen, R. G. Crispen, and V. K. Moses. 1986. Tuberculosis in physicians: a continuing problem. *Am. Rev. Respir. Dis.* **133:**773–778.

Good, R. C. 1968. Biology of the mycobacterioses. Simian tuberculosis: immunologic aspects. *Ann. N.Y. Acad. Sci.* **154:**200–213.

Greenberg, P. D., K. G. Lax, and C. B. Schechter. 1991. A decision analysis comparing the tuberculin screening strategy with the BCG vaccination. *Am. Rev. Respir. Dis.* **143:**489–495.

Greenwood, M. 1928. Professor Calmette's statistical study of BCG vaccination. *Br. Med. J.* **1:**793–795.

Grzybowski, S. 1980. Epidemiology of tuberculosis and the role of BCG. *Clin. Chest Med.* **1:**175–187.

Guérin, C. 1957. The history of BCG, p. 48–53. *In* S. R. Rosenthal (ed.), *BCG Vaccination against Tuberculosis*. Little, Brown & Co., Boston.

Hank, J. A., J. K. Chan, M. L. Edwards, D. Muller, and D. W. Smith. 1981. Influence of the virulence of *Mycobacterium tuberculosis* on protection induced by Bacille Calmette-Guerin in guinea pigs. *J. Infect. Dis.* **143:**734–738.

Hart, P. D. 1967. Efficacy and applicability of mass BCG vaccination in tuberculosis control. *Br. Med. J.* **1:**587–592.

Hart, P. D., and I. Sutherland. 1977. BCG and vole bacillus vaccines in the prevention of tuberculosis in adolescence and early adult life. *Br. Med. J.* **22:**293–295.

Hart, P. D., I. Sutherland, and J. Thomas. 1967. The immunity conferred by effective BCG and vole bacillus vaccines, in relation to the induced tuberculin sensitivity and to technical variations in the vaccines. *Tubercle* **48:**201–210.

Kaufmann, S. H. E. 1988. CD8⁺ T lymphocytes in intracellular microbial infections. *Immunol. Today* **9:**168–174.

Kaufmann, S. H. E. 1993. Immunity to intracellular bacteria. *Annu. Rev. Immunol.* **11:**129–163.

King, C. H., S. Mundayoor, J. T. Crawford, and T. M. Shinnick. 1993. Expression of contact-dependent cytolytic activity by *M. tuberculosis* and isolation of the genomic locus that encodes the activity. *Infect. Immun.* **61:**2708–2712.

Kirschner, R. A., Jr., B. C. Parker, and J. O. Falkinham III. 1992. Epidemiology of infection by nontuberculous mycobacteria. *Am. Rev. Respir. Dis.* **145:**272–275.

Lallemant-Le Coeur, S., M. Lallemant, D. Cheynier, S. Nzingoula, J. Drucker, and B. Larouze. 1991. BCG immunization in infants born to HIV-1 seropositive mothers. *AIDS* **5:**195–199.

Langermann, S., S. Palaszynski, A. Sadziene, C. K. Stover, and S. Koenig. Induction of sustained systemic and mucosal immunity by a single intranasal immunization with recombinant BCG. Submitted for publication.

Legranderie, M., P. Ravisse, G. Marchal, M. Gheorghiu, V. Balasubramanian, E. H. Weigeshaus, and D. W. Smith. 1993. BCG induced protection in guinea pigs vaccinated and challenged via the respiratory route. *Tuberc. Lung Dis.* **74:**38–46.

Lex, A., K. H. Wiesmuller, G. Jung, and W. G. Bessler. 1986. A synthetic analogue of *Escherichia coli* lipoprotein, tripalmitoylpentapeptide, constitutes a potent immune adjuvant. *J. Immunol.* **137:**2667–2681.

Lotte, A., H. G. ten Dam, and R. Henderson. 1988. Second IUATLK study on complications induced by intradermal BCG-vaccination. *Bull. Int. Union Tuberc.* **63:**47–83.

Lotte, A., O. Wasz-Hockert, N. Poisson, N. Domitrescu, M. Verron, and E. Covet. 1984. BCG complications. Estimates of the risks among vaccinated subjects and statistical analysis of their main characteristics. *Adv. Tuberc. Res.* **21:**107–193.

Lubeck. 1935. *Die Sauglingstuberkulose in Lubeck.* Springer, Berlin.

Lurie, M. B. 1964. *Resistance to Tuberculosis. Experimental Studies in Native and Acquired Defense*, 391 p. Harvard University Press, Cambridge, Mass.

Mackaness, G. B., D. J. Auclair, and P. H. Lagrange. 1973. Immunopotentiation with BCG. I. Immune response to different strains and preparations. *J. Natl. Cancer Inst.* **51:**1655–1667.

McAdam, R. A., T. Weisbrod, J. D. Cirillo, and W. R. Jacobs, Jr. Genetic analysis of IS1096: a study of transposition in *M. bovis*-BCG. *Mol. Microbiol.*, in press.

McDonough, K. A., Y. Kress, and B. R. Bloom. 1993. Pathogenesis of tuberculosis: interaction of *Mycobacterium tuberculosis* with macrophages. *Infect. Immun.* **61:**2763–2773.

Medical Research Council. 1972. BCG and vole bacillus in the prevention of tuberculosis in adolescence and early adult life. *Bull. W.H.O.* **46:**371–385.

Middlebrook, G. 1961. Immunological aspects of airborne infection: reactions to inhaled antigens. *Bacteriol. Rev.* **25:**331–346.

Milstien, J. B., and J. J. Gibson. 1989. *Quality Control of BCG Vaccines by the World Health Organization: a Review of Factors That May Influence Vaccine Effectiveness and Safety*, 30 p. Publication WHO/EPI/Gen/89.1. World Health Organization, Geneva.

Mitchison, D. A. 1964. The virulence of tubercle bacilli from patients with pulmonary tuberculosis in India and other countries. *Bull. Int. Union Tuberc.* **35:**287–293.

Momotoni, E., D. L. Whipple, A. B. Thiermann, and N. F. Cheville. 1988. Role of M cells and macrophages in the entrance of *Mycobacterium paratuberculosis* into domes of ileal Peyer's patches in calves. *Vet. Pathol.* **25:**131–137.

Murray, C. J. L., K. Styblo, and A. Rouillon. 1990. Tuberculosis in developing countries: burden, intervention, and cost. *Bull. Int. Union Tuberc.* **65:**6–24.

Narain, R., S. S. Nair, G. Ramanatha Rao, and P. Chandrasekhar. 1966. Distribution of tuberculous infection and disease among households in a rural community. *Bull. W.H.O.* **34**:639–654.

Onyebujoh, P., and G. A. W. Rook. 1991. *Mycobacterium vaccae* immunotherapy. *Lancet* **338**:1534.

Orme, I. M., and F. M. Collins. 1984. Adoptive protection of the *Mycobacterium tuberculosis* infected lung: dissociation between cells that passively transfer protective immunity and those that transfer delayed-type hypersensitivity to tuberculin. *Cell. Immun.* **84**:113–120.

Osborn, T. W. 1983. Changes in BCG strains. *Tubercle* **64**:1–132.

Packe, G. E., and J. A. Innes. 1988. Protective effect of BCG in infant Asians: a case-control study. *Arch. Dis. Child.* **63**:277–281.

Padungchan, S., S. Konjanart, S. Kasiratta, S. Karamas, and H. G. ten Dam. 1986. The effectiveness of BCG vaccination of the newborn against childhood tuberculosis in Bangkok. *Bull. W.H.O.* **64**:247–258.

Palmer, C. E. 1957. Contribution to Symposium on Value of Tuberculin Reactions for the Selection of Cases for BCG Vaccination and Significance of Post-Vaccination Allergy. *Bull. Int. Union Tuberc.* **27**:106–111.

Palmer, C. E., and M. W. Long. 1966. Effects of infection with atypical mycobacteria on BCG vaccination and tuberculosis. *Am. Rev. Respir. Dis.* **94**:553–568.

Parronchi, P., D. Macchia, M. Piccinni, P. Biswas, C. Simonelli, E. Maggi, M. Ricci, A. Asari, and S. Romagnani. 1991. Allergen and bacterial antigen-specific T-cell clones established from atopic donors show a different profile of cytokine production. *Proc. Natl. Acad. Sci. USA* **88**:4538.

Pönnighaus, J. M., P. E. M. Fine, J. A. C. Sterne, R. S. Wilson, E. Msosa, P. J. K. Gruer, P. A. Jenkins, S. B. Lucas, G. Liomba, and L. Bliss. 1992. Efficacy of BCG against leprosy and tuberculosis in northern Malawi. *Lancet* **339**:636–639.

Rich, A. R. 1951. *The Pathogenesis of Tuberculosis*, 2nd ed, 1,028 p. Charles C Thomas, Publisher, Springfield, Ill.

Rodrigues, L. C., V. K. Diwan, and J. G. Wheeler. Protective effect of BCG against tuberculous meningitis and miliary tuberculosis: a meta-analysis. *Int. J. Epidemiol.*, in press.

Rodrigues, L. C., N. Gill, and P. G. Smith. 1991. BCG vaccination in the first year of life protects children of Indian subcontinent ethnic origin against tuberculosis in England. *J. Epidemiol. Community Health* **45**:78–80.

Rodrigues, L. C., and P. G. Smith. 1990. Tuberculosis in developing countries and methods for its control. *Trans. R. Soc. Trop. Med. Hyg.* **84**:739–744.

Rosenthal, S. R. 1980. *BCG Vaccine: Tuberculosis-Cancer*, 404 p. PSG Publishing, Littleton, Mass.

Rosenthal, S. R., E. Loewinsohn, M. L. Graham, D.

Liveright, M. G. Thorne, and V. Johnson. 1961. BCG vaccination against tuberculosis in Chicago: a twenty-year study statistically analyzed. *Pediatrics* **28**:622–641.

Rosenthal, S. R., J. T. McNery, and N. Raisys. 1968. Aerogenic BCG vaccination against tuberculosis in animal and human subjects. *J. Asthma Res.* **5**:309–323.

Salgame, P., J. Abrams, C. Clayberger, H. Goldstein, J. Convit, R. L. Modlin, and B. R. Bloom. 1991. Differing lymphokine profiles of functional subsets of human CD4 and CD8 T-cell clones. *Science* **254**:279–282.

Schurr, E., D. Malo, D. Radzloch, E. Buschman, K. Morgan, P. Gros, and E. Skamene. 1991. Genetic control of innate resistance to mycobacterial infections. *Immunol. Today* **12**:42–45.

Silva, C. L., and D. B. Lowrie. A single mycobacterial protein (hsp60) expressed by a transgenic antigen-presenting cell vaccinates mice against tuberculosis. *Immunology*, in press.

Singh, I. G., R. Mukherjee, and G. P. Talwar. 1991. Resistance to intravenous inoculation of *Mycobacterium tuberculosis* H37Rv in mice of different inbred strains following immunization with a leprosy vaccine based on *Mycobacterium W*. *Vaccine* **9**:10–14.

Smith, D. W., E. H. Wiegeshaus, R. N. Stark, and G. E. Harding. 1972. Models for potency assay of tuberculosis vaccines, p. 205–218. *In* E. C. Chamberlayne (ed.), *Status of Immunization in Tuberculosis in 1971*. Department of Health, Education and Welfare, Washington, D.C.

Smith, P. G. 1982. Assessment of the efficacy of BCG vaccination against tuberculosis, using the case control method. *Tubercle* **62**:23–35.

Smith, P. G. 1988. Epidemiological methods to evaluate vaccine efficacy. *Br. Med. Bull.* **44**:679–690.

Smith, P. G. BCG vaccination. *In* P. D. O. Davies (ed.), *Tuberculosis*, in press. Chapman & Hall, Ltd., London.

Stead, W. W. 1992. Genetics and resistance to tuberculosis. Could resistance be enhanced by genetic engineering. *Ann. Intern. Med.* **116**:937–941.

Stead, W. W., J. P. Lofgren, J. W. Senner, and W. T. Reddick. 1990. Racial differences in susceptibility to infection with *M. tuberculosis*. *N. Engl. J. Med.* **322**:422–427.

Stover, C. K., V. F. de la Cruz, T. R. Fuerst, J. E. Burlein, L. A. Benson, L. T. Bennett, G. P. Bansal, J. F. Young, M. H. Lee, G. F. Hatfull, S. B. Snapper, R. G. Barletta, W. R. Jacobs, Jr., and B. R. Bloom. 1991. New use of BCG for recombinant vaccines. *Nature* (London) **351**:456–460.

Styblo, K. 1991. Epidemiology of tuberculosis. *Selected Papers R. Netherland Tuberc. Assoc.* **24**:1–136.

Styblo, K., and J. Meijer. 1976. Impact of BCG vaccination programmes in children and young adults on the tuberculosis problem. *Tubercle* **57:**17–43.

Sutherland, I. 1981. The epidemiology of tuberculosis—is prevention better than cure. *Bull. Int. Union Tuberc.* **56:**127–134.

Sutherland, I., and I. Lindgren. 1979. The protective effect of BCG vaccination as indicated by autopsy studies. *Tubercle* **60:**225–231.

Sutherland, I., and V. H. Springett. 1987. Effectiveness of BCG vaccination in England and Wales in 1983. *Tubercle* **68:**81–92.

Tang, D. C., M. DeVit, and S. A. Johnston. 1992. Genetic immunization is a simple method for eliciting an immune response. *Nature* (London) **356:**152–154.

ten Dam, H. G. 1984. Research on BCG vaccination. *Adv. Tuberc. Res.* **21:**79–106.

ten Dam, H. G. 1993. BCG vaccination, p. 251–269. *In* L. B. Reichman and E. S. Hershfield (ed.), *Tuberculosis.* Marcel Dekker, New York.

ten Dam, H. G., and A. Pio. 1988. Pathogenesis of tuberculosis and effectiveness of BCG vaccination. *Tubercle* **63:**226–233.

ten Dam, H. G., K. I. Toman, K. L. Hitze, and J. Guld. 1976. Present knowledge of immunization against tuberculosis. *Bull. W.H.O.* **54:**255–269.

Tidjani, O., A. Amedome, and H. G. ten Dam. 1986. The protective effect of BCG vaccination of the newborn against childhood tuberculosis in an African community. *Tubercle* **67:**269–281.

Tuberculosis Prevention Trial, Madras. 1980. Trial of BCG vaccines in South India for tuberculosis prevention. *Indian J. Med. Res.* **72**(Suppl.):1–74.

Vandiviere, H. M., M. Dworski, I. G. Melvin, K. A. Watsonk, and J. Begley. 1973. Efficacy of Bacillus Calmette-Guerin and isoniazid-resistant Bacillus Calmette-Guerin with and without isoniazid chemoprophylaxis from day of vaccination. II. Field trial in man. *Am. Rev. Respir. Dis.* **108:**301–313.

Vidal, S. M., D. Malo, K. Vogan, E. Skamene, and P. Gros. 1993. Natural resistance to infection with intracellular parasites: isolation of a candidate for BCG. *Cell* **73:**469–485.

Von Reyn, C. F., et al. 1987. Human immunodeficiency virus infection and routine childhood immunization. *Lancet* **ii:**669–672.

Wang, B., K. E. Ugen, V. Srikantan, M. G. Agadjanyan, K. Kang, Y. Refaeli, A. I. Sato, J. Boyer, W. V. Williams, and D. B. Weiner. 1993. Gene inoculation generates immune responses against human immunodeficiency virus 1. *Proc. Natl. Acad. Sci. USA* **90:**4156–4160.

Weigeshaus, E. H., and B. W. Smith. 1989. Review of the protective potency of new tuberculosis vaccines. *Rev. Infect. Dis.* **11**(Suppl. 2):484–490.

Weill-Hallé, B. 1980. Routes and methods of administration: oral vaccination, p. 175–181. *In* S. R. Rosenthal (ed.), *BCG Vaccine: Tuberculosis-Cancer.* PSG Publishing, Littleton, Mass.

Weltman, A. C., and D. N. Rose. 1993. The safety of Bacille Calmette-Guerin vaccination in HIV infection and AIDS. *AIDS* **7:**149–157.

Woods, G. L., and J. A. Washington II. 1987. Mycobacteria other than *Mycobacterium tuberculosis*: review of microbiologic and clinical aspects. *Rev. Infect. Dis.* **9:**275–294.

World Health Organization. 1966. *Expert Committee on Biological Standardization.* Technical report series no. 329. World Health Organization, Geneva.

World Health Organization. 1987. Expanded program on immunization: joint WHO/UNICEF statement on immunization and AIDS. *Weekly Epidemiol. Rec.* **62:**53–54.

World Health Organization. 1992. *Expanded Program for Immunization. Program Report.* World Health Organization, Geneva.

Youmans, G. P. 1979. Relationship between delayed-type hypersensitivity and immunity in tuberculosis, p. 302–316. *In* G. P. Youmans (ed.), *Tuberculosis.* The W. B. Saunders Co., Philadelphia.

Tuberculosis: Pathogenesis, Protection, and Control
Edited by Barry R. Bloom
© 1994 American Society for Microbiology, Washington, DC 20005

Chapter 32

Strategies for New Drug Development

Douglas B. Young

The emergence of strains of *Mycobacterium tuberculosis* resistant to existing drugs has focused attention on the urgent need for development of new antimycobacterial agents. Such agents have not been perceived as a high priority by pharmaceutical companies over the last 30 years, and a coordinated effort to screen general antimicrobial compounds developed during this time for activity against *M. tuberculosis* may well prove worthwhile. The recent development of genetic tools for monitoring the viability of *M. tuberculosis* provides a rapid approach for this type of screening (Jacobs et al., 1993). From a broader perspective, molecular genetic tools for study and manipulation of mycobacteria provide access to a vast amount of new information about the biochemistry and metabolism of *M. tuberculosis*, and exploitation of this information has important potential in the rational development of a new generation of antimycobacterial agents and perhaps in the design of improved strategies for use of existing drugs. This chapter focuses on the prospects for using a fundamental molecular approach to identification of novel lead compounds for new drug development. Further important steps in drug development, such as toxicity testing, optimization of pharmacokinetics, etc., are not addressed in this review.

In selecting targets for antimicrobial agents, it is clearly advantageous to avoid bacterial enzymes with closely related counterparts in mammalian cells. In addition, to avoid disruption of normal microbial flora during the prolonged course of tuberculosis therapy and to limit possible transfer of resistance factors from other bacterial genera, it is preferable that new drug targets be specific for mycobacteria. Drugs must act on a target that is essential for bacterial survival, and ideally, they should be effective against bacteria throughout their growth cycle both inside and outside mammalian cells during infection. In this section, we first review existing and potential drug targets in *M. tuberculosis*. We then discuss distinctive features of mycobacteria relevant to drug design, and finally, we consider experimental approaches applicable to rational drug discovery programs.

DRUG TARGETS IN *M. TUBERCULOSIS*

Most antibacterial agents inhibit biosynthetic pathways involved in the production of macromolecules (proteins, nucleic acids, or cell wall polymers). Several of the broad-spectrum antibacterial agents are effective

Douglas B. Young • Department of Medical Microbiology, St. Mary's Hospital Medical School, Norfolk Place, London W2 1PG, United Kingdom.

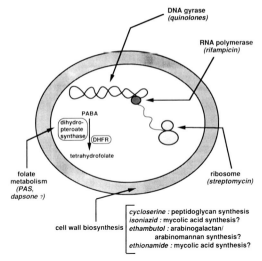

Figure 1. Sites of action of antimycobacterial agents. PABA, p-aminobenzoic acid; DHFR, dihydrofolate reductase; PAS, p-aminosalicylic acid.

against mycobacteria (Fig. 1), and the sites of action of these existing drugs clearly represent potential targets for new drug development.

Protein Synthesis

Streptomycin, the first antibiotic available for widespread use in treatment of tuberculosis, is a member of the aminoglycoside family that disrupts bacterial protein synthesis. As in other bacteria, streptomycin resistance in *M. tuberculosis* is conferred by mutations that alter the ribosomal protein S12 or the ribosomal 16S RNA molecule (Finken et al., 1993). Kanamycin, a related aminoglycoside with a similar mode of action, and its semisynthetic derivative amikacin are also used in tuberculosis therapy. While protein synthesis is clearly an important drug target in *M. tuberculosis*, other families of protein synthesis inhibitors (tetracycline, chloramphenicol, and the macrolides [e.g., erythromycin]) have no clinical use against tuberculosis. The intensive effort that has gone into development of protein synthesis inhibitors and the rather limited spectra of those agents found

to be effective against tuberculosis suggest that the ribosome may not be a particularly attractive target for new antituberculous drug design.

Nucleic Acids

Sulfonamides, which were the first clinically effective antibacterial agents, are structural analogs of p-aminobenzoic acid that inhibit biosynthesis of tetrahydrofolic acid, thus blocking production of the purine and pyrimidine bases required for nucleic acid synthesis. The antituberculous drug p-aminosalicylic acid (Fig. 2) was initially designed as a competitive inhibitor of salicylic acid and may act on the tetrahydrofolate pathway as well as on the salicylate-dependent biosynthesis of mycobactins that are required for iron transport. An important strategy for enhancing the activity of sulfonamides against some bacteria has been their use in combination with trimethoprim, a drug that inhibits a subsequent step in the tetrahydrofolate pathway catalyzed by the enzyme dihydrofolate reductase. Although trimethoprim is not active against mycobacteria, a considerable amount of structural information is available concerning bacterial and mammalian dihydrofolate reductases, and a detailed study of *M. tuberculosis* enzymes from the tetrahydrofolate pathway may provide a

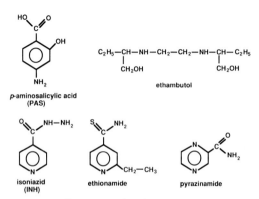

Figure 2. Structures of antimycobacterial agents.

basis for rational design of novel synergistic drug combinations.

The fluoroquinolones (ofloxacin, ciprofloxacin, sparfloxacin) are broad-spectrum antibacterial agents that disrupt the bacterial chromosome by inhibiting the supercoiling activity of DNA gyrase. The fluoroquinolones are increasingly important in treatment of mycobacterial diseases, and the genes encoding both subunits of the DNA gyrase enzyme of *M. tuberculosis* have been cloned (Takiff, personnal communication). Pharmaceutical companies have invested considerable effort in development of gyrase inhibitors, and it may be of interest to screen for evidence of specificity for the mycobacterial enzyme among such compounds.

Rifampin is a key drug in mycobacterial therapy that has a broad antibacterial spectrum and a well-defined target. In this case, transcription is inhibited by an interaction with the β subunit of the bacterial RNA polymerase molecule. In mycobacteria, as in other bacteria, resistance is conferred by point mutations in the *rpoB* gene (Telenti et al., 1993).

Cell Wall Biosynthesis

Broad-spectrum antibacterial agents

Biosynthesis of cell wall peptidoglycan provides targets for a large number of antibacterial agents. Cycloserine inhibits incorporation of D-alanine into the peptidoglycan precursor, while the glycopeptide drugs vancomycin and teicoplanin inhibit assembly of the precursors by binding to the terminal D-Ala–D-Ala residues. Members of the extensive family of β-lactams (penicillins and cephalosporins) inhibit a series of carboxypeptidases and transpeptidases (the penicillin-binding proteins) required for cross-linking of the peptidoglycan units. Among all of the agents, it is striking that only cycloserine (a drug associated with serious side effects) is effective in antimycobacterial therapy. The ineffectiveness of the other drugs is almost certainly due to their failure to get access to the appropriate target enzymes rather than to any fundamental difference in the core structure or biosynthesis of mycobacterial peptidoglycan (Jarlier et al., 1991). As discussed below, permeability is a crucial factor in determining the efficacy of antimycobacterial agents.

New cell wall targets

While the complex cell wall structure of mycobacteria probably confers the permeability barrier that underlies their resistance to many existing antibacterial agents, the same unique structure contains a series of potential targets for novel mycobacterium-specific inhibitors. A considerable amount of information concerning the polysaccharide and lipid structures that make up the mycobacterial cell wall is available. The peptidoglycan backbone is covalently attached to an arabinogalactan polymer (Daffe et al., 1990), and it is probable that inhibition of steps involved in arabinogalactan biosynthesis would prove lethal to the cell. The hydrophobic, wax-like character of the mycobacterial cell wall is conferred by a family of long-chain α-branched fatty acids (the mycolic acids) that are in turn covalently associated with the cell wall arabinogalactan. The mycolic acids are unique to the mycobacteria, and again, it can be envisaged that their synthesis and assembly into the cell wall entail a series of enzymes, each representing a potentially attractive target for antibacterial action. A further series of noncovalently associated components contributes to the cell wall structure. Lipoarabinomannan molecules are thought to traverse the cell wall in a manner analogous to lipoteichoic acids of the gram-positive bacteria and are able to trigger cytokine release by mammalian cells in a manner reminiscent of the action of gram-negative lipopolysaccharide (Chatterjee et al., 1992). Long-chain fatty acyl dialcohols (phthiocerol dimycocerosate) and sulfated and nonsulfated trehalose esters add further complexity to the outer surface of *M. tuberculosis* and may contribute both to bacterial permeability and to interactions with mammalian cells during infection. While the exact contribution of each of these components to mycobacterial viability is unknown, it is attractive to suggest that maintenance of this overall cell wall structure is a crucial factor in survival and pathogenicity of *M. tuberculosis* and that any drugs capable of disrupting synthesis and assembly of cell wall components may have some potential as antimycobacterial agents.

Ethambutol, isoniazid, and ethionamide

There are several indications that some existing antituberculous drugs may indeed act on the cell wall biosynthetic pathways. Identification of the precise targets of such drugs may allow design of novel inhibitors of the same enzyme or of related steps in the same pathway.

Ethambutol (Fig. 2) has a polyamine-like structure and was originally thought to interfere with RNA synthesis. More recent evidence from metabolic labeling experiments with ethambutol, however, suggests inhibition of glucose incorporation into arabinogalactan and arabinomannan polymers as an early event in drug action (Takayama and Kilburn, 1989). Although the biochemistry of such an activity is far from clear, the ability to transfer ethambutol resistance between mycobacterial strains by using cloned DNA fragments (Inamine, personal communication) will provide an important new approach to this problem.

Isoniazid (INH; Fig. 2) has a very high degree of specificity for *M. tuberculosis*, and there is a vast literature concerning its proposed mode of action (see Zhang and Young [1993] for a recent review). INH susceptibility is dependent on the presence of a catalase-peroxidase enzyme that may convert the drug to an activated intermediate within the bacterial cell. As in the case of ethambutol, metabolic labeling experiments monitoring the earliest detectable effects of INH provide evidence for action on cell wall biosynthesis, with mycolic acid synthesis being the most likely target (Winder and Collins, 1970). A point mutation in a locus termed the *inhA* gene is associated with INH resistance in *M. smegmatis* (Bannerjee and Jacobs, personal communication), and it is attractive to propose that this gene encodes an enzyme involved in mycolic acid synthesis. Interestingly, the same mutation confers resistance to ethionamide. Ethionamide, which is structurally related to INH (Fig. 2), may also inhibit mycolic acid biosynthesis, although in this case, the catalase-peroxidase step is not required, and some INH-resistant isolates show enhanced sensitivity to ethionamide (Winder, 1982).

ADDITIONAL FACTORS RELEVANT TO DRUG DESIGN

Permeability and Transport

As noted above, access of drugs to their target molecules appears to be a key factor in determining mycobacterial susceptibility and resistance. Strains of *M. avium-M. intracellulare* are significantly more resistant than *M. tuberculosis* to most antibacterial agents, for example, and this resistance is thought to reflect a general decrease in the organism's permeability to the drug. It has been proposed that the mycolic acids and surface-associated lipids of mycobacteria form a permeability barrier analogous to the outer membranes of gram-negative bacteria (Jarlier and Nikaido, 1990; see also chapter 22 of this volume), and discovering means of transporting drugs across this hydrophobic barrier may hold the key to improved antimycobacterial therapy. At present, we have only a few hints concerning the nature of transport systems in mycobacteria. Trias et al. (1992) detected a small amount of a porin-like molecule in cell wall preparations from *M. chelonae*, siderophores (mycobactins) and exochelins required for iron acquisition have been found (Ratledge, 1982), and an *M. tuberculosis* lipoprotein resembling a periplasmic binding protein required for phosphate transport has been characterized (Andersen et al., 1990). Detailed analysis of the uptake mechanisms required for transport of nutrients across the putative outer membrane, the intervening cell wall region, and the inner bacterial cell membrane may yield valuable insights. Drugs could be designed to take advantage of active uptake by such transport systems, for example, and transporters specific for essential nutrients could themselves be targets for novel inhibitors.

Prodrugs

M. tuberculosis isolates with defects in the *katG* gene encoding a catalase-peroxidase enzyme develop resistance to INH, indicating a possible role for the enzyme in intracellular activation of the drug (Zhang et al., 1992). Similarly, resistance to pyrazinamide (Fig. 2) is generally associated with the loss of a pyrazinamidase enzyme, and it is probable that pyrazinoic acid is the active form of the drug within the bacteria (Konno et al., 1967). The concept of using a prodrug, which is subsequently converted to an active form within the bacteria, may represent a useful mechanism for achieving efficient drug uptake. Sensitivity to pyrazinamide is dependent on the conditions of bacterial growth. Growth at acidic pH is necessary to demonstrate in vitro susceptibility of *M. tuberculosis*, while in vivo susceptibility is thought to reflect conditions encountered within intracellular phagocytic vesicles (Mackaness, 1956; Crowle et al., 1991). For other bacterial pathogens, it is broadly appreciated that key phenotypic

changes occur during adaptation to the host environment (Miller et al., 1989), and further analysis of the final target of pyrazinamide may provide useful insights into intracellular adaptation of *M. tuberculosis*. Features specific to the in vivo phenotype represent possible drug targets, and pyrazinamide provides a clear illustration of the importance of studying drug action in vivo as well as in simple bacterial cultures.

Drug Combinations

It has been demonstrated empirically that certain drug combinations (INH and pyrazinamide, for example) are synergistic, and it is attractive to propose rational strategies for the design of potentially useful combinations. Inhibition of sequential steps in a single pathway is a promising approach (e.g., sulfonamide and trimethoprim), and the association between INH resistance and loss of catalase activity suggests that drugs capable of generating oxidative radicals might usefully be combined with INH therapy. Inhibitors that disrupt some aspect of cell wall biosynthesis may not be lethal in themselves but might affect the permeability barrier in such a way as to increase the effectiveness of other drugs given in combination therapy. It has been suggested that ethambutol may have such an action in enhancing the susceptibility of *M. avium* to other drugs (Hoffner et al., 1987; Rastogi et al., 1990).

Outside the Cell Wall

An alternative strategy for circumventing the permeability barrier is to select targets that are present outside the cell wall. These could be hydrolytic enzymes or transport molecules required for bacterial nutrition or molecules involved in specific interactions with host cells. In culture, *M. tuberculosis* exports an array of proteins that are under intensive study in relation to their antigenic properties but are poorly understood in terms of biochemical function. Several fibronectin-binding proteins have been identified (Abou-Zeid et al., 1991), but it remains to be determined whether these have a functionally important interaction with the mammalian extracellular matrix or an as-yet-undetected enzymatic role important for mycobacterial growth. Some of the surface and secreted proteins are found as lipoproteins (Young and Garbe, 1991), with additional evidence of glycosylation in some instances (Fifis et al., 1991; Garbe et al., 1993). Posttranslational modification probably occurs on the outer side of the cell membrane, and identification of the relevant enzymes could provide interesting targets for antimycobacterial agents that might affect transport systems and growth of *M. tuberculosis*. Although it lacks characteristic secretion signals, superoxide dismutase (SOD) is found in culture filtrates of *M. tuberculosis* (Zhang et al., 1991). It is proposed that extracellular SOD protects *Nocardia asteroides* from exogenous superoxide radicals generated within the phagolysosome (Beaman and Beaman, 1990), and extracellular SOD may similarly be required for intracellular survival of mycobacterial pathogens. Extensive conservation between bacterial SOD and the corresponding mitochondrial enzyme in mammalian cells represents a significant barrier in relation to drug targeting, although the availability of a crystal structure for the *M. tuberculosis* enzyme may allow development of such an approach (Cooper et al., in press). Supernatant fluid from *M. tuberculosis* cultures contains several proteins (SOD and the DnaK and GroES chaperones, for example) that are considered to be cytoplasmic proteins in *Escherichia coli* (Young et al., 1990). It remains to be determined whether the presence of these proteins is due to a signal peptide-independent system for protein export or simply reflects a limited degree of leakage from dead or damaged cells. Should *M. tuberculosis* prove to have a specific protein export system, it would be important to consider the possibility that there are additional efflux systems that behave synergistically with the permeability barrier in conferring drug resistance.

Dormancy and Persisters

The greatest challenge for development of new drugs against tuberculosis is to design strategies that will reduce the duration of treatment. Current therapies kill actively growing bacteria within a few days but have to be continued for many months in order to finally eliminate persisting bacteria, which are thought to survive either by reaching a site that is inaccessible to drugs or by entering a state of dormancy with much-reduced metabolic activity. It is widely recognized that when bacterial cultures are starved for nutrients, they enter a stationary phase in which cells stop dividing and develop an ability to survive under conditions that would be lethal during the actively growing phase (Matin et al., 1989). We know nothing of the physiological state of the persisting tubercle bacilli, but entry into such a state of generalized stress resistance would be consistent with the ability of some organisms to survive during drug therapy and then reactivate in a fully drug-susceptible form.

Detailed study of stationary-phase changes in *E. coli* and other bacteria has shown that stress resistance is not simply due to a reduced metabolic activity but actually requires the programmed synthesis of a set of stress proteins (Siegele and Kolter, 1992). In *E. coli*, this synthesis is achieved by changes in transcriptional patterns associated with particular RNA polymerase sigma subunits. In addition to the α and β subunits required for polymerization of the ribonucleotide units, the bacterial RNA polymerase contains a σ subunit that directs the enzyme to transcribe particular genes. Most *E. coli* genes are transcribed by an RNA polymerase carrying a 70-kDa σ subunit (RpoD), but in response to stress, changes in the levels of minor σ subunits can direct an alteration in transcriptional patterns. Genes associated with stationary-phase stress resistance are controlled by a novel σ subunit, the product of the *rpoS* (or *katF*) gene (Hengge-Aronis, 1993). The critical importance of this form of transcriptional regulation in determining bacterial cell survival is dramatically demonstrated by the observation that bacteria carrying *rpoS* mutations can readily be selected on the basis of their ability to compete with wild-type cells during selection under starvation conditions (Zambrano et al., 1993). Elucidation of corresponding pathways in *M. tuberculosis* might allow us to think in terms of designing reagents that would interfere with development of generalized stress resistance by targeting specific σ subunits or perhaps by interrupting relevant signaling pathways, for example. While such a strategy is entirely speculative at present, it can readily be envisaged that the current intense interest in studying molecular mechanisms of mycobacterial virulence will open up quite novel opportunities for rational drug design.

EXPERIMENTAL STRATEGIES

From the above discussion, it is clear that an extensive list of potential drug targets in *M. tuberculosis* can be compiled with relative ease. Conversion of such a list into an actual drug discovery program will demand considerably greater effort and imagination. Progress will require a combination of biochemical and genetic skills, but for the purpose of outlining potential experimental approaches to rational drug design, we will address these two strategies independently.

Biochemical Approaches

Enzymes involved in synthesis of the complex cell wall components represent attractive potential drug targets. Although the structures of many of these components have been determined, the relevant biosynthetic pathways remain largely unknown. Isolation and characterization of biosynthetic intermediates represent an important strategy for defining such pathways and also provide an approach to drug discovery. By synthesizing structural analogs of these intermediates, it may be possible to identify inhibitory molecules that could provide lead compounds for new drugs. Development of cell-free systems for monitoring biosynthesis of cell wall components will play an important role both in elucidating the biochemical pathways and in screening for inhibitors. Identification of compounds that are active in cell-free systems could be followed by synthesis of related structures designed to enhance uptake into intact mycobacteria. At a further level of sophistication, purification of individual enzyme targets will simplify screening of large numbers of potential inhibitors, and resolution of three-dimensional enzyme structures will ultimately allow exploitation of the full power of rational drug discovery techniques.

Genetics and Sequencing

The recent development of molecular genetic systems for mycobacteria opens a range of novel opportunities for drug discovery. In the case of the existing antimycobacterial agents discussed above (INH, ethambutol, etc.), gene transfer experiments can be used to identify and clone the corresponding drug targets by monitoring appropriate transfer of drug resistance or susceptibility. In addition, the generation of extensive amounts of sequence information from mycobacterial genome projects will undoubtedly play an increasingly dominant role in identification of genes encoding potential drug targets. The key experimental challenge will be to design techniques to allow expression of genes or gene clusters in functional assays suitable for drug screening. While conventional *E. coli* expression systems may be suitable for some enzymes, it is likely that expression in rapidly growing mycobacterial hosts will prove advantageous, particularly when multiple genes encoding sequential enzymes within a single pathway are to be studied. In addition to development of recombinant cell-free systems as discussed above, it can be envisaged that gene replacement technology could be used to construct rapidly growing mycobacteria that utilize specific *M. tuberculosis* enzymes to catalyze individual steps involved in key biosynthetic pathways. Such chimeric organisms could provide a basis for the development of novel drug screening assays.

REFERENCES

Abou-Zeid, C., T. Garbe, R. Lathigra, H. G. Wiker, M. Harboe, G. A. W. Rook, and D. B. Young. 1991. Genetic and immunological analysis of *Mycobacterium tuberculosis* fibronectin-binding proteins. *Infect. Immun.* **59:**2712–2718.

Andersen, A. B., L. Ljungqvist, and M. Olsen. 1990. Evidence that protein antigen b of *Mycobacterium tuberculosis* is involved in phosphate metabolism. *J. Gen. Microbiol.* **136:**477–480.

Bannerjee, A., and W. R. Jacobs. Personal communication.

Beaman, L., and B. L. Beaman. 1990. Monoclonal antibodies demonstrate that superoxide dismutase contributes to protection of *Nocardia asteroides* within the intact host. *Infect. Immun.* **58:**3122–3128.

Chatterjee, D., A. D. Roberts, K. Lowell, P. J. Brennan, and I. M. Orme. 1992. Structural basis of capacity of lipoarabinomannan to induce secretion of tumor necrosis factor. *Infect. Immun.* **60:**1249–1253.

Cooper, J. B., H. P. C. Driessen, S. P. Wood, Y. Zhang, and D. Young. Crystallization and preliminary X-ray analysis of the superoxide dismutase from *Mycobacterium tuberculosis. J. Mol. Biol.*, in press.

Crowle, A. J., R. Dahl, E. Ross, and M. H. May. 1991. Evidence that vesicles containing living virulent *Mycobacterium tuberculosis* or *Mycobacterium avium* in cultured human macrophages are not acidic. *Infect. Immun.* **59:**1823–1831.

Daffe, M., P. J. Brennan, and M. McNeil. 1990. Predominant structural features of the cell wall arabinogalactan of *Mycobacterium tuberculosis* as revealed through characterization of oligoglycosyl alditol fragments by gas chromatography/mass spectrometry and by ^{1}H and ^{13}C NMR analyses. *J. Biol. Chem.* **265:**6734–6743.

Fifis, T., C. Costopoulos, A. J. Radford, A. Bacic, and P. R. Wood. 1991. Purification and characterization of major antigens from a *Mycobacterium bovis* culture filtrate. *Infect. Immun.* **59:**800–807.

Finken, M., P. Kirschner, A. Meier, A. Wrede, and E. C. Bottger. 1993. Molecular basis of streptomycin resistance in *Mycobacterium tuberculosis*: alteration of the ribosomal protein S12 gene and point mutation within a functional 16S ribosomal RNA pseudoknot. *Mol. Microbiol.* **9:**1239–1246.

Garbe, T., D. Harris, M. Vordermeier, R. Lathigra, J. Ivanyi, and D. Young. 1993. Expression of the *Mycobacterium tuberculosis* 19-kilodalton antigen in *Mycobacterium smegmatis*: immunological analysis and evidence of glycosylation. *Infect. Immun.* **61:**260–267.

Hengge-Aronis, R. 1993. Survival of hunger and stress: the role of *rpoS* in early stationary phase gene regulation in *E. coli. Cell* **72:**165–168.

Hoffner, S. E., S. B. Svenson, and G. Kallenius. 1987. Synergistic effects of antimycobacterial drug combinations on *Mycobacterium avium* complex determined radiometrically in liquid medium. *Eur. J. Clin. Microbiol.* **6:**530–535.

Inamine, J. Personal communication.

Jacobs, W. R., R. G. Barletta, R. Udani, J. Chan, G. Kalkut, G. Sosne, T. Kieser, G. J. Sarkis, G. F. Hatfull, and B. R. Bloom. 1993. Rapid assessment of drug susceptibilities of *Mycobacterium tuberculosis* by means of luciferase reporter phages. *Science* **260:**819–822.

Jarlier, V., L. Gutmann, and H. Nikaido. 1991. Interplay of cell wall barrier and β-lactamase activity determines high resistance to β-lactam antibiotics in *Mycobacterium chelonei. Antimicrob. Agents Chemother.* **35:**1937–1939.

Jarlier, V., and H. Nikaido. 1990. Permeability barrier to hydrophilic solutes in *Mycobacterium chelonei. J. Bacteriol.* **172:**1418–1422.

Konno, K., F. M. Feldmann, and W. McDermott. 1967. Pyrazinamide susceptibility and amidase activity of tubercle bacilli. *Am. Rev. Respir. Dis.* **95:**461–469.

Mackaness, G. B. 1956. The intracellular activation of pyrazinamide and nicotinamide. *Am. Rev. Tuberc.* **74:**718–728.

Matin, A., E. A. Auger, P. H. Blum, and J. E. Schultz. 1989. Genetic basis of survival in nondifferentiating bacteria. *Annu. Rev. Microbiol.* **43:**293–316.

Miller, J. F., J. J. Mekalanos, and S. Falkow. 1989. Coordinate regulation and sensory transduction in the control of bacterial virulence. *Science* **243:**916–922.

Rastogi, N., K. S. Goh, and H. L. David. 1990. Enhancement of drug susceptibility of *Mycobacterium avium* by inhibitors of cell envelope synthesis. *Antimicrob. Agents Chemother.* **34:**759–764.

Ratledge, C. 1982. Nutrition, growth and metabolism, p. 185–271. *In* C. Ratledge and J. Stanford (ed.), *The Biology of the Mycobacteria*, vol. 1. Academic Press, London.

Siegele, D. A., and R. Kolter. 1992. Life after log. *J. Bacteriol.* **174:**345–348.

Takayama, K., and J. O. Kilburn. 1989. Inhibition of synthesis of arabinogalactan by ethambutol in *Mycobacterium smegmatis*. *Antimicrob. Agents Chemother.* **33:**1493–1499.

Takiff, H. Personal communication.

Telenti, A., P. Imboden, F. Marchesi, D. Lowrie, S. Cole, M. J. Colston, L. Matter, K. Schopfer, and T. Bodmer. 1993. Detection of rifampicin-resistance mutations in *Mycobacterium tuberculosis*. *Lancet* **341:**647–650.

Trias, J., V. Jarlier, and R. Benz. 1992. Porins in the cell wall of mycobacteria. *Science* **258:**1479–1481.

Winder, F. G. 1982. Mode of action of the antimycobacterial agents and associated aspects of the molecular biology of the mycobacteria, p. 353–438. *In* C. Ratledge and J. Stanford (ed.), *The Biology of the Mycobacteria*, vol. 1. Academic Press, London.

Winder, F. G., and P. B. Collins. 1970. Inhibition by isoniazid of synthesis of mycolic acids in *Mycobacterium tuberculosis*. *J. Gen. Microbiol.* **63:**41–48.

Young, D., T. Garbe, R. Lathigra, and C. Abou-Zeid. 1990. Protein antigens: structure, function and regulation, p. 1–35. *In* J. McFadden (ed.), *Molecular Biology of the Mycobacteria*. Surrey University Press, London.

Young, D. B., and T. R. Garbe. 1991. Lipoprotein antigens of *Mycobacterium tuberculosis*. *Res. Microbiol.* **142:**55–65.

Zambrano, M. M., D. A. Siegele, M. Almiron, A. Tormo, and R. Kolter. 1993. Microbial competition: *Escherichia coli* mutants that take over stationary phase cultures. *Science* **259:**1757–1760.

Zhang, Y., B. Heym, B. Allen, D. Young, and S. Cole. 1992. The catalase-peroxidase gene and isoniazid resistance of *Mycobacterium tuberculosis*. *Nature* (London) **358:**591–593.

Zhang, Y., R. Lathigra, T. Garbe, D. Catty, and D. Young. 1991. Genetic analysis of superoxide dismutase, the 23 kilodalton antigen of *Mycobacterium tuberculosis*. *Mol. Microbiol.* **5:**381–391.

Zhang, Y., and D. B. Young. 1993. Molecular mechanisms of isoniazid: a drug at the front line of tuberculosis control. *Trends Microbiol.* **1:**109–113.

Tuberculosis: Pathogenesis, Protection, and Control
Edited by Barry R. Bloom
© 1994 American Society for Microbiology, Washington, DC 20005

Chapter 33

Molecular Epidemiology of Tuberculosis

Peter M. Small and Jan D. A. van Embden

Phenotypic markers that distinguish between strains of *Mycobacterium tuberculosis*, such as unusual antibiotic resistance patterns and mycobacterial phage susceptibility, have long been employed in the investigation of point source outbreaks of *M. tuberculosis* (Gruft et al., 1984). These investigations have provided much of the understanding of the transmission and pathogenesis of tuberculosis upon which the current approach to disease control is based.

More recently, these phenotypic markers have been replaced with molecular techniques such as DNA fingerprinting. Use of these novel techniques in conjunction with conventional investigation is providing increased insight into the current epidemiology of tuberculosis. Such approaches may permit more precise targeting of conventional control measures. For example, the characterization of specific populations that are at particularly high risk of developing tuberculosis as a result of reactivated latent disease would direct chemoprophylaxis programs. Alternatively, a more complete understanding of the factors associated with secondary transmission would identify patients who are particularly prone to spreading tuberculosis ("dangerous disseminators") and suggest which populations would benefit from increased efforts at case finding and treatment. These approaches may even provide sufficient understanding of the specific environmental and social factors that influence tuberculosis transmission to permit the design of a new tuberculosis control strategy, i.e., the identification and alteration of settings that foster the spread of disease.

Molecular epidemiology is the integration of molecular techniques to track specific strains of pathogens with conventional epidemiologic approaches to understanding the distribution of disease in populations (Small and Moss, 1993; van Embden et al., 1992). This chapter describes the genetic elements of *M. tuberculosis* that may be exploited as strain-specific markers, the strain-typing methods that are based on these elements, and some of the DNA fingerprinting results obtained to date and speculates on future directions in this field.

Peter M. Small • Division of Infectious Diseases and Geographic Medicine, Beckman Center, Room 251, Stanford University, Stanford, California 94305-5425. *Jan D. A. van Embden* • Unit Molecular Microbiology, National Institute of Public Health and Environmental Protection, P.O. Box 1, 3720 BA, Bilthoven, The Netherlands.

GENETIC ELEMENTS IN *M. TUBERCULOSIS* THAT CONTRIBUTE TO DNA POLYMORPHISM

M. tuberculosis complex bacteria constitute a remarkably homogeneous group, as

Table 1. Insertion sequences and repetitive DNA in *M. tuberculosis*

Element	Size (bp)	Source	Host range	Copy no.	Related to[a]	Reference
IS*6110*	1,355	*M. tuberculosis*	*M. tuberculosis* complex	0–25	IS*3* family of *Entero-bacteriaceae*	McAdam et al., 1990; Thierry et al., 1990; Hermans et al., 1991
IS*1081*	1,324	*M. bovis*	*M. tuberculosis* complex *M. xenopi*	5–7	IS*256* of *S. aureus*	Collins and Stephens, 1991; van Soolingen et al., 1992
DR	36	BCG	*M. tuberculosis* complex	10–50		Groenen et al., in press; Hermans et al., 1991
MPTR	10	*M. tuberculosis*	*M. tuberculosis* complex *M. gordonae* *M. kansasii* *M. asiaticum* *M. gastri* *M. szulgai*	>100	Chi and REP from *E. coli*	Hermans et al., 1992
PGRS	30	*M. tuberculosis*	*M. tuberculosis* complex	>100		Ross and Dwyer, 1993

[a] Chi, *E. coli* recombination signal; REP, repetitive extragenic palindrome.

revealed by the inability of multilocus enzyme electrophoresis to differentiate individual strains (Crawford, personal communication) and the minimal DNA polymorphism in restriction fragments of randomly chosen chromosomal DNA fragments (Collins et al., 1993; Palittapongarnpim et al., 1993c).

In contrast, various repetitive DNA elements that contribute to strain variation have been discovered in *M. tuberculosis* (Table 1). Two of these are insertion sequences (IS), and the remainder are short repetitive DNA sequences with no known function or phenotype.

IS*6110*

IS*6110* is a 1,355-bp IS that was initially identified in *M. tuberculosis* (Thierry et al., 1990) and subsequently found to be distributed throughout the *M. tuberculosis* complex (Cave et al., 1991; Hermans et al., 1990; van Soolingen et al., 1991; Zainuddin

and Dale, 1989). It is a member of the IS*3* family of insertion elements, a family initially discovered in gram-negative bacteria (McAdam et al., 1990). The DNA sequences of the three different copies of IS*6110* that have been determined differ in only a few base pairs (see chapter 14). In general, 5 to 20 copies are present in various positions in the genomes of clinical isolates of *M. tuberculosis*, although some strains with no IS*6110* copies have been identified. There appears to be limited variability in the genomic location of strains with only a few copies of IS*6110* (Collins et al., 1993; Hermans et al., 1990, 1991; van Soolingen et al., 1991, 1993).

IS*1081*

The only other transposable element known in *M. tuberculosis* is IS*1081*. This is a 1,324-bp sequence discovered by Collins while attempting to clone *M. bovis*-specific DNA sequences (Collins and Stephens,

1991). The element is related to the IS*256* family of insertion elements originally found in *Staphylococcus aureus*. This IS is found in all species of the *M. tuberculosis* complex as well as in *M. xenopi* (van Soolingen and Collins, personal communication). In contrast to IS*6110*, IS*1081* is distributed rather homogeneously in different *M. tuberculosis* strains, with five to seven copies frequently present in the same sites. Therefore, IS*1081* is not a useful marker for distinguishing between strains of *M. tuberculosis*. However, because IS*1081* is present on a characteristic *Pvu*II fragment in *M. tuberculosis*, it may be used to differentiate BCG from other strains of *M. tuberculosis* (van Soolingen et al., 1992).

DR Sequence

The direct repeat (DR) sequence is a directly repeating sequence of 36 bp clustered in one region of the genome that are interspersed by nonrepetitive DNA, with each nonrepetitive segment being 36 to 41 bp in length (Hermans et al., 1991). The number of copies of the DR sequence has been determined to be approximately 10 to 50 in a variety of *M. tuberculosis* complex strains. The vast majority of *M. tuberculosis* strains contain one or more IS*6110* elements in the DR-containing region of the genome. It appears that a significant fraction of *M. tuberculosis* strains from Asia and Africa carry a single copy of IS*6110* in the chromosomal DR region, primarily on a 1.8-kbp *Pvu*II fragment. Thus, this locus is thought to be a "hot spot" for the integration of IS*6110* (Groenen et al., in press; Hermans et al., 1991; van Soolingen et al., 1993). In the majority of such strains, which have only a single copy of IS*6110* located within the DR region, there remains DNA sequence polymorphism. This diversity is generated by differences in the copy number of DRs plus spacer sequences, suggesting that homologous recombination between DR sequences is a major driving

force for the DR-associated DNA polymorphism (Groenen et al., in press). Because there appears to be considerable polymorphism within a relatively small part of the chromosome, this region is well suited for a polymerase chain reaction (PCR)-based fingerprinting technique.

MPTRs

Major polymorphic tandem repeats (MPTRs) are 10-bp repeating sequences invariably separated by unique 5-bp spacer sequences. These sequences have been identified in *M. tuberculosis* complex as well as in a number of other mycobacteria (Hermans et al., 1992). The 10-bp repeat is heterogeneous in sequence, with at least 5 bases conserved. Self-hybridization experiments suggest that this sequence is the major repetitive DNA in *M. tuberculosis*. Because this MPTR sequence is partially homologous to the repetitive extragenic palindromic sequence and the recombination signal Chi of *Escherichia coli*, it is speculated that the MPTR sequence might play a role in genetic rearrangements and gene regulation. Because there are over 100 copies of this element in the genome of *M. tuberculosis*, MPTR is not commonly being used for strain differentiation.

PGRS

The polymorphic GC-rich repetitive sequence (PGRS) is a short sequence present in multiple chromosomal clusters composed of many nonperfect repeats, like the MPTRs. Though initially identified in *M. tuberculosis* complex, its host range is now known to include *M. kansasii*, *M. gastri*, and *M. szulgae*, a host range that resembles that of the MPTR (Doran et al., 1992; Dwyer et al., 1993; Ross et al., 1992). The similarities in structure and host range of the PGRS and the MPTR suggest that these elements belong to a related family of repetitive DNA. The mechanism that generates PGRS-associated polymorphism is not known.

TECHNIQUES FOR DEMONSTRATING POLYMORPHISM

The concept of clonality is relevant to epidemiologists in so far as it can be used to understand the origin of different isolates. For such purposes, clones may be defined as bacterial cultures isolated independently from different sources at different times but showing so many identical phenotypic and genotypic traits that the most likely explanation for this identity is a recent common ancestor. An ideal DNA fingerprinting technique for detecting clonal relations between strains would be rapid and logistically simple and would generate a discrete pattern that would be stable over time. The degree of clonal variability revealed by this technique would be diverse enough so that epidemiologically unrelated strains would be unique but sufficiently stable that strains isolated from patients infected in point source outbreaks would be identical.

The earliest DNA fingerprinting techniques that were applied to mycobacteria used ethidium bromide staining of electrophoretically separated restriction fragments of genomic DNA (Collins and de Lisle, 1984). However, as mentioned before, the mobilities of the vast majority of the restriction fragments overlap, and thus at least four different restriction enzymes are needed to obtain a reasonable strain differentiation (Collins, personal communication). In addition, the large number of fragments generated with this method makes computerized comparison of results extremely difficult. Use of restriction enzymes with long AT-rich recognition sequences (Mazurek et al., 1991) generates fewer fragments, but separating such large fragments can be accomplished only by using the cumbersome technique of pulsed-field gel electrophoresis.

Most investigators use the technique of Southern blotting to exploit the presence of the above-described genetic elements to reveal restriction fragment length polymorphisms (RFLP) among *M. tuberculosis* strains. There are only three critical parameters with such an approach: (i) the choice of the restriction enzyme, (ii) the selection of the specific sequence of the genetic element used for probing the membrane, and (iii) the use of appropriate molecular weight standards to permit comparison between different gels. A standardized protocol, agreed upon at a small international meeting in 1991 (van Embden et al., 1993), permits the comparison of results obtained from different laboratories around the world. The establishment of a central database of standardized IS*6110* fingerprints is in preparation, and these data will be made available to the scientific community, analogous to sequence libraries (van Embden et al., unpublished data).

Because the preparation of Southern blots is laborious and requires the isolation of microgram quantities of DNA from cultured bacteria, attempts are under way to develop in vitro DNA amplification-based methods for strain differentiation. Such an approach could potentially provide rapid results and may even permit the simultaneous detection and strain differentiation of *M. tuberculosis*.

Polymorphic banding patterns have been obtained by utilizing PCR amplification from as little as 10 pg of target DNA with oligonucleotide primers homologous to the ends of the IS*6110* sequence. Sequencing of the product demonstrated that the amplified products resulted from priming between one IS*6110* copy and nonspecific priming sites on the *M. tuberculosis* genome (Ross and Dwyer, 1993). PCR with arbitrary oligonucleotide primers has also been shown to produce polymorphic banding patterns that confirm the relationship between isolates in several clusters of tuberculosis cases (Palittapongarnpim et al., 1993b).

IS amplityping (Plikaytis, personal communication), another PCR-based approach, uses primers based on the MPTR sequence and nested primers in the IS6110 sequence. This approach yields reproducible banding patterns directly from sputum samples, demonstrating its suitability for generating rapid results from clinical samples.

Mixed-linker PCR (Haas et al., 1993) is another PCR-based approach in which one primer specific for IS6110 and a second primer complementary to a linker are ligated to the restricted genomic DNA. In one strand, the linker contains uracil in place of thymidine, and specific amplification is obtained by elimination of this strand with uracil N-glycosylase. This method has the advantage of generating the same banding patterns as those generated by Southern blotting. In an analogous technique, a non-phosphorylated BamHI-compatible linker is used to specifically generate amplimers from IS6110-containing fragments (Palittapongarnpim et al., 1993a). This technique has also yielded promising preliminary results but is not as well characterized as mixed-linker PCR.

Another PCR-based method exploits polymorphism within the DR region. This method is a variant of the digital DNA-typing method used for human DNA (Jeffreys et al., 1991). The technique as adapted for M. tuberculosis generates sequences from in vitro-amplified DNA in the DR region. The sequences correspond to the 5' nucleotides in consecutive spacer DNAs that separate the DRs. Such DNA sequences may allow analysis of the phylogenetic relatedness of different isolates by existing DNA computer software (Groenen et al., in press).

Although the theoretical potential and the preliminary data obtained with these rapid strain-typing methods are encouraging, in 1994 there is vastly more experience with the internationally standardized Southern blotting-based technique. In addition to refining the technical aspects of these other approaches, the global diversity and temporal stability of their results will need to be established before these methods can be rationally applied as epidemiologic tools.

IS6110 AS A TOOL FOR STRAIN DIFFERENTIATION

Southern blotting of genomic M. tuberculosis DNA with IS6110 as a probe has become the most widely used technique for strain differentiation, and consequently, much has been learned about the method's strengths and weaknesses. While much less cumbersome than phage typing, it remains somewhat laborious and time-consuming. In our laboratories, a trained technician working full time may evaluate only approximately 30 to 60 strains each week. The turnaround time can be reduced to 2 weeks by directly scraping bacteria from a Lowenstein-Jensen slant with heavy visible growth. However, results are delayed if subculturing is required. The patterns generated with this technique are relatively simple and are amenable to computerized analysis and comparison, and the degree of polymorphism generated appears well suited to epidemiologic investigations. Numerous outbreak investigations have shown that epidemiologically unrelated isolates have unique patterns whereas those of related strains generally demonstrate identical patterns. The assertion of clonality is weaker for low-copy strains (van Soolingen et al., 1993), because the M. tuberculosis chromosome seems to have preferred sites of IS integration where the element may become "locked in" (Groenen et al., in press; Hermans et al., 1991; van Soolingen et al., 1993).

Because IS6110 is an IS that has the theoretical capacity to transpose ("a jumping gene"), it is to be expected that DNA fingerprint patterns based on this element change over time. In fact, the duplication of 3 bp in DNA flanking the element suggests that such transpositions are the source of IS6110-based RFLP (McAdam et al., 1990; Mendiola et al., 1992). However, the only direct evidence of IS6110 transposition is from Fomukong and Dale (submitted), who reported transposition of IS6110 in *M. smegmatis* when artificial composite transposons containing selectable drug resistance markers were used. Though precise data regarding the degree of temporal stability of these patterns is lacking, laboratory investigations of this phenomenon suggest that IS6110 patterns are relatively stable. These patterns are stable during 6 months of serial passage in liquid media (van Soolingen et al., 1991). The most striking example of the stability of IS6110-based DNA fingerprints is BCG. This vaccine strain has been propagated separately in different laboratories for over 6 decades. Nonetheless, all 35 strains tested have been found to carry the IS element designated IS987, invariably at a unique chromosomal locus. Only three of these strains have one additional element, all of them at a common chromosomal position (Fomukong et al., 1992; van Soolingen et al., 1993). The laboratory strains H37Ra and H37Rv demonstrate the greatest degree of polymorphism within an isogenic strain. These two strains were derived from a common progenitor strain (H37R) and have been maintained separately for decades. Although both strains contain 14 copies of IS6110, 6 of these copies are present in different restriction fragments (Mazurek et al., 1991).

In vivo data also suggest that although IS6110-based DNA fingerprints may vary slightly over time, such changes do not invalidate their use as an epidemiologic tool. When the strains were serially passaged in guinea pigs for 2 months, no changes were detected in the patterns (van Soolingen et al., 1991). As shown in Fig. 1, serial isolates from patients with chronic tuberculosis have been fingerprinted and found either to be unchanged or to have patterns that differed by only the addition or loss of a single band (Otal et al., 1991; Small et al., 1993b). The stability of these patterns can also be determined by comparing the pattern of the index and secondary cases in point source outbreaks. Virtually all such comparisons have shown identical patterns; however, single additional bands have been reported in some outbreaks (Daley et al., 1992; van Soolingen et al., 1991; Yuen et al., 1992).

The degree of polymorphism in a population of *M. tuberculosis* is a crucial component of DNA fingerprinting. Clonality is most convincingly demonstrated when there is considerable background diversity in a population such that finding isolates with identical patterns implies an epidemiologic connection. This assertion can be demonstrated empirically when DNA fingerprinting results corroborate those obtained from conventional epidemiology. Investigations conducted to date have demonstrated that IS6110 results are highly significant in this regard. However, this may not be true for all patterns. As mentioned above, strains exist (particularly in Asia and Africa) that have only a single copy of IS6110, generally located on a similarly sized *Pvu*II restriction fragment, thus limiting strain differentiation based on this element (van Soolingen et al., 1993). In fact, strains with identical single-banded RFLP patterns have been isolated from residents of San Francisco whose only epidemiologic link is that they had immigrated from Asia and who were clearly otherwise not epidemiologically connected (Small, unpublished observation). Very rarely, *M. tuberculosis* strains from the Far East that do not harbor IS6110 have been encountered (Das et al., 1993; van Soolingen et al., 1993). Such strains may be differentiated by Southern blotting using either DR or PGRS DNA as a probe (Groenen et al., in press; van Soolingen et al., 1993). Preliminary data suggest that the power to resolve such differences is approximately the same with either probe.

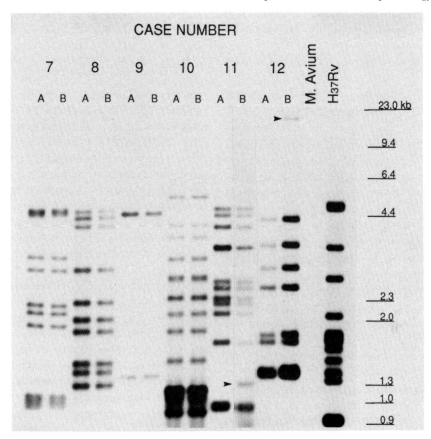

Figure 1. IS6110-based DNA fingerprinting results of initial (lanes A) and subsequent (lanes B) isolates of *M. tuberculosis* from patients with tuberculosis isolated from serial sputum samples. In each patient, the time interval between samples was 7 to 29 months, and subsequent isolates demonstrated increasing antimicrobial resistance. Serial RFLP patterns either are identical or differ by one additional band (arrow). The last two lanes contain negative and positive control DNA. (Reprinted by permission of the *New England Journal of Medicine* [Small et al., 1993b].)

ESTABLISHED USES OF THESE TECHNIQUES

Confirmation of Epidemiologically Suspected Transmission

Investigations of point source outbreaks of *M. tuberculosis* have provided important insights into the transmission and pathogenesis of tuberculosis. Such studies have been aided by the utilization of strain-specific markers such as unusual antibiotic susceptibility patterns and phage typing (Gruft et al., 1984), but previously employed techniques had serious limitations. Since 1990, IS6110-based RFLP has been used by researchers to better understand tuberculosis transmission, and this method is increasingly becoming a standard tool of public health investigators. DNA fingerprinting has been used to identify clonal transmission between neighbors (Godfrey-Fausett et al., 1992) and in a congregate-living facility (Daley et al., 1992), prisons (Centers for Disease Control, 1992), outpatient clinics (Hermans et al., 1990) and many hospitals (Beck-Sagué et al., 1992; Centers for Disease Control, 1991; Dooley et al., 1992; Edlin et al., 1992; Fischl et al., 1992). The strong evidence of nosocomial infections obtained by DNA typing often has led to the implementation of more stringent control measures.

Detection of Epidemiologically Unsuspected Transmission in a Group

DNA fingerprinting has been used in Seattle, Washington, to investigate an increase in tuberculosis among noninstitutionalized human immunodeficiency virus (HIV)-infected persons (Tabet et al., submitted). Analysis of strains from HIV-infected patients and random controls showed that six HIV-infected patients who were infected with the same strain had contact at specific bars, thus demonstrating a community outbreak of tuberculosis among HIV-infected persons who had not been previously linked following conventional investigation. Dwyer et al. (1993) and van Soolingen et al. (1992) showed that particular strains were disseminated among homeless people in Melbourne and Amsterdam, respectively. Prompt recognition should facilitate arresting such microepidemics.

Detection of Laboratory Errors

Episodes of cross-contamination in mycobacteriology laboratories have been reported when conventional and radiometric methodologies were used (Aber et al., 1980; Vannier et al., 1988). Such errors may have profound implications, since the isolation of even a single positive culture for *M. tuberculosis* frequently serves as the basis of a presumptive diagnosis of tuberculosis. Selective application of RFLP typing may be used in the investigation of suspected laboratory cross-contamination, the prompt identification of which may be helpful in identifying problematic laboratory procedures and altering clinical care (Small et al., 1993a).

FUTURE USES OF MOLECULAR EPIDEMIOLOGY

Population-Based Surveillance

If there is sufficient genetic diversity in a population, finding a group of individuals infected with *M. tuberculosis* strains that have the same RFLP pattern suggests that this group is epidemiologically connected, having been infected by each other or from a common source. This contention has been substantiated in San Francisco (Small, unpublished data), where RFLP analysis has been done for almost 500 isolates of *M. tuberculosis* cultured in the city between 1991 and 1992. Most isolates have unique RFLP patterns, demonstrating that there is considerable clonal diversity among *M. tuberculosis* in the city and that most patients are infected with unique strains. However, approximately one-third of the patients are infected with strains that have also been isolated from at least one other person. The most prevalent strain was isolated from 30 individuals. Twelve of these were known to be connected as residents of an AIDS housing facility; however, no connection had been suspected between these patients and the 18 others. Intensive epidemiologic investigation of this group revealed that there were very plausible connections between these individuals and demonstrated that the strain of *M. tuberculosis* initially isolated from one noncompliant patient now accounts for over 5% of the tuberculosis in the city. This suggests that population-based screening of isolates may detect previously unsuspected transmission.

Utilization of this approach in Switzerland has suggested that there is considerable ongoing transmission of tuberculosis in certain segments of the population (Genewein et al., in press). RFLP of 165 strains isolated from patients in Bern showed that one strain was highly prevalent in a group characterized as homeless drug users, and there was ''spillover'' into the general population. The application of molecular techniques in this setting suggests that tuberculosis control efforts should be focused on this population to prevent the emergence and spread of multidrug-resistant (MDR) tuberculosis in Europe.

If the basic assumptions and premises upon which these studies are based are confirmed and validated in other settings, then selected applications of these techniques may have broader applicability. It must be remembered, however, that these are only techniques and that they should not compete with standard control approaches for resources. Instead, they should be fully integrated into these activities, both as a tool for detecting point source outbreaks and as a method for monitoring the efficacy of tuberculosis control programs.

Determination of Contribution of Transmitted versus Reactivated Infections

The degree of polymorphism in a population of *M. tuberculosis* may serve as a proxy for the relative contribution of newly acquired and reactivated infection. If there is considerable newly acquired infection as a result of ongoing transmission, there will be limited polymorphism in the population, but if disease results from reactivated latent infection, there may be considerable diversity, reflecting the diversity of the times and places that the patients were infected. This concept has been validated in San Francisco, where the prevalence of clustered strains is greater in patients who are epidemiologically at high risk of having tuberculosis as a consequence of recent infection (such as young American-born minority group patients) and lower in those who are likely to have tuberculosis as a result of reactivated latent infection (such as elderly immigrants from countries with a high prevalence of tuberculosis) (Small et al., submitted). DNA fingerprinting of selected strains from a community may thus identify which populations develop tuberculosis as

a consequence of reactivated latent infection and thus may benefit from chemoprophylaxis.

Etiology of MDR Emergence

If RFLP diversity is a true proxy for recently transmitted disease, then it may help explain why MDR is emerging and may help focus control efforts. MDR can result from the emergence of resistance in a noncompliant patient's original strain or from the clonal dissemination of that strain. Demonstrating significant RFLP diversity among MDR strains would imply that MDR is emerging from multiple noncompliant patients and would suggest specific control measures such as directly observed therapy. However, limited RFLP diversity among MDR strains suggests that clonal dissemination of a few strains is occurring as a result of delayed diagnosis and treatment of infectious cases and that the focus of control should be on improved case finding and treatment. Preliminary data suggest that most MDR strains in San Francisco have unique RFLP but that diversity among MDR strains in New York City is limited (Small and Kreiswirth, unpublished observations). This is consistent with the observation that case finding and treatment completion are problematic in New York (Brudney and Dobkin, 1991). A detailed investigation of the temporal trends of MDR tuberculosis in one New York City hospital during a period of increasing HIV seroprevalence demonstrated that most HIV-associated MDR tuberculosis in 1991 was due to strains that had previously been isolated from HIV-negative patients (Shafer et al., submitted). This demonstrates the urgency of enacting good tuberculosis control in populations that have increasing HIV seroprevalence.

Relapse or New Infection

The possibility that patients will be exogenously reinfected with *M. tuberculosis* has been debated ever since the infectious etiology of tuberculosis was first recognized. This phenomenon has now been conclusively demonstrated to have occurred in a group of AIDS patients in New York City who were exogenously reinfected with MDR *M. tuberculosis* either during or shortly after successful therapy for the original infecting strain (Small et al., 1993b). This reinfection occurred in these patients as a result of their inability to develop protective immunity following infection and their continued exposure to *M. tuberculosis*. The incidence of this phenomenon in a population depends on the degree of immunocompetence of the individuals that make up that population and the exposure to *M. tuberculosis* in their environment. The reported cases occurred in a group of profoundly immunocompromised patients who were heavily exposed to *M. tuberculosis*. The frequency, settings, and specific risk factors for exogenous reinfection remain to be determined. If future studies demonstrate that reinfection is common, then it is not acceptable to simply treat patients and return them to an infectious environment; greater emphasis will need to be placed on eliminating *M. tuberculosis* from these environments. In addition, reinfection will complicate the evaluation of clinical trials of chemotherapeutic and chemoprophylactic regimens. It is currently assumed that relapses after therapy result from inadequacies in regimen efficacy or patient compliance. However, if exogenous reinfection is common, then relapse may reflect the reinfection of patients whose initial regimen was completely adequate.

Global Spread

The exquisite impact that social disruption has on tuberculosis is demonstrated by the observation that tuberculosis death rates in Western Europe doubled during the 4 years of World War I (Ryan, 1993). In addition, increased international travel fa-

vors the efficient transmission of pathogens across political boundaries (Lederberg et al., 1993). Thus, the persistence of tuberculosis and the emergence of drug-resistant strains in any geographic region constitute a global threat. It is hoped that a molecular epidemiologic approach will provide an understanding of the details of the global spread of tuberculosis and will suggest effective methods of curtailing such transmission in the face of the social disruption that faces the world today. Fingerprinting of strains from different countries has shown an association between DNA type and geographic origin (Godfrey-Fausset and Stoker, 1992; van Soolingen et al., 1991, 1993). Within the European community, a concerted action to collect fingerprints from many different countries and store these in a computer database together with clinical and bacteriological data has recently been initiated (van Embden, unpublished data). Once established, this database may provide clues about issues such as the impact of HIV, migration, drug use, and resistance or BCG vaccination on the transmission of tuberculosis within countries and across country borders.

Strain-Specific Phenotypic Characteristics

In many infectious diseases, such as salmonellosis, understanding strain-to-strain variability has yielded important insights into pathogenesis and has had implications for treatment and control. The identification of specific mycobacterial strains that differ in pathogenicity or tissue tropism may be similarly helpful. For example, genetic analysis of strains with a specific tropism for the lymphatic tissues may yield insight into the molecular mechanism of attachment, invasion, or intracellular persistence. This understanding may be exploited to define new therapeutic interventions or vaccines. It is even conceivable that molecular markers will be used to prioritize tuberculosis control and that special precautions will be required to control highly transmissible strains.

DNA Polymorphism Reflecting Molecular Clocks

The presently available data on genetic markers of *M. tuberculosis* have not yet led to attempts to establish phylogenetic relatedness between strains. Studies of *Escherichia coli* K-12 derivatives have shown that IS elements can in principle be used successfully for this purpose (Lawrence et al., 1989). Differences in the genetic stabilities of such genetic elements can be used to exploit these elements as molecular clocks in the evolution of divergent strains. This process can be conceptualized as a branching tree in which each branching point represents a single genetic event, such as a transposition in the case of IS elements. The pace at which these genetic events are occurring determines the number of different types revealed in a group of isolates with a common ancestor.

It is anticipated that the "best" DNA fingerprinting technique will be that which is based on genetic events occurring in synchrony with the time scale of the epidemiologic situation. Thus, different epidemiologic questions will be best addressed by different techniques. For example, tracing the spread of tuberculosis in a residential facility over weeks, in a city over years, and around the globe over decades will be done best by different techniques. If the genetic events are occurring considerably faster than the epidemiologic events, epidemiologically related strains will appear to be unrelated, whereas if the genetic events are occurring slower than the epidemiologic events, then unrelated strains will appear to be related. A major future challenge of DNA fingerprinting of *M. tuberculosis* will be to determine the paces of change of the various elements and to match these to study specific epidemiologic questions.

Acknowledgments. This work was financially supported by the World Health Organization Programme for Vaccine Development and the Commission of the European Communities Programme for Science Technology and Development (J.D.A.V.E.) and NIH grant K08 AI01137-01 (P.M.S.).

REFERENCES

Aber, V. R., B. W. Allen, D. A. Mitchison, P. Ayuma, E. A. Edwards, and A. B. Keyes. 1980. Quality control in the tuberculosis laboratory. 1. Laboratory studies on isolated positive cultures and the efficiency of direct smear examination. *Tubercle* **61:** 123–133.

Beck-Sagué, C., S. W. Dooley, M. D. Hutton, J. Otten, A. Breeden, J. T. Crawford, A. E. Pitchenik, C. Woodley, G. Cauthen, and W. R. Jarvis. 1992. Hospital outbreak of multidrug-resistant *Mycobacterium tuberculosis* infections. *JAMA* **268:**1280–1286.

Brudney, K., and J. Dobkin. 1991. Resurgent tuberculosis in New York City: human immunodeficiency virus, homelessness, and the decline of tuberculosis control programs. *Am. Rev. Respir. Dis.* **144:**745–749.

Cave, M. D., K. D. Eisenach, P. F. McDermott, J. H. Bates, and J. T. Crawford. 1991. IS*6110*: conservation of sequence in the *Mycobacterium tuberculosis* complex and its utilization in DNA fingerprinting. *Mol. Cell. Probes* **5:**73–80.

Centers for Disease Control. 1991. Nosocomial transmission of multidrug resistant tuberculosis among HIV-infected persons, Florida and New York, 1988–1991. *Morbid. Mortal. Weekly Rep.* **40:**585–591.

Centers for Disease Control. 1992. Transmission of multidrug-resistant tuberculosis among immunocompromised persons in a correctional system. New York 1991. *Morbid. Mortal. Weekly Rep.* **41:**507–509.

Collins, D. M. Personal communication.

Collins, D. M., and G. W. de Lisle. 1984. DNA restriction endonuclease analysis of *Mycobacterium tuberculosis* and *Mycobacterium bovis* BCG. *J. Gen. Microbiol.* **130:**1019–1021.

Collins, D. M., S. K. Erasmuson, D. M. Stephens, G. F. Yates, and G. W. de Lisle. 1993. DNA fingerprinting of *Mycobacterium bovis* strains by restriction fragment analysis and hybridization with insertion elements IS*1081* and IS*6110*. *J. Clin. Microbiol.* **31:** 1143–1147.

Collins, D. M., and D. M. Stephens. 1991. Identification of insertion sequence, IS*1081*, in *Mycobacterium bovis*. *FEMS Microbiol. Lett.* **83:**11–16.

Crawford, J. T. Personal communication.

Daley, C. L., P. M. Small, G. F. Schecter, G. K.

Schoolnik, R. A. McAdam, W. R. Jacobs, Jr., and P. C. Hopewell. 1992. An outbreak of tuberculosis with accelerated progression among persons infected with the human immunodeficiency virus: an analysis using restriction fragment length polymorphisms. *N. Engl. J. Med.* **326**:231–235.

Das, S., S. L. Chan, B. W. Allen, D. A. Mitchison, and D. B. Lowrie. 1993. Application of DNA fingerprinting with IS*986* to sequential mycobacterial isolates obtained from pulmonary tuberculosis patients in Hong Kong before, during and after short-course chemotherapy. *Tuberc. Lung Dis.* **74**:47–51.

Dooley, S. W., M. E. Villarino, M. Lawrence, et al. 1992. Nosocomial transmission of tuberculosis in a hospital unit for HIV-infected patients. *JAMA* **267**:2632–2634.

Doran, T. J., A. L. M. Hodgson, J. K. Davies, and A. J. Radford. 1992. Characterization of a novel repetitive DNA sequence from *Mycobacterium bovis*. *FEMS Microbiol. Lett.* **96**:179–186.

Dwyer, B., K. Jackson, K. Raios, A. Sievers, E. Wilshire, and B. Ross. 1993. DNA restriction fragment analysis to define an extended cluster of tuberculosis in homeless men and their associates. *J. Infect. Dis.* **167**:490–494.

Edlin, B. R., J. I. Tokars, M. H. Grieco, J. T. Crawford, J. Williams, E. M. Sordillo, K. R. Ong, J. O. Kilburn, S. W. Dooley, K. G. Castro, W. R. Jarvis, and S. D. Holmberg. 1992. An outbreak of multidrug-resistant tuberculosis among hospitalized patients with the acquired immunodeficiency syndrome. *N. Engl. J. Med.* **326**:1514–1521.

Fischl, M. A., R. B. Uttamchandani, G. L. Daikos, et al. 1992. An outbreak of tuberculosis caused by multiple-drug resistant tubercle bacilli among patients with HIV infection. *Ann. Intern. Med.* **117**:177–183.

Fomukong, N. G., and J. W. Dale. Transpositional activity of IS*986* in *M. smegmatis*. Submitted for publication.

Fomukong, N. G., J. W. Dale, T. W. Osborn, and J. M. Grange. 1992. Use of gene probes on the insertion sequence IS*986* to differentiate between BCG vaccine strains. *J. Appl. Bacteriol.* **72**:125–133.

Genewein, A., A. Telenti, C. Bernasconi, C. Mordasini, S. Weiss, A. Maurer, H. Rieder, K. Schopfer, and T. Bodmer. 1993. Molecular approach to identifying route of transmission of tuberculosis in the community. *Lancet* **342**:841–844.

Godfrey-Faussett, P., P. R. Mortimer, P. A. Jenkins, and N. G. Stoker. 1992. Evidence of transmission of tuberculosis by DNA fingerprinting. *Br. Med. J.* **305**:221–223.

Godfrey-Faussett, P., and N. G. Stoker. 1992. Aspects of tuberculosis in Africa. 3. Genetic fingerprinting for clues to the pathogenesis of tuberculosis. *Trans. R. Soc. Trop. Med.* **86**:472–475.

Groenen, P. M. A., A. E. van Bunschoten, D. van Soolingen, and J. D. A. van Embden. 1993. Nature of DNA polymorphism in the direct repeat cluster of *Mycobacterium tuberculosis*; application for strain differentiation by a novel method. *Mol. Microbiol.* **10**:1057–1065.

Gruft, H., R. Johnson, R. Claflin, and A. Loder. 1984. Phage-typing and drug-resistance patterns as tools in mycobacterial epidemiology. *Am. Rev. Respir. Dis.* **130**:96–97.

Haas, W. H., W. R. Butler, C. L. Woodley, and J. T. Crawford. 1993. Mixed-linker polymerase chain reaction: a new method for rapid fingerprinting of isolates of the *Mycobacterium tuberculosis* complex. *J. Clin. Microbiol.* **31**:1293–1298.

Hermans, P. W. M., D. van Soolingen, E. M. Bik, P. E. W. de Haas, J. W. Dale, and J. D. A. van Embden. 1991. The insertion element IS*987* from *Mycobacterium bovis* BCG is located in a hot spot integration region for insertion elements in *M. tuberculosis* complex strains. *Infect. Immun.* **59**:2695–2705.

Hermans, P. W. M., D. van Soolingen, J. W. Dale, A. R. Schuitema, R. A. McAdam, D. Catty, and J. D. A. van Embden. 1990. Insertion element IS*986* from *Mycobacterium tuberculosis*: a useful tool for diagnosis and epidemiology of tuberculosis. *J. Clin. Microbiol.* **28**:2051–2058.

Hermans, P. W. M., D. van Soolingen, and J. D. A. van Embden. 1992. Characterization of a major polymorphic tandem repeat in *Mycobacterium tuberculosis* and its potential use in the epidemiology of *Mycobacterium kansasii* and *Mycobacterium gordonae*. *J. Bacteriol.* **174**:4157–4165.

Jeffreys, A. J., A. MacLeod, K. Tamaki, D. L. Neil, and D. G. Monckton. 1991. Minisatellite repeat coding as a digital approach to DNA typing. *Nature* (London) **354**:204–209.

Lawrence, J. G., D. E. Dykhuizen, R. F. Dubose, and D. L. Hartl. 1989. Phylogenetic analysis using insertion sequence fingerprinting in *Escherichia coli*. *Mol. Biol. Evol.* **6**:1–14.

Lederberg, J., R. E. Shope, and E. J. Oaks. 1993. *Emerging Infections: Microbial Threats to the Health of the United States*, p. 1. National Academy Press, Washington, D.C.

Mazurek, G. H., M. D. Cave, K. D. Eisenach, R. J. Wallace, Jr., J. H. Bates, and J. T. Crawford. 1991. Chromosomal DNA fingerprint patterns produced with IS*6110* as strain-specific markers for epidemiologic study of tuberculosis. *J. Clin. Microbiol.* **29**:2030–2033.

McAdam, R. A., P. W. M. Hermans, D. van Soolingen, Z. F. Zainuddin, D. Catty, J. D. A. van Embden, and J. W. Dale. 1990. Characterization of a *Mycobacterium tuberculosis* insertion sequence belonging to the IS*3* family. *Mol. Microbiol.* **4**:1607–1613.

Mendiola, M. V., C. Martin, I. Otal, and B. Gicquel.

1992. Analysis of regions responsible for IS*6110* RFLP in a single *Mycobacterium tuberculosis* strain. *Res. Microbiol.* **143:**767–772.

Otal, I., C. Martin, V. Vincent-Lévy-Frébault, D. Thierry, and B. Gicquel. 1991. Restriction fragment length polymorphism analysis using IS*6110* as an epidemiological marker in tuberculosis. *J. Clin. Microbiol.* **29:**1252–1254.

Palittapongarnpim, P., S. Chomic, A. Fanning, and D. Kunimoto. 1993a. DNA fingerprinting of *Mycobacterium tuberculosis* by ligation-mediated polymerase chain reaction. *Nucleic Acids Res.* **3:**761–762.

Palittapongarnpim, P., S. Chomic, A. Fanning, and D. Kunimoto. 1993b. DNA fragment length polymorphism analysis of *M. tuberculosis* isolates by arbitrarily primed polymerase chain reaction. *J. Infect. Dis.* **167:**975–978.

Palittapongarnpim, P. S., S. Rienthong, and W. Panbangred. 1993c. Comparison of restriction fragment length polymorphism of *M. tuberculosis* isolated from cerebrospinal fluid and sputum: a preliminary report. *Tuberc. Lung Dis.* **74:**204–207.

Plikaytis, B. B. Personal communication.

Ross, B. C., and B. Dwyer. 1993. Rapid, simple method for typing isolates of *Mycobacterium tuberculosis* by using the polymerase chain reaction. *J. Clin. Microbiol.* **31:**329–334.

Ross, C., K. Raios, K. Jackson, and B. Dwyer. 1992. Molecular cloning of a highly repeated element from *Mycobacterium tuberculosis* and its use as an epidemiological tool. *J. Clin. Microbiol.* **30:**942–946.

Ryan, F. 1993. *Tuberculosis: the Greatest Story Never Told*, p. 173. Swift Publishers, Bromsgrove, Worchestershire, England.

Shafer, R. W., P. M. Small, C. Larkin, S. P. Singh, P. Kelly, M. F. Sierra, G. K. Schoolnik, and K. D. Chirgwin. Temporal trends and transmission patterns during the emergence of multidrug-resistant tuberculosis in New York City: a molecular epidemiological assessment. Submitted for publication.

Small, P. M., P. C. Hopewell, S. P. Singh, A. Paz, J. Parsonnet, D. C. Ruston, G. F. Schecter, C. L. Daley, and G. K. Schoolnik. The contemporary urban epidemiology of tuberculosis: a population-based study using conventional and molecular methods. Submitted for publication.

Small, P. M., and B. Kreiswirth. Unpublished observations.

Small, P. M., N. McClenny, S. P. Singh, G. K. Schoolnik, L. S. Tomkins, and P. A. Mickelsen. 1993a. Molecular strain typing of *Mycobacterium tuberculosis* to confirm cross-contamination in the mycobacteriology laboratory and modification of procedures to minimize occurrence of false-positive cultures. *J. Clin. Microbiol.* **31:**1677–1682.

Small, P. M., and A. Moss. 1993. Molecular epidemiology and the new tuberculosis. *Infect. Agents Dis.*

2:132–138.

Small, P. M., R. W. Schafer, P. C. Hopewell, S. P. Singh, M. J. Murphy, E. Desmond, M. F. Sierra, and G. K. Schoolnik. 1993b. Exogenous reinfection with multidrug-resistant *M. tuberculosis* in patients with advanced HIV infection. *N. Engl. J. Med.* **328:**1137–1144.

Tabet, S. R., G. M. Goldbaum, T. M. Hooton, K. D. Eisenach, M. D. Cave, and C. M. Nolan. 1994. Restriction fragment length polymorphism analysis detecting a community-based tuberculosis outbreak among persons infected with human immunodeficiency virus. *J. Infect. Dis.* **169:**189–192.

Thierry, D., M. D. Cave, K. D. Eisenach, J. T. Crawford, J. H. Bates, B. Gicquel, and J. L. Guesdon. 1990. IS*6110*, an IS-like element of *M. tuberculosis* complex. *Nucleic Acids Res.* **18:**188.

van Embden, J. D. A. Unpublished data.

van Embden, J. D. A., M. D. Cave, J. T. Crawford, J. W. Dale, K. D. Eisenach, B. Gicquel, P. W. M. Hermans, C. Martin, R. McAdam, T. M. Shinnick, and P. M. Small. 1993. Strain identification of *Mycobacterium tuberculosis* by DNA fingerprinting: recommendations for a standardized methodology. *J. Clin. Microbiol.* **31:**406–409.

van Embden, J. D. A., P. M. Small, and B. Gicquel. Unpublished data.

van Embden, J. D. A., D. van Soolingen, P. M. Small, and P. W. M. Hermans. 1992. Genetic markers for the epidemiology of tuberculosis. *Res. Microbiol.* **143:**385–391.

Vannier, A. N., J. J. Tarrand, and P. R. Murray. 1988. Mycobacterial cross contamination during radiometric culturing. *J. Clin. Microbiol.* **26:**1867–1868.

van Soolingen, D., and D. M. Collins. Personal communication.

van Soolingen, D., P. E. W. de Haas, P. W. M. Hermans, P. M. A. Groenen, and J. D. A. van Embden. 1993. Comparison of various repetitive DNA elements as genetic markers for strain differentiation and epidemiology of *Mycobacterium tuberculosis*. *J. Clin. Microbiol.* **31:**1987–1995.

van Soolingen, D., P. W. M. Hermans, P. E. W. de Haas, D. R. Soll, and J. D. A. van Embden. 1991. The occurrence and stability of insertion sequences in *Mycobacterium tuberculosis* complex strains; evaluation of insertion sequence-dependent DNA polymorphism as a tool in the epidemiology of tuberculosis. *J. Clin. Microbiol.* **29:**2578–2586.

van Soolingen, D., P. W. M. Hermans, P. E. W. de Haas, and J. D. A. van Embden. 1992. Insertion element IS*1081*-associated restriction fragment length polymorphism in *Mycobacterium tuberculosis* complex species: a reliable tool for recognizing *Mycobacterium bovis* BCG. *J. Clin. Microbiol.* **30:**1772–1777.

Yuen, L. K., B. C. Ross, K. M. Jackson, and B. Dwyer.

1992. Characterization of *Mycobacterium tuberculosis* strains from Vietnamese patients by Southern blot hybridization. *J. Clin. Microbiol.* **31**:1615–1618.

Zainuddin, Z. F., and J. W. Dale. 1989. Polymorphic repetitive DNA sequences in *Mycobacterium tuberculosis* detected with a gene probe from a *Mycobacterium fortuitum* plasmid. *J. Gen. Microbiol.* **135:** 2347–2355.

Tuberculosis: Pathogenesis, Protection, and Control
Edited by Barry R. Bloom
© 1994 American Society for Microbiology, Washington, DC 20005

Chapter 34

Issues in Operational, Social, and Economic Research on Tuberculosis

Christopher J. L. Murray

Many definitions of social, economic, and operational research have been proposed by the agencies, institutions, and individuals involved with these forms of research. Debates over the specific boundaries of operational research often consume considerable intellectual energy without clear benefits. For tuberculosis control, we define operational research as research that contributes to one of the following objectives: (i) to convince governments, funding agencies, and health care providers that tuberculosis is a large health problem and that effective interventions are available to deal with a large share of this burden; (ii) to provide the scientific basis for adapting successful control strategies to a wide variety of economic, social, institutional, cultural, and epidemiological conditions; and (iii) to investigate new approaches or alternatives for tuberculosis control.

This chapter is organized into four sections: the burden of tuberculosis, BCG immunization, chemoprophylaxis, and case identification and treatment. In each section, the emphasis is on briefly reviewing relevant past work, identifying key con-

straints for effective tuberculosis control, and suggesting ways that operational research may provide answers. Of the four topics, the most important is case identification and cure.

BURDEN OF TUBERCULOSIS

For most infectious diseases, the standard approach to measuring prevalence or incidence is a community survey. Rates estimated from community surveys can be compared with the number of cases detected each year by the health system. Such comparisons provide an objective assessment of the efficacy of case detection. In contrast, sampling surveys have been less useful in tuberculosis control. Tuberculosis cases are relatively uncommon in the community. In developing countries with a moderate problem, incidence of smear-positive tuberculosis will range from 50 to 100 per 100,000 population. In the absence of treatment programs, the prevalence will be approximately twice the incidence, or 100 to 200 per 100,000 population (Styblo, 1991). With good treatment programs, as cases are detected, they are rapidly placed on effective therapy, and prevalence may be lower than incidence. In a country with moderate incidence, even a large survey

Christopher J. L. Murray • Harvard Center for Population and Development Studies, Harvard School of Public Health, 9 Bow Street, Cambridge, Massachusetts 02138.

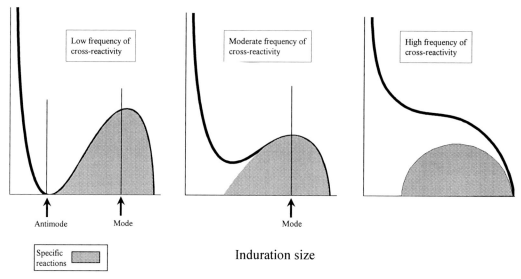

Figure 1. Frequency distributions of induration sizes: general patterns for three frequencies of atypical mycobacterial cross-reactivity. Source: Bleiker et al. (1989).

that screened 10,000 people by sputum microscopy or miniature chest radiographs would detect only 10 to 20 cases. Confidence intervals for the estimated prevalence rate in the community from such a survey would be very wide because of the small absolute number of cases. Identifying significant differences in the prevalence of tuberculosis by age and sex would require extremely large and necessarily costly surveys.

Because of these inherent measurement problems, the focus of tuberculosis epidemiology has been on measuring infection instead of disease. Infection is more than 2 orders of magnitude more common than disease and is thus much more amenable to surveying. Purified protein derivative (PPD), the refined form of Koch's *Mycobacterium tuberculosis* filtrates, was developed into a skin test for detecting past infection. Skin-testing doses and methods have been extensively studied and standardized by the World Health Organization (WHO) (see, for example, WHO [1963]). Individuals who have been exposed to *M. tuberculosis* develop cell-mediated immu-

nity that leads to a positive skin test when they are exposed to PPD. Positive tests thus imply at least past infection with mycobacteria (*M. tuberculosis*, *M. bovis*, BCG strains, or atypical mycobacteria). Canetti (1939, 1972) suggests that nearly everyone who develops cell-mediated immunity still harbors viable bacilli in walled-off granulomata, most often in the lungs.

Interpreting the results of skin tests both in the individual and at the population level is complicated by cross-reactivity with atypical mycobacteria and/or BCG strains. In parts of the world where there is considerable environmental exposure to atypical mycobacteria, individuals may have positive skin tests although they are not infected with *M. tuberculosis*. One can attempt to determine the true prevalence of *M. tuberculosis* infection by examining the population results of skin testing aggregated by induration size. Three general patterns of reactivity by induration size are found. Figure 1 illustrates that when the frequency of atypical mycobacterial cross-reactivity is low, there will be a clear mode and antimode (Bleiker et al., 1989). In such a case, the cutoff of induration size defining infection can be chosen as the antimode. Where the frequency of atypical mycobacterial cross-reactivity is greater, estimating the prevalence of infection is more complicated. With a moderate number of atypical cases, there will still be no clear antimode to define the cutoff for infection (Fig. 1). A reasonable estimate of prevalence can be derived by assuming that all PPD responses with an induration size greater than the mode indicate true *M. tuberculosis* infections. By doubling this number, one can indirectly estimate the number of infections present among those with an intermediate PPD induration size. From this discussion, it should be apparent that the appropriate induration size defining infection with a certain specificity will vary from community to community and within the same community over time. The relative nature of the appropriate induration cutoff defining infection with a reasonable specificity is in stark contrast to the routine clinical interpretation of PPD tests, in which standard cutoffs such as 10 mm are used for nearly all patients. In areas with high exposure to atypical mycobacteria, there may be a continuum of reaction diameters such that the discrimination between sensitization by *M. tuberculosis* infection and atypical mycobacteria becomes very difficult (Huebner et al. [1993]).

Skin test surveys provide figures on the prevalence of infection by age. Figure 2 (reproduced from Roelsgaard et al. [1964]) shows the prevalence of infection by age for a series of African countries surveyed between 1955 and 1960. (The characteristic drop-off of prevalence over age 40 in most surveys is not due to historically rising annual risks of infection such that younger age groups have had a higher cumulative exposure to tuberculosis. Nor is there convincing evidence that the mortality of PPD-positive patients compared to that of PPD-negative patients is high enough to explain such a drop-off in prevalence rates [Narain

et al., 1970]. Rather, there appears to be increasing anergy with age.) Prevalence curves reflect the cumulative experience of different cohorts over their lifetimes; meaningful direct comparisons of prevalence curves are difficult (e.g., Nyboe, 1957). The major breakthrough in tuberculosis epidemiology came in the 1960s, when the Tuberculosis Surveillance Research Unit developed simple methods for estimating the annual risk of becoming infected or superinfected with tuberculosis from the data on prevalence of infection by age (Styblo et al., 1969b; Sutherland et al., 1971; Sutherland, 1976, 1991; Tuberculosis Surveillance Research Unit, 1966). The observed prevalence of infection at a given age must be equal to the annual risks of infection experienced by that cohort since birth. Sutherland and Styblo examined the prevalence of infection in military recruits in The Netherlands. They found that the annual risk of infection appeared to decline exponentially at about 13% per year from 1940 to 1966 and 10.4% per year from 1967 to 1979; prior to World War II, the annual risk of infection declined about 5% per year. Assuming that the annual risk of infection declines at an exponential rate, Sutherland derived equations to estimate the prevalence of infection at any age for any rate of decline. Styblo et al. [1969b] proposed a simple approximation for the exponential decline in the annual risk of infection that provided for an integrable solution to the cumulative prevalence problem. In many ways, it is Sutherland's approximation that facilitated the spread of using risk of infection as a standard monitoring tool for tuberculosis control.) With these methods available, the annual risk of infection has become the standard approach to epidemiological monitoring in most parts of the world. (Remarkably, the United States is one of the few countries in the world in which the annual risk of infection has not been widely used as an epidemiological tool. Most analyses in the United States are based solely on re-

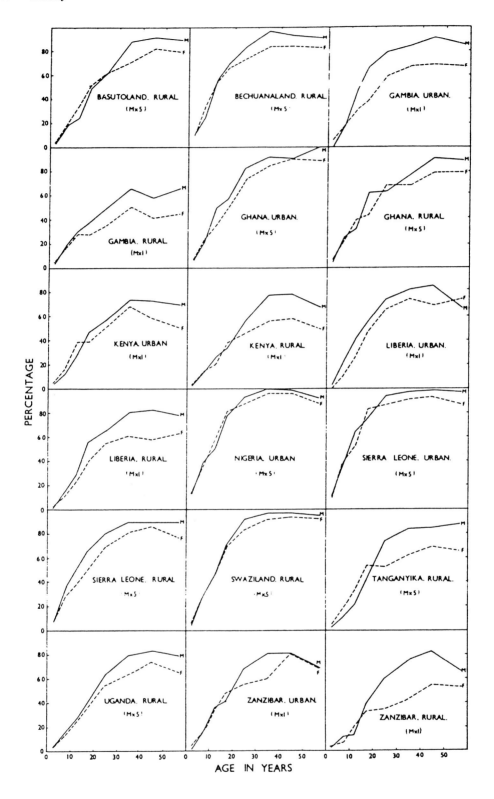

Table 1. Estimated risks of tuberculous infection and their trends in developing countries, 1985 to 1990[a]

Area	Estimated risk of tuberculous infection (%)	Estimated annual decrease in risk (%)
Sub-Saharan Africa	1.50–2.50	1–2
North Africa and western Asia	0.50–1.50	4–5
Asia	1.00–2.00	1–3
South America	0.50–1.50	2–5
Central America and Caribbean	0.50–1.50	1–3

[a] Source: Murray et al. (1993) based on Cauthen et al. (1988).

ported case numbers.) Cauthen et al. (1988) reviewed the available skin test surveys since 1975. On the basis of that review, Murray et al. (1993) estimated the average annual risk of infection for the major regions of the world (Table 1).

Unfortunately, the very success of tuberculosis epidemiologists in developing a monitoring tool for tuberculosis control from tuberculin skin tests contributed to an isolation of tuberculosis from the mainstream of international public health. For nearly two decades, tuberculosis was ignored as an international health priority. For example, at one point in 1988, WHO had only one staff person working on tuberculosis. In the last 5 years, there has been a resurgence of international interest in tuberculosis due to many factors such as the human immunodeficiency virus (HIV) epidemic and the resurgence of tuberculosis in Western countries. One factor may have been the World Bank effort to quantify the burden of all major diseases and the cost-effectiveness of interventions in a comparable fashion (Jamison et al., 1993). To demonstrate the burden of tuberculosis in terms comparable to those used for other health problems, it was essential to estimate the number of cases and deaths due to tuberculosis in various regions of the world. Murray et al. (1990) and subsequently Sudre et al. (1992) used known epidemio-

logical relationships to estimate incidence of and mortality from tuberculosis.

As might have been expected from the transmission dynamics of tuberculosis, a close relationship between the annual risk of infection and the incidence of smear-positive tuberculosis was found (Styblo, 1985). A 1% annual risk of infection is associated with an annual incidence of 50 smear-positive cases per 100,000 population (95% confidence interval of 39 to 59 cases per 100,000). As the annual risk of infection declines to very low levels, such as in the United States or The Netherlands, the relationship between incidence and the annual risk of infection is attenuated. The proportion of cases due to progressive primary disease decreases as the annual risk of infection declines, and concomitantly, the proportion due to reactivation of remote infection increases. When the majority of cases are due to reactivation, one would not expect a strong relationship between incidence and the annual risk of infection.

Using the relationship between the annual risk of infection and incidence, the number of cases each year has also been estimated. From information on case-fatality rates and the percentage of patients receiving adequate therapy, deaths from tuberculosis have also been estimated. These figures suggest that tuberculosis is

Figure 2. Estimated prevalence of tuberculosis infection by age and sex in 11 sub-Saharan African regions. Basutoland is present-day Lesotho, and Bechuanaland is present-day Botswana. Reprinted with permission from Roelsgaard et al. (1964).

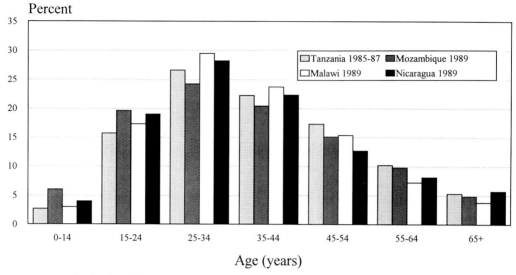

Percent

Figure 3. Age-distribution of smear-positive tuberculosis in four developing country programs. Sources: for Tanzania, Chum et al. (1988); for other countries, government registry data.

the largest single infectious cause of death in the world, causing 2.6 million deaths a year. The tremendous social and economic burdens of tuberculosis are magnified by concentration of the disease in young adults (Fig. 3). In fact, 26% of adult avoidable deaths are due to tuberculosis (Murray et al., 1990).

Based on the data in Table 1, one can estimate that approximately 50% of the population in the age groups which are heavily afflicted with HIV in Africa has been previously infected with tubercle bacilli. Consequently, coinfection with HIV and tuberculosis in adults aged 15 to 49 years is common in Africa. The WHO Global Programme on AIDS (GPA) has estimates of the seroprevalence of HIV infection in each sub-Saharan African country. The number of cases of tuberculosis can be estimated by assuming, on the basis of the data of Selwyn et al. (1989) for New York City and Attonucci et al. (1992) for Italy, that there is an annual risk of breakdown from tuberculosis infection to disease of 5 to 10%. In total, 287,000 extra cases are predicted for Africa. The Global

Programme on AIDS currently projects large increases in HIV seroprevalence over the next decade for India. If these increases eventuate, the number of tuberculosis cases in India due to HIV could be 180,000.

Tuberculosis, long thought to be disappearing in the West, has been making a comeback. Detected case rates are up in Austria, Denmark, Ireland, Italy, The Netherlands, Norway, Switzerland, and the United States (Raviglione et al., 1993). Figure 4 shows the number of cases in the United States over the last decade (Bloom and Murray, 1992). The increase in industrialized countries can be attributed to at least four factors. First, individuals dually infected with HIV and tuberculosis have a greatly increased breakdown rate, 5 to 10% per year compared to a lifetime risk of 10% (Selwyn et al., 1989; Attonucci et al., 1992). Second, certain groups such as the homeless, intravenous drug abusers, and homosexuals have an increased risk of contact with infectious cases and thus a higher effective annual risk of infection. These are often the same groups that have increased rates of HIV infection. Third, there has

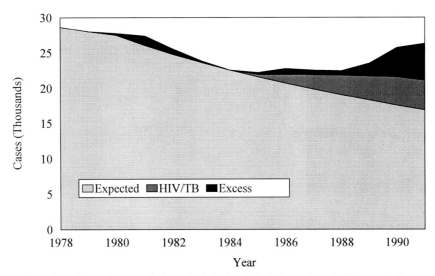

Figure 4. Estimated numbers of cases of tuberculosis in the United States from 1978 to 1991 disaggregated into cases expected on the basis of trends in the risk of infection, cases of HIV and tuberculosis coinfection, and excess cases. Source: Bloom and Murray (1992).

been in some cases increased immigration from high-prevalence countries. This probably accounts for most of the increase in countries such as Denmark, The Netherlands, Norway, and Switzerland. Finally and most disturbingly, some treatment programs in, for example, New York City have very high dropout and failure rates (Brudney and Dobkin, 1991; Bloom and Murray, 1992). While programs in poor developing countries such as Malawi, Mozambique, and Tanzania have excellent treatment completion rates, some urban programs in industrialized countries lag behind these standards.

While there is a growing international awareness of the burden of tuberculosis, in many countries tuberculosis is still seen as a disease of old men that is difficult to treat and is consequently not a priority. In many countries, there is a need for operational research to change decision makers' attitudes about the burden of tuberculosis and the potential for intervention. In fact, defining the burden of tuberculosis in each country by using either existing or new data sets is a priority for operational research. Estab-

lishing burden, as the previous discussion has demonstrated, is not simple. Where BCG prevalence is not high, the most attractive option is skin test surveys in children 0 to 14 years of age. In many countries, because of the success of the Expanded Programme of Immunization, BCG coverage exceeds 80%. Recent skin test surveys in countries with high BCG coverage have yielded strange results (Maganu et al., 1990). Methods of measuring the burden of disease in countries with high BCG coverage are an area for operational research. One possible research avenue would be to use a prevalence survey linked with questions on the duration of respiratory symptoms to impute incidence. This approach would still necessitate costly prevalence surveys, including the use of a laboratory capable of a considerable volume of cultures with high standards.

Little has been written on the differential impact of tuberculosis on men and women. Annual risk of infection estimates, case registration data, and cohort analysis results rarely provide information by sex. In industrialized countries, tuberculosis mor-

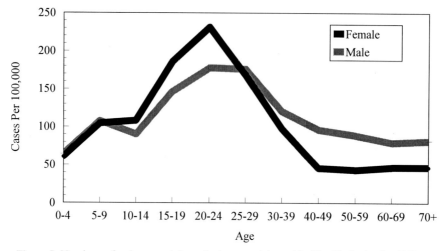

Figure 5. Numbers of pulmonary tuberculosis cases detected in The Netherlands, 1951.

tality rates among young adults 15 to 44 years of age were higher in women than in men (Fig. 5 shows incidence rates by sex for The Netherlands in 1951). With the decline in the risk of infection in these countries, tuberculosis shifted from being a disease of young women to a disease of old men. The age-sex pattern of tuberculosis must be traced to infection, breakdown, and case-fatality rates. The cumulative experience of PPD skin test surveys has shown that in most situations, the prevalence of infection is higher in men than in women, beginning in adolescence (Roelsgaard et al., 1964; Styblo, 1991; Sutherland, 1976; Sutherland and Fayers, 1975). The higher prevalence of infection in young men than in young women implies a higher annual risk of infection in young adult males. While the annual risk of infection and the cumulative prevalence of infection are higher in young men than in women, the incidence of clinical disease in many countries with moderate or high risks of infection is equal or even greater in women. Equal or higher incidence rates in women than in men suggest that for ages 15 to 44 years, the breakdown rate for women may be higher than that for men. Perhaps higher breakdown rates for women in this age

group are related to reproductive physiology. There is an old clinical observation that pregnancy and tuberculosis are related, which supports the notion that breakdown rates during the reproductive period may be higher. An alternative explanation is that a larger share of women aged 15 to 44 years are not infected and, thus, the number susceptible to progressive primary infection is greater.

Is the epidemiology of tuberculosis the same in developing countries today as it was in industrialized countries when they had a similar risk of infection? While there are not many data, as a working hypothesis it seems reasonable to expect that in young adults (15 to 34 or 44 years of age) the sex ratio of new cases should be close to equal. If it is, then there must be considerable variance between case detection rates for young men and women. Figure 6 shows that while the number of infected men and women detected in Nicaragua in these age groups is approximately equal, the number of infected men detected in Tanzania far outweighs the number of infected women. As it is unlikely that the basic distribution of incidence by sex would vary so widely, the male case detection rate in Tanzania is apparently much higher than the female

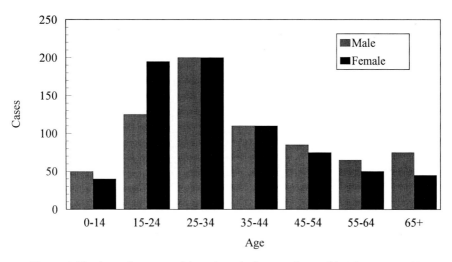

Figure 6. Numbers of smear-positive tuberculosis cases detected in Nicaragua, 1989.

case detection rate. Low case detection rates for women in some countries may be due to a variety of social, economic, and cultural factors that need to be investigated and understood in order to design interventions to raise the female case detection rate. Obstacles to female access to tuberculosis diagnosis and adequate treatment probably exist at the levels of both the community and the health services. The importance of tuberculosis as a particular problem of young women has been recently demonstrated by Murray and Lopez (1994) in a study of the global causes of mortality by age and sex. In developing regions, tuberculosis is the number two cause of mortality in women 15 to 44 years of age, causing an estimated 313,000 deaths. Clearly, tuberculosis should be on the agenda of any government or agency concerned with women and mothers. Further work documenting the incidence, case detection rate, treatment results, and death rate from tuberculosis in young women is urgently needed. If the problem is as great as this simplistic analysis suggests, considerable operational research effort may need to be devoted to the problem of tuberculosis and women.

BCG IMMUNIZATION

BCG is the most widely used vaccine in the world. The United Nations Children's Fund (UNICEF) estimates that coverage with BCG is greater than 80% in each region of the world (Table 2). The success of BCG vaccination programs is largely attributable to the organizational, financial, and technical success of the Expanded Programme of Immunization. It is not possible to review the role of operational research in ensuring this success to date, but we can note that much of the operational research was closely integrated with the management and application of the program by

Table 2. BCG coverage by region: percentage of children immunized by 12 months of age with BCG vaccine[a]

Region	Coverage (%)
Sub-Saharan Africa	79
North, South, and Central America and the Caribbean	83
North Africa and western Asia	84
Europe	75
Southeast Asia	85
East Asia and Pacific	94
Global total	85

[a] Source: WHO (1992).

UNICEF and the WHO. Remaining operational issues in expanding coverage of BCG to even higher levels are the same as for the rest of the Expanded Programme of Immunization: ensuring access by difficult-to-serve populations, taking advantage of maternal/child health service contacts, and maintaining high-quality vaccine supplies.

While the coverage of BCG is extremely high, the efficacy of the vaccine remains a source of contention (see chapter 31; Fine, 1988; Clemens et al., 1983; Rodrigues and Smith, 1990; Colditz et al., 1993). A summary of the results of the major controlled trials and case-control studies is presented in Table 1 and Fig. 1 of chapter 31. A recent meta-analysis of selected trials (Colditz et al., 1993) concluded that BCG is about 50% effective in preventing cases of tuberculosis. An alternative explanation is that it is variably effective in different environments and that we are unable to predict in which environments it is effective. Both the controlled trials and the case-control studies have demonstrated that BCG has variable effectiveness. In some environments, such as Britain, a significant protective effect has been seen in both controlled trials and case-control studies. In other environments, such as South India, BCG has had little or no effect in two controlled trials. The largest and most important trial in the developing world, the Chingleput trial, in which 360,000 people were enrolled, showed negative effectiveness. While the protective effect of BCG for pulmonary tuberculosis will undoubtedly always remain controversial, there is a greater consensus that BCG is effective in preventing miliary tuberculosis and tuberculous meningitis in children (Ten Dam and Hitze, 1980). For this reason, studies have shown that BCG is probably quite cost-effective (Barnum et al., 1980; Murray et al., 1991).

From an operational research point of view, two issues are worth stressing. First, various theories have been proposed to explain why BCG appears to be effective in some environments and not others. These theories include different strains of BCG, the presence of atypical mycobacteria in the environment, various levels of virulence in local *M. tuberculosis* strains, differences in nutritional status of the hosts, and others. Understanding the reasons for variable protection of BCG in different environments would probably provide clues to the immunology of tuberculosis. From an operational research perspective, however, developing a method to predict in which environments BCG will or will not protect would be helpful in assessing the importance of increasing BCG coverage. If such an assessment tool was truly reliable, one could even argue that BCG coverage should be reduced to save on costs. If ever such a conclusion was reached, it would have to be tempered by the increasing prospects that BCG may be an efficient vector for new antigens (Stover et al., 1992). Second, even in those environments where BCG is effective, the protective effect appears to wane by 10 to 15 years after vaccination. Figure 7 summarizes those trials that reported protection as a function of time since vaccination. Of the trials with an aggregate protective efficacy of greater than 50%, only one, the British Medical Research Council trial, monitored patients for 15 years or more, and it showed that the protective effect of BCG fell to zero after 15 years. Styblo and Meijer (1976) made the landmark observation that BCG vaccination would not have a major epidemiological impact on tuberculosis because it is delivered at birth but any effect is gone by age 15. Because children rarely have sputum smear-positive tuberculosis, they do not play a large role in transmitting the disease. The highest breakdown rates and risks of infection are in young adults, exactly the age group in which BCG vaccination at birth will have no significant effect. Figure 6 shows the concentration of smear-positive cases in a typical developing country in young adults. Styblo and Meijer

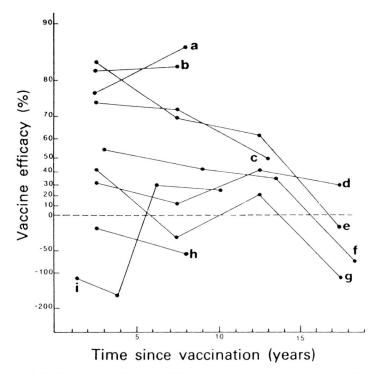

Figure 7. Variations in BCG protective efficacy at different times after vaccination in controlled trials. Reprinted with permission from Rodrigues and Smith (1990).

(1976) concluded that efforts to accelerate the decline in tuberculosis must concentrate on decreasing infectious sources in the community, namely, case detection and timely cure.

Why not repeat BCG vaccination just before the period of highest risk for developing smear-positive pulmonary tuberculosis? The obvious logic of delivering a second dose of BCG to school leavers or at some age before 15 must be tempered with the lack of any data on the efficacy of such revaccination. Several countries (including Chile and a number in Eastern Europe) have delivered repeat vaccination with BCG. One case-control study (Sepulveda et al., 1992) suggests only 10% efficacy. The prospects of getting definitive answers on the efficacy of BCG revaccination and ultimately the cost-effectiveness of this strategy are slim. Prospective trials, which

would probably be necessary to convince a wider audience of the benefits of this strategy, would take many years to provide answers. The large sample sizes required will probably make such studies prohibitively expensive. Nevertheless, case-control studies in populations practicing repeat vaccination would be interesting and potentially convincing if a wide array showed a similar impact. A similar logic has recently led to calls for BCG vaccination of health care providers in the United States (Jordan et al., 1991a).

CHEMOPROPHYLAXIS

While the first studies indicating the benefits of treating those infected with *M. tuberculosis* with isoniazid, known as chemoprophylaxis, were published in 1954 (Lincoln et al., 1954), the role for chemo-

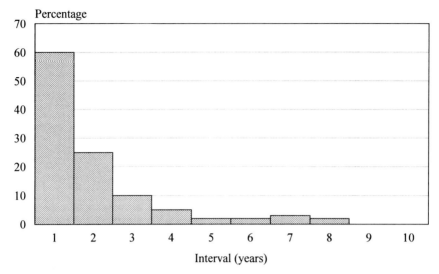

Figure 8. Intervals from conversion to onset of tuberculosis disease. Source: Styblo (1991).

prophylaxis has remained unclear. It was heralded as a method of decreasing the burden of latent infection and thus future incidence. Chemoprophylaxis has not lived up to this promise, and its role in developing countries is minor. The following discussion is divided into sections on the direct and indirect effects of chemoprophylaxis in immunocompetent hosts, the adverse effects of chemoprophylaxis, net benefits and decision analyses, net benefits in immunocompromised hosts, cost-effectiveness of chemoprophylaxis, and potential overall role in developed and developing countries, including the conflict between the HIV-infected community and the tuberculosis-infected community.

Direct and Indirect Effects of Chemoprophylaxis in Immunocompetent Hosts

Treatment of individuals who are known to be infected with *M. tuberculosis* on the basis of 12 months of skin tests with isoniazid is effective in preventing subsequent breakdown to clinical tuberculosis (Ferebee, 1969). For those who take the com-

plete course of chemoprophylaxis, the incidence of tuberculosis is reduced by greater than 90% (International Union Against Tuberculosis Committee on Prophylaxis, 1982). Early studies showing effectiveness indicated a relationship between the duration of therapy and the proportion of breakdown prevented. The breakdown rate of tuberculosis declines exponentially from the onset of infection, reaching a stable long-term breakdown rate between 5 or 7 years. Figure 8 shows the breakdown rate in new PPD converters as a function of the time since conversion recorded in the British Medical Research Council BCG trial (Sutherland, 1971). Long-term breakdown rates after the first 5 to 7 years are in the range of 10 to 200 per 100,000 individuals (Horwitz et al., 1969; Chiba, 1959; Meyer, 1949). The natural history of tuberculous infection defines high- and low-risk populations for chemoprophylaxis: those with recent infection and those with distant infection (more than 5 years past). Given the efficacy of chemoprophylaxis, one must treat 12 people in the high-risk population to prevent one case of tuberculosis. In the low-risk population, more than 50 people must be treated to prevent one case of tuberculosis.

Direct benefits are the benefits to the individual, while the indirect benefits include interrupting all the transmission that an infectious case would cause in the absence of chemoprophylaxis. Quantifying the indirect effects of chemoprophylaxis is more complicated. The total number of cases of secondary transmission per smear-positive case depends on the natural history of smear-positive cases in different environments. In a setting with no treatment, total transmission due to a case can be estimated on the basis of the long-established natural history of the disease. Berg (1939), for example, provides detailed 20-year follow-up data on untreated pulmonary tuberculosis. Styblo (1991) has reviewed the extensive literature on the epidemiology of tuberculosis when no treatment is provided. On average, an untreated patient survives for 2 years and during each year will infect 10 to 15 other individuals with the bacillus. Murray et al. (1993) have used all available information to estimate the outcome of untreated pulmonary tuberculosis.

In most communities, some of the transmission that would occur in the absence of treatment is avoided because cases are detected and chemotherapy is instituted. How much treatment is provided becomes a key determinant of the indirect benefits of chemoprophylaxis. The amount of transmission that is prevented by chemoprophylaxis depends not only on the proportion of cases that receive treatment but also on two key parameters: first, the average delay from the onset of symptoms, or more precisely, infectiousness until the institution of adequate therapy; and second, the number of secondary infections caused by an infectious host as a function of time since the onset of infectiousness.

As we discuss below, these two issues are also critical factors in assessing the indirect benefits of case treatment and thus

deserve careful review. Considerable research has been undertaken to measure the average time from the onset of respiratory symptoms to the institution of effective treatment, and this work is discussed more fully in the section on case diagnosis. In countries such as The Netherlands, where most patients are diagnosed with a short average delay and more than 80% will complete chemotherapy, how much transmission still occurs? In other words, what are the indirect benefits of chemoprophylaxis in such environments? The number of secondary infections caused by a case on average may change with the time since the onset of infectiousness. Figure 9 shows several possible shapes for the curve defining the number of secondary infections caused by a smear-positive case as a function of time since the onset of infectiousness. If individuals came in contact with each other at random, like gas molecules in a box, the number of secondary infections would be expected to be constant over time. Alternatively, if individuals came into contact with only a small number of household members, then the number of secondary infections would initially be high and then drop rapidly once those close contacts were all infected. For most individuals, their true pattern of mixing will be some combination of high rates of contact with household members and workmates and random exposure to the rest of the community.

Real data on the shape of this curve are hard to obtain. Nevertheless, the shape of this curve is probably the single most important epidemiological aspect of tuberculosis influencing control strategies. The scant evidence available can be summarized in a few sentences. First, in Africa, prior to the widespread application of chemotherapy, Anderson and Geser (1960) found in a multicountry survey program that only 13% of smear-positive patients had at least one child under 5 years of age who was infected. In other words, most of

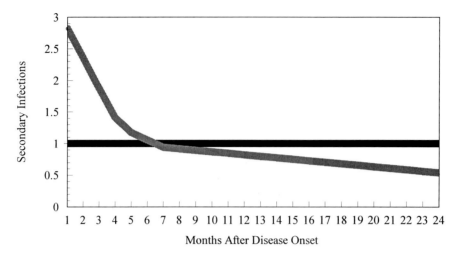

Figure 9. Alternative models of tuberculosis transmission.

the 20 or more secondary infections required to maintain tuberculosis case incidence at a relatively constant rate must have been occurring outside the household. Second, in Saskatchewan, Grzybowski et al. (1976) found nearly as many secondary infections in casual contacts such as workmates as in close household contacts. Taking into account the transmission outside of known contacts through general mixing, the majority of transmission must be occurring outside the household. Third, new data from restriction fragment length polymorphism (RFLP) studies in San Francisco and New York City show that a large share of cases are due to active transmission, most of which is outside the group of close household contacts (Small et al., 1993; Alland et al., 1994). There is probably some increased probability of transmission in the first few months due to close contact with household members, but transmission continues at a significant rate as long as the patient is excreting the bacillus in sputum. Establishing the true nature of this curve is a research priority both for the cost-effectiveness analysis of chemoprophylaxis and for developing case treatment strategies. Creative methods will be required to estimate secondary transmissions as a function

of time since the onset of disease in an ethically appropriate manner.

Adverse Effect of Chemoprophylaxis

Isoniazid chemoprophylaxis can be complicated by hepatitis, which can at times be fatal (Kopanoff et al., 1978; Moulding et al., 1989, Black et al., 1975). The risk of isoniazid-related hepatitis appears to increase with age. Reports of hepatitis due to isoniazid emerged early in the drug's use against tuberculosis. A U.S. Public Health Service multicenter study showed considerable incidence and mortality, but seven of eight deaths were in alcoholics at one center (Snider et al., 1986). More recently, clinical case reports have raised the question of whether the risk of isoniazid hepatitis may be higher for young black women (Jordan et al., 1991b). The reports of and interest in adverse outcomes are at odds with experience in sub-Saharan Africa and other developing countries, for which there are few reports of isoniazid hepatitis. Withdrawal of therapy because of hepatitis is a rare event in these national programs. The difference in experience could be due to heightened sensitivity in the United States to drug hepatitis, more frequent testing of liver function, the detection of subclinical hepatitis, missing the diagnosis of hepatitis in the developing country programs, or the concentration of tuberculosis in the United States in groups such as alcoholics, who have higher risks of adverse outcomes. For some groups, the risk of isoniazid hepatitis may outweigh the benefits of chemoprophylaxis.

Decision Analyses of Chemoprophylaxis

The existence of an adverse effect, namely, isoniazid hepatitis, has spawned a continuing series of decision analyses of when to use chemotherapy in the United States. Informal and formal analyses that examine the age at which the benefits of chemoprophylaxis outweigh the risk of isoniazid-related hepatitis (Colice, 1990; Comstock and Edwards, 1975; Tsevat et al., 1988; Taylor et al., 1981; Rose et al., 1986) have had conflicting results. Younger individuals have a higher cumulative lifetime risk of breakdown to clinical disease and a lower risk of isoniazid hepatitis. The lack of consensus on the age below which chemoprophylaxis should be recommended stems from the wide range of assumptions on the case-fatality rate for tuberculosis, the incidence of isoniazid hepatitis, and the case-fatality rate for isoniazid hepatitis. The debate on the role of chemoprophylaxis in U.S. clinical practice has only broadened with analyses suggesting that recommendations be tailored to ethnic group and gender (Jordan et al., 1991b) and that all intravenous drug abusers except tuberculin-negative black women have chemoprophylaxis (Jordan et al., 1991a).

Notably, most of these studies have not included the benefits of decreased transmission, thus ignoring one of the major components of the possible benefit. This neglect may reflect the widespread belief in the United States that nearly all tuberculosis is caused by reactivation and that active transmission is a minor issue. In analyzing the benefits of chemoprophylaxis for high-risk groups in developing countries, the indirect benefits of transmission may be larger than the direct benefits.

Cost-Effectiveness of Chemoprophylaxis

Decision analyses indicate the net benefits from a particular medical intervention. Cost-effectiveness analysis can provide information on whether the net benefits warrant the investment of scarce health resources. Cost-effectiveness analysis is a method of evaluating the cost per health benefit, which is denominated in some health status measure, such as years of life saved. Cost-benefit analysis estimates the cost per health benefit as well, but health benefits are converted into monetary terms by attaching a dollar value to each type of health outcome.

The interpretation of cost-effectiveness results clearly depends on the level of resources available in different environments. Chemoprophylaxis may not be cost-effective in developing countries because of the large number of individuals who must be treated with a long drug regimen in order to prevent a single case. In addition, wider use of chemoprophylaxis, especially in developing countries, may be limited by the feasibility of identifying individuals who would benefit from chemoprophylaxis. Many tuberculosis programs in industrialized countries and a few programs in developing countries conduct contact tracing and offer chemoprophylaxis to PPD-positive contacts. No studies of the cost-effectiveness of this very simple approach to identifying a high-risk group have been undertaken. Nevertheless, few developing-country programs have been able to institute and maintain effective case contact tracing programs. More aggressive screening programs to identify high- or low-risk groups have not been successfully implemented in developing countries. In much of the developing world, nearly half the adult population is infected with the tubercle bacilli. General population screening would simply be infeasible because of the enormous number of PPD-positive individuals who would be found. Screening programs targeted on groups at high risk for recent infection or at high risk for breakdown would in principle be more feasible. Even the cost-effectiveness of screening programs such as hospital employee screening in industrialized countries has been challenged (Le, 1984).

Third, even where it is desirable and feasible to identify high-risk groups who should receive chemoprophylaxis, such identification may not be cost-effective. Two studies have examined the cost-effectiveness of isoniazid chemoprophylaxis in the United States. Rose et al. (1988) found that it cost $14,820 to save a year of life with isoniazid chemoprophylaxis. (They actually reported that a year of life could be saved for $12,625 in 1985 dollars. We have adjusted these estimates to 1990 dollars by using the gross domestic product [GDP] deflator.) Snider et al. (1986) examined the cost-effectiveness of different durations of isoniazid. They concluded that the cost per year of life gained was $5,450 with a 24-week regimen and $12,350 with a 52-week regimen. The cost per marginal year of life saved with the longer regimen was $64,910. (Costs in the Snider et al. [1986] study were in 1983 dollars and have been adjusted to 1990 dollars by the authors.)

Chemoprophylaxis in Immunocompromised Hosts

Each of the foregoing issues must be reassessed for immunocompromised hosts, most obviously HIV-positive patients in developing and industrialized countries. First, the direct benefits of chemoprophylaxis appear to be similar in HIV-positive patients and immunocompetent hosts (Pape et al., 1993). Second, the indirect benefits depend critically on the contact patterns for HIV-positive patients and their average survival times with and without treatment. Arguments can be made in different societies that HIV-positive individuals will have higher contact rates, as in New York City intravenous drug abusers, or lower rates due to social segregation in some sub-Saharan communities.

Several studies, including studies from Zambia and Kenya, have tried to define the infectivity of HIV-positive cases of tuberculosis. Defining the infectivity of an HIV-positive case of tuberculosis will be confounded by uncertainty over the average duration of infectiousness and symptoms in an HIV-positive case compared to an HIV-negative case. The number of secondary infections caused by an HIV-positive case of tuberculosis will also depend critically on that person's survival time with and without treatment. In the United States, HIV-positive cases of multidrug-resistant (MDR) tuberculosis have had very short survival times in some small series (Fischl et al., 1992). Are these cases a good proxy for the survival time of untreated HIV-positive patients with clinically active tuberculosis in a developing country? Evidence from studies in sub-Saharan Africa suggests that AIDS patients survive on average less than 1 year.

Third, adverse effects due to isoniazid appear to be similar for HIV-positive and HIV-negative patients. The same conclusion cannot be reached for treatment with thiacetazone (discussed below).

Fourth, the feasibility and costs of implementing chemoprophylaxis for HIV-positive patients is affected by two issues. First, the high prevalence of PPD anergy in HIV-positive patients makes the identification of those infected more difficult or at least decreases the sensitivity of the test. High rates of anergy in HIV-positive patients has led several authors to recommend chemoprophylaxis for all HIV-positive patients in a high-tuberculosis-prevalence country (Raviglione et al., 1993; Attonucci et al.,

1992). Second, a strategy of targeting chemoprophylaxis to HIV-positive patients requires a system for identifying HIV-positive people in the community. Population screening for HIV to identify coinfected patients is, for ethical and financial reasons, unlikely to be undertaken. Selective screening of high-risk groups would perhaps be more feasible, but serious ethical questions would remain. The most likely use of chemoprophylaxis for HIV-positive patients would be for those patients identified through voluntary testing programs. WHO sponsored a trial in Uganda (Raviglione et al., 1993) of such a program; the results were disappointing, demonstrating that only 6% of patients identified as coinfected completed chemoprophylaxis. Cost-effectiveness studies have not been undertaken to date.

Potential Role

What is the potential impact of chemoprophylaxis as a control tool in developing and industrialized countries? In developed countries, the role is severely limited by the small population of the infected for whom chemoprophylaxis is considered a net benefit and the difficulty of ensuring compliance with a long regimen in an asymptomatic population. In developing countries, the role is even more limited. With half the population or more infected, chemoprophylaxis for those with distant infections is simply infeasible. Cost-effectiveness analysis has not yet been undertaken to show that screening particular high-risk groups and providing chemoprophylaxis are good investments. One of the only high-risk groups that may warrant more active screening measures in industrialized and developing countries is HIV-positive individuals. Several studies are currently testing the cost-effectiveness of isoniazid or rifampin chemoprophylaxis in sub-Saharan Africa. As noted above, the Centers for Disease Control and Prevention recom-

mends that in the United States, HIV-positive individuals be screened for tuberculosis and that if they are PPD positive, they receive chemoprophylaxis.

The above discussion was based on the known effectiveness of chemoprophylaxis in preventing disease due to infection with conventional *M. tuberculosis*. The effectiveness of chemoprophylaxis against drug-resistant strains and particularly MDR strains is far less clear (Snider et al., 1986), and developing appropriate preventive strategies represents a daunting problem.

CASE IDENTIFICATION AND TREATMENT

The most important tools for combating tuberculosis are the timely identification of cases and then their cure. Because treatment for tuberculosis requires long durations of therapy, tuberculosis control programs in many environments have been notoriously unsuccessful. For a variety of reasons, several national tuberculosis control programs in the last decade have achieved remarkable success in the diagnosis and treatment of tuberculosis. The following section highlights the key analytical issues around broadening this success story and some future issues. The discussion is divided into sections on the type of tuberculosis, case detection, and case treatment.

Distinction between Smear-Positive and Smear-Negative and Extrapulmonary Disease

One of the fundamental tenets of tuberculosis control is the primary importance of diagnosing and treating pulmonary sputum smear-positive tuberculosis. Smear-positive patients transmit the disease, and thus identifying and treating the infectious sources in the population have the indirect benefit of reduced transmission to the rest of the community. Pulmonary smear-negative culture-positive, pulmonary smear-

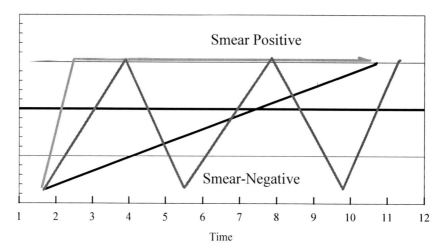

Figure 10. Progression of tuberculosis.

negative culture-negative X-ray suggestive, and extrapulmonary tuberculosis can all be lumped together as "other tuberculosis" in terms of their transmission potential. The compelling logic of focusing on smear-positive patients has pervaded nearly all aspects of tuberculosis control policy and operational research.

While tuberculosis cases can be neatly categorized into various clinical types at the time of presentation, a more dynamic perspective is required. There is no reason to expect smear-negative tuberculosis to remain smear negative if it goes untreated. On the other hand, the Bangalore longitudinal epidemiological study (Olakowski et al., 1973) demonstrated that nearly one-third of tuberculosis patients, including smear-positive cases, are cured spontaneously. Figure 10 is a schematic of the natural history of tuberculosis. One can imagine at least three models of progression. First, cases destined to become smear positive may progress rapidly through a smear-negative phase, while all other cases remain smear negative throughout their lifespan. This model would fit most closely with the current heavy emphasis on the distinction between smear-positive and smear-negative cases. Second, tuberculosis may

progress slowly through a smear-negative phase and, as the burden of the bacillus increases, ultimately become smear positive and stay that way. In this model, positive smears are a later manifestation of the disease. Negative smears, or a portion of them, would be the positive smears of the future, and thus diagnosing and treating smear-negative patients would have the significant indirect benefit of reduced transmission. In fact, as discussed above, if smear-negative patients did progress to become smear positive at some appreciable rate, their treatment would prevent the prediagnosis transmission that inevitably occurs if one waits to diagnose smear-positive cases. Finally, because of the cavitary nature of some forms of the disease, tuberculosis cases may oscillate between smear-positive and smear-negative status on a random basis. Today's smear-positive patients may be smear negative in a month and vice versa. If so, the distinction between smear-positive and smear-negative patients would no longer be significant at a population control level.

Evidence on the natural history of smear-negative pulmonary tuberculosis is limited. The Bangalore epidemiological study provides one of the few sources for estimating these parameters (Olakowski, 1973). Of 304 persons considered to have active or probably active tuberculosis according to radiological findings who were smear and culture negative, 13% became bacteriologically positive over 5 years of observation. If half of these were smear positive, that would be 6.5% of X-ray-suggestive patients who go on to become infectious smear-positive patients. This percentage is the product of the specificity of the original X-ray diagnosis and the probability of true smear-negative patients progressing to become smear positive. If diagnosis was only 50% specific, then 13% of the true smear-negative patients would have progressed to become smear positive. This figure is the minimum estimate, as smear-negative culture-positive patients were excluded from the analysis. Short-course chemotherapy trials in Hong Kong have shown in a much more medically sophisticated setting that 56% of X-ray-suggestive patients went on to develop bacteriologically positive or clinically active disease over a 60-month period (Hong Kong Chest Service, Tuberculosis Research Centre, Madras, British Medical Research Council, 1984).

Defining the natural history of smear-negative tuberculosis and potentially redefining international tuberculosis control dogma is a major priority. Opportunities to study the natural history of smear-negative pulmonary tuberculosis are severely limited, because it is unethical to deny smear-negative patients treatment for the purpose of research. Natural experiments, however, do exist. Currently, smear-negative treatment in China is not free, and reports indicate that about 50% of diagnosed smear-negative patients refuse treatment because of the cost of drugs. Retrospective analysis of this population may provide some information on the fate of smear-negative patients. Creative approaches are needed to define more precisely the natural history of smear-negative tuberculosis.

Case Detection

The importance of case detection and operational research on improving case detection remains contentious after nearly four decades of policy debate. There are two basic viewpoints. One argues that where case treatment programs do not ensure the cure of 80% or more of patients, diagnosing more cases is not a priority. In fact, improving the quality of case treatment and outcomes will naturally lead to greater consumer confidence in the tuberculosis program and increased diagnosis. The other viewpoint, widely held in India, is that little can be done to improve case treatment results, so the only mechanism for increasing the population impact of the tuberculosis control program is to increase the volume of patients moving through the system. In the following section, we do not resolve this debate, but we highlight the limitations of the technologies available for diagnosis, various diagnostic algorithms, and the relative merits of active and passive screening strategies, and we examine the importance of diagnostic delay. Four major diagnostic technologies are currently being used to detect clinical disease due to tuberculous infection.

Microscopy

Detection by microscopy of acid-fast bacilli (nearly always identical with tubercle bacilli) in sputum and other specimens (e.g., gastric washings) is the most important tool in detecting infectious cases of tuberculosis. There is strong evidence (Rouillon et al., 1976; Styblo, 1984) that those patients whose sputa contain sufficient bacilli to be detected by microscopy are highly infectious. These cases are referred to as smear positive.

Culture

The culture of specimens for mycobacteria detects, in about 4 to 6 weeks, tubercle

Table 3. Yield in cases from concurrent smear and culture examinations of eight consecutive sputum specimens from each of 194 persons with lung X-ray shadows and prolonged chest symptoms suggesting tuberculosis[a]

Bacteriological category[b]	No. of cases								
	Total	According to no. of specimen yielding first positive result							
		I	II	III	IV	V	VI	VII	VIII
S+, C+	46	34	7	1	1	0	0	1	2
S+, C−	7	2	2	0	0	0	1	1	1
Total	53	36	9	1	1	0	1	2	3
C+, S+	46	34	7	1	1	0	0	1	2
C+, S−	22	9	7	1	1	1	1	2	0
Total	68	43	14	2	2	1	1	3	2

[a] Source: Toman (1979).
[b] S+ and S−, smear positive and smear negative, respectively; C+ and C−, culture positive and culture negative, respectively.

bacilli in sputum containing insufficient bacilli to be detected by microscopy. Cases that are sputum smear negative but culture positive are then classified as smear-negative culture-positive pulmonary tuberculosis. Patients whose sputa are smear negative and culture positive are about 10 times less infectious than smear-positive patients (van Geuns et al., 1975). Newer culture methods such as BACTEC allow more rapid detection of growth (in approximately 3 weeks). These methods, which are more expensive, have not yet been widely implemented.

X ray

Pulmonary lesions due to tuberculosis can often be detected on chest X ray. In some regions of the world, such as South Asia and China, clinical judgment and X-ray diagnosis are the dominant methods used. By WHO definitions, cases that are smear and culture negative but have suspicious chest X-ray changes should be called pulmonary suspect cases because of the low specificity of X-ray diagnosis (Toman, 1979).

Culture or histology

Extrapulmonary tuberculosis is often diagnosed by biopsy, urine sample, or lumbar puncture and culture or histological examination of the specimen (for patients with tuberculous meningitis, lymphadenitis, genitourinary tuberculosis, etc.). It is important to stress that either extrapulmonary tuberculosis is noninfectious or the degree of infectivity is very low.

The "gold standard" definition of a case of pulmonary tuberculosis is most often accepted as a positive culture. Even this definition should be qualified to take into account cultures that are only scantily positive, perhaps because of contamination (Aluoch et al., 1985). A more rigorous definition of a case is a positive culture with at least three colonies of growth (Narain et al., 1968). Widespread differences in the definition of a case of pulmonary tuberculosis in national programs remain, clouding international comparisons and analysis (Research Institute of Tuberculosis, 1993; American Thoracic Society-Centers for Disease Control, 1990). Given the gold standard definition of a case of tuberculosis, what are the sensitivity and specificity of sputum examination? Toman (1979) reanalyzed a study by Nair et al. (1976), the results of which are shown in Table 3. The question must be qualified by the number of smears used. Most programs use two or three sputum examinations as the standard. By this definition, smear was 60% sensitive and 94% specific. The specificity, of course, depends on the definition of a positive culture. Nair et al.'s study (1976) also indicates the marginal yield of further sputum examinations: 89% of smear-positive culture-positive cases were detected after two examinations, but 6% were detected on the seventh and eighth examinations. Of note, 84% of culture-positive patients were detected on the first two cultures, but the remaining 16% were nearly evenly distributed across the next six cultures. Toman (1979), reporting unpublished data from a study by Nagpaul et al. (1970), provides a summary of the sensitivity and specificity of X-ray diagnosis in South India. Chest X ray as applied in study conditions was 88% sensitive and 96% specific. Even in this population, with a high prevalence of tuberculosis and experienced X-ray readers, the positive predictive value was only 62%. In other words, 38% of those diagnosed with tuberculosis by clinical judgment and X ray did not have tuberculosis. One would expect the positive predictive value of chest X ray in routine conditions in India and many other developing countries to be substantially lower.

New diagnostic technologies based on the polymerase chain reaction to amplify *M. tuberculosis* DNA, which can then be detected by a DNA probe, are under development (for background, see Bloom [1989]). These methods could provide a sensitivity equivalent to that of culture and results available in days rather than weeks. Some laboratories in developed countries have already started to use these methods on an experimental basis. While their role in routine diagnosis in developing countries is unclear, they may be more directly useful as a substitute for culture and sensitivity testing in national reference laboratories. Their impact on diagnostic methods awaits more extensive development, testing, and cost analysis.

Many tuberculosis control programs use various diagnostic technologies and clinical assessment in combination. For example,

the diagnostic algorithm used in many parts of China includes screening of symptomatic individuals with fluoroscopy. Positive individuals then get a chest X ray, and those with an X-ray abnormality get two or three sputum examinations. The aggregate effect of using such screening algorithms on sensitivity and specificity has been poorly studied. The first step in the diagnostic algorithm is the entry criterion, or the set of clinical signs and symptoms that indicates that a patient should be screened for tuberculosis. Some early work in South India (Baily et al., 1967) indicated that screening patients who had had a cough for more than 2 weeks would detect 84% of cases in a group of symptomatic individuals. Screening patients with a cough of shorter duration would necessitate a much greater workload, as the number eligible would double, but the yield in this group would be low. Few subsequent studies have examined the utility of combinations of clinical signs and symptoms that could be used to increase sensitivity or increase the yield of cases per 100 screened. Because of the growing HIV epidemic in sub-Saharan Africa and in Asia, the clinical spectrum of tuberculosis may be altered. New studies examining the signs and symptoms that could be used to qualify patients for tuberculosis screening would be useful. Studies examining the mix of technologies used in diagnosis and their aggregate sensitivity and specificity are also needed. Ultimately, the diagnostic algorithm, including the entry criterion for screening, should be chosen on the basis of cost-effectiveness analysis. Maximal sensitivity can be purchased but at extremely high costs. Cost-effectiveness analysis of alternative diagnostic algorithms should be part of any new study of case detection methods.

The second main issue in case detection is the choice of active or passive screening strategies. Active detection means attempts to screen the population at large or to target populations such as military recruits for evidence of tuberculosis. Passive case detection means screening and diagnosing only those patients who present to a health service provider because of symptoms suspicious of tuberculosis. In the 1950s and 1960s, the choice between active and passive detection in developed and developing countries was a controversial topic (Styblo et al., 1969a; Meijer et al., 1971; WHO, 1974; Styblo and Meijer, 1980; Toman, 1979). In the last two decades, a consensus for passive case detection of tuberculosis in all countries has developed; both the WHO and the International Union Against Tuberculosis and Lung Disease (IUATLD) advocate this policy.

Three assumptions underlie the wide acceptance of passive case detection as the primary strategy in tuberculosis control. First, 90% of patients with smear-positive pulmonary tuberculosis have objective symptoms such as cough, fever, loss of weight, sputum, or hemoptysis. These symptoms develop quite soon after the onset of the disease, in theory prompting the patient to seek medical advice. Second, the great majority of sputum smear-positive tuberculosis cases develop in a shorter time than the shortest feasible interval between two mass radiography survey rounds (Styblo et al., 1967). That is why smear-positive tuberculosis cases were detected by the regular health services that patients can consult when ill usually earlier than the periodic case-finding campaigns. Third, first-line diagnosis should be available through the primary health care system. The validity of these assumptions depends on local conditions, cultural perception of disease, access to care, and the efficacy of health services.

Various case-finding methods were studied extensively in Kenya over a decade and a half (Nsanzumuhire et al., 1977, 1981; Aluoch et al., 1978, 1982, 1984, 1985, 1987). Methods examined included interrogation of household heads, interrogation of village elders, repeated questioning of village elders every 3 months, screening of all patients with a previous diagnosis of tuberculosis in the past 10 years, screening of contacts of past tuberculosis cases, screening of patients with chronic cough at peripheral health facilities, screening of all symptomatic individuals with cough lasting more than 1 month at district hospitals, and interrogation of women at maternal and child welfare clinics. Taken together, this body of work demonstrated a consistent pattern. The greatest yield of cases was from asking household heads if anyone in their household had respiratory symptoms and subsequent sputum examination and culture of specimens from these individuals. Given that 2 to 6% of the population had a cough at any one time, the volume of sputum examinations was too great for this to be a practical method of screening. Formal cost-effectiveness studies, however, were not undertaken. Questioning elders detected about one-third of cases, and the yield per person screened was nearly twice as high (about 4/100 screened). More than 80% of cases, however, reported that they visited the health services for their complaints. The average number of visits in one study was nearly five per patient, but most had never been screened for tuberculosis. Paradoxically, efforts to ensure that all patients presenting at peripheral health facilities with chronic cough were registered and screened detected less than 10% of cases. The investigators then studied the yield of cases by focusing on district hospitals, where the quality of diagnosis was presumably higher, and estimated that about 40% of cases could be detected at that level. The majority of the cases detected, however, lived within 15 km of the hospital. Efforts to use the more extensive network of maternal and child welfare clinics to identify symptomatic individuals in the households of the women attending the clinics and to then encourage them by letter to present for screening detected less than 4% of cases.

Taken together, most tuberculosis practitioners have interpreted these studies to mean that the emphasis in case detection should be on improving the quality of diagnosis in the primary health care system, as most patients present repetitively to the health services. This interpretation must be tempered with several observations. In India, for example, two studies have shown that only 50% of patients detected by mass screening have already contacted the health services (Banerji and Andersen, 1963; Narayan et al., 1979). Second, there is little evidence to date of interventions that have successfully improved the performance of case diagnosis in peripheral health facilities. The studies in Kenya have led to a district hospital-based strategy that probably detects less than half of the cases. With increasing interest in case treatment of tuberculosis as a cost-effective intervention, it may be time to reexamine strategies such as using village leaders to identify symptomatic individuals on a regular basis in conjunction with efforts to improve peripheral health facility diagnosis. Third, in regions such as Asia where X ray is used extensively, there may be a problem of simultaneous overdiagnosis of smear-negative patients and underdiagnosis of smear-positive patients. The role of alternative case detection strategies in regions that use X ray extensively will most likely be different. Studies of the roles of various screening strategies must include a careful assessment of the full costs of different methods. The strategy in each community that identifies cases at up to a reasonable cost per true case diagnosed should be chosen.

The fourth major issue in case detection, which is closely related to the technology and screening strategy used, is delay to diagnosis. Diagnostic delay is defined as the duration of time from the onset of symptoms to the institution of effective therapy (Mori et al., 1992). Diagnostic delay has been divided into two components: (i) patient's delay from the onset of symptoms to seeking care and (ii) doctor's delay from first presentation to the institution of adequate therapy. If transmission of tuberculosis continues throughout the period that a patient is excreting bacilli in sputum, then long delays mean increased transmission of tuberculosis. A program that detects 80% of cases may have only a small epidemiological impact if the average delay to diagnosis is many months. The duration of delay has been studied in a number of countries, including Japan, The Netherlands, Korea, Chile, and Bolivia, and in some U.S. population groups (Baas et al., 1983; Aoki et al., 1982; Allan et al., 1979; Mori, 1982; Acuna et al., 1981; Rubel and Garro, 1992). In well-functioning programs, median delay is under 2 months; Fig. 11 provides the results for Chile. In contrast, programs with lower treatment completion and case detection rates have much longer median delays (Fig. 12). Not only is the median delay longer, but there is also a significant minority of patients with extremely long periods of symptoms prior to diagnosis. The data from Bolivia indicate that diagnostic delay is much longer for women, but in Korea, delay is equal in the two sexes (Mori et al., 1992). Studies of delay have not found consistent predictors of delay. Further research is urgently needed on the extent of delay, determinants of delay, and most important, interventions to reduce delay. Ultimately, diagnostic delay may become as important an indicator of the quality of a program as the case treatment completion rate or the case detection rate.

Treatment Completion

Despite the availability of powerful and potentially effective antituberculosis drugs, tuberculosis treatment programs in most developing and, more recently, some industrialized countries have not been very successful. Overall cure rates for most national programs in poor developing countries are below 50%. During the 1960s and 1970s in

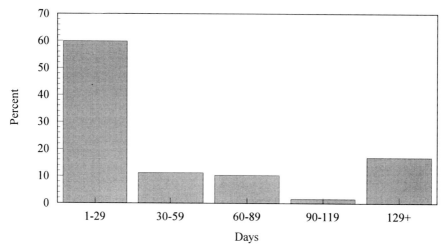

Figure 11. Delay from symptoms to diagnosis in Chile, 1985 to 1986. Source: Tabilo et al. (1987).

many poor developing countries in Africa, many parts of Southeast Asia, and certain parts of Latin America, signs of improvement in the epidemiological situation of tuberculosis were the exception, despite widespread attempts at disease control. The most important reason for the failure of such control programs was the low cure rate.

Poor cure rates, or in the majority of cases, poor treatment completion rates, in many programs are due largely to the long duration of tuberculosis treatment required to cure tuberculosis. Organizing and ensuring the delivery of effective chemotherapeutic agents for 6 to 18 months is a major challenge in any environment. Figure 13, based on the results of the Botswanan National Tuberculosis Programme, shows the essential problem: patients in any program have a rising probability of stopping treatment during the course of treatment.

The thrust of this section is the major challenges and research questions around

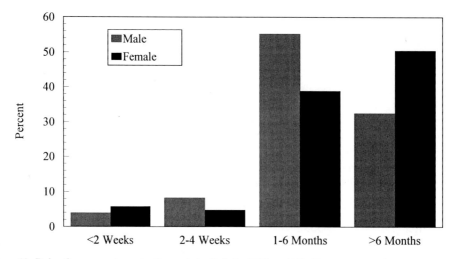

Figure 12. Delay from symptoms to diagnosis in Bolivia, 1988 to 1989. Source: Rojas and Lanza (1989).

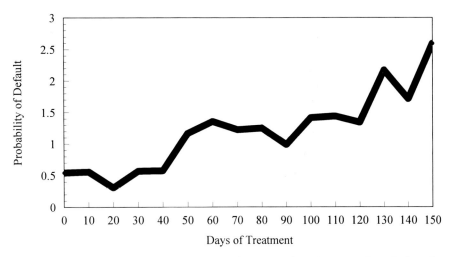

Figure 13. Probability of default for each 10-day period of treatment for pulmonary tuberculosis patients in four districts of Botswana, 1987 to 1990.

achieving a high cure rate for newly diagnosed cases. Somewhat arbitrarily, the discussion is divided into sections on the measurement of treatment outcome, regimen choice, methods to enhance compliance, program management and evaluation, and cost-effectiveness analysis of treatment strategies.

Measuring treatment outcomes

The literature on the performance of treatment programs is confused by a profusion of indicators used to measure treatment outcome. Sumartojo (1993) reviewed 15 studies reporting on treatment completion, but nearly every study used a different measure for treatment outcome. National programs differ in the indicators of treatment performance; for example, the Centers for Disease Control and Prevention use a measure of the continuity of chemotherapy, the definition of which has changed in the last decade (Bloom and Murray, 1992). Fortunately, the WHO (1992), modifying a method used by the IUATLD in a number of national programs, has proposed a standard method of reporting treatment outcomes. Six categories are defined as follows.

(i) Cured. Treatment is completed, and smear results are negative on two or more consecutive occasions at 5 months and at the end of treatment.

(ii) Treatment completed. Treatment is completed; there is no or only one positive smear result at month 5 or later.

(iii) Died. Patient is known to have died from any cause whatsoever.

(iv) Failure. Patient is smear positive at 5 months or more, or stopped treatment for more than 2 months before month 5 and was smear positive at last sputum examination, or smear-negative patient became smear positive by month 2 sputum smear examination.

(v) Defaulted. Patient has not collected drugs for more than 2 months but became (or remained) smear negative before defaulting.

(vi) Transferred out. Patient has been transferred to another district.

The cure rate is the number cured over the total number in the cohort. The treatment completion rate is the number cured plus the number with treatment completed divided by the total number in the cohort. Several important subtleties must be noted in any comparison of program results.

First, the definitions of failure and defaulted depend on the method of supervision used. In a program in which chemotherapy is supervised daily, including during the continuation phase, the definition of default is different from that in a program in which the continuation phase is self-administered. Second, treatment completion rates reported in studies sometimes exclude deaths from the denominator, thus artificially inflating performance compared to that in programs that use the standard definitions. Third, depending on the regimen in use, the thresholds for defining the completion of chemotherapy may be different. Some programs, such as the Indian National Tuberculosis Programme, use a very relaxed definition whereby a patient can miss up to 8 weeks of treatment and still be defined as completing treatment. Other programs in which chemotherapy is supervised daily, such as in Botswana, have a strict definition of missing fewer than 20 days of treatment in a 180-day course. Great care must be taken to standardize this definition when results are being compared. Fourth, reported cure rates depend on the classification of sputum examination results at the end of treatment. Many patients cannot produce sputum at the end of therapy, and as sputum induction is not widely practiced in most programs, the examination at the end of treatment is of saliva. Some programs, such as in China, report saliva as negative sputum at the end of treatment, while others, such as in Botswana, report saliva as "no sputum examination performed." Fostering a wider debate and analysis of the determinants of treatment program success requires a common vocabulary. The standard definitions of treatment completion and cure rates encouraged by the WHO and the IUATLD are important steps in the right direction. Nevertheless, further efforts are required to standardize all aspects of the definition, because there is still latitude in the defini-tions for substantial variation in reporting practices.

Treatment regimens

It is beyond the scope of this chapter to review the clinical literature on the treatment of tuberculosis or the various drug regimens that may be used for different pulmonary and extrapulmonary forms of the disease (see WHO [1993], Iseman et al. [1993], American Thoracic Society [1993], and Cohn et al. [1990] for recent reviews). The choice of regimen, however, has a direct bearing on treatment outcomes and supervision strategies. The major drugs used and developments in treatment regimens over the last two decades are briefly reviewed. Four areas for operational research are raised.

Since the first official use of streptomycin in 1947, five drugs have emerged as first-line agents for the treatment of tuberculosis: isoniazid, rifampin, pyrazinamide, ethambutol, and streptomycin. In many developing-country programs, a second-line drug, thiacetazone, is used because it is inexpensive. Tuberculosis drug regimens are divided into two phases: the intensive phase of treatment, during which the aim is to kill the population of bacilli that are dividing, and the continuation phase, during which the aim is to kill bacilli that are more dormant. More drugs are commonly used in the intensive phase, which lasts 1 to 2 months, than in the continuation phase, which lasts 4 to 10 months.

In the 1960s, 2STH/10–16TH became the standard regimen used in most national control programs. (Tuberculosis drug regimens are reported by using a standard code. The number is the duration of treatment [in months] with a particular set of drugs. The letters stand for antituberculosis drugs [H for isoniazid, T for thiacetazone, R for rifampin, S for streptomycin, E for ethambutol, and Z for pyrazinamide]. Some regimens have subscripts that indicate that the drug is given intermittently, with the subscript denoting the number of days the drug is given each week.) Since the introduction of streptomycin, there has been extensive research on the clinical efficacy of different drug regimens (D'Esopo, 1982). In the 1970s, a series of trials were undertaken in many countries that demonstrated that tuberculosis could be treated in 6 to 8 months with regimens containing multiple drugs in the intensive phase. These trials demonstrated that the most important drug in the new short-course regimens was rifampin. In 1993, both the WHO (1993) and the American Thoracic Society (1993) recommend similar regimens. The most widely recommended is 2HRZE/4HR; common substitutions include streptomycin for ethambutol in the intensive phase and 6HE or 6HT in the continuation phase.

Despite the higher drug costs of short-course regimens, it is now widely accepted that short-course chemotherapy is desirable at least for all smear-positive patients. The broad consensus for short-course chemotherapy is based on several observations. First, the proportion cured by short-course chemotherapy at each point in the drug regimen is greater than that for long-course (otherwise known as standard) chemotherapy (2STH/10–16TH). Patients who default from treatment are more likely to be cured on short-course than on long-course chemotherapy, despite not completing therapy. Second, the probability of selecting for resistance when four drugs are given is much lower. For example, Chonde (1989) has shown that in Tanzania over the past decade, there has been virtually no increase in drug resistance while short-course chemotherapy has been introduced. Third, if all other things are held constant, the shorter duration of therapy automatically increases the proportion of patients who will complete treatment. Multiple studies have shown a continuing and often rising probability of default throughout the duration of chemotherapy (Murray et al., 1993).

Fourth, despite the increased cost of drugs, short-course chemotherapy has been shown to be more cost-effective than standard chemotherapy per year of life saved (Murray et al., 1991, 1993).

While a consensus is emerging on the optimal regimen for treating smear-positive pulmonary tuberculosis, at least five operational research issues in the area of drug regimens remain.

(i) Efficacious regimens shorter than 6 months. Because the probability of default appears to climb over time, a shorter regimen will probably lead to a higher treatment completion rate and thus a higher cure rate. Research on the drug treatment for *M. leprae* has led to ultrashort regimens. Currently, 2- and 3-month regimens are being tested (Davidson, 1990). Four-month regimens for pulmonary smear-negative culture-positive tuberculosis have been used successfully (Hong Kong Chest Service, Tuberculosis Research Centre, Madras, British Medical Research Council, 1984). Unfortunately, four-drug 3-month regimens for smear-positive tuberculosis have had unacceptably high relapse rates (Tuberculosis Research Centre, Madras, and National Tuberculosis Institute, Bangalore, 1986). New regimens that last less than 6 months will have to await the development of new agents that are effective against *M. tuberculosis*. Nevertheless, if effective new drugs become available, it will be worthwhile testing shorter regimens.

(ii) Drug regimens for HIV-positive patients with pulmonary tuberculosis. Studies on the treatment of HIV-positive patients with smear-positive tuberculosis, while limited, have shown that short-course chemotherapy is as effective in them as in HIV-negative patients (Small et al., 1993). Treatment of HIV-positive patients with regimens that do not include rifampin has not been as successful (Perriens et al., 1991). Recently, Nunn et al. (1992) reported a high rate of tuberculosis in HIV-positive patients treated with 2SH/6HE that may be due to relapse or reinfection. In some sub-Saharan African countries, HIV-positive patients have been treated with regimens containing thiacetazone in the continuation phase. Clear evidence has emerged that thiacetazone carries a high risk of Stevens-Johnson syndrome, a severe adverse reaction, in HIV-positive patients (Pozniak et al., 1992). Research is urgently needed on cost-effective treatment strategies for HIV-positive patients that can address the importance of rifampin-containing intensive and continuation phases of treatment and the need for maintenance therapy after a normal regimen of treatment has been completed.

(iii) Drug regimens for the treatment of MDR tuberculosis. Current recommendations for the treatment of MDR tuberculosis are based on limited experience in certain referral centers (Iseman et al., 1993). If the volume of MDR tuberculosis increases dramatically in developing countries or the industrialized countries, cost-effective strategies for managing drug-resistant tuberculosis will need to be formulated for different settings depending on resources available.

(iv) Multidrug preparations and metered-dose delivery systems. Short-course regimens are theoretically less likely to select for resistance if the patient takes all drugs prescribed at the same time. If drug use is variable, providing access to rifampin and other short-course drugs may create conditions fostering resistance, as have been observed in New York City over the last 5 years. Combination preparations that contain, for example, isoniazid, rifampin, and pyrazinamide can be used so that patients either receive all three or not and do not receive a subset of drugs. Evaluation of the benefits of combination preparations in terms of increased compliance and decreased selection of drug resistance is needed. Also, if depot preparations akin to those of Depo-Provera for contraception could be prepared, part of the problem of patient noncompliance could be solved.

Compliance

Maintaining patient compliance with long antituberculous regimens is the fundamental challenge of tuberculosis control programs. Figure 13 demonstrates that throughout the course of treatment, patients tend to drop out of treatment. The data from Botswana demonstrate that the probability per week of dropping out of treatment increases over time. There is an extensive literature on medical compliance (also called adherence in U.S. literature) in general and on tuberculosis compliance in particular (Haynes et al., 1979; Fox, 1983a, b, 1985; Sbarbaro, 1979; WHO Tuberculosis Chemotherapy Centre, 1963; Reichman, 1987). Two recent reviews provide an extensive treatment of the subject (Sumartojo, 1993; Rubel and Garro, 1992); here, only a few major observations are provided.

In programs such as Botswana's, where every day's treatment is observed by a health worker during both the intensive and the continuation phases, defining and measuring compliance is a simple question of good bookkeeping. No similar unambiguous gold standard of measurement is available for self-administered chemotherapy. Various methods have been used, including patient self-reports (Barnhoorn and Adrianase, 1992), urine tests for isoniazid and rifampin (Burkhardt and Nel, 1980), and sophisticated electronic devices in medication bottles (Cheung et al., 1988). Despite these attempts, assessment of compliance with self-administered chemotherapy is problematic, with an inherent bias to underestimate noncompliance. The ultimate test of compliance is the result of treatment at the end of a completed course of chemotherapy. In a program in which a high proportion of patients are reported to complete therapy but smear conversion at the end of treatment is lower than expected, the measure of compliance must be questioned. Many of the factors that one might expect to influence patient compliance with antituberculosis drug regimens, such as the severity of side effects, have not been empirically observed. There is a clear consensus, however, that the duration of treatment adversely affects compliance (Haynes, 1979). Moodie (1967), in unusual circumstances in Hong Kong, found that most noncompliers dropped out in the first 3 weeks, but all other studies have observed a steady dropout over time (East African and British Medical Research Council, 1977, 1979). Improved net compliance due to a shorter regimen is a major advantage of short-course chemotherapy over standard chemotherapy. Other factors, such as age, sex, and education, have not emerged as universal determinants but have been significant in one study or another (Alcabes et al., 1989; Armstrong and Pringle, 1984; Barnhoorn and Adrianase, 1992; Bell and Yach, 1988). Some studies have examined more complex social and cultural variables such as social support systems, knowledge of the disease process, and initial intention to take therapy (Alcabes et al., 1989; Barnhoorn and Adrianase, 1992; Rubel and Garro, 1992). A number of unpublished investigations by national tuberculosis programs have elicited similar responses from patients when they are questioned about reasons for default. Common responses relate to lack of time at home, beliefs that they are no longer ill, difficulty obtaining medications, required movement, holiday celebrations, and others.

Research on the determinants of noncompliance is helpful to control programs only if it leads to interventions that enhance treatment outcomes. Objective analysis of this subject is complicated by three trends. First, many of the trials and published studies of incentives, enablers, and supervision strategies to improve compliance are from small projects run by nongovernmental agencies. Some of these agencies have a strong vested interest in demonstrating success to their funders. In addition, most of the published reports on these small-scale efforts are for tiny patient populations (e.g., Miles and Maat, 1984; Farmer et al., 1991). Second, many creative efforts at improving compliance, even on a relatively large scale in Bolivia and India, have gone unrecognized in the international literature. Information on these experiments is often available only in unpublished reports within local program offices. Third, several national programs, including those in Benin, Botswana, China (10 provinces), Malawi, Mozambique, Nicaragua, and Tanzania, have achieved impressive treatment completion rates (Murray et al., 1991). Because the number of patients in these programs is large and the administrative, social, economic, and cultural variations within each country are great, these achievements are perhaps more informative.

Various small-scale studies have examined the use of incentives to and "enablers" of patients and service providers in improving treatment outcomes. Methods such as financial payments to patients (Morisky et al., 1990), bonds paid back at the end of treatment (Chowdhury et al., 1992), blister packs (Valeza and McDougall, 1990), education and motivation of patient and family (Seetha et al., 1981; Wobeser et al., 1989), and "comprehensive interventions," including at times health care, food, financial assistance, and home follow-up (e.g., Farmer et al., 1991), have been tried with reported success. As reviewed by Sumartojo (1993), none of these studies report comparable results in terms of the WHO-defined cure or treatment completion rates. At a large-scale level, outside the domain of small, highly motivated organizations working in one or two communities, incentives and enhancers for self-administered chemotherapy have not been demonstrated to increase the treatment

Table 4. Results of chemotherapy for smear-positives in three sub-Saharan African programs

Outcome	Malawi	Mozambique	Tanzania
Cured	87.2	70.8	76.9
Treatment completed	0	7.3	0
Failed	1.3	1.5	2.4
Died	6.5	1.5	6.5
Defaulted	2.2	11.3	9.9
Transferred out	2.7	7.8	4.2

completion rate up to the WHO target of 80%. Developing methods applicable on a large scale to enhance self-administered-treatment completion rates remains a daunting but critical operational research priority for many countries and regions. While large-scale success with self-administered chemotherapy has been difficult to achieve, there are now multiple examples with hundreds of thousands of patients enrolled in national or provincial programs with treatment completion rates of over 75%, including programs in Benin, Botswana, China (10 provinces), Malawi, Mozambique, Nicaragua, and Tanzania. Treatment results from three of these programs are illustrated in Table 4. These successful national efforts have one thing in common: they invest heavily in the supervision of chemotherapy. Within these programs, there is a spectrum of supervised chemotherapy from hospitalization throughout therapy, to hospitalization during the intensive phase and supervised ambulatory therapy in the continuation phase, to totally ambulatory supervised chemotherapy as in China. Success in supervised treatment in developing countries has usefully influenced policies in the United States, recommending directly observed therapy in high-prevalence areas.

No one supervision strategy is applicable to all countries, regions, or communities. Ambulatory supervised therapy can work in urban and rural areas if a cadre of health worker exists that can be motivated to supervise chemotherapy. Hospitalization may be necessary for patients who live too far from a health facility to receive supervised outpatient care or for patient subgroups who are chronically noncompliant. The key messages are that supervision is costly but works and that the specific supervision strategy must be locally designed, taking patient and health system characteristics into account. Experience from Tanzania and China shows that proposed supervision strategies should be tested in pilot areas and then expanded once a successful model is established.

Cost-Effectiveness of Chemotherapy

The cost-effectiveness of treating smear-positive tuberculosis will be addressed first. In general, the cost per death averted directly or indirectly will be lowest for smear-positive tuberculosis, higher for other kinds of tuberculosis, and highest for retreatment cases. While this statement may run counter to intuitive notions of the clinical costs of treating each type of tuberculosis, the rationale is based on the effect of interrupting transmission, as explained more fully below.

Few studies have examined the cost-effectiveness of tuberculosis treatment in developing countries (Barnum, 1986; Joesoef et al., 1989; Feldstein et al., 1973; Murray et al., 1990). Two of these investigations reported that per case cured, short-course chemotherapy was more cost-effective. They did not, however, report figures on the cost per death averted or per year of life saved. To fill the gap in information on the cost-effectiveness of short-course and WHO standard chemotherapy, the national tuberculosis programs in Malawi, Mozambique, and Tanzania have been studied by Murray et al. (1991).

Before detailing the costs per case treated, some unit cost definitions are needed. Program costs in these three countries can be divided into three components.

Table 5. Estimated average incremental cost per patient treated in low- and middle-income countries[a]

Country GDP/capita ($)	Avg incremental cost/patient treated ($)			
	Short-course hospital	Short-course ambulatory	Standard hospital	Standard ambulatory
150	136	63	113	41
250	181	70	159	48
500	296	87	274	64
750	411	104	389	82
1,000	526	122	504	100
1,250	641	139	619	117
1,500	756	156	734	134

[a] Source: Murray et al. (1993). Short-course hospital refers to short-course chemotherapy with 60 days of hospitalization during the intensive phase, short-course ambulatory refers to short-course chemotherapy with daily supervision during the intensive phase, standard hospital refers to standard chemotherapy with 60 days of hospitalization during the intensive phase, and standard ambulatory refers to standard chemotherapy with daily supervision during the intensive phase.

First, there are variable costs, which are a direct function of the number of patients treated and include costs such as drugs, reagents for diagnosis, and food during hospitalization. Second, there are fixed costs associated with the tuberculosis program itself, such as the salaries of district and regional tuberculosis coordinators, capital costs of vehicles, and administrative costs of the tuberculosis unit. Finally, there are also fixed costs incurred through use of elements of the primary health care infrastructure such as clinics and district hospitals. Three unit costs can also be defined. Marginal costs are here defined as the average variable costs per case, average program costs are variable costs plus the fixed tuberculosis program costs per case, and average costs are total costs including the fixed costs outside the tuberculosis program per case.

Results of costs from low-income countries cannot easily be generalized to other developing countries with incomes per capita that are substantially higher than those in Malawi, Mozambique, and Tanzania. Some treatment costs require foreign currency or internationally traded goods; other costs are local costs that can be paid in local currency and not traded commodities. By separating external costs from domestic costs, we can generate more representative estimates of the cost of treating patients in countries with different incomes per capita. The external component of the cost is assumed to be the same in all countries, while the domestic component is assumed to be proportional to GDP per capita. Our best estimates for the costs of chemotherapy in countries with different levels of income are in Table 5. (This method is a modification of that of Barnum and Greenberg [1993], who have calculated unit costs in terms of the percentage of GDP per capita. External costs or the costs of internationally traded goods, whether they are domestically produced or not, vary in proportion to GDP per capita. Local costs of nontraded goods, most notably labor, will in all probability change in proportion to GDP per capita. The distinction between external and domestic costs not only leads to different estimates of unit costs but also can alter the relative costs of different interventions. As discussed above, the cost of an intervention with a higher percentage of domestic costs per total cost will rise at a faster rate than the cost of an intervention with a higher percentage of external costs. Thus, in a low-income country, one intervention with a large domestic component may be cheaper than an alternative with a large external component. The relative cost-effectiveness rank could, however, reverse as income per capita rises.)

The benefits of chemotherapy can be divided into direct benefits in terms of cure and a reduced death rate for the patient and the indirect benefit of reduced transmission. A life table for the prognosis of smear-positive pulmonary tuberculosis based on the most detailed study of the prognosis of untreated pulmonary tuberculosis by Berg (1939) was calculated. The Bangalore epidemiological study confirms the general case-fatality rates in a developing-country context (National Tuberculosis Institute, Bangalore, 1974; Olakowski, 1973). For each program, the cohort results of chemotherapy have been used to construct an alternative life table of the fate of cases treated by the program. Comparison of the treatment life table and natural-progression life table allows us to quantify the marginal benefits of treatment. A model based on the principle that in an untreated population one case of tuberculosis will lead to one case of smear-positive tuberculosis has been constructed. Transmission benefits have been counted for four transmission cycles that occur over the next 18.5 years. Deaths averted and years of life saved have been discounted at 3%. In the model, it is assumed that passive case detection will lead to diagnosis after 3 months of symptoms and that the rate of transmission during the first 3 months before diagnosis is 50% higher than in the subsequent period. This captures the increased rate of transmission to close household contacts during the period before diagnosis. The false-positive diagnosis rate has been studied in Tanzania and is less than 5%. The study results are based on an assumed false-positive rate for all three programs of 5%.

The cost-effectiveness ratios for short-course and standard chemotherapy with and without hospitalization during the intensive phase are summarized in Table 6. Four ratios are provided for each intervention: the cost per case cured; the cost per direct death averted; the cost per total death averted, which includes deaths averted due to decreased transmission over the next 18.5 years; and the cost per year of life saved, including transmission benefits. Three conclusions follow from the cost-effectiveness ratios. First, chemotherapy for smear-positive tuberculosis is extremely cost-effective. The average program cost per year of life saved ranges from $1 to $4. Second, short-course chemotherapy is preferable to standard chemotherapy in virtually all situations. The absolute difference in the cost per unit benefit is not large, but the cost-effectiveness ratios do not tell the whole story. The cure rate with short-course chemotherapy in all three countries is approximately 25% higher than that with standard chemotherapy. In economic terms, the depth of the margin is much greater with short-course chemotherapy than with standard chemotherapy. There are also several other unquantified benefits to short-course chemotherapy. Rates of secondary drug resistance with short-course treatment are much lower, and the cost of retreating failures has not been built into the comparison. With standard chemotherapy, many more patients will require the expensive retreatment regimens.

In countries with poorly trained microscopists or frequent atypical mycobacterial infections, the positive predictive value of sputum positivity could be lower than 95%. The potential of wasting scarce resources on patients without tuberculosis puts a high premium on training health workers and microscopists to diagnose tuberculosis correctly.

Cost-Effectiveness of Chemotherapy for Smear-Negative Pulmonary Tuberculosis Patients

The cost-effectiveness of chemotherapy for smear-negative pulmonary tuberculosis patients is much more difficult to assess. As

Table 6. Average incremental unit costs in the intensive phase for Malawi, Mozambique, and Tanzania[a]

Therapy[a]	Avg incremental cost[b]		
	Malawi[c]	Mozambique	Tanzania
Short course with hospitalization			
Per cure	165	232	202
Per direct death averted	200	267	236
Per total death averted	38	57	47
Per year of life	1.7	2.6	2.1
Standard with hospitalization			
Per cure	215	301	270
Per direct death averted	187	272	227
Per total death averted	54	76	68
Per year of life	2.4	3.4	3.1
Ambulatory short course[d]			
Per cure	107	81	101
Per direct death averted	130	94	117
Per total death averted	25	20	23
Per year of life	1.1	0.9	1.1
Ambulatory standard[d]			
Per cure	111	82	107
Per direct death averted	96	74	90
Per total death averted	28	21	27
Per year of life	1.3	0.9	1.2

[a] Source: Murray et al. (1993).

[b] In 1989 dollars.

[c] For Malawi, the estimates of standard chemotherapy with hospitalization, ambulatory standard chemotherapy, and ambulatory short-course chemotherapy are not based on actual program results but on estimates of the likely cost of ambulatory chemotherapy. Results of treatment are the average results achieved in Tanzania and Mozambique.

[d] The results for ambulatory treatment are based on the overall results of the programs for each country, not on specific results for ambulatory chemotherapy. As such, they are applicable only to those urban areas where high compliance can be maintained with daily supervised chemotherapy in the intensive phase.

discussed above, the criteria for both diagnosis and effective therapy are less objective. Cost-effectiveness can be discussed only in hypothetical terms, using realistic values from a variety of studies for the key parameters. Four factors are the major determinants of the cost-effectiveness of chemotherapy for smear-negative pulmonary tuberculosis: the positive predictive value of X-ray diagnosis, the case-fatality rate of untreated smear-negative cases or X-ray-suggestive cases, the effective cure rate of chemotherapy, and perhaps most important, the percentage of X-ray-suggestive tuberculosis cases that would progress to smear-positive tuberculosis if left untreated. Using the average program unit cost for ambulatory therapy in Malawi, Mozambique, and Tanzania and a cheap short-course regimen for smear-negative

patients costing $16 per course, we will calculate the hypothetical cost-effectiveness. We will assume a positive predictive value of 50% for active disease detected on X ray. The true value will be locally specific and could well range between 25 and 75%. For true smear-negative cases, we will assume a case-fatality rate of 40%. Because the regimen proposed is ambulatory and the symptoms of smear-negative tuberculosis are often less severe, we will assume that the effective cure rate would be on the order of 50%. With this set of assumptions, the cost per death averted is $450, or nearly 10 times the cost per death averted for short-course chemotherapy with hospitalization for smear-positive patients and 20 times the cost for ambulatory short-course therapy.

If a percentage of smear-negative cases

do not progress to become smear positive, then the costs of treating smear-negative patients are nearly an order of magnitude greater than that of treating smear-positive patients. However, on the basis of the Bangalore data, we expect that at least 10 to 15% of patients would progress to become smear positive. Treating smear-negative patients who go on to become smear positive cuts out the prediagnosis transmission that cannot be affected with chemotherapy for smear-positive patients. This prediagnosis transmission bonus accounts for nearly one-fifth of total transmission. If 15% of cases progress to become smear positive, the cost per death averted by treating smear-negative patients is reduced to $185; the cost is $155 if 20% become infectious. This is still 3.5 to 8 times more expensive than treating smear-positive patients. However, in comparison to many other health sector interventions, this is relatively inexpensive per death averted or year of life saved. If the positive predictive value of X-ray diagnosis can be increased to 70%, if the cure rate can be increased to 65, and if 20% of cases go on to be smear negative, then the cost per death averted could be as low as $85.

CONCLUSIONS

Operational research will continue to be critical to the success of tuberculosis control. While substantial progress has been made in developing a successful control strategy with short-course chemotherapy, many issues remain to be addressed in order to achieve success in assessment and design of more effective control strategies. Four broad topics may be summarized as follows.

Burden of Tuberculosis

Tuberculin skin test results have been successfully utilized to estimate the annual risk of infection and, from this, tuberculosis

incidence and mortality. Locality-specific operational research remains necessary to estimate the burden of tuberculosis and to convince decision makers of its rising severity. One neglected research area is the incidence of tuberculosis in young women.

BCG Immunization

Varying results from controlled trials of BCG leave the vaccine's efficacy controversial. Research could perhaps shed light on the range of factors influencing the vaccine's effectiveness and could supplement the scant existing data on the efficacy of revaccination in adolescents.

Chemoprophylaxis

While the direct effects of tuberculosis chemoprophylaxis are clear, the importance of its indirect effect of decreasing transmission (as opposed to decreasing prevalence of disease) will remain unclear until data are obtained on transmission before the onset of disease. Given the risk of isoniazid-related hepatitis, chemoprophylaxis may not be beneficial to all infected individuals. Decision analysis studies have weighed the risk of hepatitis against the direct benefits of chemoprophylaxis, i.e., reduced incidence of disease in infected individuals. Most of these studies, however, have not addressed the indirect benefit, i.e., reduced transmission, which in some developing countries may surpass the direct benefits. Cost-effectiveness analyses hint that chemoprophylaxis is feasible only for certain high-risk groups, such as HIV-positive patients. Research on transmission and cost-effectiveness, particularly on cost-effectiveness of chemoprophylaxis for cases of tuberculosis and HIV coinfection, is needed.

Case Identification and Treatment

While methods of detection for individuals are established, there is not a consensus among decision makers on population-based detection. Operational research is needed to determine a cost-effective diagnostic algorithm for screening, to select between passive and active screening strategies, and to investigate the nature and prevention of diagnostic delay. Several issues in treatment require further research. While some consensus exists on treatment regimens, further research is required for generating effective regimens of less than 6 months and for treating MDR cases as well as tuberculosis in HIV coinfected cases. The fundamental challenge for research here is to increase patient compliance, about which most data are from small-scale or questionable studies. Several successful programs in developing countries indicate that supervision of chemotherapy is the best method for reducing noncompliance. Cost-effectiveness studies indicate that short-course regimens are less expensive than full regimens for sputum smear-positive cases. Additional research is needed in estimating cost-effectiveness of treatments for smear-negative cases, which are significantly more expensive than treatments for smear-positive cases.

REFERENCES

Acuna, D., X. Ferrer, B. Galvez, L. Mujica, L. M. Maureira, A. Soto, and L. Rojas. 1981. Tuberculosis pulmonar: tiempo transcurrido entre el inicio de los sintomas respiratorios y el tratamiento. *Rev. Med. Chile* 109:628–633.

Alcabes, P., P. Vossenas, R. Cohen, C. Braslow, D. Michaels, and S. Zoloth. 1989. Compliance with isoniazid chemoprophylaxis in jail. *Am. Rev. Respir. Dis.* 140:1194–1197.

Allan, W. G., D. J. Girling, P. M. Fayers, and W. Fox. 1979. The symptoms of newly diagnosed pulmonary tuberculosis and patients' attitudes to the disease and to its treatment in Hong Kong. *Tubercle* 60:211–223.

Alland, D., G. E. Kalkut, A. Moss, R. A. McAdam, J. A. Hahn, W. Bosworth, E. Drucker, and B. R. Bloom. 1994. *Transmission of Tuberculosis in New York City: an Analysis by DNA Fingerprinting and Conventional Epidemiological Methods.* Montefiore Medical Center, New York.

Aluoch, J. A., E. A. Edwards, and H. Stott. 1982. A fourth study of case finding methods for pulmonary tuberculosis in Kenya. *Trans. R. Soc. Trop. Med. Hyg.* 76:679–691.

Aluoch, J. A., K. H. Karuga, and H. Nsanzumuhire. 1978. A second study of the use of community leaders in case-finding for pulmonary tuberculosis in Kenya. *Tubercle* 59:223.

Aluoch, J. A., D. Oyoo, O. B. Swai, and D. Kwamanga. 1987. A study of the use of maternity and child welfare clinics in case-finding for pulmonary tuberculosis in Kenya. *Tubercle* 68:93–103.

Aluoch, J. A., O. B. Swai, and E. A. Edwards. 1984. Study of case-finding for pulmonary tuberculosis in outpatients complaining of a chronic cough at a district hospital in Kenya. *Am. Rev. Respir. Dis.* 129:915–920.

Aluoch, J. A., O. B. Swai, E. A. Edwards, H. Stott, J. H. Darbyshire, W. Fox, and R. J. Stephens. 1985. Studies of case-finding for pulmonary tuberculosis in outpatients at 4 district hospitals in Kenya. *Tubercle* 66:237–249.

American Thoracic Society. 1993. Initial therapy for tuberculosis in the era of multidrug resistance. Recommendations of the Advisory Council for the elimination of tuberculosis. *Morbid. Mortal. Weekly Rep.* 42(RR-7):1–8.

American Thoracic Society-Centers for Disease Control. 1990. Diagnostic standards and classification of tuberculosis. *Am. Rev. Respir. Dis.* 142:725–735.

Andersen, S., and A. Geser. 1960. The distribution of tuberculous infection among households in African communities. *Bull. W.H.O.* 22:39–60.

Aoki, M., T. Mori, and M. Matsuzaki. 1982. Studies on patient's delay, doctor's delay and total delay of tuberculosis case-finding in Japan, p. 115–127. *In Tuberculosis Surveillance Research Unit of the IUAT. Progress Report 1982.* The Hague.

Armstrong, R. H., and D. Pringle. 1984. Compliance with anti-tuberculosis chemotherapy in Harare City. *Central Afr. J. Med.* 30:144–148.

Attonucci, G., E. Girardi, O. Armgnacco, S. Salmaso, and G. Ippulito. 1992. Tuberculosis in HIV-infected subjects in Italy: a multicentre study. *AIDS* 6:1007–1013.

Baas, M. A., H. A. van Geuns, H. S. Hellinga, J. Meijer, and K. Styblo. 1983. Surveillance of diagnostic and treatment measures of bacillary pulmonary tuberculosis reported in the Netherlands from 1973 to 1976. *Sel. Pap.* 22:41–80.

Baily, G. V. J., D. Savic, G. D. Gothi, V. B. Naidu, and S. S. Nair. 1967. Potential yield of pulmonary tuberculosis cases by direct microscopy of sputum in a district of South India. *Bull. W.H.O.* 37:875–892.

Banerji, D., and S. Andersen. 1963. A sociological study of awareness of symptoms among persons with pulmonary tuberculosis. *Bull. W.H.O.* **29**:665–683.

Barnhoorn, F., and H. Adrianase. 1992. In search of factors responsible for noncompliance among tuberculosis patients in Wardha district, India. *Soc. Sci. Med.* **34**:291–306.

Barnum, H., and E. R. Greenberg. 1993. Cancers, p. 529–560. *In* D. Jamison, W. H. Mosley, A. R. Measham, and J. L. Bobadilla (ed.), *Disease Control Priorities in Developing Countries.* Oxford University Press, Oxford.

Barnum, H. N. 1986. Cost savings from alternative treatments for tuberculosis. *Soc. Sci. Med.* **23**:847–850.

Barnum, H. N., D. Tarantola, and I. F. Setaidy. 1980. Cost-effectiveness of an immunization programme in Indonesia. *Bull. W.H.O.* **58**:499–503.

Bell, J., and D. Yach. 1988. Tuberculosis patient compliance in the western cape. *S. Afr. Med. J.* **73**:31–33.

Berg, G. 1939. *The Prognosis of Open Pulmonary Tuberculosis. A Clinical-Statistical Analysis.* Acta Tuberculosea, Scandinavica Supplementum IV.

Black, M., J. R. Mitchell, H. J. Zimmerman, K. G. Ishak, and G. P. Epler. 1975. Isoniazid-associated hepatitis in 114 patients. *Gastroenterology* **69**:289–302.

Bleiker, M. A., I. Sutherland, K. Styblo, H. G. Ten Dam, and O. Misljenovic. 1989. Guidelines for estimating the risks of tuberculous infection from tuberculin test results in a representative sample of children. *Bull. Int. Union Tuberc. Lung Dis.* **64**:7–12.

Bloom, B. R. 1989. Vaccines for the Third World, *Nature* (London) **342**:115–120.

Bloom, B. R. 1989. An ordinary mortal's guide to the molecular biology of tuberculosis. *Bull. Int. Union Tuberc. Lung Dis.* **64**:50–58.

Bloom, B. R., and C. J. L. Murray. 1992. Tuberculosis: commentary on a reemergent killer. *Science* **257**:1055–1064.

Brudney, K., and J. Dobkin. 1991. Resurgent tuberculosis in New York City—human immunodeficiency virus, homelessness, and the decline of tuberculosis control programs. *Am. Rev. Respir. Dis.* **144**:745–749.

Burkhardt, K. R., and E. E. Nel. 1980. Monitoring regularity of drug intake in tuberculosis patients by means of simple urine tests. *S. Afr. Med. J.* **57**:981–985.

Canetti, G. 1939. *Les Reinfections Tuberculeuses Latentes du Poumon.* Vigot Edit, Paris.

Canetti, G. 1972. Endogenous reactivation and exogenous reinfection. Their relative importance with regard to development of non-primary tuberculosis. *Bull. Int. Union Tuberc.* **47**:116–122.

Cauthen, G. M., A. Pio, and H. G. ten Dam. 1988.

Annual Risk of Tuberculous Infection. Publication no. WHO/TB/88.154. World Health Organization, Geneva.

Cheung, R., J. Dickens, P. W. Nicholson, A. S. C. Thomas, H. Hillas Smith, H. E. Larson, A. A. Deshmukh, R. J. Dobbs, and S. M. Dobbs. 1988. Compliance with anti-tuberculosis therapy: a field trial of a pill box with a concealed electronic recording device. *Eur. J. Clin. Pharmacol.* **35**:401–407.

Chiba, Y. 1959. *Development of Tuberculosis.* Hekendojinsha, Tokyo.

Chonde, T. M. 1989. The role of bacteriological services in the national tuberculosis and leprosy programme in Tanzania. *Bull. Int. Union Tuberc. Lung Dis.* **64**:37–39.

Chowdhury, A. M. R., A. Alam, S. A. Chowdhury, and J. Ahmed. 1992. Tuberculosis control in Bangladesh. *Lancet* **339**:1181–1182.

Chum, H. J., K. Styblo, and M. R. A. van Cleef. 1987. Eight-years' experience of the National Tuberculosis and Leprosy Programme in Tanzania. *In XXVI IUAT World Conference on Tuberculosis and Respiratory Diseases.* Professional Post Graduate Services, Tokyo.

Clemens, J. D., J. J. H. Chung, and A. R. Feinstein. 1983. The BCG controversy. A methodological and statistical reappraisal. *JAMA* **249**:2362–2369.

Cohn, D. L., B. J. Catlin, K. L. Peterson, H. N. Judson, and J. A. Sbarbaro. 1990. A 62-dose, 6-month therapy for pulmonary and extrapulmonary tuberculosis. *Ann. Intern. Med.* **112**:407–415.

Colditz, G. A., T. Brewer, C. Berky, M. Wilson, E. Burdick, H. V. Fineberg, and F. Mosteller. 1993. *The Efficacy of BCG in the Prevention of Tuberculosis: Meta-Analyses of the Published Literature.* Technology Assessment Group, Harvard School of Public Health, Boston.

Colice, G. L. 1990. Decision analysis, public health policy, and isoniazid chemoprophylaxis for young adult tuberculin skin reactors. *Arch. Intern. Med.* **150**:2517–2522.

Comstock, G. W., and P. Q. Edwards. 1975. The competing risks of tuberculosis and hepatitis for adult tuberculin reactors. *Am. Rev. Respir. Dis.* **111**:573–577.

Davidson, P. T. 1990. Treating tuberculosis: what drugs, for how long? *Ann. Intern. Med.* **112**:393–395.

D'Esopo, N. D. 1982. Clinical trials in pulmonary tuberculosis. *Am. Rev. Respir. Dis.* **125**(Suppl.):85–93.

East African and British Medical Research Council. 1977. Tuberculosis in Tanzania: a follow-up of a National Sampling Survey of drug resistance and other factors. *Tubercle* **58**:55–78.

East African and British Medical Research Council. 1979. Tuberculosis in Kenya: follow-up of the Second National Sampling Survey and a comparison with the follow-up data from the First (1964) National Sampling Survey. *Tubercle* **60**:125–149.

Farmer, P. H., S. Robin, S. L. Ramilus, and J. Y. Kim. 1991. Tuberculosis, poverty and "compliance": lessons from rural Haiti. *Semin. Respir. Infect.* **6**:254–260.

Feldstein, M. S., M. A. Piot, and T. K. Sundaresan. 1973. Resource allocation model for public health planning. A case study of tuberculosis control. *Bull. W.H.O.* **48**(Suppl.):1–110.

Ferebee, S. H. 1969. Controlled chemoprophylaxis trials in tuberculosis: a general review. *Adv. Tuberc. Res.* **17**:29–106.

Fine, P. E. M. 1988. BCG vaccination against tuberculosis and leprosy. *Br. Med. Bull.* **44**:704–716.

Fischl, M. A., G. L. Daikos, and R. B. Uttamchandani. 1992. Clinical presentation and outcome of patients with HIV infection and tuberculosis caused by multi-drug-resistant bacilla. *Ann. Intern. Med.* **17**:184–190.

Fox, W. 1983a. Compliance of patients and physicians: experience and lessons from tuberculosis. I. *Br. Med. J.* **287**:33–35.

Fox, W. 1983b. Compliance of patients and physicians: experience and lessons from tuberculosis. II. *Br. Med. J.* **287**:101–105.

Fox, W. 1985. Short-course chemotherapy for pulmonary tuberculosis and some problems of its programme application with particular reference to India. *Bull. Int. Union Tuberc.* **60**:40–49.

Grzybowski, S., K. Styblo, and E. Dorken. 1976. Tuberculosis in Eskimos. *Tubercle* **57**(Suppl.):1–58.

Haynes, R. B. 1979. Determinants of compliance: the disease and mechanics of treatment, p. 46–92. *In* R. B. Haynes, D. W. Taylor, and D. L. Sackett (ed.), *Compliance in Health Care.* Johns Hopkins University Press, Baltimore.

Haynes, R. B., D. W. Taylor, and D. L. Sackett (ed.). 1979. *Compliance in Health Care.* The Johns Hopkins University Press, Baltimore.

Hong Kong Chest Service, British Medical Research Council. 1991. Controlled trial of 2, 4, and 6 months of pyrazinamide in 6-month, three-times-weekly regimens for smear-positive pulmonary tuberculosis, including an assessment of a combined preparation of isoniazid, rifampin, and pyrazinamide. *Am. Rev. Respir. Dis.* **143**:700–706.

Hong Kong Chest Service, Tuberculosis Research Centre, Madras, British Medical Research Council. 1984. A controlled trial of 2-month, 3-month and 12-month regimens of chemotherapy for sputum smear-negative pulmonary tuberculosis. *Am. Rev. Respir. Dis.* **130**:23–28.

Hong Kong Chest Service, Tuberculosis Research Centre, Madras, British Medical Research Council. 1989. A controlled trial of 3-month, 4-month, and 6-month regimens of chemotherapy for sputum-smear-negative pulmonary tuberculosis. Results at 5 years. *Am. Rev. Respir. Dis.* **139**:871–876.

Horwitz, O., E. Wilbek, and P. A. Erickson. 1969. Epidemiological basis of tuberculosis eradication. *Bull. W.H.O.* **41**:95.

Huebner, R. E., M. F. Schein, and J. B. Bass. 1993. The tuberculin skin test. *Clin. Infect. Dis.* **17**:968–975.

International Union Against Tuberculosis Committee on Prophylaxis. 1982. Efficacy of various durations of isoniazid preventive therapy for tuberculosis: five years of follow-up in the IUAT trial. *Bull. W.H.O.* **60**:555–564.

Iseman, M. D., D. L. Cohn, and J. A. Sbarbaro. 1993. Directly observed treatment of tuberculosis. *N. Engl. J. Med.* **328**:576–578.

Jamison, D. T., W. H. Mosley, A. R. Measham, and J. L. Bobadilla (ed.). 1993. *Disease Control Priorities in Developing Countries.* Oxford University Press, New York.

Joesoef, M. R., P. L. Remington, and P. Tjiptoherijanto. 1989. Epidemiological model and cost-effectiveness analysis of tuberculosis treatment programmes in Indonesia. *Int. J. Epidemiol.* **18**:174–179.

Jordan, T. J., E. M. Lewit, R. L. Montgomery, and L. B. Reichman. 1991a. Isoniazid as preventive therapy in HIV-infected intravenous drug abusers. A decision analysis. *JAMA* **265**:2987–2991.

Jordan, T. J., E. M. Lewit, and L. B. Reichman. 1991b. Isoniazid preventive therapy for tuberculosis. Decision analysis, considering ethnicity and gender. *Am. Rev. Respir. Dis.* **144**:1357–1360.

Kopanoff, D. E., D. E. Snider, and G. J. Caras. 1978. Isoniazid-related hepatitis: a US Public Health Service Cooperative Surveillance Study. *Am. Rev. Respir. Dis.* **117**:991–1001.

Le, C. T. 1984. Cost-effectiveness of two-step skin test for tuberculosis screening of employees in a community hospital. *Infect. Control* **5**:570–572.

Lincoln, N. S., E. B. Bosworth, and D. W. Alling. 1954. The after-history of pulmonary tuberculosis. III. Minimal tuberculosis. *Am. Rev. Respir. Dis.* **70**:15–31.

Maganu, E. T., M. R. Moeti, P. Khulumani, B. S. Koosimile, and C. Sentle. 1990. *The Annual Risk of Tuberculosis Infection in Botswana. Report of a survey, 1989.* Ministry of Health, Gabarone.

Meijer, J., G. D. Barnett, A. Kubik, and K. Styblo. 1971. Identification of sources of infection. *Bull. Int. Union Tuberc.* **45**:5–50.

Meyer, N. 1949. *Statistical Investigation of the Relationship of Tuberculosis Morbidity and Mortality to Infection.* Munksgaard, Copenhagen.

Ministry of Health and Family Welfare, India. 1986.

Health Atlas of India, 1986. Directorate General of Health Services, New Delhi.

Miles, S. H., and R. B. Maat. 1984. A successful supervised outpatient short-course tuberculosis treatment program in an open refugee camp on the Thai-Cambodian border. *Am. Rev. Respir. Dis.* **130:** 827–830.

Moodie, A. S. 1967. Mass ambulatory chemotherapy in the treatment of tuberculosis in a predominantly urban community. *Am. Rev. Respir. Dis.* **95:**384–397.

Mori, T. 1982. Validity of delays as indices for effectiveness of case-finding, p. 98–107. *In Tuberculosis Surveillance Research Unit of the IUAT. Progress report, 1982.* International Union Against Tuberculosis, The Hague.

Mori, T., T. Shimao, B. W. Jin, and S. J. Kim. 1992. Analysis of case-finding process of tuberculosis in Korea. *Tuberc. Lung Dis.* **73:**225–231.

Moriskey, D. E., C. K. Malotte, P. Choi, P. Davidson, S. Rigler, B. Sugland, and M. Langer. 1990. A patient education program to improve adherence rates with antituberculosis drug regimens. *Health Educ. Q.* **15:**253–267.

Moulding, T. S., A. G. Redeker, and G. C. Kanel. 1989. Twenty isoniazid-associated deaths in one state. *Am. Rev. Respir. Dis.* **140:**700–705.

Murray, C. J. L., E. DeJonghe, H. G. Chum, D. S. Nyangulu, A. Salomao, and K. Styblo. 1994. Cost-effectiveness of chemotherapy for pulmonary tuberculosis in three sub-Saharan African countries. *Lancet* **338:**1305–1308.

Murray, C. J. L., and A. D. Lopez. 1994. Quantifying the burden of disability: data, methods, and results. *Bull. W.H.O.* **73**.

Murray, C. J. L., K. Styblo, and A. Rouillon. 1990. Tuberculosis in developing countries: burden, intervention and cost. *Bull. Int. Union Tuberc. Lung Dis.* **65:**2–20.

Murray, C. J. L., K. Styblo, and A. Rouillon. 1993. Tuberculosis, p. 233–260. *In* D. Jamison, W. H. Mosley, A. R. Measham, and J. B. Bobadilla (ed.), *Disease Control Priorities in Developing Countries.* Oxford University Press, Oxford.

Nagpaul, D. R., M. K. Vishwanath, and G. Dwarakanath. 1970. A socio-epidemiological study of outpatients attending a city tuberculosis clinic in India to judge the place of specialized centres in a tuberculosis control programme. *Bull. W.H.O.* **43:**17–34.

Nair, S. S., et al. 1976. *Indian J. Tuberc.* **23:**152.

Narain, R., K. Naganna, P. Chandrasekhar, and L. Pyare. 1970. Crude mortality by size of tuberculin reaction. *Am. Rev. Respir. Dis.* **101:**897–906.

Narain, R., S. S. Nair, K. Naganna, P. Chandrasekhar, G. Ramanatha Rao, and P. Lal. 1968. Problems in defining a "case" of pulmonary tuberculosis in prevalence surveys. *Bull. W.H.O.* **39:**701–729.

Narayan, R., S. Prabhakar, S. Thomas, and P. Kumari. 1979. A sociological study of awareness of symptoms and action taking of persons with pulmonary tuberculosis (a resurvey). *Indian J. Tuberc.* **26:**136–146.

National Tuberculosis Institute, Bangalore. 1974. Tuberculosis in a rural population of India: a five-year epidemiological study. *Bull. W.H.O.* **51:**473–488.

Nsanzumuhire, H., E. W. Lukwago, and E. A. Edwards. 1977. A study of the use of community leaders in case-finding for pulmonary tuberculosis in the Machakos district of Kenya. *Tubercle* **58:**117–128.

Nsanzumuhire, H., J. A. Aluoch, and W. K. Karuga. 1981. A third study of case-finding methods for pulmonary tuberculosis in Kenya, including the use of community leaders. *Tubercle* **62:**79–94.

Nunn, P., R. Brindle, L. Carpenter, J. Odhiambo, K. Wasunna, R. Newnham, W. Githui, S. Gathua, M. Omwega, and K. McAdam. 1992. Cohort study of human immunodeficiency virus infection in patients with tuberculosis in Nairobi, Kenya. *Am. Rev. Respir. Dis.* **146:**849–854.

Nyboe, J. 1957. Interpretation of tuberculous infection age curves. *Bull. W.H.O.* **17:**319–339.

Olakowski, T. 1973. *Assignment Report on a Tuberculosis Longitudinal Survey, National Tuberculosis Institute, Bangalore.* Publication no. SEA/TB/129. World Health Organization Regional Office for South East Asia, Manila, Philippines.

Pape, J. W., S. S. Jean, J. L. Ho, A. Hafner, and W. D. Johnson. 1993. Effect of isoniazid prophylaxis on incidence of active tuberculosis and progression of HIV infection. *Lancet* **342:**268–272.

Perriens, J. H., R. L. Colebunders, and C. Karahunga. 1991. Increased mortality and tuberculosis treatment failure rate among human immunodeficiency virus (HIV) seropositive compared with HIV seronegative patients with pulmonary tuberculosis treated with 'standard' chemotherapy in Kinshasa, Zaire. *Am. Rev. Respir. Dis.* **144:**750–755.

Pozniak, A., G. MacLeod, M. Maheri, W. Legg, and J. Weinberg. 1992. The influence of HIV status on single and multiple drug reactions to antituberculosis therapy in Africa. *AIDS* **6:**809–814.

Raviglione, M. C., P. Sudre, S. Spinaci, and A. Kochi. 1993. Secular trends of tuberculosis in Western Europe. *Bull. W.H.O.* **71:**295–306.

Reichman, L. B. 1987. Compliance in developed nations. *Tubercle* **68:**25–29.

Research Institute of Tuberculosis, Japan. 1993. *Tuberculosis Statistics in the World, 1993.* Research Institute of Tuberculosis, Tokyo.

Rodrigues, L. C., and P. G. Smith. 1990. Tuberculosis in developing countries and methods for its control. *Trans. R. Soc. Trop. Med. Hyg.* **84:**739–744.

Roelsgaard, E., E. Iverson, and C. Blocher. 1964.

Tuberculosis in tropical Africa—an epidemiological study. *Bull. W.H.O.* **30**:459–518.

Rojas, C., and O. Lanza. 1989. *Consideraciones sobre la Eficiencia de Intervenciones en Diferentes Periodes de la Evolucion de Tuberuclosis, previos a la Quimoterapia.* Accion Internacional Para la Salud, La Paz, Bolivia.

Rose, D. N., C. B. Schechter, M. L. Fahs, and A. L. Silver. 1988. Tuberculosis prevention: cost-effectiveness analysis of isoniazid chemoprophylaxis. *Am. J. Preventive Med.* **4**:102–109.

Rose, D. N., D. B. Schechter, and A. L. Silver. 1986. The age threshold for isoniazid chemoprophylaxis: a decision analysis for low-risk tuberculin reactors. *JAMA* **256**:2709–2713.

Rouillon, A., S. Perdrizet, and R. Parrot. 1976. Transmission of tubercelle bacilli: the effects of chemotherapy. *Tubercle* **57**:275–299.

Rubel, A. J., and L. C. Garro. 1992. Social and cultural factors in the successful control of tuberculosis. *Public Health Rep.* **107**:626–636.

Sbarbaro, J. A. 1979. Compliance: inducements and enforcements. *Chest* **76**(Suppl.):750–756.

Seetha, M. A., N. Srikantaramu, K. S. Aneja, and H. Singh. 1981. Influence of motivation of patients with their family members on the drug collection by patients. *Indian J. Tuberc.* **28**:182–190.

Selwyn, P. A., D. Harteri, V. A. Lewis, E. E. Schoenbaum, S. H. Vermund, R. S. Klein, A. T. Walker, and G. H. Friedland. 1989. A prospective study of the risk of tuberculosis among intravenous drug users with human immunodeficiency virus infection. *N. Engl. J. Med.* **320**:545–550.

Selwyn, P. A., B. M. Sckell, and P. Alcabes. 1992. High risk of active tuberculosis in HIV-infected drug users with cutaneous anergy. *JAMA* **268**:504–509.

Sepulveda, R. L., C. Parcha, and R. U. Sorensen. 1992. Case control study of the efficacy of BCG immunization against pulmonary tuberculosis in young adults in Santiago, Chile. *Tubercle Lung Dis.* **73**:372–377.

Small, P. M., R. W. Shafer, P. C. Hopewell, S. P. Singh, M. J. Murphy, E. Desmond, M. F. Sierra, and G. K. Schoolnik. 1993. Exogenous reinfection with multidrug-resistant mycobacterium tuberculosis in patients with advanced HIV infection. *N. Engl. J. Med.* **328**:1137–1144.

Snider, D. E., G. J. Caras, and J. P. Koplan. 1986. Preventive therapy with isoniazid. Cost-effectiveness of different durations of therapy. *JAMA* **255**:1579–1583.

Stover, C. K., V. F. de la Cruz, G. P. Bansal, M. S. Hanson, T. R. Fuerst, W. R. Jacobs, and B. R. Bloom. 1992. Use of recombinant BCG as a vaccine delivery vehicle. *Adv. Exp. Med. Biol.* **327**:175–182.

Styblo, K. 1984. *Epidemiology of Tuberculosis.* VEB Gustav Fischer Verlag Jena, The Hague.

Styblo, K. 1985. The relationship between the risk of tuberculosis infection and the risk of developing infectious tuberculosis. *Bull. Int. Union Tuberc.* **60**:117–119.

Styblo, K. 1991. *Epidemiology of Tuberculosis.* Royal Netherlands Tuberculosis Association, The Hague.

Styblo, K., D. Dankova, and J. Drapela. 1967. Epidemiological and clinical study of tuberculosis in the district of Kolin, Czechoslovakia. *Bull. W.H.O.* **37**:819–874.

Styblo, K., D. Dankova, J. Drapela, J. Galliova, Z. Jezek, J. Krivanek, A. Kubik, M. Langerova, and J. Radkovsky. 1969a. Epidemiological and clinical study of tuberculosis in the district of Kolin, Czechoslovakia. *Bull. W.H.O.* **37**:819–874.

Styblo, K., and J. Meijer. 1976. Impact of BCG vaccination programmes in children and young adults on the tuberculosis problem. *Tubercle* **57**:17–43.

Styblo, K., and J. Meijer. 1980. The quantified increase of the tuberculosis infection rate in a low prevalence country to be expected if the existing MMR programme were discontinued. *Bull. Int. Union Tuberc.* **55**:3–8.

Styblo, K., J. Meijer, and I. Sutherland. 1969b. The transmission of tubercle bacilli, its trend in a human population, TSRU. *Bull. Int. Union Tuberc.* **42**:5–105.

Sudre, P., G. Ten Dam, and A. Kochi. 1992. Tuberculosis: a global overview of the situation today. *Bull. W.H.O.* **70**:149–159.

Sumartojo, E. 1993. When tuberculosis treatment fails: a social behavioral account of patient adherence. *Am. Rev. Respir. Dis.* **147**:1311–1320.

Sutherland, I. 1971. The effect of tuberculin reversion upon the estimate of the annual risk of tuberculosis infection. *Bull. Int. Union Tuberc.* **45**:115–118.

Sutherland, I. 1976. Recent studies in the epidemiology of tuberculosis based on the risk of being infected with tubercle bacilli. *Adv. Tuberc. Res.* **19**:1–63.

Sutherland, I. 1991. On the risk of infection. *Bull. Int. Union Tuberc.* **66**:189–91.

Sutherland, I., and P. M. Fayers. 1975. The association of the risk of tuberculosis infection with age. *Bull. Int. Union Tuberc.* **50**:70–81.

Tabilo, F., M. D. Casasempere, and A. Guzman. 1987. TBC pulmonar: intervalos entre consulta, diagnostico y tratamiento servicio de salud metropolitano sur-oriente. *Bol. Epidemiol. Chile* **14**:33–40.

Taylor, W. C., M. D. Aronson, and T. L. Delbanco. 1981. Should young adults with a positive tuberculin test take isoniazid? *Ann. Intern. Med.* **94**:808–813.

Ten Dam, H. G., and K. L. Hitze. 1980. Does BCG vaccination protect the newborn and young infants? *Bull. W.H.O.* **58**:37–41.

Toman, K. 1979. *Tuberculosis Case-Finding and Chemotherapy.* World Health Organization, Geneva.

Tsevat, J., W. C. Taylor, J. B. Wong, and S. G. Pauker. 1988. Isoniazid for the tuberculin reactor: take it or leave it. *Am. Rev. Respir. Dis.* **137:**215–220.

Tuberculosis Research Centre, Madras, and National Tuberculosis Institute, Bangalore. 1986. A controlled clinical trial of 3- and 5-month regimens in the treatment of sputum-positive pulmonary tuberculosis in South India. *Am. Rev. Respir. Dis.* **134:**27–33.

Tuberculosis Surveillance Research Unit. 1966. *Progress Report.* International Union Against Tuberculosis, The Hague

Valeza, F. S., and A. C. McDougall. 1990. Blister calendar packs of treatment of tuberculosis. *Lancet* **335:**473.

van Geuns, H. A., J. Meijer, and K. Styblo. 1975. Results of contact examination in Rotterdam. *Bull. Int. Union Tuberc.* **50:**107–121.

Wobeser, W., T. To, and V. H. Hoeppner. 1989. The outcome of chemoprophylaxis on tuberculosis prevention in the Canadian Plains Indian. *Clin. Invest. Med.* **12:**149–153.

World Health Organization. 1963. *The WHO Standard Tuberculin Test.* World Health Organization, Geneva.

World Health Organization. 1974. *WHO Expert Committee on Tuberculosis, Ninth Report.* Technical report series 552. World Health Organization, Geneva.

World Health Organization. 1992. *Proposed Tuberculosis Control Programme Work Plan and Budget: 1992–1993.* World Health Organization, Geneva.

World Health Organization. 1993. *Managing Tuberculosis at District Level. A Training Course.* World Health Organization, Geneva.

World Health Organization Tuberculosis Chemotherapy Centre. 1963. Drug acceptability in domiciliary tuberculosis control programmes. *Bull. W.H.O.* **29:** 627–639.

Index

ABC transporter, 345
Abdominal tuberculosis, 42–43
Access control, laboratory, 68–69, 86
AccuProbe, 97–98, 100
Acetyl coenzyme A, 354, 356
N-Acetylglucosamine-phosphoryl-polyprenol, 372
Acid-fast staining procedure, 91
Acquired immunity, 20–21, 114
Acquired resistance, 389–415, 476–477
Active transport, 344–349
Acyl carrier protein, 376
Acyl-CoA carboxylase, 378
Adenopathy, 28, 30–31
S-Adenosylmethionine, 375–376
Adjuvant, 494, 496, 549
Adoptive transfer, 114, 142, 448
Adrenal dysfunction, 492
Aeration, culture of M. tuberculosis, 74, 78–80
Africa, 5, 15–16, 51–57, 503–513, 583–621
Agarase gene, 264
Agar-based medium, 77, 94
Age
    distribution of smear-positive tuberculosis, 588
    extrapulmonary tuberculosis and, 33
    incidence of tuberculosis and, 9–10, 56
    prevalence of infection and, 585–587
Agitation, culture of M. tuberculosis, 78–82
AIDS, see Human immunodeficiency virus infection
Airborne transmission, 18, 48–49, 472
    guinea pig model, 137
    laboratory, 61–71
L-Alanine dehydrogenase, 315, 317
Alkaline lysis procedure, 187–188
Alkaline phosphatase reporter gene, 264
α antigen, 245, 420, 425
Amikacin, 560
Amino acids
    biosynthesis, 314–315
    D isomers, 346
    metabolism, 356
    transport, 343, 346–347
Aminoglycosides
    resistance, 342–343
    self-promoted uptake, 341–342
5-Aminolevulinate synthase, 399
p-Aminosalicylic acid (PAS), 367
    mechanism of action, 369, 560
    movement into cells, 340
    resistance, 342
    structure, 560
Ammonia, production by M. tuberculosis, 393–394, 406, 488
Anemia, 27, 35
Anergy, 54–55, 419, 428, 443–444, 491–494, 508, 585, 598
Animal model

guinea pig, 135–147
historical aspects, 20
inoculation of animals, 78
mouse, 113–134
rabbit, 149–156
Annual risk of infection, 4, 585, 587, 590
Antibody detection tests, 518
Antibody response, 451
    genetics, 441–442
Antigen(s)
    identification and isolation, 518
        classic methods, 309–310
        monoclonal antibodies and recombinant DNA techniques, 310–311
        M. tuberculosis, 307–332, 424–426, 438–441, 493–494, 549
    recognition by T cells, 420
    strategies for selection, 311–314
    T-cell, 402–403
Antigen 5, 446
Antigen 6, see α antigen
Antigen bank, 311, 549
Antigen 85 complex, 245, 325–326, 425, 440–441, 444
Antiport, 344–345
β-D-Arabinofuranosyl-1-phosphodecaprenol, 289
Arabinogalactan, 275, 279, 293, 296–297, 333–335, 377, 561–562
    attachment of mycolic acids, 276, 373–376
    metabolism, 371–373
Arabinomannan, 298, 562
L-Arginine-dependent cytotoxic mechanism, 406
aroA gene, 314–315
Arteritis, 41
Arthritis, adjuvant, 449–450
Ascitic fluid, 42
AsnI restriction profile, 229
Atelectasis, 29, 473
ATP production, 354, 356
Attenuated Mycobacterium tuberculosis vaccine, 547–548
Attenuation indicator lipid, 286, 291
Atypical mycobacteria, see Environmental mycobacteria
Auramine O stain, 91–92
Autoimmune disease, 449–450, 495–497
Autopsy findings, tuberculosis in HIV-infected patient, 505–506
Auxotrophic mutants, 262–263
    in vivo expression assay, 265–266
Auxotrophic vaccine, 548
Avirulent mutants, see Virulence mutants

B cells, 437–458
Bacille Calmette-Guérin, see BCG
BACTEC 12B vial, 94–95
BACTEC TB-460 system, 94

BACTEC test
  indirect qualitative test for drug susceptibility, 107
  MIC determination, 107–108
Bacteriophage, *see* Mycobacteriophage
Bail, O., 390
BCG, 25, 494
  historical aspects, 21
  infection, 391
    rabbit model, 154–155
  insertion mutations, 262–263
  isolation, 256
Bcg gene, 405–406, 464, 540
BCG vaccine, 154–155, 213, 256, 322, 403, 437, 531–
    557, 589, 616
  case-control studies, 536–537
  cohort studies, 536–537
  cost-effectiveness, 552, 592
  development, 136–140
  effect on establishment of pulmonary lesions, 479
  future trials, 550–551
  groups targeted for, 550–551
  heterogeneity, 539
  in HIV-infected persons, 533
  impact, 551–552
  long-term duration of immunity, 551–552
  mechanism of protection, 544–547
  observational studies, 534–537
  origins, 531–532
  parent strains, 532
  production, 532
  protective efficacy, 534–538, 591–593
    duration, 592–593
  randomized control trials, 534–538
  recombinant, 246–248, 547
  repeated vaccination, 552, 592–593
  route and dose of immunization, 549–550
  safety, 533
  variation in protective efficacy, 592
    difference between vaccines, 539
    environmental mycobacterial infections, 542–544
    genetic differences in human populations, 540
    methodological flaws in studies, 538–539
    protection against endogenous and exogenous
      infection, 541–542
    virulence of *M. tuberculosis* strains, 540–541
  viability, 532
  worldwide usage, 591–593
BCG-a antigen, 425
BCG-osis, 533
Biological safety
  biosafety level 2, 86, 88
  biosafety level 3, 62, 86–88
  community standards, 69
  containment, 62–69
  emergency response guidelines, 69–70
  experimental tuberculosis laboratory, 61–71
  laboratory practices, 63–64
  medical surveillance, 70
  mycobacteriology laboratory, 85–89
  safety guidelines, 62
  safety training, 63, 86
Biological safety cabinet, 64–68, 86, 88
  spills within, 69–70

Bioremediation, 246
Blood specimen, 97–98
Bone, *see* Skeletal tuberculosis
Bovine tuberculosis, 51, 448
Breath sounds, 29
Bronchiectasis, 28
Bronchoalveolar lavage, 32, 34–35
Broncholithiasis, 28
Bronchopneumonia, 473, 478
Bronchoscopy, 32, 35
Brontë family, 19–20
Burden of tuberculosis, 583–591, 616

Calcification, 474
Calcitriol, *see* 1,25-Dihydroxyvitamin D
Calcium uptake, 348–349
Calmette, A., 531–532
Camel, 158–159
Capsule, 276–277
Carbohydrates
  M. tuberculosis, 285–306
  metabolism, 356
Carbon source, 354
D D-Carboxypeptidase, 372
Cardiolipin, 337
Carrier-mediated transport, 343–346
Case detection, 52, 569, 592, *see also* Diagnosis of
    tuberculosis
  gender differences, 590
Case identification, 599–617
Caseous lesion, 152–154, 459, 463, 467–472, 478, 495,
    507
Caseous necrosis, 155, 459–460, 464–466, 469–470,
    496
Cat, 158, 161
Catalase, plasmid-encoded, 192
Catalase test, heat-stable, 103–104
Cattle, 157–158, 189, 448
Cavity formation, 29–30, 460, 471–478, 506
Cell division, 280–281
Cell envelope
  biosynthesis, 359
    components on cell surface, 378–379
  fractionation, 273
  growth rate and, 358–359
  lipids, 285–306
  lipoglycans, 296–300
  metabolism, 370–378
  models, 277–279
  nature, 272–273
  ultrastructure, 271–284
Cell lysis, 186, 520
Cell membrane, *see* Plasma membrane
Cell wall, 272, 300, 321
  biosynthesis, drug targets, 561–562, 565
  lipoglycans, 296–300
  model, 334–335
  paired fibrous structures, 279–280
  permeability, 343
  proteins, 280–281, 323–324
  structure, 333–337
  ultrastructure, 275–277
Cell wall skeleton, 275

Cell wall-deficient forms, 186, 193
Cell-mediated immunity, 476–478, 485–487
Cellular immunity, 476–477
Central nervous system tuberculosis, 26–27, 33, 40–42
Centrifuge, containment equipment, 67–68, 88
Cephalosporins
    movement into cells, 337–339
    resistance, 342
Chase, Merrill, 21, 114, 390
Chemical-energy coupling, direct, 345
Chemiosmotic coupling, 344–345
Chemoprophylaxis, 517–518, 569, 578, 593–599, 616
    adverse effects, 596
    cost-effectiveness, 597–598
    decision analyses, 597
    direct and indirect effects, 594–596
    immunocompetent hosts, 594–596
    immunocompromised hosts, 598–599
    potential role, 599
Chemotherapy, 52, 616–617
    combination preparations, 610
    completion, 606–607
    compliance, see Compliance
    cost-effectiveness, 612–616
    duration, 564
    evaluation in mouse model, 114
    HIV-positive patients, 609
    measuring outcomes, 606–608
    multidrug resistant tuberculosis, 609–610
    regimens, 608–610
    self-administered, 610–611
    short-course, 608–610, 614
    smear-negative tuberculosis, 615–616
    supervised, 611–612
Chest radiograph
    disseminated tuberculosis, 35
    pulmonary tuberculosis, 28–32, 601–603
Chloramphenicol resistance, 242
Chopin, Frederick, 16–17
Choroidal tubercle, 35
CIE technique, see Crossed-immunoelectrophoresis technique
Ciprofloxacin
    mechanism of action, 561
    movement into cells, 341
    resistance, 342
Claisen-type condensation reaction, 293
Cleared-lysis technique, 187
Clinical tuberculosis, 25–46, 417–418
    HIV-infected patients, 53–55, 505
    infection versus, 47
    risk of, 48–51
    signs and symptoms, 603–604
    site of involvement, 25–26
    systemic and remote manifestations, 26–27
Clofazimine, 340
Clonal relationships, 569–581
Cloning, 310
Cloning vector
    mycobacteriophage, 165–170, 239–240
    plasmid, 176, 185–186, 192–195, 240–241
Codon usage, 243

Colony-forming unit, 81
Colony morphology, 101
Communal living, 56, 575–576
Community survey, 583
Complement component C5a, 463
Complement receptors, 393, 396, 399
Complementation analysis, 256–259
Compliance, 56, 577, 588, 610–612
    incentives and enhancers, 611
Conjugation, 195, 241
"Consumption," 17
Contact tracing, 52, 446, 597
Containment
    biological safety cabinet, 64–68
    experimental tuberculosis laboratory, 62–69
    facility design, 68–69
    mycobacteriological laboratory, 85–89
Contig mapping, 228, 230–231
Control strategies, 52, 583–621
Copper resistance, 191
Cord factor, 289, 293, 377, 446, 490
Cord formation, 92, 96, 101, 289
Corynebacterium-based shuttle vector, 195
Cosmid library, 228, 230–231
Cosmid pJRD215, 196
Cosmid pYUB18, 230
Cosmid pYUB178, 257
Cosmid pYUB328, 231
Cosmid TBC2, 234–235
Cost-effectiveness
    BCG vaccine, 552, 592
    chemoprophylaxis, 597–598
    chemotherapy, 612–616
Cough, 27–28, 35
    screening patients with, 603–604
Coughing, 48, 472
Crohn's disease, 496
Cross-contamination, laboratory, 576
Crossed-immunoelectrophoresis (CIE) technique, soluble antigens, 309–310, 325, 438
α-Crystallins, 438–439
Cultivation
    aeration, 74, 78–80
    agitation, 78–82
    M. tuberculosis, 73–83
    measurement of growth, 80–82
    medium, see Culture medium
    temperature, 78
    viability of cultures, 80
Culture filtrate, 440–441
    protein profile, 125–126
Culture medium, 74, see also specific types of media
    detergent in, 76, 79
    glycerol in, 75, 77, 79
    inoculation, 78, 94
    liquid, 75–77
    solid, 77–78, 94
Cure rate, 607–608
Cycloserine
    mechanism of action, 560–561
    movement into cells, 340
Cycloserine-treated cells, 186–188

Cytokines, 26–27, 312–313, 390, 417–437, 487, 489, 495, *see also specific cytokines*
  excessive release, 490–491
  guinea pig model, 142
  immunotherapeutic agents, 429
  mouse model, 114, 117, 122–128
  protection and immunopathology, 427

Dangerous disseminators, 569
Dapsone
  mechanism of action, 560
  movement into cells, 340
Decontamination
  of laboratory, 64, 67, 69–70, 88
  of specimen, 90–91
Dehydroepiandrosterone sulfate (DHEA-S), 492
Delayed-type hypersensitivity (DTH) reaction, 308, 313, 326, 421, 426, 439, 441–446, 460
Δ5 desaturase, 376
24:0 desaturase, 375
Detergent, culture medium, 76, 79
Detergent lysis, 187
Developing countries, 49, 582–621
  HIV infection, 5–6, 503
  tuberculin skin test, 494
  tuberculosis incidence and mortality, 4–5
DHEA-S, *see* Dehydroepiandrosterone sulfate
2,3-Di-*O*-acyltrehalose, 291–292
Diagnosis of tuberculosis, 85–100
  antibody detection, 518
  antigen detection, 518
  conventional tests, 101–104
  culture of specimen, 601–606
  detection of infected persons, 517–518
  diagnostic algorithm, 603
  ELISPOT test, 444, 518
  extrapulmonary, 33–35
  gas-liquid chromatography, 96, 100–101
  gene amplification methods, 520–522
  heat-stable catalase test, 103–104
  high-performance liquid chromatography, 95–96, 99–100, 519
  histologic, 602–606
  HIV-infected patient, 27, 510–511
  immunodiagnosis, 446–448
  interference by nontuberculous mycobacteria, 95–97
  laboratory confirmation of infections, 518–519
  microscopy, 601
  molecular approaches, 517–530
  NAP test, 95, 99
  niacin test, 101–102
  nitrate reduction test, 101–102
  nucleic acid probes, 95–98, 519–520
  polymerase chain reaction, 96, 98–99, 520, 603
  pulmonary, 27–32
  pyrazinamide test, 101–103
  rapid diagnostic procedures, 519–524
  reporter mycobacteriophage, 524
  serodiagnosis, 446–448
  species identification of cultured organisms, 519
  strand displacement amplification assay, 520–521
  TCH susceptibility test, 101, 103

  thin-layer chromatography, 96
  transcription-mediated amplification assay, 522–524
  tuberculostearic acid analysis, 519
  X ray, 601–603
Diagnostic delay, 605–606
Diaminopimelic acid, 296, 372
Diaminopimelic acid decarboxylase, 314–315
Diffusion
  across cell wall, 340
  facilitated, 344, 346
  passive, 344
Digestion of specimen, 90
1,25-Dihydroxyvitamin D, 392, 422, 427, 486, 492
Direct repeat (DR) sequence, 570–571, 573
Disseminated tuberculosis, 26, 30, 33–36, 41, 53, 417, 428, 447, 508
  HIV-infected patient, 504–506
DNA gyrase, 561
DNA polymorphisms
  genetic elements that contribute to, 569–572
  molecular clocks, 579
  techniques for demonstrating, 572–573
DNA probe, *see* Nucleic acid probe
DNA repair, 217–226
DNA vaccine, 549
DnaJ protein, 360
DnaK protein, 316, 320–321, 360, 438, 564
Dog, 158, 161
Domestic mammals, 157–162
Dormancy, 564–565
  M. tuberculosis in unstirred culture, 81–82
  persisters, 495, 564–565
Dot blot, plasmid detection, 188
DR sequence, *see* Direct repeat sequence
DR1 haplotype, 444–445
DR3 haplotype, 444–445
DR5 haplotype, 444–445
*Dra*I restriction profile, 229–230, 254–255
Droplet nuclei, 48, 61–62, 137
Drug(s)
  permeability of cell wall, 337–343
  prevention of iron acquisition, 369
  testing with guinea pig model, 136
Drug abuser, 53–56, 576, 588, 597–598
Drug development, 559–567
  biochemical approaches, 565
  drug synergisms, 563
  drug targets, 559–562
  factors relevant to drug design, 562–565
  genetic and sequencing approaches, 565–566
  rapid tests for determining activity, 526–527
  screens using reporter mycobacteriophage, 182, 526–527
  therapeutic trials, 32–33
Drug resistance, 9–10, 104, *see also* Multidrug resistance; *specific drugs*
  acquired, 9, 105
  definition, 104
  differences among species of mycobacteria, 342–343
  initial (primary), 105
  mechanism, 245–246

mutation, 104
permeability factors in, 337–343
plasmid-encoded, 192
porins and, 280–281
primary, 9
selectable marker, 241–242
Drug screens, 378–379
Drug susceptibility testing, 87
 BACTEC indirect qualitative test in 12B broth, 107
 definitions, 104–105
 direct, 105–107
 functional approach, 525–526
 genetic approach, 524–525
 7H11 agar plates by proportion method, 106–107
 indirect, 105–107
 principles, 105–106
 pyrazinamide MIC determination, 108
 quantitative BACTEC test for MIC, 107–108
 rapid, 524–526
 using reporter mycobacteriophage, 179, 525–526
DTH reaction, see Delayed-type hypersensitivity reaction
Dubos liquid medium, 76
Dubos oleic albumin agar, 77
Dust-associated particles, 48

Eastern Europe, 5, 14
Economic impact, 3
Economic research, 583–621
Egg-based medium, 77, 94, 96
Ehrlich, Paul, 18
Electroduction, 195
Electron microscopy, 271–284
Electroporation, 170, 194–195, 241, 256
Elephant, 158–159
ELISA, see Enzyme-linked immunosorbent assay
ELISPOT test, 444, 518
Elongation factor EF-Tu, 315
Emergency response guidelines, 69–70, 89
Empyema, 37–38
Energy source, 354
5-Enolpyruvylshikimate-3-phosphate synthetase, 314–315
Enteritis, 42
Enterobactin, see Enterochelin
Enterochelin, 362
Envelope, see Cell envelope
Environmental (atypical) mycobacteria, 584–585
 infection, protection against tuberculosis, 542–544
 vaccine, 548
Enzyme(s), amino acid and protein biosynthesis, 314–315
Enzyme-linked immunosorbent assay (ELISA), 446–447
Epidemic spread, 13–15
Epidemiology, 47–59
 annual risk of infection, 4, 585, 587, 590
 drug resistance, 9
 epidemiological model, 48–51
 future trends, 9–10
 HIV-associated tuberculosis, 5–10, 23, 53–57, 503, 576

industrialized countries, 7–9
 molecular, 569–581
 prevalence of infection, 4
 trends in tuberculosis rates, 51–52
 tuberculosis incidence and mortality, 4–5
 worldwide burden of tuberculosis, 3–11, 578, 583–591, 616
Epoxymycolates, 293, 295
Erythromycin, 341
Escherichia coli, surrogate host for cloning virulence genes, 259–260
Establishment of tuberculosis, 462
 rabbit model, 150–151
Ethambutol
 mechanism of action, 372–373, 560, 562–563
 resistance, 342
 structure, 560
 treatment regimens, 608–610
Ethionamide
 mechanism of action, 560, 562
 resistance, 524, 562
 structure, 560
Evolution, 578–579
Exochelin, 348, 357, 362–367, 563
Exochelin receptor, 367–369
Exotic mammals, 157–162
Experimental tuberculosis laboratory, 61–71
Expression vector
 extrachromosomal and integrating modes of replication, 241
 phage-based, 239–240
 plasmid-based, 240–241
 selectable markers, 241–242
 transcription and translation initiation, 242–243
Extrachromosomal vector, 241
Extrapulmonary tuberculosis, 33–44, 447
 diagnosis, 33–34
 HIV-infected patients, 34, 53, 504–508, 511
 smear-negative, 599–601
 smear-positive, 599–601

Facilitated diffusion, 344, 346
Facility design, 68–69, 87–88
Fatty acid(s)
 biosynthesis, 374–377
 metabolism, 377
 short-chain, gas-liquid chromatography, 100–101
Fatty acid synthase, 375–377
Fatty acyl elongase, 375–377
Fc receptor, 142, 393, 396
Ferric citrate, 369
Ferritin, 361, 363, 399
Fever, 27, 35
Fibronectin-binding protein, 325–326, 425, 441, 444, 447, 563–564
Fibrotic lesion, 474–475
Fluoroquinolone
 mechanism of action, 560–561
 movement into cells, 341
Fluoroscopy, 603
Foreign genes
 expression in BCG, 246–248
 expression in mycobacteria, 239–252

expression vector, 241–243
introduction and maintenance
    phage-based systems, 239–240
    plasmid-based systems, 240
    transformation, 241
    recombinant vaccines, 246–249
Foreign proteins, 243–245
    export, 244–245
    posttranslational modifications, 244–245
    translational efficiency, 243–244
Fracastoro, H., 17
Freeze-etching technique, 277
Freeze-fracture technique, 277
Fungus ball, 28

β-Galactosidase, 151–152, 263–264, 463, 468, 473–474
Gamma interferon (IFN-γ), 119–120, 123, 126–129,
    313, 390–391, 395–397, 402, 404, 418, 421–429,
    437, 441–444, 448–449, 468, 486–487, 490–491,
    497, 509, 545–547
Gas-liquid chromatography (GLC), identification of
    M. tuberculosis, 96, 100–101
Gender, differential impact of tuberculosis, 589–591
Gene expression
    foreign genes in mycobacteria, *see* Foreign genes
    mycobacteriophage L5, 178
Gene knockout techniques, 219–220
Gene mapping, 231–232
Gene-disrupted mouse model, 116, 129
Generation time, 74
Genetics
    antibody response, 441–442
    rabbit model, 155
    susceptibility to tuberculosis, 405–406, 462, 540
Genitourinary tuberculosis, 26, 33, 37–39
Genome sequencing, 227–238
    cosmid TBC2, 234–235
    data management, 233–234
    future prospects, 235
    large-scale, 231–235
    sequence analysis, 234
    sequence production, 233
Genome technology, 231–233
Gen-Probe MTD Test, 522–524
Gen-Probe Rapid Diagnostic System, 525
GLC, *see* Gas-liquid chromatography
Global burden, 3–11, 578, 583–591, 616
Glucocorticoid, 492
Glutamate transport, 346
Glycerol
    culture medium, 75, 77, 79
    movement into cells, 343
Glycolipids, 246
    phenolic, 286, 292, 377–378, 395–396
    wall-associated, 278–279
Glycolysis, 354, 356
Glycosylation of proteins, 440, 564
Glycosylphosphopolyisoprenols, 288
Glycosyltransferase, 372
GM-CSF, *see* Granulocyte macrophage-colony-
    stimulating factor
Goat, 158, 160
Granulocyte macrophage–colony-stimulating factor
    (GM-CSF), 123, 126, 418, 421, 427, 545

Granuloma, 34, 36, 44, 122, 141, 153, 389
    formation, 120, 391, 404, 437, 490
    liquefaction, 404
    productive, 402, 404
GroEL protein, 316, 320–322, 360, 438
GroES protein, 317, 320–321, 360, 438, 564
Group translocation, 345
Growth
    cell envelope and, 358–359
    dynamics, 81–82
    limiting factors, 357–360
    M. tuberculosis, 74
    measurement, 80–81
    nucleic acid synthesis and, 358
    rates, 357–360
    stationary-phase changes, 564–565
    stress response and, 359–360
    temperature dependence, 78, 191–192
Growth factors, 357
Guérin, C., 531–532
Guinea pig model, 135–147, 158
    application to clinical and experimental
      tuberculosis, 135–137
    application of immunological techniques, 141–143
    BCG in, 540–541
    drug testing, 136
    historical aspects, 135
    nonpulmonary tuberculosis, 143
    protective immunity, 449
    pulmonary tuberculosis, 137–141
    vaccination, 137–139

7H10 agar, 97
7H11 agar, 94–97
    drug susceptibility testing, 106–107
H-2 locus, 441, 443
Handwashing, 64, 88
Health care facility, screening for tuberculosis, 604–
    605
Heat shock proteins, 309, 316–317, 320–321, 359–
    360, 425, 438–439, 496–497
    in autoimmunity, 449–450
    hsp10, 438–439
    hsp60, 126–128, 445–446, 449
    hsp65, 438–439, 442–445, 450, 496–497
    hsp70, 438–439
    hsp71, 446–447
    hsp90, 438
    promoters, 243
Heating plate, 88
Heat-stable catalase test, 103–104
Helmholtz, H., 390
Hematogenous dissemination, 152–154, 417, 466–469
Hematologic abnormalities, 27
Hematuria, 39
Hemin, 357
Hemoglobin, 361, 398–399
Hemolytic activity, tubercle bacillus, 393–394, 547
Hemoptysis, 28, 473
HEPA filter, *see* High-efficiency particulate air filter
Hepatic tuberculosis, 42–43
Hepatitis, isoniazid, 596–597
Herd immunity, 13

Hexokinase, 346
High-efficiency particulate air (HEPA) filter, 65–66, 88
High-molecular-weight high-iron protein (HIP), 367–369
High-performance liquid chromatography (HPLC), identification of *M. tuberculosis*, 95–96, 99–100, 519
HIP, *see* High-molecular-weight high-iron protein
History of tuberculosis, 13–24
    and dawning of biomedical science, 16–22
    early, 13–16
    failed conquest, 22–23
HLA-DR15(DR2), 441–442
Homeless shelter, *see* Communal living
Homogenization of specimen, 90
Homosexual men, 53–54
Horse, 158, 160
Host resistance, genetics, 405–406
Host tissue, as nutrient source, 354–355
HPLC, *see* High-performance liquid chromatography
2HRZE/4HR regimen, 608
Human immunodeficiency virus (HIV) infection
    BCG vaccine in infected persons, 533
    effect of tuberculosis on HIV disease, 509
    mouse model, 128–129
    nontuberculous mycobacterial infection and, 97
    population screening, 598
    tuberculin skin test in, 25
    tuberculosis associated with, 5–10, 23, 50–57, 420, 428, 462, 467, 588
        advanced HIV disease, 508
        autopsy findings, 505–506
        cause of death, 508–509
        chemoprophylaxis, 510, 598–599
        clinical disease, 53–55, 505
        diagnosis, 510–511
        early HIV infection, 506–507
        epidemiology, 503, 576
        extrapulmonary, 34, 36, 40, 504–508, 511
        histopathology, 506–508
        HIV with moderate immunosuppression, 506–508
        immunopathogenesis, 509
        meningitis versus visceral AFB densities, 508
        multidrug resistant, 56
        pathogenesis, 503–513
        pediatric, 510
        primary disease, 53–55
        pulmonary, 30–32, 504–506
        reactivation, 503–504, 510
        reinfection, 55, 503–504, 510, 577–578
        site of infection, 26
        treatment, 509–510, 609
Hydrogen peroxide, 390, 395
Hygromycin resistance, 242
Hypercalcemia, 492
Hyperglobulinemia, 428
Hyponatremia, 27, 35

Identification of *Mycobacterium tuberculosis*, *see* Diagnosis of tuberculosis
Idiopathic disease, 495–497

IFN, *see* Interferon
IL, *see* Interleukin
Immigration, 7–8, 14–15, 23, 51, 578, 588
Immune response, 389–415
    cytokines, 417–435
    helpful and harmful effects, 479–480
    historical aspects, 20–21
    macrophage-activating, 459–463
    mouse model, 116–128
    specificity and function of T- and B-cell recognition, 437–458
    tissue-damaging, 459–463
Immunodeficient mouse model, 128–130
Immunodiagnosis, 446–448
Immunoglobulin G, glycosylation, 496
Immunosenescent mouse model, 129–130
Immunotherapy, 429
In vivo expression technology, 265–266
Incidence, 583–584, 587
Indigenous peoples, 15, 405
Inducer exclusion, 345–346
Inducer expulsion, 345–346
Industrialized countries, 49, 51, 583–621
    drug-resistant strains, 9
    tuberculosis incidence and mortality, 5, 7–9
Infection, 584–585
    clinical disease versus, 47
    primary, 49
    risk of, 48–51
Ingestion of tubercle bacilli, 48
INH, *see* Isoniazid
inhA gene, 245, 562
Inoculation
    culture medium, 78, 94
    experimental animals, 78, 115–118
Insertion sequence (IS), 199, 203–204, 579
    M. avium, 204–206
    M. intracellulare, 204–205
    M. paratuberculosis, 204–206
    M. smegmatis, 207–209
    M. tuberculosis, 206–207
Insertion sequence (IS) amplityping, 572
Insertion sequence IS3, 208–209
Insertion sequence IS900, 204–206, 211–212
Insertion sequence IS901, 204–206
Insertion sequence IS987, 574
Insertion sequence IS1081, 204, 206–207, 570–571
Insertion sequence IS1096, 204, 207–209, 211–212, 263
Insertion sequence IS1137, 204, 207–209
Insertion sequence IS1141, 204–209
Insertion sequence IS3411, 208–209
Insertion sequence IS6100, 204, 209–212
Insertion sequence IS6110, 204, 206–212, 229–230, 521–522, 570–575
Insertion sequence IS6110-IS986, 204
Insertion sequence IS6120, 204, 207–209, 211–212
Insertion sequence IS*myco*, 204
Insertional mutagenesis, 203, 212, 260–263
Integrating vector, 241
Integrin, 396, 399–400
    $\alpha_v\beta_3$, 399
Intein, 221–225

Interleukin-1 (IL-1), 126, 142, 391, 397, 418–421, 427, 545

Interleukin-2 (IL-2), 123, 127, 142, 391, 418–424, 429, 443, 449, 491–492, 509, 545–546

Interleukin-2 (IL-2) receptor, 419, 423, 443

Interleukin-3 (IL-3), 418, 421

Interleukin-4 (IL-4), 119, 126, 391, 397, 418, 421–424, 428, 442, 444, 491–492, 509, 545

Interleukin-4 (IL-4) knockout mouse model, 129

Interleukin-5 (IL-5), 142, 418, 421–422, 424, 428, 492, 509

Interleukin-6 (IL-6), 126, 391, 418–421, 428

Interleukin-8 (IL-8), 142, 391, 418, 427, 464

Interleukin-10 (IL-10), 126, 391, 397–398, 418–424, 427–429, 442, 491, 495, 509, 545

Interleukin-12 (IL-12), 126, 391–392, 423, 491, 545

International travel, 578

Intestinal tuberculosis, 42, 506

Intracellular mycobacteria, 92, 281–282, 357, 392–399, 546

Invasin, 400

Invasin gene, 259

IREP, see Iron-regulated envelope protein

Iron
  acquisition, 348, 360–370, 563
  functions, 360–361
  metabolism, 360–370, 398–399
  reduction, 366

Iron-regulated envelope protein (IREP), 367–369

IS, see Insertion sequence

Isolation, primary, M. tuberculosis, 94–95

Isoniazid (INH)
  hepatitis related to, 596–597
  historical aspects, 22
  mechanism of action, 294, 376, 560, 562
  movement into cells, 340
  prophylactic, 593–599
    in HIV-infected patients, 510
  resistance, 10, 245, 325, 342, 524–525, 562–563
  structure, 560
  treatment regimens, 608–610

Kanamycin
  mechanism of action, 560
  resistance, 242, 256

katG gene, 245, 563

Keats, John, 19

Ketomycolates, 293–294

Killed vaccine, 548

"King's Evil," 16

Koch, Robert, 17–21, 113–114, 253, 308, 389–390, 485

Koch phenomenon, 308, 485–487, 489–490, 493–494

Koch's molecular postulates, 253–254

Koch's old tuberculin, 308, 485, 489

Koch's postulates, 17–18, 135, 253–254

Laboratory errors, 576

Laboratory risk, 62

Laboratory-acquired tuberculosis, 61–71, 85–89, see also Biological safety

β-Lactam(s), 337–339, 372, 561

β-Lactamase, 337–339, 372

Lactoferrin, 361, 365–366

Laennec, Theophile, 17

LAM, see Lipoarabinomannan

Langhans giant cells, 470, 506–508

Latent tuberculosis, 25, 29, 47, 50

Leader sequence, see Signal peptide

Lectin, 373–374

Lipids, 74–75
  exogenous, 354–356
  M. tuberculosis, 285–306
  membrane-associated, 337
  metabolism, 354–356
  wall-associated, 278–279
    gas-liquid chromatography, 100–101

Lipoarabinomannan (LAM), 123, 127, 273, 277–279, 377, 419–420, 447, 561
  immunoregulatory functions, 298
  incapacitation of oxygen radical, 393, 395, 398
  mannose-capped, 298–299, 398
  structure, 297–300

Lipoglycans, 296–300

Lipooligosaccharide, 292

Lipoproteins
  associated with surface structures, 323–324
  membrane, antigenic, 439–440, 450

Lipoylation of peptides, 440

Liquefaction, 153, 459, 471–476, 496

Livestock, 157–162
  vaccines, 249

Lobar pneumonia, 473

Local immunity, 480

Lowenstein-Jensen slant, 94, 97, 101

Luciferase, 263–264

Luciferase reporter phage, 179–182, 379, 524–527

Lumbar puncture, 41

Lung biopsy, transbronchial, 32, 34–35

Lupus vulgaris, 16, 489

Lurie, Max B., 20, 149–156, 390, 461

Lymphadenitis, 36, 401, 511

Lymphatic dissemination, 152–153, 467, 469

Lymphatic tuberculosis, 26, 33, 36, 504, 506

Lymphokines, 471, 486–487, 492, 495

Lymphotoxin, 418, 421–422, 491, 545

lysA gene, 314–315

Lysogenic cycle, mycobacteriophage L5, 177–178

Lysosome, 392–394, 488

Mackaness, G. B., 390

Macrophage(s), 390, 419
  activated, 152, 459–474, 477–480, 486, 506–507, 545
  alveolar, 150, 153–154, 157, 403–404, 418, 423, 427, 459, 462–465, 479
  antimycobacterial effector functions, 392–399
  antimycobacterial functions, 390–392
  direct toxicity, 487–489
  entering liquefied caseum, 475
  entering lungs from bloodstream, 463–465
  incompetent, 466–468, 473
  intracellular mycobacteria, 92, 281–282
  in vitro activation, 390–392
  mouse model, 125–128

Macrophage–colony-stimulating factor, 126

mAGP, *see* Mycolyl-arabinogalactan-peptidoglycan complex
Major histocompatibility complex (MHC), 419, 486
　class I molecules, 400, 403–404, 437, 546
　class II molecules, 400, 403–404, 437, 487, 546
Major polymorphic tandem repeat (MPTR), 570–572
Malnutrition, 140–141
Mannophosphoinositides, 337
Mannose receptor, 393, 399
Mannose-capped lipoarabinomannan (Man-LAM), 298–299, 398
Mannosylphosphopolyprenols, 288–289
Mannosyltransferase, 372–373, 375–376
Mapping, 227–238
　contig, 228, 230–231
　future prospects, 235
　gene, 231–232
　pulsed-field gel electrophoresis, 228–230
Marble, Alice, 21–22
Marten, Benjamin, 17
MCP-1, *see* Monocyte chemoattractant protein
Medium, *see* Culture medium
Membrane anchor, 298
Meningitis, 40–42, 53, 143, 447, 511, 519, 541, 592
　HIV-infected patient, 504–506
Mercury resistance, 191, 242
Meromycolate chain, 374–375
Metabolism
　general, 354–358
　M. tuberculosis, 353–385
Metal analog, growth effects, 369–370
Metchnikoff, E., 390
Metered-dose delivery system, 610
Methoxymycolates, 293–294
Methylglucolipopolysaccharide, 296
Methylmannose polysaccharide, 296, 376–377
3-*O*-Methyltransferase, 375–376
MHC, *see* Major histocompatibility complex
MIC, *see* Minimum inhibitory concentration
β2-Microglobulin-deficient mouse model, 121–122, 129, 400–401, 486–487, 546
Microscopy, diagnosis of tuberculosis, 601
Middlebrook 7H9 broth, 94, 97
Middlebrook 7H12 broth, 94
Middlebrook media, 77
Middlebrook-Cohn 7H10 agar, 94
Migration inhibition factor, 120
Miliary tuberculosis, 417, 428, 467–469, 478, 507–508, 511, 541, 592
Milk, *see* Pasteurization of milk
Minimum inhibitory concentration (MIC)
　pyrazinamide, 108
　quantitative BACTEC test, 107–108
Mixed-linked polymerase chain reaction, 572–573
Molecular chaperones, 320, 438
Molecular clocks, 579
Monkey, 158, 160
Monoclonal antibody TB72 competition test, 447
Monoclonal antibody techniques, 310–311, 438
Monocyte(s)
　BCG-induced antimycobacterial activity, 545
　direct toxicity, 487–489
Monocyte chemoattractant protein (MCP-1), 142, 463

Mononuclear phagocytes, 418–426, 466, 471
Mortality, 4–6, 14, 587–591
Morton, Robert, 17
Mouse lung, as "culture media," 77
Mouse model, 113–134, 158
　activated macrophages, 486
　adoptive immunity, 114
　αβ-T-cell-deficient, 400
　drug evaluation, 114
　evolution, 113–115
　experimental infection of mice,115–118
　gamma interferon knockout mouse, 129
　γδ knockout mouse, 129
　γδ T cells, 445
　gene-disrupted mouse, 116, 129
　genetics, 441–442
　　of disease resistance, 405–406
　host response to tuberculosis, 116–128
　immunodeficient mouse, 128–130
　immunosenescent mouse, 129–130
　interleukin-4 knockout mouse, 129
　β2-microglobulin-deficient, 121–122, 129, 400–401, 486–487, 546
　nude mouse, 128
　protective immunity, 449
　retroviral infection, 128–129
　scid mouse, 128
　target antigens in immune response, 124–126
　T-cell repertoire, 442–443
　TXB mouse, 128
　TxCD4⁻ mouse, 128–129
MPB70 protein, 440, 448
MPT51 protein, 441
MPTR, *see* Major polymorphic tandem repeat
Multidrug preparations, 610
Multidrug resistance, 7–9, 23, 551–552, 598
　chemotherapy, 609–610
　definition, 104
　etiology of emergence, 577
　HIV and, 56
　safe handling, 87
Multiplex sequencing, 231–233
Mummies, 15–16
Mutagenesis
　insertional, 203, 212, 260–263
　reverse, 203
　transposon, 212–213
MycDB (database), 228, 233, 235
Mycetoma, 28
Mycobacterial envelope, *see* Cell envelope
Mycobacterial membrane, *see* Plasma membrane
Mycobacterial wall, *see* Cell wall
Mycobacteriology laboratory
　biological safety, 85–89
　detection of laboratory errors, 576
Mycobacteriophage, 165–183
　cloning vector, 165–170, 239–240
　genome, 167–168
　introduction of foreign DNA in mycobacteria, 167–169
　luciferase reporter, 179–182
　molecular genetic systems, 166
　optimizing DNA uptake, 166–167

Mycobacteriophage D29, 171, 196
Mycobacteriophage I3, 170–171
Mycobacteriophage L1, 170–171
Mycobacteriophage L5, 171–179
    attachment site, 172, 175–176
    clear-plaque mutants, 177
    excisionase gene, 176–177
    gene expression, 178
    genome
        essential and nonessential regions, 178–179
        structure, 171–174
    host range, 171
    immunity genes, 177–178
    integrating plasmids based on, 195
    regulation of lysogeny, 177–178
    site-specific integration, 175–177
    transposon delivery, 213
    tRNA genes, 172, 176
    virion structure and assembly, 174–175
Mycobacteriophage phAE40, 181
Mycobacteriophage TM4, 168–170, 181
Mycobacterium avium
    infection, protection against tuberculosis, 542–543
    insertion sequences, 204–206
    plasmids, 188–190
Mycobacterium bovis, virulence mutants, 256
Mycobacterium bovis BCG, *see* BCG
Mycobacterium fortuitum
    infection, protection against tuberculosis, 542–543
    plasmids, 190
Mycobacterium gauss, 542–543
Mycobacterium intracellulare, insertion sequences, 204–206
Mycobacterium kansasii, infection, protection against tuberculosis, 542–543
Mycobacterium leprae, *recA* gene, 222–223
Mycobacterium microti vaccine, 543, 548–549
Mycobacterium paratuberculosis, insertion sequences, 204–206
Mycobacterium scrofulaceum, plasmids, 190
Mycobacterium smegmatis
    insertion sequences, 207–209
    plasmid transformation, 193–194
Mycobacterium tuberculosis
    antigens, 307–332, 424–426, 438–441, 493–494, 549
    auxotrophs, 265–266
    carbohydrates, 285–306
    cultivation, 73–83
    drug targets, 559–562
    general characteristics, 73–75
    insertion mutations, 262–263
    insertion sequences, 206–207
    intracellular, 281–282, 392–399
    invasion of nonphagocytic cells, 399–400
    lipids, 285–306
    membrane permeability, 333–352
    metabolism, 353–385
    plasmids, 188
    primary isolation, 94–95
    proteins, 307–332
    strain differences in virulence, 540–541
    transport into cells, 333–352
    ultrastructure, 271–274

    virulence mutants, 256
Mycobacterium vaccae, immunotherapeutic agent, 429, 494, 548
Mycobacterium W, 548
Mycobactin, 295, 348, 357, 362–368, 399, 563
Mycocerosate synthase, 378
Mycocerosic acids, 286–287, 370
α-Mycolates, 293–295, 375
α'-Mycolates, 293
Mycolic acids, 275–276, 289–297, 333–335, 370, 519
    attachment, 374–377
    biosynthesis, 374–377
    drug targets, 561–562
    high-performance liquid chromatography, 99–100
    structure of cell wall, 277–279
Mycolipanolic acids, 291–292
Mycolipenic acids, 291
Mycolyl-arabinogalactan-peptidoglycan complex (mAGP), 296–297
Mycolyltransferase, 373–374, 377

NADH-dependent reductase, 366
NALC-NaOH method, specimen processing, 90–91
NAP test, 95, 99
Native Americans, 15, 405
Natural history of tuberculosis, 49–51, 54–55, 594–595, 599–601
    mouse model, 115–116
Natural killer (NK) cells, 392, 402, 404, 545
Necrotizing lesion, 389–390
Needle aspiration biopsy, lung, 32
Negative staining, cell envelope, 279
Neutrophil activation protein-1, 142
Niacin test, 101–102
Nitrate reduction test, 101–102
Nitric oxide synthase, 396–399
Nitrogen oxides, *see* Reactive nitrogen oxides
Nitrogen source, 356
NK cells, *see* Natural killer cells
Nocardiosis, 510–511
Noncompliance, *see* Compliance
Nontuberculous mycobacteria, 96–97
North America, 7–8, 14–15
Nosocomial tuberculosis, 8, 55–56, 575
Nramp phenotype, 405–406
Nucleic acid(s), biosynthesis, 358, 379
    drug targets, 560
Nucleic acid probe, diagnosis of tuberculosis, 95–98, 519–520
Nutrient
    in host tissues, 354–355
    transport, 343
        amino acids, 346–347
        carrier-mediated, 343–346
        regulation, 345–346
        sugars, 347–348
Nutritional immunity, 369
Nutritional status, T cells and, 140–141

Ofloxacin
    mechanism of action, 561
    susceptibility testing, 106
Oleic acid, culture medium, 191–192

Operational research, 583–621
Outbreak, 7–8, 55
Ovatransferrin, 361
Overcrowding, 15
Oxaloacetate, 354
Oxidative burst, *see* Respiratory burst
Oxygen requirement, 357

PANTA, 94
Paracentesis, 42
PAS, *see* *p*-Aminosalicylic acid
Passive diffusion, 344
Pasteurization of milk, 51, 157
Pathogenesis
  mechanism, 485–501
  pulmonary tuberculosis, 459–483
    stage I: onset, 461–462, 465
    stage II: symbiosis, 462–465
    stage III: caseous necrosis, 464–466
    stage IV: tissue-damaging and macrophage-
      activating immune response, 466–471
    stage V: liquefaction and cavity formation, 471–
      476
  tuberculosis in HIV-infected patient, 503–513
Paucibacillary infection, 447, 518
PCR, *see* Polymerase chain reaction
Pediatric tuberculosis, 510
Pellicle formation, 74–75
Penicillin-binding protein, 372, 561
Penta-arabinan motif, 377
Pentose phosphate pathway, 354, 356
Pentoxifylline, 428
Peptidoglycan, 272, 275–279, 288, 296–297, 333, 371–
  373, 561
Pericardial tuberculosis, 43–44
Pericarditis, 43
  chronic fibrotic, 43–44
Peritoneal tuberculosis, 26
Peritonitis, 42
Permeability, 358–359
  drug development and, 562–563
  drug susceptibility and, 337–343
  M. tuberculosis, 333–352
  membrane, 333–352
Permease, 344–347
Peroxynitrite anion, 397
Persisters, 495, 564–565
PFGE, *see* Pulsed-field gel electrophoresis
PGRS, *see* Polymorphic GC-rich repetitive sequence
Phage, *see* Mycobacteriophage
Phage typing, 165
Phagolysosome, 488, 546–547
Phagosome, 281–282, 392–394
Phasmid, *see* Shuttle phasmid
Phenolic glycolipids, 286, 292, 377–378, 395–396
Phenolphthiocerols, 286–287
Phenotypic characteristics, strain-specific, 578
PhoS protein, 317, 440
Phosphate transport, 323–324, 440, 563
Phosphatidylethanolamine, 337
Phosphatidylinositol, 287, 298
Phosphatidylinositol dimannoside, 288
Phosphatidylinositol hexamannoside, 288

Phosphatidylinositol mannoside (PIM), 273, 278–279,
  288, 299, 370–371
Phosphatidylinositol pentamannoside, 288
Phosphodiacylglycerols, 287
Phospholipase, 370
Phospholipids, 287–289
  membrane-associated, 370
  metabolism, 370–371
  wall-associated, 278
Phthiocerols, 286–287, 377–378, 562
Phthiodiolone, 286
Phthiotriols, 286
"Phthisis," 16
Pig, 158, 160–161, 189
PIM, *see* Phosphatidylinositol mannoside
Plasma membrane, 272
  metabolism, 370–371
  permeability, 333–352
  proteins associated with, 323–324
  structure, 333–337
  transport across, 321–322
  ultrastructure, 273–275
Plasmid(s), 176, 185–198, 256
  cloning vector, 185–186, 192–195, 240–241
  conditionally replicative, 212
  detection by dot-blot hybridization, 188
  evolution, 190
  functions coded by, 185
  gram-negative, inherited stably by mycobacteria,
    196
  isolation from mycobacteria, 186–187
  M. avium, 188–190
  M. fortuitum complex, 190
  M. scrofulaceum, 190
  M. tuberculosis, 188
  plasmid-encoded functions
    background, 190–191
    catalase, 192
    drug resistance, 192
    effect of oleic acid, 191–192
    growth temperature, 191–192
    mercury and copper resistance, 191
    restriction and modification, 191
    virulence, 192
  rapid screening methods, 187–188
  transfer
    conjugation, 195
    electroduction, 195
    electroporation, 194–195
    problems, 193
    transformation of *M. smegmatis*, 193–194
Plasmid pAL5000, 167, 170, 186, 240
  characterization, 192–193
  cloning vector, 195
  temperature-sensitive inheritance, 193
Plasmid pB4, 193
Plasmid pIJ666, 194, 196
Plasmid pLR7, 189–190
Plasmid pMSC1, 195
Plasmid pMSC262, 195
Plasmid pMV261, 195, 240–241
Plasmid pMV361, 195, 240
Plasmid pMY10, 195

Plasmid pRR3, 195
Plasmid pSGMU37, 194, 196
Plasmid pVT2, 189–190
Plasmid pYT72, 195
Plasmid RSF1010, 195–196
Pleural biopsy, 37
Pleural effusion, 143
Pleural tuberculosis, 26, 36–37
Pleuritis, 37, 44, 143, 417–422, 425, 428
Pneumonia, 473–474, 478
Polymerase chain reaction (PCR)
    diagnosis of tuberculosis, 96–99, 520–522, 603
    epidemiologic studies, 572–573
    insertion sequence amplityping, 572
    mixed-linked, 572–573
Polymorphic GC-rich repetitive sequence (PGRS),
    570–571
Polymorphonuclear granulocytes, 402
Polysaccharide, cell wall, 272, 275
Population density, 13–16
Population-based surveillance, 576–577
Porin, 279–280, 336, 338, 340, 342, 359, 563
Posttranslational modification, 564
    foreign proteins, 244–245
Pott's disease, *see* Spinal tuberculosis
PPD, *see* Purified protein derivative
Pregnancy, 590
Prehistoric peoples, 15–16
Prevalence of infection, 583–585, 590
    by age, 585–587
Primary tuberculosis, 28, 49–50, 417, 424, 427–428
    BCG vaccine and, 541–542
    HIV-infected patients, 53–55
    risk of, 55
Prison, *see* Communal living
Prodrugs, 563
Progression of tuberculosis, 600
    rabbit model, 151–152
Progressive primary tuberculosis, 29, 49, 427–428,
    587
Proline transport, 346–347
Promoter, expression vector, 242–243
Prophylaxis, *see* Chemoprophylaxis
Proportion method, drug susceptibility testing, 106–
    107
Proskauer and Beck medium, 75–76
Prostaglandins, 492, 495
Protective clothing, 64, 70, 86, 88–89
Protective immunity, 426, 448–449, 485–487
Protein(s)
    antigenic, 124–126
    associated with cell membrane or wall, 278–281,
        323–324
    biosynthesis, 314–315
        drug targets, 560
    M. tuberculosis, 307–332
    secreted/exported, 124–126, 312–313, 321–326, 425,
        438–441, 450
        drug targets, 563–564
        localization index, 322
        SDS-PAGE, 311–312
    structure and functions, 314–321
Protein kinase C, 395

Protein MPB64, 326
Protein splicing
    other genes, 222
    recA gene, 221–225
    selection for, 223–225
Protoplast, 167, 170, 193–194
Psychological disorders, 27
Public health measures, 18, 23
Pulmonary tuberculosis, 26, 418, 428, 441–442, 446–
    447
    bacteriologic evaluation, 31–33
    BCG vaccine and, 541
    case definition, 602
    chest radiographs, 28–32
    guinea pig model, 137–141
    HIV-infected patient, 30–32, 504–506
    pathogenesis, 459–483
    symptoms and physical findings, 28–29
    untreated, 595
Pulsed-field gel electrophoresis (PFGE)
    mapping by, 228–230
    virulence genes, 254
Purified protein derivative (PPD), 308, 419, 426, 443–
    446, *see also* Tuberculin
    master batch (RT23), 309
    PPD-B, 542–543
    PPD-S, 308
Pyrazinamidase, 563
Pyrazinamide (PZA)
    MIC determination, 108
    movement into cells, 340
    resistance, 103, 563
    structure, 560
    susceptibility testing, 106
    treatment regimens, 608–610
Pyrazinamide (PZA) test, 101–102
Pyridine nucleotide transhydrogenase, 315
Pyuria, 39
PZA, *see* Pyrazinamide

Rabbit model, 149–156
    BCG infection, 154–155
    genetic studies, 155
    historical aspects, 149–150
    pathogenesis of pulmonary tuberculosis, 459–477
    resistance to establishment of tuberculosis, 150–
        151
    resistance to progress of tuberculosis, 151–152
    tuberculosis caused by bovine-type bacilli, 152–153
    tuberculosis caused by human-type bacilli, 153–154
Rasmussen's aneurysm, 28
Reactivation, endogenous, 47–52, 417, 428, 462, 577,
    587
    BCG vaccine and, 541–542
    guinea pig model, 143
    HIV-infected patients, 54, 503–504, 510
Reactive nitrogen oxides (RNI), 393, 396–399, 406,
    422, 427, 486–490, 540, 545
Reactive oxygen intermediates, 489–490
recA gene, 217–226, 259
    intein, 221–223
    structure, 220–225
    virulence and, 220

RecA protein
  DNA repair, 218
  homologous recombination, 218–219
  SOS response, 217–218
  structure, 220–221
Recombinant DNA techniques, 438
  antigen identification and isolation, 310–311
Recombinant vaccine, 246–249, 547
Recombination, homologous, 217–226, 259
  as laboratory tool, 219–220
  RecA protein in, 218–219
Reinfection, exogenous, 49–50, 426, 466, 477–478
  BCG vaccine and, 541–542
  epidemiologic studies, 577–578
  guinea pig model, 143
  HIV-infected patient, 55, 503–504, 510, 577–578
Renal tuberculosis, 39
Repetitive DNA elements, 569–571
Reporter genes, 263–264
Reporter mycobacteriophage, 524
  drug screens, 526–527
  drug susceptibility testing, 525–526
Repressor, mycobacteriophage L5, 177
Respirator, dust/mist, 67–68
Respiratory burst, 390, 393–397
Restriction analysis, 254–255
Restriction enzyme, 229, 572
Restriction fragment length polymorphism (RFLP),
    see also DNA polymorphisms
  epidemiologic studies, 572
Restriction-modification system, plasmid-encoded,
    191
Retroviral infection, mouse model, 128–129
Reverse mutagenesis, 203
RFLP, see Restriction fragment length
    polymorphism
Rheumatoid arthritis, 495–497
Ribosomal RNA, 525
Rifampin
  mechanism of action, 560–561
  resistance, 10, 524–525, 561
  treatment regimens, 608–610
Rifamycin
  movement into cells, 340
  resistance, 342
RNA polymerase, 358, 524–525, 561, 564–565
RNI, see Reactive nitrogen oxides
Rotary shaker, flask culture, 79–80
Ruthenium red staining, 276–277

Safety, see also Biological safety
  BCG vaccine, 533
Salicylic acid, 362, 364, 366–367
Sampling survey, 583
Sanatoria, 22, 51
Saranac Lake, New York, 18
Sarcoidosis, 495–496
Screening for tuberculosis
  active or passive strategies, 603–604
  case-finding methods, 604
  entry criterion for, 603
  at health care facility, 604–605
"Scrofula," 16, 20

SDA, see Strand displacement amplification
Secondary gene products, 246
Secondary infection, 595–596, 598
Secondary transmission, 596
Seed pool, 78
Selectable markers, 241–242, 256
Septi-Chek AFB system, 94
Serodiagnosis, 446–448
Seronegative tuberculosis, 451
2SH/6HE regimen, 609
Sheep, 158, 160–161
Shock, tuberculin, 491
Short-course chemotherapy, 608–610, 614
Shuttle phasmid, 168–170, 239–240, 255–256
  phAE1, 240
  TM4, 169–170
Shuttle plasmid pAL8, 194
Shuttle vector, 241
  Corynebacterium-based, 195
Shwartzman reaction, 489
Siderophore, 348, 361–370, 398–399, 563
  extracellular, 363
  intracellular, 362
Signal peptide, 321, 323, 440–441
Skeletal tuberculosis, 15, 26, 39–40
Skin tuberculosis, 16, 489
S-layer glycoprotein, 280
Smear examination, 91–94
Smear preparation, 91
  biological safety, 87
Smear-negative tuberculosis, 599–601, 615–616
Smear-positive tuberculosis, 50–52, 95, 599–601
Sneezing, 48
Social impact, 3
Social research, 583–621
Socioeconomic development, 51–52
SOD, see Superoxide dismutase
SodA protein, 317, 360
SOS response, 217–218
South America, 15, 53, 587
Southern blotting, epidemiologic studies, 572–575
Sparfloxacin, 561
Species identification, 519
Specimen collection, 89–90
Specimen processing, 90–91
  biological safety, 87
Specimen shipment, 88, 90
Specimen transport, 89–90
Spills (laboratory accident), 69–70, 89
Spinal tuberculosis, 39–40
  prehistoric peoples, 15–16
Sputum specimen, 31, 34–35
  AFB-positive, 95
  collection, 89–90
  examination, 602–606
  gene amplification, 520
  induced, 90
    technique for collection, 31–32
  smear preparation, 91
Staining, 91–94
Stevens-Johnson syndrome, 609
Stevenson, Robert Louis, 19
2STH/10–16TH regimen, 608–609

Strand displacement amplification (SDA), 520–521
Streptomycin
  historical aspects, 22
  mechanism of action, 560
  resistance, 560
  treatment regimens, 608–610
Stress response, 313–314, 320–321, 359–360, 425,
    438–439, 449–450, 564–565, *see also* Heat shock
    proteins
Stringent response, 359–360
Subtractive mRNA library, 259
Subunit vaccine, 451, 549
Sugar transport, 343, 347–348
Suicide vector, 212, 262–263
Sulfatides, 290–291, 393–396
Sulfolipids, 377
Sulfonamides
  mechanism of action, 560
  resistance, 242
Superantigen, 426
Superoxide dismutase (SOD), 324–325, 360, 440, 564
Surveillance, 3
  laboratory personnel, 70, 89
  population-based, 576–577
Suter, E., 390
Sylvius, Franciscus, 17
Symport, 344–345
Systemic immunity, 480

T cells, 311–313, 389, 468, 478, 480, 486
  acquired resistance, 400–403
  activated, 119
  αβ, 400, 404–405, 420, 427, 448–449
  antigen recognition, 420, 424–426
  antigens, 402–403
  CD4, 119–121, 126–127, 400–404, 420–423, 428,
      437, 445, 448–449, 489, 493, 509, 545
    blood count, 504–505, 508
    cytokines produced by, 421–423
    Th1, 421–423, 437, 442, 489, 491–495, 509, 545
    Th2, 421–423, 437, 442, 489, 491–493, 495, 509,
      545
  CD8, 121–126, 400–404, 423–424, 437, 445, 448,
      487, 491, 493–494, 509, 545–546
  CD44, 119
  CD45RA, 421
  CD45RB, 119
  cytokines and, 417–435
  cytolytic, 119, 126, 402, 423, 439, 486–487, 546–
      547
  delayed-type hypersensitivity effector, 117, 119
  functions, 402
  γδ, 122–126, 400–405, 420, 424, 427, 437, 445–446,
      449, 487
  guinea pig model, 140–143
  memory, 117, 120–121, 313, 420–421, 426–427
  mouse model, 114, 116–126, 128, 130
  nutritional status and, 140–141
  protective, 117, 119–120
  repertoire, 442–445, 451
  specificity and function in tuberculosis, 437–458
  subsets, 404–405, 426
TB Broth Base, 76–77

TCH susceptibility test, 101, 103
Teicoplanin, 561
Temperature effect, growth of *M. tuberculosis*, 78
Tetracycline, 340
Tetrahydrobiopterin, 397, 486
Tetrahydrofolate pathway, 560
TGF-β, *see* Transforming growth factor beta
Thalidomide, 428–429, 490
Therapeutic vaccine, 551
Thiacetazone, 598, 608–610
Thin-layer chromatography, identification of
    M. tuberculosis, 96
Thiophene-2-carboxylic acid hydrazide, *see* TCH
    susceptibility test
Thoracentesis, 37
Thyroiditis, 496
Ticarcillin, 342
Tissue damage, 459–463, 485–491
TMA, *see* Transcription-mediated amplification
TNF, *see* Tumor necrosis factor
Training, laboratory safety, 63, 86
Transcription, expression vector, 242–243
Transcription-mediated amplification (TMA), 522–524
Transduction, 165
Transfection, 165–167
Transferrin, 361, 363, 365–366, 399
Transformation, 166, 176, 193–194, 241, 256
Transforming growth factor beta (TGF-β), 391, 397–
    398, 418–419, 428–429, 495
Translation, expression vector, 242–243
Transmission, 48
  associated with HIV infection, 55–57
  confirmation with molecular techniques, 575–576
  detection of unsuspected transmission in group,
      576
  diagnostic delay, 605–606
  prevention by chemoprophylaxis, 595–596
  reactivation versus, 577
  secondary, 569
  unsuspected, 576
Transport
  across cell membrane, 321–322
  carrier-mediated, 343–346
  drug, 562–563
  M. tuberculosis, 333–352
  regulation, 345–346
Transposable element, 199, *see also* Insertion
    sequence; Transposon
  general uses, 202
  genetic studies in mycobacteria, 211–214
  mycobacterial, 203–211
  pathogenic bacteria, 202–203
  structure and occurrence, 199–200
Transposition, 199–216
Transposon, 199–200
  delivery systems, 212–213
  pathogenic bacteria, 202–203
  reporter, 263–264
  from *Streptomyces*, 203
Transposon library, 262
Transposon mutagenesis, 212–213
Transposon Tn610, 204, 209–211
Transposon trap, 263

Treatment of tuberculosis, 599–616, *see also*
    Chemotherapy
    categories of treatment outcome, 607
    duration, 564
    historical aspects, 21–22
    HIV-infected patient, 509–510
    immunotherapy, 429, 494
Trehalose 2'-sulfate, 290–291
Trehalose 6,6'-dimycolate, *see* Cord factor
Trehalose esters, 289–292, 562
Trehalose mycolyltransferase, 373
Triacylglycerols, 287
Tricarboxylic acid cycle, 354, 356
Trimethoprim, 560
Trudeau, Edward Livingston, 18
Tubercle
    exudative, 468, 470, 478
    guinea pig model, 137, 141
    proliferative, 468, 470, 478
    rabbit model, 153–154
Tuberculin, 308–309
    standardization, 136
Tuberculin shock, 491
Tuberculin skin test, 25, 47–50, 308, 426, 446, 493,
        517–518, 544–545, 584
    cattle, 448
    developing countries, 494
    disseminated tuberculosis, 35
    false-positive, 50
    guinea pig, 137
    HIV-infected patients, 54
    induration size, 584–585
    laboratory personnel, 70, 89
    negative, 419, 426
    positive, 417, 427–428
    significance in healthy people, 494–495
    significance in patients with active tuberculosis,
        495
    surveys, 4, 589
Tuberculoma, 40–42
Tuberculostearic acid, 370, 519
Tuberculous lesions, 476, 478
tuf gene, 315
Tumor necrosis factor (TNF), 119–120, 126–127, 142,
        312, 399, 404, 418–421, 427–429
Tumor necrosis factor alpha (TNF-α), 26, 143, 390–
        392, 396–398, 422, 427, 486–491, 509, 545, 547
Tumor necrosis factor beta (TNF-β), *see*
    Lymphotoxin
Tween 80-albumin medium, 76

Ultrastructure
    limitations of studies, 271–272
    M. tuberculosis, 271–284
United States, 7–8, 14, 57, 588–589
    age distribution of tuberculosis, 56
    AIDS and tuberculosis, 53
    chemoprophylaxis, 597–598
Urinalysis, 39

US-Japan reference system, antigens, 309

Vaccination, guinea pig, 137–139
Vaccine, 312, 493, 531–557
    antituberculosis, 429–430
    attenuated *M. tuberculosis*, 547–548
    auxotrophic, 548
    BCG, *see* BCG vaccine
    DNA, 549
    effect on establishment of pulmonary lesions, 479
    environmental mycobacterial, 548
    killed, 548
    M. microti, 543
    recombinant, 246–249, 547
    subunit, 451, 549
    therapeutic, 551
    for use in livestock, 249
Vancomycin, 561
Ventilation system, laboratory, 64, 68–70, 88
Viability
    BCG vaccines, 532
    estimation, 379–380
    mycobacterial cultures, 80
Villemin, 17
Virulence
    culture medium and, 75
    *Dra*I polymorphism and, 230
    elucidation of determinants, 245
    genotype, 253–255
    guinea pig model, 136, 139
    molecular genetic strategies for identifying
        determinants, 253–268
    phenotype, 255
    plasmid-encoded factors, 192
    rabbit model, 150–151
    recA gene and, 220
    strain differences, 540–541
Virulence genes, 213, 253–255
    homologs in other genera, 259–260
    identification
        using *E. coli* as surrogate host, 259–260
        using reporter screens, 263–264
        using transposon mutagenesis, 260–261
Virulence mutants, 255
    complementation analysis, 256–259
    M. bovis, 256
    M. tuberculosis, 256

Wasting, 490
Waxes, 286–287
Wax-ester mycolates, 293
Weight loss, 27
Wells, William, 18
Western Europe, 8, 14–15
Wild animals, 157–162
Wild strain, 104

Ziehl-Neelsen stain, 91–93
Zimmermann-Rosselet method, 337–339, 343